MEDICAL ASPECTS OF CHEMICAL WARFARE

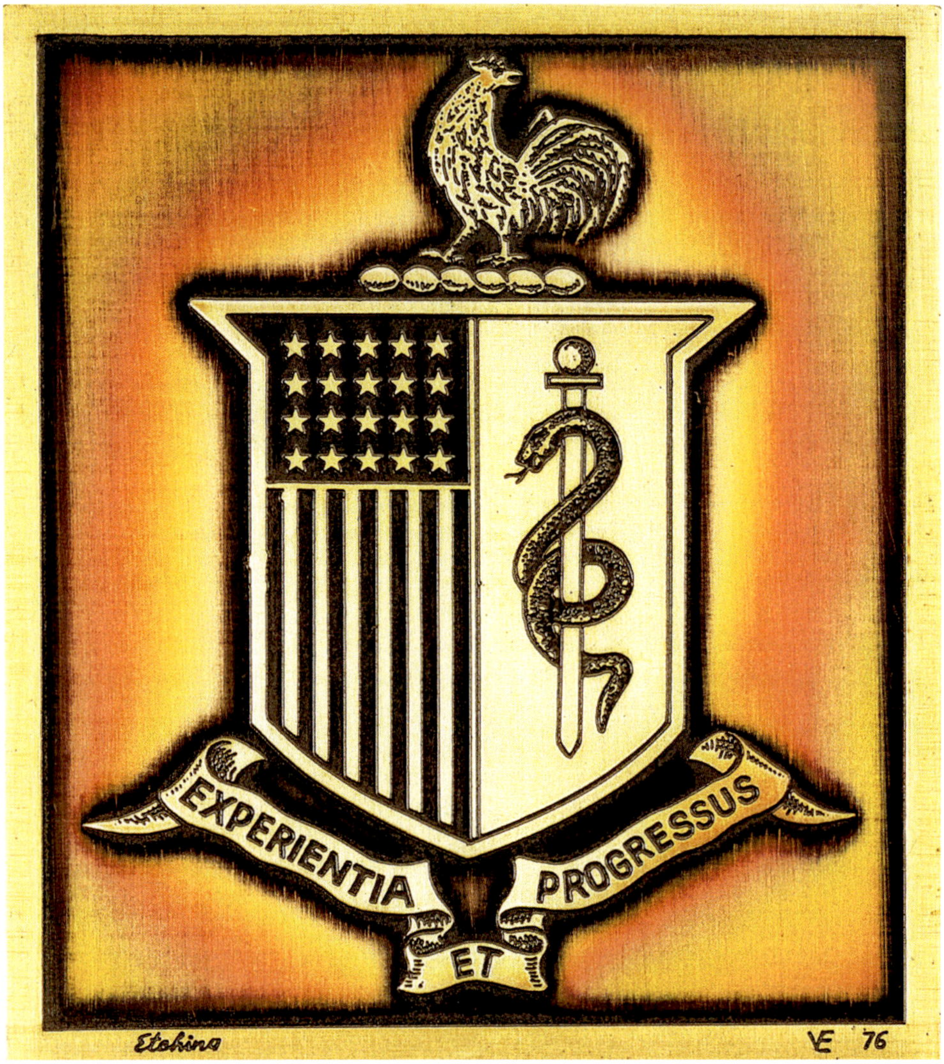

The Coat of Arms
1818
Medical Department of the Army

A 1976 etching by Vassil Ekimov of an
original color print that appeared in
The Military Surgeon, Vol XLI, No 2, 1917

The first line of medical defense in wartime is the combat medic. Although in ancient times medics carried the caduceus into battle to signify the neutral, humanitarian nature of their tasks, they have never been immune to the perils of war. They have made the highest sacrifices to save the lives of others, and their dedication to the wounded soldier is the foundation of military medical care.

Textbooks of Military Medicine

Published by the

Office of The Surgeon General
Department of the Army, United States of America

and

US Army Medical Department Center and School
Fort Sam Houston, Texas

Editor in Chief
Martha K. Lenhart, MD, PhD
Colonel, MC, US Army
Director, Borden Institute
Assistant Professor of Medicine
F. Edward Hébert School of Medicine
Uniformed Services University of the Health Sciences

For sale by the Superintendent of Documents, U.S. Government Printing Office
Internet: bookstore.gpo.gov Phone: toll free (866) 512-1800; DC area (202) 512-1800
Fax: (202) 512-2104 Mail: Stop IDCC, Washington, DC 20402-0001

ISBN 978-0-16-081532-4

The *TMM* Series

Published Textbooks

Medical Consequences of Nuclear Warfare (1989)

Conventional Warfare: Ballistic, Blast, and Burn Injuries (1991)

Occupational Health: The Soldier and the Industrial Base (1993)

Military Dermatology (1994)

Military Psychiatry: Preparing in Peace for War (1994)

Anesthesia and Perioperative Care of the Combat Casualty (1995)

War Psychiatry (1995)

Medical Aspects of Chemical and Biological Warfare (1997)

Rehabilitation of the Injured Soldier, Volume 1 (1998)

Rehabilitation of the Injured Soldier, Volume 2 (1999)

Medical Aspects of Harsh Environments, Volume 1 (2001)

Medical Aspects of Harsh Environments, Volume 2 (2002)

Ophthalmic Care of the Combat Casualty (2003)

Military Medical Ethics, Volume 1 (2003)

Military Medical Ethics, Volume 2 (2003)

Military Preventive Medicine, Volume 1 (2003)

Military Preventive Medicine, Volume 2 (2005)

Recruit Medicine (2006)

Medical Aspects of Biological Warfare (2007)

Medical Aspects of Chemical Warfare (2008)

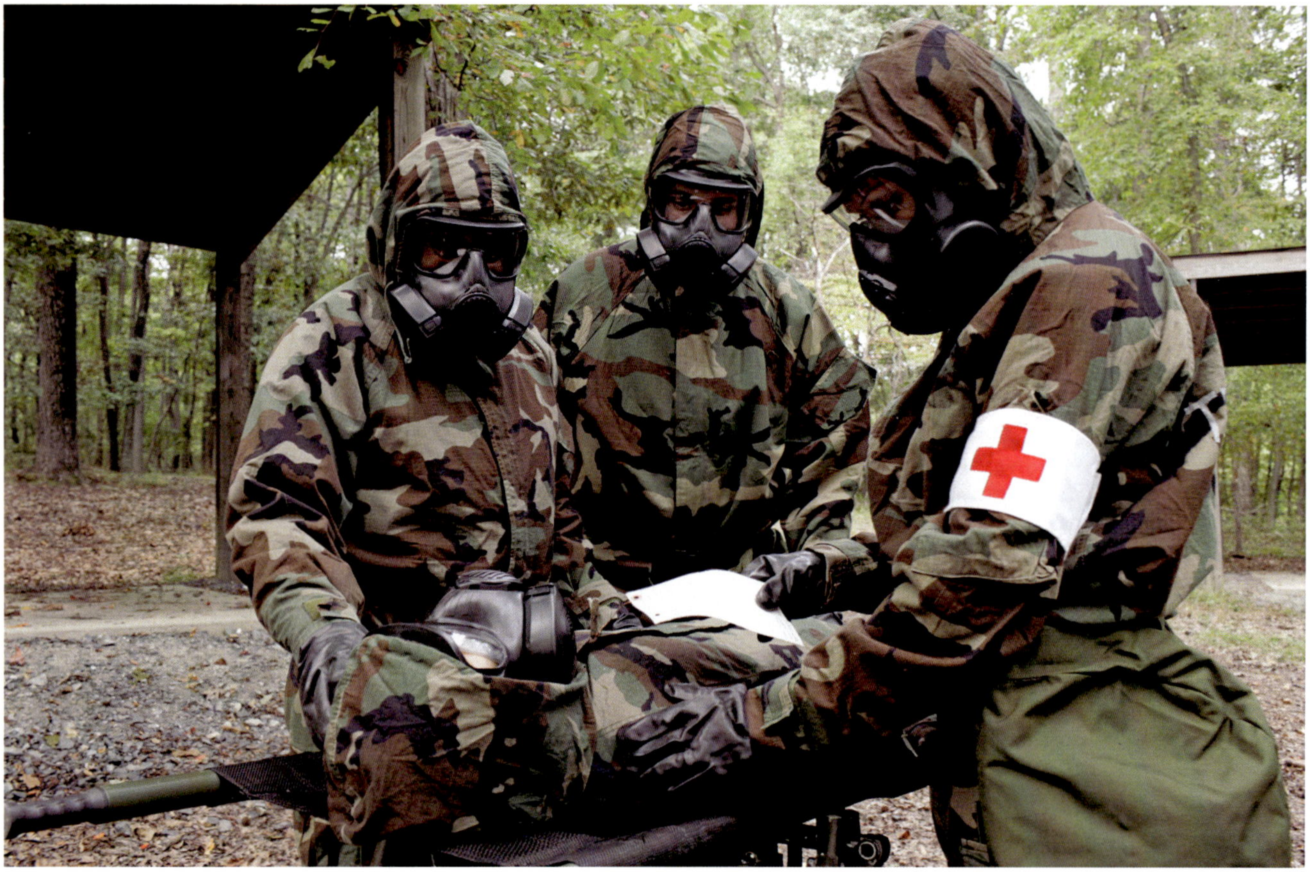

Medical Management of Chemical Casualties Field Training Site, Aberdeen Proving Ground, Edgewood Arsenal, Edgewood, Maryland. US Army healthcare professionals training for medical management of chemical casualties. The healthcare professionals are equipped with the latest protective equipment: the Joint Service Lightweight Integrated Suit Technology and the M50 protective mask.

Photograph by Stephanie R. Froberg, US Army Medical Research Institute of Chemical Defense, 2007.

MEDICAL ASPECTS OF CHEMICAL WARFARE

Senior Editor

Shirley D. Tuorinsky, MSN
Lieutenant Colonel, AN, US Army
US Army Medical Research Institute of Chemical Defense

Office of The Surgeon General
United States Army
Falls Church, Virginia

Borden Institute
Walter Reed Army Medical Center
Washington, DC

2008

Editorial Staff: Joan Redding
Senior Production Editor

Ronda Lindsay
Volume Editor

Vivian Mason
Technical Editor

Marcia Metzgar
Technical Editor

Douglas Wise
Senior Layout Editor

Bruce Maston
Illustrator

This volume was prepared for military medical educational use. The focus of the information is to foster discussion that may form the basis of doctrine and policy. The opinions or assertions contained herein are the private views of the authors and are not to be construed as official or as reflecting the views of the Department of the Army or the Department of Defense.

Dosage Selection:

The authors and publisher have made every effort to ensure the accuracy of dosages cited herein. However, it is the responsibility of every practitioner to consult appropriate information sources to ascertain correct dosages for each clinical situation, especially for new or unfamiliar drugs and procedures. The authors, editors, publisher, and the Department of Defense cannot be held responsible for any errors found in this book.

Use of Trade or Brand Names:

Use of trade or brand names in this publication is for illustrative purposes only and does not imply endorsement by the Department of Defense.

Neutral Language:

Unless this publication states otherwise, masculine nouns and pronouns do not refer exclusively to men.

Published by the Office of The Surgeon General at TMM Publications
Borden Institute
Walter Reed Army Medical Center
Washington, DC 20307-5001

Library of Congress Cataloging-in-Publication Data

Medical aspects of chemical warfare / senior editor, Shirley D. Tuorinsky.
p. ; cm. -- (Textbooks of military medicine)
Rev. ed., in part, of : Medical aspects of chemical and biological warfare. 1997.
Includes bibliographical references and index.
1. Chemical agents (Munitions)--Toxicology. I. Tuorinsky, Shirley D. II. United States. Dept. of the Army. Office of the Surgeon General. III. Borden Institute (U.S.) IV. Medical aspects of chemical and biological warfare. V. Series.
[DNLM: 1. Chemical Warfare Agents--adverse effects. 2. Chemical Warfare. 3. Military Medicine--methods. QV 663 M4875 2008]

RA648.M427 2008
363.34--dc22

2008048629

PRINTED IN THE UNITED STATES OF AMERICA

20, 19, 18, 17, 16, 15, 14 5 4 3

Contents

Contributors

MICHAEL ADLER, PhD
Research Pharmacologist, Neurobehavioral Toxicology, Department of Neurobehavioral Toxicology, US Army Medical Research Institute of Chemical Defense, 3100 Ricketts Point Road, Aberdeen Proving Ground, Maryland 21010

JAIME ANDERSON, DVM, PhD
Division Chief, Analytical Toxicology Division, Department of Neurobehavioral Toxicology, US Army Medical Research Institute of Chemical Defense, 3100 Ricketts Point Road, Aberdeen Proving Ground, Maryland 21010

GERALD P.H. BALLOUGH, PhD
Professor of Biology, La Salle University, 1900 West Olney Avenue, Philadelphia, Pennsylvania 19141

DAVID J. BARILLO, MD
Colonel, Medical Corps, US Army; Surgical Intensivist and Chief, Burn Flight Team/Special Medical Augmentation Response Team—Burn (SMART-B), US Army Institute of Surgical Research, 3400 Rawley E. Chambers Avenue, Fort Sam Houston, Texas 78234

JOHN R. BARR, PhD
Lead Research Chemist, Centers for Disease Control and Prevention, 4770 Buford Highway, Mailstop F47, Atlanta, Georgia 30341

STEVEN I. BASKIN, PhD
Deputy Research Coordinator, Cyanide Medical Countermeasures, Analytical Toxicology Division, US Army Medical Research Institute of Chemical Defense, 3100 Ricketts Point Road, Aberdeen Proving Ground, Maryland 21010

CHARLES H. BOARDMAN, MS, ORR/L
Lieutenant Colonel, Biomedical Sciences Corps, US Air Force; Instructor/Air Force Liaison and Occupational Therapist, US Army Medical Research Institute of Chemical Defense, 3100 Ricketts Point Road, Aberdeen Proving Ground, Maryland 21010

DANIEL E. BOEHM
Field Medical Education Specialist, US Army Medical Research Institute of Chemical Defense, 3100 Ricketts Point Road, Aberdeen Proving Ground, Maryland 21010-5400

CAROL A. BOSSONE, DVM, PhD
Lieutenant Colonel, US Army; Director of Toxicology, US Army Center for Health Promotion and Preventive Medicine, 5158 Blackhawk Drive, Aberdeen Proving Ground, Maryland 21010

ERNEST H. BRAUE, Jr, PhD
Scientist, US Army Medical Research Institute of Chemical Defense, 3100 Ricketts Point Road, Aberdeen Proving Ground, Maryland 21010

CLARENCE A. BROOMFIELD, PhD
Research Chemist, Research Division, Department of Pharmacology, US Army Medical Research Institute of Chemical Defense, 3100 Ricketts Point Road, Aberdeen Proving Ground, Maryland 21010

JAMES BROSELOW, MD
Clinical Associate Professor, Emergency Medicine, University of Florida College of Medicine, 1329 SW 16th Street, Suite 2204, Gainesville, Florida 32610

DUANE C. CANEVA, MD
Commander, US Navy;Head, Medical Plans and Policy, Navy Medicine Office of Homeland Security, 2300 E Street, NW, Washington, DC 20372

BENEDICT R. CAPACIO, PhD
Chief, Medical Diagnostic and Chemical Branch, Analytical Toxicology Division, US Army Medical Research Institute of Chemical Defense, 3100 Ricketts Point Road, Aberdeen Proving Ground, Maryland 21010

PATRICIA ANN CAPLE, RN
Lieutenant Colonel, Nurse Corps, US Air Force; Chemical Casualty Care Division, US Army Medical Research Institute of Chemical Defense, 3100 Ricketts Point Road, Aberdeen Proving Ground, Maryland 21010

DOUGLAS M. CERASOLI, PhD
Research Microbiologist, Research Division, Department of Physiology and Immunology, US Army Medical Research Institute of Chemical Defense, 3100 Ricketts Point Road, Aberdeen Proving Ground, Maryland 21010

MATTHEW G. CLARK, PhD
Major, Medical Service Corps, US Army; Chief, Neurobehavioral Toxicology Branch, Analytical Toxicology Division, US Army Medical Research Institute of Chemical Defense, 3100 Ricketts Point Road, Aberdeen Proving Ground, Edgewood Arsenal, Maryland 21010

THOMAS R. DASHIELL
Formerly, Director, Environmental and Life Sciences , Office of the Director of Defense Research, Office of the Secretary of Defense, Department of Defense, Washington, DC; Deceased

KENNETH DESPAIN, DVM
Lieutenant Colonel, US Army; Commander, Rocky Mountain District Veterinary Command, 1661 O'Connell Boulevard, Building 1012, Fort Carson, Colorado 80913-5108

BHUPENDRA P. DOCTOR, PhD
Director, Division of Biochemistry, Walter Reed Army Institute of Research, 503 Robert Grant Avenue, Silver Spring, Maryland 20910

MARGARET G. FILBERT, PhD
Special Assistant to the Commander, US Army Medical Research Institute of Chemical Defense, 3100 Ricketts Point Road, Aberdeen Proving Ground, Edgewood Arsenal, Maryland 21010

BRENT R. GIBSON, MD, MPH
Captain, Medical Corps, US Army; Army Medical Department Center and School, 3151 Scott Road, Suite 3507, Fort Sam Houston, Texas 78234

RICHARD K. GORDON, PhD
Chief, Department of Biochemical Pharmacology, Biochemistry Division, Walter Reed Army Institute of Research, 503 Robert Grant Road, Silver Spring, Maryland 20910

JOHN S. GRAHAM, PhD
Research Biochemist, Medical Toxicology Branch, Analytical Toxicology Division, US Army Medical Research Institute of Chemical Defense, 3100 Ricketts Point Road, Aberdeen Proving Ground, Maryland 21010-5400

ROBERT GUM, DO, MPH
Chief of Bio Surety, Barquist Army Health Clinic, 1434 Porter Street, Fort Detrick, Maryland 21702

BRADFORD W. GUTTING, PhD
Toxicologist; Naval Surface Warfare Center; Dahlgren Division (NSWCDD); Chemical, Biological, Radiological Defense Division (Code B54); Dahlgren, Virginia 22448

JULIAN R. HAIGH, PhD
Research Scientist, Department of Biochemical Pharmacology, Biochemistry Division, Walter Reed Army Institute of Research, 503 Robert Grant Road, Silver Spring, Maryland 20910

CLAUDIA L. HENEMYRE-HARRIS, PHD
Major, Medical Service Corps, US Army; Physiology and Immunology Branch, US Army Medical Research Institute of Chemical Defense, 3100 Ricketts Point Road, Aberdeen Proving Ground, Maryland 21010

BENJAMIN A. HILL, Jr, DO, MS, MEd
Lieutenant Colonel, Medical Corps, US Army; Physician Faculty, Chemical Casualty Care Division, US Army Medical Research Institute of Chemical Defense, 3100 Ricketts Point Road, Aberdeen Proving Ground, Maryland 21010

COREY J. HILMAS, MD, PhD
Research Physiologist and Pharmacologist, Analytical Toxicology Division, Department of Neurobehavioral Toxicology,US Army Medical Research Institute of Chemical Defense, 3100 Ricketts Point Road, Aberdeen Proving Ground, Maryland 21010

ELORA HILMAS, PharmD, BCPS
Clinical Pediatric Pharmacist and Pharmacy Practice Residency Coordinator, Department of Pharmacy, Alfred I. DuPont Hospital for Children, 1600 Rockland Road, Wilmington, Delaware 19803

JOSEPH J. HOUT
Researcher, Uniformed Services University of the Health Sciences, 4301 Jones Bridge Road, Bethesda, Maryland 20814

CHARLES G. HURST, MD
Colonel (Retired), Medical Corps, US Army; Director, Chemical Casualty Care Division, US Army Medical Research Institute of Chemical Defense, 3100 Ricketts Point Road, Aberdeen Proving Ground, Maryland 21010

WILLIAM L. JACKSON, MD, PhD
Commander, US Public Health Service; Centers for Disease Control and Prevention Quarantine Station, Honolulu International Airport, 300 Rodgers Boulevard, Terminal Box 67, Honolulu, Hawaii 96819; formerly, Assistant Chief Medical Officer, US Coast Guard Personnel Command, Arlington, Virginia

JAMES B. KELLY
Research Chemist, US Army Medical Research Institute of Chemical Defense, 3100 Ricketts Point Road, Room 92, Aberdeen Proving Ground, Edgewood Area, Maryland 21010

JAMES S. KETCHUM, MD
Colonel, Medical Corps, US Army (Ret); Clinical Assistant Professor of Psychiatry, University of California, Los Angeles, 2304 Fairbanks Drive, Santa Rosa, California 95403; formerly, Chief, Substance Abuse Program, Brentwood / UCLA VA Hospital, Los Angeles, California

ALLART B. KOK, MS
Biomedical Scientist, Science Applications International Corporation, 3465 Box Hill Corporate Center Drive, Abingdon, Maryland 21085

TIMOTHY A. KLUCHINSKY, Jr, PhD, MSPH
Manager, Health Hazard Assessment Program, Directorate of Occupational Health Sciences, US Army Center for Health Promotion and Preventive Medicine, 5158 Blackhawk Road, Aberdeen Proving Ground, Maryland 21010

DAVID E. LENZ, PhD
Research Chemist, Research Division, US Army Medical Research Institute of Chemical Defense, 3100 Ricketts Point Road, Aberdeen Proving Ground, Maryland 21010

ERIC S. LEVINE, PhD
Assistant Program Manager, Science Applications International Corporation, 3465 Boxhill Corporate Center Drive, MS 23, Abingdon, Maryland 21009

THOMAS P. LOGAN, PhD
Chemist, Medical Diagnostics Branch, Analytical Toxicology Division, United States Army Medical Research Institute of Chemical Defense, 3100 Ricketts Point Road, Building E3081, Room 293, Aberdeen Proving Ground, Maryland 21010

BRIAN LUKEY, PhD
Colonel, Medical Service Corps, US Army; Commander, US Army Medical Research Institute of Chemical Defense, 3100 Ricketts Point Road, Aberdeen Proving Ground, Maryland 21010

ROBERT C. LUTEN, MD
Professor, Emergency Medicine, University of Florida College of Medicine, 1329 SW 16th Street, Suite 2204, Gainesville, Florida 32610; Attending, Pediatric Emergency Medicine, Department of Emergency Medicine, Shands Jacksonville Medical Center, 655 W 8th Street #1, Jacksonville, Florida 32209

BEVERLY I. MALINER, DO, MPH
Colonel, Medical Corps, US Army; Director, Department of Occupational and Environmental Medicine, US Army Center for Health Promotion and Preventive Medicine, 5158 Blackhawk Road, Building E1930, Aberdeen Proving Ground, Maryland 21010

JOHN D. MALONE, MD, MSPH
Captain, US Navy; Professor of Medicine, Uniformed Services University of the Health Sciences, Bethesda, Maryland 20814; formerly, Commanding Officer, Medical Treatment Facility, USNS Mercy

AL MAURONI, MS
Senior Policy Analyst, Northrop-Grumman Information Technology, 8211 Terminal Road, Suite 1000, Lorton, Virginia 22079

DONALD M. MAXWELL, MS
Research Chemist, Research Division, Department of Pharmacology, US Army Medical Research Institute of Chemical Defense, 3100 Ricketts Point Road, Aberdeen Proving Ground, Maryland 21010

JOHN H. MCDONOUGH, PhD
Major, Medical Service Corps, US Army (Ret); Research Psychologist, Pharmacology Branch, Research Division, US Army Medical Research Institute of Chemical Defense, Room 161A, Building E-3100, 3100 Ricketts Point Road, Aberdeen Proving Ground, Maryland 21010

MELANIE L. MURROW
Safety and Occupational Specialist, Safety, Surety, and Security Office, Office of the Commander, United States Army Medical Research Institute of Chemical Defense, 3100 Ricketts Point Road, Building E3101, Room 104, Aberdeen Proving Ground, Maryland 21010

JONATHAN NEWMARK, MD
Colonel, US Army; Deputy Joint Program Executive Officer, Medical Systems, Joint Program Executive Office for Chemical/Biological Defense, Skyline #2, Suite 1609, 5203 Leesburg Pike, Falls Church, Virginia 22041; Adjunct Professor, Department of Neurology, F. Edward Hébert School of Medicine, Uniformed Services University of the Health Sciences, Bethesda, Maryland

MICHAEL R. O'HERN
Sergeant First Class, US Army (Ret); PO Box 46, Aberdeen, Maryland 21010; formerly, Noncommissioned Officer in Charge, Chemical Casualty Care Office, US Army Medical Research Institute of Chemical Defense, Aberdeen Proving Ground, Maryland 21010-5425

JOHN P. PETRALI, PhD
Research Anatomist, Comparative Pathology Branch, Comparative Medicine Division, US Army Medical Research Institute of Chemical Defense, 3100 RicketTs Point Road, Aberdeen Proving Ground, Edgewood Arsenal, Maryland 21010

GENNADY E. PLATOFF, Jr, PhD
Colonel, US Army (Retired); Scientific Advisor, Office of Biodefense Research, National Institute of Allergies and Infectious Disease, National Institutes of Health, 6610 Rockledge Drive, Room 4069, Bethesda, Maryland 20892-6612

LAUKTON Y. RIMPEL
Sergeant First Class, US Army (Ret); Consultant, Battelle Scientific Program Office, 50101 Governors Drive, Suite 110, Chapel Hill, North Carolina 27517

GARY A. ROCKWOOD
Research Coordinator, Cyanide Medical Countermeasures, Analytical Toxicology Division, US Army Medical Research Institute of Chemical Defense, 3100 Ricketts Point Road, Aberdeen Proving Ground, Maryland 21010

MICHELLE C. ROSS, DVM, PhD
Colonel, US Army; Director of CBRN Medical Defense Policy, Office of the Assistant Secretary of Defense for Health Affairs, 5111 Leesburg Pike, Skyline 5, Falls Church, Virginia 22041

HARRY SALEM, PhD
Chief Scientist for Life Sciences, US Army Edgewood Chemical Biological Center, 5183 Blackhawk Road, Aberdeen Proving Ground, Maryland 21010

ASHIMA SAXENA, PhD
Chief, Division of Biochemistry, Department of Molecular Pharmacology, Walter Reed Army Institute of Research, 503 Robert Grant Avenue, Silver Spring, Maryland 20910

ALFRED M. SCIUTO, PhD
Research Physiologist, Analytical Toxicology Division, Medical Toxicology Branch, US Army Medical Research Institute of Chemical Defense, 3100 Ricketts Point Road, Aberdeen Proving Ground, Maryland 21010

FREDERICK R. SIDELL, MD
Formerly, Chief, Chemical Casualty Care Division, and Director, Medical Management of Chemical Casualties Course, US Army Medical Research Institute of Chemical Defense, 3100 Ricketts Point Road, Aberdeen Proving Ground, Maryland 21010; Deceased

JEFFERY K. SMART, MA
Command Historian, US Army Research, Development, and Engineering Command, 5183 Blackhawk Road, Aberdeen Proving Ground, Maryland 21010

J. RICHARD SMITH
Chemist, Medical Diagnostic and Chemical Branch, Analytical Toxicology Division, US Army Medical Research Institute of Chemical Defense, 3100 Ricketts Point Road, Aberdeen Proving Ground, Maryland 21010

WILLIAM J. SMITH, PhD
Chief, Cellular and Molecular Biology Branch, Research Division, US Army Medical Research Institute of Chemical Defense, 3100 Ricketts Point Road, Aberdeen Proving Ground, Maryland 21010

THOMAS B. TALBOT, MD, MS
Major, Medical Corps, US Army; Chief of Operations Branch, Chemical Casualty Care Division, US Army Medical Research Institute of Chemical Defense, 3100 Ricketts Point Road, Aberdeen Proving Ground, Maryland 21010

MARY FRANCES TRACY
Research Scientist, Chemical, Biological, Radiological & Nuclear Defense Information Analysis Center, Aberdeen Proving Ground, Maryland 21010-5425

SHIRLEY D. TUORINSKY, MSN
Lieutenant Colonel, AN, US Army; Executive Officer, Combat Casualty Care Division, US Army Medical Research Institute of Chemical Defense, 3100 Ricketts Point Road, Aberdeen Proving Ground, Maryland 21010

JOHN S. URBANETTI, MD
Lecturer, Pulmonary Disease, Yale University School of Medicine, New Haven, Connecticut 06510

KEITH VESELY, DVM, PhD
Colonel, US Army; Joint Product Manager, Medical Identification and Treatment Systems, Chemical Biological Medical Systems Joint Project Management Office, 64 Thomas Johnson Drive, Frederick, Maryland 21702

SCOTT WILLENS, DVM, PhD
Major, Veterinary Corps, US Army; Chief of Department of Neurobehavioral Toxicology, Analytical Toxicology Division, Department of Neurobehavioral Toxicology, US Army Medical Research Institute of Chemical Defense, 3100 Ricketts Point Road, Aberdeen Proving Ground, Maryland 21010

PATRICK WILLIAMS, MS
Research Biologist, Department of Neurobehavioral Toxicology, US Army Medical Research Institute of Chemical Defense, 3100 Ricketts Point Road, Aberdeen Proving Ground, Maryland 21010

CSABA K. ZOLTANI, PhD
Research Physicist, Army Research Laboratory, Building 394, Aberdeen Proving Ground, Maryland 21005

Foreword

The US military has been concerned with the risk of chemical warfare for decades. By the end of the twentieth century, however, scenarios for the use of chemical weapons expanded beyond the battlefield as terrorist organizations began employing them against civilian populations. This development is not surprising, given that a great percentage of the world's population now has the ability and knowledge to develop weapons of mass destruction, particularly chemical weapons.

In 1995, Aum Shinrikyo, a well-funded Japanese religious cult with chemical expertise, released sarin, a deadly nerve agent, in five separate subway cars in downtown Tokyo. The attack not only caused panic, but also overwhelmed the medical response system. In Baghdad, Iraq, on May 18, 2004, a small amount of sarin was dispersed by a shell that exploded near a US military convoy, and on April 6, 2007, a chemical, first weaponized during World War I, reappeared when a suicide bomber in Baghdad detonated a truck loaded with chlorine gas, killing 20 people and wounding 30 others.

Although the events of September 11, 2001, did not involve chemical weapons, they did underscore terrorists' willingness to use unconventional weapons and shocked the United States into awareness of its own vulnerability to terrorist attacks. The use of chemical agents by terrorist groups is now a recognized threat to the American population and to US troops deployed abroad. We know terrorist groups have the knowledge and the financial support to design and disperse chemical weapons. Also, as our world becomes more highly industrialized, chemicals, some of which are highly toxic, are used in numerous manufacturing processes; the world's population is at risk of exposure to these lethal chemicals through their inadvertent release from manufacturing plants and accidents during their transportation or intentional release by terrorists.

Medical Aspects of Chemical Warfare is the most comprehensive source of information available on chemical agents. This text is strongly recommended reading for all military medical personnel. It should be placed in the reference libraries of every military medical treatment facility. It will serve to both enhance the knowledge and skills, and increase the level of preparedness and response capability, of those responsible for chemical casualty care. Many civilian medical professionals will also find this textbook to be a valuable reference as their hospitals prepare for the possibility of treating casualties of an accidental or deliberate exposure.

Lieutenant General Eric B. Schoomaker
The Surgeon General
US Army

Washington, DC
January 2008

Preface

A significant concern for the United States and its allies is that an ever-growing number of terrorist organizations will employ chemical warfare agents in an attack on military forces or civilians. As a result, efforts to prepare for such an attack have expanded and are now supported by the Department of Health and Human Services and Department of Homeland Security, as well as the Department of Defense.

Since its initial publication in 1997, this textbook has provided military physicians, nurses, physician assistants, and medics with the knowledge and skills to medically manage chemical agent casualties. This expanded second edition will not only continue to be an essential reference tool for military personnel, but should also become a requisite guide for civilian healthcare providers, first responders, and government agencies responsible for emergency preparedness, response, and management. Its 23 chapters will prepare these individuals and organizations to manage casualties from first chemical exposure to hospital discharge. In addition to detailed explanations of chemical agent detectors, personal protection equipment, and decontamination stations, this edition contains expanded discussions of the cutting-edge science behind countermeasure development, as can be seen in Chapter 7, Nerve Agent Bioscavenger: Development of a New Approach to Protect Against Organophosphorus Exposure. The textbook also addresses topics of particular interest to civilian healthcare providers, with chapters on the threat posed by toxic industrial chemicals and domestic preparedness.

I would like to offer my sincere thanks to the physicians, nurses, scientists, and support personnel who have contributed to this textbook either directly or indirectly. These professionals are recognized worldwide and are the foremost experts in the medical aspects of chemical warfare. Their overall goal is to provide the medical force with the understanding of the chemical agent threat, how to respond, and how to deliver quality chemical casualty care.

Major General George Weightman
Medical Corps, US Army
Commanding General, US Army Medical Research and Materiel Command

Fort Detrick, Maryland
January 2008

Prologue

The original edition of *Medical Aspects of Chemical and Biological Warfare* has been a tremendous resource for the past 10 years. Much has transpired, however, since its publication; in particular the terrorist attacks of September 11, 2001. As a result, this revised edition covers solely chemical warfare, and information on biological warfare is now published in a separate volume. Also, while the earlier edition focused on medical management of patients, a conscious effort was made in this edition to include discussions of cutting-edge science that has led to significant medical therapeutic advances.

This expanded edition covers four themes: (1) the history of chemical warfare; (2) medical diagnosis and treatment for chemical casualties; (3) the mechanisms and science behind treatments and advances in therapy; and (4) homeland security. The book addresses innovative new technologies, such as nerve agent bioscavenger enzymes, as well as advances in personal decontamination, wound healing, protective equipment, and more.

I would like to recognize and thank Lieutenant Colonel Shirley D Tuorinsky of the Army Nurse Corps, who served as the senior editor for this book. Her 2 years of thoughtful and relentless effort have resulted in a quality product of which we can all be proud.

Colonel Timothy K. Adams
Veterinary Corps, US Army
Commander, US Army Medical Research Institute of Chemical Defense

Fort Detrick, Maryland
February 2008

Acknowledgments

BOARD SUBJECT MATTER EDITORS

Lieutenant Colonel Shirley D. Tuorinsky, CRNA
Colonel (Ret) Charles G. Hurst, MD
Colonel (Ret) Gennady E. Platoff Jr, PhD
Colonel (Ret) Ernest T. Takafuji, MD, MPH
Colonel (Ret) Roger G. McIntoch, MD, MOH
Major Thomas B. Talbot, MD, MS, FAAP

PEER REVIEW BOARD

Colonel Beverly I. Maliner, OD, MPH
Lieutenant Colonel Patricia A. Caple, MSN
Lieutenant Colonel Charles H. Boardman, IV, MS, ORR/L
Margaret G. Filbert, PhD
Colonel (Ret) David H. Moore, DVM
Major Kimberly A. Whitten, DVM
Major Claudia L. Henemyre-Harris, PhD
Captain Denise M. Milhorn, PhD

EDITOR

Cindy A. Kronman

GRAPHIC DEPARTMENT

Theresa M. Tezak-Reid
Stephanie R. Froberg
Peter A. Hurst

LIBRARY

Leanna E. Bush

OPERATION SECURITY

Lloyd R. Roberts
Debra J. Coffman (MRMC)

Chapter 1

INTRODUCTION TO THE CHEMICAL THREAT

THOMAS B. TALBOT, MD*; BRIAN LUKEY, PHD†, AND GENNADY E. PLATOFF JR, PHD‡

*Major, Medical Corps, US Army; Chief of Operations Branch, Chemical Casualty Care Division, US Army Medical Research Institute of Chemical Defense, 3100 Ricketts Point Road, Aberdeen Proving Ground, Maryland 21010

†Colonel, Medical Service Corps, US Army; Commander, US Army Medical Research Institute of Chemical Defense, 3100 Ricketts Point Road, Aberdeen Proving Ground, Maryland 21010

‡Chemical, Biological, Radiological, and Nuclear Scientific Advisor, Office of Biodefense Research, National Institute of Allergy & Infectious Diseases, 6610 Rockledge Drive, Room 4069, Bethesda, Maryland 20892

INTRODUCTION

It has been nearly 90 years since the United States Armed Forces last encountered chemical weapons on the battlefield. Despite this long respite, images of poisonous chemical clouds and descriptions of sudden and horrifying death continue to foment apprehension and terror. The mention of chemical weapons elicits outrage and fear of the unknown. Soldiers confronted with even a nonspecific threat of a chemical environment must bear the inefficiencies of cumbersome and hot protective garments. Medical personnel face an unseen pathogen and the prospect of managing mass chemical casualties they are inexperienced in treating.

Chemical weapons are a classic model of weapons of mass destructive effect that result in substantial contamination of personnel and equipment. Chemical weapons are the original weapons of mass destruction, and they are ideally suited as agents of great psychological effect. Although the law in the United States prohibits using chemical weapons against an adversary, this policy is not shared by all nations or by nonstate entities; therefore, to be effective, military medical personnel must be knowledgeable and trained to deal with a chemical weapon attack.

In a chemical environment, military healthcare providers must be:

- prepared to handle military and civilian casualties resulting from chemical agents;
- cognizant of what constitutes a chemical threat and the military tactics that could be employed against the force because they may be called on to render advice from both individual and public health perspectives;
- familiar with the acute and chronic medical effects of chemical agent exposure in order to plan appropriate medical support; and
- knowledgeable of the diagnostic tools available to identify specific chemical agents to which their patients may have been exposed and aware of the most effective treatments for acute intervention and prevention of long-term sequelae.

The chemical threat may involve overt or clandestine use of single or multiple agents. Some of these may be classic chemical agents developed for military applications. Other agents may be highly toxic industrial compounds that are produced in great quantities and can have comparable effects; increased interest in the training, education, and research of toxic industrial compounds is now emphasized in both the military and civilian populations. Additionally, the advent of more formidable nonstate entities and terrorist organizations interested in the mass lethality and the powerful psychological effects of these agents has resulted in an increased concern for the potential use of chemical weapons.

Chemical warfare agents need not be lethal to be disruptive. The resultant mass casualty scenario, psychological effects, diversion of medical resources, need for decontamination, and impairment of fighting ability are all desirable outcomes for those that might deploy these agents. In a situation where there are few physical indicators of a chemical attack, the medical practitioner may be the first to recognize the effects of chemical exposure. An increased incidence of symptoms consistent with nerve, vesicant, blood, or respiratory agent exposure should raise immediate suspicion of poisoning. Healthcare providers must be familiar with the signs and symptoms of a chemical exposure or the possibility of the combined use of chemical and biological warfare agents in both military and civilian settings.

The offensive use of chemical agents continues to be an attractive alternative to some nations and nonstate entities. One reason for this is that chemical agents can be dispersed over large areas and can penetrate well-defended positions. They can be employed against specific targets (eg, headquarters control centers) with effects that include delayed or immediate incapacitation, disorientation, or death.

The goal of this chapter is to provide an encapsulated historical overview of chemical weapons, discuss the current chemical threat, and guide readers in the organization of this textbook.

A TIMELINE OF CHEMICAL WARFARE AGENTS

Early Chemical Weapons

The modern era of chemical weapons began during World War I with the 1915 introduction of chlorine gas on the battlefield of Ypres, Belgium. Chemical weapons were effective in this theater because of the fixed positions of highly concentrated troop formations. Initial lethal weapons of concern included pulmonary agents such as chlorine and phosgene, for which countermeasures were initially inadequate or nonexistent. As the use of chemical weapons increased, the gas mask was developed as an initial countermeasure. The mask was refined and improved upon during the course of World War I, and newer models are still being developed today.

The use of mustard agent during World War I was ultimately responsible for the majority of casualties from the war. By targeting the skin, eyes, and lungs, mustard rendered a large number of soldiers ineffective as part of the fighting force. The grotesque pattern of injury that resulted from exposure had a major psychological impact, demonstrating that a chemical weapon need not be lethal to be strategically effective. During this period, mustard agent became known as "the king of war gases."

In 1918 lewisite was produced in the United States, but large-scale production and stockpiling came too late for it to be used in the war. However, lewisite eventually became the primary vesicant stockpiled by the Soviet Union. Meanwhile in France and Austria, experiments with cyanide produced mixed results. Cyanide was novel because it produced nearly instant incapacitation and was highly lethal. However, its non-persistent properties and low specific gravity made it unsuitable for the open field and trench environment of the day.

By World War II, Germany had made tremendous progress with the innovation of agents toxic to the nervous system. The G-series nerve agents, such as tabun (North Atlantic Treaty Organization [NATO] designation: GA) and sarin (NATO designation: GB), featured the instant incapacitation and lethality of cyanide and were effective at much lower concentrations. The G-series agents also had superior dispersal characteristics. These new nerve agents were not used during the war, though, and the Allies discovered them and developed countermeasures only after the conflict.

From the Cold War to Disarmament

During the Cold War, the United Kingdom invented the V-series nerve agents, which were weaponized by the United States and Soviet Union. V-series nerve agents are toxic in even smaller doses than G agents and are persistent in the environment. They were considered an ideal area denial weapon by both the western powers and the Eastern Bloc.

The 1960s was a period of experimentation using incapacitating and psychedelic agents that impaired combat performance without being lethal. During the 1970s and 1980s, the Soviet Union continued to increase the size of its chemical stockpile and initiated a massive program named "Foliant" to produce newer and deadlier agents.

During the Reagan administration, the United States produced a binary chemical weapon deterrent. Binary weapons are chemically identical to traditional nerve agents, but differ in that the final chemical reaction occurs only after a projectile is fired, allowing safe storage and transportation of the weapon.[1] Simultaneously, during the Iran/Iraq war, mustard agent returned to the battlefield, and an incapacitating agent similar to 3-quinuclidinyl benzilate (often called "BZ," a glycolate anticholinergic) named "Agent 15" was developed.

The Current Age

The results of the 1993 Paris Convention, known as the "Chemical Warfare Convention," were in effect by 1997 and resulted in a period of disarmament by nation-states. Meanwhile, terrorist organizations developed interests in chemical weapons and had some success in producing and employing them. The most recent public application of chemical warfare occurred in 2002 at the Nord-Ost Moscow theater. In an attempt to free 850 hostages being held by Chechen rebels, the Russian government used a supposedly opiate-based incapacitating agent called Kolokol-1, which resulted in the deaths of 42 terrorists and at least 129 hostages. Another concerning development was noted when dissident scientist Vladimir Mirzayanov publicly stated that his country was circumventing the Chemical Warfare Convention by developing a new generation of nerve agents.[2–4]

Readers interested in more information on the historical aspects of chemical warfare can find the information in chapters 2 through 4. These chapters offer a thorough review of the history of chemical warfare, the medical management of chemical casualties, and the chemical threat.

THE CURRENT THREAT OF CHEMICAL PROLIFERATION

The Chemical Warfare Convention now includes 181 signatory countries.[5] Since it became effective in 1997, some progress destroying large chemical arsenals has been made.

Managing the Stockpile

The global declared stockpile of chemical weapons is about 70,000 tons. Of this, the stockpile declared by the United States is 30,599 tons of unitary agent and 680 tons of binary components.[6] As of 2007, about half of the US stockpile has been destroyed: two of seven chemical demilitarization facilities have completed their destruction missions.[7] Russia has had a more difficult time destroying its declared 40,000 tons of agent, which consists largely of nerve agent and lewisite.[8] The reportedly poor security of storage facilities and the very slow pace of demilitarization pose a challenge for both Russia and the international community.[9] These conditions may present an unintended proliferation risk.[10] Further details about the global stockpile and demilitarization are presented in Chapter 4.

The Terrorist Threat

It is well known that terrorists have a strong interest in chemical weapons. For example, in 1995 several followers of the Aum Shinrikyo cult carried out a nerve agent attack with sarin in the Tokyo subway system. The media has reported that Al Qaeda and its operatives have also had a fascination with weapons of mass destruction, including chemical weapons. Of particular concern are revelations that Al Qaeda had plans to employ cyanide devices against civilians in New York City subways.[11] Several cyanide plots have been thwarted prior to execution, yet plans for a crude but potentially effective cyanide dispersal device have been posted on jihadist Web sites since 2005.[12] Because the next chemical attack may occur in the civilian arena, there are implications for both the civilian first responder and for the armed forces. The military may be called upon for consultation or response in such a situation, making it necessary for it to work with civilian populations.

The Future Chemical Threat

There are myriad toxic chemicals that could be considered agents of concern for the future chemical threat. Also, the possibility that existing classes of agents may be enhanced for more lethal effects must always be considered so that countermeasures are developed. The potential future chemical threat is as wide ranging as an adversary's imagination and budget allow.

JOINT MEDICAL LIFECYCLE MANAGEMENT

In 2003 the US Army was made the executive agent for the chemical/biological program to coordinate and integrate all research, development, and acquisition programs for all the services. As of 2007 the program includes the Joint Program Executive Office (JPEO), the Joint Science and Technology Office, the Joint Test and Evaluation Executive Office, the Joint Combat Developer, and the Joint Requirements Office. These offices are dedicated to delivering joint fighting capabilities, including medical treatment.

To counter the chemical threat, sustain combat power, and maintain a healthy force, the military established the JPEO in April 2003. The JPEO integrates a systems approach to address agent delivery, doses on target, downwind dispersal, dose absorbed, and symptoms. The Chemical Biological Medical Systems Joint Project Management Office is specifically responsible for medical systems. It addresses chemical casualty medical pretreatment and posttreatment, medical surveillance, and medical diagnostics to counter the threat and leverage the joint services research and development programs for combat personnel.

The Chemical Biological Medical Systems Joint Project Management Office is responsible for developing, procuring, fielding, and sustaining premier medical protection and treatment capabilities against chemical and biological warfare agents. Medical products are submitted through the US Food and Drug Administration for licensing or approval. The management office is composed of a headquarters and support element and two joint product management offices: the Joint Vaccine Acquisition Program (which focuses on developing, testing, producing, and storing vaccines) and Medical Identification and Treatment Systems.

Medical Identification and Treatment Systems manages the development, acquisition, and fielding of products used for the prophylaxis, treatment, and diagnosis of chemical and biological warfare agent exposure in US service members. Medical Identification and Treatment Systems products range from specific hardware devices that enable medical personnel to diagnose biological warfare agent exposure to drugs that prevent or mitigate the actions of chemical or biological agents.

Science and technology (research and development) is overseen by the Defense Threat Reduction Agency chemical/biological directorate. The Defense Threat Reduction Agency must interact at many levels, including with the executive agent or the Army acquisition executive (who takes direction from the defense acquisition executive), the Joint Requirements Office (which addresses user community needs and requirements), the deputy assistant to the secretary of defense for chemical and biological programs (which provides program oversight), the Joint Staff, the US Army Chemical School, the joint program managers, and the JPEO. The medical mission of the Defense Threat Reduction Agency is to safeguard America and its allies from weapons of mass destruction (chemical, biological, radiological, nuclear, and high-yield explosives) by providing medical capabilities to reduce, eliminate, and counter the threat and mitigate its effects. The Defense Threat Reduction Agency manages the medical research and development programs and funding, including the Department of Defense medical missions at the US Army Medical Research Institute of Infectious Diseases and the US Army Medical Research Institute of Chemical Defense (USAMRICD).

THE ROLE OF THE US ARMY MEDICAL RESEARCH INSTITUTE OF CHEMICAL DEFENSE

USAMRICD is the lead Department of Defense laboratory dealing with the medical aspects of chemical defense. It focuses on medical research, training, and education for medical chemical defense. USAMRICD activity involves basic research, clinical studies, therapeutics, and other areas of research. USAMRICD also partners with major military and civilian organizations throughout the country and abroad.

Development of Medical Countermeasures

USAMRICD builds on basic research to support soldiers through the development of medical countermeasures and therapeutics. Current projects include the use of both simple and catalytic bioscavengers for prophylaxis and treatment of nerve agent casualties. Additional research areas of interest include the new oximes and neuroprotective compounds that mitigate the effects of nerve agent exposure. Studies investigating the use of midazolam as a new generation nerve anticonvulsant are in advanced stages. There is an increase in medical vesicant research to indentify the specific biochemistry of injury as well as to develop novel protectants and treatments. Cyanide and pulmonary agent research has been increasing in pace as well. Other work at USAMRICD involves developing medical diagnostics and personnel decontamination research. Work on equipment and detection gear is conducted by USAMRICD's partner institute, the Edgewood Chemical Biological Center.

Education and Educational Products

The chemical casualty care division is responsible for training military medical personnel in the practice of medical defense, medical decontamination, and triage. It also provides education for other military branches, civilians, government agencies, and foreign nationals. Courses are accredited as continuing medical education for physicians, nurses, and emergency medical technicians, and for college credit.

The courses taught onsite at the chemical casualty care division include the Medical Management of Chemical and Biological Casualties Course, which is produced jointly with the US Army Medical Research Institute of Infectious Diseases. The course consists of lectures, a field exercise, and a unique primate lab experience. It has been recognized as the gold standard for this type of training by the Office of The Surgeon General and the Government Accountability Office. Other courses include the Field Management of Chemical and Biological Casualties, which targets front echelon care. This course includes multiple field exercises to encourage proficiency in the field medical decontamination station. The Hospital Management of Chemical Biological Radiological Nuclear and Explosives Course is a preparatory course for mass casualty chemical, biological, radiological, nuclear, and explosives events. It includes instruction on regulations regarding these events and cooperation with civilian and military authorities at other echelons.

The chemical casualty care division is responsible for a large volume of educational products. These products include publication content for educational materials as well as pocket manuals for the field management of chemical casualties and medical management of chemical casualties. The chemical casualty care division produces several software products, such as reference materials, distance and online training courses, educational games, and interactive simulations.

ORGANIZATION OF THIS VOLUME

Awareness and interest in weapons of mass destruction, medical chemical defense research, and education and training of military personnel and civilians has increased dramatically in the last few years. The need for an updated and resultant text dedicated to the medical aspects of biological and chemical weapons would not fit into a single textbook. Hence, this text differs from the earlier version of the *Textbooks of Military Medicine: Medical Aspects of Chemical and Biological Warfare* because biological and chemical agents are discussed in separate volumes. This text is primarily relevant to military medicine; however, due to the increased interest in chemical casualty treatment that now exists within civilian communities, the information provided within this text can be considered an excellent resource for both military and civilian healthcare providers.

Chapters 2 through 4 offer greater depth concerning the history of chemical warfare and the basic principles of chemical warfare. "History of Chemical Warfare" takes a broad view of the historical context and significant events in the field. "History of the Chemical Threat" breaks the 20th century down into decade-long segments and provides a fresh perspective on prior military and political developments. "The Medical Aspects of Medical Management" chapter has radically changed over the years and presents this history from multiple perspectives. It includes detailed accounts of the chemical warfare management experience in the United States, as well as a revealing exploration of British, Canadian, French, Russian, and German experiences.

Chapters 5 through 7 concentrate on nerve agents. Chapter 5 is a comprehensive treatise on the present research, countermeasures, physiology, and management of nerve agent casualties. The chapter on neuroprotection (Chapter 6), new to this volume, reviews developments in protective adjuncts to classic nerve agent antidote therapy. Chapter 7, also new, examines the emerging field of therapeutics that may represent the next advancement in therapy for these casualties.

Chapters 8 through 15 cover the remaining categories of threat agents. Vesicants are presented in historical, clinical, and physiological detail in Chapter 8, and Chapter 9 has been updated with the most current clinical data in the field. Given the increased nonstate and terrorist threat from chemical weapons, the chapter on toxic industrial chemicals has been broadened (Chapter 10). Cyanide appears to be of major interest to terrorists and the civilian population, so Chapter 11 has been expanded in size and scope. Two chapters devoted to nonlethal agents are also covered in this section.

Chapters 16 through 19 are concerned with the field management, triage, and decontamination procedures within the US military. Current and new equipment are described in detail. The final section of the book relates to partnering, acquisition, and preparedness and includes an entirely new chapter dedicated to the medical management of pediatric casualties. There is also a chapter devoted to medical diagnostics (Chapter 22).

SUMMARY

The chemical warfare threat to the United States has changed dramatically in recent years, becoming less obscure. Chemical weapons that are being destroyed under the Chemical Warfare Convention by major nation -states are increasingly attractive to pariah states and terrorists. In the current environment, the United States may experience a higher likelihood of a chemical attack on its military forces and civilian population, more so than ever before in the history of chemical warfare and terrorism.

Given the changing chemical threat, this textbook has broadened in scope and depth and now encompasses an entire volume. This expanded text attempts to be a comprehensive guide to the full spectrum of these agents and to provide information on the state of the art in medical therapeutics.

REFERENCES

1. Tucker Jonathan B. *War of Nerves: Chemical Warfare from World War I to Al-Qaeda*. New York, NY: Pantheon Books; 2006: 245.

2. Englund W. Ex-Soviet scientist says Gorbachev's regime created new nerve gas in '91. *Baltimore Sun*. September 16, 1992:3A.

3. Englund W. Russia still doing secret work on chemical arms. Research goes on as government seeks U.N. ban. *Baltimore Sun*. October 18, 1992:1A.

4. Smithson AE, Mirzayanov VS, Lajoie R, Krepon M. *Chemical Weapons Disarmament in Russia: Problems and Prospects*. Washington, DC: Henry L. Stimson Center; October 1995. Report No. 17.

5. The United States Department of State, Bureau of International Security and Nonproliferation, and the United States Department of Commerce, Bureau of Industry and Security. The United States Chemical Weapons Convention Web site. Convention on the Prohibition of the Development, Production, Stockpiling and Use of Chemical Weapons and on their Destruction. Available at: http://www.cwc.gov. Accessed June 12, 2007.

6. United States Office of the Assistant Secretary of Defense, "Chemical weapons stockpile information declassified," news release, January 22, 1996. Document 024-96.

7. US Army. US Army Chemical Materials Agency Web site. Available at: http://www.pmcd.army.mil. Accessed December 2006.

8. Russian Munitions Agency Web site. Available at: http://www.munition.gov.ru/eng/zapasho.html. Accessed November 2006.

9. US House Armed Services Committee. "GAO finds Russia lacks plan for destruction of poison gas stockpile." News release, April 27, 2004.

10. Suskind R. The untold story of al-Qaeda's plot to attack the subways. *Time*. June 19, 2006.

11. Salama S. Special report: manual for producing chemical weapon to be used in New York subway plot available on al-Qaeda websites since late 2005. *WMD Insights: Issues and Viewpoints in the International Media*. 2006;7.

Chapter 2

HISTORY OF CHEMICAL WARFARE

COREY J. HILMAS, MD, PhD*; JEFFERY K. SMART, MA†; and BENJAMIN A. HILL, Jr, DO, MS, MEd‡

*Research Pharmacologist and Physician, Neurobehavioral Toxicology Branch, US Army Medical Research Institute of Chemical Defense, 3100 Ricketts Point Road, Aberdeen Proving Ground, Edgewood Arsenal, Maryland 21010-5400

†Command Historian, US Army Chemical and Biological Defense Command, 5183 Blackhawk Rd, Aberdeen Proving Ground, Edgewood Arsenal, Maryland 21010-5423

‡Lieutenant Colonel, US Army Medical Corps; Physician Faculty, Chemical Casualty Care Division, US Army Medical Research Institute of Chemical Defense, 3100 Ricketts Point Road, Aberdeen Proving Ground, Maryland 21010-5400

INTRODUCTION

A chemical agent is a substance "intended for use in military operations to kill, seriously injure, or incapacitate man because of its physiological effects."[1(p1-1)] Chemical warfare agents cause injuries directly by irritation, burning, or asphyxiation, and indirectly by contaminating ground so that it cannot be safely occupied, creating smoke screens to obscure operations or reduce the accuracy of an enemy's firepower, and damaging an enemy's equipment by incendiary action. In short, chemical warfare is the use of any synthetic compound or material designed and used for the purpose of harming others. In the modern era, chemical agents have been divided into five categories: nerve agents, vesicants, choking agents, blood agents, and incapacitants. Excluded from consideration in this chapter are riot control agents, chemical herbicides, and smoke and flame materials.

Chemical warfare evolved from studies of plant poisons by ancient Egyptian and Indian civilizations to the studies of Aristotle, Mithridates, Galen, da Vinci, and Nobel scientists at the turn of the 20th century.[2] The concept that chemicals can be used as deadly poisons on a small scale has been understood since the start of written civilization, and evidence of their use has pervaded myth and history for thousands of years. Some scholars suggest that the English colonists at Jamestown were poisoned with arsenic trioxide by Spanish operatives intent on maintaining a monopoly in the New World. Throughout history, individuals used plant poisons and chemicals to remove romantic and political rivals, despotic rulers, prisoners, and even unwanted spouses. Despite these small-scale uses of chemical poisons before the 20th century, military use of chemicals was rare. In the early 20th century, World War I changed the face of warfare with the use of chemicals on a massive scale.

This chapter, the first in a series of three chapters on the history of chemical warfare, focuses on the historical development of chemical warfare, its large-scale use during World War I, post–World War I incidents of chemical warfare, legislative efforts to ban chemical agent use, chemical warfare plans during World War II, and chemical warfare and terrorism today. The discussion will emphasize the historical experiences of the United States on the battlefields of Europe, Asia, and North Africa. It will be followed by Chapter 3, History of the Medical Management of Chemical Casualties, and Chapter 4, History of the Chemical Threat, Chemical Terrorism, and the Implications for Military Medicine.

CHEMICAL CONCOCTIONS USED IN BATTLE

Toxic Smokes

The first recorded history from civilizations in Egypt, Babylon, India, and China contain references to deadly poisons. The first pharaoh, Menes, cultivated, studied, and accumulated poisons from plants, animals, and minerals in 3000 BCE. Egyptians also investigated the lethal effects of hydrocyanic acid.[2] Beginning in 2000 BCE, the great dynasties in India used smoke screens, toxic sleep-inducing fumes, and incendiary devices on a large scale during battle.[2,3] Chinese writings from 1000 BCE contain recipes for the production of poisonous, noxious, and irritant vapors for use in war, including arsenic-containing "soul-hunting fog." The Chinese also developed stink bombs of poisonous smoke and shrapnel, along with a chemical mortar that fired cast-iron "stink" shells.[4]

The powerful city-states of ancient Greece also experimented with chemical concoctions. During the First Sacred War in 590 BCE, Athens and Sicyon plotted to lay siege to the fortified city of Kirrha in retaliation for the harassment of pilgrims to the Oracle of Apollo at Delphi. Solon, the sage of Athens, had the River Pleistos, the main water supply to Kirrha, poisoned with hellebore roots, causing diarrhea that led to the defeat of the besieged city (as described by Pausanias in 150 BCE). Thucydides described the first use of chemical warfare in Western civilization, by Sparta against Athens, in his *History of the Peloponnesian War* (431–404 BCE). During the siege of Plataea in 428 BCE, wood was saturated with pitch and sulfur to generate arsenic smoke, and then burned under the walls of the city to produce poisonous choking fumes (as well as fear and panic). A rainstorm minimized the effect, but the strategy was successfully employed again by Sparta and its allies during the siege of Delium, an Athenian fortification, in 424 BCE. Dating from the 4th century BCE, Mohist sect manuscripts in China describe chemical tactics employed against entrenched, well-defended armies in caves and tunnels, using bellows to pump smoke from burning balls of mustard and other toxic plants.[3,4]

Chemical warfare was also practiced during the time of the Roman empire. About 200 BCE, the Carthaginians left mandrake root in wine to sedate the enemy.[4] Inhabitants of Ambracia in Epirus used toxic smoke to deter the Romans from breaching their walls.[5] Between 82 and 72 BCE the Romans used a toxic smoke that caused blindness and choking pulmonary symptoms when inhaled, similar to phosgene.[6] This tactic allowed the Romans to defeat the Spanish Charakitanes in only 2 days. During the 15th century CE, arsenic smokes were used by Christians against the invading Turks at the siege of Delium. Austrian historian von Senfftenberg wrote about the arsenic cloud: "It was a sad business. Christians must never use so murderous a weapon against other Christians. Still, it is quite in place against Turks and other miscreants."[7(p7)]

Greek Fire and Flaming Concoctions

The Greeks found ways to use their static burning concoctions of pitch, sulfur, tow, and resinous wood chips with incendiary arrows, flaming pots shot from catapults, and fire cannons mounted on boats. The most famous of all the ancient methods of chemical warfare, Greek fire, helped ensure the success of the Byzantine Empire. Although the exact formula for Greek fire has been lost to history, the ingredients included resin, pitch, sulfur, naphtha or petroleum, quicklime, and saltpeter. Discharged from tubes in the bows of ships, the mixture ignited on contact with water and burned on the surface of the sea. Greek fire was invented by Kallinikos (sometimes called Callinus), who arrived in Constantinople in 668 CE after fleeing Muslim-occupied Syria. The Byzantines had used naphtha siphons and squirt guns in 513, but Kallinikos's idea to pump pressurized naphtha through bronze tubes to ignite enemy ships broke the Muslim siege of Constantinople in 677 CE, enabling the Byzantine navy to rule the seas and the Byzantine empire to flourish for many years.[3]

Poison Projectiles in Siege Warfare

The Renaissance spawned an interest in novel war machines and chemical weaponry. Leonardo da Vinci proposed a machine in the 15th century to fire shells filled with a powder mixture of sulfur, arsenic, and verdigris (copper acetate).[8] Aimed at ships' galleys, the projectiles poisoned the lungs of anyone in the vicinity of the dispersed powder. In the 1600s incendiary shells filled with sulfur, tallow, rosin, turpentine, saltpeter, and antimony were used to start fires in sieges. Similar toxic smoke projectiles were designed and used during the Thirty Years War (1618–1648). In 1672, during his siege of the city of Groningen, Christoph Bernhard van Galen, the Bishop of Münster, employed several different explosive and incendiary devices containing belladonna alkaloids intended to produce toxic fumes. In response to the use of poison projectiles, the French and Germans signed the Strasbourg Agreement just 3 years later on August 27, 1675. This was the first documented international agreement to ban the use of "perfidious and odious" toxic devices.[4] In addition to their use as gaseous poisons, militaries also used chemicals to gain an advantage under the cover of thick haze. In 1701 Charles XII of Sweden used chemical smoke screens to obscure his crossing of the Dvina River under a gas cloud.[9]

In 1854 Lyon Playfair, a British chemist, proposed a cacodyl cyanide artillery shell for use against enemy ships as a way to resolve the stalemate during the siege of Sevastopol. Although British Prime Minister Lord Palmerston considered the idea, the British Ordnance Department rejected it, calling it as "bad a mode of warfare as poisoning the wells of the enemy."[10(p22)] Playfair's response was used to justify chemical warfare into the next century:

> There was no sense in this objection. It is considered a legitimate mode of warfare to fill shells with molten metal which scatters among the enemy, and produced the most frightful modes of death. Why a poisonous vapor which would kill men without suffering is to be considered illegitimate warfare is incomprehensible. War is destruction, and the more destructive it can be made with the least suffering the sooner will be ended that barbarous method of protecting national rights. No doubt in time chemistry will be used to lessen the suffering of combatants, and even of criminals condemned to death.[10(pp22–23)]

A few years later, citizens of the fragmenting United States began considering the first American proposals for chemical warfare.

CHEMICAL WARFARE PROPOSALS IN THE US CIVIL WAR

New York schoolteacher John Doughty is credited with developing the first American proposal for chemical warfare. Pitching his idea to the War Department in 1862, Doughty advocated the offensive use of chlorine gas by launching an artillery shell filled with 2 to 3 quarts of liquid chlorine. After the shell exploded, the chlorine gas would rout "an entrenched enemy" or ward "off the attacks of iron-clad vessels and steam rams."[9(p6)] Doughty added:

> If the shell should explode over the heads of the enemy, the gas would, by its great specific gravity, rapidly fall to the ground: the men could not dodge it, and their first intimation of its presence would be by its inhalation, which would most effectually disqual-

> ify every man for service that was within the circle of its influence; rendering the disarming and capturing of them as certain as though both their legs were broken.[11(p27)]

Although Secretary of War Edwin M Stanton apparently never answered it, Doughty's letter was later published in the *Journal of the American Military Institute*.[9] The idea was one of many suggestions and inventions flooding the War and Navy Offices during the time, including a proposal by Joseph Lott of Hartford, Connecticut, for using hand-pumped fire engines to spray chloroform on Confederate garrisons to anesthetize troops prior to their capture.[12] Over 50 years after Doughty's original proposal, the German army developed chlorine gas cylinders and eventually chlorine bombs to combat trench warfare in World War I.

During the 1864 siege of Petersburg, General Ulysses Grant's army was stalled outside the city. Forrest Shepherd, a professor of agricultural chemistry at Western Reserve University, proposed mixing hydrochloric and sulfuric acids to create a toxic cloud to defeat the entrenched Confederate defenders.[11] Because chemical warfare was viewed as inhumane at the time, Grant never acted upon the plan. Other such ideas were recorded during the war. Union Army Captain EC Boyton proposed the use of a cacodyl glass grenade for ship-to-ship fighting.[11] Lieutenant Colonel William W Blackford, a Confederate engineer, designed a sulfur cartridge for use as a counter tunneling device.[13] The Confederates also considered using Chinese stink bombs against the Union troops. With the possible exemption of Blackford's cartridge, none of the proposals were applied on the battlefield.

WORLD WAR I

Chemical Warfare Use by France, Great Britain, and Germany

Most casualties in warfare from the Middle Ages until the First World War were the result of cold steel, wooden projectiles, and fast-moving metals propelled by explosives. World War I ushered in a new style of fighting involving stalemates of trench warfare (Figure 2-1), and synthetic chemists tested new chemical weapons in the arena of "no man's land." Trenches made bullets less useful and reduced mobility, but poison gas could uproot a well-entrenched enemy.

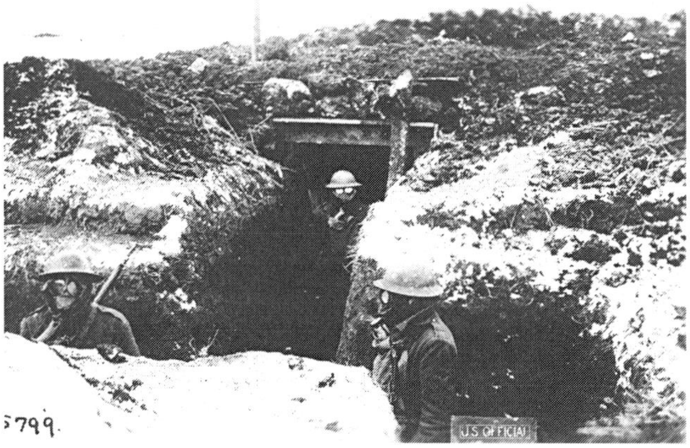

Fig. 2-1. Trench warfare. American Expeditionary Forces Second Division soldiers alerted to the sounds of gas alarms. US Signal Corps photograph.
Photograph: Courtesy of US Army Military History Institute, Carlisle, Pa.

All of Europe was caught in the crisis of 1914 after the murder of Archduke Francis Ferdinand at Sarajevo. Declarations of war among Austria-Hungary, Serbia, Germany, France, Russia, and Great Britain soon followed (Figure 2-2). The United States remained neutral for several years under President Woodrow Wilson's policy. Although few expected the 19th century chemical proposals to become instrumental in tactical operations on the battlefield, the highly skilled research scientists and chemists of the principal combatants quickly adapted chemicals as primary weapons. Early in the war, French intelligence and captured German prisoners warned the Triple Entente (the United Kingdom, France, and Russia) of the numerous German factories being built along the Rhein that were capable of synthesizing vast quantities of toxic chemicals for use on the battlefield. Despite international efforts to restrict chemical weapons in the late 19th and early 20th centuries (see Chapter 4, History of the Chemical Threat, Chemical Terrorism, and Its Implications for Military Medicine), as both sides became rooted in their labyrinth of trenches in the early stages of World War I, the armies turned to chemical warfare.

Early Allied Chemical Warfare Plans

Despite the long-held belief that Germany was the first to use chemical agents during World War I, the French were actually the first; in August 1914, they fired toxic gas from rifles in the form of ethyl bromoacetate tear gas grenades. The French had tested

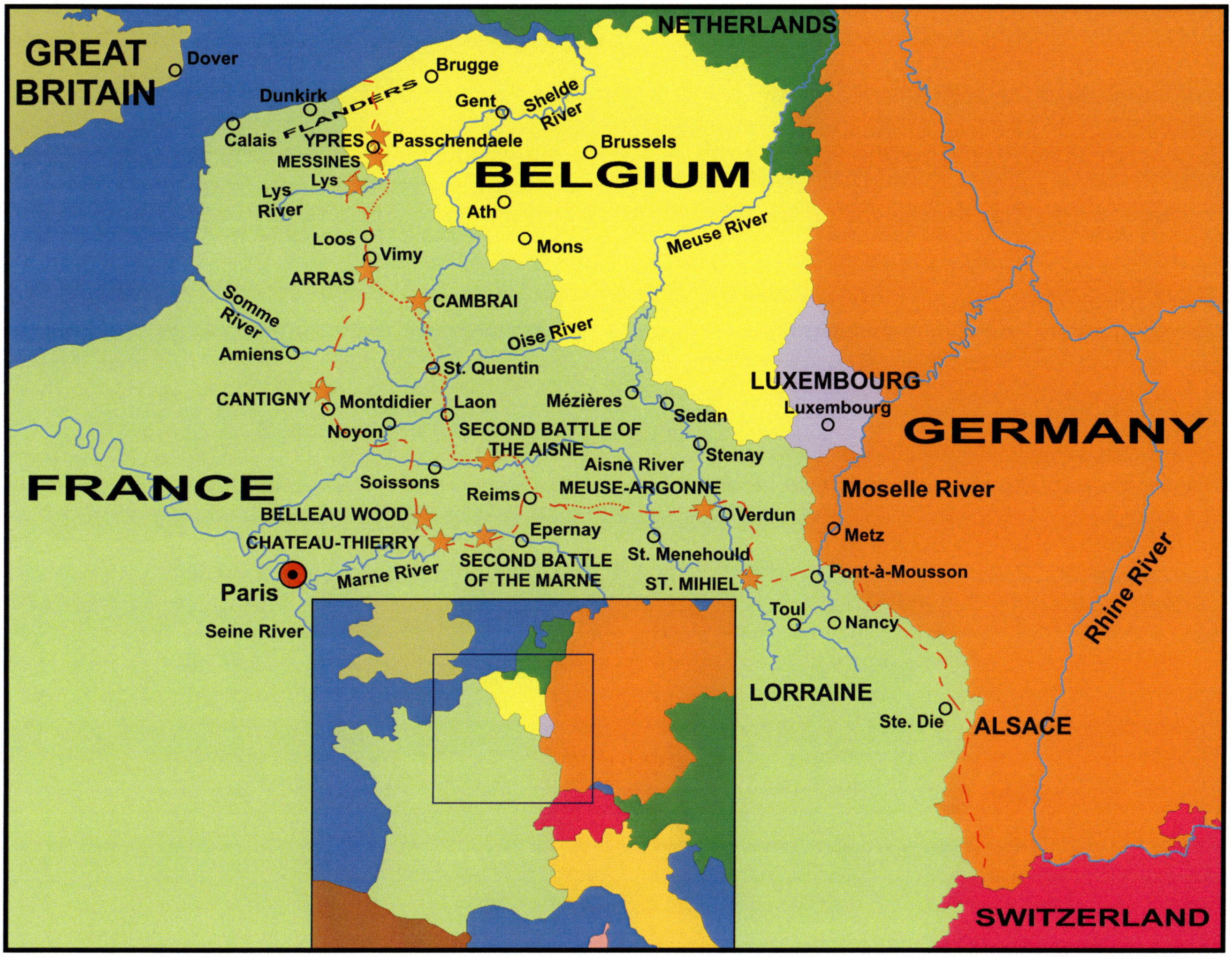

Fig. 2-2. Map of western Europe in World War I. Symbols depict major cities, lines indicating the furthest extent of German occupation, and battles where the American Expeditionary Forces engaged German lines in chemical warfare.
Map: Courtesy of Dr Corey J Hilmas, United States Army Medical Research Institute of Chemical Defense.

ethyl bromoacetate grenades before the war, and they continued to use tear agents against the Germans throughout the conflict. However, the ineffectiveness of these weapons caused poison agents to remain unnoticed until the Second Battle of Ypres in 1915.

The British also examined their chemical technology for battlefield use in the early stages of the war, investigating tear agents but later turning to more toxic chemicals. In January 1915 several chemists at the Imperial College gassed a representative of the War Office, successfully demonstrating the use of ethyl iodoacetate as a tear gas. A suggestion for using sulfur dioxide as a chemical weapon, after being rejected for the army by Field Marshal Lord Kitchener, was presented to Winston Churchill at the admiralty in March 1915. The proposal included a plan to use a sulfur dioxide cloud against the Germans, a smoke screen to provide cover, and gas-proof helmets for British troops. Churchill rejected the plan but formed a committee the following month to discuss the use of smoke on land and sea.[14]

German Chemical Warfare Plans

Possibly aware of the Allied interest in chemical weapons, the Germans also pursued war applications for chemical technology. The strong German dye industry and the plethora of scientists in Berlin created an ideal situation for developing offensive chemical weapons. Professor Walther Nernst, recipient of the 1920 Nobel Prize in chemistry, suggested placing trinitrotoluene (TNT) in a 105-mm shrapnel shell with dianisidine chlorosulphonate, an agent known to cause irritation to the mucous membranes.[15] Germans called these "Nernst Ni-Shrapnel" or "ni-shells," partly derived from the German word for sneezing powder, "niespulver." After the French deployed tear gas, Germany saw no reason to refrain from using its own chemical weapons.

Western Front: The Battle at Neuve-Chapelle

Germany first tested the Nernst weapon on the western front. On October 27, 1914, 3,000 of these shrapnel irritant shells fell on British and Indian troops near Neuve-Chapelle in Northern France. Although the British were unprepared for such an attack, the soldiers suffered no ill effects. The Germans remained convinced that chemicals had merit, however, and continued to experiment with new gas formulations.[15]

Eastern Front: T-Shells at the Battle of Bolimov

Three months after Neuve-Chapelle, the Germans tried xylyl bromide (a form of tear gas) on the Russian front in Poland. The Battle of Bolimov, launched on January 31, 1915, preliminary to the Second Battle of the Masurian Lakes, was the site of the German army's first extensive use of poison gas. Germany employed a new gas shell ("Tappen-shell," "T-shell," or "T-Stoff") that contained an explosive charge for producing a duel shrapnel and poison effect, designed by Professor Hans von Tappen of the Kaiser Wilhelm Institute for Physical Chemistry and Electrochemistry in Berlin. For the new weapon, von Tappen made two improvements to Nernst's shells. First, he stabilized the chemical liquid within the shell casing to reduce tumbling when fired from a standard 15-cm howitzer, increasing the shell's accuracy and range. Second, he designed a shell casing to prevent accidental mixing of the extremely reactive chemical substances inside. Each shell contained 7 lb of xylyl bromide, a burster charger for splinter effect, and a lead lining to prevent contact between the burster charge and the chemical payload.[15,16]

However, the firing of 18,000 shells at Russian positions around Bolimov proved entirely unsuccessful. The Russians easily repulsed the overconfident German attack and the German gas failure halted any further assaults on Bolimov. The chemical failed for several reasons. The winter weather was too cold to cause the liquid to vaporize to the gaseous state, and the agent was either blown back towards the German lines or fell harmlessly to the ground. Also, xylyl bromide was a weakly irritating tear gas, and the liquid could not be dispersed in sufficient concentration to cause damage. Although aware that the Germans had attempted an attack with poison gas, the Russians did not widely report it to their Western allies because of its failure. The Germans again attempted to use T-shells on the western front at Nieuport in March 1915, with similar results.[14,17,18] Although unsuccessful, these experiments provided Germany with the experience to improve future attempts. Poison gas next appeared with much greater success on the western front in April 1915, during the Second Battle of Ypres .

Development of Chlorine

Fritz Haber, professor at the Kaiser Wilhelm Physical Institute of Berlin (and later the 1918 Nobel Laureate in chemistry), directed German field operations involving chemical warfare (Exhibit 2-1). Haber is credited with the concept of creating a toxic cloud from chemical cylinders in late 1914. Learning the lessons from von Tappen's T-shells, Haber suggested the use of large commercial gas cylinders as a delivery system instead of artillery shells, which were in short supply. He also postulated that gas from storage cylinders would cover a far broader area than gas dispersed from artillery shells. In addition, neither the T-shell nor the chlorine gas cylinders technically violated the Hague ban on projectiles. Haber selected chlorine because it was readily available from the German dye industry and satisfied requirements for military application: it was lethal, immediately effective, nonpersistent, and volatile. Chlorine could form a toxic gas cloud dense enough to resist dilution in a moderate wind but with no prolonged influence over the terrain.[15]

The Second Battle of Ypres

During October and November 1914, the French, British, and Belgian forces had stopped the advance of Germany's Schlieffen Plan, at great costs to both sides. The First Battle of Ypres had resulted in a stalemate, with each side entrenched. Germany selected the front of the Fourth Army facing the French at Ypres as the location for a gas attack (see Figure 2-2). On March 10, 1915, Pioneer Regiment 35, under Haber's guidance, placed 1,600 large and 4,130 small cylinders (containing a total of 168 tons of chlorine) opposite the Allied troops defending Ypres.[15] The chosen site was a sector between Bixschoote and Langemarck in Belgium (Figure 2-3), a tactical weak point where French and British forces joined.[9] The English-speaking troops consisted of Canadians and the British 28th Division. The French troops were the 87th Territorial and 45th Algerian Divisions.[9] Pioneer Regiment 35 waited for winds to shift to the west toward Allied trenches before the actual gas attack was delivered late in the afternoon on April 22,[14,15,17,19]

EXHIBIT 2-1

WAR OF THE CHEMISTS

During World War I, chemists on both sides investigated over 3,000 chemical substances for potential use as weapons. The war between the nations was just as much a war between the chemists. Germany had two future Nobel Laureates in chemistry on their side, and France had one as well. The adoption of poison gas by the Germans in World War I is attributed to Professor Walther Hermann Nernst, a well-known physical chemist in Berlin. In recognition for his services to the German Empire, he was made a count late in the war. However, World War I was the setting for a strategic match between rival chemists, with Germany's Fritz Haber pitted against his French counterpart, Victor Grignard.
Fritz Haber played a major role in the development of chemical warfare in World War I. He developed early gas masks with absorbent filters and masterminded the first chlorine attacks at Ypres, Belgium. In his studies of the effects of poison gas, Haber discovered a simple mathematical relationship between the concentration (C) of the gas and the amount of time (t) it was breathed in, expressed as $C \times t = k$, where k is a constant. In other words, exposure to a low level of gas for a long time can cause the same result (eg death) as exposure to a high concentration for a short time. This relationship is known as "Haber's rule."

Haber's rival was Francois Auguste Victor Grignard, a French chemist and professor at the University of Nancy. During World War I, he was transferred to the new field of chemical warfare and worked on the manufacture of phosgene and the detection of mustard gas. His Nobel Prize in chemistry was awarded for devising a new method for creating carbon-carbon bonds in organic synthesis termed "the Grignard reaction," which allowed the means of synthesizing larger organic compounds from smaller starting materials.

Haber's wife opposed his work on poison gas and committed suicide with his service weapon after he personally oversaw the first use of chlorine in Ypres, Belgium. Haber defended gas warfare against accusations that it was inhumane, saying that death was death, by whatever means it was inflicted. In the 1920s he developed the cyanide gas formulation Zyklon B, which was used as an insecticide, especially as a fumigant in grain stores. The Nazis later used Zyklon B (hydrogen cyanide) gas chambers disguised as shower stalls beginning with the first and longest running Schutzstaffel camp at Dachau. In 1934, the Nazis forced Haber, a German Jew, to emigrate. Haber was a patriotic German who was proud of his service in World War I, for which he was decorated. He struggled to cope with the new reality that his enormous contributions to German industry were disregarded during his vilification by the Nazi regime. He died in exile in Basel after a grave illness.

Data sources: (1) Haber LF. *The Poisonous Cloud: Chemical Warfare in the First World War*. Oxford, England: Clarendon Press; 1986: 15–40. (2) Heller CE. No. 10 chemical warfare in World War I: the American experience, 1917–1918. In: *The Leavenworth Papers*. Fort Leavenworth, Kan: Combat Studies Institute, US Army Command and General Staff College; 1984: 6–7. (3) Szöllösi-Janze M. Pesticides and war: the case of Fritz Haber. *Eur Rev*. 2001;9:97–108. (4) Harris R, Paxman J. *A Higher Form of Killing: the Secret History of Chemical and Biological Warfare*. New York, NY: Random House; 2002.

when the weather and wind patterns were ideal for a toxic cloud (Figure 2-4).

The Allies claimed that 5,000 troops fell victim to the chlorine cloud (although this number was probably inflated for propaganda purposes).[9,20] The gas attack was successful, but the Germans grossly underestimated the chlorine's effects and, lacking sufficient supplies and reserves for an assault, failed to capitalize on the retreating Allied positions.[14,15,17,19] Any further possible German advance was stopped by Canadian troops at Kitchener's Wood while the British and French hastily organized a defensive front during the next 48 hours.[9]

Two days later, Germans conducted a second chlorine gas attack against the Canadian First Division northeast of Ypres, near Saint Julien, and four more cylinder gas attacks during May in the Ypres sector. The German gas-aided capture of Hill 60 on May 5 was a significant blow to the Allies.

Although the Allies expressed great indignation about this inhumane and unfair weapon (despite their own development of chemical weapons), the Germans believed their use of nonprojectile shells to form gas clouds was within the guidelines of the Hague ban. The comments of General von Deimling, commanding general of the German Fifteenth Corps at Ypres, written sometime after the war, reflected the reason for initiating chemical warfare:

> I must confess that the commission for poisoning the enemy, just as one poisons rats, struck me as it must any straight-forward soldier: it was repulsive to me. If, however, these poison gases would lead to the fall of Ypres, we would perhaps win a victory which

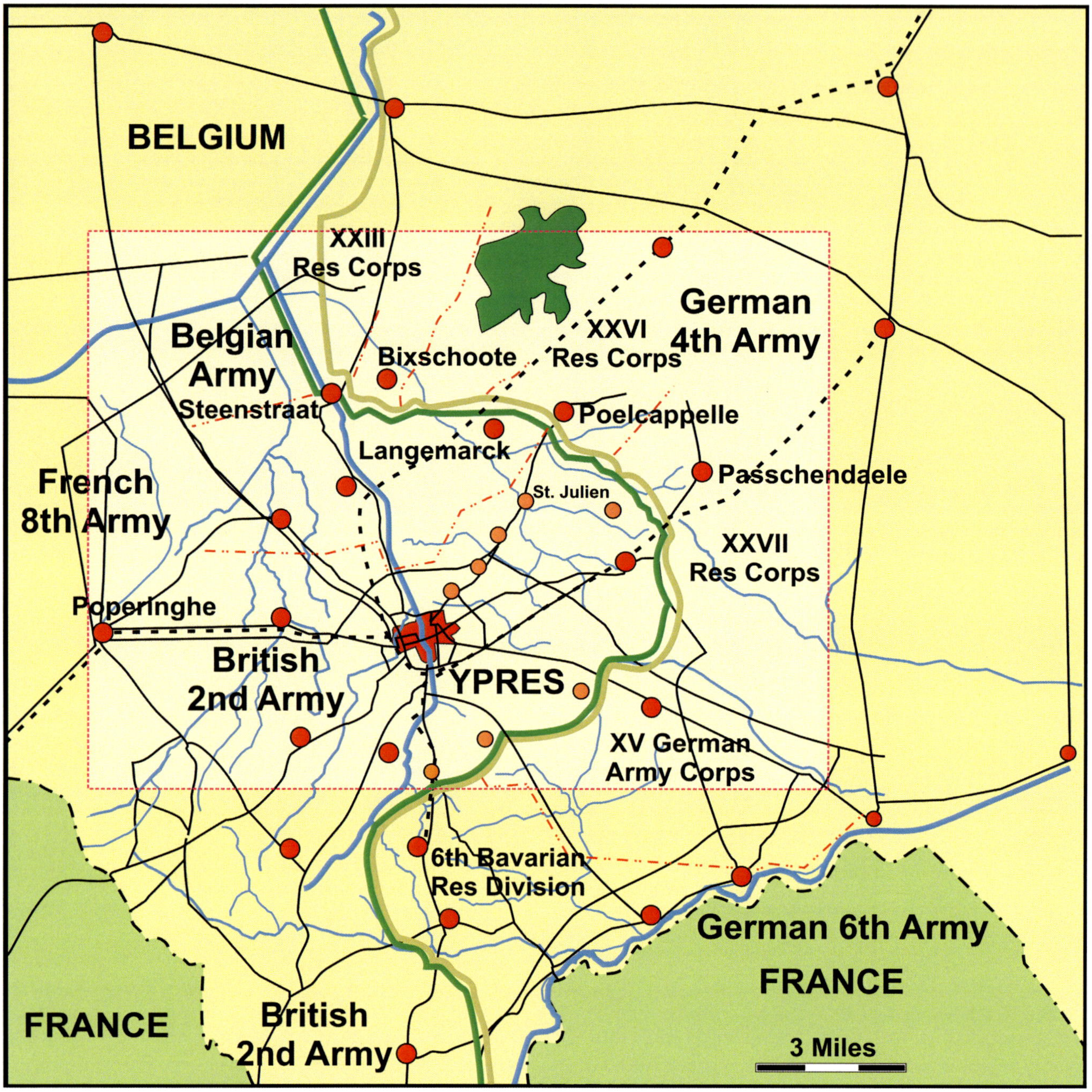

Fig. 2-3. Map of Belgian-French border showing the location of the French, Belgian, British, and German armies at the time of the Second Battle of Ypres.
Map: Courtesy of Dr Corey J Hilmas, United States Army Medical Research Institute of Chemical Defense.

> might decide the entire war. In view of such a high goal, personal susceptibilities had to be silent.[21(p5)]

Despite the numbers of Allied casualties and prisoners, the battle was a mixed success. The Germans failed to take advantage of their success, but the Allies, made aware of the pending gas attack when British pilots spotted the gas cylinders in the German trenches, were also unprepared.[21] One British soldier remarked:

> Nobody appears to have realized the great danger that was threatening, it being considered that the enemy's attempt would certainly fail and that whatever gas reached our line could be easily fanned

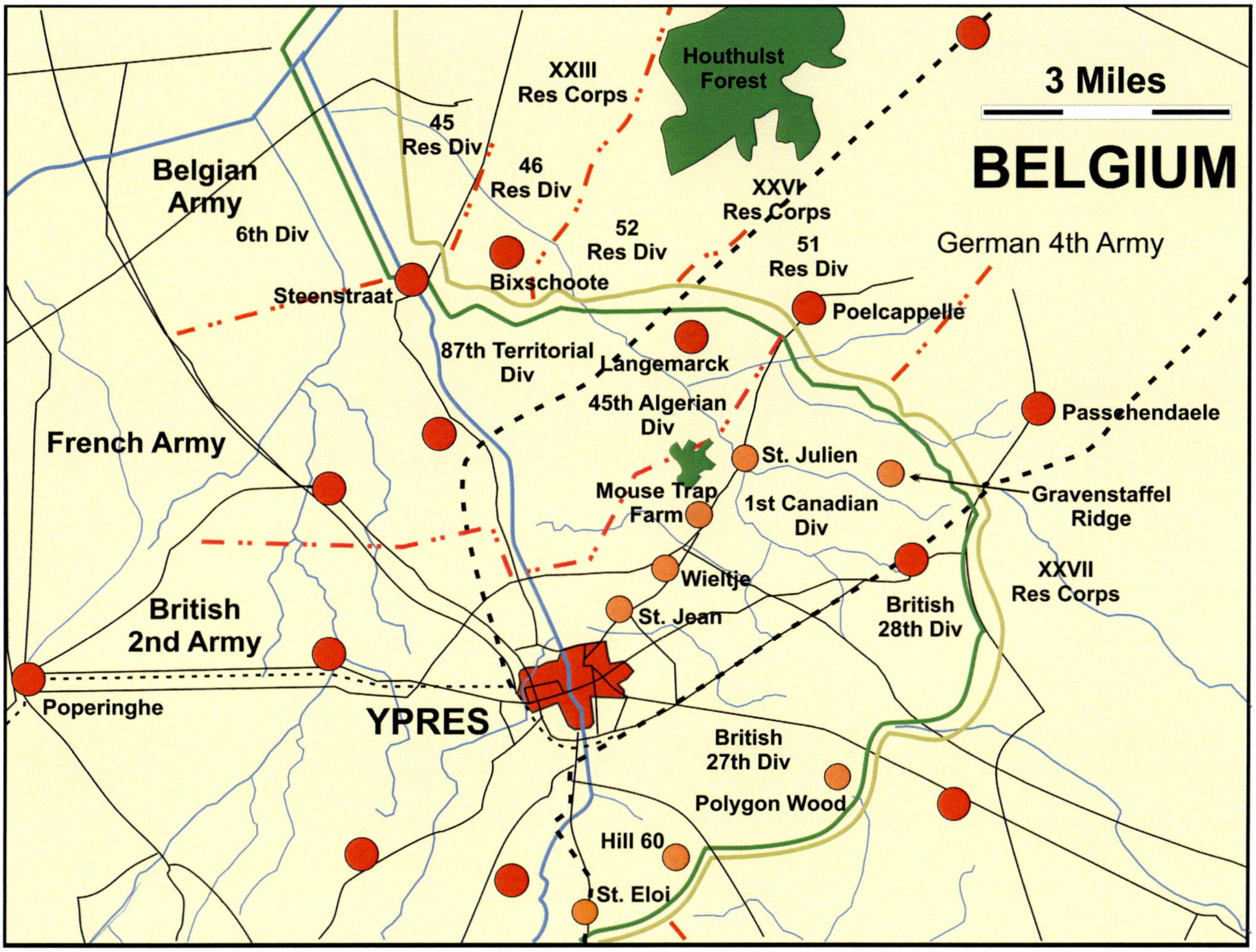

Fig. 2-4. Detailed map of Ypres, depicting the German, British, Canadian, and French fronts along the outskirts of town. This was the location of each major division prior to the release of chlorine shells on April 22, 1915.
Map: Courtesy of Dr Corey J Hilmas, United States Army Medical Research Institute of Chemical Defense.

> away. No one felt in the slightest degree uneasy, and the terrible effect of the gas came to us as a great surprise.[22(p3)]

Another observer, however, realized a profound change had occurred: "The most stupendous change in warfare since gunpowder was invented had come, and come to stay. Let us not forget that."[23(p3)]

Although chlorine had its disadvantages and the German attack against Ypres halted short of its objective, chemical warfare became a mainstay of German assaults and Allied counterattacks on the Ypres salient throughout the rest of the war (Figure 2-5). The Ypres sector became an experimental stage for the Germans to develop and test new gases on other battlefronts. A third battle occurred at Ypres in 1917 (at which the young Adolf Hitler was seriously wounded during an Allied chlorine gas attack).

After the success at Ypres, Haber turned German attention back to the eastern front to atone for the failure of xylyl bromide T-shells. In May 1915 German troops again attacked Russians at Bolimov, releasing 263 tons of chlorine gas from 12,000 cylinders along a 7.5-mile line, killing 6,000 Russian soldiers. Two more gas cloud attacks on the same positions caused 25,000 more Russian casualties.[15] The Russians had initially devoted few resources to the development of chemical protective equipment. Consequently, they were more vulnerable to gas attacks than the British and French and suffered the greatest number of chemical casualties in World War I.

All of the first chemical attacks of World War I were in the form of chemical vapor clouds projected from cylinders, totaling nearly 200 by the end of the

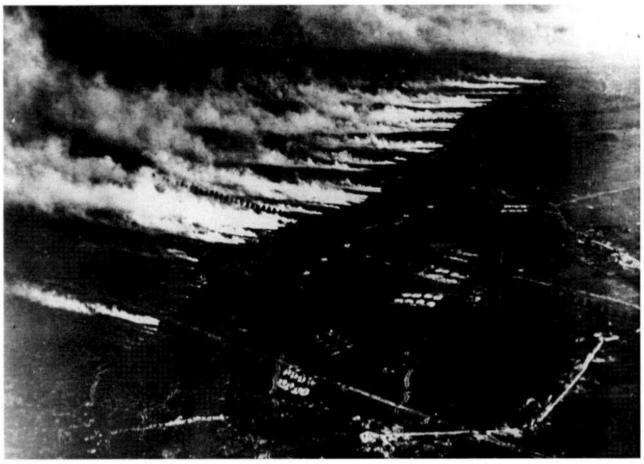

Fig. 2-5. A French cylinder attack on German trenches in Flanders. The critical importance of the wind is apparent. Condensation of water vapor caused the cloud-like appearance of the gas.
Photograph: Courtesy of Chemical and Biological Defense Command Historical Research and Response Team, Aberdeen Proving Ground, Md.

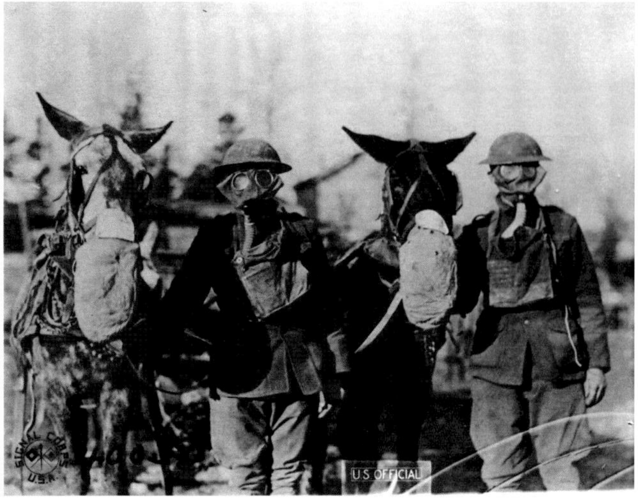

Fig. 2-6. Prevention of animal casualties during gas warfare was a concern. Photograph depicts gas masks on mule and soldier. Dun sur Meuse, Meuse, France. November 21, 1918. US Signal Corps photograph. Photograph: Courtesy of US Army Military History Institute, Carlisle, Pa.

war. Although the largest chlorine attack occurred in October 1915 at Reims, when the Germans released 550 tons of chlorine from 25,000 cylinders, chemicals delivered by artillery shells soon became the norm.[9,15] The Germans learned that a vapor cloud was dependent on wind direction and strength, neither of which could be predicted with any amount of accuracy. These initial chemical attacks also proved that an infantry attack synchronized with a discharged vapor cloud was extremely dangerous.

Allied Chemical Warfare Retaliation

Only weeks after recognizing the potential of chemical weapons at Ypres, the British and French began planning a chemical retaliation, which became a three-pronged strategy to develop their own (1) protective devices for troops (Figure 2-6); (2) offensive toxic gas weapons; and (3) systems to deliver the toxic gases to enemy lines. The Allies developed their first protective mask the day after the first German chlorine attack, and in September 1915 they launched their own chlorine attack against the Germans at Loos, Belgium. These moves initiated a deadly competition to develop better protective masks, more potent chemicals, and long-range delivery systems to disperse the agents more widely. The Germans quickly replaced chlorine with phosgene, which was more effective. In May 1916 the Germans started using diphosgene, and 2 months later the French tried hydrogen cyanide (HCN), then cyanogen chloride. In July 1917 the Germans introduced mustard agent to provide a persistent vesicant that attacked the body in places unprotected by gas masks. Both sides also mixed agents and experimented with camouflage materials to prevent quick agent identification.[4]

The Battle of Loos

In the aftermath of Ypres, it became apparent that lacking an offensive gas capability would impair troop morale, and the British cabinet approved the use of chemical agents. It took 5 months to plan the large-scale gas attack at Loos, which involved chlorine-filled cylinders clustered in batteries along the front rather than spaced far apart in one continuous line. The British had a major numerical advantage against the Germans, reaching 7-to-1 in some places along the front. British commander General Douglas Haig began the offensive with a 4-day artillery bombardment by six divisions, planning to follow the bombardment with the release of 5,500 cylinders containing 150 tons of chlorine gas from the British front line.[15(p11),20(p14–17)]

The gas attack occurred on September 24 with only minimal success. Unfavorable and shifting winds reduced the effectiveness of the chlorine gas cloud, the number of chlorine cylinders was insufficient to cover the front line, and inadequate reserve divisions were available to exploit a breakthrough (a lesson learned by the Germans at Ypres).[20] A British shell shortage also

EXHIBIT 2-2

PHOSGENE

Chlorine's deficiencies were overcome with the introduction of phosgene, first used by Germany in December 1915. Phosgene, also known as carbonyl chlorine ($COCl_2$), is a highly toxic gas first synthesized by the chemist John Davy (1790–1868) in 1812 by exposing equal quantities of carbon monoxide and chlorine to sunlight. "Phosgene" comes from Greek, literally meaning "generated by light." Phosgene is colorless and 18 times more potent than chlorine. It is often only detected by its characteristic "moldy hay" odor. One disadvantage of phosgene as a chemical warfare agent was that it was lightweight and readily dissipated, but this problem was surmounted by addition of the heavier chlorine. The chlorine supplied the necessary vapor to help eject phosgene from containers. The British employed a chlorine-phosgene mixture they codenamed "white star," which was used heavily during the Battle of the Somme. Phosgene is a particularly insidious poison, as exposure often has no initial symptoms. Symptoms usually appear within 24 hours, but can take up to 72 hours to manifest. The gas combines with water in the tissues of the respiratory tract to form carbon dioxide and hydrochloric acid. The acid then dissolves the membranes in the lungs. Fluid fills the lungs, and death results from a combination of blood loss, shock, and respiratory failure. Phosgene was far more lethal than any other common-use gas weapon; 85% of western front soldiers were killed as the result of chemical attack by phosgene.

prevented sustained artillery barrages.[15] On the other hand, British Commander-in-Chief Sir John French acknowledged that although it failed to penetrate the German lines, the "gas attack met with marked success, and produced a demoralizing effect in some of its opposing units."[15,16,23,24]

Ultimately, both sides recognized the need to avoid vapors blowing backward and learned to launch chemicals beyond a trench line using grenades, mortar bombs, and artillery shells. These realizations led to the introduction of the Livens projector and the Stokes mortar, critical advancements to chemical warfare. Both sides also achieved satisfactory protection against chlorine and began looking for newer, deadlier chemicals.

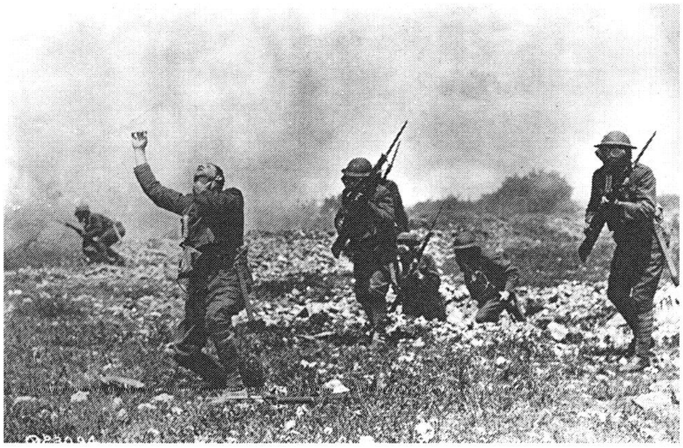

Fig. 2-7. "Gassed," a purportedly staged photograph under the direction of Major Everts Tracy, Engineer Corps, to illustrate the choking effects of phosgene. Location unknown. US Signal Corps photograph. Photograph: Courtesy of US Army Military History Institute, Carlisle, Pa.

Phosgene

Phosgene was the next chemical to debut on the western front at the close of 1915 (Exhibit 2-2). The British, warned by intelligence in midsummer 1915 that Germany planned to use a new choking gas (Figure 2-7), had several months to make defensive preparations, including development of a new gas mask. The phosgene attack took place on December 11, 1915,[9] near the Wieltje ruins of the Ypres salient. The British were ready for the new gas, and the Germans lost a major opportunity to gain a decisive victory. Although gas masks could protect troops against its harmful effects, phosgene proved to be a very effective gas throughout the war, causing more deaths than any other gas in World War I.

The Germans may have used phosgene earlier, in late May and early June 1915, against Russian troops in the vicinity of Bzura and Rawka, and they used it extensively at Verdun in 1916.[15] The "white star" mixture of phosgene and chlorine (chlorine supplied the necessary vapor to carry phosgene) was commonly used on the Somme. When newer gas masks gave adequate protection against chlorine and phosgene, both sides realized that the vapor clouds were better suited as psychological

EXHIBIT 2-3

DIPHOSGENE

Trichloromethyl chloroformate ($ClCO_2CCl_3$) was developed soon after the first use of phosgene in World War I. Like phosgene, it was also known as "green cross" because of the distinct markings on German shells containing the choking gas. The official German name was "perstoff." The British used it under the name "superpolite" or "diphosgene," while the French called it "surpalite." It is a colorless, oily liquid with a distinct odor. It is similar to phosgene because it can break down under certain conditions to form two molecules of phosgene, but it does have an added tear-gas effect. Diphosgene, classified as moderately persistent, remains at the point of release for over 10 minutes.

weapons to create panic in the lines.

Diphosgene

The Germans introduced diphosgene, another pulmonary agent, to their growing deadly arsenal in May 1916. This effective lung irritant and choking gas was dispersed via "green cross" shells, named for the shells' distinct markings. As poisonous as phosgene and sometimes considered more toxic (Exhibit 2-3), diphosgene was developed because the vapors could destroy the gas mask filters in use at the time, and it had greater persistence in the environment than phosgene. Germany eventually deployed combinations of phosgene, diphosgene, and diphenylchlorarsine.

Mustard Gas

Remaining consistently ahead in gas warfare development, Germany introduced mustard gas (sometimes referred to as "Yperite") on July 12, 1917, against Canadian troops near Ypres. Mustard gas was distinguished by the serious blisters it caused both internally and externally several hours after exposure. Protection against mustard gas proved more difficult than against either chlorine or phosgene (Figure 2-8). The first large-scale mustard gas attack occurred just over a week after its first use, when the Germans attacked the British at Nieuport, resulting in over 14,000 casualties, 500 of whom died within 3 weeks. The next month the Germans fired 100,000 mustard shells, marked with a yellow cross, against the French Second Army, causing 20,000 casualties.[25]

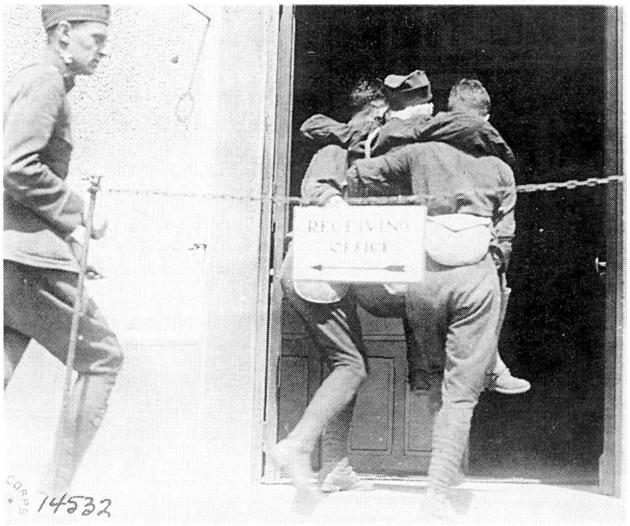

Fig. 2-8. American casualty from mustard being carried into gas hospital. US Signal Corps photograph.
Photograph: Courtesy of US Army Military History Institute, Carlisle, Pa.

In September 1917 Germany employed mustard-laden artillery shells against the Russians at Riga. The Allies did not use mustard until that November at Cambrai, after the British captured a large stock of German yellow cross shells. It took nearly a year for the British to reach large-scale mustard production on their own; they then used it extensively in breaking the Hindenburg line in September 1918.[25]

Major General Amos A Fries, head of the Gas Service of the American Expeditionary Forces (AEF) in France and later chief of the Army's Chemical Warfare Service (CWS), recognized that mustard gas completely changed gas warfare. Although it was first used to produce casualties and fragment enemy troop concentrations, mustard caused 20,000 casualties in only 6 weeks after its introduction. Despite remaining potent in soil for weeks after release, making capture of infected trenches a dangerous undertaking, sulfur mustard lived up to its nickname as "king of the war gases" on the battlefield (Exhibit 2-4). The Germans caused 5,000 French casualties alone in a matter of 10 days during shelling of Verdun in September 1917. Germany continued to use mustard gas to great advantage throughout the winter of 1917–1918, producing casualties, creating confusion, and lowering morale among enemy ranks. In March 1918, during the last great German offensive (Operation Michael), the German army used mustard to neutralize the strongly defended city

EXHIBIT 2-4

MUSTARD: "KING" OF THE WAR GASES

Sulfur mustard was used extensively because it caused more casualties than any other chemical in World War I. The countermeasures against mustard were ineffective because gas masks did not afford protection against skin absorption.

Mustard takes its name from the unpurified form, which is yellow-brown with an odor resembling mustard, garlic, or horseradish. Other names for mustard are "yellow cross," "sulfur mustard," "hun stoffe (HS)," "Distilled Hun (HD)," "senfgas," "blister agent," "Yperite," "S-LOST," or "Kampfstoff LOST." LOST is derived from Lommel and Steinkopf, who developed the process for mass producing mustard during wartime use at the German company Bayer AG. Mustard is a thioether with the formula $C_4H_8Cl_2S$. The compound eliminates chloride ion by intramolecular nucleophilic substitution to form a cyclic sulfonium ion. This reactive intermediate is detrimental to cells of the body as a mutagen and carcinogen because it can bind to the guanine nitrogen in DNA strands, leading to cell death, cancer, and genetic alterations.

The term "mustard gas" is a misnomer; the agent is not a true gas. Dispersed as an aerosol, mustard is not water-soluble but contains high lipid solubility, contributing to its rapid absorption into the skin. Blister agent exposure over more than 50% body surface area was fatal during World War I; however, mustard was lethal in only 1% of cases. As a persistent agent, mustard can remain in the environment for days and continue to cause casualties. This property enabled its use as an area-denial weapon, forcing soldiers to abandon heavily contaminated positions. Contaminated clothing from one soldier could spread to others during battle.

Mustard gas is perhaps best known for the Bari disaster. A US stockpile on the SS *John Harvey* was bombed in Bari, Italy, in 1943 during World War II. This disaster exposed thousands of civilians and Allied troops to the chemical agent.

of Armentieres. During the battle, mustard was said to have "run in the gutters like water."[9(p15)]

Although the first gas attack on a US unit did not involve mustard exclusively, American soldiers feared mustard the most. Despite the many warnings, mustard agent injured over 27,000 Americans.[25]

US Experience with Chemical Warfare

The use of chemical warfare at Ypres in April, followed by the sinking of the Lusitania by a German U-boat off the Irish coast on May 7, 1915, rocked the United States. Americans began to take greater interest in the nature of warfare taking place in Europe and elsewhere. In May 1915 President Wilson proposed that Germany halt chemical warfare in exchange for the British ending their blockade of neutral ports. Both Germany and Great Britain refused to comply.[26]

US Declaration of War

Isolationism left the United States outside what was initially perceived as a European conflict. However, German mistakes resulted in America throwing its weight toward the Allies. Early in 1917 Germany resumed its policy of unrestricted submarine warfare. The Zimmerman telegram, a proposal to the Mexican government initiated by Germany to form an alliance against the United States, was intercepted by the British, leading to public indignation and hastening the entry of the United States into the war. President Wilson asked Congress for a formal declaration of war on Germany on April 2, 1917. Congress declared war on Germany on April 6, and on Austria-Hungary in December 1917.

US Preparation for Chemical Warfare

The United States entered the war a full 2 years after the German army's first successful chlorine gas attack against the Allies. Although the US Army was aware of the increasing use of chemicals on both fronts, it made no effort to prepare for gas warfare until 2 months before the American declaration of war. As a result, the Army began the war with no doctrine or adequate training program for chemical warfare, depending on the Allies for gas-related equipment. However, once begun, preparations advanced quickly.

Only a day after Wilson's call to war, Congress established a subcommittee on noxious gases under the leadership of the director of the US Bureau of Mines. The subcommittee included Army and Navy ordnance and medical officers as well as two members of the chemical committee of the National Research Council. Its mission was to investigate noxious gases, the generation of chemical warfare agents, and the discovery of antidotes for war purposes.[19,27,28] Within a short time, the subcommittee began organizing chemical agent research at universities and industries across the nation, while mobilizing a large portion of the chemists in the country. This initial phase laid the groundwork that later led to the establishment of the CWS, the precursor to the Chemical Corps.

The country's civilian scientists, engineers, and chemistry professors played a significant role in preparing the Army for chemical warfare. Eventually, the War Department also began to plan for chemical warfare, spreading responsibilities initially among the Medical Department, Ordnance Department, and Corps of Engineers. When General John J Pershing began organizing the AEF in France, however, he placed responsibility for all phases of gas warfare in a single military service and recommended that the War Department at home do likewise. On September 3, 1917, the AEF established a centralized Gas Service under the command of Lieutenant Colonel Amos A Fries.[27,28]

Creation of the Chemical Warfare Service

In the spring of 1918 the US government began centralizing gas warfare functions in the War Department under a senior Corps of Engineers officer, Major General William L Sibert. President Wilson transferred the Bureau of Mines research facilities to the War Department, and on June 28, 1918, the CWS was formally established under Sibert as part of the National Army (the wartime Army, as distinguished from the Regular Army), with full responsibility for all facilities and functions relating to toxic chemicals.

The CWS was organized into seven main divisions: (1) The research division, responsible for most of the weapons and agent research during the war, was located at American University near Washington, DC. (2) The gas defense division, responsible for the production of gas masks, had a large plant in Long Island City, New York. (3) The gas offense division was responsible for the production of chemical agents and weapons, its main facility located at Edgewood Arsenal, Maryland. (4) The development division was responsible for carbon production and pilot plant work on mustard agent production. (5) The proving ground division and (6) the training division were located together at Lakehurst, New Jersey. (7) The medical division was responsible for the pharmacological aspects of chemical defense.

The AEF's offensive chemical unit, the 1st Gas Regiment (formerly the 30th Engineers), was organized at American University under the command of Colonel EJ Atkisson in 1917, and sent to France in early 1918 (Exhibit 2-5).[19,27] The US Army finally had an organization that controlled offensive chemical production, defensive equipment production, training, testing, and basic research, along with a new chemical warfare unit unified under a single commander. This organization helped lead the AEF to victory, although much of its work, including the construction of facilities for producing toxic gas, filling plants, and producing gas masks, was only partially completed by the end of the war.

America entered the Great War in bleak circumstances. The failed French offensive in the spring gave

EXHIBIT 2-5

EARLIEST REPORTED DESCRIPTION INVOLVING CHEMICAL WARFARE ON THE AMERICAN EXPEDITIONARY FORCES

The Germans attacked on February 2, 1918, using a bombardment of 25 phosgene or diphosgene shells. The shells were recognized by their "swish and wobbly sound in passage," fired harmlessly by the German army near the 6th Field Artillery in Hazelle woods in the late afternoon. The first American offensive instruction to attack with gas was issued that same day by Major General Bullard. The 1st Division engaged in a long barrage of 6,750 high explosive shells, with the German artillery in retaliation, and fired 80 gas shells on seven German batteries, consisting of No. 4 (cyanogen chloride) and No. 5 (phosgene) gas shells. The French disapproved of this tactic because the firing was fast and long-lasting. This marked the first gas volley between German and US armies. Several days later, on February 6, 1918, the Germans fired one shell containing mustard gas along with numerous high explosive shells, marking the first time that mustard was used on American forces. The first gas casualties were tallied from that shell; three soldiers of the 6th Field Artillery, Battery A, were evacuated with acute conjunctivitis the following day, and a gunner with a burned buttock was evacuated 2 days later.

Data source: Spencer EW. *The History of Gas Attacks Upon the American Expeditionary Forces During the World War, Part I.* Edgewood Arsenal, Md: Chemical Warfare Service, US War Department; 1928: 32–33.

TABLE 2-1

WORLD WAR I AMERICAN EXPEDITIONARY FORCES IN OFFENSIVE AND DEFENSIVE BATTLES INVOLVING CHEMICAL WARFARE

Date	Battle	Participants
November 20–December 4, 1917	Cambrai (France)	11th, 12th, and 14th Engineers
March 21–April 6, 1918	Somme defensive (France)	3rd Division; 12th, 14th Engineers; 2nd, 3rd, 4th Pursuit Groups
April 9–27, 1918	Lys (Belgium)	11th, 16th Engineers; 3rd Pursuit Group
May 27–June 26, 1918	Aisne-Marne defensive (France)	2nd Division, 3rd Division
June 9–13, 1918	Montdidier-Noyon defensive (France)	1st Division
July 15–18, 1918	Champagne-Marne defensive (France)	3rd, 26th, 28th, 42nd Divisions; 369th Infantry; 66th Field Artillery Brigade; 42nd, 44th Artilleries; 1st Corps Artillery Park; 322nd Field Signal Battalion; 406th Telegraph Battalion; 1st Corps Observation Squadron; 3rd, 5th Corps Observation Groups; 1st Pursuit Group; 1st Corps Balloon Group
July 18–August 13, 1918	Aisne-Marne offensive (France)	1st Division; 2nd Division; 3rd Division; 4th Division; 26th Division; 28th Division; 32nd Division; 42nd Division; 369th Infantry; 66th Field Artillery Brigade; 1st Corps Artillery Park; 1st Gas Regiment (B & D Companies); 1st Battalion Trench Artillery; 2nd Cavalry; 308th, 322nd Field Signal Battalions; 14th, 29th, 40th, 308th Engineers; 1st Pioneer Infantry; 52nd, 406th, 411th Telegraph Battalion; 1st, 3rd, 5th Corps Observation Groups; 1st Pursuit Group; 1st, 3rd Corps Balloon Groups
August 8–November 11, 1918	Somme offensive (France)	27th Division; 30th Division; 33rd Division; 318th Field Signal Battalion; 412th Telegraph Battalion; 301st Battalion Tank Corps
August 18–September 17, 1918	Oise-Aisne (France)	28th Division; 32nd Division; 77th Division; 370th Infantry, 57th Field Artillery Brigade; 1st, 2nd Corps Artillery Parks; 55th, 56th Artilleries; 308th Field Signal Battalion; 14th, 308th Engineers; 1st Pioneer Infantry; 52nd Telegraph Battalion
August 19–November 11, 1918	Ypres-Lys offensive (Belgium)	27th Division, 30th Division, 37th Division, 91st Division, 412th Telegraph Battalion
September 12–16, 1918	Saint Mihiel offensive (France)	1st, 2nd, 3rd, 4th, 5th, 26th, 30th, 33rd, 36th, 42nd, 78th, 80th, 82nd, 89th, and 90th Divisions; others (organizations not assigned to divisions); 1st Gas Regiment (A, B, C, D, E, and F Companies)
September 26–November 11, 1918	Meuse-Argonne offensive (France)	1st, 2nd, 3rd, 4th, 5th, 6th, 26th, 27th, 28th, 29th, 30th, 32nd, 33rd, 35th, 36th, 37th, 42nd, 77th, 78th, 79th, 80th, 81st, 82nd, 89th, 90th, 91st, and 92nd Divisions, and others
October 24–November 4, 1918	Vittorio Veneto (Italy)	332nd Infantry

way to mutinies within the ranks. The British attacks on Messines Ridge, Ypres, and Cambrai failed in their primary objectives, leading to significant casualties and low unit morale (Table 2-1). Initially, the British and French primarily wanted US infantry to reinforce the lines, but General John J Pershing resisted breaking up American units and using them simply as reinforcements. The first American units, members of the AEF 1st Division, arrived in France in July 1917. Ill-prepared to use or defend themselves against chemical weapons, the American troops found gas warfare an inescapable fact of life in the trenches, with chemicals contaminating clothing, food, water, equipment, and the trenches themselves. American officers were reluctant to employ chemical agents for fear of inviting German retaliation.

Cambrai

Three American engineer regiments, the 11th, 12th, and 14th, were engaged in construction activity behind British lines at Cambrai in November 1917 when they became the first AEF units to experience conditions in the trenches. (Even before the Cambrai offensive began, two AEF soldiers from the 11th Engineers became the first American battle casualties in France when they were wounded by German artillery shells on September 5, 1917.[29]) On November 30 German gas shelling intensified in the vicinity of the three AEF regiments. British officers ordered a withdrawal, but the AEF engineers were taken by surprise. Some hid in dugouts trapped behind the German advance while others used their picks and hand tools to fight. Most of the AEF units returned to take up defensive positions to halt the German advance. Six soldiers of the 11th Engineers were killed from shelling (high explosive and gas), 11 were wounded, and 13 were taken prisoner.[29] These casualties were counted as British gas casualties in the final statistics because they would not

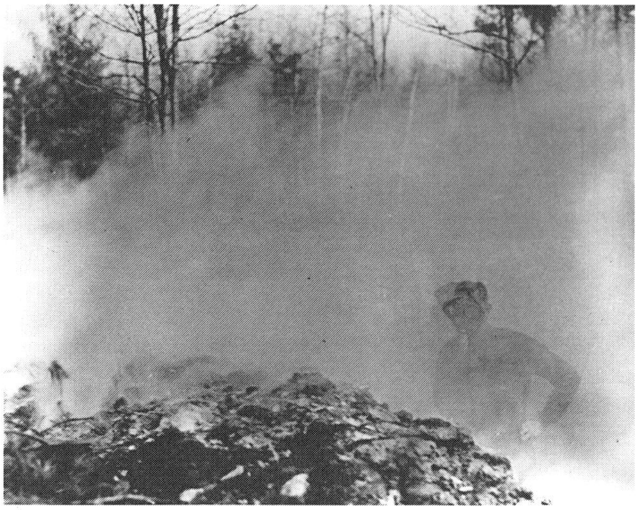

Fig. 2-10. Proper gas training to avoid becoming a casualty was routine for the American Expeditionary Forces in World War I. US Signal Corps photograph.
Photograph: Courtesy of US Army Military History Institute, Carlisle, Pa.

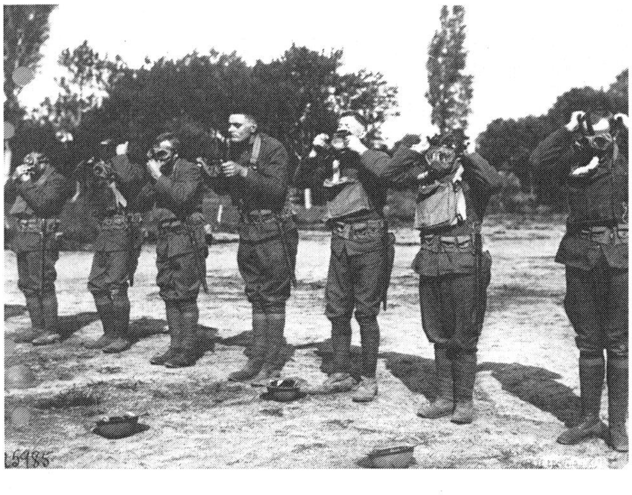

Fig. 2-9. US troops receiving gas mask instruction in 1918 before entering the trenches. 329th Infantry. US Signal Corps photograph.
Photograph: Courtesy of US Army Military History Institute, Carlisle, Pa.

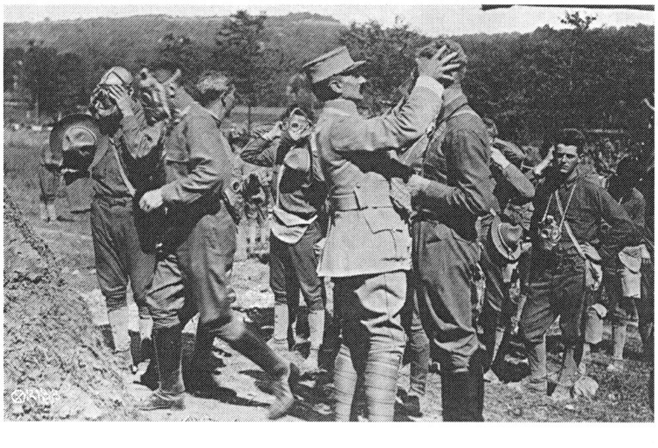

Fig. 2-11. US soldiers receiving instructions from French officers in early 1918 on quickly donning gas masks. US Signal Corps photograph.
Photograph: Courtesy of US Army Military History Institute, Carlisle, Pa.

have been funneled through American field hospitals. Cambrai represented the first participation by the AEF in active fighting.

Sommervillier and Ansauville

Pershing sought an area near Lorraine where the AEF could concentrate, train in gas warfare with help from the French (Figures 2-9, 2-10, and 2-11), and eventually fight. The 1st Division trained in gas defense exercises from September 1917 to January 1918, and a preliminary gas organization was set up in the division in December 1917.[30,31] As it began training in the practice trenches at Gondrecourt, the division was issued both the French M-2 gas mask and the British small box respirator (Figure 2-12). The French warned the Americans about Germany's use of mustard gas and the importance of using their respirators. After additional training in the Sommervillier section in Lorraine with units of the 18th French Division, the 1st Division relieved part of the 1st Moroccan Division in the Ansauville sector, where it experienced the first reported gas attack on the AEF.

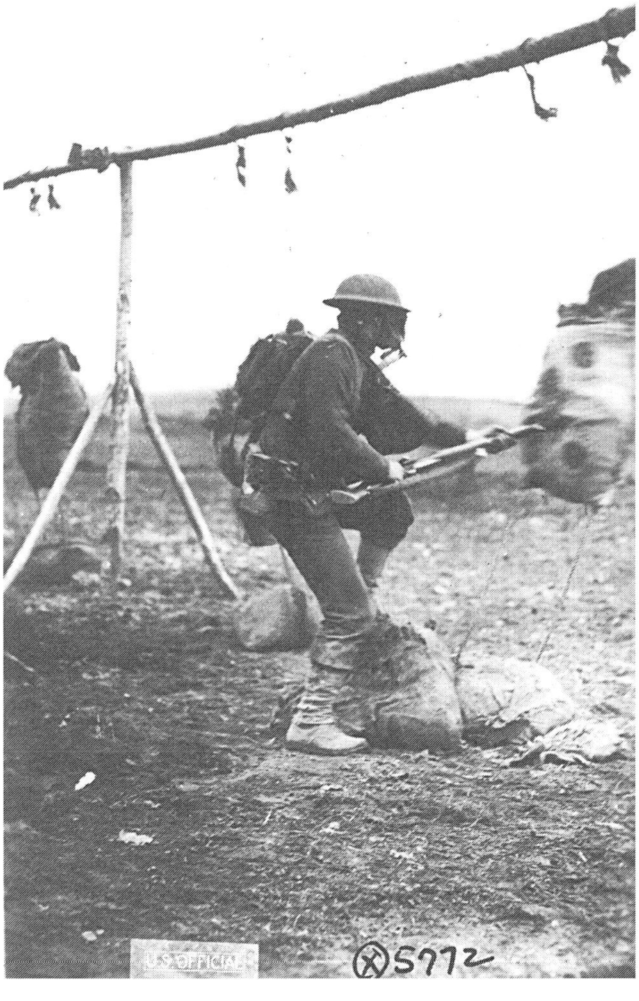

Fig. 2-12. Early American Expeditionary Forces training in 1917. American Expeditionary Forces soldier training with a bayonet while wearing the British small box respirator. US Signal Corps photograph.
Photograph: Courtesy of US Army Military History Institute, Carlisle, Pa.

The attack took place on February 26, 1918, between 1:20 and 1:30 AM, when the Germans fired some 150 to 250 phosgene and chloropicrin projectiles against the Americans near Bois de Remieres, France (Exhibit 2-6). Some projectiles exploded in the air, others on the ground. A second, similar attack occurred about an hour later. However, a discrepancy appears in the literature over the type and number of projectors and trench mortar bombs involved. Sources state that phosgene and chlorine were employed, but contain varying accounts of the number of projectors involved.[30]

Although the 1st Division received the most rigorous combat and gas training of any American division, inexperience still led to mistakes. Major General Robert Bullard, head of the 1st Division, remarked on the gas training his division received at Ansauville:

> Gas is such an intangible thing that men are only with great difficulty made to guard themselves against it. A state of instruction adequate against the danger is extremely hard to obtain. . . . Our gas officers were almost hysterical in their efforts to teach and impress our new troops; but knowledge and real efficient training came only after hard experience.[32(p5)]

The Americans suffered 85 casualties, including eight deaths—approximately a third of their battalion—in the aftermath of the attack. Although reports stated that from the time the bright lights of the crashing projectiles hit to the elaboration of gas, soldiers had no time to don either the M2 or British small box respirator, the majority of the casualties were preventable through better discipline. The lack of discipline was the result of four factors. First, some soldiers could not find their gas masks in time (Exhibit 2-7). Second, some noncommissioned officers let soldiers remove their masks too quickly, only a half hour after the last shell fell. Third, other soldiers switched from the effective but uncomfortable small box respirator to the more comfortable but less effective French M2, receiving gas in the process. Fourth, soldiers continued to work unmasked in the woods as late as 48 hours after the attack, despite the odor of phosgene in the air.[33] Determined not to be caught by such an attack again in the Ansauville sector, the 1st Division made

EXHIBIT 2-6

FIRST PROJECTOR ATTACK ON THE AMERICAN EXPEDITIONARY FORCES

The earliest written account of an attack involving projectors and trench mortar chemical bombs on the American Expeditionary Forces occurred on February 26, 1918. A projector was a device that lobbed a football-sized gas projectile into enemy trenches. The objective was to get the gas as far from friendly forces as possible before releasing it. Two attacks involving trench mortar bombs and projectiles occurred between 1:20 and 1:40 AM. The trench mortar attack consisted of two salvos of phosgene bombs. The projectiles used were mixtures of phosgene and possibly chloropicrin, based on their odors. General Bullard stated that two volleys, each consisting of 100 18-cm shells, mostly phosgene, crashed "with a loud explosion and bright flare of light." Rudolf Hanslian and records of the 78th Reserve Division in Germany indicated a much larger gas assault by the 35th Pioneer Battalion, involving 810 projectors loaded with phosgene flasks and 10 with the new diphenylchloroarsine gas, along with 80 high explosives, to produce casualties with almost 14 tons of phosgene. This discrepancy in the number of projectiles can be explained from the accounts of two German prisoners, who deserted on March 20. They reported that 900 projectors were employed, "one half of which fell in their own front lines," keeping them out for 2 days. The 35th Pioneer Regiment never completed the elaborate raid, code-named "Einladung," that immediately followed the projector attack on the American Expeditionary Forces.

Data source: Spencer EW. *The History of Gas Attacks Upon the American Expeditionary Forces During the World War, Part I.* Edgewood Arsenal, Md: Chemical Warfare Service, US War Department; 1928: 37–51.

continuous efforts to spot projector installations and neutralize them.

Lys Defensive

General Erich Ludendorff, deputy chief of the general staff for Germany, still hoped to destroy the hard-hit British army before it had a chance to recover from the effects of the Somme drive. This was the purpose of a new German attack launched April 9, 1918, on a narrow front along the Lys River in Flanders. The Germans committed 46 divisions to the assault and quickly scored a breakthrough. Chemical warfare with gas shells was a major component in this German offensive. These "Hutier tactics" involved brief but significant artillery shelling of enemy front and rear lines with high explosive and chemical weapons, followed by light infantry advancement. The British situation was desperate for some days, but Ludendorff called off the offensive on April 29. About 500 Americans participated in the campaign, including members of the 16th Engineers, 28th Aero Squadron, and 1st Gas Regiment.[34,35] Chemical casualty statistics are poor for this period; however, AEF divisions suffered higher

EXHIBIT 2-7

FIRST AIRPLANE GAS ATTACKS ON AMERICAN FORCES

Although some historians erroneously state that chemical warfare involving aircraft did not occur in World War I, German forces did drop chemical bombs from airplanes during the conflict. The first gas attacks on American Expeditionary Forces from German planes took place in the village of Seicheprey, part of the 1st Division sector. Up to that point, chemical warfare involving planes had never been described. At Ansauville, a German plane dropped gas balloons, described as balls 18 inches in diameter and filled with liquid mustard, on 1st Division batteries entrenched across Hill 246 on March 19, 1918. A second airplane gas attack occurred on March 23, 1918, as part of a series of daily mustard gas attacks on the town from March 21 to March 25. American Expeditionary Forces watched a German airplane drop gas bombs over the Beaumont-Jury road and release gas balloons that exploded in the air, liberating a reddish-blue cloud. It was later reported that neither the gas balloons nor the bombs seem to have caused any casualties.

Data source: Cochrane RC. The 1st Division at Ansauville, January–April 1918; study number 9. In: *Gas Warfare in World War I. US Army Chemical Corps Historical Studies.* Army Chemical Center, Md: US Army Chemical Corps Historical Office; 1959.

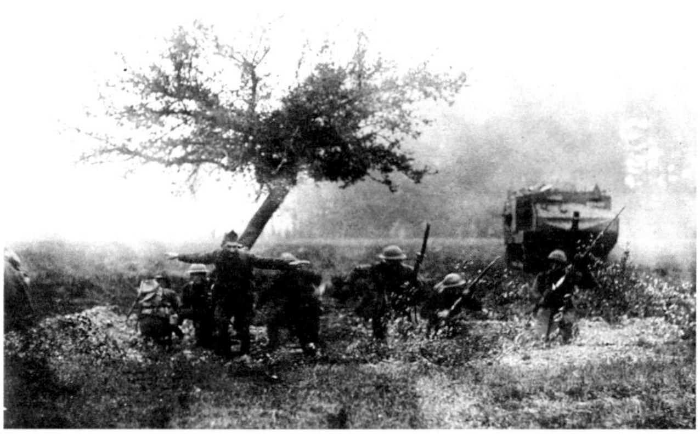

Fig. 2-13. Members of the 26th Infantry, 2nd Brigade, 1st Division, leaving a trench to go over the top during Battle of Cantigny, May 1918. US Signal Corps photograph.
Photograph: Courtesy of US Army Military History Institute, Carlisle, Pa.

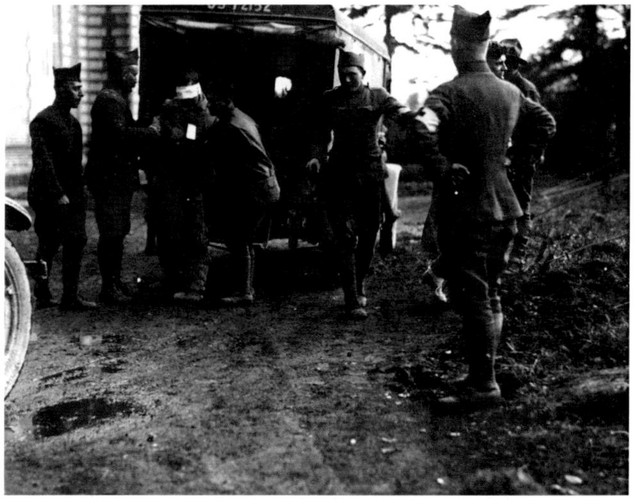

Fig. 2-14. US gas casualties from the 1st Division evacuated after the Battle of Cantigny, May 29, 1918. US Signal Corps photograph.
Photograph: Courtesy of US Army Military History Institute, Carlisle, Pa.

chemical casualties in the early months of the war compared to the later months.

First American Victory: the Battle of Cantigny

The first sustained American offensive of the war, although a minor action, was fought between May 3 and June 8, 1918, by the AEF 1st Division under Major General Bullard. The Battle of Cantigny was part of the Third Battle of the Aisne, a large-scale German offensive to win the war before the full build-up of US troops in France. Chemical attacks inflicted major casualties on the AEF 1st Division's assault and repulsion of numerous German counterattacks (Figure 2-13). Pershing initially tasked the 18th Infantry to take Cantigny, but it was so decimated by mustard shells (around 15,000) at Villers-Tournelle between May 3 and 4 (when the 1st Division suffered close to 900 chemical casualties among its ranks, predominantly in the 18th Infantry, in a single night) that it was unable to carry out the mission. Consequently, Pershing charged the 28th Infantry to take Cantigny instead.[36] On May 28 the 1st Division captured the village of Cantigny, held by the German 18th Army and commanded and strongly fortified as a German advance observation point by General Oskar von Hutier.

Rexmond Cochrane summarizes there was a total of between 2,199 and 2,708 chemical casualties at Cantigny (Figure 2-14).[36] Chemical warfare played a significant role in the prelude to battle, capture, and defense of Cantigny. The number of high explosive

EXHIBIT 2-8

AN ATTACK ON A PLATOON OF THE 28TH DIVISION

An entire platoon of infantry in the 28th Division became gas casualties before reaching the front. While moving forward toward Chateau-Thierry, the soldiers stopped to rest in shallow shell craters near the road, a common occurrence, before decontaminating them. The obvious garlic smell, emanating from holes made by yellow cross shells, was diluted from recent rains. Unbeknownst to them, the holes were contaminated by mustard. The soldiers awoke with backs and buttocks so badly burned that the skin appeared to be flayed.

Data sources: (1) Spencer EW. *The History of Gas Attacks Upon the American Expeditionary Forces During the World War, Parts I-III*. Edgewood Arsenal, Md: Chemical Warfare Service, US War Department; 1928. (2) Cochrane RC. The 3rd Division at Chateau Thierry, July 1918; study number 14. In: *Gas Warfare in World War I. U.S. Army Chemical Corps Historical Studies*. Army Chemical Center, Md: US Army Chemical Corps Historical Office; 1959: 1–4, 84, 86.

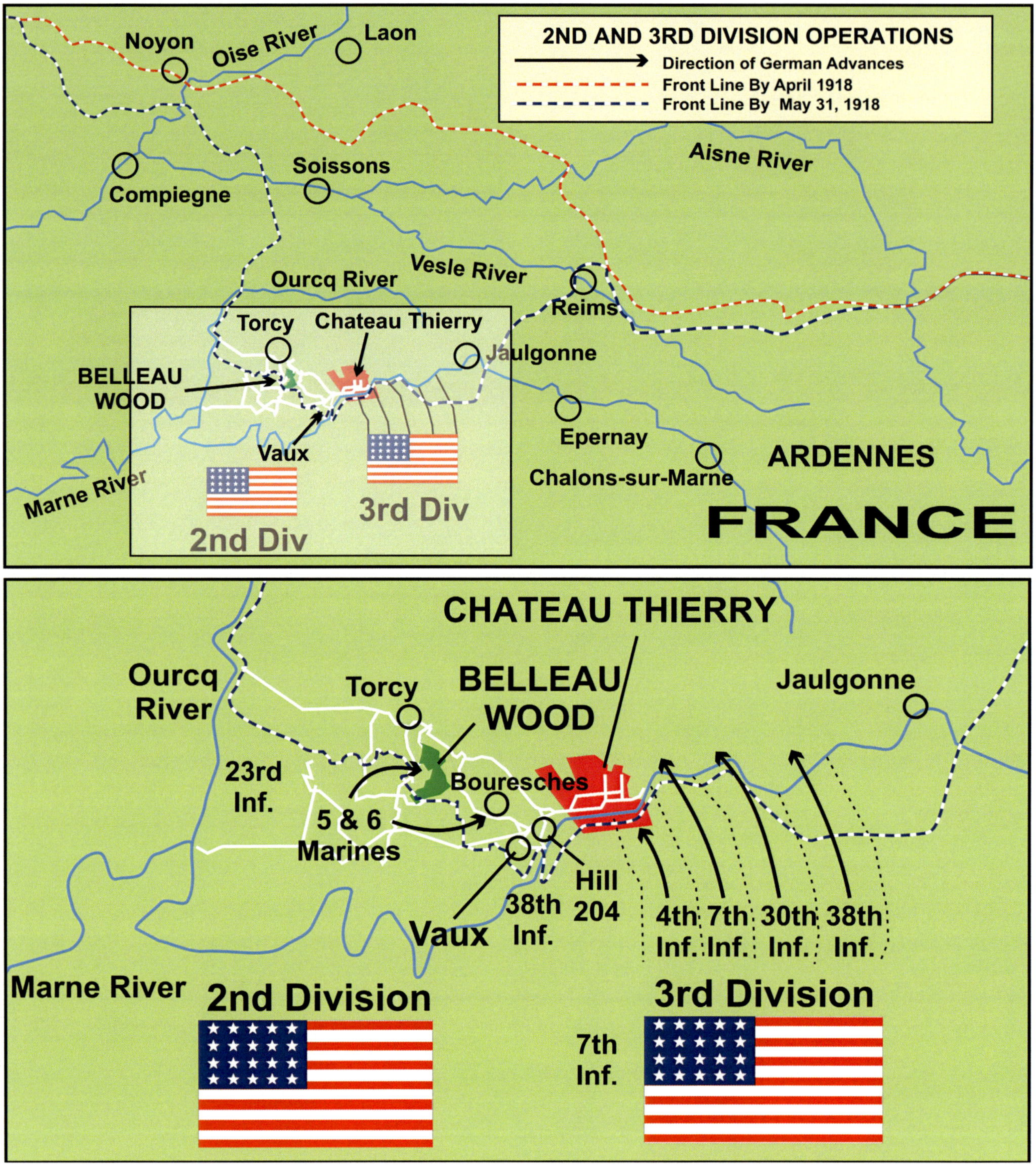

Fig. 2-15. Overview and detailed maps of 2nd and 3rd Division operations in Chateau-Thierry and Belleau Wood. Map: Courtesy of Dr Corey J Hilmas, United States Army Medical Research Institute of Chemical Defense.

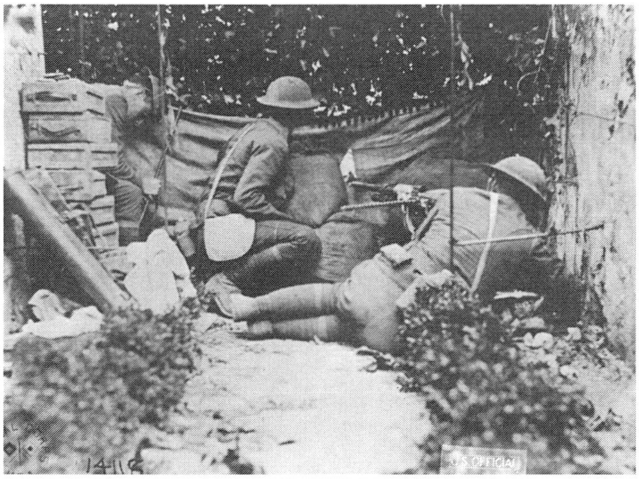

Fig. 2-16. Company A, Seventh Machine Gun Battalion, guarding the Marne from Chateau-Thierry, France. At the time this photograph was taken, Chateau-Thierry was under bombardment from German lines across the river. June 1, 1918. US Signal Corps photograph.
Photograph: Courtesy of US Army Military History Institute, Carlisle, Pa.

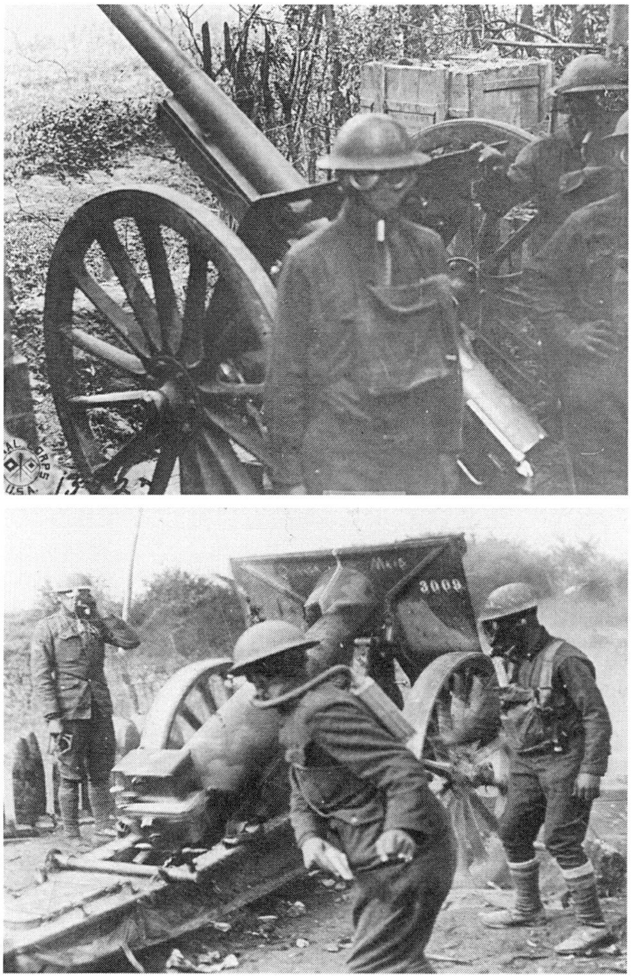

Fig. 2-17. US Field Artillery, 2nd Division sending over French 75-mm gas shells into the Bois de Belleau, France, during the Battle at Belleau Wood. June 30, 1918. US Signal Corps photograph.
Photographs: Courtesy of US Army Military History Institute, Carlisle, Pa.

shells used against the 1st Division was 7-fold that of gas shells, and the reported chemical and wounded casualty statistics were similar. The Germans predominantly used chlorine, bromine arsenic, mustard, and phosgene shells on the AEF at Cantigny.

Aisne Defensive

The significance of the Cantigny victory was overshadowed by the battle along the Aisne, some 50 miles to the northwest, where the Germans broke through nine British and French divisions with the aid of gas and captured 50,000 Allied soldiers (Exhibit 2-8). The French and British defenders were taken by surprise, and their positions were quickly overrun on a 40-mile front. The German army progressed rapidly, capturing Aisne bridges completely intact along the way. Their thrust toward Rheims failed, but Soissons was taken, and by May 31, the German army reached the outskirts of Chateau-Thierry on the Marne, less than 40 miles from Paris (Figure 2-15). If the AEF had not quickly plugged the breach in this line at Chateau-Thierry and Belleau Wood, the Germans would have marched the 40-mile track to Paris unchallenged along the Paris-Metz Road.[35,37,38]

Chateau-Thierry

Chateau-Thierry formed the tip of the German advance towards Paris. The AEF's 2nd and 3rd divisions (Figures 2-16, 2-17, and 2-18) launched a counterattack on June 3–4 with the assistance of the French 10th Colonial Division. This offensive pushed the Germans back across the Marne to Jaulgonne.[35,38] During the defense of Chateau-Thierry, the 3rd Division suffered 1,777 chemical casualties.[37]

Belleau Wood

The 2nd Division (5th and 6th Marine regiments) captured the Bois de Belleau Wood under heavy gas shelling, mostly mustard, from June 6 to 26. The casualties on the first day of the assault (Figure 2-19) were the highest in Marine Corps history until the capture of Japanese-held Tarawa in November 1943.[35,38,39]

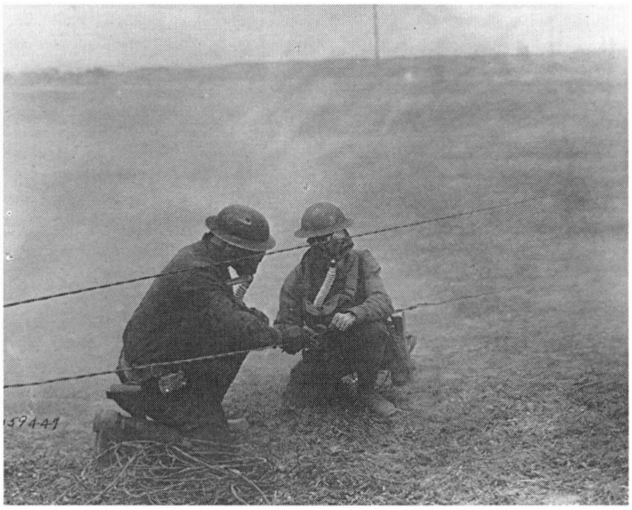

Fig. 2-18. Linemen of the 5th Field Signal Brigade, 3rd Division, repair broken wire during a gas attack. Chateau-Thierry, France, June 21, 1918. US Signal Corps photograph.
Photograph: Courtesy of US Army Military History Institute, Carlisle, Pa.

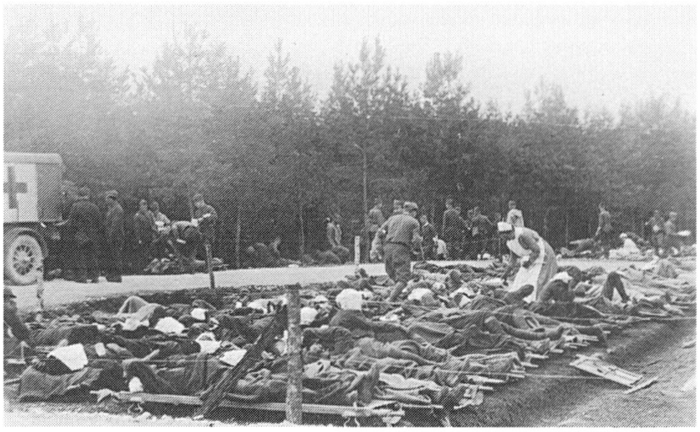

Fig. 2-19. Treating American gas casualties, mainly mustard, during the attack of Belleau Wood. 1918. US Signal Corps photograph.
Photograph: Courtesy of US Army Military History Institute, Carlisle, Pa.

The Germans took back the sector, which changed hands six times before the Germans were expelled. The 2nd Division suffered 3,152 chemical casualties in the Chateau-Thierry sector during the capture of Belleau Wood, Vaux, and Bouresche,[39] and the French renamed the wood "Bois de la Brigade de Marine," in its honor.

Champagne-Marne Defensive

The Allies were prepared for the two-pronged German assault on each side of Rheims on July 15 (Figure 2-20). Plans for the attack had leaked out of Berlin, and Allied airplanes had detected unusual activity behind the enemy front. Marshal Ferdinand Foch, commander of the Allied forces, had time to draw up reserves, and Henri Philippe, the French commander, skillfully deployed his troops in defense-in-depth tactics.[35,41] Consequently, the German drive east of Rheims fell far short of its objective. The attack west of the city succeeded in pushing across the Marne near Chateau-Thierry once again, but was checked there by French and American units. The primary AEF units involved in this action were the 3rd and 42nd divisions, with support from the 26th and 28th divisions and the 369th Infantry.[41] (The 3rd Division's 38th Infantry became known as the "rock of the Marne" at this battle.[35,41]) The 3rd and 28th Divisions suffered 789 and 378 chemical casualties, respectively, during the defense.[37] The 42nd incurred the largest number of chemical casualties here (1,246).[40] By July 18 the German offensive was halted once more, and the initiative passed to the Allies. The German war effort never recovered from the tremendous psychological blow of this failure.

Aisne-Marne Offensive

Several days before the Germans launched their abortive Champagne-Marne drive, the French high command made plans for a general converging offensive against the Marne salient. France issued orders on July 12 for the attack to begin on the 18th, with five French armies taking part. Five divisions of the French XX Corps, accompanied by the American 1st and 2nd AEF divisions (see Figure 2-20), led the assault.[35,41,42] Early on July 18 the two American divisions and a French Moroccan division launched the main blow at the northwest base of the salient near Soissons. By July 28 the American contingent included the 3rd, 4th, 28th, 32nd, and 42nd divisions (see Figure 2-20). The Germans retreated across the Aisne and Vesle rivers, resolutely defending each strong point as they went. By August 6 the Aisne-Marne offensive and the German threat to Paris were over. The eight AEF divisions in the action spearheaded much of the advance, demonstrating offensive gas capabilities that helped inspire new confidence in the war-weary Allied armies (Figures 2-21 and 2-22). About 270,000 Americans took part in the battle. Heavy losses were incurred by the 3rd Division (2,146 chemical casualties) and 28th Division (1,092 chemical casualties).[37] The 32nd Division suffered nearly 1,300 chemical casualties in the taking of Fismes, the key to the advance from the Vesle to the Aisne River.[42]

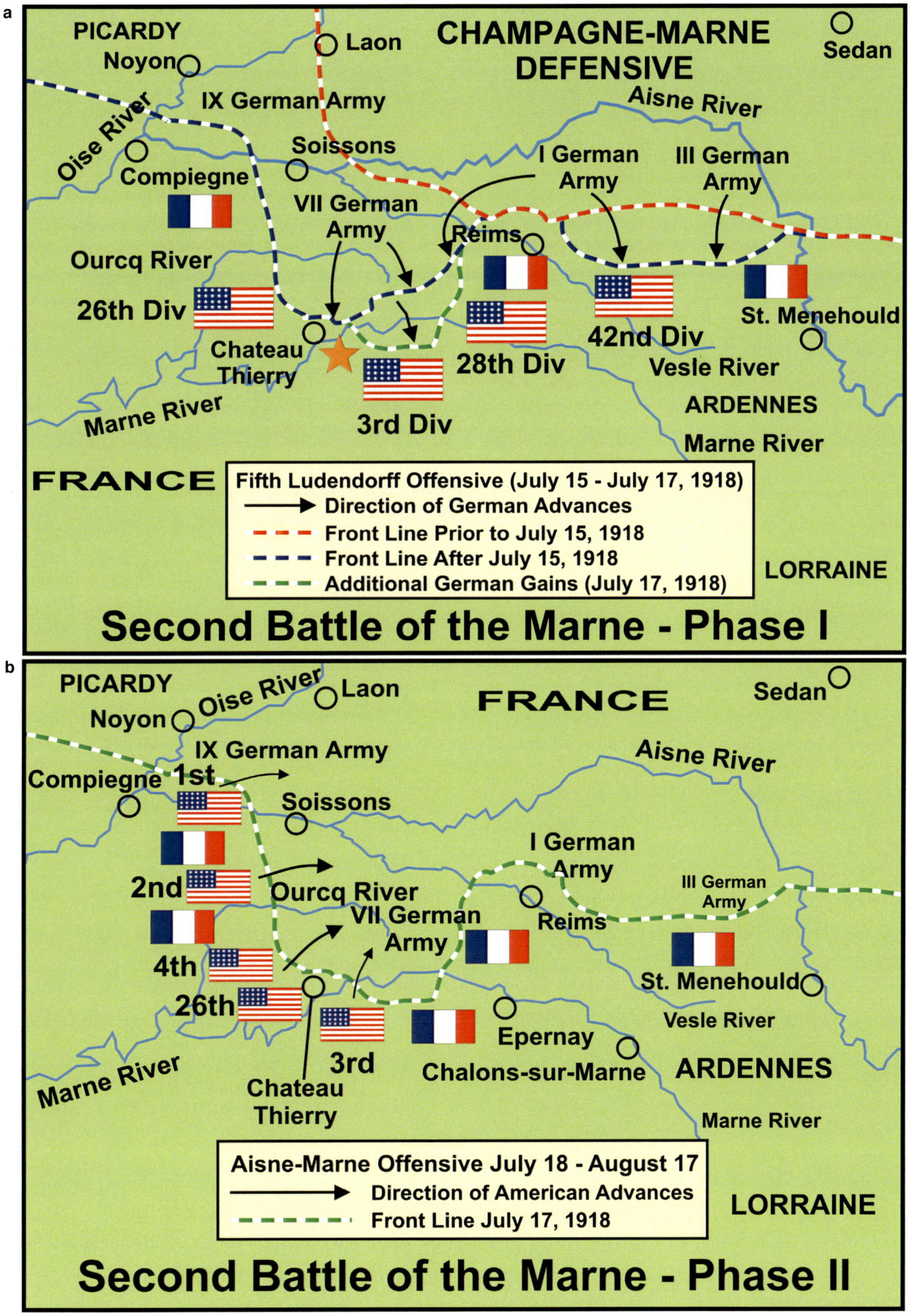

Fig. 2-20. US participation in the Second Battle of the Marne. (**a**) Champagne-Marne defensive . (**b**) Aisne-Marne offensive. Map: Courtesy of Dr Corey J Hilmas, United States Army Medical Research Institute of Chemical Defense.

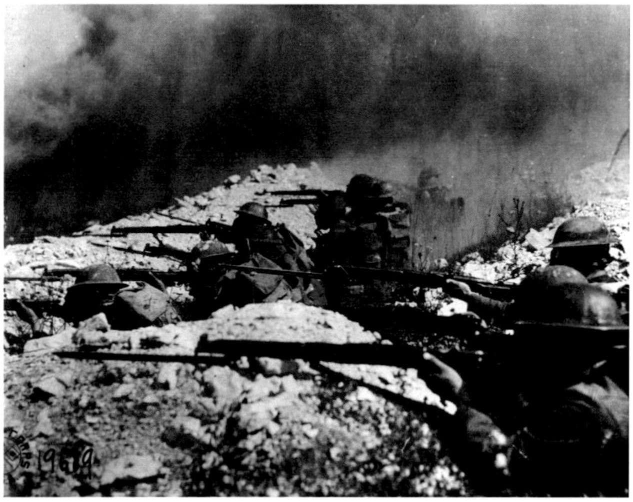

Fig. 2-21. American troops firing on German positions while under heavy gas attack in the trenches of France during the Aisne-Marne offensive. US Signal Corps photograph.
Photograph: Courtesy of US Army Military History Institute, Carlisle, Pa.

Oise-Aisne Offensive

In mid August, the French started a series of drives on their front, which extended about 90 miles from Reims westward through Soissons to Ribecourt on the Oise River (Figure 2-23).[35,43] Coordinating with the British, five French armies advanced on the Somme to the north and the Americans advanced to the east. The AEF's 32nd Division and part of the French 10th Army spearheaded the penetration of the enemy's main line on August 22 and captured the town of Juvigny, a key high ground, on August 30. The 32nd completely breached the German front, forcing them to abandon the Vesle River line.[35] The American III Corps (28th and 77th divisions) fought with the French 6th Army east of Soissons, which, in late August, held the western part of the Vesle River sector extending from Braine to Courlandon. As the Germans retreated from the Vesle northward to the Aisne valley in early September, the III Corps took part in the aggressive pursuit operations. During the Oise-Aisne offensive, the AEF suffered 2,776 casualties, 573 of which were attributable to chemical agents.[44]

Saint Mihiel

By September 1918, with both the Marne and the Amiens salients eliminated, one major threat to lateral rail communications behind the Allied lines remained: the old Saint Mihiel salient near the Paris-Nancy line (see Figure 2-2). American units from Flanders to Switzerland were shifted into the area near the salient.[35,43,45] Fourteen American and four French divisions assigned to the First Army for the operation contained ample infantry and machine-gun units for the attack; however, because of the earlier priority given to shipping infantry (at the urging of the British and French), the First Army was short of artillery, tank, air, and other support units essential to a well-balanced field army. At Pershing's insistence, this was the first major operation carried out by an independent American force, but it was subordinated to the much larger Meuse-Argonne offensive in late September.[43,45]

The Saint Mihiel offensive began on September 12 with a 3-fold assault on the salient. The main attack was made against the south face by two American corps. On the right was the I Corps, on the left, the

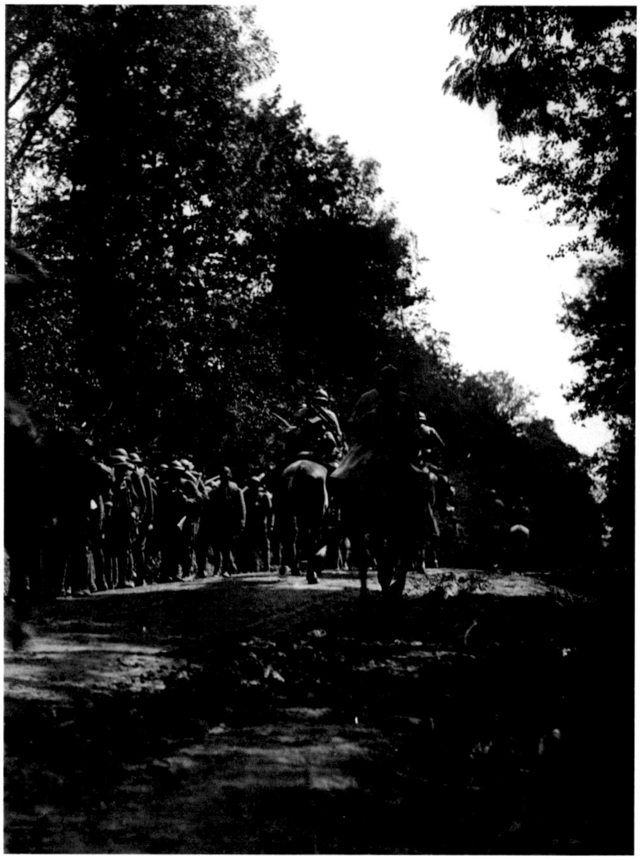

Fig. 2-22. American infantrymen of the 167th Infantry, 42nd "Rainbow" Division marching through German gas wearing Boche gas masks and box respirators near Bouvardes, France. July 29, 1918. The mounted soldiers in the counter-marching procession are French dragoons returning from patrol. US Signal Corps photograph.
Photograph: Courtesy of US Army Military History Institute, Carlisle, Pa.

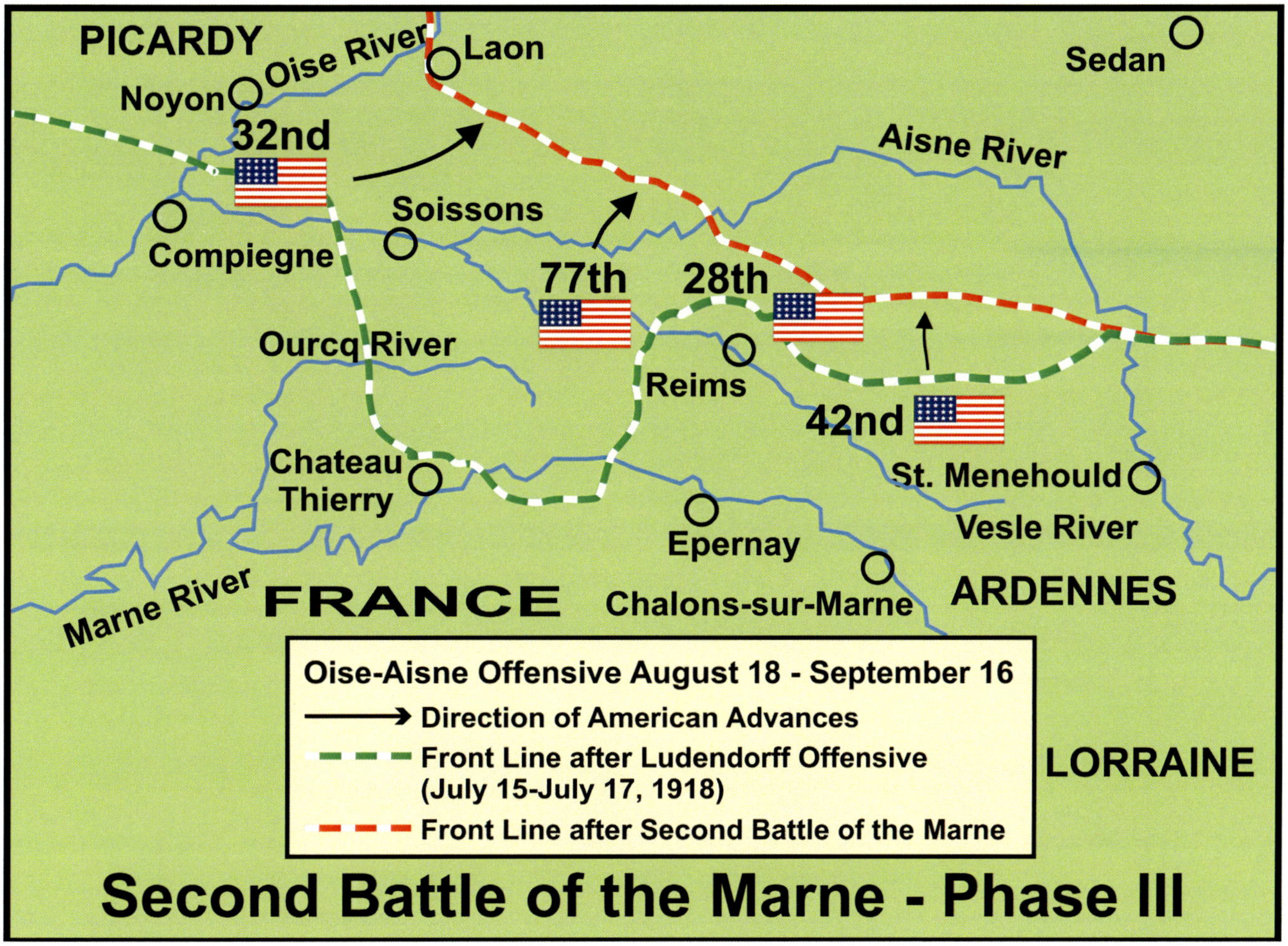

Fig. 2-23. US participation in the Oise-Aisne offensive.
Map: Courtesy of Dr Corey J Hilmas, United States Army Medical Research Institute of Chemical Defense.

IV Corps (Figure 2-24). A secondary thrust was carried out against the west face along the heights of the Meuse by the V Corps. The AEF used scant offensive gas because shelling would have negated their surprise attack, but it suffered significant casualties from German gas. Data from the division gas hospitals state that the 90th Division alone experienced 1,390 chemical casualties (460 mustard and the rest from lachrymators [tear gasses] and sternutators [sneezing agents]) during the 5-day battle, compared to 275 from the 26th Division.[45,46]

Meuse-Argonne

At the end of August, Marshal Foch submitted plans to the Allied commanders for a final offensive along the entire western front (see Figure 2-2, Figure 2-25). Pershing and the AEF struck a zone about 20 miles wide between the heights of the Meuse on the east near Verdun and the western edge of the high, rough, and densely wooded Argonne Forest (Figure 2-26).[38,50] Pershing hoped to launch an attack with enough momentum to drive the elaborate German defense lines at Montfaucon, Cunel, and Barricourt into an open area beyond and, in a coordinated drive with the French Fourth Army on the left, effectively cut off the Sedan-Mézières railroad. The Meuse-Argonne offensive operated over four phases because of stalled gains and the replacement of exhausted and depleted divisions. By November 11, 1918, the AEF closed up along the Meuse and, east of the river, advanced toward Montmédy, Briny, and Metz, ending hostilities.[35,47]

General Pershing summarized the results of the Meuse-Argonne campaign, the greatest battle in American history up to that time, in his final report:

> Between September 26 and November 11, 22 Ameri-

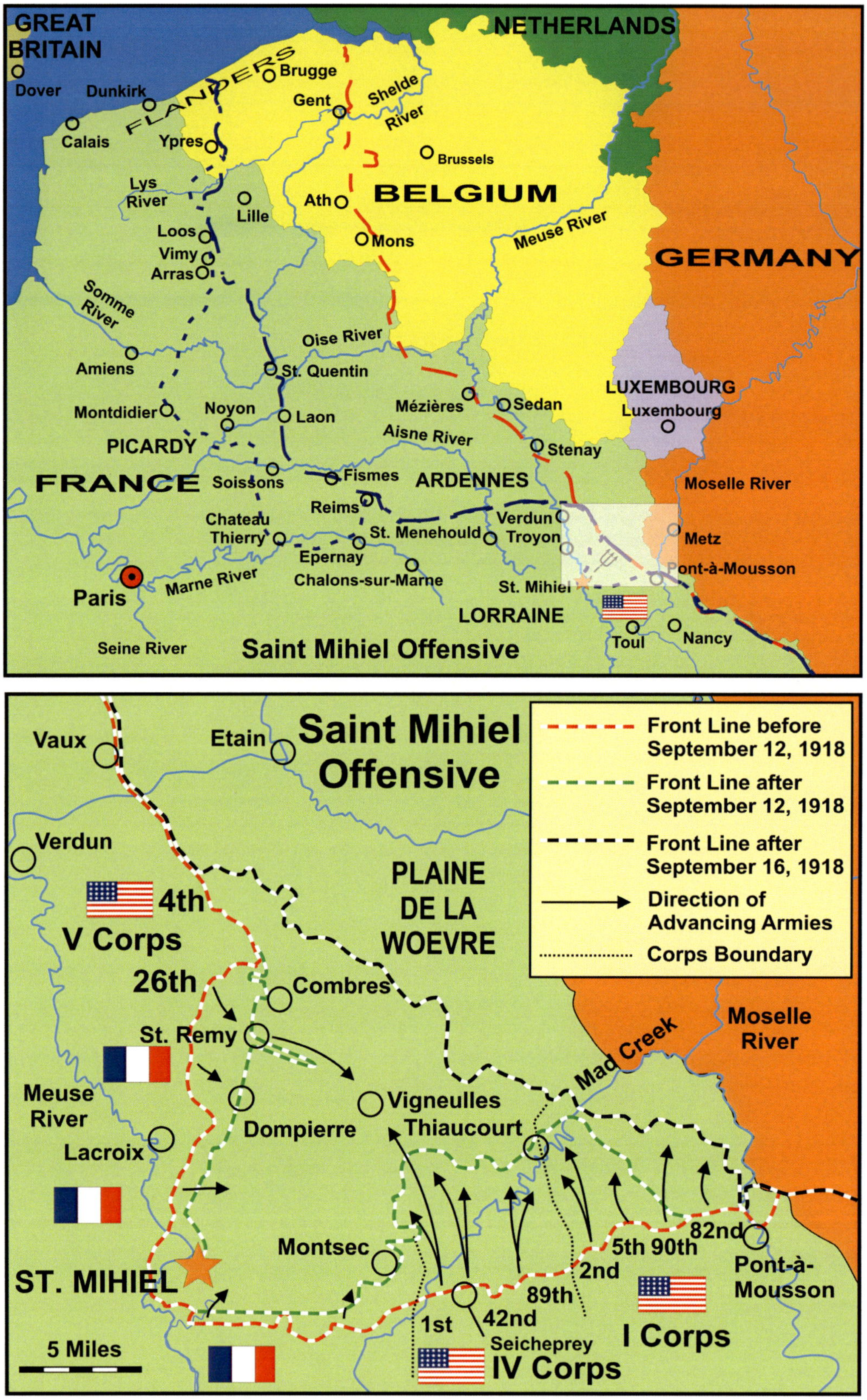

Fig. 2-24. Overview and detailed map of US participation in the Saint Mihiel offensive.
Map: Courtesy of Dr Corey J Hilmas, United States Army Medical Research Institute of Chemical Defense.

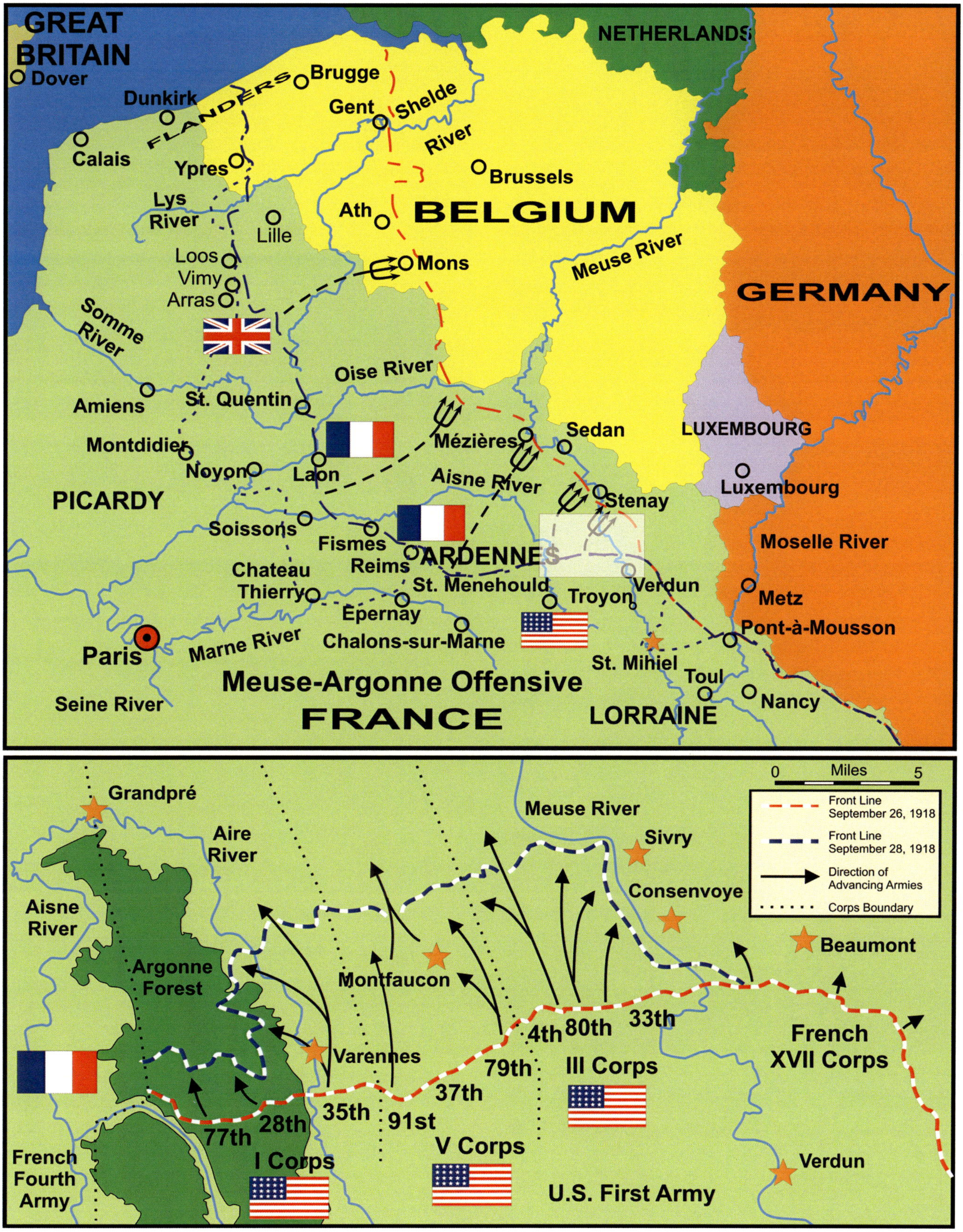

Fig. 2-25. Overview of Meuse-Argonne offensive.
Map: Courtesy of Dr Corey J Hilmas, United States Army Medical Research Institute of Chemical Defense.

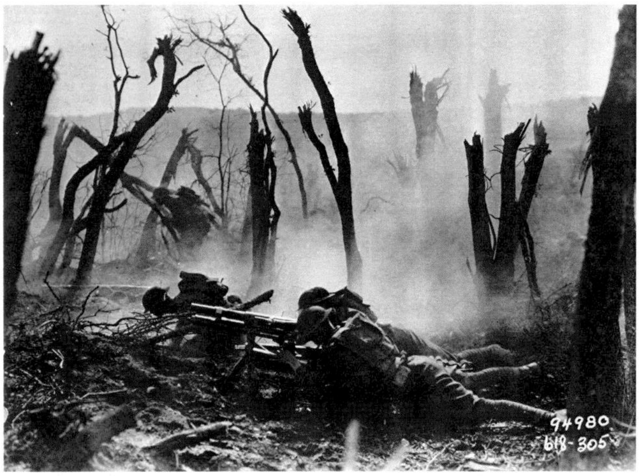

Fig. 2-26. US infantry advancing under gas bombardment against German entrenched positions. US Signal Corps photograph.
Photograph: Courtesy of US Army Military History Institute, Carlisle, Pa.

> can and 4 French divisions, on the front extending from southeast of Verdun to the Argonne Forest, had engaged and decisively beaten 47 different German divisions, representing 25 percent of the enemy's entire divisional strength on the western front.

The First Army suffered a loss of about 117,000 in killed and wounded. It captured 26,000 prisoners, 847 cannon, 3,000 machineguns, and large quantities of material.[48]

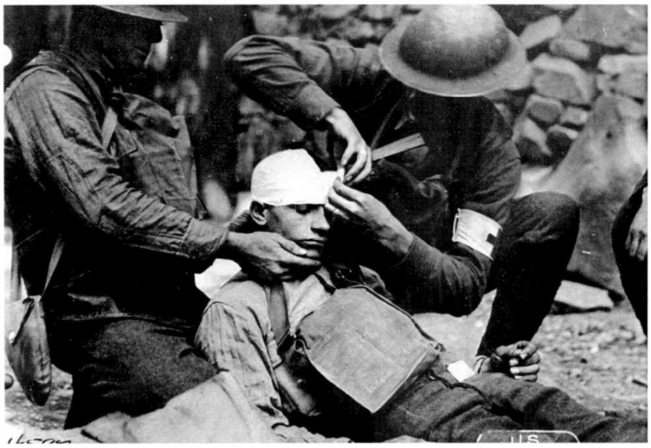

Fig. 2-27. American doctors treating a soldier wounded in head, 1918. US Signal Corps photograph.
Photograph: Courtesy of US Army Military History Institute, Carlisle, Pa.

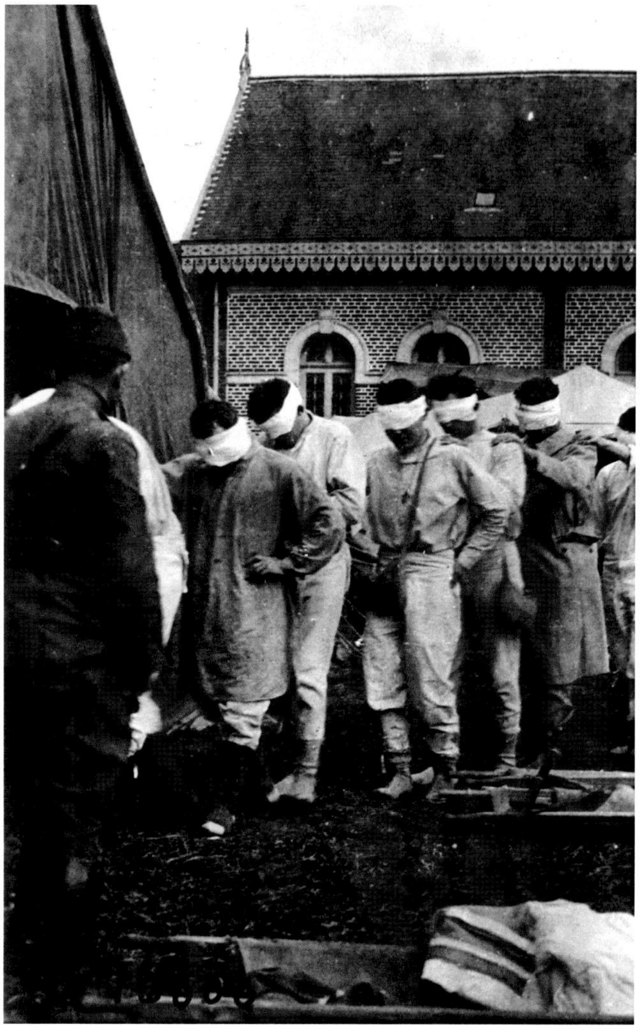

Fig. 2-28. Blinded by sulfur mustard. Gassed American Expeditionary Forces soldiers with eyes bandaged, at Field Hospital No. 13. Near Caply, France. July 2, 1918. US Signal Corps photograph.
Photograph: Courtesy of US Army Military History Institute, Carlisle, Pa.

Approximately 20,000 chemical warfare casualties were reported among the divisions of the First Army during the Meuse-Argonne campaign (Figure 2-27).[49] Gas casualties accounted for 22% of all casualties in the campaign. The 3rd Division suffered 1,237 chemical casualties, the 26th Division 1,942,[46] and the 33rd Division 2,400.[50]

Aftermath of Battle

The armistice of November 1918 ended the world's first chemical war. Of the approximately 26 million casualties suffered by the British, French, Russians,

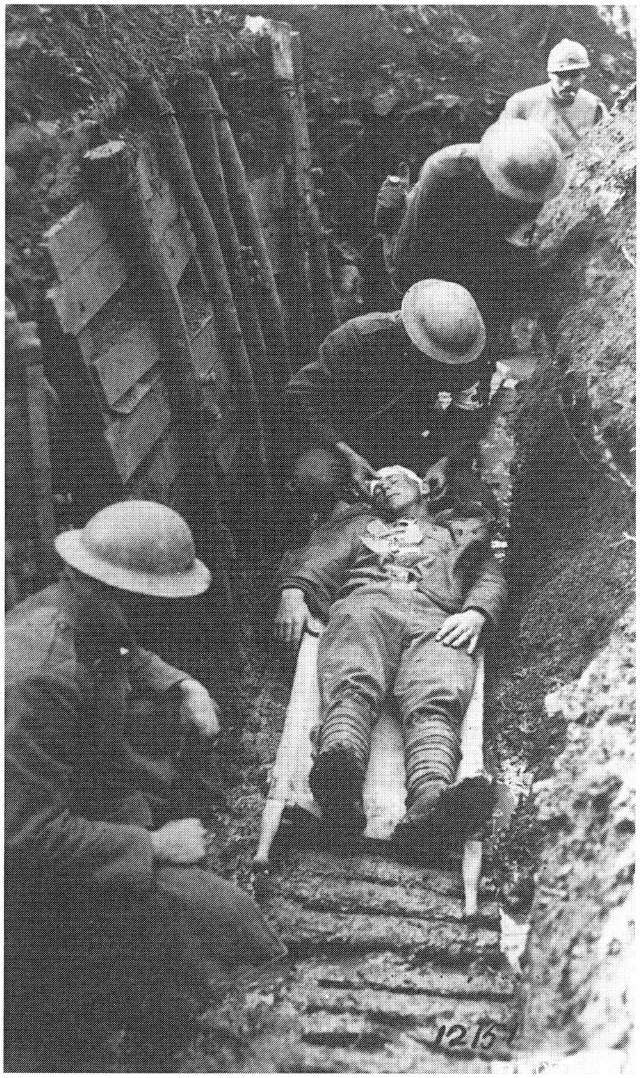

Fig. 2-29. An American gas casualty in the front line trenches of the Toulon Sector in France. March 21, 1918. US Signal Corps photograph.
Photograph: Courtesy of US Army Military History Institute, Carlisle, Pa.

Italians, Germans, Austro-Hungarians, and Americans, around a million were gas casualties. Of the total 272,000 US casualties, over 72,000, or about one fourth, were gas casualties (Figure 2-28). Of the total US gas casualties, approximately 1,200 either died in the hospital or were killed in action by gas exposure. No casualties or deaths were attributed to biological warfare, which was also used in World War I.[25] With the aid of the CWS, the US Army successfully recovered from its early poor performance and survived repeated toxic chemical attacks against its troops (Figure 2-29). Likewise, by the end of the war, the 1st Gas Regiment and numerous US artillery units successfully used toxic chemical agents in retaliation and during offensive operations (Figure 2-30). At the end of the war, the United States had developed the best protective mask, abundant munitions, and trained troops (Figure 2-31). The CWS had 1,680 officers and 20,518 enlisted personnel controlling the Army's chemical warfare program.[27]

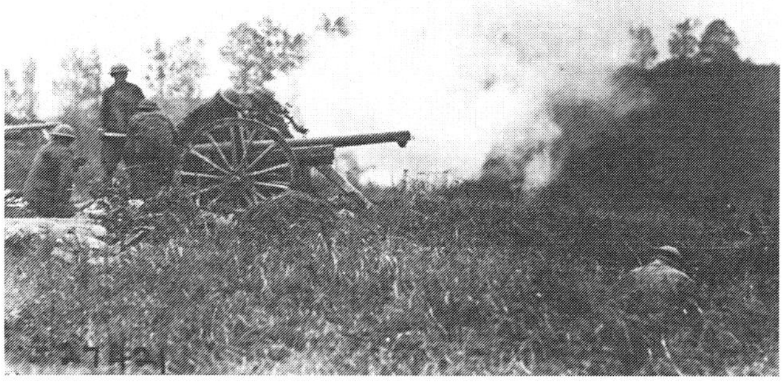

Fig. 2-30. Members of the Sixth Field Artillery, first Division, in action among bursting shells near Exermont, Ardennes, France. October 4, 1918. US Signal Corps photograph.
Photograph: Courtesy of US Army Military History Institute, Carlisle, Pa.

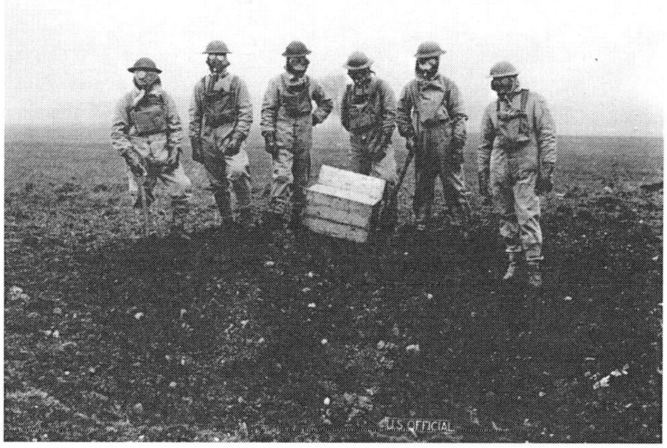

Fig. 2-31. Members of the Chemical Warfare Service decontaminating a typical mustard-laden shell hole near Hanlen Field, Marne, France. December 4, 1918. US Signal Corps photograph.
Photograph: Courtesy of US Army Military History Institute, Carlisle, Pa.

TABLE 2-2

HISTORICAL SUMMARY OF CHEMICAL WARFARE AGENTS USED IN WORLD WAR I

Type of Agent	Chemical Agent	Common Names and Shell Markings	Chemical Formula	Date Introduced	Comments
Sneezing/ vomiting, respiratory irritant, or sternutating agents	Dianisidine chlorosulphonate	Niespulver	$C_{14}H_{16}N_2O_2ClSO_3$	October 27, 1914 (Germany)	Used in Ni-Shell at Battle of Neuve-Chapelle
	Diphenyl chloroarsine	Sternite; DA; Clark I; Blue Cross	$(C_6H_5)_2AsCl$	July 10, 1917 (Germany)	Discovered in 1881 by Michaelis and LaCoste; introduced at same time as mustard gas
	Diphenyl cyanoarsine	Sternite; DC; CDA; Clark II; Blue Cross No. 1	$(C_6H_5)_2AsCN$	May 1918 (Germany)	Developed in May 1918 as an improvement over Clark I
	Ethylcarbazol		$(C_6H_4)_2NC_2H_5$	July 1918 (Germany)	Introduced at the Battle of the Marne
	Diphenylamine-chloroarsine	DM; Adamsite	$(C_6H_4)_2NHAsCl$	Never used on battlefield	Patented by Leverkusen Farb werk in 1915; synthsized by German chemist Wieland during WWI; discovered by American chemist Major Roger Adams during war
	Phenyldichloroarsine	Sternite; Blue Cross No. 1	$C_6H_5AsCl_2$	September 1917 (Germany)	
	Ethyl dichloroarsine	Dick; ED; Blue Cross	$C_2H_5AsCl_2$	March 1918 (Germany)	First called Yellow Cross 1 but not as effective as a vesicant, later incorporated into Green Cross 3 artillery shells
	Ethyl dibromoarsine		$C_2H_5AsBr_2$	September 1918 (Germany)	Used only as a mixture with ethyl dichloroarsine in Green Cross 3
	Methyl dichloroarsine	Methyldick; MD; Blue Cross	CH_3AsCl_2	Never used on battlefield	
Tearing or lacrimatory agents	Ethyl bromoacetate		$CH_2BrCOOC_2H_5$	August 1914 (France)	First combat gas used in WWI
	Xylyl bromide	T-Stoff; White Cross	$C_6H_4CH_3CH_2Br$	January 1915 (Germany)	First used in artillery shells fired against Russians at Bolimov
	Benzyl bromide	Cyclite; T-Stoff; White Cross	$C_6H_5CH_2Br$	March 1915 (Germany)	
	Bromomethylethyl ketone	Homomartonite; Bn-Stoff; White Cross	CH_3COCH-$BrCH_3$	July 1915 (Germany)	
	Ethyl iodoacetate	SK (South Kensington, England)	$CH_2ICOOC_2H_5$	September 1915 (Great Britain)	Principal lacrimator used by British; first used at Battle of Loos September 24, 1915
	Benzyl iodide	Fraissite	$C_6H_5CH_2I$	November 1915 (France)	

(**Table 2-2** *continues*)

Table 2-2 *continued*

	Bromobenzyl-cyanide	Camite; CN	$C_6H_5CHBrCN$	July 1918 (France)	Only tear gas manufactured by CWS in any quantity during WWI
	Chloroacetophe-none	CN	$C_6H_5COCH_2Cl$	Postwar (United States)	Discovered by Graebe in 1869
	Chloroacetone	Tonite; A-Stoff; White Cross	CH_3COCH_2Cl	November 1914 (France)	Substitute for ethyl bromoacetate in hand/rifle gas grenades
	Bromoacetone	Martonite; BA; B-Stoff; White Cross	CH_3COCH_2Br	July 1915 (Germany)	
	Iodoacetone	Bretonite	CH_3COCH_2I	August 1915 (France)	
	Acrolein	Papite	CH_2CHCHO	January 1916 (France)	
	Chloropicrin	Nitrochloroform; Aquinite; PS; NC; Klop	CCl_3NO_2	July 1916 (Germany); August 1916 (Russia)	Lacrimator
	Phenylcarbylam-ine chloride	Phenylisocyanide chloride	$C_6H_5CNCl_2$	May 1917 (Germany)	Lacrimator
Pulmonary agents (lung irritants or choking gases)	Chlorine	Bertholite; Red Star; Chlor	Cl_2	April 22, 1915 (Germany)	
	Methylsulfuryl chloride	Villantite; C-Stoff	$ClSO_3CH_3$	June 1915 (Germany)	First to be successfully used in projectiles (trench mortar bombs & hand grenades)
	Ethylsulfuryl chloride	Sulvanite	$ClSO_3C_2H_5$	June 1915 (France)	
	Chlormethyl-chloroformate	Palite; K-Stoff; C-Stoff	$ClCOOCH_2Cl$	June 18, 1915 (Germany)	K-Stoff when used in shells, C-Stoff when used in trench mortars and projector bombs
	Dimethyl sulfate	Rationite; D-Stoff	$(CH_3)_2SO_4$	August 1915 (Germany)	
	Perchlormethyl-mercaptan	Carbon tetrachlorsul-fide; Clairsite	$SCCl_4$	Septem-ber 1915 (France)	Introduced at Battle of Champagne; first use of gas shell by French army
	Phosgene	Carbonyl chloride; Collongite; CG; D-Stoff; White Star (Phosgene + Chlorine); Green Cross	$COCl_2$	December 19, 1915 (Germany), possibly earlier in May 1915 against Russia	White Star used extensively by British in 1916 Battles of the Somme

(**Table 2-2** *continues*)

Table 2-2 *continued*

	Diphosgene	Trichlormethylchloroformate; Surpalite; Superpalite; Perstoff; Green Cross	$ClCOOCCl_3$	May 1916 (Germany)	First used at Verdun in retaliation of French phosgene used February 1916
	Thiophosgene	Lacrimite; Green Cross			
	Chloropicrin	Nitrochloroform; Aquinite; PS; NC; Klop	CCl_3NO_2	July 1916 (Germany & Allies); August 1916 (Russia)	Discovered by English chemist Stenhouse in 1848; British called it "vomiting gas"
	Phenylcarbylamine chloride	Phenyl isocyanide chloride	$C_6H_5CNCl_2$	May 1917 (Germany)	
	Dichlorodimethyl ether & dibromodimethyl ether	"Labyrinthic substances"; Bibi; Cici	$(CH_2Cl)_2O$ $(CH_2Br)_2O$	January 1918 (Germany)	Exerts a peculiar action on the labyrinth of the ear, altering equilibrium
	Phenyldichloroarsine	Sternite	$C_6H_5AsCl_2$	September 1917 (Germany)	The first toxic lung-injuring agent
	Ethyldichloroarsine	Dick; ED	$C_2H_5AsCl_2$	March 1918 (Germany)	
	Phenyldibromoarsine		$C_6H_5AsBr_2$	September 1918 (Germany)	
Vesicants or blister agents	Dichlorethylsulphide	Sulfur mustard; LOST; Yperite; HS; Yellow Cross	$S(CH_2CH_2)_2Cl_2$	July 12, 1917 (Germany)	
	Ethyldichloroarsine	Dick; ED	C2H$_5$AsCl2	March 1918 (Germany)	
	Chlorvinyldichloroarsine	Lewisite	$CHClCHAsCl_2$	Never used on battlefield	The major American contribution to the chemical weapon inventory but never used in war time; developed by Captain Winford Lee Lewis of the CWS in 1917; Germans claim they manufactured it in 1917 prior to the American discovery
	Methyldichloroarsine	Methyldick; MD; Blue Cross	CH_3AsCl_2	Never used on battlefield	Discovered by Baeyer in 1858; Americans studied it intensely at the end of WWI; not used by either side
	Dibromoethyl sulfide	Brom LOST	$S(CH_2CH_2)_2Br_2$	Never used on battlefield	Studied by Germany in the closing days of the war
Systemic or blood agents	Hydrogen cyanide	Hydrocyanic acid; Vincennite; Manganite; Forestite	HCN	July 1, 1916 (France)	Exclusively used by French in WWI; usually mixed with other chemicals (arsenic trichloride, stannic chloride, and chloroform) to increase its stability and make it heavier

(**Table 2-2** *continues*)

Table 2-2 *continued*

Cyanogen bromide	Ce (Austrians); CB (British); Campillit; Campilite; E-Stoff	CNBr	September 1916 (Austria)	
Cyanogen chloride	Vitrite; Mauginite	CNCl	October 1916 (France)	Maybe used as early as July 1916; exclusively used by French army in WWI; often mixed with arsenic trichloride
Phenylcarbylamine chloride	Phenylisocyanide chloride	$C_6H_5CNCl_2$	May 1917 (Germany)	

CWS: Chemical Warfare Service
WWI: World War I

However, the potential for future chemical wars now loomed, as expressed by one US Army officer:

> Gas was new and in an experimental stage throughout the war and hence the man who plans for future defense must consider the use of gas to have been in its infancy. He must draw very few lessons for the future use of gas based on past performances. He must only use those lessons as pointing the way and not as approaching a final result. The firing of steel as shell passed its zenith with the passing of the Argonne fight. Never again will the world see such a hail of steel on battlefields, but in its place will be concentrations of gas and high explosives as much greater than the World War as that was greater than the Civil War.[51(p4)]

In contrast, Fritz Haber, the Nobel laureate chemist who, more than anyone else, was responsible for the development and fielding of chemical weapons for use by Kaiser Wilhelm II's army, downplayed the importance of chemical warfare as a weapon of mass destruction. In an interview published in New York in 1921, he concluded, "Poison gas caused fewer deaths than bullets."[52(p10)] General Pershing summed up his opinion of the new chemical warfare shortly after the conclusion of World War I, saying, "Whether or not gas will be employed in future wars is a matter of conjecture, but the effect is so deadly to the unprepared that we can never afford to neglect the question."[48(p77)]

A comprehensive list of chemical warfare agents used by and against the AEF during World War I, along with their dates of introduction, is provided in Table 2-2. A more humorous description of the major gases experienced by the AEF in World War I can be found in Major Fairfax Downey's poem, *How to Tell the Gases* (Exhibit 2-9).[9]

EXHIBIT 2-9

HOW TO TELL THE GASES, BY MAJOR FAIRFAX DOWNEY, FIELD ARTILLERY

Grandma smelled geranium,
Started feeling kind of bum,
Sure, you guessed the trouble right—
Grandma whiffed some lewisite.

Don't you find my odor sweetish?
Said flypaper to the fly.
I smell just like chloropicrin,
And you'll think you'd like to die.

Maud Miller on a summer day,
Smelled the odor of new-mown hay,
She said to the Judge who was turning green,
"Put on your mask! That there's phosgene!"

Apple blossoms, fresh and dewy?
Normandy and romance? Hooey!
For the charming fragrance then known,
Now is chloracetophenone.

Never take a chance if
Garlic you should strongly sniff.
Don't think Mussolini's passed,
Man, you're being mustard-gassed.

Reproduced with permission from: Waitt AH. *Gas Warfare: the Chemical Weapon, its Use, and Protection Against it.* New York, NY: Duell, Sloan, and Pearce; 1943: 4–9.

American Expeditionary Forces Chemical Warfare Casualties

Gas was responsible for approximately 2% of the deaths in World War I, but it caused considerably greater numbers of battlefield casualties (Figure 2-32). Nevertheless, it is difficult to account for the total num-

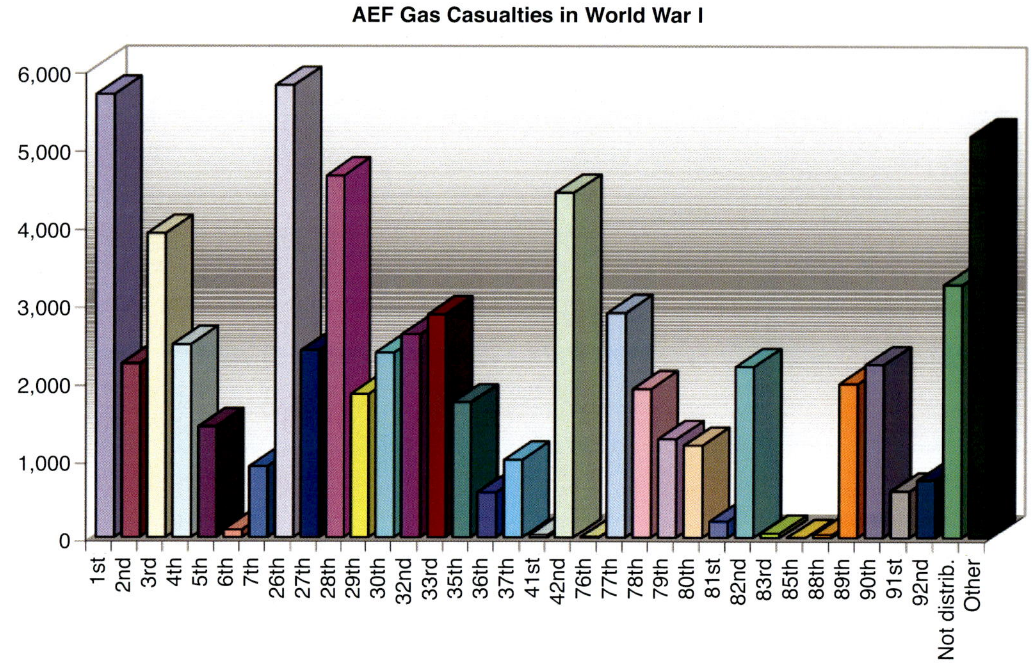

Fig. 2-32. American Expeditionary Forces gas casualties in World War I. Casualty statistics reflect those Americans treated in American, French, British, and Belgian field hospitals. The categories "Not Distributed" and "Other" reflect those American units not organized into divisions.

ber of gas cases in the surgeon general's records. Base hospitals of the French and British divisions received many of the early AEF chemical casualties. Therefore, these American casualties were either not statistically recorded as chemical casualties or were counted under British or French statistics.

In addition, gas officers, who were responsible for compiling chemical casualty statistics, arrived in Europe after the first few AEF divisions. Consequently, they were unable to tally chemical casualty statistics early in the war, when lack of discipline in the trenches caused the greatest numbers of chemical casualties.

Also, chemical casualties from inhalation were difficult to prove because only pulmonary signs and symptoms were evident. Medical personnel viewed soldiers with no clear dermatological signs and symptoms as neurotic malingerers feigning illnesses to leave the front lines. Although pulmonary intoxication from chemical weapons was common, death was often the result of influenza, a major problem in World War I. Chemical toxicity as the result of inhalational or dermal exposure to agents often led to bacterial infection and death. Base hospitals underestimated the effects of chemicals on casualties because many mortalities were tallied as death secondary to influenza, rather than from the initial chemical insult. The majority of the gas casualty reports filed included immediate deaths only (most likely due to a combination of shrapnel and gas); they often did not include deaths from gas exposure that occurred days or weeks later. Chemical shelling was also the cause of many cases of "psychoneuroses." Food contamination from dispersed chemicals in the air was a major paranoia among World War I soldiers.

THE 1920s

An international push to ban chemical weapons followed the conclusion of the war (see Chapter 4). Despite the treaties, rumors of chemical warfare attacks plagued the world throughout the 1920s. Besides the United States and the major World War I powers, several other countries began to develop chemical warfare capabilities, and some countries put their capabilities into operation. During the Russian civil war and Allied intervention in the early 1920s, both sides had chemical weapons and isolated chemical attacks were reported.

Later accounts accused the British, French, and Spanish of using chemical warfare at various times during the 1920s.[4,53] The Berber-led resistance movement against French and Spanish colonialism in

North Africa had resulted in key victories against the Spanish army, forcing their retreat to the Moroccan coastline by 1924. The following year, France forged a counterattack with Spain to subdue the rebellion. Fighting lasted a year, with the alleged use of mustard gas by Spain and France against the Berbers, who were eventually defeated.[54] Also in 1924, the Italians established the Centro Chemico Militaire, a unified chemical warfare service, and began producing chemical agents, which attracted US attention.[55–57]

Survival of the Chemical Warfare Service

The CWS, originally organized by the Army as a temporary war measure, was part of the National Army only, not the Regular Army. Its temporary status was due to expire within 6 months after the end of the war (later extended to June 30, 1920). However, if the CWS disbanded, the US Army would almost certainly forget the extensive experience of chemical offense, defense, and preparedness gained during the war. During congressional hearings, Secretary of War Newton D Baker testified, "We ought to defend our army against a gas attack if somebody else uses it, but we ought not to initiate gas."[58(p3)] Baker and Chief of Staff General Peyton C March used this philosophy to recommend abolishing the CWS and outlawing chemical warfare by a treaty.[59] Even General Sibert, when asked about the need for a permanent CWS and the possibility of chemical warfare in the future, replied, "Based on its effectiveness and humaneness, [chemical warfare] certainly will be an important element in any future war unless the use of it should be prohibited by international agreement. As to the probability of such action, I cannot venture an opinion."[60(p87)]

Several prominent civilian and military leaders lobbied for a permanent chemical warfare organization (Figure 2-33). Lieutenant Colonel Fries, one of the strongest proponents of a permanent organization,

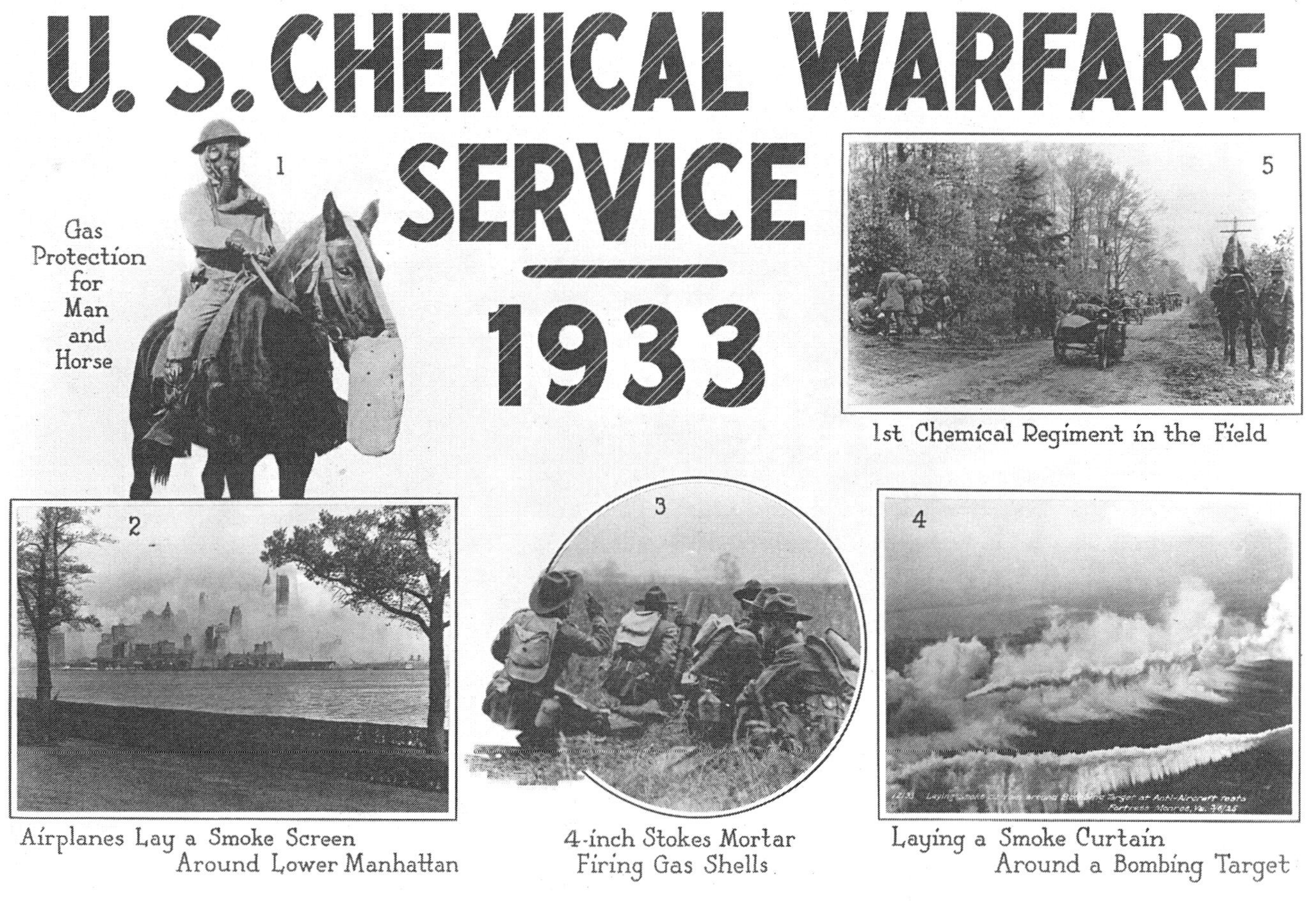
U. S. CHEMICAL WARFARE SERVICE
1933
1
Gas Protection for Man and Horse
5
1st Chemical Regiment in the Field
2
Airplanes Lay a Smoke Screen Around Lower Manhattan
3
4-inch Stokes Mortar Firing Gas Shells
4
Laying a Smoke Curtain Around a Bombing Target

Fig. 2-33. Advertisement for the US Chemical Warfare Service.
Photograph: Courtesy of US Army Military History Institute, Carlisle, Pa.

stressed the need for a central establishment, one that covered all aspects of chemical warfare. He drew on the lessons learned from the Great War, saying:

> Had there been a chemical Warfare Service in 1915 when the first gas attack was made, we would have been fully prepared with gases and masks, and the Army would have been trained in its use. This would have saved thousands of gas cases, the war might easily have been shortened six months or even a year, and untold misery and wasted wealth might have been saved.[61(p4)]

Fries also disagreed with the premise that treaties could prevent warfare:

> Researches into poisonous gases cannot be suppressed. Why? Because they can be carried on in out-of-the-way cellar rooms, where complete plans may be worked out to change existing industrial chemical plants into full capacity poisonous gas plants on a fortnight's notice, and who will be the wiser?[23(p3)]

Although Fries's comments were persuasive and eloquent, a young lieutenant more graphically expressed the opinion of those who understood the nature of chemical warfare in a 1919 poem:

> There is nothing in war more important than gas
> The man who neglects it himself is an ass
> The unit Commander whose training is slack
> Might just as well stab all his men in the back.[62(cover iv)]

Proponents for a chemical warfare service won the debate. On July 1, 1920, the CWS became a permanent part of the Regular Army. Its mission included developing, procuring, and supplying all offensive and defensive chemical warfare material, together with similar functions in the fields of smoke and incendiary weapons. In addition, the CWS was made responsible for training the Army in chemical warfare and for organizing, equipping, training, and employing special chemical troops.[27,63]

Lean Years for the Chemical Warfare Service

Despite having gained permanent status, the years after 1920 were lean ones for the CWS and the Army as a whole. The CWS was authorized 100 Regular Army officers but never actually achieved that number. The low point was 64 officers in 1923. Enlisted strength dropped to a low of 261 in 1919 and averaged about 400 the rest of the decade. Civilian employees numbered less than a thousand. The low point in funds was in 1923, when the budget was $600,000.[27]

After 1919 almost all the work of the CWS moved to Edgewood Arsenal, Maryland, with only the headquarters remaining in Washington, DC. Edgewood became the center of training, stockpiling, and research and development. Initially, the CWS was authorized to train only its own troops in all aspects of chemical warfare while other Army elements were permitted defensive training only. The CWS protested this limitation and finally in May 1930, the judge advocate general ruled that both offensive and defensive training was allowed for all troops.[64]

Leftover stocks of chemicals from World War I were deemed sufficient for the Army's stockpile. In 1922, to comply with the Limitation of Arms Conference, the War Department ordered that "the filling of all projectiles and containers with poisonous gas will be discontinued, except for the limited number needed in perfecting gas-defense appliances."[65] The CWS was only allowed to continue limited research and development based on predictions of future wars.[65,66]

At the close of the 1920s, the CWS formalized the standardization of chemical agents. Seven chemical agents and smokes were selected as the most important. The seven, with their symbols, were as follows:

- mustard agent (HS; "H" for Hun-Stoffe, "S" for the 25% solvent added to form crude mustard. "D" later replaced the "S," signifying distilled or purified mustard);
- methyldifluorarsine (MD);
- diphenylaminechlorarsine (DM);
- chloroacetophenone (CN);
- titanium tetrachloride (FM);
- white phosphorus (WP); and
- hexachlorethane (HC).

Phosgene (CG) and lewisite (L) were considered less important. Chloropicrin (PS) and chlorine (Cl) were rated the least important.[4]

New US Policy

Further international attempts to ban not only the use of chemical weapons but also all research, production, and training elicited a response that developed into a new US policy on chemical warfare. Army Chief of Staff General Douglas MacArthur stated the policy in a letter to Secretary of State Henry L Stimson in 1932:

> In the matter of chemical warfare, the War Department opposes any restrictions whereby the United States would refrain from all peacetime preparation or manufacture of gases, means of launching

gases, or defensive gas material. No provision that would require the disposal or destruction of any existing installation of our Chemical Warfare Service or of any stocks of chemical warfare material should be incorporated in an agreement. Furthermore, the existence of a War Department agency engaged in experimentation and manufacture of chemical warfare materials, and in training for unforeseen contingencies is deemed essential to our national defense.[59(p118)]

THE 1930s: GROWING THREAT OF CHEMICAL WARFARE

The use of chemical weapons in the name of imperialist expansion awakened the international community during the 1930s, when Italy and Japan deployed their offensive chemical stockpiles against unprotected neighbors. In addition, a new chemical threat emerged with the discovery of nerve agents, poisons of extraordinary potency, by Dr Gerhard Schrader in Germany. While some countries used chemical weapons, others stockpiled them. No international attempts to ban chemical warfare occurred during the 1930s.

Italian-Ethiopian War

The first major use of chemical weapons after World War I came in 1935 during the Italian-Ethiopian War. Italy's fascist dictator, Benito Mussolini, launched an invasion of Ethiopia from its neighbors Eritrea, an Italian colony, and Italian Somaliland, that lasted approximately 7 months starting October 3. Viewed as a prelude to World War II, the Italian-Ethiopian War proved the effectiveness of chemical weapons and the ineffectiveness of the League of Nations.

Ethiopia protested the invasion to the League of Nations, which in turn imposed limited economic sanctions on Italy. These sanctions, although not crippling, put pressure on Italy to either win the war or withdraw. The initial Italian offensive from Eritrea was not pursued with enough vigor in Mussolini's opinion, and the Italian commander was replaced. The new commander, Marshal Pietro Badoglio, was ordered to finish the war quickly. He resorted to chemical weapons to defeat the Ethiopian troops led by Emperor Haile Selassie. Despite the Geneva Protocol of 1925, which Italy had ratified in 1928 (followed by Ethiopia in 1935), the Italians dropped mustard bombs and occasionally sprayed mustard from airplane tanks. They also used mustard agent in powder form as a "dusty agent" on the African desert sands to burn the unprotected feet of the Ethiopians. There were rumors of phosgene and chloropicrin attacks, but these were never verified. The Italians attempted to justify their use of chemical weapons by citing the exception to the Geneva Protocol restrictions that referred to acceptable use for reprisal against illegal acts of war, stating that the Ethiopians had tortured or killed their prisoners and wounded soldiers.[67–79]

The chemical weapons devastated the unprepared and unprotected Ethiopians, who had few antiaircraft guns and no air force. Selassie described the situation to the League of Nations:

> Special sprayers were installed on board aircraft so they could vaporize over vast areas of territory a fine, death-dealing rain. Groups of 9, 15, or 18 aircraft followed one another so that the fog issuing from them formed a continuous sheet. It was thus that, as from the end of January 1936, soldiers, women, children, cattle, rivers, lakes, and pastures were drenched continually with this deadly rain. In order more surely to poison the waters and pastures, the Italian command made its aircraft pass over and over again. These fearful tactics succeeded. Men and animals succumbed. The deadly rain that fell from the aircraft made all those whom it touched fly shrieking with pain. All those who drank poisoned water or ate infected food also succumbed in dreadful suffering. In tens of thousands the victims of Italian mustard gas fell.[72(pp151–152)]

By May 1936 Italy's army had completely routed the Ethiopian army. Italy controlled most of Ethiopia until 1941, when British and other allied troops reconquered the country. The US Army closely followed the war and sent Major Norman E Fiske to observe with the Italian army, and Captain John Meade to observe with the Ethiopian army. Their different conclusions as to the role of chemical warfare in the conflict reflected the sides they observed. Major Fiske thought the Italians were clearly superior and that victory for them was assured. The use of chemical agents in the war was nothing more than an experiment. "From my own observations and from talking with [Italian] junior officers and soldiers," Fiske reported, "I have concluded that gas was not used extensively in the African campaign and that its use had little if any effect on the outcome."[77(p20)] His opinion was supported by others who felt that the Ethiopians had made a serious mistake in abandoning guerrilla operations for a conventional war.

On the other hand, Captain Meade thought that chemical weapons were a significant factor in winning the war. They had been used to destroy the morale of the Ethiopian troops, who had little or no protection, and to break up any attempts at concentrating forces. "It is my opinion that of all the superior weapons possessed by the Italians, mustard gas was the most effective," Meade said. "It caused few deaths that I observed, but it temporarily incapacitated very large numbers and so frightened the rest that the Ethiopian resistance broke completely."[77(p20)]

Major General JFC Fuller, also assigned to the Italian army, highlighted the Italian use of mustard agent to protect the flanks of columns by denying ridgelines and other key areas to the Ethiopians. He said that "in place of the laborious process of picketing the heights, the heights sprayed with gas were rendered unoccupiable by the enemy, save at the gravest risk. It was an exceedingly cunning use of this chemical."[74(p143)]

Still another observer stated:

> I think [where mustard] had [the] most effect was on animals; the majority of the Ethiopian armies consisted of a number of individual soldiers, each with his donkey or mule on which he carried rations. These donkeys and mules ate the grass and it killed them, and it was that which really broke down morale more than anything.[75(p81)]

BH Liddell Hart, another military expert, reconciled the two schools of thought, concluding that "the facts of the campaign point unmistakably to the conclusion that mechanization in the broad sense was the foundation on which the Italians' military superiority was built, while aircraft, the machine gun, and mustard gas proved the decisive agents."[76(p330)]

All observers seemed to agree that the Italian military superiority would eventually have won, whether chemical agents were used or not. In general, the US Army learned little from this war. The CWS annual report for 1937 stated that "situations involving the employment of chemical agents have been introduced into a greater number of problems."[78] The CWS Chemical Warfare School concluded that "the use of gas in Ethiopia did not disclose any new chemical warfare tactics,"[79] but only reconfirmed existing tactical use expectations. One senior Air Corps officer, perhaps noting Italy's successful use of spray tanks, commented on the school's class for Army Air Corps personnel, "We want that course repeated again and again until all of our people are thoroughly awake to the necessity for training and preparation."[80(p153)]

Japanese Invasion of China

The next war that drew the interest of chemical warfare experts began when the Japanese invaded China in 1937. In addition to their biological warfare program, the Japanese had an extensive chemical weapons program and produced agent and munitions in large numbers by the late 1930s. During the war with China, Japanese forces reportedly began using chemical shells, tear gas grenades, and lacrimatory candles, often mixed with smoke screens. By 1939 the Japanese had reportedly escalated to using mustard agent and lewisite. The weapons proved effective against the untrained and unequipped Chinese troops. The Chinese reported that their troops retreated whenever the Japanese used smoke, thinking it was a chemical attack.[53,81]

Organophosphorus Compounds

After the Italian-Ethiopian War, the possibility of war in Europe became the primary concern of the US Army. The CWS closely studied the chemical warfare capabilities of Germany and Italy, but it clearly overlooked the secret German development of nerve agents. Although largely isolationist in policy, the United States began gradually increasing its military posture because of the deteriorating political situation in Europe. Official policy, however, remained against the employment of chemical warfare, and initially the CWS met with much resistance. Public opinion continued to be solidly opposed to any chemical weapon use, and President Franklin D Roosevelt refused to permit the redesignation of the CWS as a "corps" in 1937. The US Army chief of staff finally approved two CWS battalions just before the beginning of World War II.[59]

While Italy and Japan employed conventional chemical weapons during their respective invasions, Germany pioneered new chemical warfare technology through the development of nerve agents. The history of nerve agent development had its roots with the Calabar bean, used initially as an ordeal poison in witchcraft trials by African tribal peoples,[82–84] and later used medicinally.[85] By 1864 the active compound, isolated by Jobst and Hesse, was termed "physostigmine."[82] This is the earliest use of a substance that works like a nerve agent through inhibition of the enzyme cholinesterase. Physostigmine, a member of the carbamate class of reversible cholinesterase inhibitors, was separately isolated in 1865 by Vee and Leven and called "eserine."[82]

The first organophosphorus (OP) cholinesterase inhibitor was tetraethyl pyrophosphate, synthesized by Wurtz and tested by Clermont in 1854.[86] Later chemists made contributions to the science of OP compounds,[87–90] but the toxic nature of such compounds was unrealized until the 1930s, when an investigation into both

EXHIBIT 2-10

ORGANOPHOSPHORUS CATEGORIZATION

Altogether, there are five organophosphorus compounds recognized as nerve agents, designated GA (tabun), GB (sarin), GD (soman), GF (cyclosarin), and VX by their North Atlantic Treaty Organization military abbreviation. The "G" series is so named because these compounds originated in Germany. The A through F designation was based on the chronological order of synthesis of each agent. Soman was termed GD rather than GC because the latter acronym had already been established in the medical literature, possibly reserved for gonococcus. GF was the fourth agent synthesized, but interest in this nerve agent declined in favor of the other organophosphorus compounds. The fifth agent (VX) was named for being venomous and was synthesized many years later at Porton Down, England, in 1952. Only tabun, sarin, and soman were categorized as the "Trilon group." The toxicity and lethality of these three nerve agents on the civilian population can be approximated based on their lethal doses. The lethal dose for oral ingestion of tabun is roughly 100 to 200 mg min/m^3, and 50 to 100 mg min/m^3 for sarin. Only 200 to 1000 mg of tabun applied to the skin is sufficient to kill an adult human. The 12,000 tons of tabun stocks alone that were reported at the end of the war could kill 60 billion individuals.

Data source: *German Munition Plants and Depots During World War II*. Aberdeen Proving Ground, Md: US Army Chemical and Biological Defense Command; 1996.

carbamate-type (eg, physostigmine-type, reversible) and OP-type (irreversible) cholinesterase inhibitors led to a series of monumental discoveries by German scientists (Exhibit 2-10).

The earliest reported incident of OP toxicity from inhalation came from the laboratory of Willy Lange at Friedrich Wilhelms University. In 1932 Lange and his student, Gerde von Krueger, prepared dialkyl monofluorophosphates and noted their toxic fumes.[84,86] They described the effects of the vapors on themselves, reporting breathing difficulties and blurred vision that lasted many hours before subsiding. Toward the close of 1936, at the chemical and pharmaceutical conglomerate IG Farbenindustrie, Gerhard Schrader accidentally discovered powerful OP compounds during his investigation into new insecticides. After preparing them, Schrader's biologist colleague, Hans Kukenthal, tested them for insecticidal activity. On December 23, 1936, Kukenthal tested the new compounds on leaf lice and noted one to be particularly potent. All of the insects died after being sprayed with a concentration of only one part in 200,000 of the deadly substance.[20,84] During preliminary manufacture of the compound, Kukenthal noticed its equally impressive effects in humans. A spilled droplet from a solution could constrict the pupils and cause labored breathing immediately. Even Schrader and his colleague felt the effects upon themselves, requiring several weeks to recover. This was the first of the nerve agents or gases, called "tabun."

In 1936 tabun was reported to the chemical weapons section of the German military prior to patenting. As a colorless, odorless poison, tabun was an ideal chemical weapon. In May 1937 Schrader demonstrated its deadly effects to Colonel Rüdiger, a German ordnance officer and director of the Heereswaffenamt (HWA [German army weapons agency]). The military was impressed with the effects of the compound on the nervous system and classified the project for further research. The military assigned various names to the new substance, including "Trilon-83," "Le100," "Präparat 9/91," "Nr 100," "Gelan," "Grünring 3," "Stoff 83," and "Stoff 100," but tabun was the name that stuck.[20,91] After World War II, the CWS designated it "GA," for "German agent A."

During a 2-year period between 1937 and 1939, the HWA assigned a large number of chemists to evaluate tabun and work on developing new nerve agents.[4,92,93] The next step was mass production by the military, so the HWA built a test plant in Münsterlager. Schrader filed a patent on August 2, 1938, but it was kept secret until September 1951.[94] Schrader continued to synthesize esters of fluorophosphoric acid, including diisopropyl fluorophosphate, which Lange and Krueger had synthesized in 1932 and 1933.

On December 10, 1938, 2 years after the discovery of tabun, Schrader discovered a second lethal agent. This nerve agent was initially designated "T-144," the building number at the Dyhernfurth plant responsible for its pilot production.[20] It also went by the codenames "Le 213," "Trilon-46," and "Grünring 4."[20,91,95] The compound was eventually dubbed "sarin" after the four individuals involved in the initial production process (Gerhard Schrader, Otto Ambros [IG Farben board member], Colonel Rüdiger [HWA], and Hans-Jürgen von der Linde [HWA]). Some believe the "R" is named for fellow German chemist Franz Ritter.[95,96] Animal testing showed sarin to be five to ten times as lethal as tabun. As the second nerve agent to be synthesized, sarin was later designated "GB," for "German agent B," by the United States.

WORLD WAR II

The start of World War II in 1939 and the rapid collapse of France in the spring of 1940 stimulated a major increase in the rate of American rearmament. No major use of chemical agents occurred, but rumors and reports of incidents of chemical warfare attracted the attention of intelligence officers. The possibility that massive chemical attacks could happen any day kept CWS officers pushing for preparedness. A newspaper article reflected the common prediction circulating in the press, saying, "European military authorities have predicted that gas would be used in the present war, if at any time the user could be sure of an immediate and all-out success from which there could be no retaliation."[97(p37)] Major General William N Porter, the new chief of the CWS, warned that Hitler was likely to use chemical weapons "at any moment." He also felt that "no weapon would be too bad to stop or defeat Hitler,"[98(p31)] and wanted to "fight fire with fire in the event an enemy chooses to use poison gas."[99(p36)]

Although much of Germany's and Japan's chemical weapons programs did not become known until after the war, their actual threat was impressive. Building on its experience in chemical agent use in China, Japan produced about 8,000 tons of chemical agents during the war, loading mustard agent, a mustard-lewisite mixture, and phosgene in shells and bombs and HCN into glass grenades and mortar and artillery shells. This effort was dwarfed by the German capability.

German Production

During the war, Germany produced approximately 78,000 tons of chemical warfare agents, including about 12,000 tons of tabun between 1942 and 1945 and about 1,000 lb of sarin by 1945. Key nerve agent weapons were the 105-mm and 150-mm shells, the 250-kg bomb, and the 150-mm rocket. The latter held 7 lb of agent and had a range of about 5 miles when fired from the six-barrel Nebelwerfer launcher. Mustard agent was produced in the greatest volume and used to fill artillery shells, bombs, rockets, and spray tanks. Phosgene, of somewhat less importance, was loaded in 250-kg and 500-kg bombs. About 2,000 tons of nitrogen mustards were produced and used in artillery shells and rockets. Germany also captured a large amount of chemical munitions from France, Poland, the Soviet Union, Hungary, and other occupied countries.[4,28]

Germany began constructing extensive factories in Germany (Raubkammer, Falkenhagen) and later Poland (Dyhernfurth) for the massive production of tabun, sarin, cyanogen chloride, hydrocyanic acid, and N-Stoff (chlortrifluoride).[20,96,100,101] Just as scientists in Berlin prepared the first samples of sarin, the German army launched its invasion of Poland in September 1939. Hitler's speech in Danzig on September 19, 1939, alluded to Germany's new weapons of war, against which enemies would be defenseless. Although the construction had begun earlier, full capacity production of the first toxic agents did not begin until May 1943.[102] The third and most deadly nonpersistent nerve agent, soman, was synthesized in 1944 by Richard Kuhn, a research director at the Max Planck Institute for Medical Research in Heidelberg. Soman is suggested to have been named after either the Greek word for "sleep" or the Latin word for "bludgeon."[84]

The resources, organization, and quality of chemists thrust into this top secret mission to synthesize nerve agents, develop new ones, and provide countermeasures against their devastating effects was on par with the American team of physicists working on the Manhattan Project. Tons of nerve agent munitions were synthesized and stockpiled in Germany during World War II, and neither the United States nor Great Britain were aware of them at the time. Meanwhile, no country on the Allied side possessed a weapon that could match the lethality of nerve gas.

British Development of Nerve Agents

While Germany was a decade ahead in the race to synthesize nerve agents, British scientists Bernard Charles Saunders and Hamilton McCombie stumbled upon the toxic effects of esters of monofluorophosphoric acid.[104] Diisopropyl fluorophosphate, a lethal inhalant, was of particular interest to Saunders and McCombie. Saunders reported his findings on the toxicity of diisopropyl fluorophosphate to the Ministry of Supply in London on December 11, 1941. Among the findings were pupillary constriction and a fast onset of action. The first American report on the mechanism of action by diisopropyl fluorophosphate came out immediately after the war.[105] Nevertheless, tons of nerve agent munitions were synthesized and stockpiled in Germany during World War II, and neither the United States nor Great Britain were aware of them at the time. Meanwhile, no country on the Allied side possessed a weapon that could match the lethality of nerve gas.

Why Germany Did Not Authorize Use of Chemical Weapons

The reason Hitler did not give an order to use nerve agents in World War II, a major blunder for Germany, remains a mystery. Nerve agents could have altered the course of the war, slowing the Allied D-Day invasion by several months, enough time for the introduction of long-range V-weapons to Great Britain. Hitler decided early in the war not to use chemical weapons on the battlefield because he initially wanted peace more than he wanted to wipe out targets. When he finally thought about using them late in 1944, he no longer possessed the air supremacy to drop poison gas bombs. The reverse scenario was true for the British, who had the means to deliver gas on the Germans. Early in the war, the British did not have enough stock produced to support a gas war. By the time they had the stocks of weapons to slow the blitzkrieg in 1944, the British were already on the offensive with air supremacy and gas could only hamper their march into France and Germany.

A popular explanation for Germany's reluctance to use gas is that Hitler, a victim of a chlorine gas attack during World War I, disliked poison gas and would only use chemical agents as a last resort. Hitler was wounded on at least two occasions in World War I when he served as a dispatch runner with the rank of corporal. In *Mein Kampf*, Hitler described his own gas experience after being blinded by a mustard gas attack in Flanders at the third battle of Passchendaele:

> In the night of October 13, the English gas attack on the southern front before Ypres burst loose; they used yellow-cross gas, whose effects were still unknown to us as far as personal experience was concerned. In this same night I myself was to become acquainted with it. On a hill south of Wervick, we came on the evening of October 13 into several hours of drumfire with gas shells which continued all night more or less violently. As early as midnight, a number of us passed out, a few of our comrades forever. Toward morning I, too, was seized with pain which grew worse with every quarter hour, and at seven in the morning I stumbled and tottered back with burning eyes; taking with me my last report of the War.
>
> A few hours later, my eyes had turned into glowing coals; it had grown dark around me. Thus I came to the hospital at Pasewalk in Pomerania, and there I was fated to experience–the greatest villainy of the century.[106(p118–119)]

When Germany surrendered, Hitler was angry, feeling that his physical pain and the deaths of his comrades were suffered in vain. However, he never states an aversion to the use of gas.

Hitler also alluded to Germany's potential to use nerve agents in public speeches. Hitler's actions and words did not give the perception that he was afraid to use nerve agents, despite his negative personal experiences with gas on the battlefields of World War I. Furthermore, Hitler ordered the output from the nerve agent factories to increase in 1943, despite the limited availability of material required to synthesize the agents. Hitler dedicated extensive resources to filling shells with nerve agents for his army and air force.

Others speculate that the German high command mistakenly believed the Allies had developed the nerve agents simultaneously and feared Allied retaliation as the Axis retreated. Albert Speer, the chief architect in Nazi Germany and minister of armament in Hitler's cabinet, and Otto Ambros were called to Hitler's eastern front headquarters in May 1943 and again in 1944 to discuss the use of gas. Ambros and Speer argued against gas. Ambros believed that the Allies could produce more traditional chemical agents than Germany. When later addressing the Nuremburg War Crimes Tribunal, Ambros said that he warned Hitler about using nerve agents.[107] Ambros's affidavit regarding his conversation with Hitler stated that the formulas for tabun and sarin were already known by the Allies because the nature of nerve agents had been disclosed in technical journals dating back to 1902. He said, "I have justified reasons to assume that tabun, too, is known abroad. I know that tabun was publicized as early as 1902, that Sarin was patented, and that these substances appeared in patents."[107(p1044)]

Ambros was aware that the Americans knew the basic precursor compounds in the years prior to the war but had not appeared to continue work in the field. The Germans may have speculated this was an attempt at censorship and a further indication that the United States had developed an arsenal equal to that of Germany. Ambros argued that assumption caused Germany to shelve nerve agents, a costly decision in light of Allied knowledge regarding nerve agents at the time. In reality, scientists at Edgewood Arsenal and Porton Down (Edgewood's British counterpart) did not know about either agent nor about the German antidote, atropine. It is unknown whether Ambros was telling the truth about his meeting with Hitler, but it is now known that tabun was kept secret until 1951 and sarin was never patented.

In his Nuremburg testimony, Speer pointed to Paul Joseph Goebbels, Hitler's propaganda minister, and Robert Ley, a former chemist and head of the German Labor Front, as the main proponents of gas. Martin Bormann, head of the Nazi party chancellery and Hitler's private secretary, and Hermann Ochsner, commanding general of all German chemical troops, were other prominent figures who advocated the instigation of chemical warfare against the Allies. When Speer was questioned about proposals to use poison gas warfare, he responded:

> I was not able to make out from my own direct observations whether gas warfare was to be started, but I knew from various associates of Ley's and Goebbels' that they were discussing the question of using our two new combat gases, Tabun and Sarin. They believed that these gases would be of particular efficacy, and they did in fact produce the most frightful results. We made these observations as early as the autumn of 1944, when the situation had become critical, and many people were seriously worried about it. . . . All sensible army people turned gas warfare down as being utterly insane, since, in view of their [the Allies] superiority in the air, it would not be long before it would bring the most terrible catastrophe upon German cities.[108(pp527–528)]

Speer also cites his concerns about protecting the German soldiers from the effects of nerve agents. On the question of nerve agent production, effects, and preparations made for use in the war, Speer shed light on the implementation of possible German plans:

> I cannot tell you that in detail. I am not enough of an expert. All I know is that these two gases both had a quite extraordinary effect, and that there was no respirator, and no protection against them that we knew of. So the soldiers would have been unable to protect themselves against this gas in any way. For the manufacture of this gas we had about three factories, all of which were undamaged and which until November 1944 were working at full speed. When rumors reached us that gas might be used, I stopped its production in November 1944. I stopped it by the following means. I blocked the so-called preliminary production, that is, the chemical supplies for the making of gas, so that the gas-production, as the Allied authorities themselves ascertained, after the end of December to the beginning of January, actually slowed down and finally came to a standstill. Beginning with a letter which is still in existence and which I wrote to Hitler in October 1944, I tried through legal methods to obtain his permission to have these gas factories stop their production. The reason I gave him was that on account of air raids the preliminary products, primarily cyanide, were needed urgently for other purposes. Hitler informed me that the gas production would have to continue whatever happened, but I gave instructions for the preliminary products not to be supplied any more.[108(p527)]

Despite nerve agent testing, manufacture, and stockpiling by the German military during World War II, chemical weapons were never deployed. Many argue that the Nazi philosophy of blitzkrieg accounted for the reluctance to use nerve agents:[109] a quick striking offense with tanks would only be slowed by an engagement using poison gas. The lessons Germany learned about chemical warfare from World War I were 3-fold. First, trench warfare necessitated the use of gas to break a stalemate, but gas led to only minimal gains in territory. Second, gas was more advantageous to defensive positions. Third, large advances were possible with lightning strikes using tanks and a highly mobile military, and this strategy would allow fewer casualties by overwhelming the opponent at the point of attack. Advancing into an area covered with persistent agents would hinder the mission. However, one could argue that defensively drenching the beaches of Normandy with nerve agent might have slowed the Allied D-Day invasion until the arrival of reinforcements. After the war, General Omar Bradley admitted his dread about such a defense, saying, "When D-Day finally ended without a whiff of gas, I was vastly relieved. For even a light sprinkling of persistent gas on Omaha Beach would have cost us our footing there. [Gas would have] forced a decision in one of history's climactic battles."[110(p237)]

Capture of German Facilities and Scientists

Upon capture of a German ammunition dump in April 1945 (Figures 2-34 and 2-35), Allied scientists at Porton Down became aware of German tabun gas and its physiological effects for the first time.[111] Only then did the Allied command believe in the existence of Hitler's new "war gas," despite intelligence gathered from a captured German scientist on May 11, 1943, in Tunisia. The captured chemist worked at the nerve agent laboratory at Spandau and provided valuable informa-

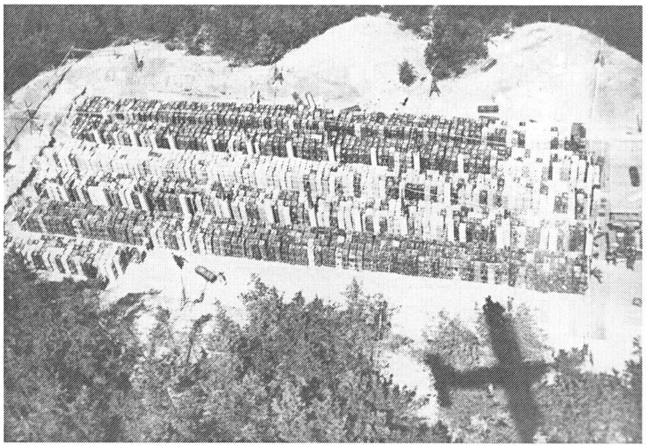

Fig. 2-34. Storage of approximately 2,000 German tabun bombs shipped into Schierling Chemical Depot after the occupation of West Germany by American troops in the aftermath of World War II. Photograph: Courtesy of Chemical and Biological Defense Command Historical Research and Response Team, Aberdeen Proving Ground, Md.

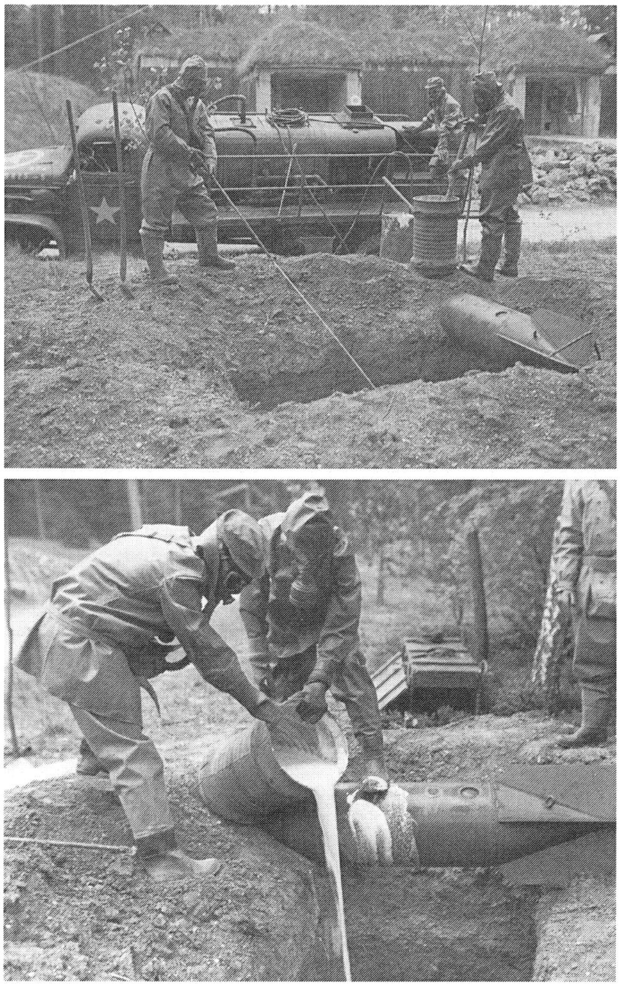

Fig. 2-35. Decontamination of weaponized nerve agents after World War II. The sequence depicts a Green Ring 3 tabun-filled aerial bomb about to be vented, drained, and decontaminated. May 1946. (**a**) Team members pour a mixture of sodium hydroxide and bleach into a pit. (**b**) The pit that will contain the fully decontaminated tabun as it drains from the bomb. Photograph: Courtesy of Chemical and Biological Defense Command Historical Research and Response Team, Aberdeen Proving Ground, Md.

tion about tabun.[20,103] Other captured German chemists also revealed the existence of the antidote, atropine.

Kuhn, who had discovered soman, was taken into custody when American troops arrived in Heidelberg. After initially denying any involvement in military research,[103] Kuhn told interrogators that all documents concerning soman were buried in an abandoned mine shaft east of Berlin. The Soviet army entered Berlin before the Americans and the documents were recovered by Soviet Colonel VA Kargin, who took them back to the Karpov Institute in Moscow.[20,103] Capturing the prized soman documents in Berlin was a major coup. The Soviet army also captured factories producing tabun and sarin, in addition to extensive documentation on the agents' research and manufacture.[20,103,109] The Soviets reassembled one of the German factories in Russia, resuming production of tabun and sarin by 1946.

Eisenhower's decision not to enter Berlin before the Soviet army seemed costly in terms of the German facilities and intelligence captured by the Soviet Union; however, the Allies capture of the majority of German scientists may have been a larger prize. The organized capture and detainment of German military scientists at Kransberg Castle was known as Operation Dustbin. Notable captured Germans included most of the chemists and technicians from Dynhernfurth, Heinrich Horlein, Gerhard Ehlers, Wilhelm Kleinhans, Werner von Braun, Albert Speer, Richard Kuhn, Walter Hirsch, Otto Ambros, and Gerhard Schrader. The Allies also captured coveted documents relating to the large-scale manufacture of nerve agents. Just prior to the fall of Falkenhagen, its director hid thousands of documents concerning Dyhernfurth, laboratory notebooks, and technical reports related to nerve agent production, which were later discovered by Allied intelligence. The British also obtained critical documents related to the tabun and sarin pilot plants at Raubkammer from German scientists there and later shipped the disassembled plants to Porton Down.[103]

Evidence of Gas Use in Germany

Although gas was not used on the battlefields of World War II, HCN gas (trade name Zyklon B), developed by Fritz Haber, was used in Nazi concentration camps first for delousing to control typhus and later for killing prisoners during the Holocaust. (The first-generation cyanide insecticide, known as Zyklon A, contained methyl cyanoformate as the active agent.) Upon exposure to air, the substrates in Zyklon B elaborated vapors of HCN. In Nazi gas chambers, Zyklon B facilities were disguised as shower and decontamination rooms. In 1941 experiments with Zyklon B were performed in Auschwitz I as well as other camps such as Dachau, the longest running concentration camp. Zyklon B was provided by the German companies Degesch and Testa, under license from patent holder IG Farbenindustrie.[103] After the war, two directors of Tesch were tried by a British military court and executed for their part in supplying the chemical.

German Plans for Gas

Both sides in the war had active plans to use chemical weapons in the event that the other side used them first. The Soviet chemical arsenal was seriously lacking compared to the stocks available to Germany, and Soviet gas masks had technical defects, which may explain Stalin's no-first-use policy.[109] During the war, the Soviets lacked chemical discipline and adequate protective equipment to instigate a chemical war. During retreats in 1941, many Soviet troops discarded their gas masks and other equipment to lighten their loads. By the end of 1941 fighting had reached a stalemate around Leningrad. Germany planned to breach the Soviet defenses by means of a chemical attack along 20 kilometers near the city, but had insufficient supplies of artillery and gas shells to carry out the maneuver.[109]

In September and December of 1942 General Hermann Ochsner, chief of Germany's chemical warfare division, carried out two attacks with a nonlethal gas to smoke out Soviet guerillas hiding in caves along the Kerch peninsula, a stretch of land forming the opening to the Sea of Azov. The Soviet government claimed the German army was responsible for thousands of deaths and had used chemical weapons in the attack.[109]

Chemical weapons were not used by either side during fierce fighting at Moscow. After defeating German troops at Moscow, Kursk, and Stalingrad, a change from defense to offense in Soviet military strategy renewed an interest in chemical weapons. Soviet intelligence before the Battle of Kursk warned of German use of the chemical weapons. Chief of Staff AM Vasil'ev wrote this directive [translated]:

> The general staff possesses information to the effect that the German command has recently heightened the preparedness of its forces for the use of chemical weapons. . . . There are enough risk takers in the German command who, relying on the fact that they could catch us by surprise, might decide on a desperate gamble and use chemical weapons against us.[112(p91)]

British Plans for Gas

Prime Minister Churchill's position on gas warfare is evident in a four-page memo sent to his chief of staff, General Hastings Ismay:

> I urge you to think very seriously over the question of poison gas. . . . It is absurd to consider morality on this topic when everybody used it [gas] in the last war without a word of complaint from the moralists or the Church. On the other hand, in the last war the bombing of open cities was regarded as forbidden. Now everybody does it as a matter of course. It is simply a question of fashion changing as she does between long and short skirts for women. . . . I want a cold-blooded calculation made as to how it would pay to use poison gas. . . . One really must not be bound within silly conventions of the mind whether they be those that ruled in the last war or those in reverse which rule in this. . . . We could drench the cities of the Ruhr and many other cities in Germany in such a way that most of the population would be requiring constant medical attention. . . . It may be several weeks or even months before I shall ask you to drench Germany with poison gas, and if we do it, let us do it one hundred per cent. In the meantime, I want the matter studied in cold blood by sensible people and not by the particular set of psalm-singing uniformed defeatists which one runs across now here now here now there.[113(p501)]

US Policy and Plans for Gas

While planning for a traditional, European-style war, the CWS also monitored Japan's use of chemical weapons in China, which increased the US Army's interest in chemical warfare preparation.[114] The CWS, however, was still unprepared to fight a major chemical war on the level of World War I. Increased budgets and personnel helped with war planning, but to actually field chemical weapons and build chemical stockpiles first required industrial mobilization and massive production.

President Roosevelt established a no-first-use policy for chemical weapons early in the war, which was reiterated in an official statement in 1943: "We shall under no circumstances resort to the use of such weapons [chemical] unless they are first used by our enemies."[115(p6)] The policy was backed up by a statement of warning: "Any use of gas by any axis power, therefore, will immediately be followed by the fullest possible retaliation upon munition centers, seaports and other military objectives throughout the whole extent of the territory of such axis country."[115(pp6–7)]

US plans for the final invasion of Japan, code-named Operation Downfall, called for the invasion of Kyushu Island in the fall of 1945, followed by an invasion of the main island of Japan in the spring of 1946. Planners predicted that the attack would lead to a major chemical conflict because Japan had already used chemical weapons against China. The Army Air Force plans called for the use of persistent 100-lb bombs (mustard gas) and nonpersistent 500-lb bombs (60% phosgene, 40% cyanogen chloride). After Germany's surrender in May 1945, the CWS contemplated augmenting their current arsenal of chemical bombs with captured stocks from Germany to address shortages based on required estimates for a chemical attack of Japan. Mustard gas, phosgene, and tabun were shipped back to the United States to be punched, drained, and used to fill American ordnance rounds.[116] It was subsequently determined that US shells were unsuitable for tabun, but German 10.5-cm projectiles could be used in US howitzers (105-mm) with worn tubes because German shells were slightly wider than US 105-mm shells.[117] In the end, Japan surrendered after nuclear bombs were dropped on Nagasaki and Hiroshima, and chemical warfare in the Pacific was averted.

Although neither Germany nor Japan chose to initiate chemical warfare with the United States, the CWS spent the war training troops; designing chemical, incendiary, smoke, explosive, and flame weapons and protective equipment; and planning for a chemical war. In addition to the M2 4.2-in chemical mortar,[4,28,118] the CWS possessed 75-mm, 105-mm, and 155-mm chemical rounds filled with mustard or lewisite. The US Air Force had 100-lb mustard agent bombs; 500-lb phosgene or cyanogen chloride bombs; and 1,000-lb phosgene, cyanogen chloride, or hydrocyanic acid bombs. In addition, the new M33 spray tank could hold 750 to 1,120 lb of mustard agent or lewisite.

None of these chemical weapons was used on the battlefield during the war,[4,119,120] but the prepositioning of chemical weapons in forward areas resulted in one major disaster and several near mishaps. The disaster occurred December 2, 1943, when the *SS John Harvey*, loaded with 2,000 M47A1 mustard agent bombs, was destroyed during a German air raid at Bari Harbor, Italy. The only members of the crew who were aware of the chemical munitions were killed in the raid. As a result of the ship's destruction, mustard agent contaminated the water in the harbor and caused more than 600 casualties, in addition to those killed or injured in the actual attack. The harbor clean-up took 3 weeks and required large quantities of lime as a decontaminant.[121]

US Lessons Learned

After the war, the phrase "had the United States been prepared for war in 1939, there would not have been a war"[122(p24)] was taken as a self-evident truth. The CWS needed to be a permanent organization that concentrated on training, research and development, and chemical warfare preparedness. This same lesson, from a slightly different angle, was reflected in the words of Under Secretary of War Kenneth C Royall to the chemical warfare specialists: "The better job you do the less likely it is that you will have to put to actual use the products of your work."[123(p41)]

Demobilization and the Creation of the Chemical Corps

The Army began demobilization activities almost immediately after the president proclaimed the end of hostilities. By early 1946 the CWS was effectively demobilized and its military strength approached prewar levels. One observer commented, "Gas warfare is obsolete! Yes, like the cavalry and horsedrawn artillery, it is outmoded, archaic, and of historical interest only. This is the atomic age!"[124(p3)]

However, CWS chief Major General Porter advocated for the CWS before an Army board considering postwar organization, resulting in the permanency long sought by the chemical program: a corps designation. The Army finally agreed that the CWS, along with the other technical services, should continue its existence as a distinct entity in the peacetime Army. On August 2, 1946, Public Law 607 changed the name of the CWS to the "Chemical Corps."[125]

After World War II, as Western defense became increasingly based on the threatened use of nuclear weapons, the Chemical Corps' mission expanded to include radiological protection as well as chemical and biological research and development. At the same

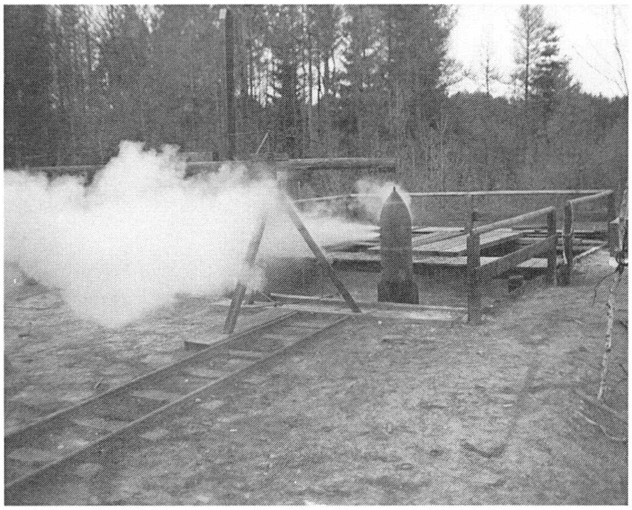

Fig. 2-36. Decontamination of captured chemical stockpiles. A 250 KC (chemical cylinder) phosgene bomb as it drops into a water tank, where the phosgene is neutralized by hydrolization. The bomb has been vented prior to decontamination, and the phosgene vapor can be seen escaping into the air. Schierling, Germany. May 1946.
Photograph: Courtesy of Chemical and Biological Defense Command Historical Research and Response Team, Aberdeen Proving Ground, Md.

time, the corps concentrated on producing and fielding nerve agent weapons and the assorted detection and decontamination equipment required.

Major General Alden H Waitt, who replaced Porter in November 1945, assessed the future of chemical warfare in 1946:

> The fact that toxic gas was not used in the late war [on the battlefield] does not justify a conclusion that it will not be used in the future. Gas has not been out-moded as a weapon. The Germans developed new gases during World War II. The magnitude of their preparedness for gas warfare is indicated by the fact that they had amassed more than a quarter of a million tons of toxic gas; their failure to use this gas against us is attributable largely to their fear of our retaliatory power. We cannot count upon other nations refraining from the use of gas when it would serve their purpose. There were numerous instances in the late war in which the use of gas might have had far-reaching results. Thus, there is no good reason for assuming that the considerations which prevented the employment of gas in World War II will prevail in the future.[126]

Demilitarization of Captured Weapons

At the end of the war, the United States was actively involved in the demilitarization of the thousands of captured munitions from German stockpiles (Figure 2-36). Following the occupation of Germany and Japan, the Allies initiated a sea-dumping and weapons disposal program to eliminate the large stockpiles of captured chemical agents. Ships containing German weapons were sunk in the North Sea as part of Operation Davy Jones' Locker, but not all the German weapons were destroyed. Between 1945 and 1947, some 40,000 of the 250-kg tabun bombs, 21,000 mustard bombs of various sizes, 2,700 nitrogen mustard rockets, and about 750 tabun artillery shells of various sizes were shipped to the United States. In addition to disposing of the enemy stockpiles, the United States dumped the US lewisite stockpile into the sea during Operation Geranium in 1948.[4,127]

THE 1950s

Korean War

With the onset of the Korean War in June 1950, the Chemical Corps participated in its first military action. The corps quickly implemented an increased procurement program to supply the Army with defensive equipment and a retaliatory chemical capability. Within a short time, however, the Army's policy on chemical warfare and the lessons learned from the past were disputed, particularly as the military situation in Korea changed. The action in Korea raised the question of whether to initiate chemical warfare to save lives. Many of the Chemical Corps' supporters favored the use of chemical weapons as humane weapons of war, particularly to offset the enemy's superior numbers. One officer stated bluntly that "the use of mustard, lewisite and phosgene in the vast quantities which we are capable of making and distributing offers the only sure way of holding Korea at the present time. We are not playing marbles. We are fighting for our lives. Let's use the best means we have to overwhelm the enemy scientifically and intelligently."[128(p3)]

Although the North Koreans and Chinese alleged that US forces employed chemical weapons on the battlefield, there is no evidence that the Chemical Corps used them, although it did use smoke and flame, as well as riot control agents to quell riots by prisoners of war. In 1968 a Czech general who defected to the United States reported that US prisoners of war were used for biological tests by the Russians in North Korea. These allegations have yet to be confirmed by the Russians and were vigorously denied by the North Koreans.[129] The United States did not change its policy about no first use of chemical weapons.

At the end of the Korean War, the Chemical Corps was in a much stronger position than it had been at the end of World War II. Although the corps slightly reduced its units and personnel and terminated many of its procurement contracts in the months following the 1953 armistice, Major General Egbert F Bullene, the new chief chemical officer, summed up the feeling of the corps regarding the Korean War and the Cold War in general: "Today, thanks to Joe Stalin, we are back in business."[130(p8)]

Changes in the Chemical Corps

During the 1950s the concept of chemical warfare continued to change radically. The phrase that one could "push a button" to start a war became popular. The lesson learned from the Korean War—that a limited war, fought without nuclear weapons and possibly against satellite states, not the "real enemy"—determined much of the Army's future planning. The fact that two wars had come and gone without the employment of chemical weapons made it necessary for successive chief chemical officers to continually remind the Army and the country that the capabilities of the Chemical Corps constituted insurance against the possibility of chemical attack in the future.

Throughout the 1950s the Chemical Corps conducted several extensive studies to improve its organization and training capabilities. A new training center at Fort McClellan, Alabama, opened in 1951 and offered more space and training options. After more than 30 years in Maryland, the Chemical School moved to Fort McClellan early in 1952.[4] The emphasis on individual training for chemical warfare resulted in the elimination of the unit gas officer, who had previously been responsible for chemical training and readiness, in 1954. After the change, troop commanders assumed the responsibility and were expected to include chemical and biological training in all their field exercises and maneuvers.[131]

Nerve Agent Production and Development

In 1950 the Chemical Corps began constructing its first full-scale sarin production complex based on pilot plant work accomplished at the Army Chemical Center (formerly Edgewood Arsenal). The production of sarin was a 5-step process divided between two sites. For the first two steps of the process, the corps constructed a plant at Muscle Shoals, Alabama, later designated "Site A," or the Muscle Shoals Phosphate Development Works, which was completed in 1953. The last three steps of the process were conducted at a new plant at Rocky Mountain Arsenal, Colorado. In 1951 the corps fully standardized sarin, and by 1953 it was producing the agent. After only 4 years of production, the plants stopped manufacturing because the stockpile requirements for the agent had been met. The plants then went into inactive status with layaway planned. The related munitions filling plants also went into standby status a year later.[4,132]

Part of the reason for the sarin plant's closure was the development of a new nerve agent. While searching for new insecticides, chemists at Imperial Chemicals Limited in the United Kingdom came across compounds extremely toxic to humans. The British shared the discovery with the United States in 1953. The Chemical Corps examined the new compounds and determined that a new series of nerve agents had been discovered that were more persistent and much more toxic than the G-series agents. This new series was designated the "V-series" in 1955 because the agents were venomous in nature. These agents enter the body through the skin, bypassing protective masks. They were 1,000-fold more toxic than sarin when applied to the skin, and 2- to 3-fold more toxic when inhaled. A drop the size of a pinhead on bare skin could cause death within 15 minutes.[4,133]

The Chemical Corps gave top priority to the investigation of these compounds. Of the compounds investigated, VX was selected in 1957 for pilot plant development and dissemination studies. It was standardized in December 1957. The annual report for that year concluded "the reign of mustard gas, which has been called the King of Battle gases since it was first used in July 1917, will probably come to an end."[134(p100)]

The corps initially planned to contract with private industry for a 10-ton-per-day production plant. A later decision put the plant at the inactivated Dana Heavy Water Plant of the Atomic Energy Commission at Newport, Indiana, within the Wabash River Ordnance Works. Construction was delayed because of a patent dispute that resulted in a restraining order. In 1959 Food Machinery and Chemical Company, the low bidder, won the contract and construction was planned for 1960. Shortly after the approval, the Chemical Corps supplemented the contract to provide for a VX weapon-filling plant.[134,135]

The remainder of the 1950s was spent developing new delivery systems and new protective gas masks and improving chemical detection systems, decontaminating methods, and treatments, as well as weaponizing sarin. Although delivery systems for VX nerve agent were initiated during the 1950s, no system was standardized. In addition, many of the sarin delivery systems took longer to develop than planned and some were never standardized.

Medical Research on Human Volunteers

Concerned with the effects of nerve and other chemical agents on soldiers, the Chemical Corps began extensive studies to determine the dangers of exposure and the proper kinds of treatment. These studies exposed soldiers to low levels of agents to demonstrate the effects of treatment and to investigate the agents' affects on humans.

Before the 1950s the use of humans in testing had been conducted on an ad hoc basis and little documentation survived. During the 1950s a more formal volunteer program was established at the Army Chemical Center that drew on local military installations and utilized a specific consent procedure, ensuring that each volunteer was briefed prior to the experiment. Between 1955 and 1975 over 6,000 soldiers participated in this program and were exposed to approximately 250 different chemicals.[136]

The Incapacitant Program

During the 1950s the Chemical Corps also became interested in developing chemical weapons that incapacitated rather than killed its targets. In 1951 the Corps awarded a contract to the New York State Psychiatric Institute to investigate the clinical effects of mescaline and its derivatives. The contractor tested 6 derivatives and the corps tested 35 derivatives. The results of the investigation indicated that mescaline and its derivatives would not be practical as agents because the doses needed to bring about mental confusion were too large.[137]

In 1955 the Chemical Corps formally established a project called "psychochemical agents." The next year, the program was redesignated "K-agents." The objective was to develop a nonlethal but potent incapacitant that could be disseminated from airplanes in all environments. The program was conducted at the Army Chemical Center and examined nonmilitary drugs like lysergic acid (LSD) and tetrahydrocannabinol (related to marijuana). None of these drugs, however, were found to be of military worth.[134,137–139]

The Growing Soviet Threat

While addressing the Communist Party Congress in Moscow in 1956, Soviet Defense Minister Georgi Zhukov warned, "[A]ny new war will be characterized by mass use of air power, various types of rocket, atomic, thermo-nuclear, chemical and biological weapons."[140(p26)] In 1959 Major General Marshall Stubbs, the new chief chemical officer, assessed the growing Soviet chemical threat, saying:

> Soviet chemical weapons are modern and effective and probably include all types of chemical munitions known to the West, in addition to several dissemination devices peculiar to the Russians. Their ground forces are equipped with a variety of protective chemical equipment and they are prepared to participate in large scale gas warfare. They have a complete line of protective clothing which will provide protection in any gas situation and a large variety of decontaminating equipment. . . . I believe that I have given you enough to make you aware that they pose a threat to the free nations of the world.[141(pp 8–9)]

The next year Major General Stubbs talked to various groups around the country about the need for greater urgency in attaining chemical preparedness. Contending that "to both military and civilian populations" the threat of chemical warfare was as great as the threat of nuclear warfare, he reported that the Soviets had about one sixth of their total munitions in chemical weapons.[142]

THE 1960s: DECADE OF TURMOIL

In January 1961 Secretary of Defense Robert S McNamara initiated about 150 projects to provide an appraisal of US military capabilities. Two of these, Project 112 and Project 80, had significant impact on the chemical and biological weapons program. Project 112's objective was to evaluate chemical and biological weapons for use as strategic weapons and for limited war applications. The result of this study was a recommendation to highlight chemical weapons and particularly to increase long-term funding, which was approved for immediate action by the deputy secretary of defense. One of the responses was the creation of Deseret Test Center, Utah, intended for extra-continental chemical and biological agent testing, including trials at sea, and arctic and tropical environmental testing. The new center was jointly staffed by the Army, Navy, and Air Force, with testing scheduled to begin in 1962.

Project 80 resulted in a committee to review the organization of the Army. The project committee eliminated the technical services and distributed their functions to various elements of the new Army organization. McNamara felt that the Chemical Corps' knowledge, experience, and training was not being "infused" into the rest of the Army because the combat troops were "structurally separated" from the corps, particularly in the areas of research, development, and training.[143]

Colonel John M Palmer, head of the Chemical Corps Training Command, reflected on the problem in 1960:

> The quickest way to reduce the effectiveness of a military training program is to train without purpose or sense of urgency. Unfortunately, for 40 years an aimless approach has largely characterized unit chemical warfare training in the U.S. Army. . . . Much of the Army still appears to visualize chemical warfare . . . as an annoying distraction from normal combat training.[144(p28)]

The 1962 Army Reorganization

Based on the problems associated with training combat troops for chemical warfare, the Defense Department ordered a far-reaching realignment of functions in 1962. Most of the technical service headquarters establishments, including that of the Chemical Corps, were discontinued, and their functions merged into three field commands. The training mission of the chief chemical officer was assigned to the Continental Army Command; the development of doctrine was assigned to the new Combat Development Command; and the logistical function, including all arsenals, laboratories, and proving grounds, was assigned to the new Army Materiel Command.[145]

The effects of the reorganization were quickly felt. Within 2 years, the chemical warfare training program had significantly improved. One junior officer, A Harrigan, described the changes:

> We have set up special 40-hour or 80-hour schools so that we can have a trained CBR [chemical-biological-radiological] officer and noncommissioned officer in every company-sized unit. We have assigned a chemical officer down to brigade, and a chemical operations sergeant down to battalion. We set aside a certain number of hours annually for classroom instruction for the troops. We set up special blocks of instruction for surveying and monitoring teams. We list CBR defense as a subject integrated into our training schedules, and we may even throw tear gas grenades or other agents at troops in the field.[145(p16)]

Harrigan, however, concluded that more realistic field training was still required to prepare soldiers for the modern battlefield with nuclear weapons and nerve agents.[145]

Beginning of the Vietnam War

The growing guerrilla war in South Vietnam made the Army again reexamine its training program, chemical warfare readiness, and no-first-use policy. In 1963 one observer stated that, "after years of almost total lack of interest, the U.S. has taken up guerrilla warfare training as though it were something new under the sun."[146(p12)] As part of that sudden interest, the role of chemical weapons again came under intense scrutiny and debate. That same year, Harrigan wrote in the *Armed Forces Chemical Journal*, "the best way for the U.S. to achieve its military aims in Southeast Asia would be to rely on chemical warfare."[146(p12)] He described how soldiers could "sanitize" a large area with gases and sprays that killed everything from vegetation to humans.[146]

In 1966 a retired US Army general suggested that mustard gas be used to clear Vietnamese tunnels. He thought the use of low-lethality chemicals would save both American and Vietnamese lives by rendering the tunnels useless.[147] Other observers and authors also recommended revising the no-first-use policy. Public opinion and national policy opposing the use of toxic chemicals was apparently the deciding factor against their employment. The Army did, however, utilize defoliants and nonlethal riot control agents in large quantities. The negative worldwide response required the Army to make clear the differences between lethal and nonlethal chemicals.

The expansion of hostilities in Vietnam caused a gradual rise in the level of development and procurement of chemical-warfare–related items. By virtue of their training and specialized equipment, Chemical Corps personnel were able to make a number of contributions, primarily in the areas of riot control and flame weapons.

Yemen Civil War

While the United States was becoming involved in the Vietnam War, a small war in the Middle East brought the subject of chemical warfare back from the hypothetical. In September 1962, just after the death of Imam Ahmad, a military coup of Yemeni dissidents overthrew the royalist monarchy and declared a republic. The new imam escaped assassination and retreated with his royalist forces into the mountains of northern Yemen, initiating a counter revolt against the republican forces. Egyptian President Gamal Abdul Nasser recognized the new republic and sent military forces to help defeat the royalist troops, who were supported by the kingdoms of Saudi Arabia, Iran, and later Jordan, straining inter-Arab tensions, mainly between Saudi Arabia and Egypt.[148,149]

Egyptian efforts to defeat the royalist forces and destroy their civilian support bases proved particularly difficult in the mountainous terrain of northern Yemen. Frustrated by the successful royalist guerrilla tactics, Egypt employed chemical weapons they had developed in the 1950s and obtained from the Soviet Union; defensive equipment was also obtained from the Soviets.[150] Egypt was the first Arab state to use chemical weapons. Despite having signed the 1925 Geneva Convention, which outlawed the use of chemical weapons, Egypt employed chloroacetophenone tear gas, mustard blistering gas, phosgene, and nerve agents repeatedly from 1963 to1967.[151]

Some of these chemical weapons were made in military plant no. 801 in Abu-Za'abal, near Cairo. Egypt received mustard-gas–filled KHAB-200 R5 aerial bombs and phosgene-filled AOKh-25 aerial bombs from the Soviet air force and secured numerous mustard-filled shells from British stocks abandoned in Egypt after World War II.[149,152,153] Some accounts attributed the chemical weapons to German scientists, usually described as Nazis, who had been brought to Egypt by President Nasser. Several sources reported that the Soviet Union, through its friendship with Egypt, used Yemen as a testing ground for its chemical research program. Other reports mentioned Communist China as the supplier.[154–161]

Egypt denied ever using chemical warfare during its support of the new republican forces, but early accounts and evidence of chemical warfare came from journalists in the area. On June 8, 1963, Soviet-made Egyptian air force airplanes dropped chloroacetophenone tear gas bombs on numerous royalist villages south of Sadah, near Saudi Arabia. Egypt allegedly used the bombs to terrorize or kill not only the village inhabitants but also the royalists hiding in caves and tunnels. An alleged attack took place in July 1963 against the village of Al Kawma and killed seven civilians. The United Nations (UN) investigated the allegation by sending an observation team to Yemen, but its report found no evidence of a chemical attack.[154]

Newspaper articles described additional chemical attacks taking place from 1963 to 1967, although most disagreed on the dates, locations, and effects of the attacks. In January 1965 Egypt used a combination of chloroacetophenone and mustard gas for the first time on villagers in the Mount Urush region. A concoction of phosgene and mustard was dropped on citizens in the Sherazeih region, northeast of Sana, between March and July. The United States, involved in its own controversy concerning the use of riot control agents in Vietnam, took little notice of the reports.

In January 1967 an attack occurred on the Yemeni village of Kitaf. During this air raid, bombs were dropped upwind of the town and produced a gray-green cloud that drifted over the village. According to newspaper accounts,[165–159] 95% of the population up to 2 km downwind of the impact site died within 10 to 50 minutes of the attack. All the animals in the area also died. The estimated total human casualties numbered more than 200. Another reported attack took place on the town of Gahar in May 1967, killing 75 inhabitants. Additional attacks occurred that same month on the villages of Gabas, Hofal, Gadr, and Gadafa, killing over 243 occupants. In addition, two villages in Saudi Arabia near the Yemen border were bombed with chemical weapons.

Shortly after these attacks, the International Red Cross examined victims, soil samples, and bomb fragments and officially declared that chemical weapons, identified as mustard agent and possibly nerve agents, had been used in Yemen. Much like the progression of chemicals used during World War I, the Egyptians allegedly started with tear gases, which were meant to terrorize more than kill, before progressing to mustard agents, which caused more serious casualties, and finally to nerve agents, which were meant to kill large numbers quickly. This was the first use of nerve agents in combat. The combination of the use of nerve agents by the Egyptians in early 1967 and the outbreak of war between Egypt and Israel during the Six-Day War in June finally attracted world attention to the events in Yemen. The Saudi government protested the Egyptian use of chemical weapons to the UN. U Thant, secretary general of the UN, sought to confirm the use of chemical weapons with the Egyptians, but they denied it. The UN apparently took little further notice of the situation. At the height of the conflict, Egypt had 75,000 troops in Yemen, but the Six-Day War with Israel and subsequent defeat in June 1967 forced it to withdraw troops from Yemen and negotiate a peace deal. The Yemen civil war officially ended with the Compromise of 1970, a political agreement between the republican and royalist factions. A republican government was formed in Yemen, incorporating members from the royalist faction but not the royal family.[154–161]

Much of what the US Army learned from the Yemen civil war was negative. Reports of possible chemical use in certain areas of the world, particularly those areas inaccessible to official and technical observers, were difficult to confirm or even condemn without accurate and verifiable information. News reports alone proved informative but unreliable. Even samples from the alleged attacks apparently did not lead to further political or military action. Most importantly, with the world distracted by the Arab-Israeli Six-Day War and events in Vietnam, politics discouraged a universal condemnation and follow-up response. In effect, the world powers let the event pass much as they had when Italy used chemical warfare against Ethiopia in the 1930s.

Six-Day War

The 1967 Arab-Israeli Six-Day War came very close to being the first major war in which both combatants openly used nerve agents and biological warfare. On June 5, 1967, fearing a pending attack from its Arab neighbors, Israel launched a preemptive strike against Jordan, Egypt, and Syria. They invaded the Sinai Peninsula, Jerusalem's Old City, Jordan's West Bank, the Gaza Strip, and the Golan Heights.

Reports soon appeared alleging that the Egyptians had stored artillery rounds filled with nerve agents in the Sinai Peninsula for use during the war. Israelis, reflecting on Egypt's possible testing of the weapons in Yemen earlier in the year, suddenly realized that their troops and cities were vulnerable to attack. The fact that chemical weapons were not used during the war was possibly due to Israel's preemptive action or to the newspaper reports of the Yemen civil war. Israel placed orders for gas masks with Western countries. However, a UN-sponsored ceasefire ended the fighting on June 10, 1967, and the potential chemical war did not occur.[73,155,156,161]

Development of Incapacitating Chemical Agents

While concern over the use of chemical agents grew during the 1960s, the United States continued its chemical agent production program. Although the Newport VX production plant was completed in 1961 and began producing agent, it operated for only 7 years before being placed on standby.[4]

The only incapacitating agent (excluding riot control agents) standardized by the Army completed development in 1962. Designated "BZ," 3-quinuclidinyl benzilate was a solid but was disseminated as an aerosol. The major problem with using the agent for military purposes was its prolonged time of onset of symptoms, estimated at 2 to 3 hours, before the enemy became confused and vulnerable. A second problem was the visible cloud of smoke produced during dissemination, which limited the element of surprise.[143]

Public Hostility Toward Chemical Weapons

The growing protests over the US Army's role in Vietnam, the use of defoliants, and the use of riot control agents both in Southeast Asia and inside the country, as well as heightened concern for the environment all gradually increased public hostility toward chemical weapons. Three events particularly galvanized public attention: the sheep-kill incident at Dugway Proving Ground, Operation Cut Holes and Sink 'Em (CHASE), and an accident with sarin at Okinawa.

Dugway Incident

The first event, according to Dugway Proving Ground's incident log, started with a telephone call on Sunday, March 17, 1968:

> At approximately 1230 hours, Dr. Bode, University of Utah, Director of Ecological and Epidemiological contract with Dugway Proving Ground (DPG), called Dr. Keith Smart, Chief, Ecology and Epidemiology Branch, DPG at his home in Salt Lake City and informed him that Mr. Alvin Hatch, general manager for the Anschute Land and Livestock Company had called to report that they had 3,000 sheep dead in the Skull Valley area.[162(pA-1)]

Skull Valley was adjacent to Dugway, one of the Army's open-air testing sites for chemical weapons. Although the findings were not definitive, the general opinion was that nerve agents had somehow drifted out of the test area during aerial spraying and had killed the nearby sheep. Whether the Army was guilty or not, the result was bad publicity and, even more damaging, congressional outrage.

Operation CHASE

The second event involved a series of sea dumps of surplus chemical warfare agents, primarily mustard agent and some nerve agent, and a problem weapon system, the relatively new M55 rocket system. Although the M55 had been standardized only 7 years before, the thin aluminum head design proved faulty for long-term storage. The problem of leaking rockets started in 1966, and a year later the Army began disposing of the rockets, sealed in concrete vaults in the hulls of ships that were then sunk in ocean-disposal sites. Operation CHASE, an ongoing program for disposing of conventional ammunition, began accepting chemical weapons in 1967. That year, CHASE 8 disposed of mustard agent in ton containers and M55 sarin rockets. In June 1968 CHASE 11 disposed of sarin and VX in ton containers, along with additional M55 sarin and VX rockets. In August 1968 CHASE 12 disposed of mustard agent in ton containers.[4]

These dumps created significant environmental concerns throughout the country, including fears of an accident during transportation of the weapons by train from storage depots to loading docks, and environmental and commercial concern about the sunken agents' effects on marine life.

Accident at Okinawa

On July 8, 1969, the Army announced that 23 US soldiers and 1 US civilian had been exposed to sarin on Okinawa. The soldiers were cleaning sarin-filled bombs preparatory to repainting them when the accident occurred.[4] Although none of the individuals died, the public announcement created two controversies. First, up until that time, the Army had kept secret the forward positioning of chemical weapons on Okinawa, and this acknowledgment created international concerns. Second, the accident pointed out the dangers of storing chemical weapons. With chemical weapons known to be stored at sites in the continental United States near cities and residential areas, the fear of an accident escalated. On July 22, 1969, in response to these concerns, the Defense Department announced that it would accelerate the previously planned removal of the chemical agents from Okinawa.[163]

Changes to the Chemical Warfare Program

In April 1969 the secretary of defense tried to explain the US chemical warfare policy to both the general public and to Congress, stating:

> It is the policy of the United States to develop and maintain a defensive chemical-biological (CB) capability so that U.S. military forces could operate for some period of time in a toxic environment if necessary; to develop and maintain a limited offensive capability in order to deter all use of CB weapons by the threat of retaliation in kind; and to continue a program of research and development in this area to minimize the possibility of technological surprise.[164(p193)]

Despite this statement, the UN released a report on chemical weapons that July condemning the production and stockpiling of weapons of mass destruction. Six days later, the United States acknowledged the Okinawa accident.[4] On July 11, 1969, Congress revealed that the Army was conducting open-air testing with nerve agents at Edgewood Arsenal (the name of the Army Chemical Center had reverted in 1963) and at Fort McClellan during training events. Shortly after the disclosure, more than 100 people protested at the gates of Edgewood Arsenal. Three days later the Army announced suspension of open-air testing at the two sites and promised to conduct a safety review of all such testing. However, the public was again displeased when the Army revealed that it had also conducted nerve agent testing in Hawaii between 1966 and 1967, something it had previously denied.[4]

In October the secretary of the Army announced that the safety review had been completed, with the following conclusion: "The lethal testing program at Edgewood Arsenal during the past two decades has compiled an enviable record for safety. The testing procedures that have been evolved are clearly effective in minimizing danger to base personnel and civilians in adjacent areas."[165(p16)] The committee's only major concern was the movement of chemical agents by truck on public roads. It recommended resumption of lethal agent open-air testing at Edgewood.[165] Before testing resumed, however, Congress passed Public Law 91-121 in November, imposing controls on the storage, testing, and disposal of agents outside the United States and the testing and transportation of chemical agents within the country. Further open-air testing of lethal chemical agents was effectively banned.[4]

In November 1969 President Richard Nixon took action against chemical warfare, effectively stopping the production of chemical weapons in the United States.[166] First, he reaffirmed the no-first-use policy for chemical weapons, saying, "I hereby reaffirm that the United States will never be the first country to use chemical weapons to kill. And I have also extended this renunciation to chemical weapons that incapacitate."[166(p5)] Second, he decided to resubmit the 1925 Geneva Protocol to the US Senate for ratification. The Senate had refused to ratify the treaty when it was first signed, and President Harry S Truman had withdrawn the treaty from the Senate in 1947. Nixon explained his future hopes: "Mankind already carries in its own hands too many of the seeds of its own destruction. By the examples that we set today, we hope to contribute to an atmosphere of peace and understanding between all nations."[166(p4)] (The US Senate did not grant Nixon's request till 1974, and President Ford officially signed the protocol on January 22, 1975, after exempting riot control agents and herbicides from the agreement.[4])

THE 1970s: THE NEAR END OF THE CHEMICAL CORPS

The events of 1969 had a severe impact on the future of the US Army chemical warfare program. In February 1970 President Nixon added toxins to the list of banned weapons and ordered all existing stocks of toxin agents destroyed. About a month later, the Army revealed it had conducted chemical testing in Alaska but reported that the testing had stopped. The Army also announced that the chemical weapons on Okinawa would be moved to Umatilla Army Depot in Oregon, which triggered a series of lawsuits that attracted the congressional concern. The next year, Public Law 91-672 prohibited the Army from moving the weapons from Okinawa to anywhere on the US mainland. Finally, Operation Red Hat moved the stockpile on Okinawa to Johnston Atoll, a small US island in the South Pacific, for long-term storage and eventual demilitarization.[167]

Because of heightened environmental concerns in the 1970s, demilitarization was not an easy project. One last sea dump took place in 1970 when, despite much negative press, CHASE 10 disposed of more M55 sarin rockets. (CHASE 10 had originally been scheduled to start earlier; although now out of numerical order, the designation was unchanged.) Two years later Public Law 92-532 prohibited the sea dumping of chemical munitions.[167]

A senior Department of Defense official reflected on the impact the restrictions had during the 1970s: "During most of the 1970s, the United States allowed its chemical retaliatory capability to decline, did little to improve chemical protection, and neglected relevant training and doctrine. The United States has not produced lethal or incapacitating chemical agents, or filled munitions since 1969."[167(p3)] The Army made plans to abolish the Chemical Corps entirely. In 1973, with the Paris Peace Accords and the end of the draft, the Army recommended reducing the Chemical Corps in size and eventually merging it with the Ordnance Corps. As the first step, the Army disestablished the chemical school at Fort McClellan and combined it with the ordnance school at Aberdeen Proving Ground. Congress, however, blocked the complete disestablishment of the corps.[168–171] Still, one observer noted: "As an additional ordnance career field, the chemical specialty almost withered and died at Aberdeen."[171(p15)]

Yom Kippur War

The Arab-Israeli Yom Kippur War lasted only from October 6 to October 24, 1973, but it brought chemical warfare preparedness back to public attention and its ramifications for the US chemical program lasted much longer. Egypt had several years to stockpile and increase its arsenal to plan an attack on Israel involving chemical weapons. Syria, Egypt's ally in the war, began stockpiling a chemical arsenal, receiving sarin from Egypt in 1972. The Egyptian and Syrian attack against Israel on Yom Kippur and the successful Israeli counterattacks ended with a ceasefire. Both sides took enormous losses in personnel and equipment. However, chemical weapons were not employed by either side.

Following the war, the Israelis analyzed the Soviet-made equipment they captured from the Egyptians and Syrians. They discovered portable chemical-proof shelters, decontamination equipment for planes and tanks, and air-filtration systems that removed toxic chemicals on most Soviet vehicles. They also found a Soviet PKhR-MV chemical agent detector kit for medical and veterinary services. The kit, which consisted of a hand pump, detector tubes, reagents in ampules, dry reagents, test tubes, and accessories, was designed to detect nerve, blister, and blood agents. US specialists determined that it could detect low concentrations of nerve agents, mustard agent, cyanide, lewisite, and heavy metals in aqueous solutions. It could also detect the same agents, plus cyanogen chloride and phosgene, in the atmosphere. However, procedures for using the kit were extremely difficult to carry out while wearing a protective suit. In addition, the glass ampules were fragile and broke easily.[172]

Overall, the experts reported finding sophisticated chemical defense materiel and a "superior quantitative capability for waging a chemical war."[173(p3-4)] The indications were that the Soviets were ready for, and might actually be planning to instigate, extensive chemical warfare in a future war. Soviet division commanders were thought to already have the authority to initiate chemical warfare.[173–176]

Restoring the Chemical Corps

The decline of the US Army Chemical Corps, combined with the discovery of sophisticated Soviet chemical defense materiel and the Soviet's capability for waging chemical war, made corrective action necessary. The Army concluded the following:

> To offset this, U.S. chemical/biological (CB) defense materiel must not only provide a protective system equivalent to or better than that of any potential enemy but the physiological and logistics burdens must be such as to permit long-term use. To cope with the hazards of any potential CB-threat environment requires the development of an integrated CB defense system. This system must contain items for individual protection, collective protection, decontamination, warning and detection, and safe devices and concepts to achieve realistic training. An effective technological base is needed from which such materiel, responsive to user needs, can be quickly developed.[173(p3–4)]

In 1976 the secretary of the Army reversed the decision to abolish the Chemical Corps, citing the heightened awareness of the Soviet Union's capability to wage chemical warfare as the primary reason. In 1977 the United States started a new effort to reach an agreement with the Soviets on a verifiable ban on chemical weapons, but the effort was unsuccessful. The chemical school was reestablished at Fort McClellan in 1979 partly as a result of this failure.[167,177–181]

Growing Danger of Chemical Warfare

Starting in about 1975, reports of the use of chemicals and toxin agents in various skirmishes and wars in Southeast Asia and Afghanistan began to attract US attention. Interviews with villagers in Laos suggested that Vietnamese and Soviet forces might have used chemical and possibly toxic weapons against the Hmong. Starting in 1978, similar reports from Kampuchea claimed that the Vietnamese and their allies had killed over 980 villagers using chemical weapons. Reports began circulating that Soviet troops were using chemical weapons against Afghan soldiers even before the Soviet invasion of Afghanistan began in December 1979.

Although they had signed the Geneva Protocol in 1928, the Soviets argued that their use of chemical weapons was legitimate because Laos, Kampuchea, and Afghanistan were not signatories. The Soviet Union, Laos, and Afghanistan signed the Biological Weapons Convention in 1975, but the allegations of toxin use were never acknowledged by the Soviets or their allies. When the Soviets signed the Biological Weapons Convention, they added, "the Soviet Union does not possess any bacteriological agents and toxins, weapons, equipment or means of delivery."[182(p6)] Other intelligence sources thought that the Soviets considered most toxins to be chemical agents, and therefore not subject to the Biological Weapons Convention. If toxins were considered chemical agents, then the Soviets would be permitted under the Geneva Protocol to use them in retaliation or against nonsignatories.[183] Their use of chemical weapons was taken as an indication that the Soviets were continuing an active chemical program.

THE 1980s: RETURN OF THE CHEMICAL CORPS

The Haig Report

Despite denials by the governments involved, the United States publicized charges that chemical warfare had been used in Southeast Asia and Afghanistan in 1980. Problems with the collection of samples and the remoteness of the sites, however, prevented definitive evidence from being obtained. Furthermore, the later identification, discussion, and media debate over the origin of possible trichothecene mycotoxins in Southeast Asia also distracted public interest from the alleged use of conventional chemical munitions.

In 1982 Secretary of State Alexander M Haig, Jr, presented a report titled "Chemical Warfare in Southeast Asia and Afghanistan" to the US Congress. After describing the evidence, he concluded:

> Taken together, this evidence has led the U.S. Government to conclude that Laos and Vietnamese forces, operating under Soviet supervision, have, since 1975, employed lethal chemical and toxin weapons in Laos; that Vietnamese forces have, since 1978, used lethal chemical and toxin agents in Kampuchea; and that Soviet forces have used a variety of lethal chemical warfare agents, including nerve gases, in Afghanistan since the Soviet invasion of that country in 1979.[182(p6)]

Based on this evidence, senior Defense Department personnel concluded that the Soviet Union "possesses a decisive military advantage because of its chemical capabilities."[167(p3)] The Haig report, however, was not able to galvanize world opinion. As in the Yemen civil war, the United States was unable to prove that chemical agents and toxins had been used in Southeast Asia and Afghanistan. Instead, the accusation became a political debate between the United States and the Soviet Union during President Ronald Reagan's administration.

Afghanistan and Iran-Iraq Wars

Afghanistan War

The US Army monitored the war in Afghanistan throughout the 1980s, often thinking of it as "the Soviet's Vietnam." The lessons learned from this war about chemical warfare provided extensive support to the US chemical defense program. The Soviets tended to use chemical weapons much like the Italians did in Ethiopia and like the US Army had used nonlethal agents in Vietnam. One military writer summed up the general lesson learned:

> The use of chemical weapons by Soviet forces in Afghanistan is also significant. The use of these weapons in Afghanistan confirms, not surprisingly, that the Soviets find them put to their best use against unprotected subjects incapable of retaliation. Afghanistan is proof positive that the Soviets do not consider these devices as special weapons. Considerations of utility and not morality will govern Soviet use of them in a future conflict.[184(p27)]

Despite the use of chemical weapons, the Soviets were unable to "win" the war and, in December 1988, met with rebel forces to discuss a withdrawal of Soviet troops from Afghanistan. In January 1989 the Soviets announced the final withdrawal, which was completed a month later.[185]

Iran-Iraq War

The United States continued to propose chemical treaties with the Soviet Union, its primary chemical warfare rival. However, the Iran-Iraq War began changing this situation. On September 22, 1980, Iraq launched an invasion against neighboring Iran. The Iraqi army, trained and influenced by Soviet advisors, had organic chemical warfare units and a wide variety of delivery systems. Neither side achieved dominance and the war quickly became a stalemate.

To stop the human-wave–attack tactics of the Iranians, the Iraqis employed their home-produced chemical agents as a defensive measure against the much-less–prepared Iranian infantry. The first reported use of chemical weapons occurred in November 1980. Throughout the next several years, additional reports of chemical attacks circulated, and by November 1983, Iran began complaining to the UN that Iraq was using chemical weapons against its troops.[186–189]

After Iran sent chemical casualties to several Western nations for treatment, the UN dispatched a team of specialists to the area in 1984, and again in 1986 and 1987, to verify the claims. The conclusion from all three trips was the same: Iraq was using chemical weapons against Iranian troops. In addition, the second mission stressed that Iraq's use of chemical weapons appeared to be increasing. The reports indicated that mustard and tabun were the primary agents used, and that they were generally delivered in bombs dropped by airplane. The third mission (the only one allowed to enter Iraq) also reported the use of artillery shells and chemical rockets and the use of chemical weapons against civilian personnel.[190–192]

In the letter of transmittal to the UN after the conclusion of the third mission, the investigators pointed out the dangers of this chemical warfare:

> It is vital to realize that the continued use of chemical weapons in the present conflict increases the risk of their use in future conflicts. In view of this, and as individuals who witnessed first hand the terrible effects of chemical weapons, we again make a special plea to you to try to do everything in your power to stop the use of such weapons in the Iran-Iraq conflict and thus ensure that they are not used in future conflicts. . . . In our view, only concerted efforts at the political level can be effective in ensuring that all the signatories of the Geneva Protocol of 1925 abide by their obligations. Otherwise, if the Protocol is irreparably weakened after 60 years of general international respect, this may lead, in the future, to the world facing the specter of the threat of biological weapons.[190]

Another analyst echoed these sentiments, saying, "In a sense, a taboo has been broken, thus making it easier for future combatants to find justification for chemical warfare, this aspect of the Iran-Iraq war should cause Western military planners the gravest concern."[193(pp51–52)]

The Iran-Iraq War failed to reach a military conclusion despite Iraq's use of chemical weapons. Roughly 5% of the Iranian casualties were caused by chemical weapons. Although Iranian use of chemical weapons was rumored, less attention was devoted to verifying those reports. In August 1988 Iraq finally accepted a UN ceasefire plan.[185]

Additional Reports of Chemical Warfare

The end of the Iran-Iraq War did not prevent new chemical warfare reports from circulating. Within a month of the war's end, the Kurds, a minority group in Iraq seeking autonomy, accused Iraq of using chemical weapons against them. Shortly before, rumors circulated that Libya had used chemical weapons obtained from Iran during an invasion of Chad. The United States rushed 2,000 gas masks to Chad in response. There were also reports of the Cuban-backed government of Angola using nerve agents against rebel forces.[194–197]

Chemical Training

In addition to establishing a retaliatory capability, the US Army significantly improved its chemical training capability by constructing a new facility at the chemical school and conducting more realistic field training. In 1987 the Chemical Decontamination Training Facility started live chemical agent training in a controlled environment. Major General Gerald G Watson, the school's commandant, was "the first American to wear the battledress overgarment in a toxic chemical environment"[198(p15)] when he entered the facility on February 19, 1987. Realistic field training, such as Operation Solid Shield 87[199] (see Chapter 3, History of the Medical Management of Chemical Casualties) was conducted, resulting in changes in Army policy.

Soviet-US Agreement

The increase in the US retaliatory and defensive capability for chemical warfare, along with internal changes in the Soviet Union, helped convince the Soviets to look closely at a new chemical weapons treaty. In 1987, after admitting possession of chemical agents for the first time, the Soviet Union announced it was halting chemical weapons production. In September 1989 the Memorandum of Understanding (MOU) Between the Government of the United States and the Government of the USSR Regarding a Bilateral Verification Experiment and Data Exchange Related to Prohibition of Chemical Weapons, otherwise known as the Wyoming MOU, started the talks between the two countries.[4] The US demilitarization program continued, despite problems (see Chapter 4).

THE 1990s: A NEW AGE OF CHEMICAL WARFARE AND TERRORISM

Persian Gulf War

Despite the ongoing political efforts to abolish chemical warfare (see Chapter 4), world events again brought chemical weapons to daily news reports. On August 2, 1990, Saddam Hussein sent Iraqi troops into

Kuwait, allegedly in support of Kuwaiti revolutionaries who had overthrown the emirate. On August 8 Iraq announced that Kuwait had been annexed and was now a part of its country. In response, President George Bush ordered US forces to be sent to Saudi Arabia at the request of the Saudi government as part of what became Operation Desert Shield, the buildup phase of the Persian Gulf War.

The US response to Iraq's invasion put the Army's chemical warfare experience, training, production program, and lessons learned in the limelight. Not since World War I had US troops been sent to face an enemy that had used chemical weapons extensively within the last few years and had publicly announced its intentions to use them against the United States. William H Webster, director of the Central Intelligence Agency, estimated that Iraq had 1,000 tons of chemical weapons loaded in bombs, artillery rounds, rockets, and missiles. Much of Iraq's biological weapons program remained unknown until after the war.[200–202]

By 1991 Iraq's production facility at al-Hakam had produced about 125,000 gallons of agents that cause botulism, anthrax, and other illnesses. After stating for years that the plant was used to produce animal feed, in 1995 the Iraqis admitted it was a biological warfare production facility. In addition to producing biological warfare agents, the Iraqis also conducted live-agent tests on animals. The Iraqis later admitted they had prepared about 200 biological missiles and bombs.[203–206]

To prepare for the military phase of the Persian Gulf War, the United States had to consider all the chemical and biological threats. Troops were given the Mark I (Meridian Medical Technologies Inc, Bristol, Tenn) nerve agent antidote kit, consisting of an atropine autoinjector and a pralidoxime chloride autoinjector to treat nerve agent poisoning. Atropine blocks the effects of nerve agent poisoning on the muscles, and pralidoxime chloride reactivates acetylcholinesterase. Pyridostigmine bromide tablets were also provided as a nerve agent pretreatment.[207] US troops moving into the area were given vaccines for anthrax and botulinum toxin.[208] All military units were fully equipped with the latest chemical and biological defensive equipment, and training was continuous.

The actual attack on Iraq on January 16, 1991, as part of the UN-mandated effort to free Kuwait, was designated Operation Desert Storm by the United States. The attack escalated fears of a new chemical war to levels not seen since World War I. The initial air attack concentrated on Iraqi chemical production facilities, bunkers, and lines of supply. While the air attacks were ongoing, daily news accounts addressed the potential for chemical and biological warfare. On January 28 Saddam Hussein told Peter Arnett of CNN News that Iraqi Scud missiles, which were already hitting Israel and Saudi Arabia, could be armed with chemical, biological, or nuclear munitions. While visiting the United Kingdom, Vice President Dan Quayle reportedly told the prime minister that the United States had not ruled out the use of chemical or nuclear weapons.[209] Likewise, the United States reportedly threatened to target Hussein personally if he used chemical weapons against UN coalition forces.[209,210] In turn, Iraq reportedly threatened to use chemical weapons against coalition forces if they continued the high-level bombings against Iraqi troops.[209]

When coalition forces began the ground war on February 23, 1991, chemical and biological defense specialists anticipated the worst. Chemical alarms frequently went off across the battlefield, but all were dismissed as false alarms. On February 27 coalition forces liberated Kuwait City and finished destroying the Iraqi divisions originally in Kuwait. No known chemical or biological attacks were made by the Iraqis.

A number of reasons surfaced after the war for why the Iraqis had not initiated large-scale chemical warfare. Vice Admiral Stanley Arthur, commander of US naval forces, thought that because the wind suddenly changed at the start of the land battle, the Iraqis realized that chemical weapons could harm their own troops. Some thought the speed of the campaign was the critical reason. Others reported that the combination of coalition bombing and the resulting Iraqi logistical chaos prevented the chemical weapons from ever reaching the front lines. General H Norman Schwarzkopf, commander of coalition forces, mentioned that Iraq might have feared nuclear retaliation.[202,209,211]

After the war, allegations of chemical exposures began to surface. The Department of Defense initially denied that any chemical exposures had taken place, but veterans of the war claimed the opposite and their ailments collectively became known as "Gulf War" syndrome. By 1996 newspapers reported that almost 60,000 veterans of the Persian Gulf War claimed some sort of medical problem directly related to their war activities. Extensive research by the Department of Defense failed to find any single cause for the problems.[212,213]

One controversial example of possible exposure occurred on March 4, 1991, at the Kamisiyah arsenal, northwest of Basra, involving the US Army 37th Engineer Battalion. After capturing the site, the engineers blew up the Iraqi storage bunkers. According to newspaper accounts, engineers claimed that their chemical agent detectors went off during the explosions. Later the same year, a UN inspection team reportedly found the remains of chemical rockets and shells in one of the bunkers in addition to traces of sarin and mustard agent. In 1996 the Department of Defense acknowledged that one of the bunkers probably contained sarin- and mustard-agent–filled munitions, and that as many as 20,000 US soldiers may have been exposed to chemical agents as a result.[214] Afterward a Pentagon spokesperson, commenting on the continuing research into the possible exposure, said, "Our understanding of this episode is still partial."[213(pA-10)]

Additional Allegations of Chemical Warfare

Shortly after the fighting between Iraq and coalition forces ended, reports circulated that Hussein was using chemical agents against rebellious Kurds and Shiite Muslims. The United States intercepted a message ordering the use of chemical weapons against the cities of Najaf and Karbala. President Bush's response was that such use of chemical weapons would result in air strikes against the Iraqi military organization using the chemicals. Thus, despite the end of fighting, Iraqi chemical weapons continued to be a problem for the world.[215,216]

US intelligence sources also detected increased chemical development activity in Libya. A Libyan chemical weapons plant at Rabta had produced about 100 tons of agent by 1990, when Libya claimed that the plant was destroyed by a fire. New disclosures surfaced in 1996 that Libya was constructing a second chemical production plant at Tarhunah. US intelligence sources claimed that this would be the largest underground chemical weapons plant in the world, covering roughly 6 square miles and situated in a hollowed-out mountain. Because Scud missiles have a range of 180 to 300 miles, Libya's neighbors were considerably threatened. Libya strongly denied the US accusation.[217,218]

PREVENTING CHEMICAL WARFARE AND TERRORISM IN THE 21ST CENTURY

Despite the signing of long-sought Chemical Weapons Convention by the United States, Russia, and other countries, and the start of large-scale chemical weapons destruction programs in the 1990s (see Chapter 4), the beginning of the 21st century saw a sudden and dramatic change in the interest in chemical warfare. The events of 2001 made US post offices, government buildings, hospitals, and media headquarters the front lines in a new war on terrorism.

Operation Enduring Freedom

The new war began on September 11, 2001, when four commercial planes were hijacked. Two crashed into the World Trade Center, one into the Pentagon, and one crashed in rural Pennsylvania before reaching its apparent target in Washington, DC. Nearly 4,000 people died in the destruction and aftermath, including many first responders. Almost immediately Al Qaeda, under the control of Osama bin Laden, was identified as the perpetrator. Although the terrorists were protected by the ruling party in Afghanistan, the Taliban, the United States began a military counterstrike.

In October 2001 the United States launched massive air attacks against Afghanistan. Special Forces troops entered the war to assist the Northern Alliance in their ongoing rebellion against the Taliban. In November Osama bin Laden notified the world that he had chemical and nuclear weapons, but would only use them if the United States used them first. A few days later, the Northern Alliance captured Kabul. During additional campaigns in Afghanistan, coalition forces discovered a chemical laboratory and training films depicting chemical agents killing dogs, but they did not discover any chemical weapons.

Russian Use of a Nonlethal Chemical Agent

Throughout 2002 Russia continued to experience terrorist incidents related to its war in Chechnya. In October Chechnyan terrorists took over a Moscow theater and held over 900 people hostage. The terrorists strapped on explosives and positioned themselves among the hostages. After failing to obtain their objectives, the terrorists began executing hostages. Russian security forces flooded the theater with a chemical agent identified in the press as fentanyl, a nonlethal gas. Russian special forces stormed the theater and most of the terrorists were killed by gunfire; however, over 118 of the hostages died from the effects of the gas.

At first the Russian government kept the identity of the gas secret from the world and from its own medical facilities. It was not until a week after the incident that the Russians finally identified the gas, leading to a strong public debate about whether Russia had violated the Chemical Weapons Convention.

Operation Iraqi Freedom

Dissatisfied with Iraq's noncompliance with the UN mandates that concluded the Persian Gulf War, the United States repeatedly bombed Iraq throughout 2000 and 2001. Of particular concern to the United States was Iraq's failure to report all its chemical warfare research and weapons productions. Iraq reportedly restricted its chemical weapons programs after

UN monitors withdrew from the country.

In 2002 both President George W Bush and British Prime Minister Tony Blair publicly warned the UN that Iraq had reinstated its weapons of mass destruction program. The UN, however, was unconvinced of the charges and debated the need for a new resolution concerning Iraq. In the meantime, the US Congress authorized President Bush to use force against Iraq if necessary. A large coalition force assembled in Kuwait in preparation for future military action. This force was well equipped with the latest chemical defense equipment.

Unable to obtain UN support for a military attack, the Unites States launched Operation Iraqi Freedom in 2003 with an unsuccessful attempt to eliminate Saddam Hussein. Allied troops then invaded Iraq, taking great precautions in case chemical weapons were used against them. Although a few Scud missiles were launched against forces in Kuwait, none contained chemical agents. The occupation of Iraq was quickly accomplished without any known use of chemical weapons. On May 1 President Bush publicly declared the end of hostilities; however, US casualties continued to occur. At least one roadside attack involved the detonation of a sarin-filled artillery projectile, but no casualties resulted.

Despite an extensive search, no large stockpiles of chemical weapons were discovered in Iraq. Investigators did find protective masks, nerve agent antidote injectors, decontamination kits, and protective clothing. Interviews with captured Iraqi scientists and other leaders indicated that the chemical weapons programs had been shut down prior to the invasion. Some commentators speculated that the Iraqis had purposely misled the world about their weapons of mass destruction as a bluff to prevent military action against them. Other reports indicated that some of the chemical weapons may have been shipped to Syria or other countries friendly to Iraq. Because the Chemical Weapons Convention prohibited the use of tear gas in combat, world debate arose when US forces used tear gas during security operations in Iraqi cities. However, the Chemical Weapons Convention allowed tear gas use in domestic riot control, which is how the United States had used it.

Iraqi insurgents stepped up terror attacks on the streets of Taji, north of Baghdad, in February and March 2007. On February 21, 2007, insurgents used conventional explosives to detonate a tanker carrying chlorine, creating a toxic cloud. Baghdad security spokesperson General Qassim Atta reported five deaths from the blast and 148 casualties from the gas. The following day, suspected Sunni Arab insurgents detonated a car carrying an explosive device attached to chlorine gas canisters on a road leading to Baghdad's airport. The gas cloud killed two and left 33 others feeling ill. The chlorine gas cloud suggested new and coordinated tactics with unconventional weapons. A raid in Fallujah in late February 2007 revealed a homegrown factory for car bombs and cylinders of toxic chlorine gas and other chemicals. This discovery caused the United States to fear future tactics with chlorine bombs, and fears were confirmed as additional attacks involving three chlorine gas car bombs were carried out in western Iraq on March 16, 2007, killing two and injuring hundreds of Iraqi civilians.

SUMMARY

Although chemical warfare has not been repeated on the scale that occurred during World War I, incidents of chemical weapons used on the battlefield have continued throughout the 20th and into the 21st century, and the potential for a major escalation remains. Terrorist attacks with chemical weapons are an even more likely scenario. To prevent such an event, US military forces must continue to learn about chemical warfare and how to accomplish their missions on chemical battlefields and chemical terrorist fronts throughout the world. In the words of General Pershing, "we can never afford to neglect the question"[48(p77)] of chemical preparedness again.

REFERENCES

1. Department of the Army. *NATO Handbook on the Medical Aspects of NBC Defensive Operations*. AMedP-6, Part 3. Washington, DC: DA; 1996: Field Manual 8-9.

2. Osius TG. The historic art of poisoning. *Med Bull (Ann Arbor)*. 1957;23:111–116.

3. Mayor A. Greek Fire, Poison Arrows, and Scorpion Bombs: Biological and Chemical Warfare in the Ancient World. Woodstock, NY: Overlook Press; 2003.

4. Smart JK. *History of Chemical and Biological Warfare Fact Sheets*. Aberdeen Proving Ground, Md: US Army Chemical and Biological Defense Command; 1996. Special Study 50.

5. Mauroni A. *Chemical and Biological Warfare: a Reference Handbook*. Santa Barbara, Calif: ABC-CLIO, Inc; 2003: 80.

6. United Kingdom Ministry of Defense Web site. Defending against the threat of biological and chemical weapons page. Available at: http://www.mod.uk/issues/cbw/history.htm. Accessed November 12, 2003.

7. Coleman K. *A History of Chemical Warfare*. Basingstoke, Houndsmills, England: Palgrave Macmillan; 2005: 6–7.

8. MacCurdy E, ed. *The Notebooks of Leonardo da Vinci*. Vol 2. London, England: Jonathan Cape; 1977: 206.

9. Waitt AH. *Gas Warfare: the Chemical Weapon, its Use, and Protection Against it*. New York, NY: Duell, Sloan, and Pearce; 1943: 4–9.

10. Browne CA. Early references pertaining to chemical warfare. *Chemical Warfare*. 1922;8:22–23.

11. Miles WD. Chemical warfare in the Civil War. *Armed Forces Chemical Journal*. 1958;12:27, 33.

12. Haydon F. A proposed gas shell in 1862. *Military Affairs*. 1938;2:54.

13. Miles WD. Suffocating smoke at Petersburg. *Armed Forces Chemical Journal*. 1959;13:34–35.

14. Haber LF. *The Poisonous Cloud: Chemical Warfare in the First World War*. Oxford, England: Clarendon Press; 1986: 15–40.

15. Heller CE. No. 10 chemical warfare in World War I: the American experience, 1917–1918. In: *The Leavenworth Papers*. Fort Leavenworth, Kan: Combat Studies Institute, US Army Command and General Staff College; 1984: 6–7.

16. Hogg IV. Gas. In: Pitt B, ed. *Ballantine's Illustrated History of the Violent Century: Weapons Book No. 43*. New York, NY: Ballantine Books; 1975: 20–23.

17. Prentiss AM. *Chemicals in War: a Treatise on Chemical Warfare*. New York, NY: McGraw-Hill; 1937.

18. Hogg I. Bolimow and the first gas attack. In: Fitzsimons B, ed. *Tanks and Weapons of World War I*. New York, NY: Beckman House; 1973: 17–19.

19. Fries AA, West CJ. *Chemical Warfare*. New York, NY: McGraw-Hill; 1921.

20. Harris R, Paxman J. *A Higher Form of Killing: the Secret History of Chemical and Biological Warfare*. New York, NY: Random House; 2002.

21. Hanslian R. The gas attack at Ypres: a study in military history, I. *Chemical Warfare Bulletin*. 1936;22:5.

22. An Account of German Cloud Gas Attacks on British Front in France. Attachment to letter dated February 11, 1922, from Major ON Solbert, military attaché, American Embassy, London, England, to chief, Chemical Warfare Service, Edgewood, Md. History of gas and development of British respirators from beginning of war to armistice. In file: Gas Warfare History (British) 1915. Located at: US Army Chemical and Biological Defense Command Historical Office, Edgewood, Md.

23. Fries AA. Gas in attack. *Chemical Warfare*. 1919;2:3,8.

24. Foulkes CH. *Gas! The Story of the Special Brigade*. Edinburgh, Scotland: William Blackwood & Sons; 1934: 24.

25. Clark DK. *Effectiveness of Chemical Weapons in WWI*. Bethesda, Md: Johns Hopkins University Operations Research Office: 1959: 99–123. Staff Paper ORO-SP-88.

26. Bancroft WD. *Bancroft's History of the Chemical Warfare Service in the United States*. Washington, DC: Research Division, Chemical Warfare Service, American University Experiment Station; May 1919: 12, 16.

27. Brophy LP, Fisher GJB. *The Chemical Warfare Service: Organizing for War*. Washington, DC: Office of the Chief of Military History; 1959: 3–18, 25–27, 424–471.

28. Brophy LP, Miles WD, Cochrane RC. *The Chemical Warfare Service: From Laboratory to Field*. Washington, DC: Office of the Chief of Military History; 1959: 2–27, 49–76, 85–86, 101–138, 268, 336, 436–453.

29. Baldwin W. Past in Review: Eleventh Engineers in World War I. *Engineer*. 1985-1986;Winter:5.

30. Cochrane RC. The 1st Division at Ansauville, January–April 1918; study number 9. In: *Gas Warfare in World War I. US Army Chemical Corps Historical Studies*. Army Chemical Center, Md: US Army Chemical Corps Historical Office; 1959: 1–27.

31. Ireland M. The 1st Division in the Sommerviller, Ansauville, and Cantigny Sectors. Chap 10. In Montdidier-Noyon Operation. In: *The Medical Department of the United States Army in the World War: Field Operations, Section II American Divisions with French Armies.* Vol 8. Washington, DC: Government Printing Office; 1925.

32. Spencer EW. *The History of Gas Attacks Upon the American Expeditionary Forces During the World War, Parts I-III*. Edgewood Arsenal, Md: Chemical Warfare Service, US War Department; 1928.

33. Spencer EW. An historical lesson. *Chemical Warfare*. 1923;9:2–10.

34. *United States Army in the World War 1917–1919: Military Operations of the American Expeditionary Forces*. Vol 4. Washington DC: US Government Printing Office, 1948.

35. US Department of the Army. American Military History 1607–1953. Washington DC: US Government Printing Office; 1956: 343–359. ROTC Manual 145-20.

36. Cochrane RC. The 1st Division at Cantigny, May 1918; study number 11. In: *Gas Warfare in World War I. U.S. Army Chemical Corps Historical Studies*. Army Chemical Center, Md: US Army Chemical Corps Historical Office; 1959: 1–4, 15, 70.

37. Cochrane RC. The 3rd Division at Chateau Thierry, July 1918; study number 14. In: *Gas Warfare in World War I. U.S. Army Chemical Corps Historical Studies*. Army Chemical Center, Md: US Army Chemical Corps Historical Office; 1959: 1–4, 84, 86.

38. *United States Army in the World War 1917–1919: Military Operations of the American Expeditionary Forces*. Vol 5. Washington DC: US Government Printing Office; 1948.

39. Cochrane RC. Gas Warfare at Belleau Wood, June 1918; study number 1. In: *Gas Warfare in World War I. U.S. Army Chemical Corps Historical Studies*. Army Chemical Center, Md: US Army Chemical Corps Historical Office; 1957: 1–10, 66.

40. Cochrane RC. The 42nd Division before Landres-et-St. Georges, October 1918; study number 17. In: *Gas Warfare in World War I. U.S. Army Chemical Corps Historical Studies*. Army Chemical Center, Md: US Army Chemical Corps Historical Office; 1960: 1–8, 77.

41. *United States Army in the World War 1917–1919: Military Operations of the American Expeditionary Forces*. Vol 6. Washington DC: US Government Printing Office, 1948: 1–4. 56-58, 77–203.

42. Cochrane RC. The 32nd Division Advances to Fismes, August 1918; study number 12. In: *Gas Warfare in World War I. U.S. Army Chemical Corps Historical Studies*. Army Chemical Center, Md: US Army Chemical Corps Historical Office; 1959: 1–15, 62, 64–72.

43. *United States Army in the World War 1917–1919: Military Operations of the American Expeditionary Forces*. Vol 9. Washington, DC: US Government Printing Office; 1948: 1–114.

44. Ireland M. The Oise-Aisne Operation, August 18 to September 17, 1918. In: *The Medical Department of the United States Army in the World War: Field Operations, Section II American Divisions with French Armies*. Vol 8. Washington, DC: Government Printing Office; 1925: Chap 8.

45. Cochrane RC. The Use of Gas at St. Mihiel, the 90th Division, September 1918; study number 5. In: *Gas Warfare in World War I. U.S. Army Chemical Corps Historical Studies*. Army Chemical Center, Md: US Army Chemical Corps Historical Office; 1957: 1–36, 49–56, 62.

46. Cochrane RC. The 26th Division in the Aisne-Marne Campaign, July 1918; study number 4. In: *Gas Warfare in World War I. U.S. Army Chemical Corps Historical Studies*. Army Chemical Center, Md: US Army Chemical Corps Historical Office; 1957: 57.

47. *United States Army in the World War 1917–1919: Military Operations of the American Expeditionary Forces*. Vol 8. Washington, DC: US Government Printing Office; 1948: 1–287.

48. Pershing JJ. *Final Report of General John J Pershing*. Washington, DC: US Government Printing Office; 1920: 77.

49. Cochrane RC. The Use of Gas in the Meuse-Argonne Campaign—September–November 1918; study number 10. In: Gas Warfare in World War I. *U.S. Army Chemical Corps Historical Studies*. Army Chemical Center, Md: US Army Chemical Corps Historical Office; 1958: 77, 79.

50. Cochrane RC. The 33rd Division Along the Meuse, October 1918; study number 8. In: *Gas Warfare in World War I. U.S. Army Chemical Corps Historical Studies*. Army Chemical Center, Md: US Army Chemical Corps Historical Office; 1958: 78.

51. Fries AA. Chemical warfare inspires peace. *Chemical Warfare*. 1921;6:4.

52. Poison gas is indispensable, says German inventor. *Chemical Warfare*. 1921;17:10.

53. Stockholm International Peace Research Institute. The rise of CB weapons. Vol 1. In: *The Problem of Chemical and Biological Warfare*. New York, NY: Humanities Press; 1971: 111–124, 141–142, 147, 214–230.

54. Woolman DS. *Rebels in the Rif: Abd el Krim and the Rif Rebellion*. Stanford, Calif: Stanford University Press; 1968.

55. Fair SD. Mussolini's chemical war. *Army*. 1985;35:47.

56. Foreign developments in chemical warfare. *Chemical Warfare*. 1923;9:19.

57. Smalley VE. *Report of the CW Status of Italy (1926–1948). Army Chemical Center, Md: Chemical Corps Technical Command*; 1948: 14, 52–53.

58. Knappen TM. Chemical warfare and disarmament. *Chemical Warfare*. 1921;7:3.

59. Brown FJ. *Chemical Warfare, a Study in Restraints*. Princeton, NJ: Princeton University Press; 1968: 74–75, 98–110, 118, 145, 193–194, 267–269, 279–281.

60. Clark EB. As chemical warfare chieftain. *Chemical Warfare Bulletin*. 1941;27:87. Editorial.

61. Fries AA. Sixteen reasons why the Chemical Warfare Service must be a separate department of the Army. *Chemical Warfare*. 1920;2:4.

62. Clapp D. Gas. *Chemical Warfare*. 1919;2:iv.

63. Barker ME. The work of the Chemical Warfare Service. *Chemical Warfare*. 1933;19:1330–1339.

64. Brophy LP. Chemical corps troops and training in the years between the two wars. *Chemical Corps Journal*. 1948;2:25–28.

65. War Department. General Orders No. 26. Washington, DC: War Department; 1922.

66. Status of chemical warfare preparedness in the US. *Chemical Warfare*. 1924;10:13.

67. Duffield M. Ethiopia: the unconquered lion of Africa. *Command Magazine*. 1990;4:10–22.

68. Neil EJ. *Use of Gas in Ethiopia*. Washington, DC: War Department. Memorandum, September 2, 1936.

69. Thuillier HF. *The Use of Mustard Gas by the Italians in the Abyssinian War*. Porton, United Kingdom. Memorandum CDR5/1793, April 25, 1941.

70. Volkart W. The Gas Weapon in the Italian–Abyssinian War 1935–1936. Translated from *Allgemeine Schweizerische Militär Zeitschrift*. Typescript prepared for Army Chemical Center, Md; 1951.

71. Murphy P. Gas in the Italo-Abyssinian campaign. *Chemical Warfare Bulletin*. 1937;23:1–8.

72. *Time*. Quoted in: Brett HH. Chemicals and aircraft. *Chemical Warfare Bulletin*. 1936;22:151–152.

73. Kohn GC. *Dictionary of Wars*. New York, NY: Facts on File Publications; 1986: 226, 433–434, 524.

74. Chemicals in Ethiopia. *Chemical Warfare Bulletin*. 1936;22:143.

75. Use of gas in Italo-Abyssinian campaign. *Chemical Warfare Bulletin*. 1937;23:81.

76. Hart L. The Abyssinian War. *Ordnance*. 1937;17:330.

77. Clark DK. *Effectiveness of Toxic Chemicals in the Italo-Ethiopian War*. Bethesda, Md: Operations Research Office; 1959: 1–21.

78. Baker WC. *Annual Report of the Chief of the Chemical Warfare Service for the Fiscal Year Ending June 30, 1937*. Washington, DC: War Department; 1937.

79. Chemical Warfare School. Use of Gas in Ethiopia–1936. Edgewood Arsenal, Md: Chemical Warfare School; 1936. Mimeo 1.

80. Brett GH. Chemicals and aircraft. *Chemical Warfare Bulletin*. 1936;22:153.

81. 5250th Technical Intelligence Company. *The Use of Poison Gas by Imperial Japanese Army in China, 1937–1945*. Tokyo, Japan: 5250th Technical Intelligence Company; 1946.

82. Koelle GB. Anticholinesterase agents. In: Goodman LS, Gilman A, eds. *The Pharmacological Basis of Therapeutics*. 5th ed. New York, NY: Macmillan; 1975: 445.

83. Davis W. *The Serpent and the Rainbow*. New York, NY: Warner Books Inc.; 1985: 36–37.

84. Sidell FR. Nerve agents. In: *Medical Aspects of Chemical and Biological Warfare*. In: Zajtchuk R, Bellamy R. *Textbook of Military Medicine*. Washington, DC: Borden Institute; 1997: 130.

85. Fraser TR. On the characters, actions, and therapeutic use of the ordeal bean of Calabar. *Edinb Med J*. 1863;9:124–132.

86. Holmstedt B. Structure–activity relationships of the organophosphorus anticholinesterase agents. In: Koelle GB, ed. *Cholinesterases and Anticholinesterase Agents*. Berlin, Germany: Springer Verlag; 1963: 429.

87. Arbuzov AE. Über die Struktur der phosphorigen Säure und ihrer Derivate. IV. Isomerisation und Übergang der Verbindungen des dreiwertigen Phosphors in solche des fünfwertigen [On the structure of phosphoric acid and its derivatives. Isomerization and transition of bonds from trivalent to pentavalent phosphorus]. Zhurnal Russkago Fiziko–Khimicheskago Obschchestva. *Russ Phys Chem Soc*. 1906;38:687.

88. Arbuzov AE. Über die Struktur der phosphorigen Säure und ihrer Derivate. IV. Isomerisation und Übergang der Verbindungen des dreiwertigen Phosphors in solche des fünfwertigen [On the structure of phosphoric acid and its derivatives. Isomerization and transition of bonds from trivalent to pentavalent phosphorus]. Abstract. *Chem Zentr*. 1906;2:1639.

89. Michaelis A, Kaehne R. Ueber das Verhalten der Jodalkyle gegen die sogen. Phosphorigsäureester oder O-Phosphine [Over the behavior of the iodine alkyls against suctions: phosphorous acid ester or o-Phosphine]. *Berichte der Deutschen Chemischen Gesellschaft*. 1898;31:1048.

90. Nylén P. The behavior of hypophosphorous acid and phosphorous acid and their monoesters with iodine. A comparative kinetic study. *Z Anorg Allgem Chem*. 1937;230:385–404.

91. Smart JK. History of chemical and biological warfare: an American perspective. In: *Medical Aspects of Chemical and Biological Warfare*. In: Zajtchuk R, Bellamy R. *Textbook of Military Medicine*. Washington, DC: Borden Institute; 1997: 30, 36.

92. Wiseman DJC. *Special Weapons and Types of Warfare*. London, England: War Office; 1951: 150.

93. Intelligence Division, Chemical Warfare Service. *German Chemical Warfare, World War II*. Washington, DC: CWS; 1945: 28–30, 115–117.

94. Gerhard Schrader, Hans Kükenthal, inventors; Farbenfabriken Bayer, Leverkusen assignees. Bekämpfung tierischer Schädlinge. German Patent (DE) 767,153. September 20, 1951.

95. Leiter des Heeresgasschutzlaboratoriums Spandau, der als Chemiker für fabrikatorische Entwicklungsfragen zuständig [Memorandum from chief of chemical weapons laboratory and chemist responsible for development, Spandau, Germany]. 1939.

96. Kahlert H. Why Hitler did not deploy nerve agent in World War II. Paper presented at: The Fifth International Conference on the History of Chemistry; September 8, 2005; Estoril, Portugal.

97. Watson M. Army is speeding chemical defense. *Baltimore Sun*. November 12, 1941. Quoted in: *CWS News Letter*. 1941;5:37.

98. Nazis may use gas, General Porter warns. *CWS News Letter*. 1941;5:31.

99. General Porter urges America to "get tough." *CWS News Letter*. 1941;5:36.

100. *German Munition Plants and Depots During World War II*. Aberdeen Proving Ground, Md: US Army Chemical and Biological Defense Command; 1996.

101. Kahlert H. Chemiker unter Hitler—wirtschaft, technik und wissenschaft der deutschen chemie 1914–1945 [Chemistry under Hitler—economy, technology, and knowledge of German chemistry 1914–1945]. *Grevenbroich*. 2001: 318.

102. DuBois JE. *The Devil's Chemists: 24 Conspirators of the International Farben Cartel Who Manufacture Wars*. Boston, Mass: Beacon Press; 1952: 3–7.

103. Tucker JB. *War of Nerves: Chemical Warfare from World War I to Al-Qaeda*. New York, NY: Pantheon Books; 2006: 44, 45, 55, 70, 74, 89–92.

104. McCombie H, Saunders BC, Wheeler CL. A process for the preparation of fluorophosphonic acids and chlorophosphonic esters. British Patent (GB) 601,210. September 15, 1943.

105. Mazur A, Bodansky O. The mechanism of in vitro and in vivo inhibition of cholinesterase activity by diisopropyl fluorophosphate. *J Biol Chem*. 163:261–276.

106. Hitler A. *Mein Kampf*. Murphy J, trans. New York, NY: Hurst and Blackett Ltd.; 1939: 118–119.

107. The "I.G. Farben Case," United States against Carl Krauch, et al. In: *Trials of War Criminals Before the Nuremberg Military Tribunals, Volume 7, Under Control Council Law No. 10*. 1947: 1044.

108. Joosten PA, ed. *Trial of the Major War Criminals Before the International Military Tribunal: Vol XVI, Proceedings 11, June 1946–June 24, 1946*. Nuremberg, Germany: Secretariat of the International Military Tribunal; 1948: 527–528.

109. Krause J, Mallory CK. *Chemical Weapons in Soviet Military Doctrine*. Boulder, Colo: Westview Press; 1992: 74, 75, 88–94, 112, 114, 115.

110. Bradley ON. *A Soldier's Story*. New York, NY: Henry Holt & Co.; 1951: 237.

111. Sidell FR. Colonel, US Army Medical Corps (Ret). Personal communication, 2004.

112. Babushkin A. The improvement of the chemical troops in the war years. *J Mil His*. 1978;7:91.

113. Weber M. Churchill wanted to "drench" Germany with poison gas. *Journal for Historical Review*. 1985–1986;6:501.

114. Japs reported using gas. *CWS News Letter*. 1941;5:33–34.

115. Ditto RC. Will Hitler's goose be cooked with gas? *Chemical Warfare Bulletin*. 1943;29:6–7.

116. Kirby R. History notes: the CWS effort to obtain German chemical weapons for retaliation against Japan. *CBIAC Newsletter*. 2004;5: 3,13.

117. Lieutenant Colonel DP Gaillard, assistant chief of ordinance, to headquarters, ASF, office, chief of Chemical Warfare Service. Letter. July 9, 1945. Located at: US Army Chemical and Biological Defense Command Historical Office, Edgewood, Md.

118. Miller GA. The development of the 4.2 chemical mortar. *Armed Forces Chemical Journal*. 1948;3:33–32; continued in 1949;3(3):35-42.

119. US War Department. *Characteristics and Employment of Ground Chemical Munitions*. Washington, DC: War Department; 1946. Field Manual 3-5.

120. US War Department. *Employment and Characteristics of Air Chemical Munitions*. Washington, DC: War Department; 1946. Field Manual 3-6.

121. Infield G. *Disaster at Bari*. New York, NY: Bantam Books; 1988: 209, 230–231.

122. Finlay WW. Why prepare? *Chemical Corps Journal*. 1946;1:24.

123. Royall KC. A tribute to the corps. *Chemical Corps Journal*. 1947;2:41.

124. King L. Exit gas warfare? *Chemical Corps Journal*. 1948;2:3.

125. *The Army Almanac*. Washington, DC: Government Printing Office; 1950: 89.

126. Waitt AH. *Chemical Warfare Organization and Policy in the Post-War Army*. Washington, DC: Chemical Warfare Service. May 9, 1946. Memorandum.

127. Office of the Chief of Chemical Corps. *The History of Captured Enemy Toxic Munitions in the American Zone, European Theater, May 1945 to June 1947*. Headquarters: Chemical Corps, European Command; 1947.

128. Baker ER. Chemical warfare in Korea. *Armed Forces Chemical Journal*. 1951;4:3. Letter.

129. Probe into biological experiments on Korean War POWs reported. *Washington Times*. August 15, 1992.

130. Bullene EF. The needs of the army. *Armed Forces Chemical Journal*. 1952;6:8.

131. Abolish unit gas officer positions. *Armed Forces Chemical Journal*. 1954;8:4.

132. Hylton AR. *The History of Chemical Warfare Plants and Facilities in the United States*. Kansas City, Mo: Midwest Research Institute, US Arms Control and Disarmament Agency: 1972; 4: 59–75. ACDA/ST-197.

133. Fielding GH. *V Agent Information Summary*. Washington, DC: US Naval Research Lab; 1960. NRL Report 5421.

134. US Army Chemical Corps. *Summary of Major Events and Problems, FY58*. Army Chemical Center, Md: US Army Chemical Center Historical Center; 1959: 97–101, 108–111, 153–158.

135. US Army Chemical Corps. *Summary of Major Events and Problems, FY59*. Army Chemical Center, Md: US Army Chemical Center Historical Center; 1960: 101–105, 112–114, 117–118, 160–162.

136. The Inspector General, Department of the Army. *Use of Volunteers in Chemical Agent Research*. Washington, DC: DA, IG; 1976. DAIG-IN 21-75.

137. US Army Chemical Corps. *Summary of Major Events and Problems, FY57*. Army Chemical Center, Md: US Army Chemical Center Historical Center; 1957: 97–98, 103.

138. US Army Chemical Corps. *Summary of Major Events and Problems, FY55*. Army Chemical Center, Md: US Army Chemical Center Historical Center; 1955: 48–49, 61–62, 133.

139. US Army Chemical Corps. *Summary of Major Events and Problems, FY56*. Army Chemical Center, Md: US Army Chemical Center Historical Center; 1956: 128–130, 133–134, 140–141.

140. Creasy WM. The forward look in the Army Chemical Corps. *Armed Forces Chemical Journal*. 1957;11:26.

141. Stubbs M. CBR—A power for peace. *Armed Forces Chemical Journal*. 1959;13:8–9.

142. Stubbs M. Untitled speech. Presented to: Directors, New York State Civil Defense Commission; Febraury 9, 1960; Hotel Thayer, West Point, NY.

143. US Army Chemical Corps. *Summary of Major Events and Problems, FY1961–62*. Army Chemical Center, Md: US Army Chemical Center Historical Center; 9–20, 124–126, 131–132.

144. Palmer JM. Chemical warfare training. *Armed Forces Chemical Journal*. 1930;14:28.

145. Anckaitis WH. Realistic CBR training. *Armed Forces Chemical Journal*. 1964;18:16.

146. Harrigan A. The case for gas warfare. *Armed Forces Chemical Journal*. 1963;17:12.

147. United Press International. Mustard gas use suggested. *Washington Post*. October 18, 1966;A-2.

148. Badeeb SM. *The Saudi-Egyptian Conflict Over North Yemen, 1962–1970*. Boulder, Colo: Westview Press; 1986: 2–41.

149. Shoham D. *Evolution of Chemical and Biological Weapons in Egypt*. Boulder, Colo: Westview Press; 1998: 3–27.

150. Cordesman A. *Chemical and Biological Warfare*. New York, NY: 1991: 55.

151. Stockholm International Peace Research Institute. The rise of CB weapons. Vol 1. In: *The Problem of Chemical and Biological Weapons*. New York, NY: Humanities Press; 1971: 86–87.

152. Bermudez R. *Concerns in Yemen*. Washington, DC: Government Printing Office; 1989: 22.

153. Thomas AR. *Growing Threat in the Middle East*. Boston, Mass: Springer: 1998: 2–5.

154. Meselson M. The Yemen. In: Rose S, ed. *CBW: Chemical and Biological Warfare*. Boston, Mass: Beacon Press; 1968: 99.

155. Pearson D, Anderson J. Egypt's use of gas in Yemen verified. *Washington Post*. June 6, 1967.

156. Childs M. Chemical warfare and a death wish. *Washington Post*. June 21, 1967; A-20.

157. How Nasser used poison gas. *US News & World Report*. July 3, 1967; 60.

158. Cromley R. Russians use Yemen as lab for "poison gas." *Washington News*. July 24, 1967.

159. Nasser stoops lower. *Chicago Daily News*. July 31, 1967.

160. Cromley R. Why Israel stocks up on gas masks. *Detroit News*. August 8, 1967.

161. Dupuy TN. *The Encyclopedia of Military History From 3500 BC to the Present*. New York, NY: Harper & Row; 1986: 1279–1280.

162. Stone WW. *Report of Investigation Concerning Sheep Deaths in Skull Valley, Utah*. Washington, DC: US Army Materiel Command; A-1.

163. Associated Press. Army speeds removal of Okinawa gas. *Washington Post*; December 3, 1969; A-3.

164. Stockholm International Peace Research Institute. CB weapons today. Vol 2. In: *The Problem of Chemical and Biological Warfare*. New York, NY: Humanities Press; 1973: 193.

165. Ward PF. *A Summary of Ecological Investigations at Edgewood Arsenal, Maryland: Fiscal Year 1970*. Edgewood, Md: Edgewood Arsenal Research Labs; 1971: 15–23. Edgewood Arsenal Special Publication 100-101.

166. Reducing the terror of war. *Commanders Digest*. 1969:4–5.

167. Wagner RL, Gold TS. Why we can't avoid developing chemical weapons. *Defense*. 1982;3.

168. Fair SD. The chemical corps: alive, well and visible. *Army*. 1972; 29–32.

169. "Preferred alternative" would move chemical training to Ft. McClellan. *APG News*. April 4, 1979; A-1.

170. Chemical Corps School. *Chemical School*. Fort McClellan, Ala: Chemical Corps School; nd.

171. Guiler DC Jr. Chemical Corps: a branch in search of an identity. *Army*. 1977; 14–15.

172. Foreign Science and Technology Center. *Foreign Materiel Exploitation Report, Detection Kit, Chemical Agent, Model PKhR-MV (Soviet) (U)*. Washington, DC: Foreign Science and Technology Center; 1975. AST-1640X-174-75.

173. US Army Armament Research and Development Command. *Laboratory Posture Report*. Dover, NJ: ARRADCOM; Fiscal Year 1978: 3–4.

174. Gas antidote. *Washington Star-News*. July 18, 1974.

175. Eifried G. Russian CW: our Achilles' heel, Europe. *Army*. 1979;29:24–28.

176. Kastenmayer WW. A rebirth of chemical R&D. *Army Research, Development & Acquisition Magazine*. 1981;22:13–15.

177. Siebert GW, Choi YH. Chemical weapons: dull swords in the US armory. *Milit Rev*. 1985;65:23–29.

178. Famiglietti G. Army may switch decision, reestablish Chemical School. *Army Times*. January 22, 1979.

179. US Army Chemical Corps School. *The Chemical Corps Regimental Activation Ceremony*. Fort McClellan, Ala: Chemical Corps School; 1986. PAM 27.

180. US Army Chemical Corps. *Wizard of Battle*. Fort McClellan, Ala: Army Chemical Corps; nd. PAM.

181. *Fort McClellan*. Fort McClellan, Ala: National Military Publications; 1983: 3. PAM.

182. Keegan RJ. Definition of policy of the USA and USSR on chemical and biological warfare. Commander's NU-CH Flash. *Bulletin of the US Army Nuclear and Chemical Agency*. 1982;9:6.

183. Haig AM Jr. *Chemical Warfare in Southeast Asia and Afghanistan*. Washington, DC: US Department of State; 1982. Special Report to Congress 98.

184. Collins JJ. The Soviet military experience in Afghanistan. *Milit Rev*. 1985;65:27.

185. Hoffman MS, ed. *The World Almanac and Book of Facts, 1990*. New York, NY: Pharos Books; 1990: 44, 46, 49, 721.

186. Spiers EM. *Chemical Weaponry: a Continuing Challenge*. New York, NY: St. Martin's Press; 1989: 121.

187. Dunn P. The chemical war: journey to Iran. *Nuclear, Biological, and Chemical Defense and Technology International*. 1986;28–35.

188. Associated Press. Iraqi gas attack on Kurds disputed. *Washington Times*. December 18, 1990.

189. Rohrbaugh DK, Ward JR, Yang Y. *Comments on the Origin of Mustard in the Gulf War*. Aberdeen Proving Ground, Md: US Army Chemical Research Development and Engineering Center; 1990: 8. Technical Report.

190. Dunn P. *Chemical Aspects of the Gulf War, 1984–1987, Investigations by the United Nations*. Ascot Vale, Australia: Materials Research Laboratories; 1987.

191. United Nations. *Report of the Mission Dispatched by the Secretary-General to Investigate Allegations of the Use of Chemical Weapons in the Conflict Between the Islamic Republic of Iran and Iraq*. New York, NY: United Nations Security Council. March 12, 1986: 19.

192. U.N. panel says Iraq used gas on civilians. *New York Times*. August 24, 1988.

193. Dingeman J, Jupa R. Chemical warfare in the Iran-Iraq conflict. *Strategy & Tactics*. 1987;113:51–52.

194. Morrison J. Angola again tied to use of nerve gas. *Washington Times*. March 11, 1988.

195. Lancaster P. Fighting guerrillas with gas. *The Middle East*. June 1, 1987; 17.

196. Wayne EA. Libya seeks chemical weapons in war against Chad, US charges. *Christian Science Monitor*. January 5, 1988:A-1.

197. Satchell M, Blaug E. A plague of "hellish poison." *US News & World Report*. October 26, 1987:30.

198. Parker C. Toxic chemical training. *Army Chemical Review*. 1987:15.

199. Polley W, Dlugopolski M, Hartzell W. 40,000 train in chemical environment. *Army Chemical Review*. 1988:26–31.

200. Reid B. Experts debating Saddam's threat to use chemicals. *Baltimore Evening Sun*. January 22, 1991.

201. Baker C. Tenacity may be Iraqi ace. *Army Times*. February 4, 1991.

202. Atkinson R. No chemical arms found on battlefields. *Washington Post*. March 7, 1991:A1.

203. Associated Press. UN arms monitors destroy Iraqi germ-weapons plant. *Baltimore Sun*. June 21, 1996:A-22.

204. Iraqi weapons plant destroyed. *Military Newswire*. 1996.

205. Smith RJ. Iraq had program for germ warfare. *Washington Post*. July 6, 1995:A-1.

206. Crossette B. Germ war plan underreported, Iraq tells U.N. *New York Times*. August 23, 1995.

207. Herbig AT. Nerve agents–their physiological effects. *Army Chemical Review*. 1990;July:9–13. PB 3-90-2.

208. Barker RB. The future of the DOD chemical/biological defense program. *Defense*. 1992;May–Jun:27.

209. Smart JK. *Desert Storm Diary*. Aberdeen Proving Ground, Md: US Army Chemical and Biological Defense Command; 1991.

210. Johnson SS. Cheney fears chemical attack possible. *USA Today*. January 28, 1991:A3

211. Gertz B. Nerve gas detected by Czechs during Gulf War. *Washington Times*. September 7, 1993.

212. Gulf War veterans link ailments to destruction of Iraqi bunker. *Baltimore Sun*. August 11, 1996:3A.

213. American soldiers may have been exposed to Iraqi chemical weapons, Pentagon says. *Baltimore Sun*. June 22, 1996:10A.

214. Lewthwaite GA. 20,000 troops may have faced gas. *Baltimore Sun*. October 23, 1996:1A.

215. Matthews M. US warns Iraq against using chemical arms. *Baltimore Sun*. March 10, 1991:16A.

216. Tyler PE. U.S. planning air strikes if Iraq uses gas on rebels: Baghdad reportedly told commanders to use chemicals. *Baltimore Sun*. March 10, 1991:1A.

217. Wines M. U.S. hints at chemical arms bunker in Libya. *New York Times*. March 7, 1991:A13.

218. Libya close to finishing huge chemical weapons plant. *Baltimore Sun*. February 25, 1996:20A.

Chapter 3

HISTORY OF THE MEDICAL MANAGEMENT OF CHEMICAL CASUALTIES

BENJAMIN A. HILL Jr, DO, MS, MEd*

Lieutenant Colonel, US Army Medical Corps; Physician Faculty, Chemical Casualty Care Division, US Army Medical Research Institute of Chemical Defense, 3100 Ricketts Point Road, Aberdeen Proving Ground, Edgewood Arsenal, Maryland 21010-5400

INTRODUCTION

Much that is known today about the medical management of chemical casualties resulted from experience with the large number of chemical casualties managed during World War I. However, because chemicals have scarcely been used on the battlefield since then, the US armed forces have yet to apply the chemical lessons learned from that war on a large scale. This chapter continues the series of history chapters in this textbook begun in Chapter 2, History of Chemical Warfare, which provides a detailed history of chemical weapons in World War I and subsequent incidents of their use on the battlefield, which gave rise to the casualties discussed here. Chapter 4, History of the Chemical Threat, Chemical Terrorism, and Its Implications for Military Medicine, will provide further insight into the subject.

Integrating the specifics of chemical casualty support within general medical and surgical support involves numerous command and staff actions. These actions interface at all command echelons and with all components of a commander's staff. For example, the ability to train the appropriate number of personnel involves personnel actions, and knowing what medical materiel needs to be emplaced requires gathering medical intelligence. World War I provided insight into how to manage all aspects of medical support in the event of a chemical attack. Specialty care personnel, physicians, nurses, and first responders required training, and how these trainees performed in the theater of combat required operations and planning action.

The medical logistics portion of a unit supplies trained troops with the specific tools and equipment to perform their specialty missions. None of these staff actions can exist without the establishment, direction, and supervision of leadership elements throughout every echelon of military organization. However, the initial management of chemical casualties did not always have the defined leadership and staff actions it does currently; the management process has been refined as the nature of chemical warfare and its resulting casualties have evolved over time. Because military physicians base treatment regimens on both the quality and quantity of the anticipated combat injuries, the main focus of this chapter is World War I, when organized paradigms were first developed to handle a potentially massive influx of chemical casualties.

HISTORY UNTIL WORLD WAR I

Although historians do not agree on what devices should be considered the first chemical weapons, the signs and symptoms of weapon-induced pathology were documented long before World War I. From the earliest times, physicians managed natural "chemical" casualties. Animal and plant agents, such as jellyfish; man-o-wars; spitting snakes; skunks; poison ivy, sumac, and oak; and stinging nettles provided physicians with a variety of casualties and clinical presentations.[1,2] Around the recorded times of early Troy (1200 BCE), weapons such as arrows were wrapped with flammable plant fibers (flax, hemp, or straw) and set afire, and military physicians used appropriate medications and therapies to treat the resulting injuries.[3] The Chinese used arsenic and sulfur tactically during 1000 to 700 BCE to produce irritating fogs, fumes, and poisonous smoke balls that affected soldiers' airways. One specific concoction that called for aconite root, wolfsbane, and croton bean engendered blisters and pustules in airways and on skin surfaces.[3] As a result, casualty types broadened from pulmonary and respiratory to dermatological (vesicant).

Around 600 BCE Solon documented that hellebore roots thrown into a river gave rise to profuse diarrhea, forcing military physicians to manage the resulting severe dehydration without intravenous fluid resuscitation.[3] In *History of the Peloponnesian War,* Thucydides described chemical warfare and the types of casualties it produced during the 5th-century BCE conflict between Athens and Sparta. Thucydides tells how Sparta's allies, the Boethians, took an Athenian fort at Delium in 424 BCE with an engine filled with lighted coals, sulfur, and pitch, which made a great blaze and set fire to the fort walls. The defenders abandoned the fort, leaving pulmonary casualties in need of medical treatment.[4] Later, Romans used mucous-membrane irritants against the Ambracians, allies of Corinth, during 193 to 189 BCE. The medical management of these casualties undoubtedly involved removing them from irritant sources and flushing irritated surfaces with copious amounts of water. In the 9th century CE, Leo IX of Byzantium, writing on warfare, described hand-thrown "vases filled with quicklime," the effects of which had been known since the Peloponnesian War. Quicklime was one of three combustible substances known in the Mediterranean at that time (the other two were sulfur and pitch). When broken, the vases of quicklime let loose an overpowering odor that suffocated anyone nearby.[5]

From that point onward, various types of chemical weaponry were engaged. Over time, military physicians developed the most effective leadership, staff organization, and curative techniques to maintain the effectiveness of the fighting force during and following a chemical attack. As 1914 drew near, chemicals used on the battlefields were primarily irritants. In the early years of World War I, the Germans employed nontoxic "ni-shells" and "T-shells," containg xylyl bromide (see Chapter 2).[6] Because these chemicals were nontoxic and their employment as weapons was tactically unsound, the combatant armies established no real medical support organization or protocol to respond—organized management of chemical casualties was not necessary because no elevated influx of chemical patients occurred.

WORLD WAR I

World War I heralded several battlefield discoveries that changed the face of warfare and the future chemical threat. In addition to causing large numbers of casualties, gas was an effective and versatile weapon because it placed an additional strain on every aspect of combat. According to British Major General Charles H Foulkes, the "appearance of gas on the battlefield . . . changed the whole character of warfare."[7(p345)] Gas permeated clothing, food, and water. It corroded human skin, internal organs, and even steel weapons. Its smell lingered in the air. Not only did soldiers have to train constantly in emerging chemical warfare, but an entire logistical network had to be established for offensive and defensive gas equipment. As a result, a new branch of the US Army came into existence, and new units, such as decontamination squads, mobile degassing units, and special gas troops, were created (Figure 3-1). Combat arms officers became gas officers in divisions, regiments, and battalions, reducing the number of combat arms personnel. The impact of gas on the Medical Department also posed tremendous problems for casualty treatment. The number of gas wounded became so great that one field hospital out of four per division was dedicated solely to the treatment of gas casualties (Table 3-1).[7]

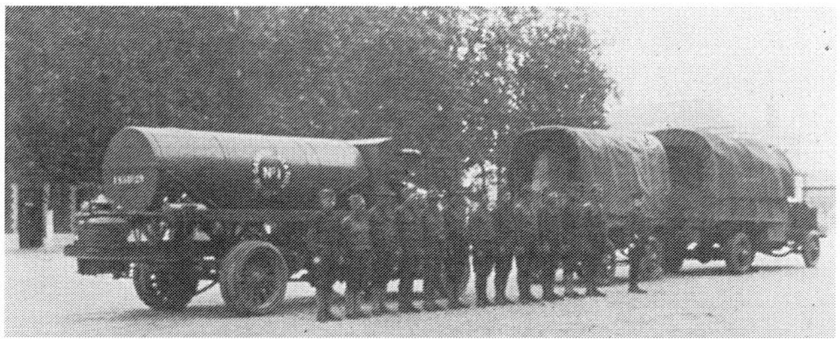

Fig. 3-1. The mobile decontamination facility was an essential part of the degassing station, and plans called for two per division. As events transpired, only one experimental mobile decontamination facility was actually constructed, and it was never used in combat. Its objective was "to give hot baths and clean clothing to those subjected to the fumes of mustard gas at the nearest possible points to where gas bombardments take place."[1] Given what is now known about the speed with which mustard injury develops, attempting to slow the progression of mustard injury by this regimen was most likely ineffective. Nevertheless, by providing a shower and clean clothing, the degassing station would have played an important role in improving the general sanitation and morale of combat troops.
(1) Gilchrist HL. Field arrangements for gas defense and the care of gas casualties. In: Weed FM, ed. *Medical Aspects of Gas Warfare*. Vol 14. In: Ireland MW, ed. *The Medical Department of the United States Army in the World War*. Washington, DC: Government Printing Office; 1926: Chap 4: 61.
Photograph: Courtesy of Chemical and Biological Defense Command Historical Research and Response Team, Aberdeen Proving Ground, Md.

Prewar Intelligence and the Second Battle of Ypres

The failure to plan for chemical warfare in World War I was a strategic error on the part of the Allies because they had sufficient intelligence to warrant preparation. In the time leading up to the first gas attack at Ypres, intelligence of chemical weaponry mounted. Trepidation existed on both sides of the trenches, however. According to the official German World War I military history, *Der Weltkrieg*, constant reports by the foreign press appeared in the early weeks of the war about new inventions and secret weapons that might

TABLE 3-1

CHEMICAL CASUALTIES IN WORLD WAR I

Country	Nonfatal Chemical Casualties	Chemical Fatalities	Percentage Fatal
Germany	191,000	9,000	4.5
France	182,000	8,000	4.2
British Empire	180,597	8,109	4.3
United States	71,345	1,462	2.0
Russia*	419,340	56,000	11.8

*The data from which these figures were derived have apparently been lost to history. However, the Russians themselves analyzed their casualty statistics from World War I. The Narkomzdrav Commission found the figures for nonfatal and fatal gas casualties to be only about one tenth as great as AM Prentiss's values, which are the ones commonly accepted in the West (total gassed casualties: 40,000–65,000; total gas fatalities: 6,340).
Data sources: (1) Prentiss AM. *Chemicals in War: A Treatise on Chemical Warfare.* New York, NY: McGraw-Hill; 1937: 653. (2) Kohn S. *The Cost of the War to Russia.* New York, NY: Howard Fertig; 1973: 136.

be used against the German army. A French chemist, Eugene Turpin, reportedly created a secret weapon that caused injury without a visible external wound.[8]

Germany's first chemical weapon was chlorine gas. In the winter of 1914–1915, German chemist and professor Fritz Haber came up with the idea of generating a chlorine gas cloud to attack the enemy line, an improvement on Walther Nernst's recommended chlorine gas artillery munitions. By blowing the chlorine from a point source, such as fixed cylinders in a front line trench, it was thought possible to create a chlorine cloud that would creep across the ground and down into the trenches in enough measure to create mass casualties (Figure 3-2). Chlorine gas was intended to render troops incapable of fighting but was not considered to have a lasting physical effect.[9]

Despite the warnings of potential chemical attack, neither the French, Algerians, British, nor Canadians prepared personal protective measures or plans for managing chemical casualties. On April 13 a German deserter, Private August Jaeger, told French authorities:

> An attack is planned for the near future against the French trenches of the above mentioned sector. With this object in view four batteries have been placed in position in the first line trenches; these batteries each have 20 bottles of asphyxiating gas. Each Company has 4 such batteries. Each battery has 5 gunners. At a given signal—3 red rockets fired by the artillery—the bottles are uncorked, and the gas on escaping, is carried by a favourable wind towards the French trenches. This gas is intended to asphyxiate the men who occupy the trenches and to allow the Germans to occupy them without losses. In order to prevent the men being themselves intoxicated by the gas, each man is provided with a packet of tow steeped in oxygen.[10(pp228–229)]

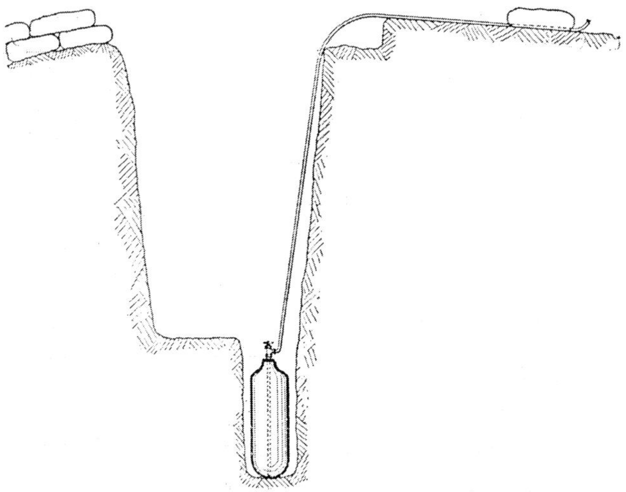

Fig. 3-2. A typical German chemical cylinder set up and ready for discharge. The discharge from thousands of cylinders created a gas cloud.
Reproduced from: Army War College. German methods of offense. Vol 1. In: *Gas Warfare*. Washington, DC: War Department; 1918: 14.

Two days later, another German deserter, Julius Rapsahl, claimed that a cotton mouth protector was issued to German soldiers for protection in the event that the Allies attacked them with gas.[10] Additionally, a reliable Belgian intelligence agent warned that German "reserves have been brought up and passages have been prepared across old trenches existing in rear of present German trenches to facilitate bringing forward artillery. Germans intended on making use of tubes with asphyxiating gas placed in Bts. [batteries] of 20 tubes for every 40 metres in front of 26th Corps."[10(p231)] The appendix in the *British Second Army War Diary* noted "it is possible that if the wind is not favourable to blow the gases over our trenches that the attack may be postponed."[10(p231)] An additional information bulletin was received by French general headquarters from the Belgian army's deputy chief of staff. According to the bulletin, a Belgian agent had sent word that the Germans had placed an urgent order at a factory in Ghent for the provision of 20,000 mouth protectors made of tulle that soldiers could carry in waterproof packets.[11]

This information was subsequently published in the French army's *Bulletin de Renseignements de la Détachement d'Armée de Belgique*. Copies were sent to the British general headquarters, and translations were circulated to the general staff, but the intelligence was essentially ignored by Allied headquarters.[12] Because chemical warfare was an unknown entity, the likelihood of the event was greatly minimized.

On the evening of April 22, 1915, during the Second Battle of Ypres, chlorine gas, released from point sources, created a large number of bewildered chemical casualties (Figure 3-3). A German soldier, part of a specialized chemical engineer unit in Ypres, Belgium, reported:

> That day was a Thursday in April 1915. Finally we decided to release the gas. The weatherman was right. It was a beautiful day, the sun was shining. Where there was grass, it was blazing green. We should have been going to a picnic, not doing what we were about to do. The artillery put up a really heavy attack, starting in the afternoon. The French had to be kept in their trenches. After the artillery was finished, we sent the infantry back and opened the valves with strings. About supper time, the gas started toward

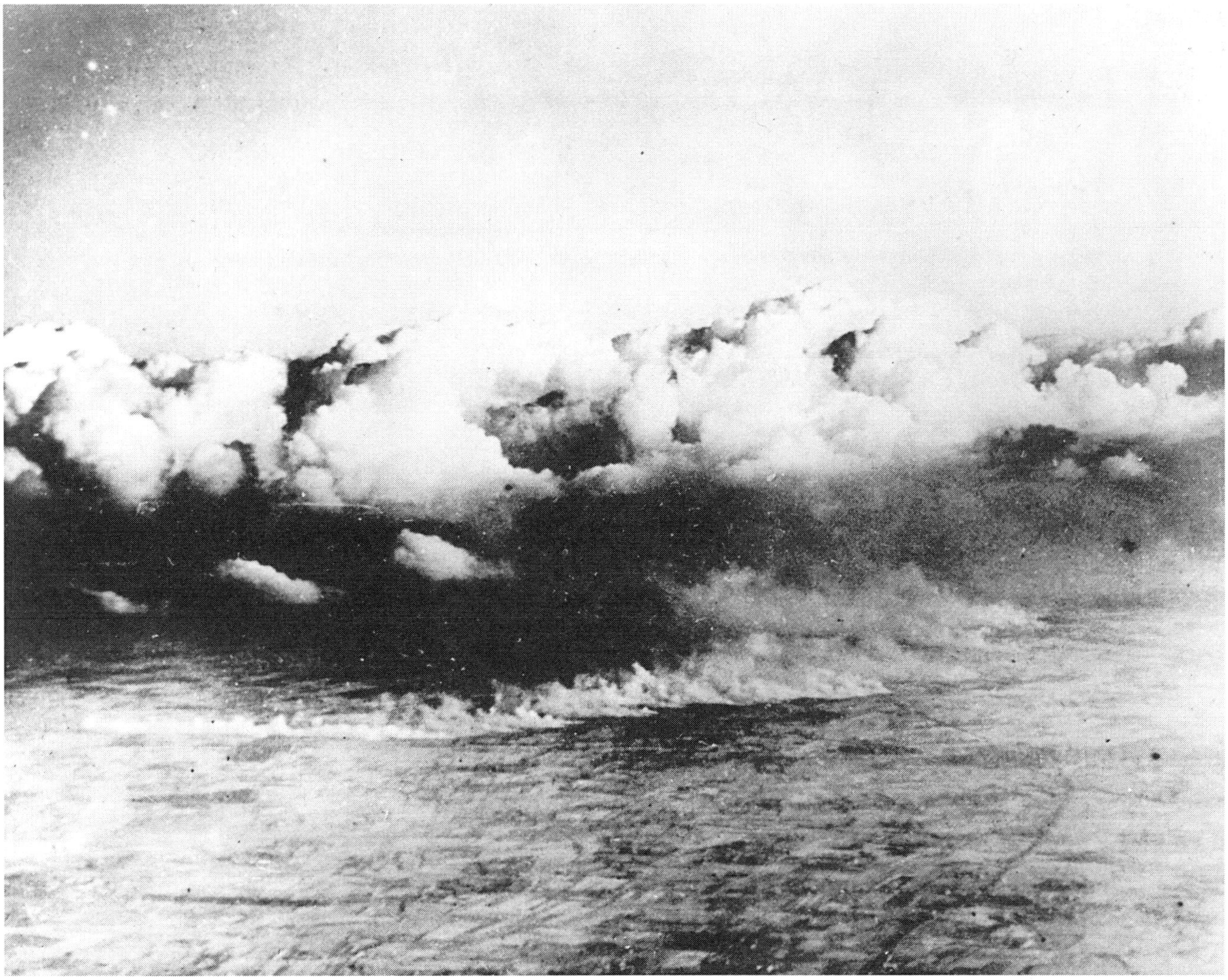

Fig. 3-3. This photograph is reputed to show the German chlorine gas cloud attack at Ypres, Belgium, on April 22, 1915. Although there is little evidence to support this claim, the photograph does show a visible cloud, probably created by a cylinder attack.
Photograph: Courtesy of Chemical and Biological Defense Command Historical Research and Response Team, Aberdeen Proving Ground, Md.

the French, everything was quiet. We all wondered what was going to happen.

As this great cloud of green gray gas was forming in front of us, we suddenly heard the French yelling. In less than a minute, they started with the most rifle and machine gun fire that I had ever heard. Every field artillery gun, every machine gun, every rifle that the French had must have been firing. I had never heard such a noise. The hail of bullets going over our heads was unbelievable, but it was not stopping the gas. The wind kept moving the gas towards the French lines. We heard the cows bawling, and the horses screaming. The French kept on shooting. They couldn't possibly have seen what they were shooting at. In about fifteen minutes, the gun fire started to quit. After a half hour, only occasional shots [were heard]. Then everything was quiet again.

In a while it had cleared and we walked past the empty gas bottles [cylinders]. What we saw was total death. Nothing was alive. All of the animals had come out of their holes to die. Dead rabbits, moles, rats, and mice were everywhere. The smell of the gas was still in the air. It hung on the few bushes that were left. When we got to the French lines, the trenches were empty. But in a half mile, the bodies of French soldiers were everywhere. It was unbelievable. Then we saw that there was some English. You could see where men had clawed at their faces, and throats, trying to get their breath. Some had shot themselves. The horses, still in the stables, cows, chickens, everything, all were dead. Everything, even the insects were dead.

We started counting the casualties. This operation was so much bigger than we had ever imagined. That night we guessed over 20,000 French soldiers, and even more town people had died. The infantry followed us but when they couldn't find any French to fight, they stopped. All of us went back to our camps and quarters wondering what we had done. What was next? We knew what happened that day had to change things.[13]

The number of French and Algerian soldiers killed that day is estimated to be about 10,000. The number of civilians and animals killed is undetermined. Even as the chemical casualties from the attack began filtering into rear areas, the response was generally denial. When the word of a chemical attack reached Harvey Cushing, an American physician working with the French at Compiegne, he responded with disbelief (Exhibit 3-1):

It was soon whispered about that this lot had come from Ypres and that they had all suffered greatly from some German gaz asphyxiant [*sic*]; but I hardly believed the tale, or thought I had misunderstood, until this evening's communiqué bears it out. Many of them were coughing; but then, as I've said, most of the wounded still come in with a bronchitis. We have heard rumors for some days of a movement of German troops in the direction of Ypres, and this attack is apparently the result.

When we got back to the Ambulance, the air was full of tales of the asphyxiating gas which the Germans had turned loose on Thursday—but it is difficult to get a straight story. A huge, low-lying greenish cloud of smoke with a yellowish top began to roll down from the German trenches, fanned by a steady easterly wind. At the same time there was a terrifically heavy bombardment. The smoke was suffocating and smelled to some like ether and sulphur, to another like a thousand sulphur matches, to still another like burning rosin. One man said that there were about a thousand Zouaves of the Bataillon d'Afrique in the lines and only sixty got back either suffocated or shot as they clambered out of the trenches to escape. Another of the men was en repos five kilometres [*sic*] away and says he could smell the gas there. He with his fellows was among those of the reserves who were called on to support the line, but by the time they got up the Germans were across the canal, having effectively followed up their smudge. They seem to have been driven out later, or at least the seamen thought they had been. We'll have to await the official communiqués, and perhaps not know even then. In any event, there's devil's work going on around Ypres, and the heralded "spring drive" seems to have been initiated by the Germans. . . .

Then we saw many of the severely "gassed" men who had come in this morning—a terrible business—one man, blue as a sailor's serge, simply pouring out with every cough a thick albuminous secretion, and too busy fighting for air to bother much about anything else—a most horrible form of death for a strong man.[14(p69)]

EXHIBIT 3-1

DR HARVEY CUSHING

Dr Harvey Cushing experienced the western front in the French and British sectors of occupation before the American Expeditionary Forces deployed medical support. His first duty was in the early spring of 1915, when he served with a Harvard unit in the American Ambulance at Neuilly, France. At that time he became familiar with the French Service de Santé. From Paris he visited the British Royal Army Medical Corps in Flanders. He managed chemical casualties during the battles for the Messines and Passchendaele ridges in Flanders at the time of the Third Battle for Ypres. His observations as an American physician gave insight into how American wartime medical management of chemical casualties compared to international standards.

Data source: Cushing H. *From a Surgeon's Journal, 1915–1918*. Boston, Mass: Little, Brown and Company; 1936.

Initial Responses

The deliberate use of tactical chemicals on an unprepared enemy created a marked change in the nature of the casualty. It was quickly learned that chemical agents had a debilitating effect on soldiers: not only did the chemicals physically injure soldiers, but they also added a psychological element that common artillery could not match. During a chemical attack, soldiers felt that other than masking, they had no real defense. This resulted in a "gas-fright" syndrome hallmarked by psychological depression and war weariness. Untrained physicians were unsympathetic to those suffering from "gas poisoning" and the battle fatigue it caused, often accusing soldiers of malingering. Unfortunately, few physicians knew how to medically manage a chemical casualty at the onset of the war (Table 3-2). In the absence of a remedy, soldiers were given bed rest with the hope that the body's intrinsic healing abilities would be adequately facilitated.

On a chemical battlefield, normal medical opera-

TABLE 3-2

SIX CHLORINE-PHOSGENE CLOUD ATTACKS: BRITISH CASUALTIES DECEMBER 1915–AUGUST 1916

Casualties	Percentage
Gas casualties as a percentage of exposed troops	4.1
Deaths from gas as a percentage of troops	0.7
Deaths from gas as a percentage of total gas casualties	23.6

Adapted with permission from: Moore W. *Gas Attack*. London, England: Leo Cooper; 1987: Appendix D.

tions were encumbered by protective gear; soldiers who did not follow the strict protective measures soon became casualties. Ultimately, half the battle casualties during the war were attributed to gas. One officer wrote of the attacks:

> When sent out into the darkness to bring in the wounded or perform other duties . . . the [soldiers] repeatedly removed the face part of the S.B.R. [small box respirator] so as to see what they were doing or where they were going. . . . Others, straining at the heavy loads of bringing in casualties found the mask painfully oppressive and removed it. [Only] one who has been under such a night bombardment can realize the difficulties attending the supervision and control of gas discipline during such a time.[15(p13)]

The early poor gas discipline was blamed on the ineffectiveness of the British small box respirator and French M2 masks, which were issued to all American Expeditionary Forces (AEF) personnel entering the theater (Figure 3-4). The adoption of a better mask was recommended early in response to the AEF's Chemical Warfare Service (CWS) and 1st Division Medical Corps complaints.[15] One soldier said of the equipment: ". . . surgeons, stretcher bearers, and runners, had found it impossible to carry on in the SBR because the arrangement of the eyepieces and the fogging of the lenses impaired vision."[15(pp19–20)]

Pulmonary agents were used first on the battlefield, and the resulting casualties were managed under the medical doctrine of the French and British medical systems. Later, the Germans developed sulfur mustard, a vesicant (blister agent) that attacked the skin, making masks less effective (Figure 3-5). Mustard was first used on July 12, 1917, just prior to the Third Battle of Ypres, and the Allies had to devise a medical response to this new type of agent.[16]

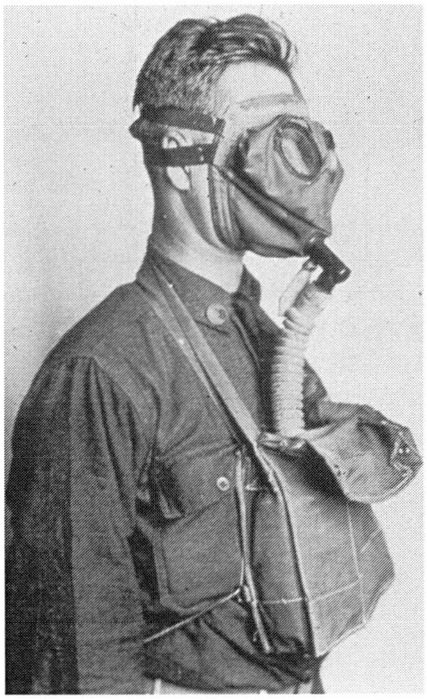

Fig. 3-4. The British small box respirator, introduced in 1916 and seen in 1918 in this photograph, was vastly more effective than the earlier British versions. The wearer breathed through a mouthpiece. Because a spring clip was applied to the nose, only air that had passed through the mouthpiece could enter the lungs. An absolute seal between the face and mask was unnecessary. The mouthpiece was connected by a tube to the canister containing neutralizing chemicals, which was worn around the trunk. Although the small box respirator was more protective than its predecessors, it was probably less user-friendly.
Reproduced from: Pictorial History, Gas Defense Division, Chemical Warfare Service. Vol 5. Edgewood Historical Files. Located at: Chemical and Biological Defense Command Historical Research and Response Team, Aberdeen Proving Ground, Md.

As World War I progressed, physicians became more adept at managing chemical casualties, though bed rest remained the most common form of treatment. Soldiers who inhaled large volumes of asphyxiating gases usually died. Mustard was probably the most difficult agent to medically manage because it temporarily blinded individuals, produced blisters on the skin, and resulted in a large number of casualties who required extensive medical treatment. As the number of chemical casualties increased, field hospitals became overburdened. Eventually, some special hospitals were erected to deal solely with soldiers suffering from chemical-related injuries. The number of chemical casualties produced was staggering, and the forward-deployed Canadian, French, and Algerian dressing stations were quickly overwhelmed.

Another setback early in the war was the abysmal field sanitation French and British troops had to deal

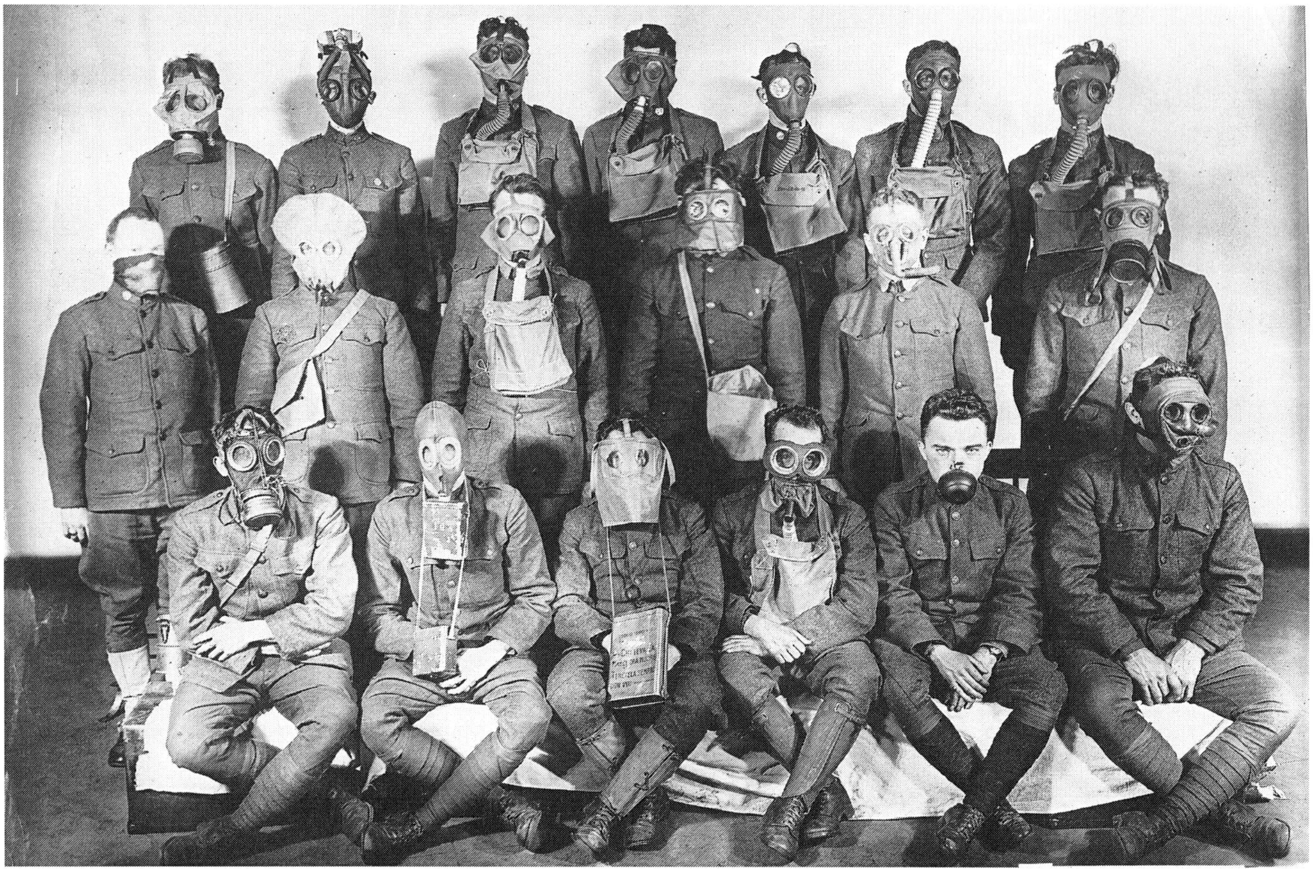

Fig. 3-5. Allied response to the use of gas was to create myriad devices designed to protect the respiratory system. By 1917 the Germans had found a way to defeat the effectiveness of these masks by introducing vesicants, agents that attacked the skin as well. Top row, left to right: US Navy Mark I mask; US Navy Mark II mask; US CE mask; US RFK mask; US AT mask; U.S. KT mask; US model 1919 mask. Middle row, left to right: British Black Veil mask; British PH helmet; British BR mask; French M2 mask; French artillery mask; French ARS mask. Bottom row, left to right: German mask; Russian mask; Italian mask; British Motor Corps mask; US Rear Area mask; US Connell mask.
Photograph: Courtesy of Chemical and Biological Defense Command Historical Research and Response Team, Aberdeen Proving Ground, Md.

with. The French trenches taken over by Canadian and American forces were found in poor condition. Personal accounts from Canadian soldiers document the overpowering stench from numerous dead French and German soldiers buried in shallow graves in or near the trenches or left unburied. Captain TC Irving, commanding officer of the Second Field Company, Canadian Divisional Engineers, reported that ". . . things were in a deplorable state from the standpoint of defence, safety and sanitation, and large quantities of disinfectant should be sent into the trenches immediately for liberal use."[10] His report continues:

> The right flank and the next portion to the left had a parapet of mud heaped up in front approximately 2 feet thick at the bottom and from 4 inches to 1 foot at the top with an occasional loophole punched through the earth. . . . The water level is about two feet down below the surface of the ground with numerous shell holes and also a section of the trench behind partially filled with water. There was a plugged drain passing between these two sections in a North Easterly direction through the German lines. In front of these sections are numerous bodies buried at a very shallow depth making it impossible for us at many places to excavate at all. There is also human excreta littered all over the place.
>
> Going to the left we next strike 650 feet of firing line completely enfiladed by the enemy's artillery, which had no traverses in it. The parapet ranged from 2 feet to 4 feet in height and from 6 inches at the top to three feet at the bottom in thickness. The ground where the men stand in the firing position is paved with rotting

bodies and human excreta. The ground behind is full of excreta and dead bodies.[10(pp235–238)]

The French army's structure was responsible for the unsanitary state seen by the arriving Canadians. The French medical service was part of the only World War I combatant army whose medical officers (MOs) were not organized in a separate corps. The absence of an independent medical service meant that medical issues were under the auspices of the French combat arms leadership and maneuver commanders. Field sanitation and troop hygiene were lower priority than tactical matters. Almost all water supplies were infected by *Salmonella typhi*. The French army experienced 50,000 cases of typhoid in the first 3 years of the war.[17,18] Because the French medical service was plagued with problems, the Americans arriving on the western front looked to the British Royal Army Medical Corps as a template for medical organization. During the early part of World War I, the US Army surgeon general assigned a number of MOs to act as observers within the French and British armies. Reports on the medical aspects of the European conflict, including the diagnosis and treatment of chemical casualties, were received by the surgeon general from 1916 onward.

Royal Army Medical Corps

The Royal Army Medical Corps had three main responsibilities during the war: (1) sanitation (physical and environmental hygiene), (2) patient transport (evacuation of the sick and wounded), and (3) hospitalization (the medical management of the sick or wounded). Chemical warfare impacted all three (Figure 3-6). Chemical casualties had to be managed in a battlefield creviced with trenches of varying depths. Some had flimsy dugouts that protected troops from the elements but not from artillery shelling. In most places the trenches did not run in a continuous line, but were instead made up of groups of shallow fire and support trenches.[10]

Collecting, Evacuating, and Distribution Zones

The Royal Army Medical Corps provided support for itself and for its attached forces. Its management scheme divided the battlefield into the collecting zone, the evacuating zone, and the distribution zone. The collecting zone was the first or forward area to which the wounded were evacuated from the battlefield (Figure 3-7). The middle area, known as the evacuating zone, encompassed the roads, railway lines, and canals along which casualties were transported to the distribution zone. The evacuating zone occasionally contained a medical supply unit or "stationary" hospital for receiving casualties who could not be advanced to the distribution zone (see Figure 3-7). The distribution zone contained the various facilities needed for definitive medical treatment, staffed by logistical and service support units dispersed in a rear area of operations of indeterminate size, including mainland Great Britain. Stationary hospitals out of theater in Great Britain were called "home hospitals," and those outside of Great Britain were called "overseas" or "base hospitals."[19]

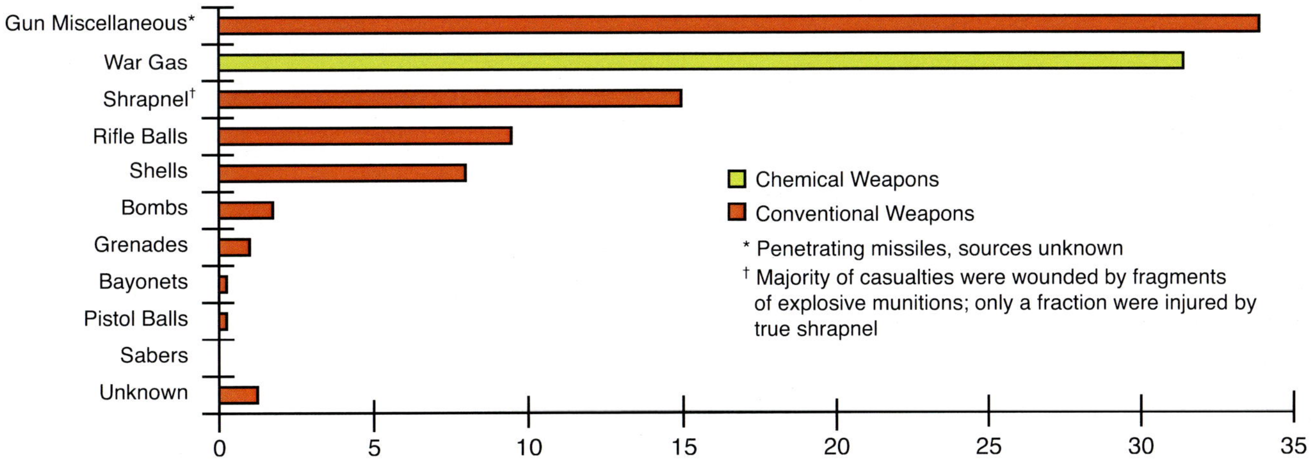

Fig. 3-6. Hospitalized casualties in World War I, in percentages by causative weapon (224,089 casualties).
Adapted from: Gilchrist HL. *A Comparative Study of World War Casualties from Gas and Other Weapons.* Chart 7. Edgewood Arsenal, Md: Chemical Warfare School; 1928:19.

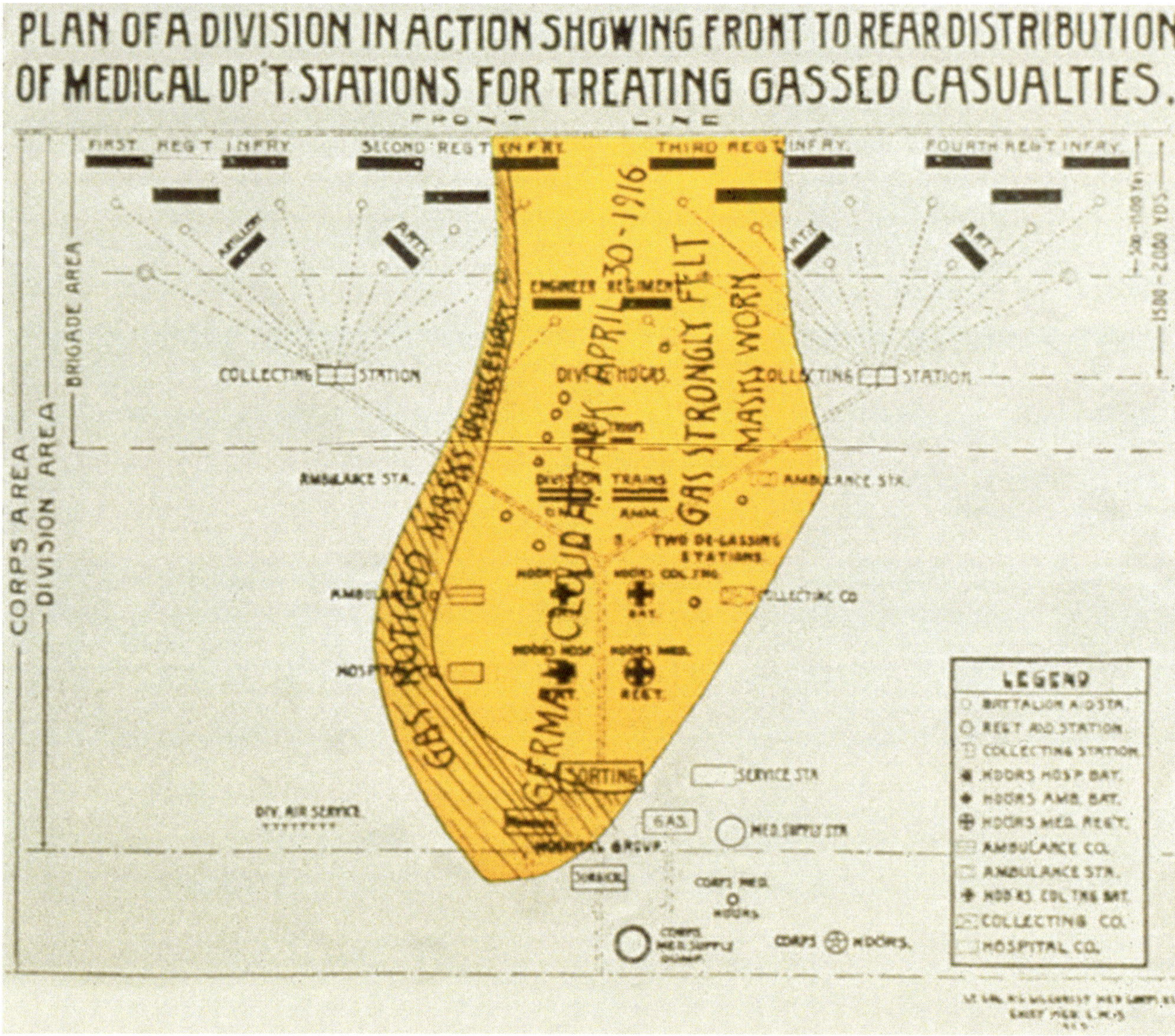

Fig. 3-7. Plan of a division in action. Colonel HL Gilchrist, medical director of the American Expeditionary Force for gas warfare, prepared this illustration for chemical warfare training purposes. The drawing is based on an actual German gas cloud in 1916 but an American division is substituted for the British division that was actually attacked. The gas cloud is seen as totally interrupting the division's medical evacuation system, as well as making its two "degassing stations" inoperative. Reproduced from: Gilchrist HL. *A Comparative Study of World War Casualties from Gas and Other Weapons*. Edgewood Arsenal, Md: Chemical Warfare School; 1928.

Regimental Aid Posts

The battalion or regimental MO was responsible for the basic design of a regimental aid post equipped for medical and surgical casualty stabilization, which often had to be rapidly established during movement. Depending on the unit's location, the aid post might have been the cellar of a ruined cottage or house, a deserted German dugout, or a shellproof annex to a communication trench. The post needed to offer protection from direct fire and, if possible, be located adjacent to a road to support evacuation. Regardless of location, the aid post had to protect casualties from further chemical compromise, which was accomplished by closing all doorway openings with blankets soaked in an antigas solution.[20,21]

The mission of the aid post was to treat for shock (by administering morphine and providing hot drinks) and protect casualties from environmental exposure. Treatment was provided in these forward areas until the casualty flow slackened. Casualties who required stabilization beyond the regimental MO's level of expertise were evacuated to the next echelon of care: the advanced dressing station. Litter-bearers who originally brought in the casualties transported them from aid posts to advanced dressing stations, or casualties were moved between the two echelons by motorized or horse-drawn ambulances.[19]

Advanced Dressing Stations

Advanced dressing stations were set up at locations accessible by the regimental aid posts. Because their locations were further rearward (albeit still in artillery range), an advanced dressing station may have been in a crypt or cellar of a building, such as a church or school. The floor plan of the advanced dressing station was like an enlarged version of a regimental aid post. Provisions were made for casualties that required increased stabilization. Because they were in artillery range, additional care had to be taken to protect staff and patients from chemical attacks. At the advanced dressing station, casualties were further stabilized for continued transport, which was the responsibility of supporting echelons from the field ambulance headquarters or main dressing station. In the presence of a high influx of casualties, the walking wounded were intercepted prior to their arrival at the advanced aid station and sequestered in a holding area called a "divisional collecting post." This collecting post was supported by a field ambulance station. From there, casualties moved to a main dressing station, if needed.[19]

Main Dressing Stations

The field ambulance headquarters formed the main dressing station, located outside of artillery range (thus defense against chemical artillery was not a major concern). Field ambulances were responsible for transporting the sick and wounded from the advanced dressing stations to the main dressing stations. Casualties might require an extended stay for treatment at the main dressing station before further evacuation to the clearing stations. Evacuation at this level was carried out by specially equipped motor ambulance convoys. Each motor ambulance car could carry six or eight sitting or four reclining casualties. Unfortunately, chemical casualties in these ambulances were exposed to heated carbon monoxide from the vehicle's exhaust fumes.[19]

Casualty Clearing Stations

Casualty clearing stations or railhead hospitals served as the final collecting zones. The casualty clearing station's primary function was to receive and evacuate casualties to the distribution zone and the stationary base hospitals. Casualty clearing station sites needed adequate ingress for casualties and adequate egress for evacuation by rail, water, or road, and had to provide sufficient interim casualty medical support. The casualty clearing station was obligated to act as a hospital only part of the time, depending on the tactical situation. In some instances, the casualty support mission became so predominant that the term "clearing hospital" evolved. Although some clearing stations were only about 6 miles from the front, many were fully functional as fixed hospitals with trained female nurses (Figure 3-8), ordinary hospital beds, operating tables equipped with electric light, and the same appliances and features found in the hospitals of large towns, such as radiograph equipment and clinical laboratories. Dr Cushing visited one such hospital in Bailleul, Belgium, and recorded Royal Army Medical Corps casualty processing at a clearing station 2 weeks after the first chemical attack (Exhibits 3-2 and 3-3).[14]

Base Hospitals

Casualties were evacuated to the base hospital by rail (ambulance train), road (motor convoy), or water (hospital barge). A typical hospital train could carry about 400 casualties. Evacuation by hospital barge was extremely slow and restricted by the availability of navigable canals. Barges traveled only by daylight, at the rate of about 3 miles per hour, taking an average 24 to 48 hours to complete an evacuation. The motor convoy, preferred when speed was essential, was the primary means of evacuation.[19]

The medical facilities to which casualties were sent within the distribution zone were also known as "gen-

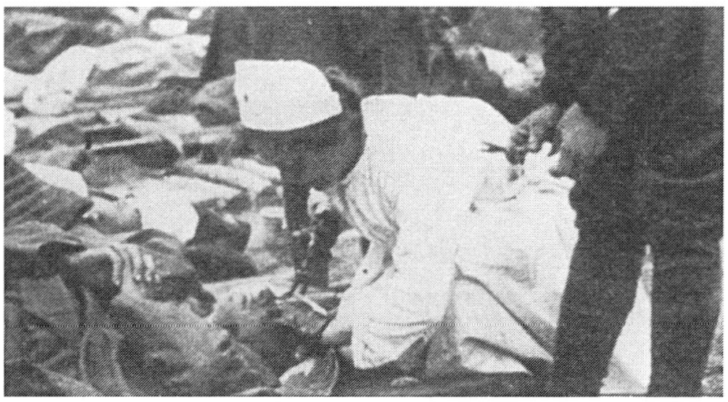

Fig. 3-8. A nurse irrigates the eyes of soldier who has a probable mustard injury. It is now known that eye irrigation would have provided only symptomatic relief because of the rapidity with which mustard damages tissue.
Reproduced from: Moore WE, Crussell J. *US Official Pictures of the World War*. Washington, DC: Pictorial Bureau; 1920.

EXHIBIT 3-2

DR HARVEY CUSHING'S ACCOUNT OF ROYAL ARMY MEDICAL CORPS CAPABILITIES, FLANDERS, BELGIUM, MAY 5, 1917

In normal times Bailleul—a typical old Flemish town—is a peaceful lace-making place of some 13,000 inhabitants with two old picturesque churches. But today, it is a bedlam, packed with motor cars of all kinds, though ambulances predominate, since, owing to the recent evacuation of the clearing station at Poperinghe, the burden has fallen heavily on this place. We visit only one of the several hospitals—an old monestary [monastery], where a long line of ambulances at the moment were being unloaded. Many of the field ambulances and stations have recently been targets for German shells, and there has been a very heavy "take-in," as they say, for several days. . . .

Through this single hospital 43,000 wounded have gone, and there are three other clearing hospitals in Bailleul! No wonder Colonel Gallie is busy with his trains to and from Boulogne. I looked at the men's tags to see where they had come from—that is, from what field hospital—and was again disturbed to see how flimsy, insecure, and illegible the labels were—attached to a button merely by a slit in the tag. There has been 300 "gassed" victims admitted here in the past twenty-four hours, and all told they have received 1,000 cases since this business began, with about 30 deaths—not so bad after all—at least for those who manage to get back this far.

I gather that the English system of evacuating the wounded, not unlike the French, corresponds with the printed regulations prepared before the war, except that at present there is no need of stationary intermediate hospitals between the clearing hospital and the temporary overseas base hospitals at Boulogne and Rouen. The wounded are either brought off the fields by the regimental stretcher-bearers, or else they make their own way at nightfall as best they can to a regimental aid post, which, like the poste de secours [relief posts] of the French, is merely a place of temporary refuge in a copse, a dugout, or the cellar of a ruined building somewhere. Here their first dressings are usually applied, or first aid, such as in rare instances may have been given on the field or in the trenches, is supplemented. Thence by hand cart, or some horse-drawn vehicle, or possibly even by motor, they reach a field ambulance or dressing station which, like the ones we are to visit at la Clytte, corresponds to the ambulance de premiere ligne [of the first line] of the French and is in the zone of battle. From there the wounded are taken in turn by motor ambulances to such a clearing hospital as this in Bailleul; thence by a hospital train to Boulogne; then via Boulogne-Folkstone by hospital ship to "dear old Blighty," to a hospital train again, to a general hospital somewhere, to a convalescent home, whence comes a final discharge, or back into service, as the case may be.

The main aim, of course, is rapid evacuation of wounded from France, and I am told that wounded have been known to reach St. Thomas's Hospital in London, eighteen hours after they have been in action. Yet in this particular sector, in which we are, it is a variable three miles or so from the aid station to the field ambulance, another six or seven to this clearing hospital, and about fifty-five from here to Boulogne. Of course, the character of work of a clearing hospital such as we have seen is largely one of classification and proper distribution, and though its capacity may be small, say 200 beds, 1,500 wounded may easily pass through in a day.

Reproduced from: Cushing H. *From a Surgeon's Journal, 1915–1918.* Boston, Mass: Little, Brown and Company; 1936: 66–68.

eral" or "stationary" hospitals. Their medical support rivaled that of large nonmilitary hospitals, accommodating 500 to 1,000 casualties. A few hospitals occupied large buildings, such as hotels and casinos. Although base hospitals were similarly well-equipped and managed relative to their civilian counterparts, they were highly specialized in the services they offered. For instance, at each base, one hospital dealt solely with infectious diseases, while the remainder accepted other aspects of specialty care, including dermatologic, maxillofacial, neurologic, ophthalmologic, orthopedic, and eventually chemical casualties. Nevertheless, these specialty care hospitals were always prepared to admit less-specialized casualties.[19]

When sulfur mustard made its first appearance, the British medical staff was unaware of the blistering effects of a vesicant, and most believed that the casualty presentation was linked to an infectious etiology (eg, scarlet fever). In his journal, Cushing noted his initial impressions when the new category of chemical agent appeared (Figure 3-9):

> Poor devils [mustard gas victims]! I've seen too many of them since–new ones–their eyes bandaged, led along by a man with a string while they try to keep to the duckboards [narrow planks laid on top of the mud]. Some of the after-effects are as extraordinary as they are horrible—the sloughing of the genitals,

EXHIBIT 3-3

EXCERPT FROM "TAKE ME BACK TO DEAR OLD BLIGHTY!"—A POPULAR BRITISH WARTIME SONG

Take me back to dear old Blighty!
Put me on the train for London town!
Take me over there,
Drop me ANYWHERE,
Liverpool, Leeds, or Birmingham, well, I don't care!
I should love to see my best girl,
Cuddling up again we soon should be,
WHOA!!!
Tiddley iddley ighty,
Hurry me home to Blighty,
Blighty is the place for me!

Reproduced from: Mills AJ, Godfrey F, Scott B. *Take Me Back To Dear Old Blighty.* London, England: Chappell Music; 1916.

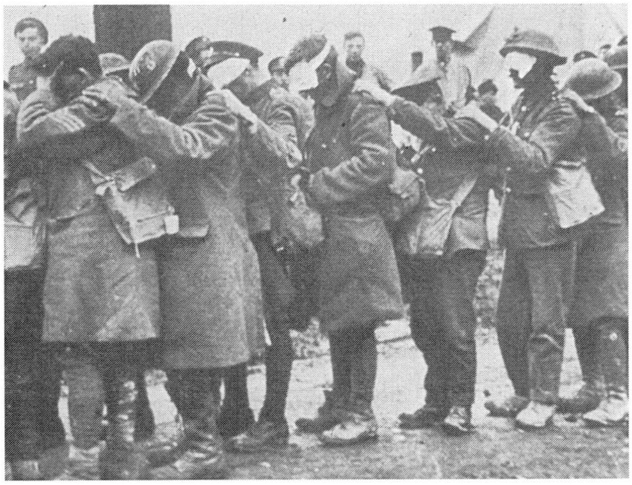

Fig. 3-9. This photograph is frequently held to show the inhumanity of chemical warfare; however, very few mustard casualties developed permanent eye injuries, let alone blindness.
Reproduced with permission from: Marshall SLA. *American Heritage History of World War I.* New York: NY: Simon and Schuster; 1964: 167.

for example. They had about twenty fatalities out of the first 1,000 cases, chiefly from bronchial troubles. Fortunately vision does not appear to be often lost.[14]

American Expeditionary Forces Medical Organization

Faced with the need to respond rapidly to the chemical battlefield, the AEF based its medical support organization on the British system. On June 13, 1917, while the general staff in the United States struggled to organize, staff, and equip an army, General John J Pershing, commander of the AEF, and his personnel arrived and settled in Paris, followed by the first American troops several weeks later. General Order No. 8, published on July 5, 1917, established the organization of the AEF general headquarters, including the "chief of the gas service."[22] The medical division originated in July 1917 when the Bureau of Mines established a laboratory for the study of toxic gases at Yale in New Haven, Connecticut, at the urging of Dr Yandell Henderson, an expert on oxygen rescue equipment. The laboratory was staffed by several scientists from around the country.[23]

On July 24, 1917, the chief of staff ordered the Medical Department to provide nine officers as instructors for a gas defense school to be organized at the infantry school of musketry at Fort Sill, Oklahoma. As a result, the Medical Department was tasked with conducting defensive gas training, placing MOs without gas warfare experience in charge of training other MOs for duty as instructors (Table 3-3).[24]

On August 17, 1917, General Pershing sent a cable to Washington requesting the organization of a gas service and the authority to appoint Lieutenant Colonel Amos A Fries of the Corps of Engineers as its chief (Figure 3-10). On August 22 Fries began building an organization based on specialized British and French units. Additionally, staff officers gave Fries a draft of a proposed General Order No. 31, which established

TABLE 3-3

MAJOR DEFENSIVE CAMPAIGNS OF THE AMERICAN EXPEDITIONARY FORCES, 1918

Dates	Campaign
March 21–April 6	Somme Defensive
April 9–April 27	Lys Defensive
May 27–June 5	Aisne Defensive (Chatieau-Thierry, Belleau Wood, Vaux)
June 9–June 13	Montdidier-Noyon Defensive
July 15–July 18	Champagne-Marne Defensive (Second Battle of Marne)

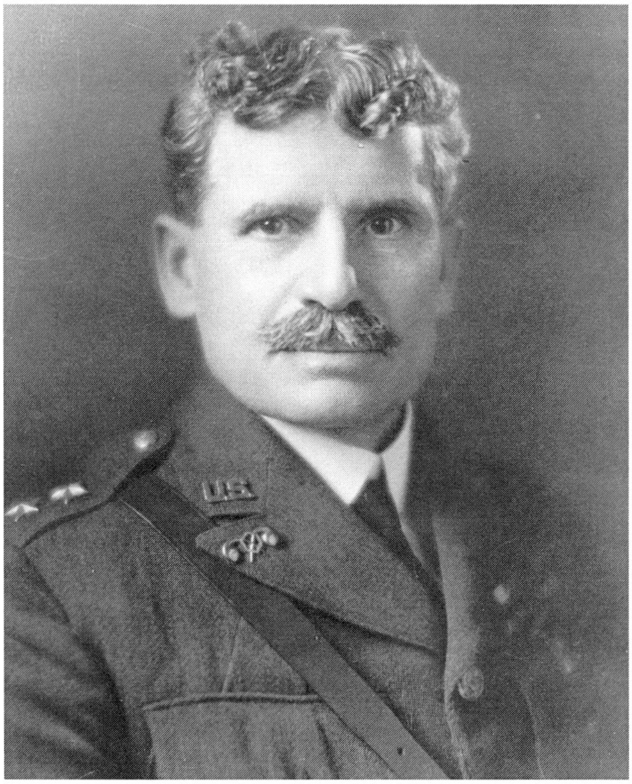

Fig. 3-10. Lieutenant Colonel Amos A Fries, shown here as a major general, was instrumental in organizing the chemical warfare service as it evolved in France.
Photograph: Courtesy of Chemical and Biological Defense Command Historical Research and Response Team, Aberdeen Proving Ground, Md.

a gas service responsible for both offensive and defensive operations, including gas personnel, gas warfare training, and gas warfare logistics in the AEF.[25]

On August 31 the surgeon general created a gas defense service composed of three sections: field supply, overseas repair, and training. He placed a Medical Corps officer in command and filled the staff with members of the Medical Department's Sanitary Corps (the equivalent of today's Medical Service Corps). The officers had no chemical warfare doctrine to guide them; only two existing War Department publications could be of use: *Notes on Gas as a Weapon in Modern War* and *Memorandum on Gas Poisoning in Warfare with Notes on its Pathology and Treatment*, both provided by the Army War College. These documents appeared to have borrowed extensively from French and British gas warfare doctrine.[26]

The US Army's CWS was established on May 11, 1918, with Major General William L Sibert as the first chief. The CWS's overseas division was known as the Gas Service, and Major JR Church was its first medical director in France. Church had assisted in the initial planning for the Gas Service, and as medical director he devoted most of his time to organizational matters. The increase in gas casualties, however, resulted in a personnel change in the position, with Lieutenant Colonel Harry L Gilchrist replacing Church (Figure 3-11). Gilchrist prepared for his new assignment by attending the British gas school in Rouen, France.[23,27]

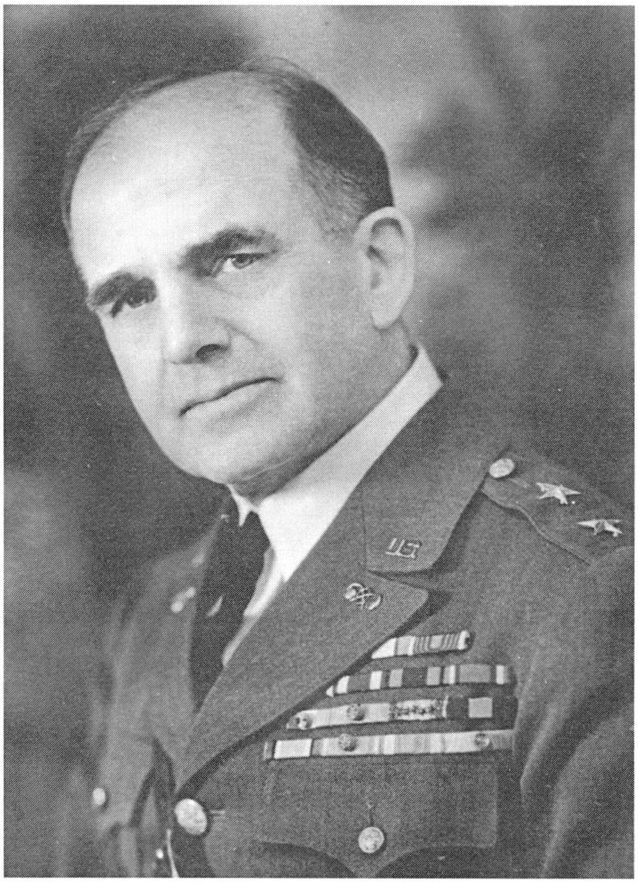

Fig. 3-11. Lieutenant Colonel Harry L Gilchrist (1870–1943), shown here as a major general in the Chemical Corps, was a preeminent figure in the history of the US Army's medical management of chemical casualties. As a Medical Corps officer, he was the second medical director of the Gas Service (overseas component) of the American Expeditionary Forces (AEF) in France in 1917–1918. He was responsible for the evolution of chemical casualty care within the AEF in Europe. Later, at Edgewood Arsenal in Maryland, he taught Medical Corps officers a course in the medical management of chemical casualties. Eventually, he transferred to the Chemical Corps, serving as its chief from 1929 to 1934.
Photograph: Courtesy of Chemical and Biological Defense Command Historical Research and Response Team, Aberdeen Proving Ground, Md.

Finding nothing to define his position when he reported for duty, Gilchrist made his first priority to spearhead chemical casualty management education for AEF MOs. On February 9, 1918, Gilchrist published a pamphlet titled "Symptomology, Pathology and General Treatment of Gas Cases," containing basic information on the medical management of chemical casualties. Following this publication, the medical director's office issued a constant stream of bulletins aimed at keeping AEF MOs current on the latest medical developments in chemical warfare. Gilchrist visited most AEF divisions and hospitals, where he lectured on chemical warfare from a medical perspective, emphasizing the prevention and treatment of chemical casualties (Figure 3-12). Gilchrist also visited the sites of battles where large numbers of gas casualties had occurred, as well as hospitals, hospital trains, and other locations, comparing their efficiency and relaying his findings to both the Gas Service chief and the Medical Department. He also assisted medical researchers in developing new treatment techniques for chemical casualties. His approach emphasized combating the effects of enemy chemicals therapeutically and prophylactically.[27]

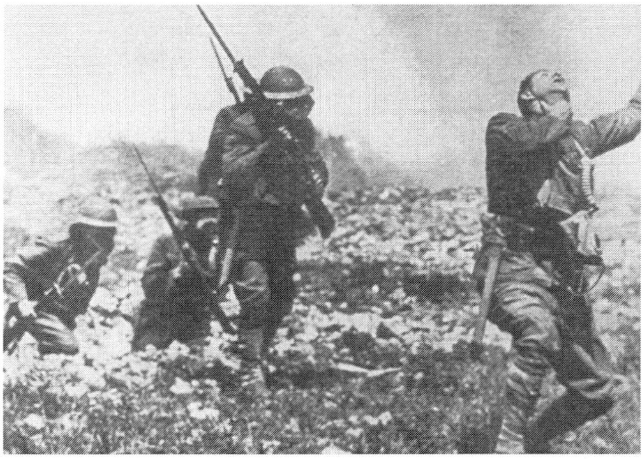

Fig. 3-12. In this posed instructional picture of a World War I gas attack, the soldier on the right has removed his small box respirator and is inhaling poison gas. This photograph reminds soldiers that removing their masks in the presence of chemical agents leads to injury. Gilchrist pointed this out in 1928: "Investigation showed that these casualties were caused by general lack of gas discipline. It was found that the standing order that 'Men will not remove the mask until ordered to do so by an officer' was absolutely disregarded by practically all units affected, and that fully 75 per cent of the casualties were due to the disobedience of this order, casualties which efficient training and discipline would have prevented."1 Gas mask discipline was the key to low chemical casualty rates in the face of chemical weapons.
(1) Gilchrist HL. *A Comparative Study of World War Casualties from Gas and Other Weapons*. Edgewood Arsenal, Md: Chemical Warfare School; 1928: 16.
Reproduced from: Moore WE, Crussell J. US Official Pictures of the World War. Washington, DC: Pictorial Bureau; 1920.

When the AEF's 1st Division began encountering German chemical attacks, no actions were initially taken to provide division medics with additional training in the treatment of chemical casualties, and they were unprepared to handle the sudden influx of chemical victims. In the confusion of organizing and placing an American army in combat, it took the AEF until October 1918 to establish a uniform procedure to handle chemical casualties.[19,28]

Because the AEF division was on the ground long before the evolution of the corps and army organizational structure, the medical structure to treat chemical casualties first evolved within the division. Later, when the AEF army and corps evolved, so did their medical organization. On March 1, 1918, the 42nd Division became the second American division to occupy a sector on the western front. Although initially the division had few chemical casualties, the divisional MOs prepared for a large influx of victims. All four of the division's field hospitals were set up to accept chemical casualties, with a total of 500 beds dedicated to such cases.[29]

At 5:30 PM on March 20, approximately 400 German mustard rounds landed on a position held by the division's 165th Infantry.[30] In the space of a few minutes, the vesicant caused 270 casualties, including one death. The initial aid station through which the casualties passed also became secondarily contaminated with chemicals. Medical personnel had to wear masks as they treated the casualties.[31,32] The weather conditions enhanced the agent's persistence; it had rained earlier and there was no breeze to dissipate the vesicant as it hung in the air. At midnight, soldiers began to suffer delayed effects. One company (Company K) lost two thirds of its effectives. A week later, Gilchrist reported 417 gas casualties from the 165th Infantry at a base hospital.[30]

As the intensity of fighting increased, so did the number of chemical casualties. Medical organization systems became taxed. Many shell-shocked soldiers suffering from exhaustion and hunger believed themselves to be chemical casualties. Some panicked after smelling shell fumes, reporting themselves gassed, and some feigned being gassed. "The symptomology of gas poisoning is so complex," observed Major William V Sommervell, a gas officer of the 3rd Division, "and at the same time so indefinite" that anyone who claimed to be gassed was immediately processed to the rear.[24(p65)] One division field hospital commander established a board to review the 251 chemical casualties in his wards. The board's report indicated that only 90 were truly chemical casualties.[24]

Division medical personnel devised several techniques to detect and thwart suspected malingerers. Because front line troops were observed to always be hungry and true chemical casualties presented with decreased appetite, one approach was to offer the alleged chemical casualty a large meal. A "chemical casualty" who devoured the food was promptly returned to the fight. Medical personnel also offered suspected malingerers a cigarette laced with diphosgene; gagging was a sign the soldier was pretending to be poisoned.[24]

As a result of continued chemical attacks, the 42nd Division, second only to the 1st Infantry Division as the most experienced American combat division of the AEF, took several measures to improve the management of chemical casualties. These measures became the standard for all AEF divisions on the line. The first measure was to dedicate one of the four division field hospitals to chemical cases. The position of a division gas MO was also created. The 42nd Division published Memorandum No. 148 on April 23, 1918, listing this officer as the instructor of medical personnel in gas defense. The gas MO also supervised gas protection of the medical dugouts, aid stations, and field hospitals, and made an early diagnosis of symptoms to treat all types of gas casualties.[32]

The AEF adopted the 42nd Division's practices when it instituted the position of division gas MO for all AEF divisions (General Order No. 144, dated August 29, 1918[33]). General headquarters took this measure in the face of mounting chemical casualties and a high incidence of related malingering throughout the AEF. As a consequence, in addition to the gas MO duties indicated in Memorandum No. 148, the AEF ordered additional duties, such as instructing all division personnel on the early symptoms and treatments of gas poisoning and instructing line officers in practical medical matters connected with chemical warfare. The orders stated that selected officers must be "live, wide-awake, energetic men, and must show a keen appreciation of the work." By the first week in October 1918, each AEF division had a gas MO who was sent to the University of Paris' gas school for a 4-day course in preparation for division duties.[24,33]

The AEF organized the First Army in the fall of 1918. The general direction of the medical service was then executed by the chief surgeon of the AEF.[34] At the level of the field army, the chief surgeon performed as an advisory officer and established the following administrative divisions: hospitalization, sanitation and statistics, personnel, supplies, records and correspondence, and gas service.[35]

Specialization was one of the issues addressed early by the chief surgeon. Specialized hospitals required many teams of personnel, including those trained to function as gas teams. These teams were usually organized from the personnel of the field hospitals themselves or were obtained from other Medical Department units of the division.

Some AEF hospitals were new and had not seen active service in combat before July 1918. Most of the mobile hospitals had been organized and equipped in Paris during July and August, and several of the evacuation hospitals did not reach France until shortly before the Saint Mihiel offensive. Although every available hospital unit in France was assembled, the inexperience of some and the limited equipment of others caused considerable apprehension about the adequacy of medical support.[36]

In the defensive position, the front line was usually little more than a line of lightly held outposts, with the remainder of the troops supporting trenches or in reserve. Sometimes, as in the 5th Division in the Vosges, a battalion held a frontage of 5 km (3 miles).[28] One battalion surgeon was usually on duty with the advance troops, while the other was in charge of the battalion aid station. Two medics were normally assigned to each company at the front and staffed what was, in effect, a company aid post located at some sheltered point and near a communicating trench to the rear.[37,38]

Company Aid Posts

The company aid post was frequently provided with equipment such as litters, splints, bandages, dressings, whale oil, sodium bicarbonate, and a few drugs. The medics were ordered to promptly adjust the respirators of chemical casualties. Those disabled on the front line were habitually brought to the company aid post (if necessary, on litters carried by company bearers), except when their wounds had been dressed where they fell and it was easier to remove them directly to a battalion aid station.[39,40]

Battalion Aid Stations

At the battalion aid station, chemical casualties were stripped of contaminated clothing, bathed, and reclothed. Normally there was one battalion aid station for each battalion, located near the communication trench to the rear in a support trench from 240 to 500 yards from the front, utilizing any shelter available.[41] One room in the aid station was for receiving casualties, one was for applying dressings and administering treatment for shock, one was for the battalion surgeon, one was for medical logistics, and one or more were for the station personnel. The aid station could accommodate 30 casualties, but rarely received more than 12.[37,38] A separate dugout at one side typically contained two rooms for the bathing, emergency treatment, and reclothing of chemical casualties. The doors to the dugouts were generally 3 feet wide and were protected by two tight-fitting blanket curtains placed at least 8 feet apart. The curtains, soaked with alkaline, glycerin, or sometimes hexamethylenamine solution, were adjusted so they would fall into place upon engaging a release. The first curtain was intended to be shut before the second was opened. It was hoped that the curtains would sufficiently gas-proof the dugout. A hand-pumped fire extinguisher filled with a sodium thiosulfate solution was used to neutralize chlorine (Figure 3-13).[20,21,37]

However, gas-proofing with two blankets made it difficult to rapidly exit a dugout, so early US manuals advised against gas-proofing front line dugouts. This advice was generally unheeded because the advantage of having a chemical-free environment in which to sleep and occasionally remove protective masks outweighed the risk. The same Army manual stated that

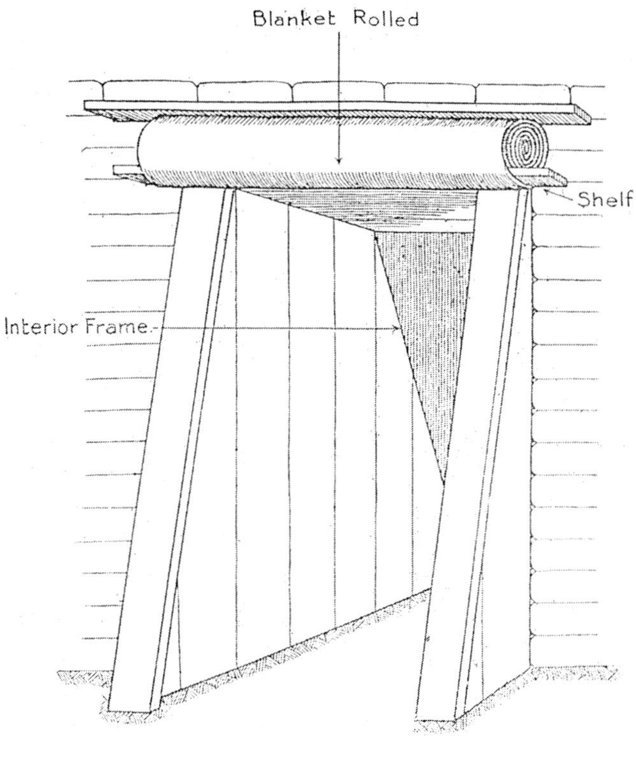

Fig. 3-13. Early attempts at collective protection during World War I included the dugout blanket, which was used to cover the doorways to dugouts.
Reproduced from: Army War College. *Methods of Defense against Gas Attacks.* Vol 2. In: *Gas Warfare.* Washington, DC: War Department; 1918.

"medical aid-posts and advanced dressing stations; Company, Regiment, and Brigade Headquarters; at least one dugout per battery position; Signal Shelters and any other place where work has to be carried out during a gas attack should always be protected."[20,21]

The personnel on duty at a battalion aid station normally consisted of an MO, a dental officer if available, and from four to six medics. These were often supplemented by two runners and a litter squad assigned from an ambulance company. The number of litter squads was increased if unusual activity was anticipated and equipment and supplies to support casualty respiration were necessary. Battalion equipment beyond that furnished by logistics tables included equipment for managing chemical casualties, such as two 500-L oxygen tanks, suits of overalls, gloves, and masks for attendants caring for chemical casualties, gas fans, alkalis, and sprayers used to clean out the galleries that chemical agents had penetrated.[42]

Aid stations were established in banked earth, abandoned cellars, or dugouts because in the offensive phase there was no time to construct elaborate shelters. For the most part, the aid stations were small, dimly lit, and poorly ventilated. Medical personnel on duty in the aid stations were continually exposed to off-gassing from the chemical casualties. When hospital facilities were limited, one small building was used for dressing purposes and another for treating chemical casualties. After treatment, casualties were managed in tents or on litters in the open.[40]

In the absence of sufficient equipment and water, an effective method was developed for bathing chemical casualties. Under a shelter, rows of inclined planes were constructed by placing litters on wooden trestles of unequal height. The litters were covered with rubber blankets that drained into buckets at their lower ends. Above, suspended from wires, were flushers for the eyes, nose, and ears. Watering pots containing a strong soap (alkaline) solution were used for the face. The staff was protected by chemical protective clothing and gloves.[43] At some hospitals, only selected casualties could be bathed and given special mouth and eye treatment because of water restrictions. Care at the battalion aid station was similar to that given at equivalent stations in the trenches: wounds were redressed and splints were adjusted, if necessary; hemorrhage was checked; and shock was controlled as much as possible. Chemical casualties were given as much relief as practicable.

Ambulance Company Dressing Station

At the minimum, the functions of an ambulance company dressing station were to receive, triage, and treat casualties (control hemorrhage, treat shock, and process chemical casualties). As in the British system, the ambulance dressing station was established at the farthest point forward that ambulances could reach with reasonable safety. Casualties were selected for evacuation to supporting hospitals at the ambulance dressing station.[30] Supported by an ambulance service, casualties were transported directly to the appropriate hospital. A regulating station was often operated in conjunction with the dressing station, and ambulances were parked nearby.[44]

Routes to dressing stations were often shelled and bombed, so ambulances began carrying chemical defense equipment. The following articles were added to the regulation equipment of the 42nd Division: coats (gas, 2 each); masks (M2 French, 4 each); mittens (gas, 2 each); and small oxygen tanks with connectors (4 each). The 42nd Division also provided three gas-proof shelters for dressing stations from 2.5 to 3 miles behind the front, each accommodating 20 casualties, with facilities for bathing and treating shock, hemorrhage, and other symptoms.[29]

The number of dressing stations in a division rear area varied from one to three, according to the width and activity of the sector. Organization of the dressing station varied considerably, being most elaborate in the comparatively few divisions that used this formation as a triage station. The station consisted of specific departments involved in chemical casualty management.[29] Casualties arrived at a receiving and forwarding department divided into two sections that addressed triage and transportation. The personnel conducting triage were, in part, the divisional consultants (eg, the divisional chief of surgery or a representative, orthopedist, psychiatrist, urologist, tuberculosis expert, and gas treatment officer).[37]

Chemical casualties, triaged into the first classification along with miscellaneous sickness, psychic disorders, venereal diseases, skin diseases, and convalescents, were separated. The gas department was located in an isolation room for wound-dressing purposes. Here, under direction of the divisional gas officer, chemical casualties were stripped, bathed, and clothed with such attire as could be obtained from the salvage section. Some chemical casualties found their way into the second classification, which ranged from malingerers to those with fatal wounds. The sick, the gassed, and those suffering from gas fright were classified as "seriously disabled," and were immediately evacuated or retained until they stabilized. In the 1st Division, dressing-station supplies were supplemented by additional chemical defense supplies, such as "antigas" suits and gloves and sodium bicarbonate (for vesicants).[45]

Division Triage Stations

Each division of the First Army established a triage station that received, classified, and distributed evacuees. Medical specialty personnel, including the division gas MO, were assigned to each triage station. Divisions triaged a large number of casualties classified as "war neuroses," varying from shell-shock cases to shell fright, gas fright, hysteria, mental and physical fatigue, malingering, and cowardice.[38] Many division hospitals employed a psychiatrist to assist with differentiating these cases.

The organization for managing chemical casualties was specific. A corps medical gas officer served as a specialty officer to the corps surgeon. As with all specialty officers, the gas officer circulated constantly throughout the divisions within the corps to aid in chemical casualty management and was responsible for supervising the division medical gas officer.[46]

Evacuation Hospitals

The evacuation hospital was located near outbound transportation routes such as paved roads or railheads. The preferable location was as close to the front as possible, yet safe from direct or indirect artillery fire—usually a distance of 15 to 25 kilometers (9 to 15 miles) from the line.[47] Mobile hospitals, including supplemental Red Cross base hospitals, were often provided for personnel. Supplementary professional groups provided for special patients in the evacuation hospitals, namely contagious, neurological, and chemical casualties. Sometimes special wards for these patients were set aside in the hospital. A registrar recorded, among other things, daily gas casualties. Chemical casualties were classified, if possible, according to the kind of chemical agent used. The classification for all patients was made according to the condition from which patients were suffering, whether they were sent out recumbent or sitting, and whether they were commissioned or enlisted. Chemical casualties could fall into any of these categories.[48]

Other than administration, distinct departments of an evacuation hospital provided specific services. Included among the receiving ward, dressing tent, preoperative ward, radiograph room, examination room, operating rooms, sterilizing room, pharmacy, laboratory, dental clinic, and shock ward were the wards for special casualties, including medical, surgical, and chemical casualties. Chemical casualties were classified as medical and were sent to the appropriate wards or to neighboring units that provided for such patients exclusively.[48,49] If casualties were retained and their conditions warranted, they were sent to their destinations via the bathhouse. There, chemical casualties were treated or bathed with alkaline soap and solution. Otherwise they were bathed in the ward. Retained patients were furnished with pajamas; evacuated patients and those returned to duty were given fresh clothing and sent to the evacuation ward.[48]

Base and Gas Hospitals

The organization of gas teams at base hospitals was authorized by the AEF's chief surgeon on June 2, 1918. Each team consisted of an officer, two nurses, and two enlisted soldiers. A course on degassing instruction was provided at the central laboratory at Dijon for officers designated to perform degassing service.[50] The gas team's mission was established as an additional duty. If the hospital received chemical casualties, degassing teams (usually three soldiers) were organized under the chief of the medical service but were under the direct supervision of another officer. Degassing teams were relatively permanent and functioned like receiving and evacuating departments.[51]

Gas hospitals had to support special treatment for chemical casualties. They were located near a water source because persistent and even nonpersistent agents clung to clothing, hair, and skin. The 2nd Division's gas hospital bath house had a portable heater and six shower heads. After admission to a hospital, soldiers stripped off their clothing and showered. Casualties with serious symptoms were bathed while still on litters. When soldiers left the showers, medics sprayed their eyes, noses, and throats with bicarbonate of soda. Depending on the diagnosis, patients might be given a special treatment of alkaline, oxygen, and, if necessary, venesection to counteract the effects of inhaled gas. Doctors prescribed olive or castor oil to coat the irritated stomach linings of soldiers who had ingested food or water contaminated by gas. When treatment failed to allow free breathing or when patients developed additional symptoms, medics immediately evacuated them to a base gas hospital.[24] Because of the shortage of medical personnel, ambulance personnel were often temporarily used to relieve overworked and understaffed gas hospitals.[52]

Division Field Hospitals

When possible, division field hospitals were located in the same general area as base and gas hospitals, with one hospital officially designated to handle chemical casualties. Soldiers were placed into one of the following categories: severely gassed (immediate or expectant); fit for duty, immediate return to unit (minimal); fit for duty in 24 hours, return to unit (delayed); or evacuate to an Army hospital. Exhausted soldiers who complained of gas symptoms but who showed no outward signs of having been gassed were held in the division rear for rest, food, and observation. If medics verified their claims of gas poisoning, they were evacuated.[32] In open warfare, field hospitals were usually located from 4.8 to 9.6 km (3 to 6 miles) from the front. This site was often determined on the basis of the routes of ingress and egress. Because in open warfare field hospitals had a paucity of fixed structures, they often operated out of tents. In many divisions, field hospitals were so near the front that they were easy targets for enemy shells.[53]

Although by design field hospitals were specialized, they were expected to care for casualties outside specializations, as seen in the May 16 report of Field Hospital No. 2, which was managing 3 sick and 189 chemical casualties (98%). Field Hospital No. 3 reportedly managed 123 sick and wounded and 159 chemical casualties (56%), Field Hospital No. 12 managed 24 sick and wounded and 43 chemical casualties (64%), and Field Hospital No. 13 managed 37 sick and wounded and 37 chemical casualties (50%).[54]

Casualties began arriving at division field hospitals shortly after the onset of the Aisne-Marne offensive in July 1918. From July 22 to August 11, one ambulance company evacuated 1,860 casualties, including medical personnel, of which four were chemical casualties. The field hospital at Ville Chamblon received chemical casualties of the 3rd Division, but only a few of these were severely affected; most of the chemical casualties that initially arrived were sneezing or vomiting from gas intoxication (riot control agents). Phosgene casualties presented later. Mustard casualties began to appear after German counterattacks.[55]

During the summer and fall of 1918, the Second Corps fought with the British in Flanders in two phases. The corps made its medical personnel familiar with conditions in the British section of the western front, providing lectures and practical demonstrations that covered the medical management of chemical casualties, methods employed for transporting the wounded, the selection and operation of lines of evacuation, the treatment of water for drinking purposes, and related topics.[56] By September 1918 the field hospitals of the 2nd Division had become specialized, and the permanent triage station carried portable baths with both tubs and showers, gas soap, soda, and extra pajamas and underwear for reissue. The remaining field hospital was equipped to medically manage chemical casualties.[57]

With the reduction of the Saint Mihiel salient, the front became so vast and the objectives so diverse that a single army could no longer manage alone, so the

AEF created the Second Army. By mid October 1918, chemical casualty management was becoming more routine. The Fourth Corps' Field Hospital No. 34 (the triage station) received 3,121 patients, including 935 chemical casualties (30%), while it operated at the front. Field Hospital No. 35 practiced routine chemical casualty management for all chemical casualties who had not been treated at the dressing stations. These casualties were undressed by personnel wearing protective ensembles. Chemical casualties' eyes were treated with a saturated solution of boric acid or a 1% solution of sodium bicarbonate, followed by liquid petrolatum. Casualties were then transferred to rooms where they were bathed first with soap and water and then with a 2% solution of sodium bicarbonate. They were dried, warmed, given hot drinks, and taken to a ward. After receiving treatment, patients usually slept for 24 hours.[58]

In the Third Corps, two companies of the 1st Gas Regiment were assigned in support of offensive chemical operations. Chemical casualties were to be sent to the gas hospital at Souhesme le Grande.[59] The few chemical casualties from corps troops were sent to an improvised gas hospital at Rambluzin.[60] In the 4th Division, one field hospital was located as far forward as possible to receive, classify, and distribute all patients from the front. A field hospital for the primary treatment of chemical casualties and one that received slightly gassed and doubtful cases were nearby. The gas hospital was augmented with a mobile degassing unit.[39]

Experience on the eastern border of the Argonne Forest demonstrated the difficulty of carrying "antigas" medical equipment to the forwardly positioned battalion aid stations, as well as the impracticality of administering antigas treatment to patients in these exposed areas. The nearest point at which such treatment could be given effectively was the more rearward dressing station. Even there, only the most acute management could be addressed. It was observed that, in many cases, chemically contaminated clothing could be removed at a dressing station, thereby preparing the chemical casualty for "clean" evacuation to the field hospital, where more elaborate antigas equipment was available.[45] The commanding officer of Field Hospital No. 328 gave the following description of his establishment at Apremont:

> The hospital in the forest 1 km southwest of Apremont was situated back about 200 yards from the main highway and connected with it by an excellent road. It occupied nine wooden buildings, a large dugout, and an abandoned ward tent. All, in excellent condition, were wired for electricity and provided with many modern conveniences. A complete laboratory and dispensary were found intact. The immediate vicinity of the hospital was strewn with equipment, dead horses, and a few dead men. During the first 24 hours 480 patients were admitted and evacuated.
>
> On October 13 Field Hospital 326 joined to act as a gas hospital, operating under canvas. With the exception of a lull of three days, the two following weeks saw an endless procession of wounded. The great majority of these were only slightly wounded and able to walk, with the result that the two wards set apart for these cases were exceptionally busy. The heaviest days were October 15–18, when the admissions and evacuations averaged one patient every one and a half minutes.[61(p34)]

Withdrawing German forces often used persistent agents to deny terrain and contaminate personnel and equipment. To handle the resulting casualties, field hospital personnel performing triage were given guidance on how to establish a departmental "gas group." It was suggested that the following personnel comprise a triage group that would work a 12-hour shift: two MOs, two noncommissioned officers, two clerks, one stenographer, twelve litter bearers, two soldiers for kitchen detail, one ward attendant for each patient tent, and two soldiers for the dispensary and dressing room (Figure 3-14).[62]

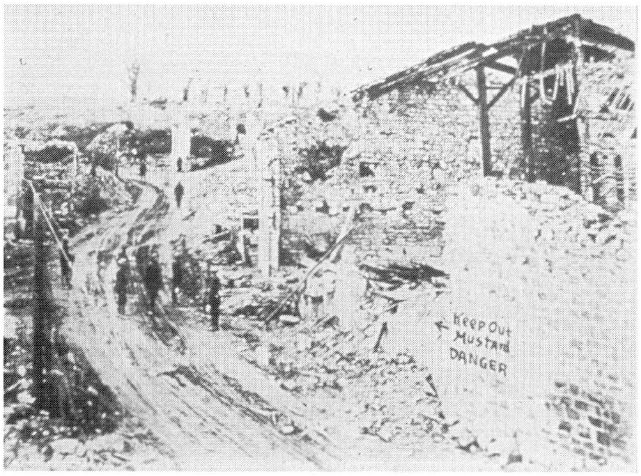

Fig. 3-14. This photograph from Gilchrist's study of World War I gas casualties has the following figure legend: "War photograph–An old ruin heavily contaminated with mustard. Warning sign on ruin; place guarded by troops to prevent entrance." Often contaminated sites were not so clearly identified.
Reproduced from: Gilchrist HL. *A Comparative Study of World War Casualties from Gas and Other Weapons*. Edgewood Arsenal, Md: Chemical Warfare School; 1928: 26.

Army-Level Hospitals

Beyond the division field hospitals, each army established its own army-level gas hospitals. The first such installation began operation on August 29, 1918. Army-level hospital personnel were casuals, or officers and enlisted personnel loaned from base or evacuation hospitals or anywhere else medical personnel could be found. To meet the demands of the Meuse-Argonne offensive, the AEF's chief surgeon established five army-level gas hospitals with a total of 1,650 beds. Colonel Gilchrist suggested three mobile 1,500-bed gas hospitals be established, one for each US corps. This plan, however, was never implemented because of insufficient personnel. Another plan called for the creation of two "emergency gas teams" to be assigned to each base hospital. The mission of these teams was to "relieve the strain" that sudden chemical attacks put on division field hospitals. The AEF general headquarters organized several emergency gas teams, each consisting of an MO, two nurses, and two orderlies. The chief surgeon of the First Army, Colonel AN Stark, however, objected to these teams on the grounds that base hospitals were too far removed from the fighting; he believed that the division field hospitals set aside for chemical casualties were sufficient. Heeding Stark's objections, the chief surgeon disbanded the teams.[24]

On August 2, 1918, a hospital center was organized west of Toul in the area called Le Rue Justice, near a railhead. The Justice Hospital Group was formed in part to meet the needs imposed by the Saint Mihiel operation, including managing chemical casualties. The provisional gas hospital was based at the Annex Caserne La Marche and was equipped with 650 beds. With the exception of Caserne Luxembourg, these barracks were situated close together on the Rue Justice, about 1.6 km (1 mile) from the center of the city of Toul.[24]

Base Hospital No. 51 arrived in Toul on August 27 tasked to treat gas casualties. It was located near Evacuation Hospital No. 14 in a centralized group of four-story barracks and other buildings. These hospitals were prepared to receive chemical casualties and were provided with some supplies from French stores. Casualties were admitted to a receiving ward, where an MO sorted them into the following three classes: (1) walking wounded (sent to the dressing room), (2) gassed and medical cases (sent to special wards), and (3) wounded on litters (the majority; sent to a second triage or preoperative ward). These patients received 80% of the professional care given in the hospital.[63]

Although the Justice Hospital Group's provisional gas hospital was formed to support the Saint Mihiel offensive, its personnel initially consisted of 3 permanent officers, 6 other officers, 14 nurses, 9 medical noncommissioned officers, and 50 soldiers from the training battalion depot at Saint Aignan. Forty more soldiers from that battalion joined on September 19. The gas hospital occupied the part of Caserne La Marche originally constructed for hospital purposes and used in peace time by the French as a hospital for the local garrison, so the buildings were perhaps better suited for hospital purposes than were other buildings of the Toul group.[64]

The four buildings gave adequate provision for the designated 650 patients, with suitable rooms for logistical stores and service. A Bessonneau tent was used as a receiving ward and sorting station. A screened-off section provided for the immediate administration of oxygen or treatment by phlebotomy for casualties intoxicated by phosgene, and mustard gas casualties were sent to a building equipped with two French portable bathing machines supplied with running water (the marked shock of phosgene casualties and the sloughing of the respiratory mucosa of mustard casualties were the most pronounced symptoms in chemical casualties). Other buildings were used for an officers' ward, a place to treat mild vesicant casualties, and rooms for convalescents recovering from the effects of phosgene. From September 10 to October 7, 1918, the unit admitted 1,336 medical and 1,351 gas cases.[64]

Evacuation Methods

The corps medical evacuation methods varied considerably between and within each corps, depending on the tactical situation (Exhibit 3-4, Figure 3-15). For example, in the 42nd Division, casualties were carried from the front line trenches by regimental medical personnel or by combat troops from the place of injury to the battalion aid post. There, casualty cards, called "diagnosis tags," were attached by the first MO or medic who treated the casualty. The forward-deployed medical personnel learned quickly to construct gas-proof dugouts in casualty care areas. This was essential for survival in a static defensive trench warfare scenario because of the prolonged nature of the attacks and the extensive employment of chemical agents. Casualties treated at aid posts were carried by litter bearers detailed from the ambulance section to the ambulance dressing station, which was located with a main dressing station.[65]

In some instances, facilities permitting, chemical casualties were separated from other wounded soldiers.[65] The ambulance crews that brought chemical casualties to the advanced dressing stations needed appropriate chemical defense equipment. Extra gas masks were

EXHIBIT 3-4

HEADQUARTERS, FIRST ARMY CORPS, MEMORANDUM ON THE EVACUATION OF SICK AND WOUNDED, 1918

Memorandum: Evacuation sick and wounded.

The following plan of evacuation of sick and wounded for each division in the corps will be put into effect at once.

AMBULANCE DRESSING STATION

. . .

2. At this ambulance dressing station will be stationed the following medical officers in addition to the personnel of the ambulance section conducting the station: division psychiatrist, division orthopedist, division medical gas officer, and a medical officer with good surgical experience and judgment. Each of these officers should have an understudy who can relieve him when necessary to secure rest or food.

****

6. The division medical gas officer will examine all gassed patients, returning to the front line all deemed fit for duty. He will return to the rear all that require hospitalization. He will also supervise the preliminary gas treatment at this point. Bathing facilities will be provided so that mustard gas patients will get the earliest possible attention and thus prevent subsequent burning.

****

8. In past experience during open warfare, it has been found that large numbers of men return from the front diagnosed as shell shock or gas casualties. The great majority of these men present neither of the above conditions, but are simply exhausted, mentally and physically. They are disabled for the time being, but should not be sent to evacuation hospitals. They must be held in divisional sanitary organizations, given the necessary food, a bath when possible, and an opportunity to thoroughly rest. It will be found that within one to four days they will be able to return to full duty at the front, thus saving a very marked loss of man power when the maintenance of the man power of a division at its full strength is most important. Any such subsequently developing serious symptoms will at once be transferred to an evacuation hospital.

9. During active operations when the number of casualties becomes very large, it will be found that the available ambulance transportation will be entirely insufficient to carry all wounded to the rear and to prevent congestion of wounded in the front areas. It therefore is necessary for division surgeons to maintain liaison with the division motor transport officer and to secure the use of as many trucks as possible to carry back slightly wounded and gassed patients. Severely wounded and gassed must be carried in ambulances only. The corps surgeon will give every possible assistance to division surgeons during such periods of stress and will utilize for this purpose all available ambulances within the corps.

FIELD HOSPITALS

. . .

3. The field hospital will be utilized as follows: (a) Gas hospital, and (b) one hospital in reserve.

4. Gas hospitals: One field hospital will be utilized as a gas hospital. To this hospital will be sent from the triage all patients who have been gassed. Therefore, facilities must be provided to give them the necessary special treatment required—proper bathing, alkaline treatment, administration of oxygen and, if necessary, venesection. As soon as the necessary treatment has been given and their condition permits, such patients as require further hospitalization will be sent to the nearest evacuation hospital. However, during open warfare, it will be found as noted before that the majority of gassed patients or the so-called gassed, will not require anything beyond a few days' rest, sleep, and food. These must not be sent to evacuation hospitals but must be retained until fit for duty (provided this does not require more than four days) and then returned to the line. At this hospital, there will also be installed a shock table for the treatment of those needing shock treatment at this point.

****

7. One field hospital in reserve: This will be used to give assistance where needed both in personnel and equipment. A detail of 1 medical officer and 10 enlisted men will be sent to the ambulance dressing station to give the necessary preliminary bathing and alkaline treatment to patients with mustard gas burns as may be deemed necessary by the division medical gas officer on duty at this station.

Reproduced from: Lynch C, Ford J, Weed F. *Field Operations*. Vol 8. In: *The Medical Department of the United States Army in the World War*. Washington, DC: Government Printing Office; 1925. Chapter 18.

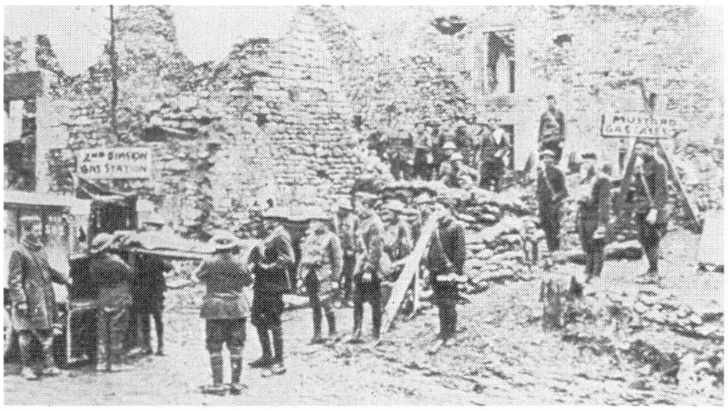

Fig. 3-15. This photograph from Gilchrist's study of WW I gas casualties has the following figure legend: "War photograph: Special gas aid station for administering to gas casualties. Here cases suffering from different gases were, when possible, segregated." The lack of protective equipment in the photograph suggests that the casualty being loaded into the ambulance was not deemed a threat, possibly because he was a victim of a respiratory agent.
Reproduced from: Gilchrist HL. *A Comparative Study of World War Casualties from Gas and Other Weapons.* Edgewood Arsenal, Md: Chemical Warfare School; 1928.

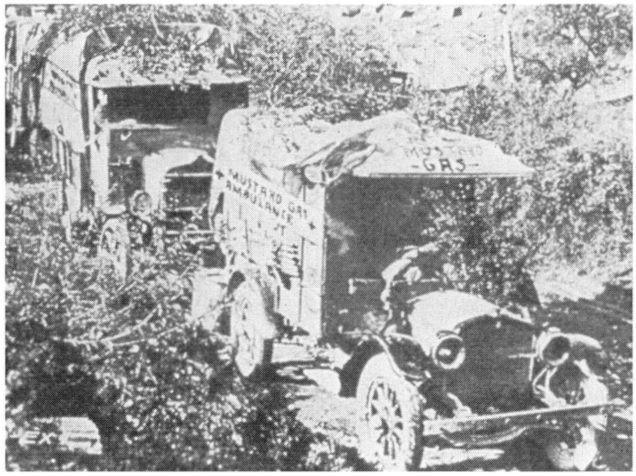

Fig. 3-16. This photograph, taken near Cheppy and Very, France, has the following figure legend: "War photograph–Special ambulances used for transporting mustard gas casualties rendered necessary due to insidiousness of mustard." These vehicles from Ambulance Company No. 13 supported the First Division.
Reproduced from: Gilchrist HL. *A Comparative Study of World War Casualties from Gas and Other Weapons.* Edgewood Arsenal, Maryland: Chemical Warfare School; 1928.

often carried in ambulances, and sometimes one or more French Tissot masks were added for the use of the driver.[66]

By the time of the southern attack of the Saint Mihiel offensive on September 12, 1918, medical support provided for the initial treatment of chemical casualties near the front. Ambulances were forbidden to speed; although it was acknowledged that casualties should be transported as rapidly as possible, their arrival condition was severely compromised if their transport was hurried or if they did not receive adequate stabilization to prepare them for an ambulance journey (Figure 3-16). This was particularly true of those intoxicated by phosgene.[67]

Throughout the occupation of the Toul sector, ambulances drove directly to battalion aid stations and carried the wounded to triage, almost without exception. Casualties tended to reach triage 1 to 3 hours earlier than expected. In one instance, casualties loaded near Norroy reached Evacuation Hospital No. 1 at Sebastopol barracks (40 miles) within 3 hours of being wounded, though it typically took an average of 4 hours to get a casualty from the place of injury to triage. Pulmonary and vesicant (inhalational) casualties who arrived without respiratory signs and symptoms in this 4-hour window had an excellent prognosis for recovery (Exhibit 3-5).[53]

Part five of the Fourth Corps plan of communication, supply, and evacuation (Annex No. 4 of Field Order No. 14, dated Sept 6, 1918) determined that the divisional medical gas officer, psychiatrist, and orthopedist would perform triage. The medical gas officer would examine all chemical casualties and advise preliminary medical management as required. Casualties would be either hospitalized or returned to duty if fit. The psychiatrist examined all cases of shock or simulated shock and other nervous conditions. All troops designated for evacuation were directed to a gas hospital at the La Marche section of the Justice Hospital Group near Toul. All nonevacuated chemical casualties were to be managed in an established field gas hospital.[36] Although no specific plan for managing chemical casualties was presented, the following quote was recorded, which placed the medical logistical mission into context:

> The difficulties to be met and overcome by the medical supply unit of a division are of a unique character. A fairly comprehensive idea of them may be formed if one will draw a mental picture of managing the only drug store in a city of 30,000 people, operating it day and night, and frequently, sometimes daily, changing its location. There are only eight clerks, for no more can be obtained, and transportation consists of two 3-ton trucks operating over congested roads. The community of which the unit forms a part is frequently bombed and shelled.[29(p107)]

Evacuation in Trench Versus Open Warfare

In open warfare, the medical management (includ-

EXHIBIT 3-5

SECRET FIELD ORDER NO. 41, ANNEX NO. 7, ISSUED BY THE FIFTH DIVISION, SEPTEMBER 9, 1918

The triage will be located at Camp-de-Cirque, eight hundred (800) meters north of the cross roads at St. Jean. Messages to the commander of the sanitary train and the director of ambulance companies will be sent to the triage by returning ambulances.

The following information will be sent:

(1) The number and location of wounded and gassed to be evacuated.

(i) Severe casualties will be evacuated by ambulance, preference being given as follows:

(1) Severe hemorrhage.

(2) Abdominal wounds, not in shock.

(3) Severely gassed.

(4) Wounds of thorax.

(5) Fractures.

****

(u) Hospital for nontransportable wounded and gassed and for slightly sick.

(1) The hospital for nontransportable wounded and gassed and for slightly sick will be located south of Domevre-en-Haye on the western side of the Manonville—Tremblecourt road. At this place there will be located Field Hospital #17 and operating team #17 for treatment of nontransportable wounded.

(2) Field Hospital #29 for treatment of gassed.

(v) Evacuation service for army and corps artillery:

Surgeons of artillery organizations operating in the 5th Division area exclusive of 5th Artillery Brigade will establish collecting stations for wounded and gassed along this road. They will notify the director of field hospitals at Domevre-en-Haye of the number of casualties and location of these collecting stations.

(a-1) Evacuation hospitals.

(2) At La Marche barracks, "The Caserne," just south of Toul. Hospital for gassed.

NOTE. Gassed and wounded patients will not be loaded in the same vehicle.

Reproduced from: Lynch C, Ford J, Weed F. *Field Operations*. Vol 8. In: *The Medical Department of the United States Army in the World War*. Washington, DC: Government Printing Office; 1925. Chapter 18.

ing evacuation) of chemical casualties on the battlefield and in field hospitals was very different from that observed when troops were in the trenches because all medical assets had to be deployed forward. Casualty evacuation required units to close in on the combat zone, placing medical assets closer to chemical weapons used by the enemy. In the beginning of the offensive against Soissons, one station within the 2nd Division was located within 50 yards of the enemy lines.[68]

The methods of the sanitary train in open warfare also differed from those in trench warfare. Difficulties were magnified by prolonged enemy fire, increased road congestion due to the movement of troops and supporting medical units, limited fixed facilities for logistics, increased numbers of wounded, a greater need for medical unit replacements, the inexperience of medical replacements upon arrival, and physical exhaustion caused by long-continued hard labor and exposure. Chemical agent casualties encountered longer evacuation times and were thus vulnerable to subsequent gas attacks.

One of the most conspicuous differences between trench and open warfare was in the way the ambulances and field hospitals conducted business. In open warfare, especially during the Meuse-Argonne operation, animal-drawn ambulances were more valuable than motorized ones and were much more frequently employed, chiefly because they could traverse routes impassable to motor vehicles and bypass road obstructions. Chemical casualties could receive timely management if they were transported by animal-drawn ambulances because chemical agents used in World War I had an overall delayed effect, unlike nerve agents or cyanide (which appeared later) in which immediate treatment was necessary.

The second phase of AEF operations was fought primarily "over the top" in the offensive. The AEF units participating in the Aisne-Marne offensive in early summer were either under French or British command (Table 3-4).[65] In the early days of the AEF offensive, it was necessary to remove all litter casualties that required transportation from the aid station to a pick-up point a kilometer (0.6 mile) or more to the rear that could be easily accessed by ambulances. As soon as ambulances could evacuate directly from aid stations, congestion was no longer an issue.[39]

Spanish Influenza

In mid June 1918 through mid July, Spanish influenza appeared on the battlefield and affected the degree of fighting during the defensive campaigns. It tapered off by the end of July, but reappeared in the offensive campaigns in October 1918.[15] Influenza's attack on the pulmonary/respiratory system seriously affected military operations twofold, first, by reducing the number of healthy soldiers, and second, by taxing the capabilities of the sanitary trains. The chemical casualty patients in sanitary train facilities had compromised and vulnerable pulmonary systems by virtue of the mechanism of action of pulmonary (phosgene) and vesicant (mustard) chemical agents. The Spanish influenza of 1918 did not stop military operations in theater, but it slowed them noticeably. When its peak was passed, reinvigoration of offensive operations increased the already heavy strain upon medical support capabilities.[67]

The First Army was hit hard by the influenza. Its chief surgeon reported 72,467 battle casualties in the Meuse-Argonne operation, of which 18,664 (25.7%) were chemical casualties.[69] It is possible that not all chemical casualties were reflected in the existing administrative records. Many chemical casualties passed through the hospital without being admitted to the gas ward. Some required surgical intervention for wounds and were categorized under other admission criteria. Others were so lightly gassed they were treated in other categories, including generalized respiratory diseases. The "gassed" category included nearly all those who had been incapacitated by mustard gas, which caused burns, conjunctivitis, laryngitis, gastroenteritis, and bronchitis.

TABLE 3-4

MAJOR OFFENSIVE CAMPAIGNS OF THE AMERICAN EXPEDITIONARY FORCES, 1918

Dates	Campaign
July 18–August 6	Aisne-Marne Offensive (Flanders Operations: Dickenbush/Scherpenberg)
August 8–November 11	The Somme Offensive
August 18–September 17 (November 11)	The Oise-Aisne Offensive
August 19–November 11	Ypres-Lys Offensive (AEF in Belgian French Sector)
September 12–September 16	Saint Mihiel Offensive
September 26–November 11	Meuse-Argonne Offensive, American Sector The Meuse-Argonne Champagne, AEF in British Sector (Phases I–III)

AEF: American Expeditionary Forces

Medical Personnel as Victims

Even medical personnel became victims of chemical attacks during the war. For example, Dr Eric P Dark, an Australian army physician, was on the receiving end of a chemical attack while managing chemical casualties (Exhibit 3-6). Dr Harvey Cushing also wrote of medical personnel who became chemical casualties:

> Poor Telfer is all bunged up with a secondhand dose of this mustard-oil gas or whatever it is. Many more of these men were brought in last night; and as the orderlies were panicky, owing to the raid, he did a lot of handling of patients himself and to-night has a bad cough, swollen and lachrymating eyes–like the men themselves. One or two others who have handled and undressed gassed Tommies have got it too in mild form.[14]

In the AEF's 78th Division, the regimental aid station of the 309th Infantry was located at Marcq, and its battalion stations were in Saint Juvin, about 1 km (0.6 mile) west, in the shelter of a hill. In this regiment, all but one of the MOs and most of the medical enlisted personnel were evacuated as chemical casualties. The regiment itself was so reduced in strength that line litter bearers could not be

EXHIBIT 3-6

THE ACCOUNT OF A CASUALTY: DR ERIC P DARK*

On the 16th [October 1917], I went up with 11 squads of bearers, and established a dressing station under a kind of lean-to against the wall of the block houses on the creek side. About midnight fairly heavy shelling began, and continued off and on till dawn, and there was a lot of general strafing all along the front. Probably the Germans were expecting an attack. Most of the German shelling must have been aimed at our field guns, but fell about 50 yards short, between the creek and the block houses. They mixed a lot of gas shells with the high explosive—one could tell the gas shell as it went off with a little plop, instead of the roar of the high explosive. Unfortunately a gentle breeze blew the gas back over our position.

Brigade, of course, had a gas sentry mounted who sounded the gas alert at appropriate times; certainly, all the men with me put on their gas masks the moment the alert sounded and did not take them off until the all clear. Looking back on it I think the sentry did not allow enough time for the gas to disperse, considering the very gentle breeze. I should probably have allowed a good margin for safety, but we had been told to depend on the sentry.

Wounded constantly came in, walking cases, and stretcher cases that the bearers brought from the forward area. No other MO. was with me so I was fully occupied with dressings. Just before dawn a heavy shell got a direct hit on one of the block houses, blowing it in, and seriously wounding two infantrymen. When I got there with a corporal, Sachs by name, and stretcher bearers, I found that both the men had compound fractures of the femurs (thighs).

We had our gas masks on, as the all clear had not yet sounded, and set about trying to fix the men up. In the conditions, with the men lying on the floor that was littered with smashed concrete, the air thick with the dust of the explosion, and our sight constantly blurred by fogged eye-pieces, it seemed impossible ever to get the wounds dressed and the fractures properly put up on Thomas's splints. After fumbling about for some time I made a decision, and told Sachs "Look Corporal we are getting nowhere; you and I will take off our masks so that we can do the job properly." He made no demur, and worked well and dexterously to help me get the men fixed and away.

It was a horrible night, and by dawn 32 of my 44 bearers were casualties, mostly gassed, ultimately 16 of them died, including Sachs, a good man, whom probably my order killed.

At dawn I went back to our advanced dressing station to report to Frazer, feeling very gloomy, there was the loss of the men, and there was my responsibility, for an officer was not supposed to let his men be gassed. Frazer did not say a word except "Bad luck; are you gassed?" He gave me extra bearers to clear the few remaining stretcher cases remaining to be shifted.

Some time about noon my relief came up as Frazer had promised (I had told him I wished to get the last cases cleared before being relieved). Abraham found me nearly blind from intense irritation and swelling of the cornea, and constantly vomiting. The gas had been a mixture of mustard and phosgene. He put me on a stretcher where I felt horribly exposed, hoisted on the shoulders of the four bearers, for shells still fell sporadically.

I reached the CCS fairly late in the afternoon, and there I was put in a small tent, and apparently forgotten, for I lay there until long after darkness came, hearing people pass, and hoping that some time someone would pick me up and put me into bed. I could still tell the difference between light and darkness, but by morning even that amount of sight was gone, and I was quite blind for four or five days; also I had a violent bronchopneumonia, spitting up quarts of thin blood-stained serous muck. They gave me other quarts of what they told me was sodium hyperchlorite, which was supposed to be helpful; anyhow it was not bad stuff. The nursing staff there were quite magnificent, constant attention, and everything I needed there on the moment.

Dr Dark was gassed during the long Paschendale offensive, which began on August 31, 1917.
Reproduced with permission from: World War I: The Medical Front Web site. The WWI military memoirs of Captain Dark, MC, Australian doctor, Great War. Available at: http://www.vlib.us/medical/dark/dark.htm. Accessed February 9, 2008.

furnished, and the regimental band augmented medical support.[70] During the Aisne-Marne offensive, 50% of the medical personnel casualties of the 3rd Division were caused by managing chemical casualties.[55]

HISTORY SINCE WORLD WAR I

Chemical Training and Research

Although World War I ended on November 11, 1918, work on chemical agent exposure continued at the Edgewood, Maryland, medical research laboratories. The Army Medical Department spent more money on chemical weapons research than anything else during the interwar years.[26,71–73] In 1922 Lieutenant Colonel Edward Vedder, a 1902 graduate of the University of Pennsylvania and a Medical Corps officer, was selected to become the chief of the medical laboratory at Edgewood (Figure 3-17, Exhibit 3-7).[74] Clinical cases were studied, animal research was performed with chemical agents, human experiments were conducted, and new treatments were tested in the Edgewood laboratories.

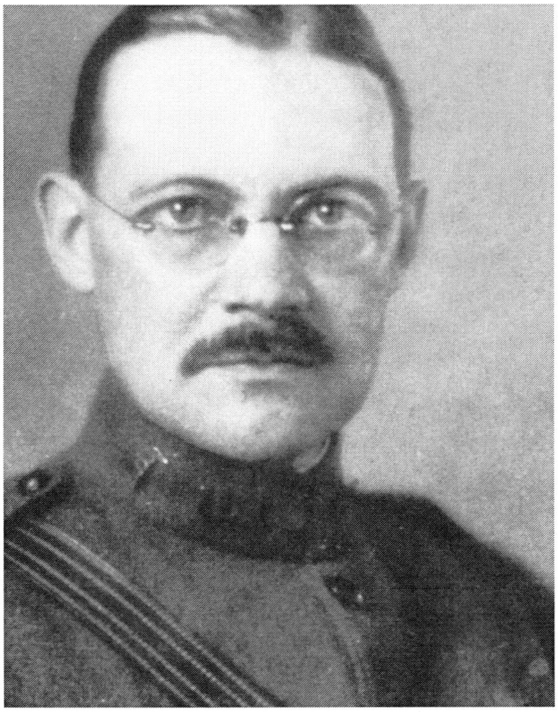

Fig. 3-17. Edward Bright Vedder (1878–1952) was director of pathology at the Army Medical School (now Walter Reed Army Institute of Research) from 1904 to 1913. During this period he wrote his seminal book on beriberi. After serving in the Philippines during World War I, Colonel Vedder returned to the Army Medical School in 1919, where he wrote a book on chemical casualties that remains relevant. From 1925 to 1929, he was chief of medical research for the chemical warfare service. He had an illustrious civilian academic career following his retirement from the Army.
Photograph: Courtesy of the National Library of Medicine. Bethesda, Md.

Chemical training for soldiers gave way to chemical casualty management training for military physicians. Vedder was the first to establish a "course for medical officers," the forerunner of today's courses taught by the Chemical Casualty Care Division of the US Army Medical Research Institute for Chemical Defense. The early course was a 5-day event covering critical information for managing chemical casualties. Instructors for the course were influential CWS members: Colonel Harry Gilchrist (later general and commander of the Chemical Corps), Captain Alden Waitt (gas officer of

EXHIBIT 3-7

LIEUTENANT COLONEL EDWARD VEDDER

Edward Vedder deferred a clinical residency for a research fellowship to study bacteriolytic serum complement. As a member of the first graduating class of the US Army's Medical School for Officers (an early version of Medical Officer's Basic Course started by Surgeon General George Sternberg), Vedder was sent to the Philippines, where he developed his research and laboratory skills in the study of malaria, amoebic dysentery, dengue, and a host of other tropical diseases. In 1910, after finishing a clinical utilization tour, he returned to the Philippines as part of the Army board for the study of tropical diseases and focused on medical research involving beriberi. In 1913 he returned to the United States, where he worked in the laboratory at the US Army Medical School and taught serology and bacteriology. The United States became involved in World War I in 1917 and, along with Dr Franklin Martin (one of the founders of the American College of Surgeons), Lieutenant Colonel Vedder was selected to serve as the Army's representative to a committee on education, where he was involved in the design of pocket manuals used to teach military physicians the medical management of war casualties (Medical War Manual No. 1, "Sanitation for Medical Officers"). In 1919 Vedder began a 3-year tour as the director of the Eighth Corps Area Laboratory housed at Fort Sam Houston, Texas. In October 1922 Army Surgeon General Merrite W Ireland established a medical research division as part of the Chemical Warfare Service at Edgewood Arsenal and selected Vedder to be its organizer and first medical director.

Data source: Vedder E. Fifty years of medicine. In: The Papers of Edward B. Vedder. Edward G Miner Library, University of Rochester Medical Center, Rochester, New York; Box 3, Folders 1–14. Chapter I.

the 29th Division and future major general and chief of the CWS), and Colonel Amos Fries (wartime chief of the overseas component of the CWS). Dr Gilchrist served as chief of the medical division of the CWS from 1922 to 1929. In 1925 Lieutenant Colonel Vedder published *Medical Aspects of Chemical Warfare*, a book containing data on the pathology and physiology of various chemical agents (particularly mustard). Much of the text is still germane. In it and his memoirs, Vedder expressed staunch support for chemical warfare:

> Gas did not maim as did missiles, the wounds of which caused the loss of arms, legs, and the distressing destruction of the jaws and other wounds of the face. Chemical Warfare therefore, appeared to do the work of dissipating the opposing Army better than did firearms, and it was at the same time more human or at least less barbarous, and more economical. It required many fewer troops and much less money to produce sufficient gas than to secure fire control.[74]

Leading into World War II, the organization for medically managing chemical casualties was based upon the World War I schemas. Despite the general expectation that chemical weapons would be used in World War II, smoke and flame were the only chemical agents used in the war (smoke was used for screening troops and movement, especially in Europe, and Americans in the Pacific used flame weapons in Japanese caves and bunkers). For reasons that historians are still debating (see Chapter 2), gas itself was not used, though the United States was prepared for a gas attack. In an address to the students of the Industrial College of the Armed Forces, Lieutenant General Alden Waitt, the CWS chief in 1946, commented on his discoveries and impressions as he visited the German heartland after the end of World War II:

> The Germans had gases that were unknown in World War I, gases which were much more potent than World War I gases. They would have used them if we had not had protection against them and had not been able to retaliate in kind. I saw the tremendous preparations which the Germans had made for waging gas warfare. . . . We in the Chemical Warfare Service who were responsible for the program had been worried because we had not turned up any German gas as we moved through France and western Germany. A few of us who were responsible for the planning and establishing the requirements wondered if questions would be raised after the war as to whether we had been thoroughly justified in spending money of the Government and insisting that there be placed over in England quantities of gas for retaliation. No gas depots showed up when we came into Normandy. No German gas appeared in France. No German gas appeared before we got to the Rhine. But after we got across the Rhine it began to show up in tremendous quantities, we discovered large stocks of gas in central Germany, scattered all through the country. The tremendous German effort and potential were apparent, once we had gotten into the central part of the country. After the surrender, when I saw these things, I realized that we had been well justified in all our preparations. As a matter of fact, we had won a gas war without firing a shot, without dropping a bomb. I saw the tremendous installations at Raubkammer—tremendous proving grounds, pilot plants, and depots. This one proving ground at Raubkammer was the equivalent of our Edgewood Arsenal and Dugway Proving Ground combined. It was equipped with splendid facilities. . . . I do not have time to tell you about them. I can only assure you that I was amazed at what I saw there. Several bomb-storage depots were located at Raubkammer. At Muna Ost, a few miles away, there was a storage depot for chemical mines and artillery and mortar shells. There was a tremendous quantity of munitions there. The Luftwaffe gas storage depot was located at Oerrel. Here I saw 175 beautifully camouflaged concrete bunkers all filled with 250-kllo and 500-kllo bombs charged with phosgene, mustard, and the new German gas, green ring 3—thousands upon thousands of bombs and all of them invulnerable against attack. We might, if we could have gotten a direct hit on one of these bunkers with a thousand pound bomb have destroyed it; but, only by a direct hit. They were beautifully hidden. As a matter of fact, we did not know of any of these installations until we got in there. They had not been located by allied intelligence. The same thing was duplicated all through central Germany. In all we located approximately a quarter of a million tons of toxic gas-munitions and bulk agent. What do you suppose they figured on doing with those quarter of a million tons–250 thousand tons, not pounds? What do you suppose they had that for? Why did they not use it?
>
> The fact that we were prepared—that we had gas overseas in England ready for instant retaliatory use, and finally, that we had the great potential of our arsenals and industry, is why they did not use gas at Normandy when we landed. I am confident of this, and it is one of the best lessons in preparedness the American people can have. We prevented a gas war by being ready!
>
> I am sure that a gas war would have set us back six months if they had dropped large quantities of gas on us when we were concentrated in small areas on the beaches in Normandy. I am just as sure of that as I am sure of anything. Had the gas appeared at Normandy, it would have delayed us seriously. It might have given the Germans time to get ready their V-3 or V-4 or whatever their next great technical development was going to be. But they did not dare to use it, because they knew if they did, their cities would have been drenched with gas.

> I am not sure they made the right decision. I am not sure that the six months' advantage might not have been worth to them the terrific shellacking they would have gotten from our gas. It was a difficult decision. They decided not to use it. I am sure the only reason they decided not to use it was because they knew we were ready, and could retaliate heavily and effectively.[75]

The Bari Disaster

Shortly after the 1943 disaster at Bari, Italy (see Chapter 2), Lieutenant Colonel Stewart Alexander of the US Army Medical Corps, the chemical warfare consultant on General Eisenhower's staff, was sent to Bari, where he made the diagnosis of mustard poisoning. He reported 6l7 cases in troops and merchant marine seamen, with a 14% fatality rate. This high fatality rate was nearly 3-fold that of the mustard fatality rate in World War I, largely because the merchant marine seamen had been thrown into the sea, where they either swallowed mustard in the water or were badly burned.[68,76] Dr Cornelius P Rhoads, another physician involved in diagnosing and treating the casualties, observed chemically induced leucopenia among the locals.

Chemical Agents in Concentration Camps

Biological and chemical casualties and fatalities from Germany's experimental testing of chemical and biological warfare agents, including cyanide, mustard, lewisite, and nerve agents, were found at Dachau and Buchenwald. Camp Natzweiller-Struthof, the only concentration camp in France, used phosgene and mustard on inmates. Sachsenhausen Camp at Oranienburg, just north of Berlin, used mustard in experimentation on inmates, and Spandau University in Berlin was believed to have used nerve agents for experimentation. At the camp in Neuengamme, mustard was given to inmates to drink. The details of this kind of chemical agent use were explored by the United States in the Nuremburg and British war trials. After the defeat of the Nazi forces along the eastern front, the Soviet Army uncovered Auschwitz-Berkinau and saw how Zyklon B, a rat poison, had been used in specially constructed gas chambers for the purpose of mass human extermination. Before settling on Zyklon B, the Nazis had experimented with specially adapted carbon monoxide gas vans to induce mass killing at the Russian front.[77]

No clearly structured chemical casualty management was established for camp inmates after liberation. All camp inmates had baseline clinical presentation consistent with food deprivation, malnutrition, and close-quartering, and all were physically, mentally, and emotionally exhausted from atrocious working and living conditions. Diseases such as typhus, tuberculosis, and dysentery were evidenced. The US military medical organization faced a multifaceted presentation for which it had no organizational adaptations.

Chemicals in Korea and Vietnam

After World War II the management of chemical casualties shifted back to research and training. The Korean War did not produce any documented chemical casualties. The organization for medically managing chemical casualties during the Vietnam era was similarly untried, though the United States did use chemical defoliants in Vietnam for canopy clearing and crop destruction. It also used tear gas for clearing tunnels and bunkers (Figure 3-18).[78] "Tunnel rats" were often Chemical Corps personnel assigned to use *o*-chlorobenzylidene malononitrile agent (known as "CS," a riot control agent) when searching for enemy

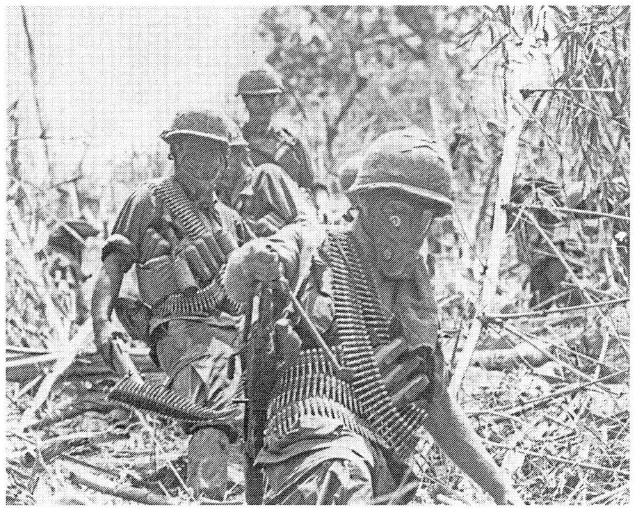

Fig. 3-18. Tear gas was used extensively by US forces in the Vietnam War, especially in clearing enemy tunnel complexes. However, the US government did not consider tear gas to be a chemical weapon and therefore did not consider its use to be banned by international law. Many others outside of government disagreed, using as evidence the fact that those who used tear gas wore protective masks. The soldiers shown here are wearing the little-known M28 protective mask. This lightweight (and perhaps more comfortable) mask was designed to be worn in situations in which the threat was not from nerve agents, and the heavy-duty protection offered by the standard masks was not necessary.
Photograph: Courtesy of Chemical and Biological Defense Command Historical Research and Response Team, Aberdeen Proving Ground, Md.

burrowers. Resulting riot control agent casualties did not engender special organizational changes to the existing management schemas. Because defoliants were not used as tactical weapons, casualties exposed to them were not managed outside the realm of usual exposure protocols.

Field Training

For realistic field preparation, the Army conducted training such as Operation Solid Shield 87, which tested how US troops performed on a chemically contaminated battlefield. Over 40,000 personnel from the US Army, Navy, Marine Corps, Air Force, and Coast Guard participated in simulated chemical attacks. Of the many conclusions drawn from the training, the impact on medical personnel trying to help both conventional and chemical casualties caused particular concern:

> Use of chemical weapons in an otherwise conventional warfare scenario will result in significant impact on the medical capability to treat and handle casualties. Many medical facilities might be located near chemical target areas and may be subject to contamination.
>
> These facilities include battalion aid stations, hospital and medical companies, casualty receiving and treatment ships, fleet hospitals, and hospital ships. Provision of medical care in a contaminated environment is extremely difficult due to the encapsulation of medical personnel in their individual protective ensembles.
>
> Medical care is best provided in an environment free of toxic agents. This environment might be provided by a collectively protected facility, or be in an uncontaminated area. Medical units ashore and afloat can expect to receive contaminated casualties and must be prepared to provide contaminated casualties with a comprehensive and thorough decontamination. This procedure is similar whether processing patients into a collectively protected facility or processing from a contaminated area to an area free of contamination.[79(p31)]

One officer summed up this new way of thinking about chemical training as demonstrated by Solid Shield 87:

> NBC warfare is not a separate, special form of war, but is instead a battlefield condition just like rain, snow, darkness, electronic warfare, heat, and so on. Units must train to accomplish their wartime missions under all battlefield conditions. Whenever NBC is separated from other training events, we condition our soldiers to regard operations under NBC conditions as a separate form of warfare.[79(p31)]

To reflect conceptual and equipment changes, the Army's field manuals were rewritten and updated to incorporate chemical warfare readiness into the Army's air–land battle doctrine. The five parts of the new doctrine called for contamination avoidance, individual and collective protection, decontamination, chemical weapons employment, and the deliberate use of smoke.[80] Military medicine had to incorporate improved overpressure systems in collective protection as part of their management of chemical casualties.

Chemical Use After Vietnam

The post-Vietnam era heralded an age of terrorism. Some states, such as Iraq, used chemical terror to control neighbors and citizens. Cyanide and mustard returned to the battlefield during the Iran-Iraq War, and nerve agents (eg, tabun) also debuted on the chemical battlefield (see Chapter 2). Iranian medical staffs were forced to manage chemical casualties during the conflict, and their atropine dosing protocols are the basis for nerve agent management today. The presence of chemical casualties within a Kurdish population in northern Iraq in 1988 did not lend itself to increased knowledge of chemical casualty management, although over 5,000 people lost their lives in an attack later confirmed by the United Nations to have involved sulfur mustard and nerve agent.[81]

In the Persian Gulf War, the Spearhead Division (3rd Armored Division [forward]) was commanded by Major General Paul E Funk, who modified the medical support organization of the cavalry elements by attaching an additional medical platoon.[82,83] On March 1, 1991, Private First Class David Allen Fisher, a cavalry soldier with the 3rd Armored Division, was medically processed (Exhibit 3-8).[84] Fisher, who had been investigating one of many munitions bunkers, presented with two 2-cm blisters on his left forearm. After Fisher was initially diagnosed with a spider bite, unit aid station personnel Chief Warrant Officer 2 Ahmed and Chief Warrant Officer 3 Wildhelm began to suspect that chemical weaponry might be involved. The warrant officers evacuated Fisher to C Company of the 45th Support Battalion, where a physician's evaluation was performed. Soon a Fox (Fuchs) vehicle was dispatched and Fox infrared analysis indicated that mustard was present at the site Fisher had been inspecting.[85]

Colonel Michael Dunn filed a medical report indicating Fisher's management by cavalry, division, and forward support battalion personnel. The medical personnel at the cavalry aid station and the physician at the 45th Forward Support Battalion were graduates of the Medical Management of Chemical

EXHIBIT 3-8

A CASE OF ACCIDENTAL EXPOSURE

AETV-TF-CC 10 June 1991

MEMORANDUM FOR RECORD

SUBJECT: Chemical Casualty Occurring During "Bunker Search and

Equipment Destruction Mission" Within the 3AD Area of Operation.

1. On 01 Mar 91, PFC David A. Fisher . . . , a 19D cavalry scout assigned to the 4/8th Cav, 3AD was performing a search and destroy mission of Iraqi equipment and bunker complexes. Somewhere among the several complexes he visited he brushed against an unknown surface which deposited a chemical agent upon his flack jacket and his Nomex suit. He was unaware of the contact with the chemical agent.

2. PFC Fisher returned back to his unit still unaware of any contact. He was assigned to morning guard duty at 0100 hrs on 02 Mar. He noticed a redness associated with skin irritation on his upper left arm which felt like a "spider bite". By 0400 the same day, blisters appeared. The blisters were in the area of his polio-immunization site. The blister size was 1/4" x 1/2". Later that morning he reported to sick call to get treatment. He was not treated for a chemical injury at that time.

3. Later that day his signs and symptoms did not go away. His blisters spread to his lower arm. He returned to sick call where he underwent skin decontamination. At this point he was processed as a chemical agent casualty and treated as such.

4. Chemical RECON (FOX) vehicles were dispatched to "sniff" the articles of clothing and to search bunkers in the AO for signs of chemical contamination. The FOX mass spectrometer tapes indicated the presence of an H-series blister agent. On 03 Mar 0940, HD chemical blister agent was reported to be found in a bunker at location QU 050072.

5. Clinical confirmation came from Col Dunn M.D., Commander of the US Army Medical Research Institute of Chemical Defense. Col Dunn stated that PFC Fisher showed a sufficient clinical history and syptomotology to classify him as a classical Mustard agent (blister) casualty. Col Dunn, further stated that if a positive urine test for thiodiglycol, a breakdown products of mustard agent, could be gathered, then the clinical diagnosis was sound. A urine specimen was taken.

6. . . . 3AD Division Surgeon, confirmed that the urine test was positive. PFC Fisher was confirmed to be a chemical "mustard blister agent" casualty. The clothing, flack jacket, and fluid from the blisters were secured from 2d BDE by . . . and 513th MI personnel for further analysis and control.

. . .

Assistant Division Chemical Officer 423

Data source: *Chemical Casualty Occurring During "Bunker Search and Equipment Destruction Mission" Within the 3AD Area of Operation*. US Department of the Army, Third Armored Division; 1991. Memorandum, 10 June 1991. Available at: http://www.gulflink.osd.mil/fisher_ii/fisher_ii_refs/n45en062/970725_sep96_decls26_0001.htm. Accessed April 15, 2008.

and Biological Casualties Course (taught by US Army Medical Research Institute of Chemical Defense) and were confident of their suspicions.

The value of chemical casualty management lies in staff coordination and communication of medical information. Russia's 2002 use of nonlethal gas against Chechnyan terrorists at a Moscow theater (see Chapter 2) provides an example of unsuccessful chemical casualty management. Had Russian special operations personnel indicated to first responders and receivers the nature of the chemical weapon used, the judicious use of nalaxone could have been easily planned. Instead, healthcare providers thought they were facing a new nerve agent and were unable to respond appropriately.

PROJECTIONS FOR THE FUTURE OF CHEMICAL CASUALTY MANAGEMENT

The historical key to the success of managing chemical casualties has unfortunately been hands-on experience. Today's military medical community has no residency or specialty training in disaster or terror medicine other than that offered at the US Army Medical Research Institute of Chemical Defense. Lieutenant Colonel Edward Vedder's "course for medical officers" has evolved into comprehensive training for all facets of the US government and allied countries as well. Modern audiovisual technologies now bring training to the battlefield. When communication elements support it, an organizational interface with medical and chemical experts in personnel, intelligence, operations, research, and logistics can provide "reach-back" capabilities for combat decision-makers and their staffs (Figure 3-19). The potential for a trained and confident chemical casualty manager exists if command is willing to engage.

As demand for specialty training increases, the medical community must modify its organization to encompass chemical casualty managers. Educational communities must consider providing residency in specialties including disaster or terror medicine and subspecialties that address the spectrum of chemical casualty management. As long as soldiers are unprepared to manage chemical casualties, sources with the capability to use chemical weapons will engage those capabilities to their best strategic and tactical advantage.

SUMMARY

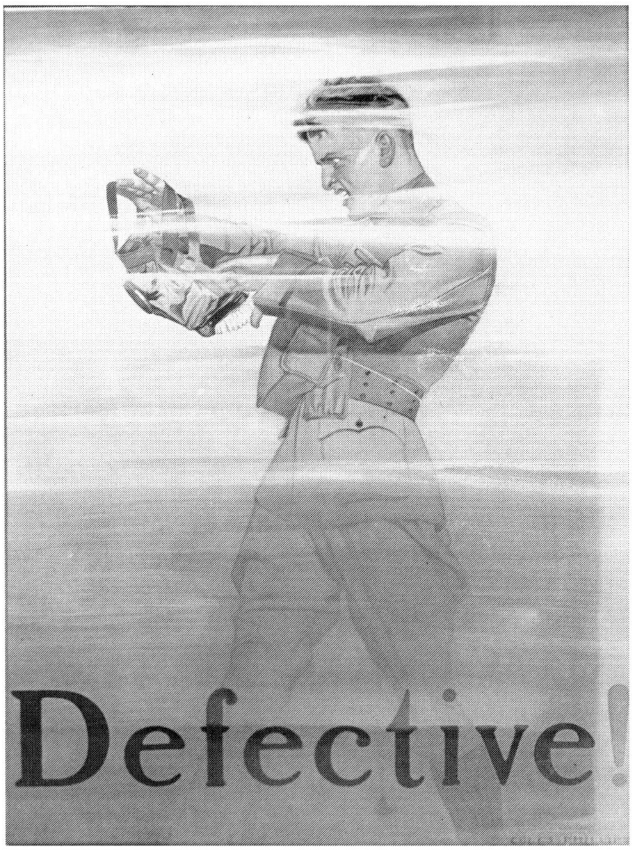

Fig. 3-19. This poster from World War I was designed to encourage enthusiasm for quality assurance among women who manufactured protective masks.
Reproduced from: Pictorial History, Gas Defense Division, Chemical Warfare Service. Vol 5. Edgewood Historical Files. Located at: Chemical and Biological Defense Command Historical Research and Response Team, Aberdeen Proving Ground, Md.

Combatants respond to a current war in the manner in which they conducted the previous one. In terms of employing medical assets on a chemical battlefield, World War I saw units on both sides of the battlefield performing reactively rather than proactively. After all the lessons learned in World War I, the chemical casualties of the Bari disaster found themselves medically managed by physicians who were still unable to meet the minimum standard of care for chemical casualties. After World War II, the fate of the chemical casualty fell into the hands of medical personnel untrained in the appropriate medical management. This disconnect among experts in chemical warfare, military medicine, and military personnel must be addressed so that casualties on the chemical battlefield have the service support system that yields the greatest chance for success. Today, when terrorists are sufficiently organized to bring chemicals to the home front, base hospitals, military medical centers, and other medical treatment facilities must be competently prepared for chemical casualties.

Lieutenant Colonel Vedder studied with medical historian Richard Shryock, who suggested that all sciences must pass through stages of development. Vedder said of Shryock:

> In his landmark work, The Development of Modern Medicine, Shryock postulates that all sciences, including medicine, must pass through four stages of development. The first is a period of minimal observation and maximal theoretical synthesis. The second is an early attempt at objectivity and measurement. The third stage sees a partial lapse of quantitative procedures due to unforeseen difficulties, while the fourth is a revival of such procedures with "a final victory for modern technology."

For North American medicine, the leap from the first stage to the second was the most difficult, because it required a change in professional modes of thinking: the medical educator (if not the average practitioner) had to come to understand and accept the importance of the scientific method for the advancement of medical knowledge. Attainment of the fourth stage, medicine's "final victory," required as well a change in American social values: the average citizen had to perceive the products of scientific investigation as important—indeed necessary.[86]

There is still much to learn about medically managing chemical casualties. Past lessons must be combined with current research and future predictions to best prepare military medical personnel for a chemical attack. The United States has not seen chemical warfare in any sizable scale since World War I, but its military medical personnel must continually be ready to respond in the event of an attack.

REFERENCES

1. Gilchrist H. Instructor notes from Gilchrist's lecture on the history of chemical warfare. *Science*. 1929;70:113–117.
2. Mueller U. *Die Chemische Waffe IM WeltKrieg Und Jetzt* [*The Chemical Weapon in the World War and Now*]. Berlin, Germany: Verlag Chemie; 1932: W10.
3. Mayor A. *Greek Fire, Poison Arrows and Scorpion Bombs*. New York, NY: Overlook; 2003.
4. Thucydides. *The History of the Peloponnesian War*. Crawley R, trans. New York, NY: Modern Library; 1934.
5. Laffout R. *The Ancient Age of Warfare: 1300BC–1650AD*. Vol 1. New York, NY: Time-Life; 1966: 45--46.
6. McWilliams JL, Steel RJ. *Gas! The Battle for Ypres, 1915*. St Catharine's, Ontario, Canada: Vanwell Publishing Ltd; 1985.
7. Foulkes CH. *Gas! The Story of the Special Brigade*. London, England: W Blackwood and Sons: 1934: 345.
8. *Der Weltkrieg 1914 bis 1918: Sommer und Herbst 1915* [*The World War 1914 to 1918: Summer and Autumn 1915*]. Vol 8. Berlin, Germany: Im Auftrage des Reichskriegsministeriums, Mittler und Sohn; 1932: 34–49.
9. Legg J, Parker G. The Great War Web site. Ypres Salient page. Available at: www.greatwar.co.uk/westfront/ypsalient/. Accessed January 9, 2008.
10. Duguid AF. *History of the Canadian Forces in the Great War, 1914–1919*. Vol I. Ottawa, Ontario, Canada: King's Printer; 1947.
11. *Les Armées Françaises dans la Grande Guerre [French Armies in the Large War]*. Ministere de la guerre, etat-major de l'armee [Director of the Large War, Army Chief of Staff]: Librairie Payet; 1913. Appendix no. 1392.
12. *British Military Operations: France and Belgium 1915*. London, England: Macmillan and Co Ltd; 1927.
13. Zapotoczny Walter S. The use of poison gas in World War I and the effect on society [Walter S Zapotoczny Web site]. Available at: http://wzaponline.com/PoisonGas.pdf. Accessed March 18, 2008.
14. Cushing H. *From a Surgeon's Journal, 1915–1918*. Boston, Mass: Little, Brown and Company; 1936.
15. Cochrane R. The First Division at Cantigny, May 1918. In: *U.S. Army Chemical Corps Historical Studies, Gas Warfare in World War I*. Washington, DC: Office of the Chief Chemical Officer, US Army Chemical Corps Historical Office; 1958. Study Number 11.
16. Prentiss AM. *Chemicals in War: a Treatise on Chemical War*. New York, NY: McGraw-Hill; 1937.
17. Gabriel RA, Metz KS. From the Renaissance through modern times (contributions in military studies). Vol. 2. In: *A History of Military Medicine*. Westport, Conn: Greenwood Press; 1992: 245.

18. Ashburn PM. *A History of the Medical Department of the United States Army*. Boston, Mass: Houghton-Mifflin; 1929: 334.

19. Gilchrist H. *A Comparative Study of World War Casualties from Gas and Other Weapons*. Edgewood Arsenal, Md: US Army Chemical Warfare School; 1928.

20. Fries AA. *Gas in Attack and Gas in Defense*. Fort Leavenworth, Kan: Army Command and General Staff College Combined Arms Research Library; 1919: 14.

21. Army War College. *Methods of Defense Against Gas Attacks*. Vol 2. In: *Gas Warfare*. Washington, DC: War Department; 1918.

22. US Department of the Army, Historical Division. Table 4, "Technical and Administration Services (Gas Service)." In: General Orders, General Headquarters, American Expeditionary Forces, General Order No. 8, July 5, 1917: Organization, of Headquarters, American Expeditionary Forces. In: *United States Army in the World War, 1917–1919*. Vol. 16. Washington, DC: US Government Printing Office; 1948: 23.

23. Chemical Warfare Service. *Report of the Director of Chemical Warfare Service*. Washington, DC: Government Printing Office; 1919: 33–34.

24. Bancroft WD, Bradley HC, Eyster JAE, et al. *Medical Aspects of Gas Warfare*. In: Lynch C, Weed F, McAfee L, eds. *The Medical Department of the United States Army in the World War*. Vol. 14. Washington, DC: US Government Printing Office; 1926.

25. Fries AA. *History of Chemical Warfare*. Letter. Carlisle Barracks, Pa: US Army Military History Institute; 1919.

26. Fries AA, West CJ. *Chemical Warfare*. New York, NY: McGraw-Hill; 1921: 34.

27. Heller, CE. Chemical Warfare in World War I: The American Experience, 1917–1918 [US Army Command and General Staff College Web site]. Available at: http://www-cgsc.army.mil/carl/resources/csi/Heller/HELLER.asp. Accessed January 25, 2008.

28. Report of Medical Department activities, Fifth Division, American Expeditionary Forces. Part 3. In: Lynch C, Ford J, Weed F. Field Operations. Vol 8. In: *The Medical Department of the United States Army in the World War*. Washington, DC: Government Printing Office; 1925: 149.

29. Report of Medical Department activities, 42nd Division, American Expeditionary Forces. Part I. In: Lynch C, Ford J, Weed F. *Field Operations*. Vol 8. In: *The Medical Department of the United States Army in the World War*. Washington, DC: Government Printing Office; 1925.

30. Persons EE. US Army Ambulance Service, with the Italian Army. In: Lynch C, Ford J, Weed F. *Field Operations*. Vol 8. In: *The Medical Department of the United States Army in the World War*. Washington, DC: Government Printing Office; 1925: 944.

31. Spencer EW. *The History of Gas Attacks Upon the American Expeditionary Force During the World War*. Book 1, Part I. Carlisle Barracks, Pa: Military Historical Institute; 1928. Bound typescript.

32. Grissinger JW. Medical field service in France. *Mil Surg*. 1927:61–63.

33. US Department of the Army, Historical Division. General Orders, American Expeditionary Forces, General Order No. 144, August 29, 1918. In: *United States Army in the World War, 1917–1919*. Vol. 16. Washington, DC: US Government Printing Office; 1948: 429–432.

34. US Department of the Army, Historical Division. General Headquarters, American Expeditionary Forces, General Orders No. 1, May 26, 1917. In: *United States Army in the World War, 1917–1919*. Vol. 16. Washington, DC: US Government Printing Office; 1992: 1.

35. US Department of the Army, Historical Division. Report of the chief surgeon, American Expeditionary Forces, to the commanding general, service of supply, April 17, 1919. In: *United States Army in the World War, 1917–1919*. Vol. 16. Washington, DC: US Government Printing Office; 1925: 218.

36. Maddux HC. Report of Medical Department activities, Toul Hospital Center. In: Lynch C, Ford J, Weed F. *Field Operations*. Vol 8. In: *The Medical Department of the United States Army in the World War.* Washington, DC: Government Printing Office; 1925.

37. Ashford BK. Report of the Medical Department activities of the combat divisions. In: Lynch C, Ford J, Weed F. *Field Operations*. Vol 8. In: *The Medical Department of the United States Army in the World War.* Washington, DC: Government Printing Office; 1925: 149.

38. Reynolds CR. Evacuation system of a field army. In: Lynch C, Ford J, Weed F. *Field Operations*. Vol 8. In: *The Medical Department of the United States Army in the World War.* Washington, DC: Government Printing Office; 1925: 219.

39. Report of Medical Department activities, Fourth Division, American Expeditionary Forces. In: Lynch C, Ford J, Weed F. Field Operations. Vol 8. In: *The Medical Department of the United States Army in the World War.* Washington, DC: Government Printing Office; 1925.

40. Report of operations, Medical Department, Second Division, American Expeditionary Forces, July 18–24, 1918, from the division surgeon to the commanding general, Second Division, February 5, 1919. In: Lynch C, Ford J, Weed F. *Field Operations*. Vol 8. In: *The Medical Department of the United States Army in the World War*. Washington, DC: Government Printing Office; 1925: 425 .

41. Report of Medical Department activities, 89th Division, American Expeditionary Forces. In: Lynch C, Ford J, Weed F. *Field Operations*. Vol 8. In: *The Medical Department of the United States Army in the World War.* Washington, DC: Government Printing Office; 1925: 149.

42. From reports of Medical Department activities of divisions in the American Expeditionary Forces. In: Lynch C, Ford J, Weed F. *Field Operations*. Vol 8. In: *The Medical Department of the United States Army in the World War.* Washington, DC: Government Printing Office; 1925: 149.

43. Report of Medical Department activities, 26th Division, American Expeditionary Forces, prepared under the direction of the division surgeon. Part I. In: Lynch C, Ford J, Weed F. *Field Operations*. Vol 8. In: *The Medical Department of the United States Army in the World War.* Washington, DC: Government Printing Office; 1925: 51.

44. Howe HE. The editor's point of view. *Indust Eng Chem*. 1932:24;121–122.

45. Report of Medical Department activities, First Division. In: Lynch C, Ford J, Weed F. *Field Operations*. Vol 8. In: *The Medical Department of the United States Army in the World War.* Washington, DC: Government Printing Office; 1925: 308.

46. Grissinger JW. Report of Medical Department activities, First Army Corps. In: Lynch C, Ford J, Weed F. *Field Operations*. Vol 8. In: *The Medical Department of the United States Army in the World War.* Washington, DC: Government Printing Office; 1925: 308.

47. Wadhams SH. Report on activities of G-4-B, medical group, fourth section, general staff, General Headquarters, American Expeditionary Forces, December 31, 1918. In: Lynch C, Ford J, Weed F. *Field Operations*. Vol 8. In: *The Medical Department of the United States Army in the World War.* Washington, DC: Government Printing Office; 1925: 51.

48. Report of Medical Department board, General Headquarters, American Expeditionary Forces, 1919. In: Lynch C, Ford J, Weed F. *Field Operations*. Vol 8. In: *The Medical Department of the United States Army in the World War.* Washington, DC: Government Printing Office; 1925: 51.

49. Cutler EC. Organization, function, and operation of an evacuation hospital. *Mil Surg*. 1920; xlvi:9.

50. Letter from the chief surgeon, American Expeditionary Forces, to the director of professional services, AEF, June 2, 1918. "Gas teams." In: Lynch C, Ford J, Weed F. *Field Operations*. Vol 8. In: *The Medical Department of the United States Army in the World War.* Washington, DC: Government Printing Office; 1925: 220.

51. Evacuation of sick and wounded. Memorandum, September 3, 1918, Headquarters, First Army Corps. In: Lynch C, Ford J, Weed F. *Field Operations*. Vol 8. In: *The Medical Department of the United States Army in the World War.* Washington, DC: Government Printing Office; 1925: 149.

52. Lyle HHM. Evacuation of the wounded in the Meuse-Argonne operation, May 10, 1921. In: Lynch C, Ford J, Weed F. *Field Operations*. Vol 8. In: *The Medical Department of the United States Army in the World War.* Washington, DC: Government Printing Office; 1925.

53. Report of Medical Department activities, 90th Division, American Expeditionary Forces. In: Lynch C, Ford J, Weed F. *Field Operations*. Vol 8. In: *The Medical Department of the United States Army in the World War.* Washington, DC: Government Printing Office; 1925: 153.

54. Memorandum from the medical representative of G-4-B, General Headquarters, American Expeditionary Forces, to the chief surgeon, AEF, May 16, 1918. In: Lynch C, Ford J, Weed F. *Field Operations*. Vol 8. In: *The Medical Department of the United States Army in the World War.* Washington, DC: Government Printing Office; 1925: 309.

55. Report of Medical Department activities of the Third Division, American Expeditionary Forces. In: Lynch C, Ford J, Weed F. *Field Operations*. Vol 8. In: *The Medical Department of the United States Army in the World War.* Washington, DC: Government Printing Office; 1925.

56. Collins CC. Report of Medical Department activities, Second Corps, American Expeditionary Forces. In: Lynch C, Ford J, Weed F. *Field Operations*. Vol 8. In: *The Medical Department of the United States Army in the World War.* Washington, DC: Government Printing Office; 1925: 893.

57. Report of Medical Department activities, Second Division, American Expeditionary Forces. Part II. In: Lynch C, Ford J, Weed F. *Field Operations*. Vol 8. In: *The Medical Department of the United States Army in the World War.* Washington, DC: Government Printing Office; 1925.

58. Report of Medical Department activities, Seventh Division, American Expeditionary Forces. In: Lynch C, Ford J, Weed F. *Field Operations*. Vol 8. In: *The Medical Department of the United States Army in the World War.* Washington, DC: Government Printing Office; 1925: 985.

59. Operations of the Third Corps, Meuse-Argonne operation, November 25, 1918. In: Lynch C, Ford J, Weed F. *Field Operations*. Vol 8. In: *The Medical Department of the United States Army in the World War.* Washington, DC: Government Printing Office; 1925: 609.

60. Bevans JL. Report of Medical Department activities, Third Army Corps. In: Lynch C, Ford J, Weed F. *Field Operations*. Vol 8. In: *The Medical Department of the United States Army in the World War.* Washington, DC: Government Printing Office; 1925: 428.

61. Report of Medical Department activities, 82nd Division, American Expeditionary Forces. In: Lynch C, Ford J, Weed F. *Field Operations*. Vol 8. In: *The Medical Department of the United States Army in the World War.* Washington, DC: Government Printing Office; 1925: 1018.

62. Operation report, Fourth Division, Meuse-Argonne operation, December 10, 1918. In: Lynch C, Ford J, Weed F. *Field Operations*. Vol 8. In: *The Medical Department of the United States Army in the World War.* Washington, DC: Government Printing Office; 1925.

63. Report of Medical Department activities, Base Hospital No. 51, American Expeditionary Forces. In: Lynch C, Ford J, Weed F. *Field Operations*. Vol 8. In: *The Medical Department of the United States Army in the World War.* Washington, DC: Government Printing Office; 1925: 520.

64. Report of Medical Department activities, gas hospital, Toul Hospital Center, American Expeditionary Forces. In: Lynch C, Ford J, Weed F. *Field Operations*. Vol 8. In: *The Medical Department of the United States Army in the World War.* Washington, DC: Government Printing Office; 1925.

65. Evacuation of sick and wounded. Letter from the division surgeon, 42nd Division, to the commanding general, 42nd Division, April 4, 1918. In: Lynch C, Ford J, Weed F. *Field Operations.* Vol 8. In: *The Medical Department of the United States Army in the World War.* Washington, DC: Government Printing Office; 1925: 149.

66. Jones PL. Report on the activities of the US Army Ambulance Service, with the French Army. In: Lynch C, Ford J, Weed F. *Field Operations.* Vol 8. In: *The Medical Department of the United States Army in the World War.* Washington, DC: Government Printing Office; 1925: 259.

67. Stark AN. Evacuation system in the Zone of the Armies. In: Lynch C, Ford J, Weed F. *Field Operations.* Vol 8. In: *The Medical Department of the United States Army in the World War*. Washington, DC: Government Printing Office; 1925.

68. Infield GB. *Disaster at Bari.* New York, NY: Macmillan; 1971.

69. Final report of the chief surgeon, First Army, American Expeditionary Forces, upon the Saint Mihiel and Meuse-Argonne operation, November 18, 1918. In: Lynch C, Ford J, Weed F. *Field Operations.* Vol 8. In: *The Medical Department of the United States Army in the World War*. Washington, DC: Government Printing Office; 1925: 809.

70. Report of Medical Department activities, 78th Division. In: Lynch C, Ford J, Weed F. *Field Operations*. Vol 8. In: *The Medical Department of the United States Army in the World War.* Washington, DC: Government Printing Office; 1925.

71. Waitt AH. *Gas Warfare.* New York, NY: Duell, Sloan, and Pearce; 1942: 9–11.

72. Vedder EB. *The Medical Aspects of Chemical Warfare.* Baltimore, Md: Williams & Wilkins; 1925.

73. Brophy LP, Miles WD, Cochrane RC. *US Army in World War II: The Chemical Warfare Service, From Laboratory to Field.* Washington, DC: US Government Printing Office; 1959: 1–27.

74. Vedder E. Fifty years of medicine. In: *The Papers of Edward B. Vedder*. Edward G Miner Library, University of Rochester Medical Center, Rochester, New York; Box 3, Folders 1–14. Chapter I.

75. Waitt A. Recent technological developments of the Chemical Warfare Service. Speech to the Industrial College of the Armed Forces, Washington, DC. May 21, 1946.

76. Alexander SF. Medical report of the Bari Harbor mustard casualties. *Mil Surg*. 1947;101:1–17.

77. Gilbert M. *The Holocaust.* New York, NY: Henry Holt; 1985.

78. Westmoreland WC. *A Soldier Reports.* New York, NY: Dell Publishing Co; 1980.

79. Polley W, Dlugopolski M, Hartzell W. 40,000 train in chemical environment. *Army Chemical Review.* 1988;26–31.

80. US Department of the Army. *Operations*. Washington, DC: DA; 1982. Field Manual 100-5.

81. British Broadcasting Network. Dutchman in Iraq genocide charges [BBC News Web site]. March 18, 2005. Available at: http://news.bbc.co.uk/2/hi/middle_east/4360137.stm. Accessed March 18, 2008.

82. US Army Third Armored Division. *Personnel Aspects of Operation Desert Storm for Historical Records.* Kuwait: Third Armored Division Headquarters; 1991. Operation Order 90-1.

83. Tucker T, Major General, US Army, US Armor Center, Fort Knox, Kentucky. Interview. November 3, 2005.

84. Englehardt JP. *Desert Shield and Desert Storm: A Chronology and Troop List for the 1990-1991 Persian Gulf Crisis.* Carlisle Barracks, Pa: Strategic Studies Institute; 1991. Strength Management Casualty Report: 3AD G1/AG.

85. Historical Report Files, G3 Chemical, 3AD Files. Located at Patton Museum Archives, Fort Knox, KY.

86. Graner JL. The primary care crisis: part I. The contribution of anti-scientism. *Humane Medicine*. 1986;2:96–99.

Chapter 4

HISTORY OF THE CHEMICAL THREAT, CHEMICAL TERRORISM, AND ITS IMPLICATIONS FOR MILITARY MEDICINE

JEFFERY K. SMART, MA*; AL MAURONI, MS†; BENJAMIN A. HILL JR, DO, MS, MED‡; AND ALLART B. KOK, MS§

*Command Historian, US Army Research, Development, and Engineering Command, 5183 Blackhawk Road, Aberdeen Proving Ground, Maryland 21010-5424

†Senior Policy Analyst, Northrop-Grumman Information Technology, 8211 Terminal Road, Suite 1000, Lorton, Virginia 22079

‡Lieutenant Colonel, US Army Medical Corps; Physician Faculty, Chemical Casualty Care Division, US Army Medical Research Institute of Chemical Defense, 3100 Ricketts Point Road, Aberdeen Proving Ground, Maryland 21010-5400

§Biomedical Scientist, Science Applications International Corporation, 3465 Box Hill Corporate Center Drive, Abingdon, Maryland 21085

INTRODUCTION

This chapter is the third in the series of historical investigations into the use of chemicals as weapons, following Chapter 2, History of Chemical Warfare, which focuses on the history of chemical warfare on the battlefield, and Chapter 3, History of the Medical Management of Chemical Casualties, which describes the organizational management of the resultant casualties. Over the last 20 years, the nature of the chemical threat dramatically changed. This chapter outlines the historical progression of chemical weapon development, summarizes how conventional and unconventional agents may be delivered in the contexts of conventional conflict and terrorism, and addreses the status of current chemcial warfare capabilities in relation to the evolution and implementaion of international chemical warfare agreements.

DEVELOPMENT OF CHEMICAL WEAPONRY

Before World War I, the United States knew little about the potential of chemical warfare, particularly in terms of preparing soldiers for future wars. By the end of the war, the large-scale chemical warfare used by and against American soldiers on the battlefield had drastically changed the situation (Figure 4-1).

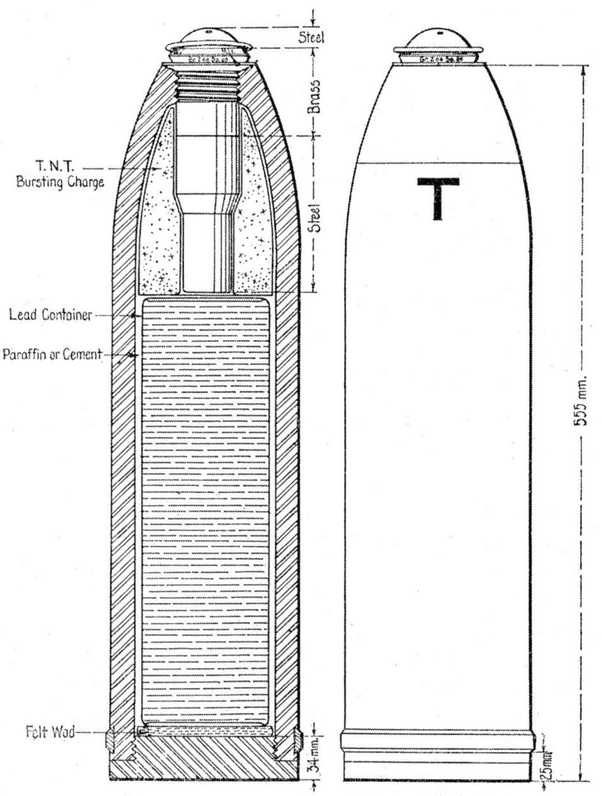

Fig. 4-1. The German 150-mm T-Shell, which mixed xylyl bromide with an explosive charge. The explosive charge was in the front and the chemical agent in the rear compartment. This design is similar to the one proposed in 1862 by John Doughty during the American Civil War.
Reproduced from: Army War College. *German Methods of Offense.*Vol 1. In: *Gas Warfare.* Washington, DC: War Department; 1918: 59.

Early History

Few of the chemical agents first used in combat during World War I were 20th-century discoveries. Many of the key agents (Table 4-1) were already known to chemists; they were actually discovered during the 18th and 19th centuries and could have been used on earlier battlefields. The 18th-century finds included chlorine (Cl_2), discovered by Carl Wilhelm Scheele, a Swedish chemist, in 1774. Scheele also determined the properties and composition of hydrogen cyanide (HCN; North American Treaty Organization [NATO] designation: AC) in 1782. In the 19th century, Charles A Wurtz first discovered cyanogen chloride (NATO designation: CK), which was synthesized in 1802 by a French chemist, Comte Claude-Louis Berthollet. In 1812 phosgene (NATO designation: CG) was synthesized by a British chemist, Sir Humphry Davy. Dichlorethylsulphide (commonly known as mustard agent, H, or HS) was synthesized by Cesar-Mansuete

TABLE 4-1

EARLY CHEMICAL WARFARE AGENTS

US Army Code	Agent
Cyanide	
AC	Hydrogen cyanide
CK	Cyanogen chloride
Lung agents	
CG (phosgene)	Carbonyl chloride
DP (diphosgene)	Trichloromethyl chloroformate
Vesicants	
HD (mustard)	*bis*-2-Chloroethyl sulfide
Tear gas	
CN	2-Chloro-1-phenylethanone
CS	2-Chlorobenzalmalononitrile
Vomiting gas	
DM (adamsite)	10-Chloro-5,10-dihydrophenarsazine

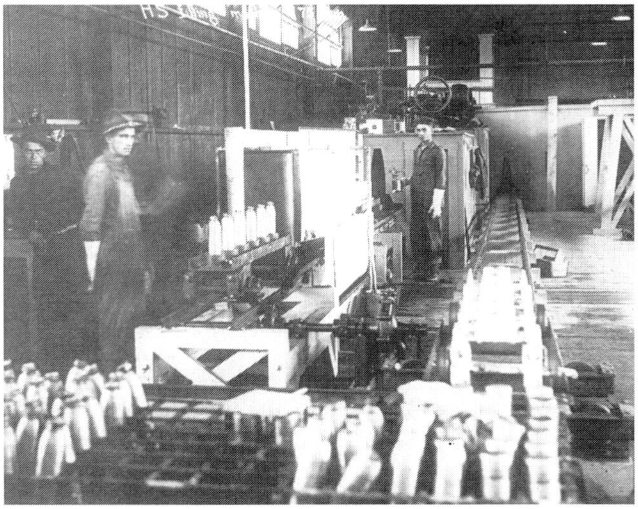

Fig. 4-2. Filling 75-mm artillery shells with mustard agent at Edgewood Arsenal, Maryland. Facilities designed to fill shells with chemical agents were notoriously hazardous. Anecdotal reports from mustard shell-filling plants indicated that over several months, the entire labor force could be expected to become ill.
Photograph: Courtesy of Chemical and Biological Defense Command Historical Research and Response Team, Aberdeen Proving Ground, Maryland.

Despretz in 1822, by Alfred Riche in 1854, and finally fully identified in 1886 by a German chemist, Victor Meyer. In 1848 chloropicrin (PS) was synthesized by a Scottish chemist and inventor, John Stenhouse.[1]

Numerous chemical weapons were used or proposed for use during campaigns and battles prior to World War I (see Chapters 2 and 3). In 1887 Germany apparently considered using lachrymators (tear agents) for military purposes. The French also began a rudimentary chemical weapons program, developing a tear gas grenade containing ethylbromoacetate and proposing to fill artillery shells with chloropicrin.[2,3]

World War I

Chemical Agent Production

Shortly after entering World War I in April 1917, the United States initiated a large-scale chemical weapons program. Chemical agent production and chemical shell filling were initially assigned to the US Army Ordnance Department, and then to the Chemical Warfare Service (CWS) when it was organized in June 1918. The primary facility for production and filling was Edgewood Arsenal, Maryland, erected in the winter of 1917–1918 (Figures 4-2 and 4-3). The facility was designed to have four shell-filling plants and four chemical agent production plants. The first shell-filling plant filled 75-mm shells with a mixture of chloropicrin and stannic chloride (designated NC) and Livens projectiles with phosgene. A second plant filled 75-mm shells with mustard agent. Two additional shell-filling plants were started but not completed before the end of the war.

The four agent production plants made the agents thought to be the highest priority for use on the western front in 1917. These were chlorine, chloropicrin, phosgene, and mustard agent. By 1918 the first two were no longer considered critical agents, although chlorine was used in phosgene production. Over 935 tons of phosgene and 711 tons of mustard agent were produced at the arsenal by the end of the war. Government contractors also produced these four agents and lewisite, named after Captain W Lee Lewis, a member of the CWS Research Division. Lewisite, however, never reached the front and was disposed of in the Atlantic after the armistice.[4,5]

Chemical Weapons

The CWS used foreign technology during the war for offensive weapons (see Chapters 2 and 3). The initial mode of offensive chemical attack was the portable chemical cylinder, designed to hold 30 to 70 lb of agent. To release the agent from the cylinders, soldiers opened a valve and relied on the wind to carry the agent in the correct direction. The resulting cloud could drift many miles behind enemy lines or, if the wind changed, contaminate friendly troops. The British improved on

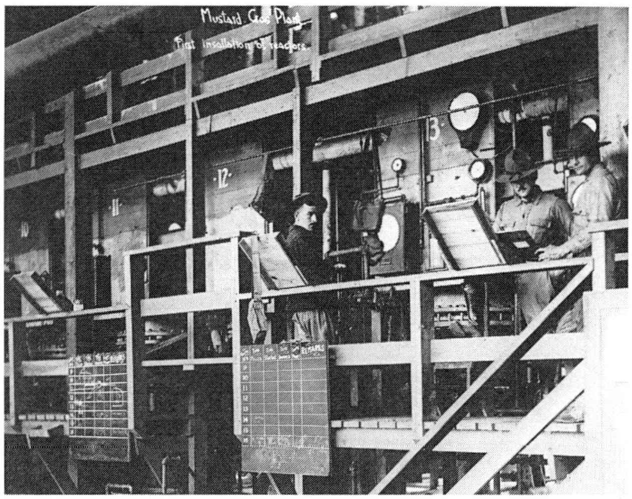

Fig. 4-3. Interior view of the mustard agent production plant at Edgewood Arsenal, Maryland. Photograph: Courtesy of Research, Development and Engineering Command Historical Research and Response Team, Aberdeen Proving Ground, Maryland.

this delivery system by developing the Livens projector, an 8-in, mortar-like tube that shot or projected a cylinder into the enemy's lines (Figures 4-4 and 4-5). Its range was 1,700 yd, with a flight time of 25 seconds. The Livens system had several problems; a battery of the projectors required extensive preparation because they were electrically fired and could not be moved once they were set up, and a battery could normally only be emplaced and fired once a day. This limited mobility required the element of surprise to prevent the Germans from taking counter measures.

British 4-in trench mortars, called "Stokes mortars" (Figure 4-6), provided a solution to some of the problems with the Livens projectors. Stokes mortars did not require extensive preparation and could be moved as needed. Because it was not rifled, the mortar's range was only 1,200 yd, which meant about a 14-second flight time. The small shell held only about 6 to 9 lb of agent, but experienced gunners could fire 25 rounds per minute. American troops used both Livens projectors and Stokes mortars during the war. An American version of the Stokes mortar failed to reach the front before the end of the war.

In addition to the special chemical weapons, the CWS fired chemical rounds from 75-mm, 4.7-in, 155-mm, and larger caliber guns. Many of these guns had ranges of 5 to 10 miles and payloads of as much as 50 lb of agent. Because of a shortage of shell parts and the late completion of US shell-filling plants, US artillery primarily fired French chemical rounds.[2,4,5]

The 1920s

The 1920s brought reports of isolated chemical attacks during the Russian civil war, as well as later accounts of the British, French, and Spanish using chemical weapons at various times during the decade (see chapter 2).[6] In addition, reports of Italy's developing chemical warfare service particularly alarmed the United States.[7–9] The CWS improved various delivery systems for chemical weapons during the 1920s. As early as 1920, Captain Lewis M McBride experimented with rifling the barrel of the Stokes mortar, and in 1924 a rifled Stokes mortar barrel was tested. Truing the inside diameter of the 4-in barrel before rifling expanded the bore's diameter to 4.2 in. This increased the range of the mortar from 1,100 yd (0.63 miles) to 2,400 yd (1.3 miles). In 1928 the improved mortar was standardized as the M1 4.2-in chemical mortar and became the CWS's prized ground weapon for delivering toxic chemical agents as well as smoke and high explosives.[5]

An expanded role for airplanes in the next chemical war was predicted in 1920:

> The dropping of gas bombs of all kinds upon assembly points, concentration camps, rest areas and the

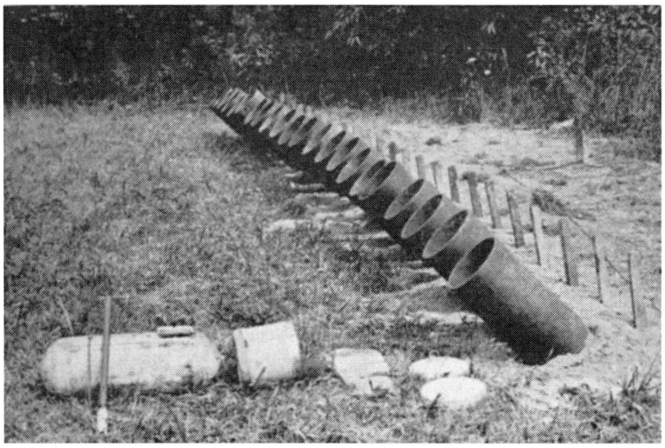

Fig. 4-4. A battery of dug-in Livens projectors, with one gas shell and its propellant charge shown in the foreground. Electrically-controlled salvo firing was the usual mode of operation. Emplacement was a slow process that limited the possibility of a surprise attack.
Photograph: Courtesy of Research, Development and Engineering Command Historical Research and Response Team, Aberdeen Proving Ground, Maryland.

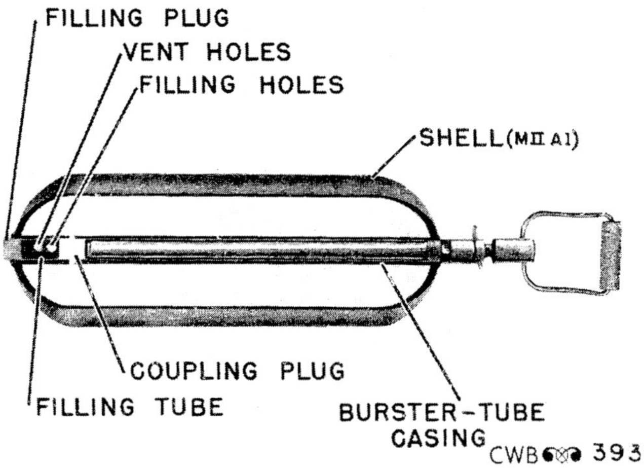

Fig. 4-5. Sectionalized view of a Livens projectile. The central tube contains a small explosive charge, which, when detonated by the contact fuse, breaks the shell, aiding in the dissemination of the chemical agent. The usual weight of the chemical agent was 30 lb; the shell weighed an additional 30 lb. Photograph: Courtesy of Research, Development and Engineering Command Historical Research and Response Team, Aberdeen Proving Ground, Maryland.

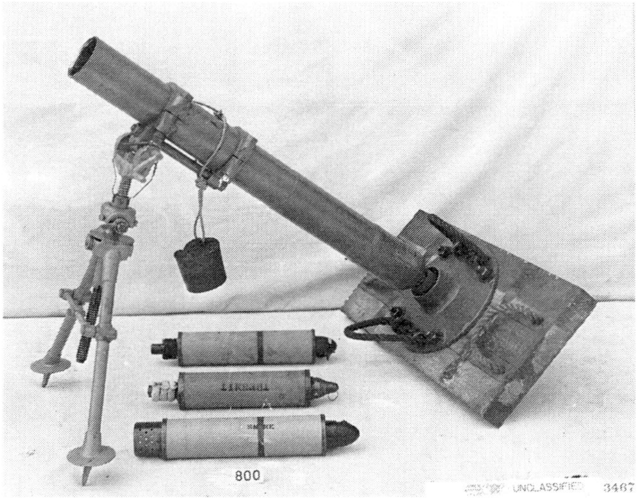

Fig. 4-6. A complete Stokes mortar with ammunition and accessories for firing.
Photograph: Courtesy of Research, Development and Engineering Command Historical Research and Response Team, Aberdeen Proving Ground, Maryland.

> like, will be so fruitful a field for casualties and for wearing down the morale of armies in the future that it will certainly be done and done on the very first stroke of war.[10(p4–5)]

In response to this prediction, the CWS standardized the M1 30-lb chemical bomb, which held only about 10 lb of agent because of its thick shell.[2] To test the use of airplanes in a chemical war, the CWS simulated chemical attacks against battleships in 1921.[11] In 1928 the CWS began stockpiling select chemical agents (see Chapter 2).[12]

The 1930s

New Chemical Agents

The CWS continued to maintain stockpiles of the key World War I chemical agents during the 1930s. In 1935 Captain Alden H Waitt, then secretary of the US Army Chemical Warfare School at Edgewood Arsenal and later chief chemical officer, summed up the CWS's planning for the next war:

> Foreign writers agree that at least for the first few months of any war, should one occur within a few years, the gases that were known at the end of the World War would be used. Of these, the opinion is unanimous that mustard gas would be the principal agent and the most valuable. Opinion in the United States coincides with this.[13(p285)]

In 1937 Edgewood Arsenal rehabilitated its mustard agent plant and produced 154 tons of mustard agent to increase its stockpile. The same year, the phosgene plant was renovated for additional production and the CWS changed phosgene from substitute standard to standard chemical warfare agent.[14]

The confidence in these selected agents resulted in the CWS overlooking the development of several key new agents. In the same article quoted above, Waitt wrote:

> Occasionally a statement appears in the newspapers that a new gas has been discovered superior to any previously known. Such statements make good copy, but not one of them has ever been verified. Today no gases are known that are superior to those known during the World War. It is unlikely that information about a new gas will be obtained until it is used in war. The chemical agent is too well adapted to secrecy. The only insurance against surprise by a new gas is painstaking research to find for ourselves every chemical agent that offers promise for offensive or defensive uses. It seems fairly safe to say that today mustard gas is still the king of warfare chemicals and to base our tactical schemes on that agent as a type.[13(p285)]

However, the reign of mustard agent was already ending. In 1935 Kyle Ward, Jr, published an article describing nitrogen mustard, an odorless vesicant agent. The CWS investigated the substance, but found it less vesicant than mustard. It was eventually standardized as HN-1, and while the United States discounted it, Germany took a great interest in the new vesicant.[5] Germany also developed tabun and sarin in the late 1930s and began production of the new agents by the time World War II began in 1939 (see chapter 2).[15,16]

New Chemical Weapons

In preparation for a future war, the CWS continued to stockpile chemical agents and weapons, primarily the Livens projectors, Stokes mortars, and portable cylinders, as well as chemical shells for 75-mm, 105-mm, and 155-mm artillery pieces. The production of the new 4.2-in chemical mortar eventually made that weapon the key ground delivery system for the CWS (Figures 4-7 and 4-8). Between 1928 and 1935 the Army attempted to make the 4.2-in a mechanized weapon by mounting it on various vehicles. The CWS also began experiments in 1934 to make the mortar a more versatile weapon by testing high explosive shells as an alternative to chemical rounds.

The improved M1A1 mortar was standardized in 1935. It had an improved barrel, an improved base-

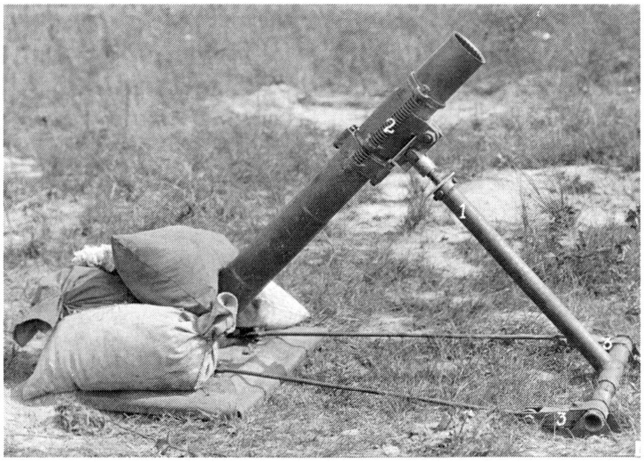

Fig. 4-7. An experimental 4.2-in chemical mortar, showing (1) the standard, (2) the barrel with the shock-absorbing mechanism, and (3) the tie rods connecting the standard to the baseplate. This weapon differed from the Stokes mortar, its predecessor, in that it was easier to set up and it was rifled; the spiral grooves can be seen on the inside of the barrel at its muzzle.
Photograph: Courtesy of Research, Development and Engineering Command Historical Research and Response Team, Aberdeen Proving Ground, Maryland.

plate, and a new standard connected to the baseplate by two tie rods for support. The M1A1 had a maximum range of 2,400 yd. Each shell held 5 to 7 lb of phosgene, mustard agent, cyanogen chloride, white phosphorus, or smoke agent.[2,5] Additional new delivery systems included the first standardized chemical land mine for mustard agent, developed in 1939. Designated the "M1," this 1-gallon, gasoline-type mine held 10 lb of mustard agent and required a detonating cord to burst the can and disseminate the agent.[5]

The 1940s: World War II and the Nuclear Age

The most important ground weapon for chemical agent delivery during the 1940s was the 4.2-in chemical mortar. In December 1941 there were only 44 chemical mortars on hand, but the supply quickly increased as the demand for the versatile weapon rose. The continued need for greater range, accuracy, durability, and ease in manufacturing resulted in the improved M2 4.2-in mortar in 1943. The M2 had a maximum range of 3,200 yd when standardized, which was later increased to 5,600 yd by modifying the propellant in test firings at Edgewood Arsenal in 1945. Despite a slow start, the M2 series 4.2-in chemical mortar rapidly became the central weapon of the CWS, not only for chemical agent delivery, but also for high explosive, smoke, and white phosphorus rounds. Over 8,000 chemical mortars were procured by the CWS for chemical mortar battalions during the war.[5,17] The other offensive weapons for chemical agent attack were to be delivered by artillery or by airplanes. The artillery had 75-mm, 105-mm, and 155-mm chemical rounds that were primarily filled with mustard agent.

In 1945 the CWS standardized the first chemical rockets: a 7.2-in version used phosgene and cyanogen chloride, fired from a 24-barrel, multiple-rocket–launcher platform, and a smaller, 2.36-in rocket fired cyanogen-chloride–filled bazooka rounds.[18] The Army Air Force had 100-lb mustard agent bombs, 500-lb phosgene or cyanogen chloride bombs, and 1,000-lb phosgene, cyanogen chloride, or hydrocyanic acid bombs. The CWS standardized the first good airplane smoke tank, the M10, for air delivery in 1940. This tank held 30 gallons of mustard (320 lb), lewisite (470 lb), or smoke material (Figure 4-9). The system was simple: electrically fired blasting caps shattered frangible seals in the air inlet and the discharge line, allowing air and gravity to force the liquid out; the plane's slipstream then broke the liquid into a spray. In addition, a newer M33 spray tank could hold 750 to 1,120 lb of mustard agent or lewisite. None of these weapons was used on the battlefield to disseminate chemical agents during the war.[19,20]

The 1950s: Heyday of the Chemical Corps

In response to the deterrence lesson learned in World War II and the growing Soviet threat (see Chapter 2), the Chemical Corps increased its chemical weapons capacity. Following the discovery of the German nerve agents after the end of World War II, the United States selected sarin for production. The first items standardized in 1954 for air delivery were the 1,000-lb M34 and M34A1 cluster bombs. These clusters held 76 M125 or M125A1 10-lb bombs, each containing 2.6 lb of sarin.[21] The corps standardized the M360 105-mm and the M121 155-mm shells for ground delivery in 1954. The smaller shell held about 1.6 lb of agent and the larger about 6.5 lb. In 1959 the corps standardized the first nonclustered bomb, designated the "MC-1 750-lb GB bomb." This was a modified general purpose demolition bomb that held about 215 lb of sarin filling and was suitable for high-speed aircraft.[22]

The 1960s

Having concentrated on sarin nerve agent bombs during the 1950s, the corps turned its attention to artillery, rocket, and other delivery systems, particularly for the newly standardized VX (O-ethyl-S-[2(diisopropylamino)ethyl]) nerve agent, in the 1960s. In 1960 the corps standardized the first nerve agent land mine, the M23 2-gallon VX mine (Figure 4-10). This mine resembled the conventional high-explosive

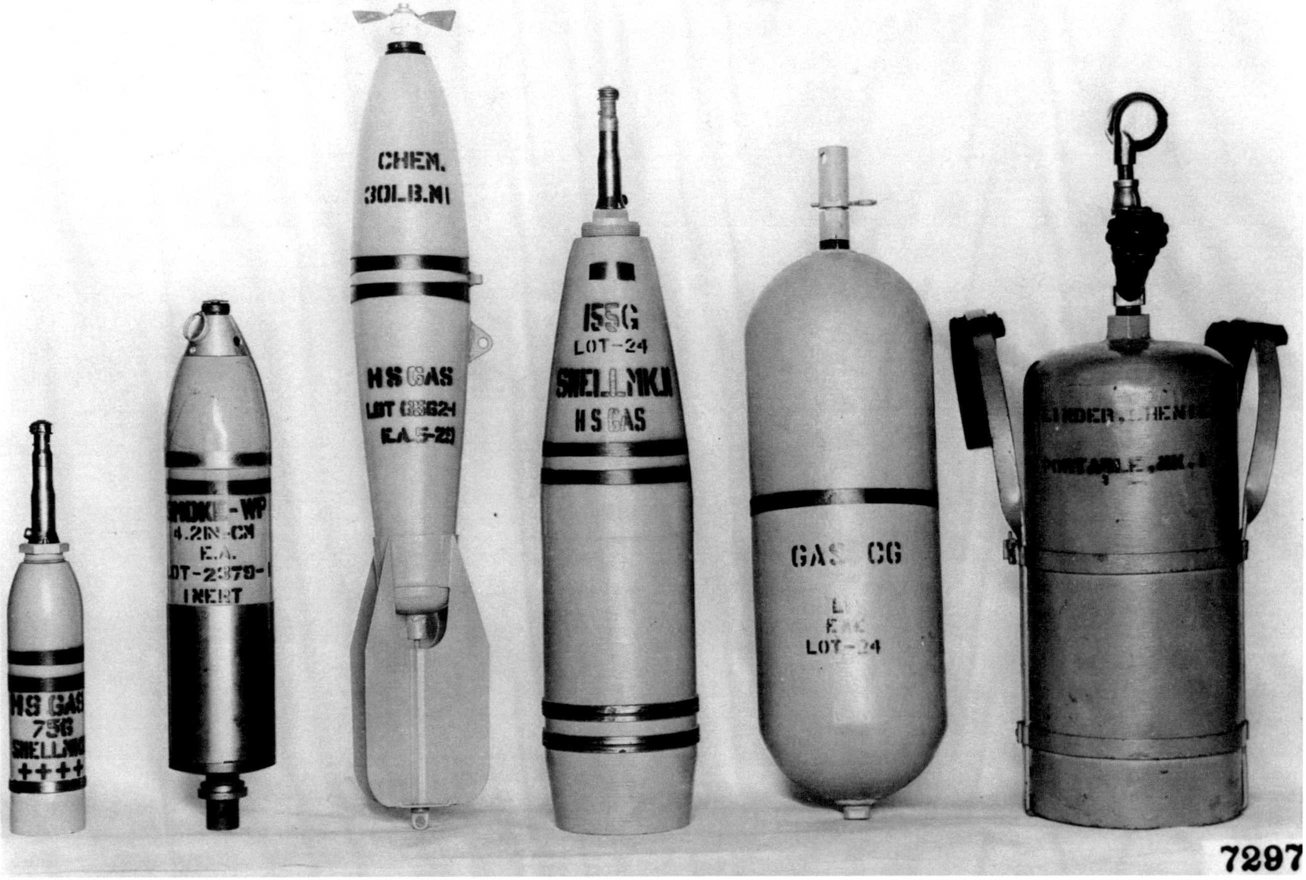

Fig. 4-8. Chemical weapons of the 1920s and 1930s. From left to right: the 75-mm mustard shell; the 4.2-in white phosphorus shell; the M1 30-lb mustard bomb; the Mk II 155-mm mustard shell; the Livens phosgene projectile; and the Mk I portable chemical cylinder.
Photograph: Courtesy of Research, Development and Engineering Command Historical Research and Response Team, Aberdeen Proving Ground, Maryland.

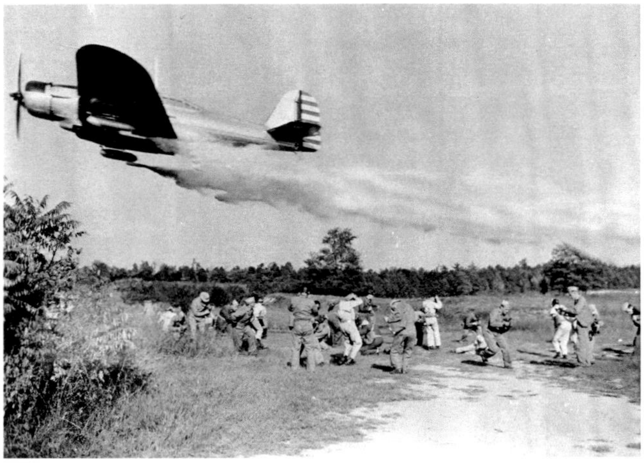

Fig. 4-9. Aerial spraying of a Chemical Warfare School class with tear gas during a training event, 1937. Photograph: Courtesy of Research, Development and Engineering Command Historical Research and Response Team, Aberdeen Proving Ground, Maryland.

land mine, but held about 11.5 lb of agent. It was designed to be activated either by a vehicle running over it or with an antipersonnel, antitampering fuse.[23]

In 1961 the corps standardized two new VX projectiles for artillery. The M121A1 was an improved version of the earlier sarin round. Each round held about 6.5-lb of agent. The M426 8-in sarin or VX projectile held over 15.5 lb of agent.

The early 1960s was the peak of the nerve agent rocket program. The program was first started at the end of World War II to duplicate the German V-2 missiles used against England. The United States eventually developed both short-range and long-range rockets. The corps standardized the M55 115-mm rocket in 1960 for short-range tactical support (Figure 4-11). Described as the first significant ground capability for the delivery of chemical agents since the 4.2-in chemical mortar, the M55 was loaded with 11 lb of VX or sarin nerve agent. When fired from the M91

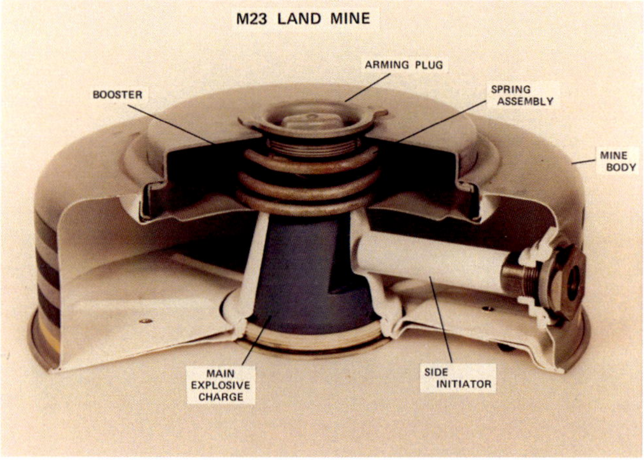

Fig. 4-10. The M23 VX land mine. Most of the interior was intended to be filled with the nerve agent VX.
Photograph: Courtesy of Research, Development and Engineering Command Historical Research and Response Team, Aberdeen Proving Ground, Maryland.

multiple rocket launcher, its range was over 6 miles. Each launcher held 45 rockets that could be fired simultaneously. The Army initially approved 40,000 sarin-filled and 20,000 VX-filled rockets, but many more were actually filled.[23]

For middle-range tactical support, the corps standardized the M79 sarin warhead for the 762-mm "Honest John" rocket in 1960 (Figure 4-12). The rocket had a range of 16 miles and the warhead held 356 M135 4.5-in spherical bomblets, each containing about 1 lb of sarin. A smaller warhead was standardized in 1964 for the 318-mm "Little John" rocket, which contained 52 of the improved M139 bomblets, each holding 1.3 lb of sarin (Figure 4-13). The first long-range rocket warhead was standardized the same year for the Sergeant missile system. The missile had a range of 75 miles and the warhead held 330 M139 sarin bomblets. Additional developmental projects added chemical warheads to other long-range missiles, such as the Pershing missile, which had a range of over 300 miles.[24]

In addition to the rocket program, the corps examined several drones for chemical agent delivery. The SD-2 drone was a slow (300 knots), remote controlled, recoverable drone that could hold over 200 lb of nerve agent. It had a range of about 100 knots and could disperse agent over about 5 to 10 knots. The SD-5 was an improvement that used a jet engine to achieve speeds of over Mach .75 and a range of over 650 knots. The added horsepower allowed it to hold about 1,260 lb of chemical agent that was discharged through a tail nozzle.[25]

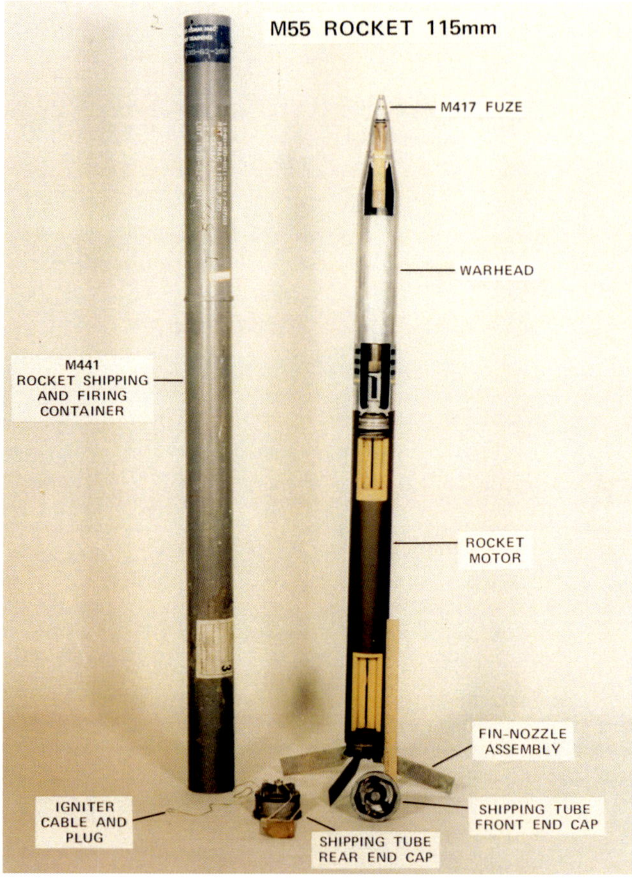

Fig. 4-11. The M55 115-mm rocket could hold the nerve agents VX or sarin, but the aluminum warhead began leaking soon after production.
Photograph: Courtesy of Research, Development and Engineering Command Historical Research and Response Team, Aberdeen Proving Ground, Maryland.

The BZ (3-quinuclidinyl benzilate) incapacitant program also reached weaponization status in the 1960s. In 1962 the corps standardized the M43 750-lb BZ bomb cluster and the M44 175-lb BZ generator cluster. The M43 held 57 M138 BZ bomblets. The M44 held three 50-lb thermal generators, each containing 42 BZ canisters.[25]

The 1970s: Emergence of Binary Weapons

The end of the chemical weapons production program, as ordered by President Richard Nixon in 1969, stopped all production but left one type of chemical retaliatory weapon still in development: binary weapons, which the Army first investigated in the 1950s. Until that time, chemical weapons were unitary chemical munitions, meaning that the agent was produced at a plant, put into the munitions, and then stored ready

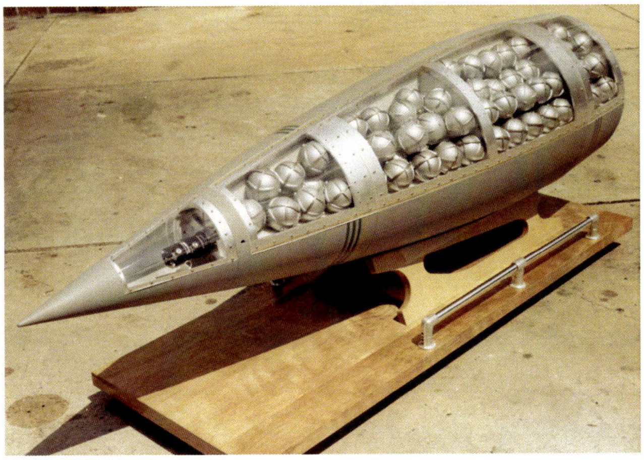

Fig. 4-12. A chemical warhead for the Honest John rocket. It was designed to break apart and disperse the spherical bomblets of nerve agent.
Photograph: Courtesy of Research, Development and Engineering Command Historical Research and Response Team, Aberdeen Proving Ground, Maryland.

to be used. Because most agents were extremely corrosive, long-term storage of unitary munitions was logistically problematic.

The idea behind binary munitions was to create nerve agent in the weapon after firing or dropping by mixing two nonlethal chemicals. The two nonlethal chemicals could be stored separately, solving the problem of long-term storage and making handling safer. The Navy initially took more interest in the binary program during the 1960s and requested a 500-lb bomb designated the "Bigeye." In the Army, however, the binary program received high priority only after the production of unitary chemical munitions was halted.

The M687 projectile used a standard M483A1 155-mm projectile to carry the chemical payload. The chemical reactants were contained in two separate, plastic-lined, hermetically sealed containers. These leak-proof canisters were loaded through the rear of the shell and fitted one behind the other in the body of the projectile. The forward canister contained methylphosphonic difluoride and the rear canister contained isopropyl alcohol and isopropylamine solution.[26,27]

M687 projectiles were shipped and stored with only the forward methylphosphonic-difluoride–filled canister in place to ensure safe handling. A fiberboard spacer occupied the cavity provided for the isopropyl alcohol and isopropylamine solution canister. Projectiles were secured horizontally on a pallet, as opposed to the conventional vertical position used for other

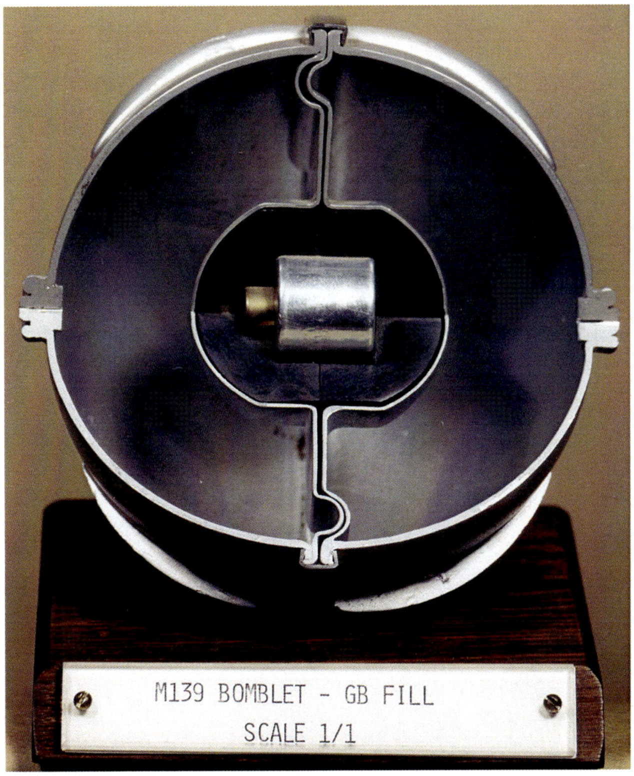

Fig. 4-13. The M139 4.5-in spherical sarin bomblet used in the Little John rocket. The vanes on the outside of the bomblet created a spin, which armed the impact fuse. The explosive burster is in the center, and sarin fills the two outer compartments.
Photograph: Courtesy of Research, Development and Engineering Command Historical Research and Response Team, Aberdeen Proving Ground, Maryland.

155-mm projectiles. This orientation permitted rapid removal of the projectile's base with a special wrench. The fiberboard spacers were removed and replaced with the isopropyl alcohol and isopropylamine solution canisters. The fuse was installed just prior to firing. Upon firing, setback and spin forces caused the facing disks on the canisters to rupture, allowing the reactants to combine to form sarin while en route to the target.[26,27]

The last open air test of lethal agents took place at Dugway Proving Ground on September 16, 1969, when a 155-mm projectile filled with sarin binary reactants was test fired. Throughout the early 1970s additional test firings took place using simulants. In 1976 the Army standardized the M687 binary GB2 155-mm projectile (Figure 4-14).

In addition to the M687, the Army also worked on the Bigeye bomb and other projectiles, including an 8-in projectile. None of these was ever standardized. Standardization of the M687 did not lead immediately

a

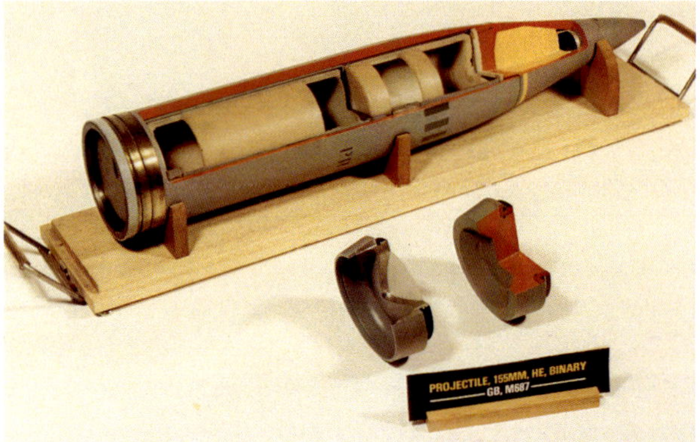

b

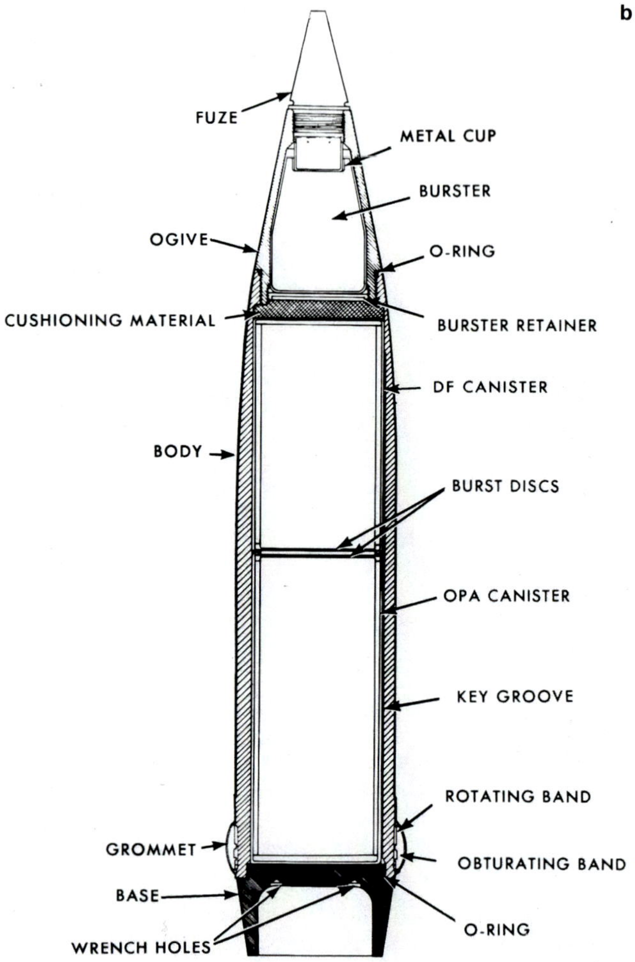

Fig. 4-14. (a) The M687 GB2 binary 155-mm projectile, which was standardized in 1976 but not produced until a decade later. **(b)** A diagram of the M687 GB2 binary 155-mm projectile.
Photograph (a): Courtesy of Research, Development and Engineering Command Historical Research and Response Team, Aberdeen Proving Ground, Md. (b) Reproduced from: Department of the Army. *Binary Chemical Munitions Program.* Aberdeen Proving Ground, Maryland: Chemical Systems Laboratory; 1981: 5. Programmatic Environmental Impact Statement ARCSL-EIS-8101.

to production. In 1976 Congress passed a Department of Defense (DoD) appropriation authorization act that restricted the development and production of binary chemical weapons unless the president certified to Congress that such production was essential to the national interest. The Army took another decade to locate the production plants, pass environmental inspection, receive presidential approval, and begin production of binary chemical weapons.

The 1980s: Production of Binary Weapons

In 1981 the secretary of defense issued a memorandum to proceed with acquiring binary chemical bombs. However, the appropriation restrictions of 1976 blocked procurement of binary munitions for several more years. In 1984 Congress created a chemical warfare review commission to consider several issues related to the military's chemical warfare preparedness. The committee visited numerous sites, interviewed experts, reviewed policy, and examined intelligence reports. Among their findings was the following:

> The Commission has concluded, however, that in spite of the approximately $4 billion that the Congress has appropriated since 1978 for defense against chemical warfare, that defense, measured either for purposes of deterrence or for war fighting utility, is not adequate today and is not likely to become so. Chemical combat as it would exist in the late twentieth century is an arena in which because defense must be nearly perfect to be effective at all, detection is so difficult, and surprise offers such temptation the offense enjoys a decisive advantage if it need not anticipate chemical counterattack. Defense continues to be important to pursue, because it can save some lives and preserve some military capabilities. But for this country to put its faith in defense against chemical weapons as an adequate response to the Soviet chemical threat would be a dangerous illusion.[28(p50)]

The answer to the problem was simply stated by President Ronald Reagan:

> The United States must maintain a limited retaliatory capability until we achieve an effective ban. We must

> be able to deter a chemical attack against us or our allies. And without a modern and credible deterrent, the prospects for achieving a comprehensive ban would be nil.[29(p23)]

In 1985 Congress passed Public Law 99-145[30] authorizing production of chemical weapons, and in 1987 President Reagan certified to Congress that all the conditions had been met to start binary chemical weapons production. The production of the M687 binary projectile began on December 16, 1987, at Pine Bluff Arsenal, Arkansas, despite public resistance incited by environmental and safety concerns. To resolve political concerns, the M20 canisters were filled and stored at Pine Bluff Arsenal, while the M21 canisters were produced and filled at Louisiana Army Ammunition Plant. The filled M21 canisters and shell bodies were then stored at Tooele Army Depot, Utah. The parts would be combined when necessary to provide the Army with a chemical retaliatory capability.[31]

In addition to the M687 round, development continued on the BLU 80/B Bigeye bomb and the XM135 multiple-launch rocket system binary chemical warhead. The Bigeye bomb was compatible with Air Force, Navy, and Marine Corps fixed-wing aircraft. The bomb dispersed persistent nerve agent VX after mixing two nonlethal chemical agents, NE and QL. The XM135 binary chemical warhead was designed as a free flight, semipersistent, nerve-agent–dispersing system. The XM135 was fired from the MLRS, a 12-round rocket launcher mounted on a tracked vehicle.[31]

The 1990s: The Threat Materializes

Despite Iraq's chemical warfare use in the 1980s (see Chapter 2), operations Desert Shield and Desert Storm were free of tactical chemical warfare operations, although an accidental chemical exposure occurred in the Army's 3rd Armored Division (see Chapter 3). Counterterrorism agencies also attempted to use some of the items developed by the Chemical Corps in the civilian world. In 1993 the Federal Bureau of Investigation (FBI) decided to use a riot control agent to attack the Branch Davidian compound in Waco, Texas. Fires broke out, destroying the complex and killing 80 occupants, though whether the fire was started from the inside or was the result of FBI tactics remains unresolved.[32]

After Waco, many state and local officials told Congress that they did not have the training or equipment to combat a chemical act of terrorism. Senator Sam Nunn of Georgia expressed his concerns, saying, "I, like many of my colleagues, believe there is a high likelihood that a chemical or biological incident will take place on American soil in the next several years."[33]

After the Aum Shinrikyo attacks of 1995 and other terrorist incidents that will be described in the next section, the use of chemical weapons for terrorism became a key concern of the Army. In 1996 Congress responded by passing a new antiterrorism training bill to prepare the United States for future chemical terrorism incidents. In addition to using military experts to equip and train local chemical response teams, the bill provided funding for former Soviet republics to destroy their own chemical weapons to keep them out of the hands of terrorists.[33,34]

HISTORY OF CHEMICAL TERRORISM

Definition of Terms

The term "terrorist" can be traced back to the French Revolution's "Reign of Terror" in the late 18th century, when the French government executed 12,000 people as enemies of the state. After World War II, colonies began to fight for independence, and acts of "terrorism" were one method of attacking the government. In the 1960s and 1970s several terrorist organizations became active, such as the Basque separatists in Spain, the Irish Republican Army in Ireland, Marxist groups in Africa and Latin America, the Baader-Meinhof Gang in West Germany, the Red Brigades in Italy, and the Japanese Red Army. A number of terrorist organizations in the Middle East began operations, most attempting to carry out attacks against Israel and its allies following the Arab-Israeli conflict of 1973. Many Middle Eastern groups, such as Hamas, Hezbollah, and Al Qaeda, have strong religious connections with extreme Islamic fundamentalism.

The DoD defines terrorism as "the calculated use of unlawful violence or the threat of unlawful violence to inculcate fear; intended to coerce or intimidate governments or societies in the pursuit of goals that are generally political, religious, or ideological."[35] Terrorists often target noncombatants to show that no one is safe and to cause the greatest amount of fear. The State Department defines "noncombatants" as civilians and military personnel who are not deployed in a war zone or a war-like setting.[36] In addition, military law defines specific members of the armed forces, such as chaplains or surgeons whose duties lie outside combat, as noncombatants. Definitions are important to distinguish true terrorist activities from those of criminal organizations, pirates, psychotics, disgruntled employees, and covert state operations. Title 22 of the US Code also identifies these key terms:

- terrorism: premeditated, politically motivated violence perpetrated against noncombatant targets by subnational groups or clandestine agents;
- international terrorism: terrorism involving citizens or the territory of more than one country; and
- terrorist group: any group practicing, or which has significant subgroups which practice, international terrorism.[37]

In addition, domestic terrorism includes activities that "involve acts dangerous to human life that are a violation of the criminal laws of the United States or of any State" that "appear to be intended to intimidate or coerce a civilian population; to influence the policy of a government by intimidation or coercion; or to affect the conduct of a government by mass destruction, assassination, or kidnapping; and occur primarily within the territorial jurisdiction of the United States."[37] While most discussions of domestic terrorism focus on the attempts by terrorist organizations to attack civilians and to influence governments along political, religious, or ideological lines, the potential also exists for lone individuals to attack symbols of the government or the civilian populace (eg, the 1995 Oklahoma City bombing incident and the 1996 Atlanta Olympics pipe bomb incident). Whether they work alone or in groups, the goal of terrorists is to intimidate.

State intimidation through terrorism, or fascism, wherein a village may be exterminated by an oppressive occupier as an example to others, was demonstrated in the 1988 indiscriminate gassing of civilians in Halabja, Birjinni, and other towns in the Kurdish region of Iraq. Over 5,000 citizens lost their lives in these attacks, which were later confirmed by the United Nations (UN) to have been poisoning by sulfur mustard and nerve agent.[38] According to Captain Kifah Ali Hassan, director of the Intelligence Center of Kalar, "During the month of March 1988, our aircraft bombed the headquarters of the sabotage bands in the villages of Saywan . . . and Balakajar . . . in a chemical strike. This resulted in the death of 50 saboteurs and the wounding of 20 other saboteurs."[39]

Despite the deaths of more than 200 Marines in the Beirut bombing in 1983, the military did not have a clear approach to addressing terrorism until the Khobar towers bombing incident in 1996. This event caused the chairman of the Joint Chiefs of Staff to appoint a deputy director for antiterrorism and force protection to lead the development of joint doctrine, training, and tactics for antiterrorism efforts. These efforts to protect individuals on military installations and in DoD-owned or leased facilities has been termed "installation preparedness." Traditionally, installation preparedness has focused on conventional forms of terrorism, such as the use of small, conventional explosives, handguns, knives, and threats of violence or kidnappings. In 2002 the Office of the Secretary of Defense directed an effort to improve the protection of US military installations and facilities against the potential effects of chemical, biological, radiological, and nuclear incidents caused by terrorists. Although each service and combatant command is responsible for addressing and executing antiterrorism efforts within its respective area of responsibility, the DoD focus directed the addition of chemical, biological, radiological, and nuclear defense equipment to installations and facilities. Following a pilot project initiated in the fall of 2002, military installations began to acquire the equipment in the fall of 2004.[40]

Incidents of Chemical Terrorism

Compared to chemical agents, biological agents are decidedly more subtle, and conventional explosives are considerably cheaper and more readily available. Biological agents offer a much wider impact than chemical ones because they can be quietly delivered and it can take days for infection to manifest. Chemical agents, however, are appealing to terrorists because compared to biologicals, chemicals are ubiquitous, inexpensive, and more stable.[41] Chlorine and cyanide are extremely common, and the technology required to produce a nerve agent like sarin is readily accessible to any moderately experienced chemist. Additionally, chemical agents used as weapons, especially nerve agents, are more dramatic than biological weapons. As history has shown, chemical agents can wreak havoc in urban settings; onlookers bear witness to the convulsive sequelae of an insidious chemical poisoning that needs no heralding of an exploding shell.

The general tendency of many terrorism experts is to declare "it's not a question of if, but when" terrorists will use chemical agents against noncombatants. This view is focused primarily on the vulnerability of unprotected civilians, increased access to education sources, and increased availability of technology with hazardous materials in a global economy. Additionally, pound for pound, chemicals are much more potent than conventional explosives, causing many experts to speculate that terrorists would naturally be interested in weapons that could cause the most casualties. However, despite documented examples of terrorist interest in chemical warfare agents and the concern of government officials about the impact of a terrorist chemical incident, the actual history of any such incident is minimal.

The Alphabet Bomber (1974)

Muharem Kurbegovic, known as the "Alphabet Bomber," may be the first lone terrorist to have sought to use chemical warfare agents against citizens on US soil. Kurbegovic, who was apparently mentally disturbed, had a background in engineering and could have posed a greater chemical threat had he not been captured. He threatened to fire chemical-laden artillery shells at Capitol Hill and mailed postcards to each of the nine Supreme Court justices, securing tiny, liquid-filled vials under the stamps and claiming that the vials contained nerve agent (which was later proven untrue). He also detonated a series of bombs in Los Angeles, leaving behind tape cassettes labeled with letters (hence his nickname) that, had he not been captured, were to eventually spell out the name of his fictitious terrorist organization, Aliens of America. A search of his apartment 2 months after his arrest revealed a hidden cache that included 25 lb of NaCN and other chemicals capable of volatilizing cyanide or being assembled to manufacture phosgene or nerve agent.[42]

The Covenant, the Sword, and the Arm of the Lord (1986)

The Covenant, the Sword, and the Arm of the Lord (CSA) was a paramilitary survivalist group numbering about a hundred people living in the Ozark Mountains in Arkansas. Their ideology was based on a movement known as "Christian identity," that in part envisioned an apocalypse that would destroy "sinners" and allow believers to survive. CSA had largely been ignored until one of its members allegedly murdered a woman and another killed a Missouri state trooper in 1985. The second incident provoked a massive search, leading to a law enforcement raid on the CSA's main complex. In addition to a sizeable amount of conventional weaponry, the task force found 30 gallons of potassium cyanide. CSA's leader initially claimed that the chemical was meant for killing pests, although the group's second-in-command admitted that the potassium cyanide was obtained to poison urban water supplies. Although the 30 gallons of poison would have been diluted in a large city reservoir, the group was convinced that God would make sure the right people died. CSA appears to have decided on potassium cyanide because it was easy to purchase. Although its initial attack with potassium cyanide would have been unsuccessful, CSA may have pursued additional attempts to use chemical weapons.[43]

Aum Shinrikyo (1995)

The story behind Aum Shinrikyo's use of sarin nerve agent in the Tokyo subway on March 20, 1995, is perhaps the most famous and repeated example of chemical terrorism. It remains the only case of a nongovernmental group successfully manufacturing a modern military chemical warfare agent and using it against unprotected civilians. Aum Shinrikyo, or "Supreme Truth," was founded around 1987 by Shoko Asahara, a partially-blind guru espousing a faith system that incorporated aspects of Buddhism, Hinduism, and Christianity. Failing to achieve legitimate political influence and reacting to outside pressures, Asahara eventually incorporated an Armageddon involving chemical agents into his teachings, and even predicted his own death by sarin.[44]

Aum Shinrikyo was well-financed, claiming to have a membership of some 40,000 by 1995, including 10,000 in Japan and 30,000 in Russia (where the recent fall of communism had left citizens vulnerable to new spiritual ideologies and charismatic leaders). Well-funded, organized, and centrally controlled terrorist groups are more likely to be capable of acquiring, developing, and implementing a sophisticated chemical warfare capability. The Aum was particularly controlling over its hierarchical structure, and members acquiesced to a "Supreme Truth" that effectively stifled any independent thought or questioning of its authoritarian spiritual leader. The Aum facilitated internal organizational control and intimidated police scrutiny and access to its members and workings in three ways: (1) demanding its members sever all family ties, (2) seeking and acquiring the status of a formal and protected religion, and (3) responding vigorously to any and all criticisms and legal challenges with defamation suits.[44] Bellicose intimidation, both externally and internally, was routine, and included murder; at least 20 of its members appear to have been killed with sarin or VX.[45]

Asahara had been interested in manufacturing both chemical and biological warfare agents since at least 1990, when cult members began to run for political office. The group researched how to manufacture sarin nerve agent and planned to build a facility capable of producing 2 tons of sarin daily. After failing to cause casualties by attacks with anthrax the group had manufactured, the Aum began using sarin in 1993. On June 27, 1994, the Aum targeted a neighborhood in Matsumoto, about 200 miles northwest of

Tokyo, where three judges were hearing a real estate lawsuit against the cult. The decision seemed likely to go against the Aum, who then decided to murder the judges. Using a modified refrigeration truck that held a heater, an electric fan, and 30 kilograms of sarin, the assassination team arrived at the courthouse too late to intercept the judges. They traveled to the judges' living quarters, an apartment complex, and released the sarin near midnight, spreading a cloud of agent over a 500 by 100-yd area. Seven people were killed and 144, including the three judges, were injured.[44,45]

In March 1995 the Japanese police planned to raid Aum's major facilities. In an attempt to disrupt the raid, cult leaders decided to attack the Tokyo subway, focusing on subway stations that served key government agencies, including the national police agency. Five teams of two cult members boarded three major lines of the subway, each with two polyethylene bags of 600 g of sarin sealed inside a second bag. Once on board the trains, the terrorists punctured the bags with umbrellas and quickly left. As the sarin evaporated, passengers at more than 15 subway stations were exposed. Twelve people died, 54 were in critical condition, and about 900 required hospitalization (including about 135 emergency responders). More than 5,500 "worried well" individuals stormed to the hospitals, demanding screening and treatments.[46]

Two HCN attacks followed the Tokyo subway incident in an attempt to cause further panic. Cult members also attempted to mix bags containing sulfuric acid and NaCN to release HCN gas in a subway restroom. Over a period of 5 years, the Aum probably attempted to release chemical agent 17 times, including squirting VX and phosgene through keyholes and mail slots.[47,48]

When police finally raided the cult's chemical agent facility at Kamikuishiki, near Mount Fuji, they found extensive amounts of agent precursors, including around 500 drums of the sarin ingredient phosphorus trichloride, several forklift pallets of sodium fluoride, and isopropyl alcohol. Other chemicals included 34 large containers of acetonitrile, cyanide compounds, and even atropine. Ultimately, around 150 tons of about 40 compounds were reported to have been found, enough to yield 50 tons of sarin. Furthermore, the Kamikuishiki facility may have been capable of manufacturing tabun. The Aum reportedly invested around $10 million to $30 million toward the development of a large-scale sarin manufacturing facility and had tried, unsuccessfully, to recruit Russian chemical weapons engineers in the fall of 1994. The building was well-equipped with state-of-the-art components from commercial sources to produce thousands of kilograms of agent per year.[49]

There may have been plans for cultists to bring sarin into the United States for attacks on Disney World; New York, New York; and Washington, DC. Investigations and hearings on the Aum Shinrikyo incident led directly to the Nunn-Lugar-Domenici Act (within Public Law 104-210, National Defense Authorization Act for FY 1997, dated September 23, 1997[50]). This act directed the DoD to initiate a domestic preparedness program that included training the emergency responders of 120 major cities, creating a rapid response force, and developing an emergency hotline and a nonemergency "helpline," among other initiatives. The FBI and the Federal Emergency Management Agency formalized Presidential Decision Directive 39, issued in June 1995, which outlined federal counterterrorism plans, and created a terrorism annex in the Federal Response Plan in 1997.

The Aum cult was short lived but enormously successful.[51] Immensely wealthy (contributions reportedly reached $1.4 billion,[52] Aum Shinrikyo was also well networked, owned extensive property, and had even won the confidence of the head of Russia's national security council. The group had bought access to Russian television and radio, purchased small arms and a retired Russian military helicopter, sought both weapons training and technology, and maintained offices around the world. If its leadership had been less impetuous and aggressive, the group might have developed a functional biological weapons capability and a better chemical agent capability. The Aum was poised to evolve into a global menace.

Cyanide Plot Against the US Embassy, Italy (2002)

In March of 2002 Italian authorities arrested a group of suspected terrorists, most of them Moroccans, apparently plotting to attack the US Embassy in Rome. The group had about 9 lb of potassium-ferrocyanide, a compound used in agriculture, and some explosive powder possibly intended to create the heat necessary to release the cyanide. They were said to possess maps of water pipes leading to the Embassy, although potassium-ferrocyanide will only release cyanide when treated with acid and high temperatures, does not readily permeate tissue cells, and was not expected to have caused significant toxicity if directly applied to the water system.[53]

William Krar (2003)

In April 2003 federal and state law enforcement agents raided the Noonday, Texas, home and storage units of William Krar and his common-law wife, Judith

Bruey, uncovering a small arsenal of ammunition, pipe bombs, machine guns, remote-controlled bombs disguised as briefcases, pamphlets on making chemical weapons, 2 lb of NaCN, and bottles of hydrochloric, nitric, and acetic acids. The search was ordered after Krar attempted to send false identification documents to a self-described militia member. It is unclear what he was intending to do with the cache found at his storage unit and who else may have been involved.[54]

Al Qaeda

Osama bin Laden, born into a wealthy Saudi Arabian family, formed Al Qaeda, or "the Base," toward the end of the Soviet Union's involvement in Afghanistan, around 1988. This organization was dedicated to opposing non-Islamic governments and to driving US armed forces out of Islamic countries such as Saudi Arabia and Somalia. Initially establishing a headquarters in Sudan in 1991, bin Laden set up a number of legitimate front companies to provide income and support to the group's members, as well as to obtain explosives, weapons, and chemicals. Although terrorist groups had been suspected of seeking to obtain and use chemical weapons for some years, it was not clear what Al Qaeda's goals were until the publication of a November 2001 interview with bin Laden. A Pakistani newspaper quoted bin Laden as saying, "I wish to declare that if America used chemical or nuclear weapons against us, then we may retort with chemical and nuclear weapons. We have the weapons as a deterrent."[55]

The US intelligence community acknowledged that Al Qaeda was seeking weapons of mass destruction but believed it possessed neither the weapons nor any means to deliver them. Yet when US forces invaded Afghanistan to attack and defeat Al Qaeda and the Taliban government in October 2002, attempts were made to identify any possible sites at which Al Qaeda might be developing chemical or biological weapons or training people to use such weapons. US Central Command, with support from other government agencies, developed "sensitive site exploitation" units to search for and collect such evidence. No weapons or agent stock were recovered, but training materials, including videos demonstrating the use of toxic industrial chemicals on dogs, were discovered. Symptoms displayed by the dogs, initially judged to be from nerve agent, were probably from cyanide poisoning,[56] a mode of killing previously revealed in Al Qaeda plots. Later in 2002 reports emerged that Al Qaeda members had acquired old Iraqi VX munitions, a proliferation of concern because UN inspectors in Iraq failed to account for some 1.5 tons of VX, of which some portion was weaponized.[57]

In April 2004 Jordanian police arrested Al Qaeda operatives in a plot involving 20 tons of chemicals, purchased for $170,000. The chemicals, which included a large amount of sulfuric acid, were speculated to be intended for deadly explosions in the city of Amman.[58]

Once openly able to attract and train Islamic militants to disseminate its terrorist missions, Al Qaeda's infrastructure has been under pursuit and, without the protection of a national benefactor, remains clandestine and unlikely to be able to establish a highly structured base of operations. Hence, the current Al Qaeda model contrasts sharply with Aum Shinrikyo in that its adherents often appear loosely connected by time spent in training camps, exposure to common indoctrination and technical manuals, and shared religious contacts and extremism. They are more likely to engage in chemical terrorism in an opportunistic way, as seen in their attempt to poison the water supply of the US Embassy in Rome. However, local Al-Qaeda–affiliated groups have shown the ability to implement coordinated attacks, and the possibility of orchestrated attacks, such as that of September 2001, cannot be discounted.[59]

Accidental Battlefield Exposure in Operation Desert Storm

An unclassified analysis by the Central Intelligence Agency[60] lists all potential chemical agent releases that may have occurred in the context of the first Persian Gulf War. In March 1991, after the conclusion of Operation Desert Storm, US Army demolition teams destroyed captured Iraqi munitions in bunkers and pits in the same way it eliminated conventional arms in similar situations. In 1996 it was determined that two Khamisiyah sites contained 122-mm rockets weaponized with a mixture of sarin and cyclosarin. Although no symptoms of nerve agent exposure were noted at the time, a considerable modeling and research effort was initiated by the DoD to evaluate possible exposure dosage and long-term health effects of low-level nerve agent exposure.

Initial 1997 atmospheric modeling studies[60] of the plume associated with the demolition indicated that the prevailing winds at the time were not directed at any large concentrations of troops and that concentrations of agent were likely many-fold lower than those required to elicit threshold agent symptoms such as miosis. Employing field studies of agent deposition, the studies determined that only shells with charges placed immediately beneath them would have ignited a rocket's aerosolizing burster tubes. Therefore, aerosolized droplets were largely removed from the model, and most agent was represented as vapor or as pooled liquid in the storage site. Meteorological data, as well as the distribution of soot deposited around the blast sites, was used in the plume model. Several Czech chemical agent detectors that had sounded alarms were not located in the vicinity of the plume.

These conclusions were met with criticism from government and public sectors. In response, further model refinements and better data on topography, ground cover, deposition of agent onto physical surfaces encountered by the plume, nerve agent stability, and soldier deployment positions were incorporated into the studies.[61] The revised models of 2000 also incorporated previously classified information on munitions and agent quantity and quality, including a revision of the number of projectiles from 500 in 1997 to 225. A potentially higher toxicity of cyclosarin (25% of the fill) was also incorporated. The outcome of the 2000 modeling study showed a narrower plume distribution and the conclusions remained effectively unchanged.[61]

Although up to 100,000 veterans were involved, epidemiological studies proved unhelpful because of the diversity of reported symptoms and the varied placement of personnel relative to the release site. No increased hospitalization rates were observed,[62,63] and demographically adjusted mortality rates were not found to be higher than those in the general population; rather, they were possibly lower.[64] Troops within 50 km of the explosions were found to fare no worse than those deployed further away. Although sarin is not known to be a carcinogen, a 1995 study found a doubling of brain cancer incidence, from 12 to 50 cases/100,000 population, among veterans in the vicinity of the demolition.[64] However, chemically induced brain cancer within 4 years of exposure is questionable; the data suggest that preexisting conditions may more likely have been the cause.[65]

Overall the general conclusion drawn from modeling studies and from reviews of a considerable number of animal studies of low-level agent effects, including one by the US Institute of Medicine,[66] provide no basis for supporting that personnel in the Khamisiyah area were affected by the detonations. While some low-level exposure impacts were observed in animal studies, many of these employed subsymptomatic exposures at levels much higher than were likely to have been present at Khamisiyah. Furthermore, considering the apparent rapid sequestration of low levels of nerve agent, the estimated low levels of these toxicants are unlikely to reach most tissues.

Chemical Weapons and the Improvised Explosive Device

In 2003 Operation Iraqi Freedom brought US ground forces back into the Iraqi theater. Beginning in May 2004, coalition forces recovered 53 chemical munitions. Based on their physical conditions and residues, all of them appeared to have been part of pre-Operation Desert Storm war logistics. These included mustard, sarin, cyclosarin, and riot control agents. Among these was a 152-mm binary sarin artillery projectile that contained a 40% concentration of sarin; insurgents had attempted to use it as an improvised explosive device. The existence of this weapon raises questions about the number of viable chemical weapons remaining in Iraq and engenders the possibility that an unknown quantity of long-lasting chemical weapons still exists, possibly in binary form.[67]

Iraqi troops uncovered a chemical facility in Fallujah and discovered instructions on how to create improvised explosives and disseminate blood agents. In addition to explosive materials, such as various nitrate salts, they found cyanide and hydrochloric acid, along with instructions on disseminating hydrogen cyanide gas and cyanogen chloride.[68] Also notable was the discovery of a warehouse in Mosul, Iraq, containing 1,500 gallons of unidentified toxic chemicals that could be used to implement an attack.[69]

CHEMICAL WARFARE CAPABILITIES

The Chemical Threat

Thus far this chapter has discussed the development of chemical weapons, as well as the groups and individuals who used (or threatened to use) them. The term "chemical threat" is an attempted measure of enemy capability considering those subjects as well as the following:

- the availability and supply of specific agents,
- the delivery systems that could be used in different battle situations,
- the facilities used to produce these agents and munitions,
- plans and procedures for the employment of such weapons, including training for weapons delivery and handling, and
- the will to use such weapons.

Historically, combatants with chemical warfare

capability were well-equipped for chemical warfare protection; they had defined procedures on decontamination, individual and equipment protection, and detection and surveillance. Because chemical warfare agents are dangerous for the user as well as the enemy, they required that offensive and defensive programs be developed simultaneously. Special military teams (eg, logistical, medical, and chemical corps teams trained to operate in a chemical environment) and the ability to monitor meteorological conditions were characteristic of nations with offensive or defensive programs. In assessing enemy capability, chemical stockpiles, production capacities, and the control of use are evaluated when an offensive or defensive posture is being determined. Such assessments are complicated by the possibility that industrial plants, manufacturing products with peaceful applications, may be "dual use"; that is, their manufacturing processes may be redirected toward chemical agent production.

Over recent decades, the chemical threat has shifted appreciably, from fully structured military offensive and defensive capabilities to more clandestine activities by rogue nations and terrorist elements. Today, the greatest chemical threat comes from the accidental or intentional release of industrial toxicants, a lesson that should be learned from the catastrophe of Bhopal,[70] and accidents involving extremely common toxicants, such as those involving chlorine in Henderson, Nevada, in 1991[71] and in Graniteville, South Carolina, in 2005.[72] Although only 11 chorine railcars are known to have been breached between 1956 and 2006, these cars are extremely common and represent a particularly significant urban threat.[73] The widespread acceptance of the Chemical Weapons Convention (CWC)—a near-global chemical weapons ban—and promotion of laws governing chemical export controls[74] have substantially reduced the risk of national chemical weapon use, though likely possessor nations, such as North Korea, must continue to be monitored for potential clandestine weapons proliferation. Modern chemical threats appear to originate most frequently from rogue groups with little or no sophisticated chemical warfare capability; hence, chemical agent employment from terrorist elements may present differently than they would from nation states. Chemical toxicants can be applied unaltered, or chemical warfare agents can be manufactured virtually undetected in relatively crude laboratories and used to create disruption. Political instability and radicalism heighten these inherent dangers.

National Chemical Warfare Capabilities of Nations

Since World War I, the reluctance of possessor states to employ chemical weapons has been relatively high. However, the Iraqi precedent, the ineffective world response to Iraq's use of chemical warfare, and the perceived effectiveness of this use all suggest that the chemical warfare threshold has been substantially lowered. The growing list of states motivated, for reasons of offense or deterrence, to develop relatively low-technology, low-cost weapons of mass destruction greatly increases the likelihood that military personnel will need to contend with casualties of chemical warfare.

On March 15, 1991, an article in *The Washington Post* described the latest annual report of the Office of Naval Intelligence, listing 14 nations with "an offensive chemical-warfare capability."[75] The list included Egypt, Israel, Pakistan, and South Korea, four nations that receive large quantities of military aid from the United States.[75] Four additional nations (Saudi Arabia, Indonesia, South Africa, and Thailand) were purported to possibly possess such a capability, and more nations were believed to be in the process of developing or seeking to develop chemical weapons. In a 1993 US House of Representatives Committee on Armed Services report, 31 nations were mentioned as possessing or having the ability to develop offensive chemical weapons.[76]

Because chemical weapons are less expensive and easier to acquire than nuclear weapons, they are a credible threat from developing nations. The adaptation and incorporation of chemical-agent–containing munitions to conventional or missile delivery systems can give a weaker nation a military threat to counterbalance neighbors with greater conventional capabilities. Nations may initially acquire a limited chemical warfare capability through the transfer or purchase of bombs or artillery-compatible chemical weapons shells. In some cases, unweaponized agent may be transferred.[77] Alternatively, nations may invest in the development of chemical industries that involve the manufacture or acquisition of chemical precursors or intermediates. In this way, wealthier nations or those under a strong, perceived threat may increase their chemical warfare potential by acquiring the technology and facilities to synthesize agents and incorporate them into munitions compatible with existing or newly acquired delivery systems. Industrial compounds such as organophosphates (pesticides), phosgene, chlorine, and cyanide are not difficult to obtain.

Inevitably, a trickle-down effect occurs in the arms world as aging munitions and weapons systems are replaced and move from the major weapons producers to their client states in developing nations, and from there to other nations. For example, the Soviet Union probably supplied a chemical warfare capability to

Egypt,[77] which in turn supplied Syria,[78] which then supplied Iran.[79] Some weapons systems, especially from the former Eastern Bloc countries, were designed to operate in a chemical warfare theater.[80]

Tactical and Strategic Use of Chemical Weapons

Chemical agents can be delivered by a range of weaponry. Liquid agents may be dispensed with land mines, spray tanks, artillery projectiles, aerial bombs, rocket and missile warheads, or even cruise missiles. This means that all battlefield areas, from front lines to rear reserves, are vulnerable to chemical warfare attack, and medical practitioners should be fully prepared to treat chemical warfare casualties from a variety of locations. Medical personnel must be similarly prepared for the possibility of isolated and spontaneous chemical attacks on both military personnel and civilians in areas subject to low-intensity conflict via acts of terrorism.

To be effective, chemical agents must be efficiently dispersed over their intended targets. Most applications call for large-scale agent distribution over large target areas occupied by, or of interest to, military units. For example, documents recovered from the former German Democratic Republic called for Warsaw Pact forces to employ heavy chemical weapons attacks early in any conflict with the West.[81] Considerable quantities of an agent may be needed to ensure adequate coverage in the face of wind, heat, or agent volatility. Effectiveness is also increased by surprising the enemy and catching them unprotected (eg, unmasked).

Chemical Agent Delivery Systems

The four methods of delivering chemical agents are (1) explosive release, (2) bulk release, (3) base ejection, and (4) spray delivery (Figure 4-15). The most common method is explosive release. Bursts from individual explosive munitions are, effectively, point sources for chemical weapons dissemination. Chemical weapons artillery shells, which serve as smaller point sources, might be laid down in a grid to cover a large area. The same effect could be accomplished with fewer missiles that carry larger payloads and have longer ranges. Agents can also be delivered from multiple explosive point sources using submunitions to cover a larger area or, if detonated in sequence, to lay the agent down along a trajectory line. Such line deliveries may be distributed directly over the target or upwind of the target, preferably perpendicular to the wind.

Bulk release, base ejection, and spray delivery also distribute chemical warfare agents along trajectory lines. In bulk release, the forward covering, or "skin," of a warhead is blown off, aerodynamically breaking up the agent via high-speed air flow. In base ejection, an explosive charge causes an internal piston-like action to force the agent out of the back of the warhead, either by pushing it through small apertures, aerosolizing it, or sending it into a high-speed air stream for aerodynamic breakup. Explosive, bulk release, and base ejection methods are primarily suited for the dispersal of liquid chemical agents. For solid agents such as the tear gas CS (2-chlorobenzalmalononitrile) and the incapacitating agent BZ (3-quinuclidinyl benzilate), effective aerosolization is often achieved by pyrotechnic munitions.

Spray delivery is more efficient than the other three methods in providing a very fine aerosolization (with average droplet diameter $< 5\ \mu m$), which can be inhaled far down into the lungs. This method is particularly suited to toxin delivery, which requires deep inhalation and differs from most chemical agents in that toxins are solids and do not vaporize. Spray delivery requires slow speeds and low altitudes, conditions that render aircraft particularly vulnerable to attack. Spray tanks could also be mounted on trucks or boats, and unpiloted aircraft could be designed to deliver agent. The increased vulnerability of spray-delivery systems makes their use more likely against unarmed or poorly equipped opponents, or on carefully targeted sites under cover of surprise. Spray delivery could also be applied to closed ventilation systems in more focal applications.

From a tactical military standpoint, explosive munitions, the dominant mode of chemical agent delivery, vary with respect to effective agent delivery (Figure 4-16). Explosion of a chemical agent shell at ground level or some height over the target site generates two products: (1) vapor and (2) droplets. Droplets (average diameter range of $100\ \mu m$ to 1 mm for pure agents) fall to the ground in a fine rain to coat the target surface with liquid.

Agent vapor, which poses the greatest threat for inhalational intoxication, derives from three sources. First, agent vaporizes from explosive burst energy, which varies with shell design and specific agent payload. Shell casing thickness, shell casing material, and the agent-to-burster ratio are all important shell design factors. Second, additional vapor is generated as falling droplets vaporize. Heat from the explosion dissipates quickly, and ambient air temperature is the most important factor driving this volatilization. Third, the liquid coating of agent on the ground evaporates, making ground temperature an important factor. Vapor produced by explosive energy and droplet vaporization is called "primary" vaporization, and that rising from the ground is called "secondary"

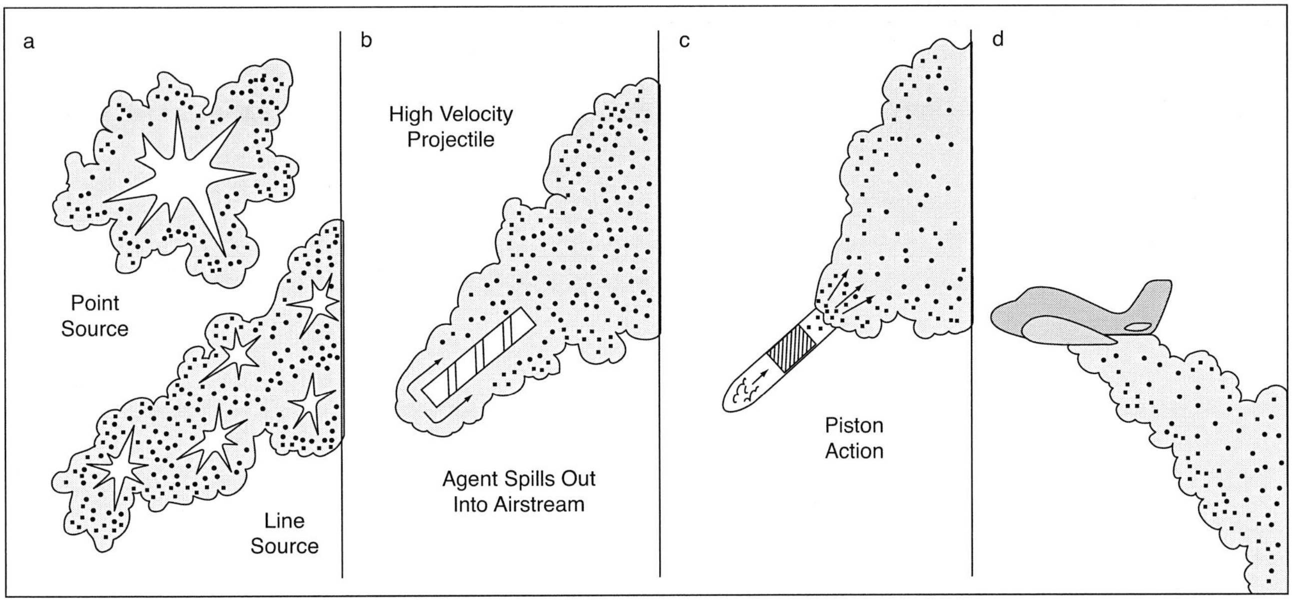

Fig. 4-15. Four modes of chemical agent release. **(a)** Explosive-release devices are predominantly represented among the major chemical warfare arsenals. While some agent is lost to decomposition, their simplicity makes these the weapons of choice. Point-source explosives are single detonation devices, and line-source munitions release a series of time-delayed explosions that lay agent toward the end of the trajectory. **(b)** Bulk-release munitions spill agent into the air stream of the projectile. **(c)** Base-ejection devices are relatively uncommon because of their cost and complexity. Like explosives and bulk-release devices, these munitions can be carried on longer-range missiles. **(d)** Spray delivery can be used to achieve large-area coverage, such as that required for terrain denial. However, because of aircraft vulnerability, spray delivery is generally limited to application on undefended territory or against a poorly defended foe.

vaporization.

A scenario in which chemical agent shells are dropped on a desert area at different times of the day can be used to demonstrate the differences in agent threat caused by liquid persistence and deposition versus vaporization. The influence of wide environmental temperature fluctuations over the 24-hour cycle, combined with the agent used, can make a substantial difference: increased surface deposition and skin-contact threat during cool nights, and a considerably increased inhalational toxicity threat during the heat of the day are expected. Successful employment of chemical agents is influenced by many variables, most notably weather, because the agent is transported by the wind and air currents when released as a vapor or an aerosol. Unfavorable meteorological conditions frequently preclude successful agent deployment because of the inordinately high number of weapons used. Once deployed, the persistence of liquid contamination is affected by temperature, sunlight, wind action, and rainfall.

Military Chemical Agents

Military chemical agents are characterized according to several features, including nature of use, persistency in the field, and physiological action. Toxic chemical warfare agents are capable of producing incapacitation, serious injury, and death. These agents are further characterized by their physiological action and are discussed in detail in their individual chapters (Table 4-2). The most common agents in modern arsenals are vesicants and nerve agents. Cyanides and pulmonary toxicants are thought to be represented in some stockpiles, but are typically less toxic and more difficult to employ because of their physical characteristics. Some cyanides and pulmonary toxicants have specific characteristics that make them appropriate for military use, such as rapid rate of action, very low persistency, and the ability to penetrate or damage protective equipment.

Other chemicals present in military arsenals include incapacitating agents, which produce physiological and mental effects, rendering individuals incapable of performing their assigned duties. Recovery may take several hours to several days, although intensive medical treatment may not be required. Riot control agents produce intense effects, such as irritation of the skin, eyes, and respiratory tract, but recovery is normally rapid when exposure is terminated. Some

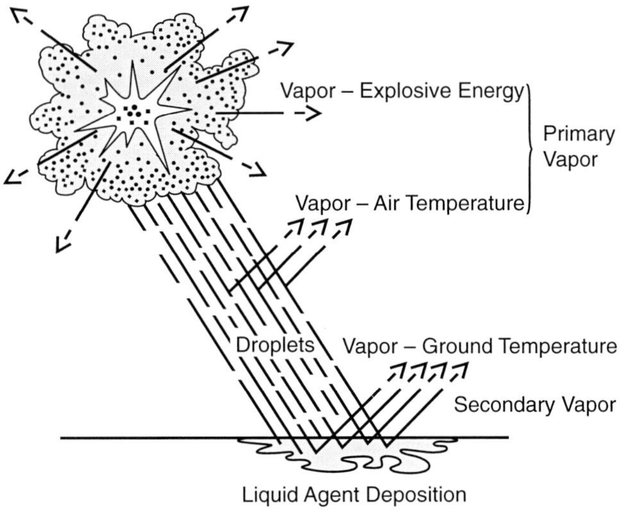

Fig. 4-16. Agent vaporization increases in proportion to energy sources, such as heat from explosive charges or from ambient heat (as measured by air or surface temperatures). Vapor persistence is then determined by weather factors such as wind and humidity. Hydrolysis rates are affected by factors such as temperature and solubility. Agents show characteristic hydrolysis rates in water, and water vapor, as described by humidity, may cause significant hydrolysis of vaporized agent. The vesicant lewisite, for example, shows relatively rapid hydrolysis in water vapor, while the nerve agent VX is more resistant to hydrolysis.

TABLE 4-2

MODERN CHEMICAL WARFARE AGENTS

US Army Code	Agent
Cyanide	
AC	Hydrogen cyanide
CK	Cyanogen chloride
Nerve agents	
GA (tabun)	Ethyl N,N-dimethyl-phosphoramido-cyanidate
GB (sarin)	Isopropyl-methylphosphonofluori-date
GD (soman)	1,2,2-Trimethylpropyl meth-ylphosphonofluoridate
GF	Cyclohexyl-methylphosphonofluori-date
VX	o-Ethyl S-[2-(diisopropylamino)ethyl] methylphosphonothiolate
Lung agents	
CG (phosgene)	Carbonyl chloride
DP (diphosgene)	Trichloromethyl chloroformate
Vesicants	
HD (mustard)	bis-2-Chloroethyl sulfide
L (Lewisite)	2-Chlorovinyl dichloroarsine
HL	Mustard-lewisite mixture
Incapacitating agents	
BZ	3-Quinuclidinyl benzilate (QNB)
Tear gas	
CN	2-Chloro-1-phenylethanone
CS	2-Chlorobenzalmalononitrile
Vomiting gas	
DM (Adamsite)	10-Chloro-5,10-dihydrophenarsazine

studies provide epidemiological data on CS, such as the 1969 and 1971 Himsworth reports.[82,83] Additionally, the National Institutes of Health provides data on carcinogen bioassays on both CS and chloroacetophenone.[84] Unfortunately, little is known about the long-term effects of many of these agents, an area of increasing medical concern. Chemical smoke agents are used to obscure objects or areas from observation or from engagement by weapons with electrooptical control systems. They are usually not toxic in field concentrations, but may cause eye or respiratory irritation in higher concentrations. Some smokes have adverse chronic exposure effects.

Other compounds with military applications include agents used in flame warfare, such as thickeners for napalm and incendiary materials, and herbicides (defoliants). Other highly toxic industrial chemicals also pose a potential risk to the military. The disaster in Bhopal, India, in December 1984, when an estimated 8,000 people died and another 30,000 were injured from breathing methylisocyanate and chlorine released in an industrial accident, is just one of many examples of the devastating effect of poisonous gases.[85]

Chlorine and phosgene are industrial compounds that have been and could again be used as military weapons. Medical personnel should be prepared for such chemical emergencies when military missions are in close proximity to industry. During World War I, the list of chemical agents was expanded to include mustard, phosgene, adamsite, and cyanide.

Physical Properties of Chemical Agents

The physical properties of an agent and its formulation also present important threat considerations. Selection of agents and agent formulations can be used to affect differential impacts with respect to droplet size and liquid deposition, agent persistence, and agent volatility. The classic chemical warfare agents have a wide range of volatility (Table 4-3), and volatility can be a determinant in deciding which agents to use.[86] Agents such as HCN and sarin are relatively volatile;

they present an immediate but short-lived threat. These agents are referred to as "nonpersistent" because they vaporize rapidly after delivery. Alternatively, agents such as VX and sulfur mustard tend to fall largely in droplets with less vaporization and remain on exposed surfaces for at least 24 hours. These agents are called "persistent."

Wind is an important consideration in determining the distribution of an agent cloud. As in any fluid-solid interface, the earth's surface exerts a drag on wind currents. Under a moving cloud, volatile agent concentrations can be expected to mix more slowly at the surface and increase in concentration with height. Vegetation further exacerbates this drag and increases the height of the protective layer in which agent concentration is low.

Formulation is also used to manipulate the fate of an agent. Soman, VX, lewisite, and sulfur mustard can be mixed with thickeners of high molecular weight to increase droplet size and thereby decrease primary vaporization. Such additives are generally used to promote efficient agent deposition on the target site. Thickeners can also increase agent persistence and may hamper decontamination efforts. Adding silica powder to sulfur mustard ("dusty mustard") can propel the agent in a dust cloud. Stabilizers increase agent shelf life.

Nonpersistent Agents

In tactical use, the threat of nonpersistent, volatile agents, such as HCN or sarin, is greatest to the respiratory systems of unprotected soldiers. A sudden, heavy bombardment of these agents may affect many casualties if unmasked soldiers are caught by surprise. When used against an unprotected force, nonpersistent agents are particularly effective in generating casualties, thereby creating breakthrough points in enemy front lines. Iraq successfully used nonpersistent nerve agent in counterattacks against Iranian forces during 1988.[81] Nonpersistent agents can be used to slow enemy advancement by forcing the enemy to wear protective equipment. They can also circumvent an enemy's protection against conventional high-explosive munitions and may be used in night attacks to harass troops.

TABLE 4-3

COMPARATIVE VOLATILITY OF CHEMICAL WARFARE AGENTS

Agent	Volatility (mg/m^3) at 25°C
Hydrogen cyanide (HCN)	1,000,000
Sarin (GB)	22,000
Soman (GD)	3,900
Sulfur mustard	900
Tabun (GA)	610
Cyclosarin (GF)	580
VX	10
VR ("Russian VX")	9

Data source: US Departments of the Army, Navy, and Air Force. *Potential Military Chemical/Biological Agents and Compounds.* Washington, DC: Headquarters, DA, DN, DAF; December 12, 1990. Field Manual 3-9. Naval Facility Command P-467. Air Force Regulation 355-7.

Persistent Agents

Given favorable weather conditions, the use of persistent agents such as mustard and VX may pose a threat for many days. Such agents can deny or interfere with enemy occupation of terrain or equipment use and could be used defensively to protect vulnerable flanks. However, although persistent agents can slow enemy movement, they can also hamper the movement of friendly forces through a contaminated area. Delayed casualties may occur even among protected troops operating in a contaminated area for an extended period. Hence, persistent agents, which can linger as coatings or in puddles for weeks, may not be the agents of choice when occupation of territory by friendly forces is imminent.

Chemical land mines that disperse persistent agent may be used in conjunction with military barrier systems to complicate breaching or clearing the barriers. The mines are typically based on high-explosive mine designs, with several pounds of agent substituted for most of the explosive charge. High-explosive land mines cause contaminated open wounds, primarily on lower extremities, that must be properly decontaminated; decontamination could be more difficult when persistent agents are used.

Sulfur mustard, a blistering agent, tends to linger on skin, promoting percutaneous absorption, and offers strategic benefits besides those considered above. It was used very effectively both during World War I and the Iran-Iraq War to generate thousands of casualties. Although deaths among unprotected sulfur mustard exposure victims are relatively few, mustard casualties can overwhelm medical treatment facilities.[87] Survivors of other agent exposures stabilize relatively quickly, but mustard lesions demand months of medical care. This was the fate of many thousands of unprepared or poorly equipped Iranian recruits exposed to sulfur mustard agent.

Underscoring the importance of ambient temperature and climate, persistence can also change greatly with temperature; sulfur mustard volatility increases nearly 40-fold between 0°C and 40°C. The threat of respiratory intoxication from sulfur mustard, which is always present, is considerably greater at higher temperatures, although its persistence is reduced.

Rapidity of action also factors into agent selection. Volatile agents such as cyanide and sarin can act very swiftly, primarily via the respiratory tract. In general, nerve agent effects follow immediately after exposure, culminating in seizures and death within a few minutes of inhalation, cutaneous dosing, or both. Other agents, such as mustard, lewisite, and phosgene, act only after a delay. For example, both the blistering and the edematous effects of skin exposure to sulfur mustard occur only many hours after contact, and skin exposure to mustard may not be noticed for quite some time. By contrast, lewisite, which is also a vesicant, heralds its presence by immediate pain and irritation.

Choice of Agent and Delivery System

By selecting the appropriate agents, formulations, and delivery systems, a well-equipped military is in a better position to achieve its tactical objectives. Field manuals, such as the now-limited US Army Field Manual (FM) 3-10, *Employment of Chemical Agents*, discuss how chemical munitions could be used separately or integrated with conventional weapons. Chemical warfare agents can be used to cause casualties, harass the enemy, and hamper or restrict the use of terrain. Although an offensive capability no longer exists, FM 3-10 provides useful information on how chemical warfare agents can be used defensively on the battlefield.[88] In his classic 1937 book, *Chemicals in War*, Brigadier General Augustin M Prentiss, a CWS officer, describes the offensive tactical uses of chemical agents that were in place following World War I.[2]

CHEMICAL WEAPONS AGREEMENTS

Although world terrorism has shown no signs of recession, the CWC has recently been implemented among nations. This ban is the product of the evolution of ideas driven by 20th-century global conflicts and imperatives. Although the idea of a global agreement to ban the use of chemical weapons actually preceded the development of effective chemical weapons, the rapid development and effective use of chemical weapons during World War I created a more favorable climate for seeking a limited international agreement to restrict agent use in war: the Geneva Protocol. This protocol served as a precursor to the much more complicated CWC treaty.

Development of the Geneva Protocol

The earliest international agreement banning chemical weaponry was the 1675 Strasbourg Agreement between France and Germany, which prohibited the use of poisoned bullets between forces. Later, 19th-century battlefield carnage led to international efforts to protect civilians and reduce the suffering of injured combatants. Initial efforts to improve medical care in the field in the 1860s were followed by the Brussels Convention of 1874, which called for a ban on the use of poison or poisoned weapons. Although never ratified, the Brussels Convention served as a model and catalyst for future international agreements and unilateral policies governing military conduct on the field.

The industrial revolution of the 19th century and technological innovations in weaponry combined to create an atmosphere of insecurity and fear resulting from the prewar buildup of weaponry among European nations. This led to the First Hague Conference of 1899, in which arms control measures were considered but never ratified. Although effective chemical weaponry had yet to emerge, negotiations included language to curb the use of chemicals in warfare: "Three propositions were . . . adopted . . . one forbidding the use of projectiles the sole purpose of which was, on bursting, to spread asphyxiating or deleterious gases. . . ."[89]

Although unsuccessful in implementing arms control, the Hague conferences of 1899 and 1907 established a permanent court of arbitration at The Hague, providing both a future venue for the potential arbitration and peaceful resolution of international disputes and an initial framework for developing multilateral entities, such as the League of Nations and the UN.

The extensive chemical industry of World War I Germany probably provided the impetus for the rapid development of chemical arms. Germany's capitulation led to the 1919 Treaty of Versailles, which imposed a unilateral ban on Germany's use, manufacture, storage, and importation of chemical agents and munitions. However, even with fresh memories of gas warfare and widespread public revulsion to chemical weapons, governments were loathe to part with their own chemical warfare capabilities for fear of having such weapons used against them.[90]

After World War I, armament stockpiles and fresh memories of carnage led the newly formed League of Nations to convene the May 1925 Conference for the Supervision of the International Trade in Arms and

Ammunition. Although the conference was unsuccessful in curbing the international arms trade, a subtext to these negotiations became the well-known Geneva Protocols. In addition to setting international rules governing the protection of civilians and wounded and captured combatants, the Geneva conventions included the first multinational agreement banning the use of chemical weapons.[90]

During negotiations, efforts to implement a ban on the export of chemical agents forwarded by the US delegation were ultimately foundered by issues such as difficulty of import and export verification, extensive and dual use in the chemical industry, and the concerns of inequity raised by nonpossessor nations or those with a less-advanced chemical infrastructure.[90] These concerns led to the adoption of compromise language, which limited chemical warfare agent use:

> Whereas the use in war of asphyxiating, poisonous or other gases, and of all analogous liquids, materials or devices, has been justly condemned by the general opinion of the civilized world; and Whereas the prohibition of such use has been declared in Treaties to which the majority of Powers of the World are Parties; and To the end that this prohibition shall be universally accepted as a part of International Law, binding alike the conscience and the practice of nations. . . .[91]

Signed June 17, 1925, for implementation on February 8, 1928, the Geneva prohibition was ultimately signed by 133 "states parties." Many signatories, including the United States, ratified the treaty on a no-first-use basis. Other nations reserved for themselves the right of first use against a nonsigning nation. Finally a number of nations, including Iraq, a 1931 signatory, limited their application of the protocol to international conflicts, retaining their internal sovereignty.

An inevitable weakness of the Geneva Protocol as a ban is that multinational agreements are difficult to enforce. Chemical weapons use by a weaker nation may elicit intervention by superior external forces, but responding to militarily powerful offenders would be difficult or impossible. Italy's use of mustard gas in its invasion of Abyssinia (Ethiopia) in 1935–1936 drew no significant repercussions from the League of Nations nor from other signatories, even though both Ethiopia and Italy had ratified the protocol prior to the invasion. The International Red Cross, wishing to retain neutrality during the conflict, declined to testify on the issue before the League of Nations,[92] and sanctions from the latter were ineffectual.

Excepting the United States and Japan, most major powers ratified the treaty soon after its development. Despite being favorably reviewed by the Senate Foreign Relations Committee in 1926, the treaty was kept from reaching a vote by opposition, and it was withdrawn from consideration by President Harry S Truman after World War II. However, like many unratified treaties, signatories generally abide by them without ratification. Warned that the Axis powers might employ chemical weapons, President Franklin D Roosevelt reaffirmed the US no-first-use policy in June 1943. Subsequent US rejections of ratification were based on a stated preference in favor of verifiable disarmament.[91] The US use of defoliant herbicides and riot control agents during the Vietnam War led to further conflicts in interpretation of the protocol and a continued reluctance to sign.

In 1969 President Nixon resubmitted the protocol, affirming a no-first-use policy and offering to ban incapacitating agents under the treaty. Ultimately the US Senate delayed ratification of the treaty until January 22, 1975, when the Ford administration proposed a version that retained a more limited use of herbicides and riot control agents, promising neither would be employed in first use in war.[91] Herbicide application was limited to defensive perimeters around military installations, and riot agents were generally limited to quelling prisoner disturbances, reducing civilian injuries, implementing rescues, and supporting rear echelon defensive responses by besieged convoys.

The United Nations Disarmament Committee

Nuclear, chemical, and biological stockpile accumulation in the context of the political and armed conflicts of the Cold War created momentum for the development of effective dialogue toward the eventual negotiation of disarmament treaties. Although conventional weapons issues and nuclear proliferation and testing took precedent over chemical weapons arms control, the implementation of the Eighteen-Nation Disarmament Committee by the UN General Assembly in 1962 provided a forum for discussions addressing all aspects of disarmament, including chemical weapons. This body, initially composed of eight nonaligned and five aligned nations each from the Eastern Bloc and Western sides, was renamed several times as membership expanded, and became instrumental in developing workable positions in support of chemical and biological arms control.[93]

The Biological Weapons Convention

Because military biological capabilities were much

less developed than chemical ones, negotiating a treaty for biological pathogens and toxins posed a much greater probability of success. Chemical weapons were already widely distributed among large and small nations as a valued retaliatory deterrent in the event of a chemical weapons attack or an attack by a stronger aggressor. Extensive and intrusive verification and assurance mechanisms would have to be developed, a challenging demand for hostile and mistrusting Cold War adversaries. Linking the seemingly intractable problem of chemical arms to the more manageable biological weapons issue caused considerable deliberative conflict, although treaty negotiations ultimately arrived at the Soviet Union's position: chemical and biological arms control would be linked as they had been in the Geneva Protocol.

In 1969 and 1970 President Nixon facilitated discussions by declaring a unilateral ban on the offensive development of biological warfare agents, including toxins. Deliberations leading up to the Biological Weapons Convention of 1972 resulted in formal language that provided an impetus for discussions toward eliminating the much more extensively developed chemical warfare capabilities of Eastern Bloc and Western nations:

> Article IX: Each State Party to this Convention affirms the recognized objective of effective prohibition of chemical weapons and, to this end, undertakes to continue negotiations in good faith with a view to reaching early agreement on effective measures for the prohibition of their development, production and stockpiling and for their destruction, and on appropriate measures concerning equipment and means of delivery specifically designed for the production or use of chemical agents for weapons purposes.[94]

The treaty, negotiated by the UN, called for confidence-building measures through the exchange of technical and scientific information and material support. It also set the framework for the provision of future data exchanges and negotiations toward the elimination of chemical weapons.

US-Soviet Weapons Destruction Agreement

With the fall of many of the communist governments in Eastern Europe and improved relations with the Soviet Union, the United States and Soviet Union signed a bilateral chemical weapons destruction agreement on June 1, 1990. In support of this agreement, the secretary of defense canceled most of the new chemical retaliatory program and the Army decided to suspend its new binary chemical production facilities in 1990.[76,95,96]

The Chemical Weapons Convention

The Eighteen-Nation Disarmament Committee was expanded in 1969 and renamed the "Conference of the Committee on Disarmament," and in 1984 renamed the "Conference on Disarmament." In 1980 a Conference of the Committee on Disarmament working group was tasked to design an acceptable text for a convention banning chemical weapons.[97] Over the 12-year period of its development, the CWC treaty involved consultation with military and chemical industry representatives, which led to carefully defining regulated chemicals and working out effective inspection and verification procedures.

A high-level state department meeting in 1989 formalized mechanisms allowing for visits, data exchanges, and challenge inspections required for a demilitarization treaty, including that for chemical weapons. On May 13, 1991, US President George Bush advanced his 1989 plan before the UN to destroy 98% of the US stockpile of chemical weapons in the first 8 years of a new, proposed treaty. Under the new treaty's conditions, Bush pledged to destroy all US chemical weapons within 10 years and never to use chemical weapons again.[98] However, anticipated difficulties in chemical weapon demilitarization and destruction might prolong the presence of chemical weapon depots. This message sent a clear challenge to other nations to eliminate their chemical weapons. The Bilateral Verification Experiment and Data Exchange Agreement, nicknamed the "Wyoming MOU" (Memorandum of Understanding), called for visits and data exchanges in 1990, followed by further data transfer and a limited number of challenge inspections in 1994. A final chemical weapons treaty draft was submitted to the UN General Assembly in June of 1992. The Organization for the Prohibition of Chemical Weapons (OPCW), located in The Hague, was to be responsible for overseeing the CWC treaty. The CWC was convened in Paris in 1993 and the treaty was implemented in April 1997. The United States ratified the treaty on April 24, 1997, a few days before it went into effect.[87]

By April 2006 178 nations, or "states parties," had ratified the CWC. Eight nonsignatory states remain, including the Syrian Arab Republic, Egypt, Iraq, Somalia, Lebanon, and North Korea (Democratic People's Republic of Korea). Eight states have signed but not ratified the treaty, including Burma (Myanmar) and Israel.[99] The treaty leaves in doubt the development and use of chemical warfare agents by developing nations or nonsigners of such agreements, most notably Libya, Iraq, and North Korea. Chemical warfare treaty ratification by nations such as Iran that border nonsignatories may prove difficult in the short term.

The CWC is a complicated document because it was designed to effect the demilitarization of chemicals that may be in widespread commercial use while minimally impacting the world's extensive chemical industries.[100,101] Its basic tenets are listed in Article I:

Article I General Obligations:

1. Each State Party to this Convention undertakes never under any circumstances:
   (a) To develop, produce, otherwise acquire, stockpile or retain chemical weapons, or transfer, directly or indirectly, chemical weapons to anyone;
   (b) To use chemical weapons;
   (c) To engage in any military preparations to use chemical weapons;
   (d) To assist, encourage or induce, in any way, anyone to engage in any activity prohibited to a State Party under this Convention.
2. Each State Party undertakes to destroy chemical weapons it owns or possesses, or that are located in any place under its jurisdiction or control, in accordance with the provisions of this Convention.
3. Each State Party undertakes to destroy all chemical weapons it abandoned on the territory of another State Party, in accordance with the provisions of this Convention.
4. Each State Party undertakes to destroy any chemical weapons production facilities it owns or possesses, or that are located in any place under its jurisdiction or control, in accordance with the provisions of this Convention.
5. Each State Party undertakes not to use riot control agents as a method of warfare.[101]

The authors of the CWC sought to implement many of the concepts discussed in the development of the Geneva Protocol and incorporate the concerns and caveats of its signatories. The CWC bans the use of chemical weapons proliferation and requires the timely destruction of all chemical weapons manufacturing facilities, weaponized and unweaponized agent, and any devices or structures specifically intended for chemical warfare. Negotiations leading to the development of the CWC involved industry representatives early in the process, creating multiple lines of communication and accommodating both industrial and arms control interests. Some of these representatives came forward to support the document's ratification in the US Senate.[100]

The CWC defines chemical capability in terms of chemical weapons and chemical weapon production facilities (Table 4-4). The term "chemical weapon" denotes everything that is specifically manufactured for conducting chemical warfare, ranging from small machined parts to bulk-stored agent and agent weaponized mines, spray tanks, and projectiles. The order of priority for chemical weapons destruction depends on the type or presence of agent. The CWC also includes riot control agents and biological toxins.

Declarations, Scheduling and Order of Destruction

Within 30 days of acceding to the CWC, a nation or "state party" must declare all of its chemical weapons and facilities that have made chemical weapons at any time since 1946, any old or abandoned chemical weapons (including those abandoned on the territory of another state party), and plans for the destruction of chemical weapons and facilities.

The CWC requires the elimination of all chemical weapons and chemical weapons facilities over a 10-year schedule (Table 4-5). Destruction of schedule-1 and non-schedule-1 manufacturing facilities must

TABLE 4-4

CHEMCIAL WARFARE CONVENTION SCHEDULE AND CATEGORY OF CHEMICALS AND CHEMICAL WEAPONS

Schedule 1 chemicals	Chemicals that have no or little purpose other than to be used in chemical warfare. Examples: nerve agents, sulfur mustard.
Schedule 2 chemicals	Chemicals that have limited commercial use or precursors, such as thiodiglycol, a precursor to sulfur mustard.
Schedule 3 chemicals	Chemicals, such as phosgene, that can either be used as weapons or in the manufacture of chemical weapons and have legitimate large-scale industrial uses.
Category 1 CWs	CWs containing schedule 1 chemicals.
Category 2 CWs	All weaponized schedule 2 and 3 chemicals.
Category 3 CWs	Unfilled munitions and CW-specific devices and equipment.

Data source: Carpenter WD. How industry came to support the CWC. *OPCW Synthesis*. November 2000.

commence by 1 year after accession and be completed 10 and 5 years later, respectively. The schedule was designed to activate at a date when a large portion of the world's nations had ratified and acceded to it to promote a mutual, gradual rate of "leveling out" over the 10-year implementation period. The time schedule allows for the development, testing, and sharing of destruction technologies, and for confidence building. Disparities in arsenal size and economies are partially reduced through international technology exchange and financial assistance. States parties can request extensions for up to 5 years.

Having agreed to the CWC in April 1997, the United States and the Russian Federation had to eliminate all category 2 and 3 chemical weapons by April 2002 and category 1 chemical weapons in phases by 2007. Nations acceding to the CWC after April 1997 must implement this time schedule relative to their implementation date.

Inspection and Verification

Over 3,200 inspections were conducted by February 2008. They are minimally intrusive, although the treaty does allow for challenge inspections in which any state party can request the immediate "challenge" inspection of the facilities of another state party. Challenge inspections cannot be refused by the state party being investigated and are done with as little warning as possible. Schedule 1, 2, and 3 site inspections are negotiated under facility agreements by the technical secretariat to be minimally inconvenient and disturbing, employing detailed, advanced scheduling and arrangements. Advanced notice is generally given between 36 and 48 hours. By December 2006 over 9 years had passed without a challenge inspection, likely due to the largely unfettered access of inspectors to declared sites.[102] The CWC language strives to reduce tensions, build confidence, and promote international liaisons and cooperation. Because this spirit is central to both process and progress, challenge inspections are deemed less an implementation tool than a last resort.

TABLE 4-5

CHEMICAL WEAPONS CONVENTION SCHEDULE OF IMPLEMENTATION PLAN

Category 1 Implementation Phase	Percentage of Category 1 Chemicals Destroyed	Years After Entry into Force	From April 1997
	Planning and testing	1–2	April 1999
1	1	3	April 2000
2	20	5	April 2002
3	45	7	April 2004
4	100	10	April 2007

Data source: Organisation for the Prohibition of Chemical Weapons Web site. Convention on the Prohibition of the Development, Production, Stockpiling and Use of Chemical Weapons and on their Destruction. Accessed April 22, 2008. Available at: http://www.opcw.org/html/db/cwc/eng/cwc_menu.html.

Noncompliance

In the event of noncompliance, article VIII of the CWC instructs the executive council to seek corrective actions by the offending state party. Depending on the latter's response, the executive council may variously involve the conference or, in the event of a crisis, it may inform but bypass the conference and bring its concerns directly to the UN General Assembly or Security Council. For example, following complaints of poor compliance with article VII, the OPCW demanded that states parties implement domestic legislation and controls consistent with the objectives of the CWC by November 2005.[103]

Issues in Implementation

An appeal was raised in 2003 by 60 former OPCW officials, diplomats, negotiators, legal scholars, and scientists to reinvigorate the unique spirit that convened to create the CWC. This public appeal, directed at the states parties and citizen observers, expressed concern over the fundamental lack of candor and the politicized direction in which the OPCW was implementing the CWC. It also protested that national governments were becoming complacent, failing to seek ratification or enact domestic laws supporting the CWC. Wealthier states parties were accused of undermining the CWC timeline by failing to provide timely support to international demilitarization efforts.[104]

A number of these criticisms and concerns were summarized and elaborated upon a few years later by Walter Krutzsch, a former technical secretariat official and CWC negotiator.[105] Krutzsch criticized the executive committee for failing to respond to CWC violations, including arbitrary misinterpretation of provisions, violations of OPCW diplomatic immunity, and failures to keep schedules. He suggested that such compliance issues could be resolved in a context of greater public transparency, claiming that the public record, OPCW's *Annual and Quarterly Reports*, diminishes overall CWC accountability by providing only aggregate summaries and fails to inform both the public and states parties of the extent of noncompliance.[105]

Krutzch went on to explain inspection and verification as described to be unduly influenced through the state parties' control of the budget, greatly limiting the ability of the technical secretariat to prioritize its mission activities. By defining, in the budget, the number of inspections to be held in each schedule category, the technical secretariat had to revisit a schedule 1 site of minimal concern six times, while large numbers of chemical production facilities were disproportionally uninspected.[105]

Progress Made Toward Compliance

Unless a nation declares its own state of progress in implementing the CWC, any effort to compile a listing of progress by state party is incomplete because the OPCW generally reports only numbers in aggregate form. Many nations, including smaller ones such as Albania, have or had modest stockpiles and may depend on foreign assistance for their elimination.[106] The OPCW scorecard shows the United States and Russian Federation declared an overall total of 64,260 metric tons of agent. The remaining 167 declarations total an additional 7,055 metric tons of agent[99] (Table 4-6).

TABLE 4-6

CHEMICAL WEAPONS CONVENTION PROGRESS, FEBRUARY 2008

Total weight of declared chemical agents	~ 71,315 metric tons
Total number of declared munitions/containers	~ 8,679,000 items
Total destroyed agent	~ 27,199 metric tons (38%)
Total destroyed munitions/containers	~ 2,930,000 items (34%)
CWPFs certified as destroyed	42 of 65 declared
CWPFs certified as converted	19
Number of states parties (as of December 2007)	183
Initial declarations received	169
Implementing legislation submitted enacted in all key areas	79

CWPF: chemical weapons production facility
Data source: Organisation for the Prohibition of Chemical Weapons Web site. Accessed: May 16, 2008. Available at: www.opcw.org/index.html.

Chemical Demilitarization

The CWC does not specify how chemicals are to be destroyed.[107] It provides language requiring that destruction be completed in a safe manner and in compliance with a state party's environmental regulations. Both incineration and various chemical elimination methods are employed. The CWC requires elimination of the offending chemical; as long as the reaction products are not CWC scheduled compounds, the agent is considered destroyed. Demilitarization is generally a multistep process. VX nerve agent hydrolysis, for example, yields a mixture of schedule 2 products based not on toxicity but on the presence of residual phosphonate alkyl groups. Hence this product is subsequently subjected to further oxidation or biodegradation. A Russian plan incorporated the unwanted products into asphalt. Concrete embedding can also be used.

US Program

The Army has been responsible for destroying leaking or obsolete chemical weapons since it began developing them. In October 1972 Army Materiel Command headquarters formalized the mission through the creation of a Program Manager for Demilitarization of Chemical Materiel, headed by Colonel Sampson Bass. This office was to plan, direct, and control the chemical demilitarization program, including the design, development, and acquisition of special equipment and facilities. Its initial projects included addressing leaking munitions and bulk agent at the nine chemical weapons stockpile sites and Dugway Proving Ground, Utah, in addition to chemical remediation efforts at Rocky Mountain Arsenal, Colorado, and finishing biological warfare agent disposal efforts at Fort Detrick, Maryland. Between 1969 and 1985 the Army destroyed nearly 15 million lb of chemical agents through neutralization and incineration technologies at Rocky Mountain Arsenal alone.

The duties and scope of disposal operations eventually prompted Army leadership to propose that a formal agency take responsibility for chemical demilitarization, which had grown to include developing disposal technologies, building permanent facilities, coordinating with interagency government offices, and running disposal operations. The US Army Toxic and Hazardous Materials Agency began operations in 1978. One of its first major efforts was to build the US Army Chemical Agent Materiel Disposal System at Tooele Army Depot, Utah, as a test facility to develop proven industrial and military processes and equipment and to demonstrate their applicability to large-scale demilitarization facilities. The test facility was the primary tool for evaluating technologies and processes to destroy chemical munitions and agents between 1979 and 1986. Based on extensive testing and evaluation, the Army decided that a reverse-assembly approach to disassembling the munitions, followed by incineration and treatment of off-gases by a pollution abatement system, should be used for constructing a pilot disposal facility at Johnston Island in the Pacific Ocean.

In the 1980s Congress tied the binary program to the chemical demilitarization program by language that directed the Army to destroy an equal amount of unitary weapons as they built the new binary weapons.[108] In 1985 Congress authorized the Army to execute the binary weapons production with a number of constraints, one of them being the elimination of the existing chemical agents and munitions by September 1994. This language also authorized the creation of a new Army management organization, headed by a general officer, to execute the disposal mission.[30,38] As a result, the Army's Program Manager for Chemical Munitions (Demilitarization and Binary) was established at Aberdeen Proving Ground on May 1, 1986. In 1987 the binary munitions project split off, and in 1988, the office was renamed the "Program Manager for Chemical Demilitarization."

The US Army Chemical Materials Agency, which assumed the responsibilities of the Program Manager for Chemical Demilitarization in 2003, employs manual and robotic technologies to carry out either high-temperature incineration or chemical elimination. Several of the agency's facilities use high-temperature incineration for agent, explosive, and propellant components. Prototype studies were conducted at Johnston Island (1990–1993), and the technology was then transferred to the Tooele, Utah, facility, which commenced operation in 1996. Public unease with incinerator-based technologies resulted in the creation of the Assembled Chemical Weapons Alternatives Program in 1997. Under this DoD program, the Pueblo Chemical Depot in Colorado will neutralize HD with hot water followed by bacterial elimination of the products. At the Bluegrass Army Depot in Kentucky, agent will be hydrolyzed and the hydrolysate subjected to fundamental decomposition under high temperature and pressure. The Newport Army Depot in Indiana became fully operational in 2005, hydrolyzing its nerve agent stocks.

Nonchemical weapons are typically rendered inoperable through mechanical means such as crushing, sawing, or detonation. Contaminated materials are incinerated or chemically decontaminated. The United States has also developed a portable, flatbed-mounted explosive destruction system to destroy old, unstable chemical warfare munitions.

From a medical perspective, the chemical demilitarization program upholds occupational safety standards enacted to protect workers and maintains public health measures to protect citizens. Both the Environmental Protection Agency (EPA) and the Centers for Disease Control and Prevention (CDC) worked with the Army surgeon general and the Army Center for Health Promotion and Preventive Medicine to develop worker and public health standards in line with similar Occupational Safety and Health Administration and National Institute of Occupational Safety and Health guidance for working with hazardous materials.

For personnel working at the stockpile sites and disposal facilities, the CDC promulgated airborne exposure levels as occupational safety standards for various timeframes and purposes. These include the following limits:

- Immediately dangerous to life or health: the maximum exposure concentration at which one could escape within 30 minutes without any escape-impairing symptoms or permanent adverse health effects.
- Short-term exposure limit: the maximum concentration at which unprotected chemical workers may be exposed for up to 15 minutes.
- Worker population limit: the maximum allowable concentration at which unprotected chemical workers may be exposed for an 8-hour workday and 40-hour workweek over 30 years.
- General population limit: the maximum concentration at which the general population may be exposed continuously, based on exposure 24 hour per day, 7 days per week, over a 70-year lifetime.[109]

In addition to protecting civilians and military employees on post, the Army's chemical demilitarization program supports the development and implementation of medical emergency response protocols for any chemical accidents or incidents that involve an off-post exposure hazard. The Chemical Stockpile Emergency Preparedness Program, established in 1988, has funded both on-post and off-post efforts to ensure that state and local emergency responders can react to chemical accidents or incidents, protecting the public living around the stockpile sites. The medical agencies at those sites work to prepare emergency medical technicians and hospitals to receive and treat potentially exposed civilians by providing advice on the procurement of personal protective equipment, decontamination equipment and practices, and stockpiling medical countermeasures such as atropine injectors.

Additionally, the National Research Council, working with the EPA and the Center for Health Promotion and Preventive Medicine, has developed public safety exposure acute exposure guidance levels (AEGLs) to guide civil decision-makers in determining whether to shelter in place or evacuate the population from the potential hazard effects of a chemical plume. AEGLs exist for hundreds of toxic industrial chemicals, but they have only recently been developed for chemical warfare agents.[110,111]

- AEGL-1: level above which nondisabling, reversible discomfort may be noted.
- AEGL-2: level above which more serious effects may occur, including possible long-lasting or escape-impairing effects.
- AEGL-3: level above which exposures may become life-threatening or result in death.[112]

As the Army's chemical demilitarization program progresses, challenges continue to emerge. With Congress's insistence that the Army use neutralization technologies at four of the eight stockpile sites, the Army must continue to work with the EPA, CDC, and other agencies on liquid waste health risks, in addition to continuing to monitor incineration emissions and comply with emissions standards. To date, the Army has met or exceeded all EPA and CDC requirements and suggestions. Although leaks and spills have occurred, as the original programmatic environmental impact statement warned, the Army's health safety and environmental record remains unblemished.

Status of US Chemical Weapons Demilitarization

In 1985 there were 29,033 metric tons of chemical agents among the nine stockpile sites and an Army depot in Germany (the contents of which were sent to Johnston Island in 1990) (Table 4-7). By 2008 demilitarization by the US Army Chemical Materials Agency and its predecessor, the Program Manager for Chemical Demilitarization, had successfully disposed of nearly 60% of the original, predeclaration stockpile without incurring serious injury or placing the public at risk. The prototype Johnson Island demilitarization facility eliminated its chemical weapons by 2000 and is now closed. The Tooele facility has eliminated over 70% of its sizeable nerve agent stockpile. Chemical agent destruction at Aberdeen, Maryland, was completed in 2007. The Anniston, Alabama, and Umatilla, Oregon, facilities came on line in 2003 and 2004, while the Pine Bluff, Arkansas, and Newport, Indiana, sites commenced operations in 2005. The United States eliminated 45% of its declared stockpile of category 1 agents in 2007, meeting its first milestone. In 2006 the United States requested an extension of the 100% destruction deadline to the treaty limit of 2012.[113,114]

TABLE 4-7

US STOCKPILE AGENT DESTRUCTION *

Site	Metric Tons Originally Declared	Percent of Stockpile	Declared Metric Tons Destroyed	Percentage Destroyed	Agents
Aberdeen, Md	1,471	5.3	1,471	100	HD
Tooele, Utah	12,121	43.9	8,705	71	GB
Anniston, Ala	2,045	7.4	867	42	GB, VX, HD
Umatilla, Ore	3,374	12.2	1,085	32	GB, VX, HD
Pine Bluff, Ark	3,492	12.7	528	15	GB, VX, HD
Newport, Ind	1,152	4.2	823	84	VX
Pueblo, Colo	2,371	8.6	0	0	HD
Lexington, Ky	475	1.7	0	0	GB, VX, HD
Closed sites	1,098	4.0	1,098	100	GB, VX, HD
Total	**27,599**	**100.0**	**9,431**	**34**	

*Status as of March 23, 2008

Status of the Russian Federation Chemical Weapons Demilitarization

By far the most challenging chemical weapon demilitarization is taking place in the Russian Federation, which inherited its chemical weapons stocks from the Soviet Union. The Russians declared 32,480 metric tons of nerve agents (sarin, soman, VX), and another 7,700 metric tons of vesicants (sulfur mustard, lewisite, and combined sulfur mustard-lewisite) at seven storage sites[115] (Table 4-8).

Russian destruction of chemical weapons employs a two-step chemical inactivation and detoxification strategy. The CWC time schedule for agent destruction applies to the first chemical step, which eliminates the agent, although the resulting product residues require further treatment.

The establishment of the Russian chemical destruction program in 1996, set to take place at seven facilities, was followed by several years of delay due to economic instability and a lack of intragovernmental coordination, which undermined the willingness of outside nations to offer financial aid. Program planning was lacking in technological detail, scheduling, and cost analysis. Further issues included poor public transparency, bureaucratic unresponsiveness, burdensome and expensive visa requirements, and contracting issues.[116] In 2002 the G8 Global Partnership against Proliferation of Weapons and Materials of Mass Destruction encouraged other nations to support Russia in eliminating its vast chemical stockpile. Since that time, with the increased obligation of foreign funds from the United States and other (mostly European) nations and the strengthening of the Russian economy, the Russian program has undergone profound development, most notably since 2004. Russia increased its investment in chemical agent demilitarization from $186 million in 2004 to real and projected spending on the order of a billion dollars each year for the 2007–2009 period. The country also met the CWC's 1% and 20% destruction milestones on schedule.[117–119]

By the end of 2007 Russia estimated that its elimination program would total about $7.18 billion, of which $2 billion would be provided by other nations. The US commitment to the overall effort, totaling just over a billion dollars, is limited to constructing a CW elimination facility at Shchuch'ye. By 2007 foreign funds had contributed about $430 million to Russia's chemical demilitarization program, with $240 million expected the following year. The country has substantially funded its own program. Of the three sites having achieved operational status by 2007, the Maradykovsky facility was entirely internally funded. Germany provided extensive support for the cost of the Kambarka and Gornyy facilities.[120]

Gornyy, now closed, was the first operational facility, and eliminated all of its stocks of lewisite, sulfur mustard, and mixed vesicants by December 2005. In June and August of 2006, the Kambarka and Maradykovsky facilities became operational, and by March and April of 2008, these had destroyed 5,279 and 4,394 metric tons of agent, or 83% and 63% of the agent stockpiles, respectively. Kambarka contained 80 metric-ton containers of lewisite, and aerial bombs containing nerve agent were stored at Maradykovsky.[116]

The US contribution to Russian chemical weapons demilitarization is mediated through the Nunn-Lugar Cooperative Threat Reduction Program, which was established under the Nunn-Lugar Act of 1991, and is focused on Shchuch'ye. Shchuch'ye was recognized as a potential site for the theft and proliferation of chemical weapons munitions because its nearly 2 million portable chemical artillery shells are surrounded by an economically impoverished population. The United States initially provided funding to help secure the facility, but has also funded one of two destruction facilities there. US release of $160 million in start-up funds was delayed until 2003. Although operations were set to begin at Shchuch'ye in 2006, they have been delayed for an estimated 2 to 3 years.[121]

Of the three remaining destruction sites in Russia, Leonidovka is reported to be under construction, while Pochep and Kizner are known to be either in the planning phase or possibly developing early infrastructure.

TABLE 4-8

RUSSIAN FEDERATION STOCKPILE DESTRUCTION *

Site	Metric Tons	Percent of Stockpile	Percentage Destroyed
Shchuch'ye	5,435	13.6	0
Gornyy	1,159	2.9	100
Kambarka	6,355	15.9	83
Leonidovka	6,874	17.2	0
Maradyk-ova	6,954	17.4	63
Pochep	7,513	18.8	0
Kizner	5,675	14.2	0
Total	**39,965**	**100**	**27**

*Status as of March/April 2008

Data source: Green Cross International Web site. Available at: http://gci.ch/index.php?option=com_frontpage&Itemid=1). Accessed August 18, 2008.

Germany, Italy, and Switzerland are assisting with the construction of Pochep, where nerve agent is stored. Switzerland is supporting construction at Leonidovka, and Canada and the United Kingdom are supporting construction at Kizner between 2007 and 2009.[122]

It has become clear that, while eliminating chemical weapons is imperative, it is a very costly and time-consuming process to design acceptable and reliable technologies to address public safety concerns and environmental impacts. Both the United States and Russian Federation have been granted the maximum 5-year extensions under the CWC (to April 2012). The CWC does not address extensions beyond that date, although it is currently anticipated that chemical weapons demilitarization will exceed that date for both nations. Either these states parties will continue chemical weapons demilitarization under a technically "noncompliant" status or components of the CWC will be modified to accommodate the delays in progress.

Status of Chemical Proliferation

With the implementation and wide acceptance of the CWC, world security has improved immensely with respect to the proliferation of chemical capability at the governmental level. Although some unpredictable countries, such as North Korea,[123] potentially posses chemical weapons, the remaining threat has largely become nongovernmental entities such as terrorist groups.

Governmental Proliferation Threat

North Korea has developed an extensive chemical weapons capability and reportedly possesses an arsenal of between 2,500 and 5,000 metric tons of agents distributed over 12 locations. Suspected chemicals in its supply include sulfur mustard, lewisite, phosgene, HCN, sarin, and V-type nerve agents. North Korea's arsenal includes agent-weaponized, long-range missile and artillery delivery systems that are forward-deployed, threatening highly populated regions of South Korea. North Korean military doctrine considers chemical weaponry an integral part of its force and has resisted joining the CWC.

Some level of government-sponsored terror is also likely to persist. Members of the Palestinian Authority have provided payments to the families of suicide bombers. Other Middle Eastern governments, such as Iran and Syria, have long been suspected of supporting terrorist organizations.[124]

Nongovernmental Proliferation

Individuals seldom present a significant threat, but well-financed, hostile groups have proven capable of recruiting the relatively common and low-level expertise required to manufacture chemical agents, as demonstrated by Aum Shinrikyo, which was in the process of developing an exceptionally large capacity for sarin production. Al Qaeda documents on the manufacture of sarin have also been recovered.[56] These well-financed groups were able to access the chemicals they desired, as were rogue governments before them.[74]

However, extensive organization and significant financial support are not mandatory prerequisites to acquiring a chemical agent capability. Many terrorist groups that form only loose networks have little difficulty acquiring chlorine, cyanide, and organophosphates. The use of improvised explosive devices demonstrates terrorists' abilities to readily develop chemical weaponry. Additionally, evidence exists that the agent used in Al Qaeda propaganda films may have been VX recovered from Iraqi munitions.[57] Incidents involving the acquisition of chemicals by subversive groups, such as Al Qaeda, or individuals prove that emergency response plans would likely benefit most by planning to respond to more accessible toxic industrial compounds, such as cyanide and chlorine.

The protection of chemical industry facilities and transport vehicles must be bolstered to prevent terrorist access and accidental exposures. Sobering lessons have been learned from accidents and incidents involving the release of commercial compounds in an urban context (eg, the 1984 Bhopal disaster).[70] In 2005 releases of chlorine in Graniteville, South Carolina (killing nine); ammonia near Salt Lake City, Utah; and hydrogen fluoride near Pittsburgh, Pennsylvania, posed challenges to the medical management of casualties. In a densely populated world dependent on industrial chemistry, attention must also be focused on chemicals positioned locally.

PRESENT AND FUTURE IMPLICATIONS FOR MILITARY MEDICINE

The milieu of the chemical battlefield is especially alien to medical personnel, whose usual professional practice includes nothing resembling the management of chemical casualties. Despite strategic or tactical justification for chemical warfare, medical providers must face the psychologically demoralizing effects and personal ethical concerns about suffering resulting from the deliberate use of chemical weapons.

Although military strategists might view chemical warfare agents as simply one means to immobilize or destroy an enemy force, others may view such weapons as abhorrent extensions of conventional warfare. Current US policy prohibits using chemical weapons against an adversary, but this policy is not shared by all other nations; therefore, to be effective, military medical personnel must be knowledgeable, trained, and prepared. Although healthcare providers are usually not involved in the political or military decisions surrounding the use of chemical weapons, they must be ready to deal with the military and civilian casualties resulting from the use of such agents, cognizant of what constitutes a chemical threat and the military tactics that could be employed against them, familiar with the acute and chronic medical effects of chemical agents to plan appropriate medical support, knowledgeable of the diagnostic tools available to identify specific etiologic agents to which their patients may have been exposed, and aware of the most effective methods of intervention and prevention.

From the standpoint of military strategy, two reasons are commonly cited for a combatant to employ chemical weapons. First, chemical weapons can be highly effective when densely applied onto concentrated, largely immobile forces or populations. This factor largely accounted for their use against entrenched troop positions during World War I. During the Cold War, military strategists anticipated similar intense chemical warfare bombardments from Warsaw Pact forces in the European theater. The second reason often used to support chemical weapon use is that chemical attacks can be initiated at lower levels to encumber an opponent with defensive equipment or to create panic and disorder among poorly trained or unprepared troops. Application onto enemy troops or civilian populations can also have a strong demoralizing effect. Therefore, the United States military must maintain a strong readiness posture in the face of a continuing chemical warfare threat.

SUMMARY

The military healthcare provider must be prepared to recognize military or civilian casualties of chemical warfare or terrorism, which requires an informed understanding of the historically based likelihood of chemical warfare agent use or threat. Providers must be able to clearly recognize agent-exposure symptoms against a varying background of typical injury and chemical exposure stress behaviors. Providers must also be informed, to the fullest extent possible, about anticipated chemical attacks by hostile forces or terrorist activities. This intelligence requires consideration of an adversary's political factors and motivation, chemical agent or toxicant possession or access, chemical warfare offensive and defensive capabilities, and any strategic advantage to be realized through agent use. As a healthcare provider manages individuals suspected to have been exposed to chemical warfare agents, initial recognition of the type of agent used may be facilitated through an understanding of tactics, modes of agent dissemination, likely routes of casualty exposure, physical agent properties, and other factors determining the persistence of these toxicants in the environment.

REFERENCES

1. Sartori M. *The War Gases*. New York, NY: D Van Nostrand Company, Inc; 1943.

2. Prentiss A. *Chemicals in War: a Treatise on Chemical Warfare*. New York, NY: McGraw-Hill Book Company, Inc; 1937.

3. Haber LF. *The Poisonous Cloud: Chemical Warfare in the First World War.* Oxford, England: Clarendon Press; 1986: 15–40.

4. Fries AA, West CJ. *Chemical Warfare*. New York, NY: McGraw-Hill Book Company Inc; 1921: 53–59.

5. Brophy LP, Miles WD, Cochrane RC. *The Chemical Warfare Service: from Laboratory to Field*. Washington, DC: Office of the Chief of Military History; 1959.

6. Stockholm International Peace Research Institute. *The Problem of Chemical and Biological Warfare*. New York, NY: Humanities Press; 1971.

7. Fair SD. Mussolini's chemical war. *Army*. 1985;35(1):47.

8. Foreign developments in chemical warfare. *Chemical Warfare*. 1923;9(9):19.

9. Smalley VE. *Report of the CW Status of Italy (1926–1948).* Army Chemical Center, Md: Chemical Corps Technical Command; 1948.

10. Fries AA. Chemical warfare—past and future. *Chemical Warfare.* 1920;5(1):4–5.

11. Chemical warfare bombing tests on warship. *Chemical Warfare.* 1921;6(10):6.

12. Chemical Warfare Technical Committee. Reference A, 3rd Indorsement, Adjutant General Office, subj: Adoption of Type (Chemical Agents). 16 Apr 1928. British National Archives, Kew, England. File WO195/16864.

13. Waitt AH. Europe looks at chemical warfare. *Army Ordnance.* 1935;15(89):285.

14. Brigham CE. Final report on status of chemical readiness by the retiring chief, 1937. National Archives Branch Depository, Suitland, Md. RG 114.

15. Wiseman DJC. *Special Weapons and Types of Warfare.* London, England: The War Office; 1951: 150.

16. Intelligence Division, Chemical Warfare Service. *German Chemical Warfare, World War II.* Washington, DC: CWS; 1945: 28–30, 115–117.

17. Miller GA. The development of the 4.2 chemical mortar. *Armed Forces Chemical Journal.* 1948;3(2):33.

18. US War Department. *Characteristics and Employment of Ground Chemical Munitions.* Washington, DC: 1946. Field Manual 3-5.

19. US Department of the Army. *Chemical Corps Equipment Data Sheets.* Washington, DC: 1961. Technical Manual 3-500.

20. US War Department. *Employment and Characteristics of Air Chemical Munitions.* Washington, DC: 1946. Field Manual 3-6.

21. US Department of the Army. *Chemical Bombs and Clusters.* Washington, DC: 1957. Technical Manual 3-400.

22. US Army Chemical Corps. *Summary of Major Events and Problems, FY59.* Army Chemical Center, Md: US Army Chemical Center Historical Center; 1960: 112–114.

23. US Army Chemical Corps. *Summary of Major Events and Problems, FY60.* Army Chemical Center, Md: US Army Chemical Center Historical Center; 1961: 154.

24. Davis S. *GB Warheads for Army Ballistic Missiles 1950–1966.* Edgewood Arsenal, Md: US Army Munitions Command; 1968: 11, 29–30.

25. US Army Chemical Corps. *Summary of Major Events and Problems, FY1961–62.* Army Chemical Center, Md: US Army Chemical Center Historical Center; nd: 123–126.

26. US Department of the Army. *Binary Chemical Munitions Program.* Aberdeen Proving Ground, Md: Chemical Systems Laboratory; 1981: 1–7. Programmatic Environmental Impact Statement ARCSL-EIS-8101.

27. Ward FP. *Construction and Operation of a 155mm M687 GB2 Binary Production Facility at Pine Buff Arsenal, Jefferson County, Arkansas.* Aberdeen Proving Ground, Md: Chemical Systems Laboratory; 1981: 3–7. Environmental Assessment ARCSL-EA-8101.

28. Chemical Warfare Review Commission. *Report of the Chemical Warfare Review Commission.* Washington DC: US Government Printing Office: 1985: 50.

29. The Chemical Strategy. *Army Chemical Review.* January 1988:23.

30. Department of Defense Authorization Act of 1985. Pub L No. 99-145. October 19, 1984.

31. *Engineering Center (CRDEC) Annual Historical Review (AHR)*. Aberdeen Proving Ground, Md: AMCCOM; Fiscal Year 1988: 8–9, 107–180.

32. Associated Press. ATF officials say they've instituted reforms since Waco. *Baltimore Sun*. November 1, 1995:A10.

33. Wire Reports. Anti-terrorism training bill clears senate on 96-0 vote. *Baltimore Sun*. June 28, 1996:A10.

34. US Congress. House. *Defense Against Weapons of Mass Destruction*. HR 3730. June 27, 1996.

35. US Department of Defense. *Department of Defense Dictionary of Military and Associated Terms*. May 9, 2005. Joint Publication 1-02.

36. State Department Web site. Country reports on terrorism. Available at: http://www.state.gov/s/ct/rls/45323.htm. Accessed April 27, 2005.

37. 18 USC §2331.

38. Dutchman in Iraq genocide charges. BBC Web site. March 18, 2005. Available at: http://news.bbc.co.uk/1/hi/world/middle_east/4360137.stm. Accessed May 22, 2008.

39. Hassan KA. Human Rights Watch Web site. Quarterly report about the saboteurs, June 7, 1988. Available at: http://www.hrw.org/reports/1994/iraq/APPENDIX.htm#TopOfPage. Accessed July 31, 2007.

40. US Department of Defense. Protecting critical bases of operations (US homeland, forces abroad, allies, and friends) and defeating CBRNE weapons and means of delivery. Annex A. In: *Defense Planning Guidance for FY 2004*. Washington, DC: DoD; 2003.

41. Purver R. *Chemical and Biological Terrorism: the Threat According to the Open Literature*. Canadian Intelligence Security Service unclassified report. June 1995.

42. Simon J. The Alphabet Bomber (1974). In: Tucker J, ed. *Toxic Terror: Assessing Terrorist Use of Chemical and Biological Weapons*. Cambridge, Mass: The MIT Press; 2000.

43. Bishop K. Witness says supremacists sought to avenge death. Feb 23, 1988. New York Times Web site. Available at: http://query.nytimes.com/gst/fullpage.html?res=940DE2D9153BF930A15751C0A96E948260. Accessed May 15, 2008.

44. Smithson A, Levy L. Rethinking the lessons of Tokyo. In: Smithson A, Levy L, eds. *Ataxia, the Chemical and Biological Terrorism Threat and the U.S. Response*. Stimson Center Report No. 35; 2000. Henry L Stimson Center Web site. Available at: http://www.stimson.org/cbw/pdf/atxchapter3.pdf. Accessed May 15, 2008.

45. Recollecting the series of Aum Shinrikyo incidents. August 30, 1996. Monterey Institute of International Studies Web site. Available at: http://cns.miis.edu/pubs/eanp/wpap.pdf. Accessed May 15, 2008.

46. Beaton R, Stergachis A, Oberle M, Bridges E, Nemuth M, Thomas T. The sarin gas attacks on the Tokyo subway—10 years later/ lessons learned. *Traumatology*. 2005;11(2):103–119.

47. Tucker JB. *Toxic Terror: Assessing Terrorist Use of Chemical and Biological Weapons*. Cambridge, Mass: The Massachusetts Institute of Technology Press; 2000.

48. Chronology of Aum Shinrikyo's CBW activities. Monterey Institute of International Studies Center for Nonproliferation Studies Web site. Available at: http://cns.miis.edu/pubs/reports/pdfs/aum_chrn.pdf. Accessed July 31, 2007.

49. Canadian Security Intelligence. *2003 Public Report*. October 28, 2004. Canadian Security Intelligence report.

50. National Defense Authorization Act for FY 1997. Pub L No. 104-210. September 23, 1997.

51. Sourcewatch Web site. Center for Media and Democracy Iraqi Insurgency page. July 2005. Available at: http://www.sourcewatch.org/index.php?title=Iraqi_insurgency. Accessed July 31, 2007.

52. Olson KB. Aum Shinrikyo: once and future threat? *Emerg Infect Dis*. 1999;15(4):513–516.

53. Croddy E, Osborne M, McCloud K. Chemical terrorist plot in Rome? March 11, 2002. James Martin Center for Nonproliferation Studies Web site. Available at: http://cns.miis.edu/pubs/week/020311.htm. Accessed May 15, 2008.

54. Associated Press. Cyanide, arsenal stirs domestic terror fear. January 30, 2004. CNN Web site. Available at: http://www.cnn.com/2004/US/Southwest/01/30/cyanide.probe.ap/. Accessed May 15, 2008.

55. Venzke B, Ibrahim A. Al-Qaeda tactic/target brief v1.5. June 14, 2002. IntelCenter Web site. Available at: http://www.intelcenter.com/QaedaTacticTarget-v1-5.pdf. Accessed May 15, 2008.

56. Robertson N. Disturbing scenes of death show capability with chemical gas. August 19, 2002. CNN Web site. Available at: http://archives.cnn.com/2002/US/08/19/terror.tape.chemical/index.html. Accessed July 31, 2007.

57. Gellman B. US suspects al Qaeda got nerve agent from Iraqis. Analysts: chemical may be VX, and was smuggled via Turkey. *Washington Post*. December 12, 2002:A1.

58. Associated Press. Jordan militants confess to chemical plot. April 26, 2004. Available at: http://www.acsa2000.net/alzarqawi.htm. Accessed July 31, 2007.

59. Katzman K. Al Qaeda, profile and threat assessment. Washington, DC: Library of Congress Congressional Records Service; Aug 15, 2005. CRS Report for Congress, RL33038.

60. Persian Gulf War Task Force. *Intelligence Update: Chemical Warfare Agent Issues During the Persian Gulf War*. April 2002. Available at: https://www.cia.gov/library/reports/general-reports-1/gulfwar/cwagents/index.htm#top. Accessed July 31, 2007.

61. US Department of Defense. Modeling and risk characterization of US demolition operations at the Khamisiyah Pit. Washington, DC: DoD; April 16, 2002. Technical Report.

62. Kang HK, Bullman TA. *Mortality Among US Gulf War Veterans Who Were Potentially Exposed to Nerve Gas at Khamisiyah, Iraq*. Washington, DC: Veterans Health Administration; 2002.

63. Defence Analytical Services Agency. *1990/1991 Gulf Conflict—UK Gulf Veterans Mortality Data: Causes of Death*. Newport, Wales, United Kingdom: DASA; 2005.

64. Bullman TA, Mahan CM, Kang HK, Page WF. Mortality in US Army Gulf War veterans exposed to 1991 Khamisiyah chemical munitions destruction. *Am J Public Health*. 2005;95(8):1382–1388.

65. Concern over chemicals brain risk. BBC Web site. November 7, 2006. Available at: http://news.bbc.co.uk/1/hi/health/6126082.stm. Accessed July 31, 2007.

66. Institute of Medicine of the National Academies, Committee on Gulf War and Health. *Gulf War and Health: Updated Literature Review of Sarin*. Washington, DC: National Academies Press; 2004.

67. Bomb said to hold deadly sarin gas explodes in Iraq. MSNBC Web site. May 17, 2004. Available at: http://www.msnbc.msn.com/id/4997808/. Accessed May 22, 2008.

68. Multinational Forces in Iraq. Fallujah update. Insurgent chemical/explosives weapons laboratory. November 26, 2004. Global Security Web site. Available at: http://www.globalsecurity.org/wmd/library/report/2004/fallujah-cw_cpic_26nov2004.ppt#602,1,Fallujah UpdateInsurgentChemical/ExplosivesWeaponsLaboratoryMULTI NATIONALFORCE – IRAQ. Accessed May 15, 2008.

69. Knickmeyer E. Iraqi chemical stash uncovered: post-invasion cache could have been for use in weapons. *Washington Post*. August 14, 2005. Available at: http://www.washingtonpost.com/wp-dyn/content/article/2005/08/13/AR2005081300530.html. Accessed May 15, 2008.

70. Dow, Inc. *A Legacy Acknowledged*. December 3, 2002. Statement. Available at: http://www.dowethics.com/r/about/corp/bhopal.htm. Accessed July 31, 2007.

71. Routley JG. Massive leak of liquefied [*sic*] chlorine gas. Henderson, Nevada (May 6, 1991). In: Sandia National Laboratories. *Identification and Analysis of Factors Affecting Emergency Evacuations*. Appendices. United States Nuclear Regulatory Commission Web site. Available at: http://www.nrc.gov/reading-rm/doc-collections/nuregs/contract/cr6864/v2/cr6864v2.pdf. Accessed May 16, 2008.

72. Brittle S. Emergency response issues: what went wrong in Graniteville. Don't Waste Arizona, Inc. Web site. Available at: http://www.chemicalspill.org/railcar.html. Accessed May 16, 2008.

73. Hess G. Chlorine makers to commit to upgrading railcars: manufacturers plan to replace their North American tank car fleets with safer, more secure cars by 2017. November 17, 2006. Chemical and Engineering News Web site. Available at: http://pubs.acs.org/cen/news/84/i47/8447railcar.html. Accessed May 16, 2008.

74. Gordon M. US companies ties to chemical sales. *New York Times*. January 30, 1989. Available at: http://query.nytimes.com/gst/fullpage.html?res=950DE4DB1F3CF932A05752C0A96F948260. Accessed May 16, 2008.

75. Smith J. Confusing data on chemical capability: US intelligence, diplomatic lists of armed nations differ. *Washington Post*. March 15, 1991:A21.

76. Browder G. *Countering the Chemical Weapons Threat in the Post-Soviet World*. Washington, DC: US Government Printing Office; February 23, 1993. Report of the special inquiry into the chemical threat of the Committee on Armed Services, US House of Representatives, 102nd Congress (2nd Session).

77. Livingstone NC, Douglass JD. *Chemical Weapons: the Poor Man's Atomic Bomb*. Cambridge, Mass: Institute for Foreign Policy Analysis; February 1, 1984. National Security Paper 1.

78. Rathmell A. Chemical weapons in the Middle East: Syria, Iraq, and Libya. *Marine Corps Gazette*. 1990;59.

79. Timmerman KR. *The Poison Gas Connection: Western Suppliers of Unconventional Weapons and Technologies to Iraq and Libya*. Los Angeles, Calif: Simon Weisenthal Center; 1990. Special Report.

80. Segal D. The Soviet Union's mighty chemical warfare machine. *Army*. 1987;37(8):26–35,38.

81. US Army Chemical School. *World-wide NBCE threat briefing*. Fort McClellan, Ala: US Army Chemical School Threat Office; March 1992. Unclassified.

82. Himsworth Committee. Enquiry into the medical situation following the use of CS in Londonderry on 13th and 14th August, 1969. In: *Report of the Enquiry into the Medical and Toxicological Aspects of CS (Orthochlorobenzylidene Malononitrile)*. Part I. London, England: Command 4173, Her Majesty's Stationery Office; 1969.

83. Himsworth Committee. Enquiry into the toxicological aspects and its use for civil purposes. In: *Report of the Enquiry into the Medical and Toxicological Aspects of CS (Orthochlorobenzylidene Malononitrile)*. Part II. London, England: Command 4775, Her Majesty's Stationery Office; 1971.

84. US Department of Health and Human Services, National Toxicology Program. *Toxicology and Carcinogenesis Studies of CS2 (94% o-chlorobenzalmalononitrile) (CAS No. 2698-41-1) in F334/N Rats and B6C3F1 Mice (Inhalational Studies)*. Research Triangle Park, NC: National Toxicology Program; 1990. NTP Technical Report 377.

85. Kurzman D. *A Killing Wind: Inside Union Carbide and the Bhopal Catastrophe*. New York, NY: McGraw-Hill; 1987.

86. US Departments of the Army, Navy, and Air Force. *Potential Military Chemical/Biological Agents and Compounds*. Washington, DC: Headquarters, DA, DN, DAF; December 12, 1990. Field Manual 3-9. Naval Facility Command P-467. Air Force Regulation 355-7.

87. Gilchrist HL. Statistical consideration of gas casualties. In: Weed FW, ed. *Medical Aspects of Gas Warfare*. Vol 14. In: Ireland MW. *The Medical Department of the United States Army in the World War*. Washington, DC: US Government Printing Office. 1926: 273–279.

88. US Departments of the Army, Navy, and Air Force. *Employment of Chemical Agents*. Washington, DC: Headquarters, DA, DN, DAF; March 1966. Field Manual 3-10. Naval Warfare Information Publication 36-2. Air Force Manual 355-4. Fleet Marine Force Manual 11-3.

89. Mahan AT. *Report of Captain Mahan, Technical Delegate of the United States to the Second Peace Conference at The Hague, to the United States Commission to the International Conference at the Hague, on Disarmament*. July 31, 1899. Report.

90. Zanders JP. The CWC in the context of the 1925 Geneva debates. *Nonproliferation Review*. 1996;3:38–45.

91. Geneva Conference for the Supervision of the International Traffic in Arms. *Protocol for the Prohibition of the Use in War of Asphyxiating, Poisonous or other Gases, and of Bacteriological Methods of Warfare* [Geneva Protocol]. Geneva, Switzerland; June 17, 1925.

92. Bridel B. Les ambulances à croix-rouge du CICR sous les gaz en Ethiopie [Ethiopia 1935–36: mustard gas and attacks on the Red Cross]. *Le Temps*. August 13, 2003.

93. Tulliu S, Schmalberger T. Negotiating arms control and disarmament agreements. January 2004. In: Tulliu S, Schmalberger T. *Lexicon for Arms Control, Disarmament and Confidence-Building*. United Nations Institute for Disarmament Research Web site. Available at: http://www.unidir.ch/pdf/articles/pdf-art2089.pdf. Accessed May 16, 2008.

94. US Department of State Web site. Convention on the Prohibition of the Development, Production and Stockpiling of Bacteriological (Biological) and Toxin Weapons and on their Destruction, Washington, Moscow, 1972 page. Available at: http://www.state.gov/documents/treaties/72296.pdf. Accessed August 6, 2007.

95. Felton J. Approval seen on chemical weapons. *Congressional Quarterly Weekly Report*. 1990;48 (23):1800.

96. Towell P. In the bag: chemical weapons pact. *Congressional Quarterly*. 1990;48(21):1664.

97. Organisation for the Prohibition of Chemical Weapons Web site. Background of Chemical Disarmament, 1980–1997. Available at: http://www.opcw.org. Accessed August 1, 2007.

98. Smith RJ, Yang YE. Bush to scrap all US chemical arms. *Washington Post*. May 14, 1991:A-1, A-12.

99. Organisation for the Prohibition of Chemical Weapons Web site. Membership of the Organisation for the Prohibition of Chemical Weapons: States Parties to the Chemical Weapons Convention as of 3 January 2008. Available at: http://www.opcw.org/html/db/members_ratifyer.html. Accessed May 16, 2008.

100. Carpenter WD. How industry came to support the CWC. *OPCW Synthesis*. November 2000.

101. Organisation for the Prohibition of Chemical Weapons Web site. Convention on the Prohibition of the Development, Production, Stockpiling and Use of Chemical Weapons and on their Destruction. Available at: http://www.opcw.org/html/db/cwc/eng/cwc_menu.html. Accessed May 16, 2008.

102. Comments from the Department of Defense. Appendix V. In: United States Government Accountability Office. *Nonproliferation: Delays in Implementing the Chemical Weapons Convention Raise Concerns about Proliferation*. Washington, DC: GAO; 2004. GAO Report to the Chairman, Committee on Armed Services, House of Representatives, GAO-04-361.

103. Javits EM. Thirty-third regular session of the Executive Council of the Organization for the Prohibition of Chemical Weapons (OPCW). June 25, 2003. US Department of State Web site. Available at: http://www.state.gov/t/ac/rls/rm/2003/22045.htm. Accessed May 16, 2008.

104. An International Appeal in Support of the Chemical Weapons Convention Web site, 2002. Available at: http://www.cwc-support.org/. Accessed August 1, 2007.

105. Krutzsch W. "Never under any circumstances": the CWC three years after its first review conference. *The CBW Conventions Bulletin*. 2005;68.

106. US Department of State. Bush earmarks funds to destroy chemical warfare agents in Albania. Washington, DC: Bureau of International Information Programs, US Department of State. Press Release. October 21, 2004.

107. Manley RG. Overview of the status of the chemical demilitarization worldwide and the way ahead. *OPCW Synthesis*. August 2000.

108. Department of Defense Authorization Act for 1984. Pub L No. 98-94. September 24, 1983.

109. US Department of Health and Human Services, Centers for Disease Control and Prevention. CDC proposed airborne exposure limits for chemical warfare agents. *Federal Register* 68, no. 140 (July 22, 2003).

110. Health effects associated with nerve agent acute exposure guideline levels (AEGLs). January 2003. US Center for Health Promotion and Preventive Medicine Web site. Available at: http://www.osha.gov/SLTC/emergencypreparedness/chemical/pdf/tier_3_nerve_aegl_health_effects_usachppm1_03.pdf. Accessed May 16, 2008.

111. US Center for Health Promotion and Preventive Medicine. *Acute Toxicity Estimation and Operational Risk Management of Chemical Warfare Agent Exposures*. Aberdeen Proving Ground, Md: USACHPPM; 2004. USACHPPM Report No.47-EM-5863-04.

112. National Advisory Committee for Acute Exposure Guideline Levels (AEGLs) for hazardous substances; proposed AEGL values. *Federal Register* 66, no. 85 (May 2, 2001). Available at: http://www.epa.gov/EPA-TOX/2001/May/Day-02/t11001.htm. Accessed May 22, 2008.

113. Reuters. Pentagon reviews pricey weapon disposal program. December 6, 2006. Green Cross/Global Green News Forum Web site. Available at: http://www.greencross.ch/news/index.php?mode=singleview&action=overview&table=news_english&language=english&id=272. Accessed May 16, 2008.

114. Emery E. Pueblo depot costs up sharply: the Pentagon says it will cost $3.6 billion, and it won't be done before 2020. *Denver Post*. January 12, 2007:B05.

115. Tucker JB. Russia's new plan for chemical weapons destruction. *Arms Control Today*. 2001;31(6).

116. Walker P, de Guzman J. *Implementing Chemical Weapons Destruction in Russia: an Investigation of Best Practices in WMD Demilitarization*. Washington, DC: Center for Strategic and International Studies, Strengthening the Global Partnership Project; 2006. Issue Brief #6.

117. World News Connection. Kholstov stresses importance of international aid at CWC conference. January 3, 2007. Green Cross/Global Green News Forum Web site. Available at: http://www.greencross.ch/news/index.php?mode=singleview&action=overview&table=news_english&language=english&id=281. Accessed May 16, 2008.

118. Itar-Tass News Agency. Russia disposes 8,456 tonnes or 20% of chemical weapons 9 days ahead of plan. April 20, 2007. Green Cross/Global Green News Forum Web site. Available at: http://www.greencross.ch/news/index.php?mode=singleview&action=overview&table=news_english&language=english&id=317. Accessed May 16, 2008.

119. World News Connection. Draft budget allocates 75 billion rubles for chemical weapons disposal in 2008–2010. June 29, 2007. Green Cross/Global Green News Forum Web site. Available at: http://www.greencross.ch/news/index.php?mode=singleview&action=overview&table=news_english&language=english&id=340. Accessed May 16, 2008.

120. Litovkin V. Commentary: United States hinders Russia's chemical disarmament. April 27, 2006. RIA Novosti News Service. Available at http://www.cwwg.org/rn04.27.06.html. Accessed May 16, 2008.

121. Arnaudo D. Progress of problems at CW destruction site? *Arms Control Today*. 2007;37(4).

122. G8 Summit 2007 Web site. Report on the G8 global partnership page. June 8, 2007. Available at: http://www.g-8.de/Content/EN/Artikel/__g8-summit/anlagen/gp-report-final,templateId=raw,property=publicationFile.pdf/gp-report-final. Accessed May 16, 2008.

123. Nuclear Threat Initiative Web site. North Korea Profile: Chemical Overview page. Available at: http://www.nti.org/e_research/profiles/NK/Nuclear/index.html. Accessed July 31, 2007.

124. The Middle East Forum. Sponsoring terrorism, U.S. Department of State. *Middle East Quarterly*. 2004;11(2).

Chapter 5

NERVE AGENTS

FREDERICK R. SIDELL, MD*; JONATHAN NEWMARK, MD†; AND JOHN H. MCDONOUGH PHD‡

*Formerly, Chief, Chemical Casualty Care Office, and Director, Medical Management of Chemical Casualties Course, US Army Medical Research Institute of Chemical Defense, Aberdeen Proving Ground, Maryland; deceased

†Colonel, Medical Corps, US Army; Deputy Assistant Joint Program Executive Officer, Medical Systems, Joint Program Executive Office for Chemical/Biological Defense, Skyline #2, Suite 1609, 5203 Leesburg Pike, Falls Church, Virginia 22041; Adjunct Professor, Department of Neurology, F. Edward Hébert School of Medicine, Uniformed Services University of the Health Sciences, Bethesda, Maryland

‡Major, Medical Service Corps, US Army (Retired); Research Psychologist, Pharmacology Branch, Research Division, US Army Medical Research Institute of Chemical Defense, Room 161A, Building E-3100, 3100 Ricketts Point Road, Aberdeen Proving Ground, Maryland 21010

INTRODUCTION

Nerve agents, secretly developed for military use before World War II, work by inhibiting cholinesterase (ChE). Though similar chemicals are used in areas such as medicine, pharmacology, and agriculture, they lack the potency of military agents, which are extremely toxic. The military stockpiles of several major world powers are known to include nerve agents, and other countries undoubtedly possess nerve agents as well. Terrorist organizations have used nerve agents to cause mass injury and death, as was the case in the 1994 and 1995 Aum Shinrikyo subway attacks in Japan. Other groups, like Al-Qaeda, have indicated strong interest in obtaining these compounds. Therefore, it is imperative that military medical personnel are familiar with these agents, their effects, and the proper therapy for treating casualties.

HISTORY

The earliest recorded use of nerve agents comes from west Africa, where the Calabar bean, from the plant *Physostigma venenosum*, was used as an "ordeal poison" to combat witchcraft. Tribal members accused of practicing witchcraft were forced to ingest the beans and if they survived, they were proclaimed innocent.[1,2] An extract, "the elixir of the Calabar bean," was later used medicinally,[3] and in 1864, the active principle was isolated by Jobst and Hesse and called physostigmine.[1] Vee and Leven independently isolated this same substance in 1865 and named it eserine,[1] resulting in its dual nomenclature.

Five organophosphorus compounds are generally regarded as nerve agents. They include tabun (North Atlantic Treaty Organization military designation GA), sarin (GB), soman (GD), cyclosarin (GF), and VX (no common name). More recently, a Soviet-developed substance closely related to VX, called VR or Russian VX, has been added to the list. The agents in the "G" series were allegedly given that code letter because they originated in Germany; the "V" in the latter series allegedly stands for "venomous." GF is an old agent, an analog of sarin, which was previously discounted by the United States as being of no interest. During the Persian Gulf War, it was believed that Iraq might have GF in its arsenal. The toxicity and speed of action of this agent still merits consideration of it as a threat.

The first organophosphorus ChE inhibitor was probably tetraethyl pyrophosphate, synthesized by Wurtz and tasted (with no ill results) by Clermont in 1854.[4] During the next 80 years, chemists such as Michaelis, Arbusow, and Nylen made advances in organophosphorus chemistry, but they did not realize the toxicity of the substances with which they were working.[4]

In the early 1930s, interest in both physostigmine-type (reversible) and organophosphorus-type (irreversible) ChE inhibitors increased. (The terms "reversible" and "irreversible" refer to the duration of binding of the compound with the enzyme ChE; see below.) The reversible type, most of which are carbamates, were developed for treating conditions such as intestinal atony, myasthenia gravis (a disorder in which the immune system attacks postsynaptic acetylcholine [ACh] receptors), and glaucoma; for example, there is a documented case from 1931 of a doctor treating gastric atony with neostigmine.[1]

Lange and Krueger reported on the marked potency of organophosphorus compounds in 1932 after noting the effects of the vapors of dimethyl and diethyl phosphorofluoridate on themselves.[1,4] Shortly thereafter, the German company IG Farbenindustrie developed an interest in using organophosphorus compounds as insecticides. On December 23, 1936, Gerhard Schrader, who headed the company's research effort, synthesized what is known today as tabun.[5,6] Like Lange and Krueger, he noted the toxicity (miosis and discomfort) of the vapors of the substance in himself.

Over a year later, Schrader synthesized a second organophosphorus compound and named it *sarin* in honor of those who were instrumental in its development and production: Schrader, Ambros, Rudriger, and van der Linde.[5] Because the German Ministry of Defense required that substances passing certain toxicity tests be submitted to the government for further investigation, these compounds were examined for possible military use.

The potential of tabun and sarin as weapons was soon realized. A large production facility was built in Dyhernfurth, Poland (part of Germany at the time), and production of tabun began in 1942.[5,6] Sarin was also produced in Dyhernfurth and possibly at another plant in Falkenhagen.[6] Late in World War II, Soviet troops captured the Dyhernfurth facility, dismantled it, and moved it, along with key personnel, to the former Soviet Union, where production of the agents commenced in 1946.[6] Some believe the Soviets insisted on placing the border between Poland and Germany as far west as the Oder-Neisse line, where it remains today, because Stalin did not want the Dyhernfurth site, located between the Oder and Neisse rivers, to be in Germany.[7]

About 10,000 to 30,000 tons of tabun and smaller quantities of sarin were produced and put into munitions by the Germans during World War II, but these weapons were never used.[6] Although it is unclear why they were never used, possible explanations include Hitler's distaste for chemical warfare given his own exposure to mustard gas in World War I; Germany's loss of air superiority on the battlefield by the time sufficient nerve agent stocks were available; and Germany's mistaken belief that the Allies had also developed nerve agents.

In the waning days of World War II, troops of the United States and the United Kingdom captured some of the German munitions, which were being stored at Raubkammer, a German testing facility. The weapons, which contained an agent unknown to scientists in the United Kingdom and the United States, were taken to the each of the countries for examination. Over a single weekend, a small group of scientists at the United Kingdom Chemical Defence Establishment, working despite miosis caused by accidental exposure to the agent vapor, elucidated the pharmacology and toxicity of tabun and documented the antidotal activity of atropine.[8]

Use of these weapons probably would have been devastating and might have altered the outcome of the war. The Germans had tested nerve agents on inmates of concentration camps, not only to investigate their intoxicating effects but also to develop antidotes.[9] Many casualties, including some fatalities, were reported among the plant workers at Dyhernfurth. However, the medical staff there eventually developed antidotal compounds.[5] The Allies were unaware of these German experiments until the close of the war, months after the initial UK studies,[8] and much of the basic knowledge about the clinical effects of nerve agents comes from research performed in the decades immediately following World War II.

Soman was synthesized in 1944 by Richard Kuhn of Germany, who was attempting to develop an insecticide.[6] Although small amounts were produced for the military, development had not proceeded far by the end of the war. The nerve agent VX was first synthesized in the 1950s by a chemical company in the United Kingdom looking for new pesticides.[6] It was then given to the United States for military development. Other potential nerve agents were synthesized by scientists in the United States and United Kingdom but were not developed for military use. For example, GF, which may have been synthesized around 1949 by a foreign chemist searching for alternative nerve agents, was studied in both the United States and the United Kingdom. It was then discarded for reasons that are not entirely clear. Possible explanations are that it was too expensive to manufacture or that there was no perceived need for an agent with its properties. The manufacturing process for GF is apparently similar to that for GB. During the Persian Gulf War (1990–1991), Iraq was believed to have switched from manufacturing GB to manufacturing GF when the precursors of GB were embargoed.

The United States began to produce sarin in the early 1950s, and VX in the early 1960s, for potential military use. Production continued for about a decade.[6] The United States placed these two nerve agents in M55 rockets; land mines; 105-mm, 155-mm, and 8-in. projectiles; 500-lb and 750-lb bombs; wet-eye bombs (which have liquid chemical ["wet"] contents); spray tanks; and bulk containers.[10] These munitions were stored at six depots within the continental United States and one outside the continent,[11] near the following locations: Tooelle, Utah; Umatilla, Oregon; Anniston, Alabama; Pine Bluff, Arkansas; Newport, Indiana; Richmond, Kentucky; and Johnston Island in the Pacific Ocean.

The United States signed the Chemical Weapons Convention in 1996, and it came into effect in 1997. Under its provisions, the United States pledged to eliminate its stockpile of chemical weapons, including the nerve agent stockpiles. The overseas stockpile, moved from Europe and Asia to Johnston Island, has been completely destroyed at the time of this writing. On-site destruction facilities either exist or are being built at all of the depots in the continental United States. The timetable for destruction of these stockpiles accelerated after the 2001 terrorist attacks because the depots are seen as potential terrorist targets. The largest stockpile was kept at Tooele, Utah, and was the first to be completely destroyed.

The former Soviet Union had a stockpile of chemical weapons, including nerve agents, estimated to be ten times the size of the US stockpile. Russia has pledged to eliminate this stockpile.

Nerve agents, although developed for World War II in Germany, were not used on the battlefield until 50 years later. During the Iran-Iraq War, Iraq used large quantities of tabun and sarin against Iranian forces, causing between 45,000 and 120,000 casualties, depending upon the source.[12] In 1995 Iraq declared to the United Nations Special Commission that the country still possessed 4 metric tons of VX and up to 150 metric tons of sarin. At the time, the United Nations Special Commission suspected that Iraq had up to 200 metric tons of each. As of this writing, no Iraqi stockpiles of chemical weapons have been found; however, in May 2004, two US soldiers were exposed to sarin in Baghdad, Iraq, in the form of an old Iraqi weapon that was being used as part of an improvised explosive device.[13] There have been reports that Iran may have developed nerve agents and used them against Iraq, but these reports have never been confirmed.

Sarin has also been used in terrorist attacks. In June 1994 members of a Japanese cult released sarin from the rear of a van in Matsumoto, Japan. Although there were almost 300 casualties, including 7 deaths, this event was not well publicized. On March 20, 1995, the same group broke open plastic containers of sarin on several Tokyo trains during the morning commute. The containers held a 30% solution of liquid sarin, which the cult members synchronously ripped open on three subway trains and allowed to spill onto the seats and floors. More than 5,500 people sought medical care; about 4,000 had no effects from the agent but 12 casualties died. This incident required a major commitment of medical resources to triage and care for the casualties. (For more information on the Aum attacks, see Chapter 2, History of Chemical Warfare and Chapter 4, History of the Chemical Threat, Chemical Terrorism, and Its Implications for Military Medicine).

PHARMACOLOGY OF CHOLINESTERASE INHIBITORS

Cholinesterase in Tissue

According to the current, widely accepted explanation, nerve agents are compounds that exert their biological effects by inhibiting the enzyme acetylcholinesterase (AChE). The cholinergic system is the only neurotransmitter system known in which the action of the neurotransmitter is terminated by an enzyme, AChE.

AChE belongs to the class of enzymes called *esterases*, which catalyze the hydrolysis of esters. ChEs, the class of esterases to which AChE belongs, have high affinities for the esters of choline. Although there are several types of choline esters, ACh, the neurotransmitter of the cholinergic portion of the nervous system, is most relevant to nerve agent activity.

AChE, found at the receptor sites of tissue innervated by the cholinergic nervous system, hydrolyzes ACh rapidly. It has one of the highest known enzyme turnover numbers (number of molecules of substrate that it turns over per unit time).[14] A similar enzyme with ACh as its preferred substrate is found in or on erythrocytes (red blood cells) and is known as red blood cell, or true, cholinesterase (RBC-ChE). Butyrylcholinesterase (BuChE, also known as serum or plasma cholinesterase and as pseudocholinesterase), another enzyme of the ChE family, uses butyrylcholine as its preferred substrate. Butyrylcholine is present in plasma or serum and in some tissues.

BuChE and RBC-ChE are the two forms of ChE in the blood. While there is a single gene for each form of ChE, the active sites are identical regardless of the physical form. However, because blood is easy to draw, the activities of each of these enzymes can be assayed by standard, relatively simple laboratory techniques, whereas tissue enzyme is unavailable for assay. The measurements obtained from the blood assay can be used as an approximation of tissue enzyme activity in the event of a known or possible exposure to an AChE inhibitor.

Cholinesterase-Inhibiting Compounds

Most ChE-inhibiting compounds are either carbamates or organophosphorus compounds. The best known among the carbamates is physostigmine (eserine, elixir of the Calabar bean), which has been used in medicine for more than a century.[3] Neostigmine (Prostigmin, manufactured by ICN Pharmaceuticals, Costa Mesa, Calif) was developed in the early 1930s to manage myasthenia gravis; ambenonium was developed later for the same purpose. Pyridostigmine bromide (Mestinon, manufactured by ICN Pharmaceuticals, Costa Mesa, Calif) has been used for decades to manage myasthenia gravis. On any given day, an estimated 16,000 patients in the United States take pyridostigmine bromide medication to treat myasthenia gravis. The US military and several other nations also field pyridostigmine bromide (manufactured by Phillips Duphar, Holland), known as PB or NAPP (nerve agent pyridostigmine pretreatment), as a pretreatment or antidote-enhancing substance to be used before exposure to certain nerve agents (see below). Today these carbamates are mainly used for treating glaucoma and myasthenia gravis. Other carbamates, such as carbaryl (Sevin, manufactured by Bayer, Leverkusen, North Rhine-Westphalia, Germany), are used as insecticides.

Recently, several anticholinesterase drugs have been used to treat Alzheimer's disease, in which cholinergic transmission is faulty. In the past few years, these have become the basis of treatment of early stages of this disease. Three are approved for this indication by the US Food and Drug Administration (FDA): donepezil, rivastigmine, and galanthamine. Rivastigmine is a carbamate, donepezil is a piperidine compound, and galanthamine is a tertiary alkaloid. All inhibit ChEs.

Most commonly used insecticides contain either a carbamate or an organophosphorus compound. The organophosphorus insecticide malathion has replaced parathion, which was first synthesized in the 1940s. The organophosphorus compound diisopropyl phosphorofluoridate (DFP) was synthesized before World War II and studied by Allied scientists before and during the war, but was rejected for use as a military agent. For a period of time, this compound was used topically to treat glaucoma, but later was deemed unsuitable because it produced cataracts. It has been widely used in pharmacology as an investigational agent.

Mechanism of Action

Nerve agents inhibit ChE, which then cannot hydrolyze ACh. This classic explanation of nerve agent poisoning holds that the intoxicating effects are due to the excess endogenous ACh; nerve agents disable the off switch for cholinergic transmission, producing cholinergic overactivity or cholinergic crisis. A detailed discussion of the chemistry of ChE inhibition is beyond the scope of this chapter and can be found in most textbooks of pharmacology,[14,15] though the relevant aspects are summarized here.

The human nervous system is made up of conducting cells, or neurons, whose primary mission is to convey information from place to place via efficient electric signals or action potentials. When a signal reaches the end of a neuron, it can only continue as a chemical signal, the secretion of a packet of neurotransmitter molecules and its diffusion across the space or synaptic cleft separating its parent neuron from the next cell in series. When the neurotransmitter molecule reaches the target cell, it interacts with specific postsynaptic receptors on the receiving cell's surface membrane, giving rise to a miniature endplate potential. Once sufficient numbers of these are generated, they summate and a new action potential is created, allowing information transmission to proceed. Each neuron in the nervous system uses only one neurotransmitter for this purpose. The neuroanatomy of each neurotransmitter system is specific; neurons in particular tracts or regions use specific neurotransmitters. Approximately 20 neurotransmitters have been identified in neurobiology. The portion of the nervous system that uses ACh as its neurotransmitter is referred to as the cholinergic system. It is the most widely distributed and best studied in neurobiology.

Cholinergic tracts are found in almost every part of the brain within the central nervous system (CNS). Within the peripheral nervous system, however, the cholinergic system is found only in very specific fiber tracts. Clinically, the most important of these are the sympathetic and parasympathetic divisions of the autonomic nervous system.

The cholinergic nervous system can be further divided into the muscarinic and nicotinic systems, because the structures that are innervated have receptors that recognize two false experimental transmitters, alkaloids muscarine and nicotine, and can be stimulated by these compounds. In the periphery, where cholinergic input is primarily autonomic, muscarinic sites are innervated by postganglionic parasympathetic fibers. In the periphery, these sites include glands (eg, those of the mouth and the respiratory and gastrointestinal systems), the musculature of the pulmonary and gastrointestinal systems, the efferent organs of the cranial nerves (including the heart via the vagus nerve), and other structures. Nicotinic sites are predominantly found at the autonomic ganglia and skeletal muscles.

The brain contains a high number of cholinergic neurons. Both muscarinic and nicotinic receptors are active in the central cholinergic system, with muscarinic receptors predominating in a ratio of roughly 9 to 1. Clinically, the most important characteristic of the central cholinergic system is that it is the most anatomically widespread of any known neurotransmitter system in human brain. Consequently, a chemical, such as nerve agent, that affects the cholinergic system as a whole will affect all parts of the brain rather than only a few, as in more restricted neurotransmitter systems such as the dopaminergic or serotoninergic systems.

When an action potential in a cholinergic neuron reaches the terminal bouton, ACh packets are released, cross the synaptic cleft, interact with postsynaptic cholinergic receptors, and cause a new action potential to be generated. The cycle continues until ACh is hydrolyzed by AChE, a membrane-bound protein. This is the mechanism that prevents cholinergic stimulation from getting out of hand (Figure 5-1).

In the cholinergic nervous system, ChE hydrolyzes the neurotransmitter ACh to terminate its activity at the receptor site (Figure 5-2). The catalytic mechanism of AChE involves first an acylation step, in which serine 203 reacts with ACh to displace the choline moiety and forming an acylated serine (the choline, having been displaced, diffuses away). This reaction is greatly facilitated by other strategically placed residues in the active site that orient the ACh to the appropriate angle for serine to displace the choline and stabilize the transition state by a three-pronged hydrogen bond (the "oxyanion hole"). In a second step, a water molecule bound to, and polarized by, another key amino acid residue, histidine 447, attacks the acyl group, displacing it from the serine to form acetic acid, which diffuses away and leaves a regenerated or reactivated enzyme that can repeat the operation.

If AChE is absent from the site, or if it is unable to function, ACh accumulates and continues to produce postsynaptic action potentials and activity in the organ. The nerve agents and other ChE-inhibiting substances

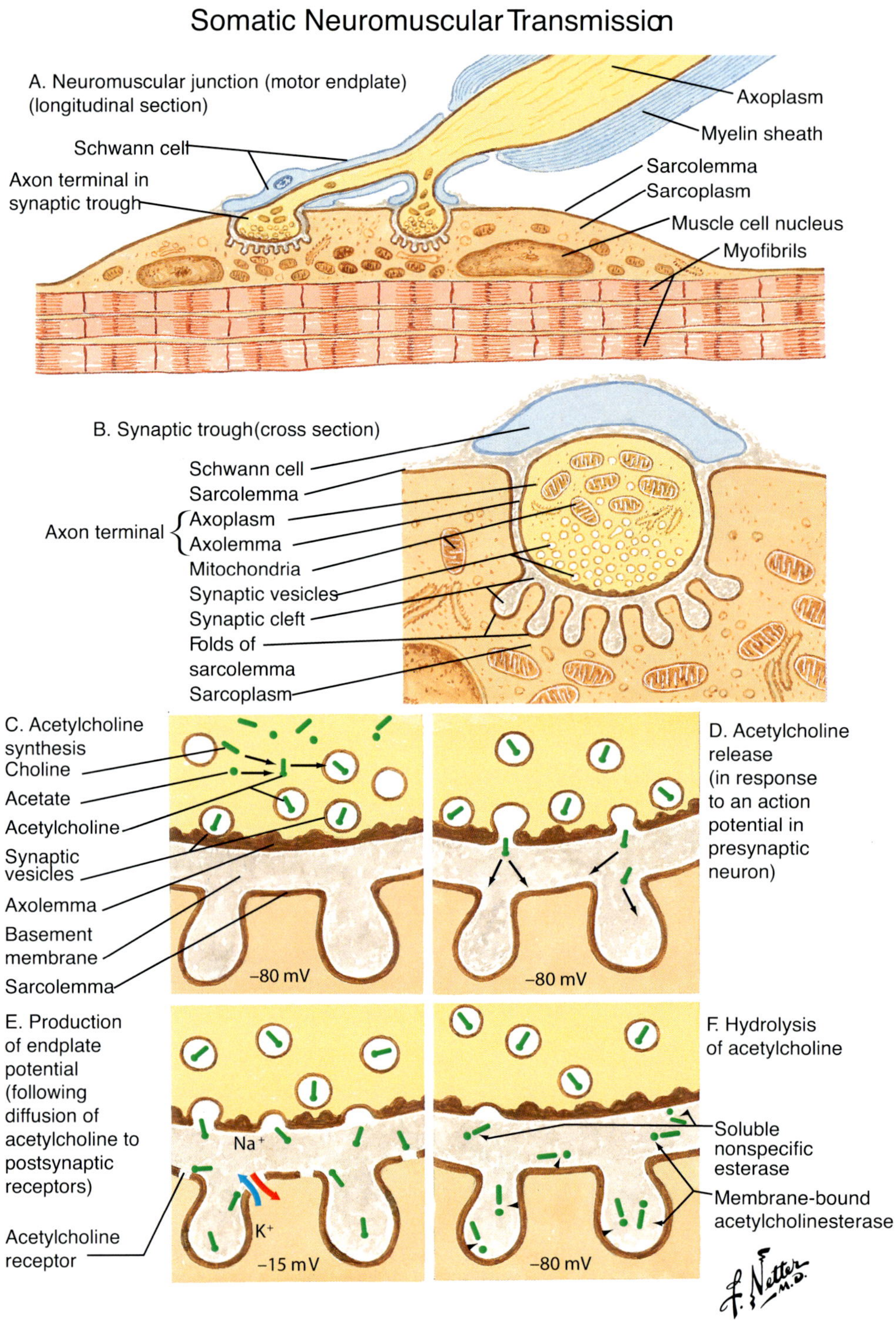

Fig. 5-1. Diagram of neuromuscular conduction. **(a)** Nerve fiber with axon terminal in synaptic trough of muscle. **(b)** Close-up of axon terminal in trough, with synaptic vesicles indicated. **(c)** Acetylcholine synthesis from acetate and choline and storage of acetylcholine in synaptic vesicles. **(d)** Release of acetylcholine from synaptic vesicles after an action potential. **(e)** Acetylcholine stimulation of endplate at receptor for site. **(f)** Hydrolysis of acetylcholine by membrane-bound acetylcholinesterase.
Reproduced with permission from: *Clinical Symposia*. 1948;1(1§8):162. Plate 3118. West Caldwell, NJ: CIBA-GEIGY Medical Education Division.

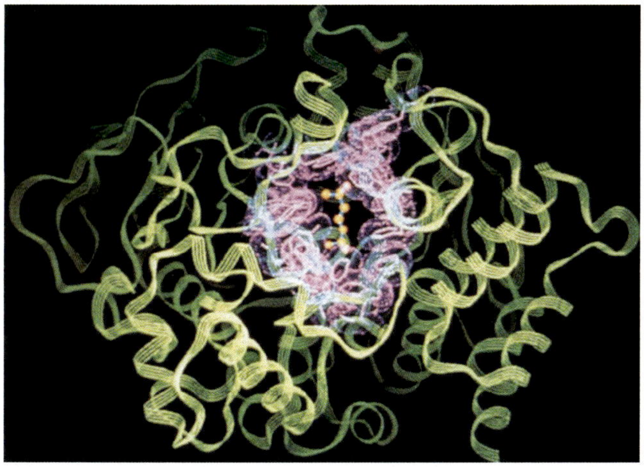

Fig. 5-2. This schematic ribbon diagram shows the structure of Torpedo californica acetylcholinesterase. The diagram is color-coded; green: the 537-amino acid polypeptide of the enzyme monomer; pink: the 14 aromatic residues that line the deep aromatic gorge leading to the active site; and gold and blue: a model of the natural substrate for acetylcholinesterase, the neurotransmitter acetylcholine, docked in the active site.
Reproduced with permission from: Sussman JL, Silman I. Acetylcholinesterase: Structure and use as a model for specific cation-protein interactions. *Curr Opin Struct Biol.* 1992;2:724.

produce biological activity by disabling (or inhibiting) AChE, an action that leads to an accumulation of ACh. The biological activity, or toxicity, of ChE inhibitors is due to this excess endogenous ACh, which is not hydrolyzed. The resulting toxidrome is referred to as cholinergic crisis.

The compounds in the two major categories of AChE inhibitors, carbamates and organophosphorus compounds, also attach to the ChE enzyme. There are some differences, however, between them and the natural substrate ACh. Carbamates attach to both the esteratic and the anionic sites. A moiety of the carbamate is immediately split off, leaving the enzyme carbamoylated at the esteratic site. Instead of hydrolysis occurring at this site within microseconds, as it does with the acetylated enzyme, hydrolysis does not occur for minutes to hours, and the enzyme remains inactive or inhibited for about an hour after reacting with physostigmine and for 4 to 6 hours after reacting with pyridostigmine.

Most organophosphorus compounds combine with the ChE enzyme only at the esteratic site, and the stability of the bond (ie, the interval during which the organophosphorus compound remains attached) depends on the structure of the compound. Hydrolytic cleavage of the compound from the enzyme may occur in several hours if the alkyl groups of the organophosphorus compound are methyl or ethyl, but if the alkyl groups are larger, cleavage may not occur. Thus, the phosphorylated form of the enzyme may remain indefinitely. In that case, enzymatic activity returns only with the synthesis of new enzyme. Functionally then, organophosphorus compounds may be said to be irreversible inhibitors of ChE, whereas the carbamates cause only temporary inhibition and are therefore referred to as reversible inhibitors.

Because most of these compounds attach to the esteratic site on AChE, a second binding compound cannot attach on that site if the site is already occupied by a molecule. A previously administered ChE inhibitor will, in a manner of speaking, protect the enzyme from a second one.[16,17] This activity forms the pharmacological basis for administering a carbamate (pyridostigmine) before expected exposure to some nerve agents to provide partial protection (lasting 6–8 h) against the more permanently bound nerve agents (see below).

After inhibition by irreversibly bound inhibitors, recovery of the enzymatic activity in the brain seems to occur more slowly than that in the blood ChE.[18,19] An individual severely exposed to soman, however, was alert and functioning reasonably well for several days while ChE activity in his blood was undetectable (Exhibit 5-1).[20] This case study and other data suggest that tissue function is restored at least partially when ChE activity is still quite low.

Blood Cholinesterases

Individuals occupationally exposed to ChE-inhibiting substances are periodically monitored for asymptomatic exposure by assays of blood-ChE activity. Those at risk include crop sprayers and orchard workers who handle ChE-inhibiting insecticides, and chemical agent depot workers or laboratory scientists who handle nerve agents. To be meaningful, such monitoring must include knowledge of physiological variation in the blood enzymes.

Individuals who work with or around nerve agents must have their RBC-ChE activity monitored periodically. Before the individuals begin work, two measures of RBC-ChE, drawn within 14 days but not within 24 hours of each other, are averaged as a baseline. At periodic intervals, the frequency of which depends on the individuals' jobs, blood is drawn for measuring ChE activity. If the activity is 90% or more of the worker's baseline, no action is taken. If the activity is below 90% of the baseline, the sample is rerun. If the second test also indicates activity below 90% of baseline, the individual is referred to the oc-

EXHIBIT 5-1

CASE REPORT: ACCIDENTAL EXPOSURE OF A MAN TO LIQUID SOMAN

This 33-year-old man [who worked at Edgewood Arsenal, Edgewood, Maryland] had been working with small amounts of soman in solution [25% (V/V) concentration, total volume <1 mL] when a syringe-needle connection broke, splashing some of the solution into and around his mouth. . . He immediately washed his face and rinsed his mouth with water and was brought to the emergency room about 9 AM, 5-10 min after the accident. He was asymptomatic until he arrived at the ER when, as he later said, he felt "the world was caving in on me," and he collapsed. His past medical history was noncontributory. Physical examination showed him to be comatose and mildly cyanotic with slightly labored respirations. Intravenous atropine sulfate (2 mg) was given and may have been partially responsible for his initial blood pressure of 180/80 and heart rate of 150. He had miosis (1-2 mm, bilaterally), markedly injected conjunctiva, marked oral and nasal secretions, moderate trismus and nuchal rigidity, prominent muscular fasciculations, and hyperactive deep-tendon reflexes. Except for tachycardia, his heart, lungs, and abdomen were normal.

Within a minute after he collapsed (about 10 min after exposure) he was given intravenous atropine sulfate and in the ensuing 15 min he received a total of 4 mg intravenously and 8 mg intramuscularly, and pralidoxime chloride (2-PAMCl) was administered (2 gm over a 30 min period in an intravenous drip). Supportive care in the first 30 min consisted of oxygen by nasal catheter and frequent nasopharyngeal suction. Bronchoconstriction and a decreased respiratory rate and amplitude were prominent; the former was more responsive to atropine therapy. He became cyanotic and attempts to insert an endotracheal tube were unsuccessful because of trismus. Since spontaneous respiration did not cease, a tracheostomy was not performed.

After the initial therapy his cyanosis cleared and his blood pressure and heart rate remained stable. He began to awaken in about 30 min and thereafter was awake and alert. Migratory involuntary muscular activity (fasciculations and tremor) continued through the day.

He improved throughout the day, but was generally uncomfortable and restless with abdominal pain and nausea throughout the day and night. Atropine (4 mg, i.v.) was required again at 11 PM (14-hr post exposure) after several episodes of vomiting. About 4 AM, he was catheterized because of urinary retention.

His restlessness and intermittent nausea continued, and about 5 AM (20 hr after exposure) he again vomited. Because the previous atropine had apparently caused urinary retention, this emesis was treated with a small dose (5 mg, i.m.) of prochlorperazine, although phenothiazines have been reported to be deleterious in anticholinesterase compound poisoning. His general condition, including his discomfort, did not change.

He vomited twice more between 7:30-8 AM (22-23 hr post exposure) and was again given atropine (4 mg, i.m.). He voided small amounts several times, but catheterization was necessary several hours later.

Several EKGs recorded on admission and during the first day showed sinus tachycardia. On the second day (25 hr after exposure and about 2 hr after atropine administration), his cardiac rhythm was irregular, and an EKG showed atrial fibrillation with a ventricular rate of 90-100 beats per min. This persisted throughout the day and evening, but his cardiac rhythm was again regular sinus the next morning.

During the second evening (about 36 hr after exposure), he again became nauseated and had recurrent vomiting. Because of the occurrences of urinary retention and arrhythmia, presumably due to atropine, he was again given prochlorperazine (5 mg, i.m.) at 10 PM and again at 2 AM. Half an hour after the first he complained of transient "tingling" feelings over his body, but there were no objective changes. After the second he rested comfortably and slept soundly for 3-4 hr, his first restful sleep since the exposure. At 11 AM the next morning, he was restless and had an expressionless face, torticollis, and athetoid movements. Diphenylhydramine hydrochloride (50 mg, i.v.) promptly relieved these symptoms and signs, which are characteristic of the extrapyramidal side effects of a phenothiazine. Throughout the remainder of his hospitalization, the patient's physical condition improved although he was treated with sulfisoxazole for three weeks for a urinary tract infection that developed after catheterization.

His psychiatric condition did not improve as rapidly as his physical condition. As the complications of the treatment for the physical effects subsided, evidence of lingering mental effects began to appear. A psychiatrist . . . who saw the subject frequently, recorded that he seem depressed, was withdrawn and subdued, admitted to antisocial thoughts, slept restlessly and fitfully, and had bad dreams. On the third day [after the exposure] the patient was given scopolamine hydrobromide (5 µg/kg, or 330 µg, i.m.) as a therapeutic trial. Psychiatric evaluation at the time of maximum scopolamine effect showed a slight but distinct improvement in mental status as he seemed more comfortable and performed better on several mental function tests (eg, serial 7s) than before scopolamine. That evening he was given 1.8 mg of scopolamine (orally) at bedtime and slept much better for most of the night.

This nighttime benefit from scopolamine may have occurred because of its sedative properties, but the improvement in mental status during the day suggested a more specific action, as scopolamine in this dose produces a slight decrease in intellectual functioning in normal subjects. [Thereafter, scopolamine and methscopolamine (which does not enter the central nervous system) were admin-

(Exhibit 5-1 *continues*)

Exhibit 5-1 *continued*

istered on randomly assigned days. The patient did better mentally (by examination) and on a written arithmetic test after receiving scopolamine than after methscopolamine.]

There was no detectable RBC-ChE until about the tenth day after exposure. . . . Apparently neither the RBC nor plasma ChE was significantly reactivated by the initial oxime therapy, which reflects the rapid irreversible phosphorylation and hence refractoriness of the soman-inhibited enzyme to reactivation by oxime.

Hematocrit, hemoglobin, white blood cell count, prothrombin time, blood urea nitrogen, bilirubin, creatinine, calcium, phosphorus, serum glutamic oxaloacetic transaminase, alkaline phosphatase, sodium, potassium, chloride, and carbon dioxide were all within normal limits the day of admission and on repeated measurements during his hospitalization.

About five weeks after his admission, the subject again received scopolamine (5 mg/kg, i.m.) and had a decrement in mental functioning, including a 25-30% reduction in NF [Number Facility] scores, which are the findings in normal subjects. This contrasts with the paradoxical improvement in mental status seen earlier.

About a week later, the psychiatrist noted that "he is probably close to his premorbid level intellectually and there is no evidence of any serious mood or thinking disorder."

A battery of standard psychological tests was given the subject 16 days, 4 months, and 6 months after the accident. He scored well on the Wechsler-Bellevue IQ test with a slight increase in score on the arithmetic section at the later testings. He had high Hs (hypochondriasis) and Hy (hysteria) scales on the Minnesota Multiphasic Personality Inventory (MMPI) on the early test and their later improvement indicated to the examiner that he had a decreased concern about bodily function. He did poorly on a visual retention task (the object of which was to remember and then reproduce a simple drawing) on first testing as he attempted to improve already correct drawings, made several major errors, and showed poor motor control; his later tests were normal. On word association, proverbs, and the ink blot he was slow and sometimes used delaying tactics, had difficulty generating verbal associations, and failed the harder proverbs, responses that in the examiner's opinion were not consistent with his IQ. The results of his later tests were faster, imaginative, and indicated full use of his intellectual facilities.

When last seen, six months after his exposure, the patient was doing well.

Reproduced with permission from Sidell FR. Soman and sarin: clinical manifestations and treatment of accidental poisoning by organophosphates. *Clin Toxicol*. 1974;7:1–17.

cupational health physician for review to determine if the depression in RBC-ChE activity is related to exposure to ChE-inhibiting substances. If RBC-ChE is depressed to 75% or below baseline, the worker is considered to have had an exposure and is withdrawn from work. Investigations are undertaken to discover how the worker was exposed. Although workers may be asymptomatic, they are not permitted to return to a work area around nerve agents until their RBC-ChE activity is higher than 90% of their baseline activity.[21] If workers have symptoms from a possible nerve agent exposure or if an accident is known to have occurred in their work area, RBC-ChE activity is immediately measured and the criteria noted above, as well as signs and symptoms, are used for exclusion from and return to work. The values of 75% and 90% were selected for several reasons, including the following: (a) the normal variation of RBC-ChE in an individual with time; (b) laboratory reproducibility in analysis of RBC-ChE activity; and (c)the lower tolerance to nerve agents with a low RBC-ChE as demonstrated in animals (see below).

In training responders to deal with acute nerve agent poisoning, little emphasis should be given to the use of laboratory diagnosis of ChE activity. Time does not permit using this determination to guide immediate treatment. On the other hand, laboratory values in patients are particularly helpful in two specific instances: (1) as a screen for exposure to a ChE inhibitor, as in agricultural workers or military personnel who may have been exposed to a nerve agent, and (2) as a way to follow exposed patients as they recover over time.

Butyrylcholinesterase

The enzyme BuChE is present in blood and throughout tissue. Its physiological role in humans is unclear[22]; however, it may be important in canine tracheal smooth muscle,[23] the canine ventricular conducting system,[24] and rat atria.[25]

BuChE is synthesized in the liver and has a replacement time of about 50 days. Its activity is decreased in parenchymal liver disease, acute infections, malnutrition, and chronic debilitating diseases, and is increased in the nephrotic syndrome.[22] This enzyme has no known physiological function in blood, but may assist in hydrolyzing certain choline esters.

People who have a prolonged paralysis caused by succinylcholine, a muscle relaxant, usually have low BuChE activity.[22] The structure of BuChE is determined by two autosomal alleles. The frequency of occurrence of the gene responsible for abnormal ChE is about 1 in 2,000 to 1 in 4,000 people. Thus, about 96% of the population have the usual phenotype, close to 4% have the heterozygous phenotype, and about 0.03% have the homozygous abnormal phenotype.[22] In addition to having the low BuChE activity in the usual assay (as a result of this genetic abnormality), people with abnormal ChE have low dibucaine numbers (the enzyme activity in an assay in which dibucaine is used as the ChE substrate). The mean dibucaine number for the normal phenotype is about 79%, that for the heterozygote is 62%, and that for the homozygous abnormal phenotype is 16%.[26] There are over 20 variants of the abnormal BuChE phenotype, each with different, low dibucaine numbers, including zero.

The relationship of BuChE activity and succinylcholine can be somewhat different. One author[27] reports on an individual whose BuChE activity was 3 times higher than normal. His dibucaine number was normal, and he was found to be relatively resistant to succinylcholine. His sister and daughter also had high BuChE activities. The author of this report suggests that this abnormality is autosomal dominant and that it represents another genetic abnormality of BuChE.

Erythrocyte Cholinesterase

RBC-ChE is synthesized with the erythrocyte, which has an average life of 120 days. The activity of this enzyme is decreased in certain diseases involving erythrocytes, such as pernicious anemia, and is increased during periods of active reticulocytosis, such as recovery from pernicious anemia, because reticulocytes have higher ChE activity than do mature cells. No other disease states are known to affect RBC-ChE activity,[22] but one report[28] describes three members of one family who had decreased RBC-ChE activity, suggesting that differences in this enzyme are genetic.

The physiological role of the enzyme in (or on the stroma of) the erythrocyte is unknown. Recovery of RBC-ChE activity after irreversible inhibition takes place only with the synthesis of new erythrocytes, or at a rate of approximately 1% per day.

Variation in Cholinesterase Activities

Butyrylcholinesterase

In longitudinal studies[29,30] lasting 3 to 250 weeks, the coefficient of variation (standard deviation divided by the mean) for an individual's BuChE activity ranged from 5% to 11.8% in both men and women. Of the ranges (the difference between the highest and lowest activities divided by the mean) for individuals in the study, the lowest was 24% and the highest was 50% over 1 year.[30]

BuChE activity does not vary with age in women[31,32] until the age of 60 years, when higher BuChE activities are seen.[32] BuChE activities in men have been reported in some studies to increase with age and in other studies to decrease with age.[20] In matched age groups, BuChE activity was higher in men than in women,[20,30] and higher in women not taking oral contraceptives than in those taking them.[32–34]

Erythrocyte Cholinesterase

RBC-ChE activity is more stable than the activity of the BuChE.[30,35,36] In a study[30] that lasted 1 year, the coefficients of variation were 2.1% to 3.5% in men and 3.1% to 4.1% in women, with ranges of 7.9% to 11.4% in men and 12.0% to 15.9% in women. This variation was less than that observed for the hematocrits of these individuals.

It is unclear whether age affects RBC-ChE activity. In one study,[31] RBC-ChE activity was unchanged with age, while in another,[32] enzyme activity increased with age from the third to the sixth decades in men, with a less marked increase through the fifth decade in women.

Inhibition of Blood Cholinesterases

Some ChE-inhibiting substances inhibit BuChE preferentially, and some inhibit RBC-ChE preferentially. Large amounts of ChE inhibitors will completely inhibit both enzymes.

The blood enzymes appear to act as effective scavengers of nerve agents while they remain in the circulation. There is little inhibition of tissue enzyme until much of the blood enzyme is inhibited because, with the exception of local tissue effects (eg, eye, respiratory tract, skin contact), the blood is the first tissue to encounter the agent. The RBC-ChE appears to correlate more closely with tissue ChE and physiological signs of poisoning than the plasma enzyme in this regard. In two studies,[37,38] a small dose of DFP in humans inhibited about 90% of the plasma enzyme activity but only 15% to 20% of RBC-ChE activity. Symptoms correlated with depression of RBC-ChE, but not with depression of BuChE (see below). In humans, some pesticides, such as parathion,[39–41] systox,[39] and malathion,[22] also preferentially inhibit the plasma enzyme, while others, such as dimefox[41] and mevinphos,[42] initially bind with the RBC enzyme. In animals, there appears to be a species difference because parathion preferentially inhibits RBC-ChE in rats and the plasma enzyme in dogs.[22]

The nerve agent VX preferentially inhibits RBC-ChE; in two studies,[43,44] a small amount caused a 70% or greater decrease in the activity of this enzyme, whereas the activity of BuChE was inhibited by no more than 20%. Sarin also preferentially inhibits the RBC-ChE; 80% to 100% inhibition of RBC-ChE activity was observed in two studies,[37,45] while BuChE was inhibited by 30% to 50%. Therefore, estimation of the RBC-ChE activity provides a better indicator of acute nerve agent exposure than does estimation of the plasma enzyme activity.

When the blood enzymes have been irreversibly inhibited, recovery of ChE activity depends on production of new plasma enzymes or production of new erythrocytes. Hence, complete recovery of BuChE activity that has been totally inhibited by sarin will occur in about 50 days, and recovery of the RBC-ChE, in 120 days (about 1% per day).[46] In humans, after inhibition by VX, the RBC-ChE activity seems to recover spontaneously at the rate of about 0.5% to 1% per hour for a few days, but complete recovery depends on erythrocyte production.[43,44]

Time Course of Inhibition

After very large amounts of nerve agent (multiple LD_{50}s [ie, multiples of the dose that is lethal to 50% of the exposed population]) are placed on the skin, signs and symptoms occur within minutes, and inhibition of blood ChE activities occurs equally quickly. However, with smaller amounts of agent, the onset is not so rapid. In studies in which small amounts of VX were applied on the skin of humans, the onset of symptoms and the maximal inhibition of blood ChE activity were found to occur many hours after application of the agent. In one study[44] in which equipotent amounts of VX were applied to the skin in different regions, the time to maximal inhibition was 5 hours for the head and neck, 7 hours for the extremities, and 10 hours for the torso. In a similar study,[47] the average time from placing VX on the skin to the onset of nausea and vomiting and maximal drop of blood ChE activity was 10.8 hours.

In a third study,[48] VX was applied to the cheek or forearm at environmental temperatures ranging from 0°F to 124°F, and 3 hours later the subjects were decontaminated and taken to a recovery area (about 80°F). In all temperature groups, the RBC-ChE activity continued to decline after decontamination, and maximal inhibition occurred at 5.6 hours after exposure at 124°F, 8.5 hours after exposure at 68°F, 10.4 hours after exposure at 36°F, and 12.2 hours after exposure at 0°F. At the two lowest temperatures, the rates of agent penetration and of decline in RBC-ChE activity increased after the subjects were taken from the cold environment and decontaminated. These results suggest that agent absorption through the skin is more rapid and complete at higher temperatures, and that even after thorough decontamination, a considerable amount of agent remains in the skin.

Inhalation of nerve agent vapor inhibits blood ChE activity and produces signs and symptoms of exposure more rapidly than does dermal contact. Although there is no correlation between ChE activity and clinical effects after exposure to small amounts of vapor, both clinical effects and ChE inhibition occur within minutes. In one study,[43] both the maximal inhibition of RBC-ChE activity and the appearance of signs and symptoms occurred about 1 hour after intravenous (IV) administration of small amounts of VX. After ingestion of VX, the interval was 2 to 3 hours.

Relation to Signs and Symptoms

The local signs and symptoms in the eye, nose, and airways caused by small amounts of vapor are due to the direct effect of the vapor on the organ. There appears to be no correlation between the severity of these effects and the blood ChE activity. Early experimental data[49–51] indicating the lack of correlation were supported by a retrospective analysis of 62 individuals seen at the Edgewood Arsenal Toxic Exposure Aid Station between 1948 and 1972. Although all individuals had physical signs or definite symptoms (or both) of nerve agent vapor exposure, there was no correlation between local effects from vapor exposure and RBC-ChE activity (Table 5-1).[52] More recently, clinical data from the Tokyo incident has shown that symptoms and signs can both be present with normal blood ChE levels.[53]

Minimal systemic effects, such as vomiting, occur in half the population when the RBC-ChE is inhibited to 25% of its control activity.[43,44] In a study[44] in which VX was placed on the skin, no vomiting occurred in 30 subjects whose minimal RBC-ChE activities were 40% of control or higher. Vomiting occurred in 9 (43%) of 21 subjects whose minimal RBC-ChE activities were 30% to 39% of control, in 10 (71%) of 14 subjects whose

TABLE 5-1

RELATION OF EFFECTS OF NERVE AGENT EXPOSURE TO ERYTHROCYTE CHOLINESTERASE ACTIVITY

Effect	Patients Affected (N=62)	Range of RBC-ChE Activity (% of Baseline*)
Miosis alone (bilateral)	22	0–100
Miosis alone (unilateral)	7	3–100
Miosis and tight chest	12	28–100
Miosis and rhinorrhea	9	5–90
Miosis, rhinorrhea, and tight chest	9	20–92
Rhinorrhea and tight chest	3	89–90

*Cholinesterase activity before nerve agent exposure.
RBC-CHE: red blood cell cholinesterase.
Data source: Sidell RF. Clinical considerations in nerve agent intoxication. In: Somani SM, ed. *Chemical Warfare Agents*. San Diego, Calif: Academic Press; 1992: 163.

minimal enzyme activities were 20% to 29% of control, and in 3 (60%) of 5 subjects whose minimal RBC-ChE activities were 0% to 19% of control. In other instances, the authors observed that patients had an RBC-ChE activity of 0% without the expected symptoms; this inhibition was acutely induced.

TABLE 5-2

RELATION OF CHOLINESTERASE ACTIVITY TO VOMITING AFTER EXPOSURE TO VX

Minimum RBC-ChE (% of Baseline*)	Patients (N=283)	Patients Vomiting	Percentage Vomiting
> 50	166	1	0.6
40–49	24	2	8.3
30–39	27	9	33.3
20–29	42	19	45.2
< 20	24	16	66.7

*Cholinesterase activity before nerve agent exposure
RBC-ChE: red blood cell cholinesterase.
Data sources: (1) Sidell FR, Groff WA. The reactivatibility of cholinesterase inhibited by VX and sarin in man. *Toxicol Appl Pharmacol*. 1974;27:241–252. (2) Sim VM. *Variability of Different Intact Human Skin Sites to the Penetration of VX*. Edgewood Arsenal, Md: Medical Research Laboratory; 1962. Chemical Research and Development Laboratory Report 3122.

Data from 283 individuals who received VX by various routes are categorized below (Table 5-2). The degree of inhibition needed to cause vomiting in these 283 people corresponds to that found in experimental data from other sources, which indicate that "to exert significant actions in vivo, an anti-ChE must inhibit from 50% to 90% of the enzyme present."[14(p446)]

Nerve Agents

Molecular models of the nerve agents tabun, sarin, soman, and VX are shown in Figure 5-3. The chemical, physical, and environmental properties of these compounds are summarized in Table 5-3. Nerve agents differ from commonly used ChE inhibitors

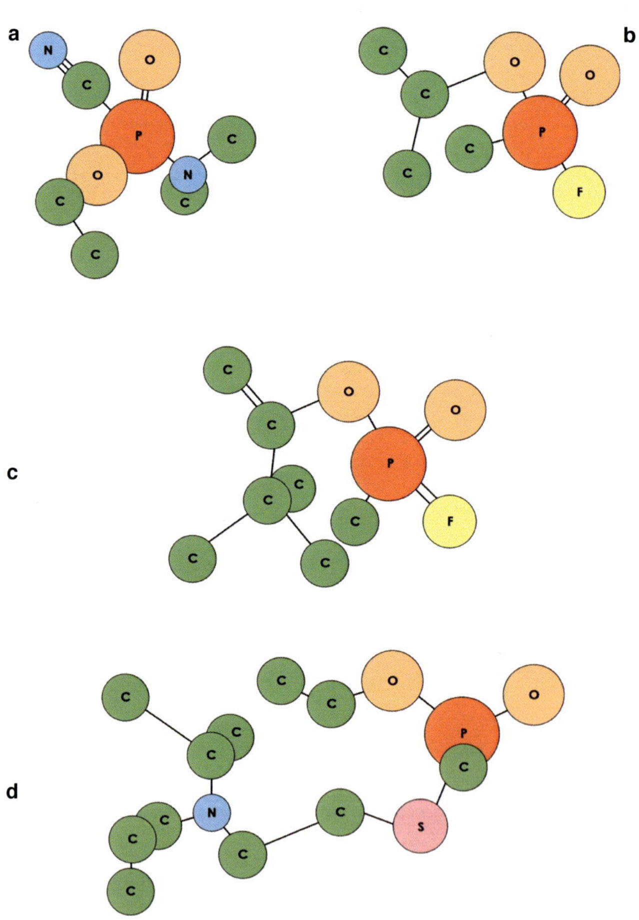

Fig. 5-3. Molecular models of **(a)** Tabun (GA), **(b)** Sarin (GB), **(c)** Soman (GD), **(d)** VX.
Molecular models: Courtesy of Office E Clark, Researcher, US Army Medical Research Institute of Chemical Defense, Aberdeen Proving Ground, Md.

TABLE 5-3

CHEMICAL, PHYSICAL, AND ENVIRONMENTAL PROPERTIES OF NERVE AGENTS

Properties	Tabun (GA)	Sarin (GB)	Soman (GD)	VX
Chemical and Physical				
Boiling point	230°C	158°C	198°C	298°C
Vapor pressure	0.037mm Hg at 20°C	2.1 mm Hg at 20°C	0.40 mm Hg at 20°C	0.0007 mm Hg at 20°C
Density				
Vapor (compared to air, air = 1)	5.6	4.86	6.3	9.2
Liquid	1.08 g/mL at 25°C	1.10 g/mL at 20°C	1.02 g/mL at 25°C	1.008 g/mL at 20°C
Volatility	610 mg/m^3 at 25°C	22,000 mg/m^3 at 25°C	3,900 mg/m^3 at 25°C	10.5 mg/m^3 at 25°C
Appearance	Colorless to brown liquid	Colorless liquid	Colorless liquid	Colorless to straw-colored liquid
Odor	Fruity	Odorless	Fruity; oil of camphor	Odorless
Solubility				
In water	9.8 g/100 g at 25°C	Miscible	2.1 g/100 g at 20°C	Miscible < 9.4°C
In other solvents	Soluble in most organic solvents	Soluble in all solvents	Soluble in some solvents	Soluble in all solvents
Environmental and Biological Detectability				
Vapor	M8A1, M256A1, CAM, ICAD	M8A1, M256A1, CAM, ICAD	M8A1, M256A1, CAM, ICAD	M8A1, M256A1, CAM, ICAD
Liquid	M8, M9 papers	M8, M9 papers	M8, M9 papers	M8, M9 papers
Persistency				
In soil	Half-life 1–1.5 days	2–24 hours at 5°C–25°C	Relatively persistent	2–6 days
On materiel	Unknown	Unknown	Unknown	Persistent
Decontamination of skin	M258A1, diluted hypochlorite, soap and water, M291 kit	M258A1, diluted hypochlorite, soap and water, M291 kit	M258A1, diluted hypochlorite, soap and water, M291 kit	M258A1, diluted hypochlorite, soap and water, M291 kit

CAM: chemical agent monitor
ICAD: individual chemical agent detector
LCt_{50}: vapor or aerosol exposure necessary to cause death in 50% of the population exposed
LD_{50}: dose necessary to cause death in 50% of the population with skin exposure
M8A1: chemical alarm system
M256A1: detection card
M258A1: self-decontamination kit
M291: decontamination kit
M8 and M9: chemical detection papers

primarily because they are more toxic (ie, a smaller amount is needed to cause an effect on an organism). For example, an in vitro study[45] with ChE from human erythrocytes, brain, and muscle showed that sarin had about 10 times more inhibitory activity than TEPP, 30 times more than neostigmine, 100 times more than DFP, and 1,000 times more than parathion.

The nerve agents are liquid at moderate temperatures (the term "nerve gas" is a misnomer). In their pure state, they are clear, colorless, and, at least in dilute solutions of distilled water, tasteless. Tabun has been reported to have a faint, slightly fruity odor, and soman, to have an ill-defined odor; sarin, cyclosarin, VR, and VX are apparently odorless.

One of the US soldiers exposed to sarin in Iraq in 2004 reported to the authors that the agent smelled like garbage, but that may have been due to impurities.

Cyclosarin (GF) and VR are not as well studied as the other agents. In animal tests GF has a toxicity intermediate between sarin and tabun, while VR has the same level of toxicity as VX.

The G agents are volatile; VX and VR have very low volatility. Sarin, the most volatile, is somewhat less volatile than water; tabun, cyclosarin, and soman are less volatile than sarin. The G agents present a definite vapor hazard; VX and VR are much less likely vaporize unless the ambient temperature is high.

EXPOSURE ROUTES

Inhalational Exposure to Vapor

The effects produced by nerve agent vapor begin in seconds to minutes after the onset of exposure, depending on the concentration of vapor. These effects usually reach maximal severity within minutes after the individual is removed or protected from the vapor, but they may continue to worsen if the exposure continues. There is no delay in onset as there is after liquid exposure.

At low *Ct* values (the concentration to which an organism is exposed to a substance times the amount of time the organism is exposed; Exhibit 5-2), the eyes, nose, airways, or a combination are usually affected. The eyes and nose are the most sensitive organs; the eyes may be affected equally or unequally. There may be some degree of miosis (with or without associated conjunctival injection and pain) with or without rhinorrhea, or there may be rhinorrhea without eye involvement (Table 5-4).

As exposure increases slightly, a combination of eye, nose, and lung involvement is usually seen. The casualty may or may not notice dim vision and may complain of tightness in the chest, possibly in the absence of physical findings. At higher exposures, the effects in these organs intensify. Marked miosis, copious secretions from the nose and mouth, and signs of moderate-to-severe impairment of ventilation are seen. The casualty will complain of mild-to-severe dyspnea, may be gasping for air, and will have obvious secretions.

In severe exposures, the casualty may not have time to report the initial effects before losing consciousness, and may not remember them on awakening. One severely exposed individual later recalled to the authors that he noticed an increase in secretions and difficulty breathing, and another said he felt giddy and faint before losing consciousness. In both instances, the casualties were unconscious within less than a minute after exposure to agent vapor. When reached (within minutes) by rescuers, both were unconscious and exhibited convulsive jerking motions of the limbs; copious secretions from the mouth and nose; labored, irregular, and gasping breathing; generalized

EXHIBIT 5-2

DEFINITIONS OF Ct, LCt_{50} AND LD_{50}

The terms *Ct* and LCt_{50} are often used to express a dose of a vapor or aerosol. However, the terms do not describe inhaled doses; they refer to the amount of compound to which an organism is exposed.

- *Ct* is used to describe an estimate of dose. C represents the concentration of the substance (as vapor or aerosol) in air (usually expressed as mg/m^3), and *t* represents time (usually expressed in minutes).
- The *Ct* value is the product of the concentration (C) to which an organism is exposed multiplied by the time (*t*) during which it remains exposed to that concentration. *Ct* does not express the amount retained within an organism; thus, it is not an inhalational dose.
- Because *Ct* is a product of C times *t*, a particular value can be produced by inversely varying the values of C and *t*. The *Ct* to produce a given biological effect is usually constant over an interval of minutes to several hours (Haber's law). Thus, an effect that is produced by an exposure to 0.05 mg/m^3 for 100 minutes is also produced by an exposure to 5 mg/m^3 for 1 minute ($Ct = 5\ mg/min/m^3$ in both cases). This generalization is usually invalid for very short or very long times, however, because an organism may hold its breath for several seconds and not actually inhale the vapor, or some detoxification may occur over many hours.
- The term LCt_{50} is often used to denote the vapor or aerosol exposure (*Ct*) necessary to cause death in 50% of the population exposed (L denotes lethal, and 50 denotes 50% of the population). In the same manner, the term LD_{50} is used to denote the dose that is lethal for 50% of the population exposed by other routes of administration.

TABLE 5-4

EFFECTS OF EXPOSURE TO NERVE AGENT VAPOR

Amount of Exposure	Effects*
Small (local effects)	Miosis, rhinorrhea, slight bronchoconstriction, secretions (slight dyspnea)
Moderate (local effects)	Miosis, rhinorrhea, slight bronchoconstriction, secretions (moderate to marked dyspnea)
Large	Miosis, rhinorrhea, slight bronchoconstriction, secretions (moderate to marked dyspnea), loss of consciousness, convulsions (seizures), generalized fasciculations, flaccid paralysis, apnea, involuntary micturition/defecation possible with seizures

*Onset of effects occurs within seconds to several minutes after exposure onset.

TABLE 5-5

EFFECTS OF DERMAL EXPOSURE TO LIQUID NERVE AGENTS

Level of Exposure	Effects
Mild	
Effects may be precipitant in onset after an asymptomatic interval of up to 18 hours	Increased sweating at the site Muscular fasciculations at site
Moderate	
Effects may be precipitant in onset after an asymptomatic interval of up to 18 hours	Increased sweating at the site Muscular fasciculations at site Nausea Diarrhea Generalized weakness
Severe	
Effects may be precipitant in onset after a 2–30 minutes asymptomatic interval	Increased sweating at the site Muscular fasciculations at site Nausea Diarrhea Generalized weakness Loss of consciousness Convulsions (seizures) Generalized fasciculations Flaccid paralysis Apnea Generalized secretions Involuntary micturition/defecation possible with seizures

muscular fasciculations; and miosis. One developed flaccid paralysis and apnea a minute or two later. The other received immediate, vigorous treatment, and his condition did not progress.

Dermal Exposure to Liquid

The early effects of a drop of nerve agent on the skin and the time of onset of these effects depend on the amount of nerve agent and several other factors, such as the site on the body, the temperature, and the humidity. After a delay during which the individual is asymptomatic, localized sweating occurs at the site of the droplet. Less commonly, there are localized fasciculations of the underlying muscle (Table 5-5). Unless the amount of the nerve agent is in the lethal range, the next effects (or perhaps the first effects, if the sweating and fasciculations do not occur or are not noticed) are gastrointestinal: nausea, vomiting, diarrhea, or a combination of these symptoms. The casualty may notice generalized sweating and complain of tiredness or otherwise feeling ill. There may be a period of many hours between exposure and the appearance of symptoms and signs. These symptoms and signs may occur even if the casualty has been decontaminated.[48]

After large exposures, the time to onset of effects may be much shorter than for smaller exposures and decreases as the amount of agent increases. For instance, two individuals were decontaminated within minutes of exposure to a drop of nerve agent. There was a 15-minute to 20-minute asymptomatic interval before the precipitant onset of effects: collapse, loss of consciousness, convulsive muscular jerks, fasciculations, respiratory embarrassment, and copious secretions. Within several minutes, the authors observed flaccid paralysis and apnea in both individuals.

The major clinical differences between the inhalational and dermal routes of exposure are the following:

- Miosis and respiratory involvement are almost invariant with inhalational exposure, but may be delayed or even absent in dermal exposure.

- The speed of onset and progression of symptoms will be far faster in inhalational exposure.
- Decontamination of dermal exposure may not occur before agent has penetrated the skin, and consequently patients who are treated for nerve agent symptoms after dermal exposure may subsequently worsen as agent becomes available systemically. This is not likely with inhalational exposure.

Exposure to nerve agent liquid through a wound will likely produce effects intermediately.

EFFECTS ON ORGANS AND ORGAN SYSTEMS

Most of the information on the effects of nerve agents on organ systems in humans is derived from studies done in the post–World War II period, from reports of people exposed to pesticides, or from clinical evaluations of accidental exposures of people who worked in nerve agent research laboratories, manufacturing facilities, or storage areas or depots (Table 5-6). Some organ systems have been studied more intensively than others. For example, there is a plethora of data from animal studies and studies in isolated neuromuscular preparations for the musculoskeletal system, but study results are difficult to apply to a human clinical situation. The two terrorist attacks using sarin in Japan in 1994 and 1995 have provided a fund of new human clinical data, but this data is all uncontrolled. The Japanese terrorist and Iranian battlefield clinical experience is summarized in a later section of this chapter.

The Eye

Nerve agents in the eye may cause miosis, conjunctival injection, pain in or around the eye, and dim or blurred vision (or both). Reflex nausea and vomiting may accompany eye exposure. These effects are usually local, occurring when the eye is in direct contact with nerve agent vapor, aerosol, or liquid, but exposure by other routes (such as on the skin) can also affect the eyes. Because eyes often react late in the course of intoxication in the latter case (exposure on the skin), they cannot be relied on as an early indication of exposure.

Systemic (such as skin or perioral) exposure to a nerve agent might be large enough to produce moderate symptoms (nausea, vomiting) without miosis. In studies[43,44,47] in which VX was placed on the skin, administered intravenously, or given orally, a significant number of subjects experienced nausea, vomiting, sweating, or weakness, but none had miosis. In 47 patients with parathion poisoning, all of the 14 severe cases had miosis, whereas 6 of 11 patients with moderate poisoning and only 5 of 22 patients with mild effects had miosis.[54] On the other hand, a vapor or aerosol exposure might cause miosis without other signs or symptoms and an exposure in one eye will cause miosis in that eye (a local effect because of a mask leak in one eyepiece or similar causes) without

TABLE 5-6

EFFECTS OF NERVE AGENTS IN HUMANS

Organ or System	Effect
Eye	Miosis (unilateral or bilateral), conjunctival injection; pain in or around the eye; complaints of dim or blurred vision
Nose	Rhinorrhea
Mouth	Salivation
Pulmonary tract	Bronchoconstriction and secretions, cough; complaints of tight chest, shortness of breath; wheezing, rales, and/or rhonchi on exam
Gastrointestinal tract	Increase in secretions and motility; nausea, vomiting, diarrhea; complaints of abdominal cramps, pain
Skin and sweat glands	Sweating
Muscular	Fasciculations ("rippling"), local or generalized; twitching of muscle groups, flaccid paralysis; complaints of twitching, weakness
Cardiovascular	Decrease or increase in heart rate; usually increase in blood pressure
Central nervous system	Acute effects of severe exposure: loss of consciousness, convulsion (or seizures after muscular paralysis), depression of respiratory center to produce apnea Acute effects of mild or moderate exposure or lingering effects (days to weeks) of any exposure: forgetfulness, irritability, impaired judgment, decreased comprehension, a feeling of tenseness or uneasiness, depression, insomnia, nightmares, difficulty with expression

affecting the other eye.

If the eye exposure is not associated with inhalation of the nerve agent, there is no good correlation between severity of the miosis and inhibition of RBC-ChE activity. RBC-ChE activity, then, may be relatively normal or may be inhibited by as much as 100% (see Table 5-1), so the severity of the miosis cannot be used as an index of the amount of systemic absorption of agent or amount of exposure. On the other hand, an early study[52] demonstrated a relationship between the C*t* of sarin and pupil size at the time of maximal miosis, and the investigator suggested that the pupil size might be used as an index of the amount of exposure. For the same reason, miosis is the most likely symptom to persist after all systemic effects of nerve agent have resolved.[52]

Unilateral miosis is sometimes seen in workers handling nerve agents or insecticides and usually occurs because of a small leak in the eyepiece of the protective mask. Again, the RBC-ChE may or may not be inhibited (see Table 5-1). The unilateral miosis has no prognostic medical significance; however, there may be problems with judging distances (depth perception). This impairment may cause difficulty in activities such as driving a car or piloting an airplane, which require stereo-visual coordination (the Pulfrich stereo effect).[22]

Miosis may begin within seconds to minutes of the start of exposure; if the concentration of agent vapor or aerosol is low, maximal miosis may not occur until an hour or longer following exposure. The duration varies according to the amount of agent. The pupils may regain their ability to react to normal levels of indoor lighting within several days after exposure, but their ability to dilate maximally in total darkness may not return for as long as 9 weeks (Figure 5-4 and Exhibit 5-3).[20,55]

The effects of nerve agents on vision have been studied for decades.[56] Characteristically, an unprotected individual exposed to nerve agent will have the signs discussed above and may complain of dim vision, blurred vision, or both.

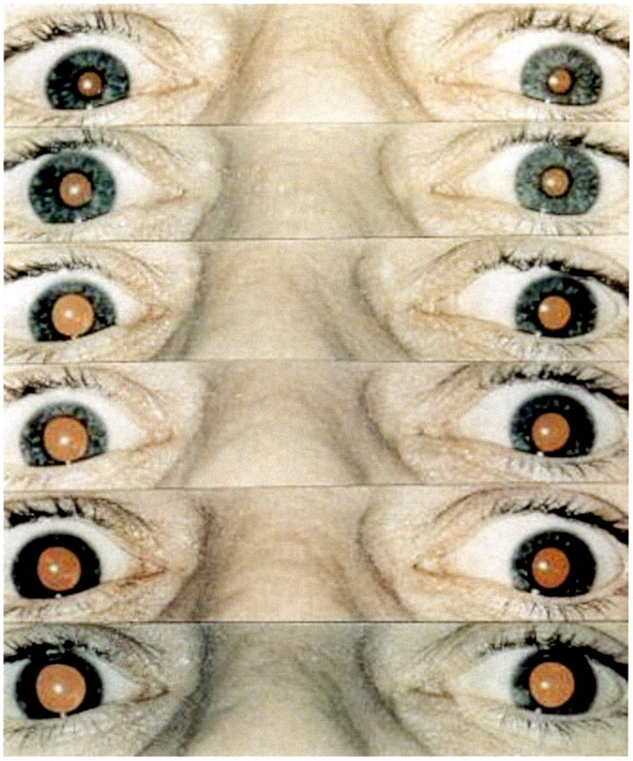

Fig. 5-4. This man was accidentally exposed to an unknown amount of nerve agent vapor. The series of photographs shows his eyes gradually recovering their ability to dilate. All photographs were taken with an electronic flash (which is too fast for the pupil to react) after the subject had been sitting in a totally dark room for 2 minutes. These photographs were taken (from top to bottom) at 3, 6, 13, 20, 41, and 62 days after the exposure. Subsequent photographs indicate that the eyes did not respond fully to darkness for 9 weeks; maximal dilation was reached on day 62 after the exposure.
Reproduced with permission from: Sidell FR. Soman and sarin: clinical manifestations and treatment of accidental poisoning by organophosphates. *Clin Toxicol*. 1974;7:11

Light Reduction

Dim vision is generally believed to be related to the decrease in the amount of light reaching the retina because of miosis. In a study[57] in which miosis was induced in one eye by instillation of sarin, the decrease in visual sensitivity correlated with the reduction in the area of pupillary aperture. Fifty-three subjects accidentally exposed to G agents reported improvements in dim vision before miosis improved, which suggests that factors other than a small pupil are responsible for the high light threshold.[58] In another study,[59] however, no change in visual threshold was measured after miosis was induced by instillation of sarin onto the eye. The light threshold increased after systemic administration of sarin vapor with the eyes protected so that miosis did not occur. The threshold was reduced to normal following systemic administration of atropine sulfate (which enters the CNS), but not after administration of atropine methyl-nitrate (which does not enter the CNS).[60] The authors suggested that the dimness of vision was due to neural mechanisms in the retina or elsewhere in the CNS.

Although the dim vision reported by individuals exposed to nerve agent vapor is generally ascribed to miosis, the above accounts suggest that central neural

EXHIBIT 5-3

CASE REPORT: EXPOSURE OF THREE MEN TO SARIN

Three men [who worked at Edgewood Arsenal, Edgewood, Maryland], ages 27, 50, and 52 years, were brought to the emergency room because of sudden onset of rhinorrhea and slight respiratory discomfort. At the onset of symptoms they were working in a large room in which some containers of sarin were stored. Although there were other workers in the room, the three patients were together at one end where a leak was later found in one of the containers.

On examination all three patients had essentially the same signs and symptoms: very mild respiratory distress, marked miosis and slight eye pain, rhinorrhea, a moderate increase in salivation, and scattered wheezes and rhonchi throughout all lung fields. No other abnormal findings were noted.

All three patients reported that their respiratory distress had decreased since its onset about 20 min before they arrived at the emergency room. The men were kept under observation for the next 6 hr, but no therapy was administered. They continued to improve and at the time of discharge from the ward they were asymptomatic except for a slight irritation in the eyes and decreased vision in dim light.

The patients were seen the next day and at frequent intervals thereafter for a period of four months. Each time they were seen, their [blood cholinesterase activities (both erythrocyte cholinesterase and butyrylcholine esterase)] were measured . . . and photographs were taken of their eyes [see Figure 5-4]. The first photographs were taken the day of the exposure, but the patients were not dark adapted. On each visit thereafter a photograph was taken by electronic flash after the man had been in a completely dark room for 2 min. . . . About 60-70% of the lost ability to dark adapt returned in two weeks, but complete recovery took two months.

Reproduced with permission from: Sidell FR. Soman and sarin: clinical manifestations and treatment of accidental poisoning by organophosphates. *Clin Toxicol.* 1974;7:1–17.

mechanisms may have equal or greater importance. In the case of the carbamate physostigmine, an increase in light sensitivity (a decreased threshold) after intramuscular (IM) administration of the drug has been reported.[61] Carbamates may differ from nerve agents in their effects on vision.

Regardless of its cause, reduction in visual sensitivity impairs those who depend on vision in dim light, individuals who watch a tracking screen, monitor visual displays from a computer, or drive a tank in the evening. Anyone whose vision has been affected by exposure to a nerve agent should not be allowed to drive in dim light or in darkness.

Visual Acuity

Individuals exposed to nerve agents sometimes complain of blurred as well as dim vision. In one study,[62] visual acuity was examined in six subjects before and after exposure to sarin vapor at a *Ct* of 15 mg/min/m^3. Near visual acuity was not changed in any of the subjects after exposure and was worsened after an anticholinergic drug (cyclopentolate) was instilled in the eyes. Far visual acuity was unchanged after sarin exposure in five of the six subjects and was improved in the sixth, who nonetheless complained that distant vision was blurred after sarin.

Two presbyopic workers who were accidentally exposed to sarin had improved visual acuity for days after exposure. As the effects of the agent decreased, their vision returned to its previous state, which took about 35 days.[55] The author suggested, as others have previously, that miosis accounted for the improvement in visual acuity (the pinhole effect).

Eye Pain

Eye pain may accompany miosis, but the reported incidence varies. A sharp pain in the eyeball or an aching pain in or around the eyeball is common. A mild or even severe headache (unilateral if the miosis is unilateral) may occur in the frontal area or throughout the head. This pain is probably caused by ciliary spasm and is worsened by looking at bright light, such as the light from a match a person uses to light a cigarette (the "match test"). Sometimes this discomfort is accompanied by nausea, vomiting, and malaise.

Local instillation of an anticholinergic drug, such as atropine or homatropine, usually brings relief from the pain and systemic effects (including the nausea and vomiting), but because these drugs cause blurring of vision, they should not be used unless the pain is severe.[62]

The Nose

Rhinorrhea is common after both local and systemic nerve agent exposure. It may occur soon after exposure to a small amount of vapor and sometimes precedes miosis and dim vision, or it may occur in the absence of miosis. Even a relatively small exposure to vapor may cause severe rhinorrhea. One exposed worker compared the nasal secretions to the flow from a leaking faucet, and another told the authors that the secretions were much worse than those produced by a cold or hay fever.

Rhinorrhea also occurs as part of an overall, marked increase in secretions from glands (salivary, pulmonary, and gastrointestinal) that follows a severe systemic exposure from liquid on the skin and, under this circumstance, becomes a secondary concern to both the casualty and the medical care provider.

Pulmonary System

The pulmonary effects of nerve agent poisoning are crucial, probably the most important component of the nerve agent poisoning toxidrome. A nerve agent death is almost always a pulmonary death, whether from bronchoconstriction, bronchorrhoea, central apnea, paralysis of the muscles of respiration, or, in most cases, a combination of all of these. Military medics are trained to focus on respiratory status as the most important parameter of the effectiveness of treatment in nerve agent poisoning.

After exposure to a small amount of nerve agent vapor, individuals often complain of a tight chest (difficulty breathing), which is generally attributed to spasm or constriction of the bronchiolar musculature. Secretions from the muscarinically innervated goblet and other secretory cells of the bronchi also contribute to the dyspnea. Exposure to sarin at a *Ct* of 5 to 10 mg/min/m^3 will produce some respiratory discomfort in most individuals, the discomfort and severity increasing as the amount of agent increases.

Several decades ago, investigators attempted to characterize pulmonary impairment caused by exposure to nerve agents by performing pulmonary function studies (such as measurements of vital capacity and maximal breathing capacity) on subjects exposed to small amounts of sarin vapor (the *Ct* values for sarin ranged up to 19.6 mg/min/m^3).[63] Some observers found increases in airway resistance[64] and other changes, while other researchers did not.[65]

Although these studies yielded conflicting results, clinical practitioners have found that the inhalation of nerve agent vapor or aerosol causes dyspnea and pulmonary changes that are usually audible on auscultation. These changes are noticeable after low *Ct* exposures (5–10 mg/min/m^3) and intensify as the *Ct* increases. The pulmonary effects begin within seconds after inhalation. If the amount inhaled is large, the effects of the agent include severe dyspnea and observable signs of difficulty with air exchange, including cyanosis. Clinically, this resembles a severe asthmatic attack.

If the amount of the inhaled agent is small, a casualty may begin to feel better within minutes after moving into an uncontaminated atmosphere, and may feel normal in 15 to 30 minutes. The authors observed that it was not uncommon, for example, for individuals who had not received atropine or other assistance to arrive at the Edgewood Arsenal Toxic Exposure Aid Station about 15 to 20 minutes after exposure and report that their initial, severe trouble in breathing had already decreased markedly. If the exposure was larger, however, relief was likely to come only after therapeutic intervention, such as administration of atropine.

Attempts to aid ventilation in severely poisoned casualties can be greatly impeded by constriction of the bronchiolar musculature and by secretions. One report[66] mentions thick mucoid plugs that hampered attempts at assisted ventilation until the plugs were removed by suction. Atropine may contribute to the formation of this thicker mucus because it dries out the thinner secretions.

A severely poisoned casualty becomes apneic and will die as a result of ventilatory failure, which precedes circulatory system collapse. Three major factors contribute to respiratory failure: obstruction of air passages by bronchoconstriction and by respiratory secretions; weakness followed by flaccid paralysis of the intercostal and diaphragmatic musculature needed for ventilation; and a partial or total cessation of stimulation to the muscles of respiration from the CNS, indicating a defect in central respiratory drive.

Older data on the relative contributions of each of these factors in causing death were summarized in a report[67] describing original studies in nine species. The authors of the report concluded that central respiratory failure appeared to dominate in most species, but its overall importance varied with the species, the agent, and the amount of agent. For example, under the circumstances of the studies, failure of the central respiratory drive appeared to be the major factor in respiratory failure in the monkey, whereas bronchoconstriction appeared early and was severe in the cat. The authors of another report[68] suggest that the presence of anesthesia, which is used in studies of nerve agent intoxication in animals, and its type and depth are also factors in establishing the relative importance of central and peripheral mechanisms.

In another study,[69] bronchoconstriction seen in the dog after IV sarin administration was quite severe compared with that in the monkey. Dogs have thick airway musculature, which may explain that finding. Differences in circulatory and respiratory effects were seen between anesthetized and unanesthetized dogs given sarin.[70] Convulsions and their associated damage were not seen in the anesthetized animals. In this study, there were no significant differences in the cardiovascular and respiratory effects when the agent was given intravenously, percutaneously, or by inhalation. In a study[71] of rabbits poisoned with sarin, bronchoconstriction appeared to be a minor factor, while neuromuscular block (particularly at the diaphragm) and central failure were the primary factors in respiratory failure.

In a review[72] describing studies in anesthetized cats given tabun, sarin, soman, or VX, the loss of central respiratory drive was found to be the predominant cause of respiratory failure with each of the agents, and the contribution of bronchoconstriction was apparently insignificant (in contrast to the severe bronchoconstriction noted in the earlier study[67]). Respiratory failure was the predominant cause of death in the species studied because significant cardiovascular depression occurred only after cessation of respiration.[71,72] When atropine was administered in adequate amounts before the failure of circulation, it reversed the central depression and bronchoconstriction but not the neuromuscular block, a finding that might be expected, because the neuromuscular effects of poisoning with these nerve agents occur at a nicotinic site.[67,71]

In one study,[73] pyridostigmine was administered to primates, which were then exposed to a nerve agent and given the standard therapeutic drugs, atropine and 2-pyridine aldoxime methyl chloride (2-PAM Cl, also called 2-pralidoxime chloride; pyridine-2-aldoxime methyl chloride; 2-formyl-1-methylpyridinium chloride; Protopam chloride, manufactured by Wyeth-Ayerst Laboratories, Philadelphia, Pa). Pyridostigmine does not appear to enter the CNS because it is a quaternary compound and thus would not be expected to protect central sites of respiratory stimulation from the effects of a nerve agent. The pretreated animals continued to breathe, however, in contrast to controls that did not receive pyridostigmine pretreatment but were otherwise treated in the same manner.

The results of this study suggest that pyridostigmine protects against the cessation of respiration. Since pyridostigmine does not appear to enter the CNS, it is suggested that peripheral mechanisms of breathing (skeletal muscles and airways) must predominate in sustaining breathing. Alternatively, the blood–brain barrier may change in the presence of a nerve agent (as with other types of poisoning or hypoxia) to allow the penetration of drugs it otherwise excludes. For example, when 2-PAM Cl, which is also a quaternary compound, is administered to animals poisoned with a ChE inhibitor, it can be found in the animals' central nervous systems, but it is not found in the brains of normal animals after they receive 2-PAM Cl.[74]

Skeletal Musculature

The neuromuscular effects of nerve agents have been the subject of hundreds of studies since nerve agents were first synthesized in 1936. Much of our information on the mechanism of action of nerve agents and potential therapeutic measures has come from these studies. Because this chapter is primarily concerned with clinical effects of nerve agent poisoning, a comprehensive review of these studies is not presented here.

The effects of nerve agent intoxication on skeletal muscle are caused initially by stimulation of muscle fibers, then by stimulation of muscles and muscle groups, and later by fatigue and paralysis of these units. These effects on muscle may be described as fasciculations, twitches or jerks, and fatigue.

Fasciculations are the visible contractions of a small number of fibers innervated by a single motor nerve filament. They are normally painless, and small fasciculations often escape the patient's notice. They appear as ripples under the skin. They can occur as a local effect at the site of a droplet of agent on the skin before enough agent is absorbed to cause systemic effects; the patient is not likely to notice these if the area affected is small. Fasciculations can also appear simultaneously in many muscle groups after a large systemic exposure. A casualty who has sustained a severe exposure will have generalized fasciculations, a characteristic sign of poisoning by a ChE inhibitor. Fasciculations will typically continue long after the patient has regained consciousness and has voluntary muscle activity.

After a severe exposure, there are intense and sudden contractions of large muscle groups, which cause the limbs to flail or become momentarily rigid or the torso to arch rigidly in hyperextension. Whether these movements, which have been described as convulsive jerks, are part of a generalized seizure or originate lower in the nervous system has been a matter of debate. Occasionally, these disturbances may be a local effect on the muscle groups below or near the site of exposure (for instance, the marked trismus and nuchal rigidity in an individual who has pipetted soman into his or her mouth; see Exhibit 5-1).[20] Nerve agents also produce convulsions that are associated with frank epileptiform seizure activity as measured by EEG recordings.[75–77] In cases of severe poisoning, convulsive movements and associated epileptiform seizure activity may stop or become episodic as respiratory status becomes compromised and oxygenation is depressed. It may be impossible to clinically distinguish convulsive activity because of frank central seizures from the purely peripheral neuromuscular symptoms of jerks and tremor.

Central Nervous System and Behavior

Behavioral and psychological changes in humans exposed to ChE-inhibiting substances have been discussed in numerous reports. The incidence of psychological effects is higher in individuals who have had more severe exposures to nerve agents, but they may occur, probably more frequently than is commonly recognized, in individuals who have received a small exposure and have no or minimal physical signs or symptoms. Although the effects may begin as late as 1 day after exposure, they usually start within a few hours and last from several days to several weeks. In the Aum Shinrikyo attacks of 1995, some patients complained of effects lasting longer, even months.[78] Whether these are direct nerve agent effects, posttraumatic stress disorder, or a combination is not known. Common complaints include feelings of uneasiness, tension, and fatigue. Exposed individuals may be forgetful, and observers may note that they are irritable, do not answer simple questions as quickly and precisely as usual, and generally display impaired judgment, poor comprehension, decreased ability to communicate, or occasional mild confusion. Gross mental aberrations, such as complete disorientation or hallucinations, are not part of the symptom complex. Several of the findings on behavioral and psychological changes that occur following exposure to nerve agents or pesticides have recently been summarized.[79,80]

Studies of Behavioral and Psychological Changes

In one of the earliest studies of the effects of ChE-inhibiting substances,[38] behavioral and psychological changes were reported in 49 of 60 subjects (of whom 50 were normal and 10 had myasthenia gravis) after daily IM doses (1.5–3.0 mg) of DFP. Changes were reported about 1 hour after dose administration. The most prominent CNS effects reported were excessive dreaming (33 subjects); insomnia (29 subjects); and jitteriness, restlessness, increased tension, emotional lability, and tremulousness (29 subjects). The authors of the study noted, without comment, that one subject reported visual hallucinations. Hallucinations are not mentioned elsewhere as an effect of ChE inhibitors. Later, similar effects were reported as sequelae of accidental exposure to nerve agent poisoning.[81,82]

One report[66] suggests that several workers accidentally exposed to sarin had some behavioral effects. Another report[72] lists "weakness" (actually tiredness), nervousness, and drowsiness as complaints from 16 of 40 workers accidentally exposed to small amounts of nerve agent vapor.

In a series[58] of 49 workers who were accidentally exposed to sarin or tabun (a total of 53 exposures), 13 workers reported sleep disturbances, 12 reported mood changes, and 10 reported easy fatigability. Overall, 51% had CNS effects. The report authors pointed out that the complex of CNS symptoms may not fully develop until 24 hours after exposure. The data on blood ChE activities (both RBC-ChE and BuChE) in these workers were scanty. The individual with the greatest ChE inhibition, however, had an RBC-ChE activity of 33% of his personal control value, which suggests that the exposures were not severe. No correlation between the presence or severity of symptoms and the degree of ChE inhibition was seen, and most of the effects of exposure disappeared within 3 days. Systemic atropine was not given to any of these individuals, which suggests that therapy is unnecessary if a paucity of physical signs exists. The report authors concluded that mild intoxication by nerve agents may cause psychological disturbances and that these disturbances might have serious consequences to the individuals and to those dependent on their judgment.[58]

In a series[83] of 72 workers exposed to sarin, two reported difficulty in concentration, five reported mental confusion, five reported giddiness, and four reported insomnia. All but two of these individuals were considered to have been exposed to a small amount of sarin; they were given 2 mg of atropine intramuscularly, and 12 others received atropine orally (0.4–0.8 mg). RBC-ChE ranged from less than 9% to more than 100% of the individual's control activity.

Behavioral changes and whole-blood ChE activities were reported in another study[84] in which VX was placed on the skin of volunteers. Since VX preferentially inhibits RBC-ChE and has relatively little effect on BuChE, the decreases in whole-blood ChE activities were assumed to indicate mainly inhibition of RBC-ChE. In subjects with whole-blood ChE activities of 10% to 40% of control (RBC-ChE activities < 20% of control), 30% reported anxiety, 57% had psychomotor depression, 57% had intellectual impairment, and 38% had unusual dreams. Of those with whole-blood ChE activities of 41% to 80% of control (RBC-ChE activities of 20%–40% of control), 8% reported anxiety, 4% had psychomotor depression, 4% had intellectual depression, and 33% had unusual dreams. Nausea and vomiting were the other symptoms noted. Some subjects had both psychological and gastrointestinal effects, with onsets often separated by several hours. Some subjects had symptoms related to only one organ system.

Overall, the onset of signs and symptoms occurred 3.5 to 18 hours after percutaneous exposure, and maximal depression in blood ChE occurred 3 to 8 hours after exposure. But no measurements were taken between 8 and 24 hours, and the maximal inhibition might have been in this period. Often it is overlooked that there may be a long delay between exposure on the skin and onset of signs or symptoms. The study authors stressed that psychological impairment might occur before the onset of other signs or symptoms or might occur in their absence.[84]

Although the frequency, onset, and duration of each reaction were not noted, some of the behavioral effects reported in the VX subjects were fatigue, jitteriness or tension, inability to read with comprehension, difficulties with thinking and expression, forgetfulness, inability to maintain a thought trend, a feeling of being mentally slowed, depression, irritability, listlessness, poor performance on serial 7s (subtracting from 100 by 7s) and other simple arithmetic tests, minor difficulties in orientation, and frightening dreams. Illogical or inappropriate trends in language and thinking were not noted, nor was there evidence of conceptual looseness. The investigators found no evidence of perceptual distortion resulting in delusions or hallucinations.

A severe, accidental exposure to soman caused one person to become depressed, withdrawn, and subdued, have antisocial thoughts, and sleep restlessly with bad dreams for several days immediately after the exposure (see Exhibit 5-1).[20] He received oral doses of scopolamine hydrobromide on 3 of the following 6 days and was given scopolamine methylbromide, which does not enter the CNS, on the other days to mimic the peripheral effects of hydrobromide salt, such as dry mouth. On the hydrobromide days, the subject was more spontaneous and alert, less depressed, and slept better; his performance on a simple arithmetic test also improved. Because scopolamine hydrobromide is more effective in the CNS than the methylbromide salt of scopolamine or atropine, it seemed likely that the drug reversed the CNS effects, at least temporarily. The subject's performance on standard psychological tests 16 days after exposure was below that expected for one of his intellectual capabilities, but it improved to his expected level of functioning when he was tested 4 months later and again 6 months later when he was discharged from further care. The author suggested that the use of scopolamine hydrobromide deserves further evaluation in patients who have these lingering effects while recovering from nerve agent poisoning.

Changes in the ability to perform certain laboratory or field tests after exposure to sarin have been reported. Generally, at the exposures used (C*t*s of 4–14.7 mg/min/m^3), there was some impairment on tasks requiring vision, hand-eye coordination, dexterity, response time, comprehension, and judgment.[85,86] No decrements were found on physical tasks[87] (at a C*t* of 14.7 mg/min/m^3). On a military field exercise,[88] most tasks were performed satisfactorily, if suboptimally, in the daylight. Nighttime performance, however, was difficult, if not hazardous due to a miosis-induced decrement in dark adaptation and subsequent visual acuity.

The behavioral effects of exposure to nerve agents or other potent organophosphorus compounds in humans can be conceptually grouped into three classes: effects on cognitive processes, effects on mood or affect, and disturbances of sleep-wakefulness. This cluster of CNS and behavioral effects of nerve agents is consistent with what is known about the role of ACh and cholinergic neurons within the brain. Central cholinergic circuits are involved in both cognition and short-term memory, as demonstrated by the effects of drugs,[89] experimentally produced lesions,[90] and naturally occurring pathological states of cholinergic insufficiency (such as Alzheimer's disease).[91] It has also been hypothesized for a number of years that depression is due to an imbalance between the cholinergic and adrenergic systems within the brain, and that depressive symptoms are associated with cholinergic hyperactivity.[92–94] Finally, sleep cycle control, specifically the initiation and maintenance of the rapid eye movement (REM) stage of sleep, the sleep stage that is associated with dreaming, is controlled by increased activity of cholinergic neurons within specific nuclei in the pontine brain stem.[95–98] Administration of carbamates, organophosphorus anticholinesterase compounds, or cholinergic agonists that act like nerve agents can induce REM sleep in both animals and humans.[98–102]

Electroencephalographic Effects

Information is scanty on the electroencephalographic (EEG) effects in humans who have been severely poisoned by ChE-inhibiting substances. In an early study,[103] DFP, administered intramuscularly daily, caused EEG changes in 19 of 23 subjects (19 normal, 4 with myasthenia gravis). The changes were

- greater-than-normal variations in potential;
- increased frequency, with increased beta rhythm; and
- more irregularities in rhythm and the intermittent appearance of abnormal waves (high-voltage, slow waves; these were most prominent in the frontal leads).

These changes usually followed the onset of CNS symptoms, they could be correlated with decreases of RBC-ChE activity (but not with BuChE decreases), and they were decreased or reversed by atropine (1.2 mg, IV).

In another study,[104] the EEG of a subject who was severely intoxicated with sarin was recorded after the loss of consciousness but before the onset of convulsions. The recording showed marked slowing of activity, with bursts of high-voltage, 5-Hz waves in the temporofrontal leads. These waves persisted for 6 days despite atropine administration.

In one study[45] in which subjects were exposed to smaller amounts of sarin, the EEG changes coincided with severity of symptoms. With mild symptoms, voltage was slightly diminished. Irregularities in rhythm, variation in potential, and intermittent bursts of abnormal waves (slow, elevated-voltage waves) occurred with moderate symptoms. These changes persisted for 4 to 8 days after the disappearance of symptoms and decreased somewhat (decreases in voltage, in irregular frequency and potential, and in slow waves) after administration of atropine (1 mg, IV).

The effects of various anticholinesterase agents (nerve agents, other organophosphorus compounds, and carbamates) on EEG activity were reviewed and the study authors proposed that a three-stage change is produced in the normal EEG of animals or humans by progressively higher doses of these compounds.[105] At Stage I an activation pattern is produced in the EEG that is characterized by a low amplitude desynchronized pattern of mixed frequencies normally seen in alert subjects. This pattern is induced regardless of the subject's behavioral state when the anticholinesterase is administered, and may last from minutes to several hours, depending upon the dose and the type of compound. This pattern is associated with an approximately 30% to 60% inhibition of RBC-AChE, which is comparable to levels of inhibition associated with minimal to mild signs or symptoms of exposure. This level of ChE inhibition may also be associated with some mild, short-term effect on REM sleep.

The Stage II EEG pattern is marked by a continuation of the activation pattern seen during Stage I, with intrusions of high-voltage, slow-frequency (delta, theta) waves and an increased amount of high frequency (beta) waves. The Stage II pattern is associated with mild to moderate signs or symptoms of intoxication in both human and animal studies. These EEG changes may persist for hours or days, depending upon the severity of the dose, and are associated with approximately 60% to 80% inhibition of RBC-AChE. Such levels of exposure are also expected to produce a moderate increase of REM.

Stage III EEG changes are associated with the most severe levels of exposure and are represented by epileptiform activity in a variety of patterns. This is typically marked by very high-voltage waves, with low-frequency delta waves being most prominent. There are marked signs of agent intoxication, as well as seizure and convulsive activity, that require immediate pharmacological treatment. Animal studies show that all nerve agents are potent convulsant compounds that can elicit prolonged seizure activity that has all the clinical and electrophysiological features of status epilepticus.[76,77,106,107] Seizure activity in human victims of severe nerve agent exposure is typically of limited duration, due to the rapid compromise in respiratory status and associated decrease in oxygenation.

Following such severe exposures, EEG changes may persist for months to years, depending upon the severity of the initial insult and possibly upon the rapidity and effectiveness of pharmacological treatment. Long-term EEG effects show up as isolated spikes, sharp waves, or both during sleep or drowsiness, or with hyperventilation.[46,103,108–110] Such severe EEG and neurobehavioral effects are associated with initial levels of RBC-AChE inhibition greater than 70%. The effects of such severe exposures on REM sleep are prominent and can persist for weeks or months after the exposure. In experimental animal studies, unchecked, nerve-agent–induced seizures can persist over a period of many hours, and can result in brain damage and long-term neurobehavioral changes. Both the brain damage and neurobehavioral effects can be blocked or minimized by rapid treatment with appropriate anticonvulsant medications.[77,111]

Long-Term Effects

Long-term effects on the human CNS after poisoning with nerve agents or organophosphorus insecticides have been reported.[20,79,80,112,113] These reports are based on clinical observations, occasionally supported by psychological studies. In general, the behavioral effects have not been permanent but have lasted weeks to several months, or possibly several years.[114] A distinction needs to be made between these more transient effects that represent reversible neurochemical changes of nerve agents on brain function and those more permanent effects described below.

In the early 1980s, several laboratories reported that animals that survived high-dose exposure to nerve agents developed brain lesions.[115–117] Similar findings had been reported by Canadian researchers in technical reports in the 1960s.[118,119] Further studies confirmed these initial findings and led to several hypotheses as to the cause of these brain lesions. First, some authors suggested that the nerve agents may produce a direct neurotoxic effect on brain neurons.[115,120] Second, the pattern of brain damage seen in these nerve-agent–

exposed animals was similar to that seen after hypoxic encephalopathy. Because nerve-agent–exposed animals exhibit varying durations of respiratory distress, several authors hypothesized that nerve-agent–induced hypoxia was primarily responsible for producing these lesions.[116,118,119] A third hypothesis was that the lesions were the consequence of the prolonged seizures experienced by the animals during the intoxication.[121]

Subsequent work both in vivo[122] and in vitro[123] has failed to demonstrate support for the hypothesis that nerve agents are directly neurotoxic. Likewise, the overwhelming evidence that effective treatment of nerve-agent–induced seizures can block or significantly reduce the extent of brain lesions argues against the direct neurotoxicity hypothesis.[77]

There is conflicting evidence regarding the possible role of hypoxia as an etiologic factor in brain damage following seizure activity, whether nerve agents or other chemoconvulsants cause this seizure activity. Rats given bicuculline convulsed for 2 hours under controlled conditions. Those given a lower percentage of oxygen in their inspired air to keep the partial pressure of arterial oxygen close to 50 mm Hg did not have brain lesions, whereas those with normal air intake and partial pressure of arterial oxygen higher than 128 mm Hg developed brain lesions.[124] Although this evidence does not eliminate the possibility of localized hypoxic areas in the brain as a factor in nerve-agent–induced damage, it does suggest that systemic hypoxia is not a factor. On the other hand, a similar study[125] (hypoxic rats with bicuculline-induced convulsions that lasted 2 h) suggested that there were slightly more brain lesions in the hypoxic animals than in normoxic animals.

The hypothesis that prolonged seizure activity is primarily responsible for nerve-agent–induced brain damage in experimental animals has now become well accepted.[77] Studies in rats have shown that brain damage development requires a minimum duration of continuous seizure activity.[124,125] Seizures terminating before 10 minutes have elapsed resulted in no observable damage. In animals that seized for 20 minutes before seizures were stopped, about 20% experienced mild amounts of damage in restricted foci. In contrast, in animals that experienced 40 minutes of seizure before seizures were stopped, over 80% experienced damage, and this damage was more severe and widespread than the 20-minute-treatment group. Studies in nonhuman primates confirm that delay in seizure control increases subsequent brain pathology.[126,127] Studies with effective drugs that can stop nerve agent seizures (benzodiazepines, anticholinergics, N-methyl-D-aspartate antagonists) by many research groups have overwhelmingly demonstrated that seizure control protects experimental animals (rats, guinea pigs, nonhuman primates) from developing brain damage.[107,128–137]

There are, however, experimental studies that show that convulsion development following nerve agent exposure does not invariably lead to brain damage and, conversely, that some animals that never display convulsions develop brain lesions. All of these studies used observational procedures to determine presence of convulsive/seizure activity following nerve agent exposure. While nonconvulsive/nonseizure-mediated neuropathology may have been observed following exposure to nerve agents, the exact neuropharmacological mechanism(s) that might produce this damage has yet to be described.

In addition to having morphologically detectable brain lesions, animals surviving severe nerve agent intoxication have been shown to have decrements in performance, as measured on a variety of behavioral tests.[136–140] These decrements were apparent in some studies for at least 4 months, when the last survivors were sacrificed. These animals, mostly rats, are reported to display other persistent behavioral changes (hyperresponsiveness, difficulties regulating body weight, spontaneous convulsions) that can also be considered consequences of the brain lesions.

In general, in untreated or inadequately treated nerve-agent–poisoned animals, convulsive (and seizure) activity usually stops shortly after respiration becomes compromised. Some of these animals die while others recover after some degree of apnea, and electrographic seizure activity, as monitored on the EEG, can resume while overt motor convulsions may no longer be apparent. Motor movements (finger twitches, repetitive arm/leg movements, nystagmus) become more subtle, of smaller amplitude, and intermittent. These bear all the same clinical characteristics as described for late-stage status epilepticus in humans.[141] In some of the reported cases of severe nerve agent intoxication in humans,[20,66,104] convulsive activity has also been brief and medical treatment was promptly available to prevent further convulsive episodes. There are several reports, however, from the Aum Shinrikyo terrorist attacks of individuals exhibiting prolonged seizure activity before adequate therapy could be delivered.[110,142] It is not known whether these victims suffered brain damage similar to that described in experimental animals, but two individuals experienced profound retrograde amnesia, one of which still displayed high-amplitude epileptiform waves in the EEG 1 year after the exposure.

Interpreting clinical studies in light of experimental results is difficult largely because the role of hypoxia is very hard to separate from any seizure-mediated nerve agent toxicity on the human brain. Because of respiratory depression, it is possible to attribute much of the reported CNS sequelae in human victims to hypoxic damage.

A major challenge in interpreting the reports of long-lasting neurobehavioral complaints in patients who have survived nerve agent exposure is separating out that part of the syndrome that is clearly psychological, including, in many cases, posttraumatic stress disorders satisfying psychiatric criteria in *The Diagnostic and Statistical Manual of Mental Disorders*, 4th edition, from that which is due to direct toxicity of nerve agent upon the nervous system itself. Some of these reports are summarized below.

Only one case has been reported of peripheral nerve damage after human nerve agent intoxication. In this one case, a victim of the Tokyo Aum Shinrikyo attack developed distal sensory axonopathy months after his exposure. Causality could not be established.[143]

Cardiovascular System

Little data exists on the cardiovascular effects of nerve agents in humans. In mild-to-moderate intoxication from nerve agents, blood pressure may be elevated, presumably because of cholinergic stimulation of ganglia or other factors, such as stress reaction.

Arrhythmias

After nerve agent exposure, the heart rate may decrease and the authors have observed that some atrial-ventricular (A-V) heart block (first-, second-, or third-degree) with bradycardia may occur because of the stimulation of the A-V node by the vagus nerve. In some cases an increase in heart rate may occur because of stress, fright, or some degree of hypoxia. Because treatment initiation is urgent in severely intoxicated patients, electrocardiograms (ECGs) have not been performed before atropine administration. However, if possible, an ECG should be done before drugs are given if the procedure will not delay therapy. In normal subjects, atropine may cause a transient A-V dissociation before the onset of bradycardia (which precedes tachycardia), and ChE-inhibiting substances may cause bradycardia and A-V block. For reasons noted above, these transient rhythm abnormalities have not been recorded in patients with nerve agent intoxication. These rhythm disturbances are probably not clinically important.

Reports of patients exposed to pesticides and the results of animal studies provide additional information about cardiovascular reactions to nerve agents. In one study,[144] dogs exposed to lethal amounts of sarin vapor had idioventricular rhythms within minutes after exposure; following atropine therapy, some of the dogs had third- degree and first-degree heart blocks before a normal rhythm returned. In another study,[145] conscious dogs had few cardiac rhythm changes after sublethal doses (0.25–0.5 LD_{50}, administered subcutaneously) of VX. Four of five anesthetized dogs receiving a 1-LD_{50} dose had arrhythmias, including first-degree heart block and premature ventricular complexes; one had torsade de pointes (a type of ventricular tachycardia). Cardiac arrhythmias are not uncommon in humans after organophosphorous pesticide poisoning.[146]

Dogs were instrumented to examine the cardiac changes occurring for a month after IV administration of 2 LD_{50} of soman.[147] Atropine and diazepam were administered shortly after soman exposure to control seizure activity. During the study period, there was increased frequency of episodes of bradycardia with ventricular escape, second-degree and third-degree heart block, and independent ventricular activity (single premature beats, bigeminy, or runs of ventricular tachycardia).

In a similar study,[148] rhesus monkeys were given the standard military regimen of pyridostigmine before exposure to soman (1 LD_{50}, IM), and atropine and 2-PAM Cl after the agent. The monkeys were monitored continuously for 4 weeks. Except for the period immediately after agent administration, the incidence of arrhythmias was the same as or less than that observed during a 2-week baseline period.

Torsade de pointes has been reported after nerve agent poisoning in animals[145] and after organophosphorus pesticide poisoning in humans.[149] Torsade de pointes is a ventricular arrhythmia, usually rapid, of multifocal origin, which on ECG resembles a pattern midway between ventricular tachycardia and fibrillation. It is generally preceded by a prolongation of the QT interval, it starts and stops suddenly, and it is refractory to commonly used therapy. It was first described as a clinical entity in the late 1960s; undoubtedly it was seen but called by another name in experimental studies with nerve agents before then. Recent studies have shown that sarin-exposed rats display pronounced QT segment prolongation for several weeks after near-lethal exposures, and that these animals showed an increased sensitivity to epinephrine-induced arrhythmias for at least 6 months after exposure.[150]

In addition to the arrhythmias described above, studies have shown that animals (rats, nonhuman primates) severely poisoned with nerve agents can develop frank cardiac lesions.[125,131,151–154] The early stage (15 minutes–several hours) of these lesions consists of hypercontraction and hyperextension of sarcomeres, focal myocytolysis, and the development of contraction bands that are the result of the breakdown of markedly hypercontracted myofibril bundles. This is followed by an inflammatory response (24 hours or less), which begins with edema and neutrophil infiltration and ends with mononuclear cell infiltration and scavenging of necrotic sarcoplasm by macrophages. This is followed by a stage of repair (72 hours or less), which begins with a proliferation of fibroblasts and ends with myofiber loss and replacement fibrosis. Some studies have shown a relationship between the development of seizures following nerve agent exposure and the occurrence and severity of cardiac lesions.[131]

Ventricular fibrillation, a potentially fatal arrhythmia, has been seen after administration of a ChE inhibitor and atropine. It can be precipitated by the IV administration of atropine to an animal that has been rendered hypoxic by administration of a ChE inhibitor.[155,156] Although this complication has not been reported in humans, atropine should not be given intravenously until the hypoxia has been at least partially corrected.

Because of the well-recognized possibility that ventricular fibrillation can occur in a hypoxic heart given atropine, many intensive care unit physicians and nurses are reluctant to give the large amounts of atropine that may be required to treat acute nerve agent poisoning. The authors have observed that this issue has come up in several training exercises. Although data are fragmentary, the literature suggests that the chance of death from acute nerve agent poisoning is greater than the chance of ventricular fibrillation from atropine on a hypoxic heart, at least in initial field management. Once the patient has reached a hospital setting where proper monitoring is possible, it should be less problematic to administer atropine safely in the amounts required while giving oxygen as necessary.

Heart Rate

Although it is frequently stated that a patient intoxicated with a nerve agent will have bradycardia, this is not proven by clinical data. In a review of the records of 199 patients seen at the Edgewood Arsenal Toxic Exposure Aid Station for mild-to-moderate nerve agent exposure (one or more definite signs or symptoms of nerve agent intoxication, such as miosis or a combination of miosis with dim vision or a tight chest), 13 presented with heart rates less than 64 beats per minute. There were 13 patients with heart rates of 64 to 69 beats per minute, 63 with heart rates of 70 to 80 beats per minute, 41 with heart rates of 81 to 89 beats per minute, 38 with heart rates of 90 to 99 beats per minute, and 31 with heart rates higher than 100 beats per minute. A heart rate of 64 to 80 beats per minute is considered normal in adults.[157] Thus, 13 patients (6.5%) had low heart rates, and 110 patients (55%) had high heart rates (69 of these patients [35%] had heart rates > 90 beats per min).

Reports of the heart rates of patients severely intoxicated by insecticides vary. In a report[158] describing 10 patients (9 of whose consciousness was moderately-to-severely impaired), 7 presented with heart rates over 100 beats per minute, and the other 3 had heart rates over 90 beats per minute (5 had a systolic blood pressure of 140 mm Hg or higher, a diastolic blood pressure of 90 mm Hg or higher, or both). In another report,[159] the heart rates of three unconscious patients were slow (one had cardiac arrest). Two acutely ill, unconscious patients were described in a comprehensive review of organophosphorus poisoning[54]; one had a heart rate of 108 beats per minute, the other 80 beats per minute. The authors of the study pointed out that cardiovascular function is usually maintained until the terminal stage and that blood pressure and heart rate increase in the acute stage but may decline later. Heart rate was not listed in their tabulation of signs and symptoms.

GENERAL TREATMENT PRINCIPLES

The principles of treatment of nerve agent poisoning are the same as they are for any toxic substance exposure: namely, terminate the exposure; establish or maintain ventilation; administer an antidote if one is available; and correct cardiovascular abnormalities. Most importantly, medical care providers or rescuers must protect themselves from contamination. If the caregiver becomes contaminated, there will be one more casualty and one fewer rescuer. Protection of the rescuer can be achieved by physical means, such as masks, gloves, and aprons, or by ensuring that the casualty has been thoroughly decontaminated. The importance of casualty decontamination should be obvious, but it is often forgotten or overlooked.

This section discusses the general principles of treating nerve agent poisoning. The specific treatment of casualties in the six exposure categories (suspected, minimal, mild, moderate, moderately severe, and severe) is addressed in the next section.

Terminating the Exposure

The first and perhaps most important aspect of treating acute nerve agent poisoning is decontaminating the patient. Decontamination is performed to prevent the casualty from further absorbing the agent or to keep the agent from spreading further on the casualty or to others, including medical personnel, who may come into contact with the casualty.

Ventilatory Support

Ventilatory support is a necessary aspect of therapy to save a casualty with severe respiratory compromise. Antidotes alone may be effective in restoring ventilation and saving lives in some instances. In animal studies,[160,161] antidotes alone, given intramuscularly at the onset of signs, were adequate to reverse the effects of agent doses of about 3 times LD_{50}, but their effectiveness was greatly increased with the addition of ventilation. Pyridostigmine, given as pretreatment and followed by the current therapy after challenges with higher amounts of two agents, appears to prevent apnea.

Breathing impairment is an early effect of exposure to nerve agent vapor or aerosol. When the exposure is small, the casualty may have mild to severe dyspnea, with corresponding physical findings, and the impairment will be reversed by the administration of atropine. If the distress is severe and the casualty is elderly or has pulmonary or cardiac disease, the antidote may be supplemented by providing oxygen by inhalation. In most other circumstances, supplementation with oxygen is unnecessary.

Severely exposed casualties lose consciousness shortly after the onset of effects, usually before any signs of respiratory compromise. They have generalized muscular twitching or convulsive jerks and may initially have spontaneous but impaired respiration. In a severely poisoned person, breathing ceases completely within several minutes after the onset of exposure.

Assisted ventilation may be required to supplement gasping and infrequent attempts at respiration, or it may be required because spontaneous breathing has stopped. In addition to a decrease in central respiratory drive, weakness or paralysis of thoracic and diaphragmatic muscles, and bronchospasm or constriction, there are copious secretions throughout the airways. These secretions tend to be thick, mucoid, and "ropy," and may plug up the airways. Postural drainage can be used, and frequent and thorough suctioning of the airways is necessary if ventilation is to be successful. In one instance, efforts to ventilate a severely apneic casualty were markedly hindered for 30 minutes until adequate suction was applied to remove thick mucoid plugs.[66]

Initially, because of the constriction or spasm of the bronchial musculature, there is marked resistance to attempts to ventilate. Pressures of 50 to 70 cm H_2O or greater may be needed. After the administration of atropine, resistance decreases to 40 cm H2O or lower, and the secretions diminish (although they may thicken), creating less obstruction to ventilatory efforts. Thus, in the unlikely but conceivable situation that a lone first responder must treat a severely poisoned casualty whose heart is still beating, IM atropine should be administered first (because it only takes a few seconds) before attempting to intubate and resuscitate the patient.

There are numerous mechanical devices, including sophisticated ventilators, that can be used to provide ventilatory assistance in an apneic casualty. None of these is available to the soldier, and only a few—the mask-valve-bag ventilation device, the RDIC (resuscitation device, individual, chemical), and a simple ventilator—are available at the battalion aid station. Whatever device is used, it must be able to overcome the initial high resistance in the airways. If a casualty is apneic or has severe respiratory compromise and needs assisted ventilation, then endotracheal intubation, which will enable better ventilation and suction of secretions, should be attempted.

Mouth-to-mouth ventilation might be considered by a soldier who wants to assist an apneic buddy when no aid station is nearby. A major drawback to this is the likelihood of contamination. Before even considering this method, the rescuer should be sure that there is no vapor hazard, which is not always possible, and that there is no liquid contamination on the individual to be ventilated. The expired breath of the casualty is a smaller hazard. Studies[162–164] involving sarin have shown that only 10% or less of inspired nerve agent is expired, and that the toxicant is expired immediately after inspiration of the agent.

When managing a mass casualty incident, planners need to understand that the period of time that ventilatory support will be necessary in nerve agent casualties is much shorter than that required for severe organophosphate insecticide poisoning. This is because organophosphate insecticides tend to be more fat-soluble than nerve agents, disappear into the fat stores, and off-gas, causing symptoms, for days. Despite the greater toxicity of nerve agents, ventilatory support should only be required for hours at most. Nerve agents also differ greatly in this respect from both pulmonary oedemagenic agents, such as chlorine and phosgene, and from sulfur mustard. Casualties of both of these types of agents may require ventilatory support for days to weeks.

In the Aum Shinrikyo subway attack in Tokyo, only four of 640 patients seen at Saint Luke's International Hospital for definite or suspected sarin poisoning required intubation for ventilatory support. Of the four patients, one died with severe hypoxic encephalopathy on hospital day 28, and was intubated throughout the course. Of the remaining three patients, representing the most severe cases who survived, intubation was required only for 24 hours or less. This shows that mechanical ventilation in essentially all cases who survive sarin poisoning is a short-term clinical concern.[165]

In summary, spontaneous respiration will stop within several minutes after onset of effects caused by exposure to a lethal amount of nerve agent. Antidotes alone are relatively ineffective in restoring spontaneous respiration. Attempts at ventilation are hindered by the high resistance of constricted bronchiolar muscles and by copious secretions, which may be thick and plug the bronchi. Ventilatory assistance may be required briefly (20–30 min) or for a much longer period. In several instances, assistance was required for 3 hours[20,66]; this seems to be the longest reported use of ventilation.

Atropine Therapy

The antagonism between the ChE-inhibiting substance physostigmine and a cholinergic blocking substance has been recognized for well over a century.[166] In the early 1950s, atropine was found to reduce the severity of effects from ChE-inhibitor poisoning, but it did not prevent deaths in animals exposed to synthetic ChE-inhibiting insecticides.[167]

Cholinergic blocking substances act by blocking the effects of excess ACh at muscarinic receptors. ACh accumulates at these receptors because it is not hydrolyzed by ChE when the enzyme is inactivated by an inhibitor. Thus, cholinergic blocking substances do not block the direct effect of the agent (ChE inhibition); rather, they block the effect of the resulting excess ACh.

Many cholinergic blocking substances have been tested for antidotal activity. Among the findings are the following:

- Almost any compound with muscarinic cholinergic blocking activity has antidotal activity.
- Atropine and related substances reduce the effects of the ChE inhibitors, primarily in those tissues with muscarinic receptor sites.
- Antidotal substances with higher lipoid solubility, which penetrate the CNS more readily, might be expected to have greater antidotal activity, since some of the more severe effects of ChE inhibitor poisoning (such as apnea and seizures) are mediated in the CNS.

Several countries use, or have proposed to use, other anticholinergic drugs as adjuncts to atropine for treating nerve agent poisoning. These anticholinergics have much more potent and rapid effects on the CNS than does atropine. For example, Israel uses a mixture of drugs known as TAB as their immediate nerve agent treatment. This mixture contains the oxime TMB-4, atropine, and the synthetic anticholinergic benactyzine. From 1975–1980 the US military also used TAB. The atropine and benactyzine combination in the TAB mixture is similar in composition to the atropine, benactyzine and 2-PAM combination antidote mixtures investigated by Yugoslav researchers in the early 1970s.[168,169] Animal studies have shown that benactyzine is much more potent and acts more rapidly to reverse the CNS effects of nerve agent intoxication than does atropine.[170,171] In addition, benactyzine is significantly less potent in inhibiting sweating or producing mydriasis than atropine, and is therefore less likely to induce heat casualties in a warm environment or compromise near vision in the case of accidental use. Military researchers in the Czech Republic have advocated the use of the synthetic anticholinergics benactyzine and trihexyphenidyl, along with the carbamate pyridostigmine, in a prophylactic mixture they have designated as PANPAL.[172] In addition, the Czechs utilize benactyzine and biperiden, as well as atropine, as postexposure antidotal treatments.[172,173]

While many countries have other anticholinergic drugs to use as adjuncts to atropine to treat nerve agent poisoning, none of these compounds have been tested or used in human clinical cases of poisoning either with nerve agents or other organophosphate or carbamate pesticides.

Nevertheless, atropine has been the antidote of choice for treating nerve agent intoxication since nerve agents were first discovered and produced during World War II. It was included in the German nerve agent first aid kits[174] and was determined to be an effective antidote by British scientists at Porton Down who first analyzed the pharmacology and toxicology of tabun obtained from captured German artillery shells. Since the 1940s, atropine has been adopted as the first-line antidote to counteract nerve agent poisoning by the armed forces of most countries. It is also almost universally used as the antidote to treat anticholinesterase poisoning by organophosphate or carbamate pesticides.[175,176]

A dose of 2 mg atropine was chosen for self -administration or buddy-administration (the AtroPen automatic injector included in the Mark I (Meridian Medical Technologies Inc, Bristol, Tenn) kit contains 2 mg; Figure 5-5) by the US and the military of several other countries because it reverses the effects of nerve agents, the associated side effects of a dose this size can be tolerated, and reasonably normal performance

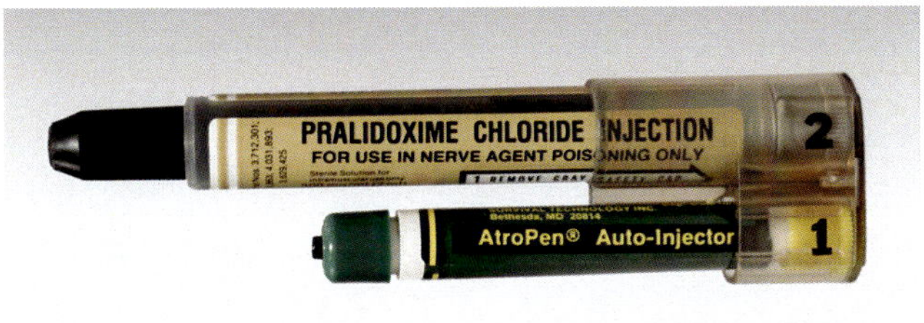

Fig. 5-5. The Mark I kit with its two autoinjectors: the AtroPen containing 2 mg atropine, labeled 1—indicating it is to be injected first—and the ComboPen containing 600 mg 2-pyridine aldoxime methyl chloride (2-PAM Cl), labeled 2—indicating it is to be injected second. The plastic clip keeps both injectors together and serves as a safety for both devices. The kit is kept in a soft black foam holder that is carried in the gas mask carrier.
Reproduced with permission from: Meridian Medical Technologies Inc, Bristol, Tenn.

can be maintained by the individual receiving it. The rationale for this choice of dose was expressed in the unclassified portion of a classified document as follows:

> The dose of atropine which the individual serviceman can be allowed to use must be a compromise between the dose which is therapeutically desirable and that which can be safely administered to a nonintoxicated person. Laboratory trials have shown that 2 mg of atropine sulfate is a reasonable amount to be recommended for injection by an individual and that higher doses may produce embarrassing effects on troops with operational responsibilities.

When given to a normal individual (one without nerve agent intoxication), a dose of 2 mg of atropine will cause an increase in heart rate of about 35 beats per minute (which is not usually noticed by the recipient), a dry mouth, dry skin, mydriasis, and some paralysis of accommodation. Most of these effects will dissipate in 4 to 6 hours, but near vision may be blurred for 24 hours, even in healthy young patients. The decrease in sweating caused by 2 mg of atropine is a major, potentially harmful side effect that may cause some people who work in heat to become casualties. For example, when 35 soldiers were given 2 mg of atropine and asked to walk for 115 minutes at 3.3 mph at a temperature of about 83°F (71°F wet bulb), more than half dropped out because of illness or were removed from the walk because of body temperature of 103.5°F or above. On another day, without atropine, they all successfully completed the same march.[177]

The 6 mg of atropine contained in the three injectors given each soldier may cause mild mental aberrations (such as drowsiness or forgetfulness) in some individuals if administered in the absence of nerve agent intoxication. Atropine given intravenously to healthy young people causes a maximal increase in the heart rate in 3 to 5 minutes, but other effects (such as drying of the mouth and change in pupil size) appear later. In one study,[178] when atropine was administered with the AtroPen, the greatest degree of bradycardia occurred at 2.5 minutes (compared with 4.3 min when administered by standard needle-and-syringe injection); a heart rate increase of 10 beats per minute occurred at 7.9 minutes (versus 14.7 min with needle-and-syringe injection); and maximal tachycardia (an increase of 47 beats per min) occurred at 34.4 minutes (compared with an increase of 36.6 beats per min at 40.7 min with needle-and-syringe injection).

Thus, the autoinjector is more convenient to use than the needle and syringe, and it results in more rapid absorption of the drug. Needle-and-syringe delivery produces a "glob" or puddle of liquid in muscle. The AtroPen, on the other hand, sprays the liquid throughout the muscle as the needle goes in. The greater dispersion of the AtroPen deposit results in more rapid absorption. It has not been determined whether the onset of beneficial effects in treating nerve agent intoxication corresponds to the onset of bradycardia, the onset of tachycardia, or to other factors.

The FDA has recently approved a combined-dose autoinjector including both atropine and 2-PAM Cl. Bioequivalence was demonstrated in animal studies. The dose of atropine in the new product, designated by the Department of Defense as the antidote treatment nerve agent autoinjector (ATNAA), is 2.1 mg (Figure 5-6). At the time of writing, this product awaits a production contract with an FDA-approved manufacturer; it is anticipated that the ATNAA will replace the older MARK 1 kit by approximately 2008. Its tactical value

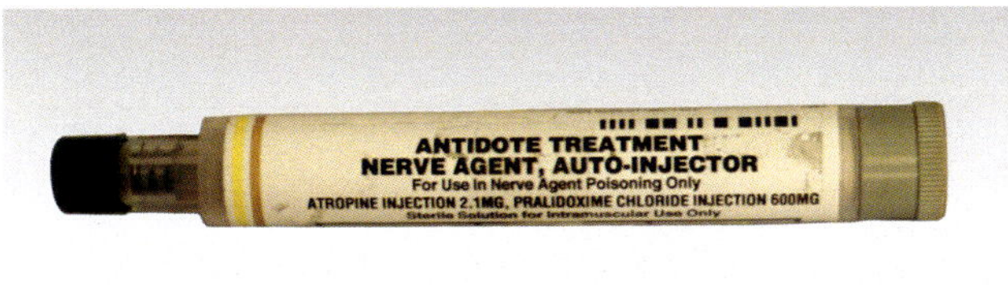

Fig. 5-6. The antidote treatment nerve agent autoinjector (ATNAA) delivers 2.1 mg atropine and 600 mg 2-pyridine aldoxime methyl chloride (2-PAM Cl). The medications are in separate compartments within the device and are expressed out of a single needle. The gray cap on the right end of the injector is the safety.
Reproduced with permission from: Meridian Medical Technologies Inc, Bristol, Tenn.

lies in halving the time to administer the two antidotes compared to the MARK 1 kit.

When administered in an adequate amount, atropine reverses the effects of the nerve agent in tissues that have muscarinic receptor sites. It decreases secretions and reverses the spasm or contraction of smooth muscle. The mouth dries, secretions in the mouth and bronchi dry, bronchoconstriction decreases, and gastrointestinal musculature become less hyperactive. However, unless given in very large doses, IV or IM atropine does not reverse miosis caused by nerve agent vapor in the eyes. A casualty with miosis alone should not be given atropine, and pupil size should not be used to judge the adequacy of atropine dosage.

The amount of atropine to administer is a matter of judgment. In a conscious casualty with mild-to-moderate effects who is not in severe distress, 2 mg of atropine should be given intramuscularly at 5-minute to 10-minute intervals until dyspnea and secretions are minimized. Usually no more than a total dose of 2 to 4 mg is needed. In an unconscious casualty, atropine should be given until secretions are minimized (those in the mouth can be seen and those in the lungs can be heard by auscultation), and until resistance to ventilatory efforts is minimized (atropine decreases constriction of the bronchial musculature and airway secretions). If the casualties are conscious, they will report less dyspnea, and if assisted ventilation is underway, a decrease in airway resistance will be noted. Secretions alone should not be the reason for administering more atropine if the secretions are diminishing and are not clinically significant. Mucus blocking the smaller airways may remain a hindrance, despite adequate amounts of atropine. In severe casualties (unconscious and apneic), 5 to 15 mg of atropine has been used before spontaneous respiration resumed and the casualty regained consciousness 30 minutes to 3 hours after exposure.[20,66] The authors have observed several recovering casualties without non-life-threatening, adverse effects (such as nausea and vomiting) 24 to 36 hours after exposure for which atropine was administered.[20] However, there appears to be no reason to give atropine routinely in this period.

In the only battlefield data that have been published, Syed Abbas Foroutan reported using atropine much more aggressively and in larger amounts.[12] After an initial IV test dose of 4 mg atropine, he waited 1 to 2 minutes. If there was no sign of atropinization, he gave another 5 mg IV over 5 minutes while checking the pulse. He titrated his dose to pulse rate, accelerating if the heart rate dropped to 60 beats per minute to 70 beats per minute and decreasing it for pulse rates over 110 beats per minute. This resulted in doses of atropine, in some cases, up to 150 mg IV in 5 minutes. US doctrine, by contrast, uses a 6-mg IM loading dose followed by 2-mg increments until IV access is established. Foroutan's protocol may reflect the pressure of having large numbers of casualties to treat, the relative lack of availability of oximes, particularly far forward, and his inability to guarantee that atropine could be continually administered during evacuation to the next echelon of medical care.

In contrast with nerve agent treatment, much larger amounts of atropine (500–1,000 mg) have been required in the initial 24 hours of treatment of individuals severely poisoned by organophosphorus pesticides.[179–181] Medical care providers must recognize that the amount of atropine needed for treating insecticide poisoning is different than the amount needed for treating nerve agent poisoning. Pesticides may be sequestered in the body because of greater fat solubility or metabolized at a slower rate than nerve agents. Whatever the reason, they continue to cause acute cholinergic crises for a much longer period (days to weeks). This point is crucial in training personnel who are used to seeing insecticide poisonings to manage nerve agent casualties. Insecticide casualties may require intensive care unit beds for days; nerve agent casualties almost never do and are usually either dead or well enough to require minimal medication within 24 hours.

There has recently been increased discussion about the endpoints of atropinization and the most efficient means to achieve it. The textbook recommendations for early atropinization from various authors have been assessed using model data of atropine dose requirements in patients severely poisoned with organophosphate pesticides.[175] These authors concluded that a dose-doubling strategy, continued doubling of successive doses, would be the most rapid and efficient way to achieve atropinization. Likewise, the treatment regimen used by Foroutan[12] would also result in a rapid atropinization. The endpoints of atropinization recommended by Army Field Manual 8-285, *Treatment of Chemical Agent Casualties*,[182] the *Medical Management of Chemical Agent Casualties Handbook*,[183] Foroutan,[12] and Eddleston et al[175] are very similar: lack of bronchoconstriction, ease of respiration, drying of respiratory secretions, and a heart rate > 80 to 90 beats per minute.

The goal of therapy with atropine should be to minimize the effects of the agent (ie, to remove casualties from life-threatening situations and make them comfortable), which may not require complete reversal of all of the effects (such as miosis). However, in a casualty with severe effects, it is better to administer too much atropine than too little. Too much atropine does far less harm than too much unantagonized nerve agent in a casualty suffering severe effects. However, a moderately dyspneic casualty given atropine 2 mg, administered intramuscularly, will report improvement within 5 minutes. A caregiver should resist the temptation to give too much atropine to a walking, talking casualty with dyspnea. In general, the correct dose of atropine for an individual exposed to a nerve agent is determined by the casualty's signs and symptoms, the route of exposure (vapor or liquid), and the amount of time elapsed since exposure.

Atropine Therapy after Inhalational Exposure to Vapor

After vapor exposure, the effects of nerve agents appear very quickly and reach their maximum activity within seconds or minutes after the casualty is removed from or protected against the vapor. In what were apparently high concentrations of nerve agent vapor, two individuals collapsed (one at Edgewood Arsenal, Maryland, in 1969 and one at Dugway Proving Ground, Utah, in 1952), unconscious, almost immediately after taking one or two breaths, and 4 to 5 minutes later they were flaccid and apneic.[20,66] Even at very low concentrations, maximal effects occur within minutes of exposure termination. Because effects develop so rapidly, antidotal therapy should be more vigorous for a casualty seen during or immediately after exposure than for a casualty seen 15 to 30 minutes later. For example, if a soldier's buddy in the field or a coworker in a laboratory suddenly complains of dim vision in an environment suspected of containing nerve agent vapor, the buddy or worker should immediately administer the contents of one Mark I antidote kit or ATNAA. There may be continuing exposure before the casualty can exit the environment or don a mask, or the effects from the exposure already absorbed may continue to develop for several minutes. On the other hand, if the casualty is seen at the medical aid station (installation or field) 15 to 30 minutes after the vapor exposure has terminated, an antidote is not needed if miosis is the only sign (atropine given intramuscularly has very little effect on miosis). Effects caused by nerve agent vapor will not progress after this time.

If a casualty is seen immediately after exposure from vapor only, the contents of one Mark I kit or ATNAA should be given if miosis is the only sign, the contents of two kits or injectors should be administered immediately if there is any dyspnea, and the contents of three kits should be given for severe dyspnea or any more severe signs or symptoms. When seen 15 to 30 minutes after an exposure to vapor alone, the casualty should receive no antidote if miosis is the only sign, the contents of one Mark I kit or ATNAA for mild or moderate dyspnea, the contents of two kits or injectors for severe dyspnea (obvious gasping), and the contents of three kits or injectors and diazepam (with additional atropine, but no more oxime) if there are more serious signs (such as collapse or loss of consciousness). If dyspnea is the most severe symptom, relief should begin within 5 minutes, and the drugs should not be repeated until this interval has passed. The aggressive therapy given immediately after the onset of effects is not for those early effects per se (eg, atropine is relatively ineffective against miosis), but is in anticipation of more severe effects within the following minutes.

Atropine Therapy after Dermal Exposure to Liquid

The therapy for an individual whose skin has been exposed to nerve agent is less clear. The onset of effects is rarely immediate; they may begin within minutes of exposure or as long as 18 hours later. Generally, the greater the exposure, the sooner the onset; and the longer the interval between exposure and onset of effects, the less severe the eventual effects will be. Effects can begin hours after thorough decontamination; the time of onset may be related to the duration of time the agent was in contact with the skin before decontamination.

The problem with treating dermal exposure is not so much how to treat a symptomatic casualty as it is deciding to treat an asymptomatic person who has had agent on the skin. Medical personnel usually have little or no information about the exposure incident, because the casualty often does not know the duration or amount of exposure.

Unlike, for example, lewisite exposure, nerve agent does not irritate the skin. The first effects of agent on the skin are localized sweating and fasciculations of underlying musculature (rippling), which usually are not observed. If these effects are noted, however, the casualty should immediately self-administer or be given the contents of one Mark I kit or ATNAA. These signs indicate that the chemical agent has penetrated the skin layers.

In general, an asymptomatic person who has had skin contact with a nerve agent should be kept under medical observation because effects may begin precipitately hours later. Caregivers should not administer the contents of a Mark I kit or ATNAA to an asymptomatic person, but should wait for evidence of agent absorption. However, if an individual is seen minutes after a definite exposure to a large amount of nerve agent on the skin ("large" is relative; the LD_{50} for skin exposure to VX is only 6–10 mg, which is equivalent to a single drop 2–3 mm in diameter), there may be some benefit in administering antidotes before the onset of effects. When the occurrence of exposure is uncertain, the possible benefits of treatment must be weighed against the side effects of antidotes in an unpoisoned individual.

Antidotes should be administered until ventilation is adequate and secretions are minimal. In a mildly to moderately symptomatic individual complaining of dyspnea, relief is usually obtained with 2 or 4 mg of atropine (the amount of atropine in one or two Mark I kits or ATNAA). In a severely exposed person who is unconscious and apneic or nearly apneic, at least 6 mg of atropine (the amount in three Mark I kits or ATNAA), and probably more, should be administered initially, and ventilatory support should be started. Atropine should be continued at appropriate intervals until the casualty is breathing adequately with a minimal amount of secretions in the mouth and lungs. The initial 2 or 4 mg has proven adequate in conscious casualties. Although 6 to 15 mg has been required in apneic or nearly apneic casualties, the need for continuing atropine has not extended beyond 2 to 3 hours (although distressing but not life-threatening effects, such as nausea and vomiting, have necessitated administering additional atropine in the following 6–36 h). This is in contrast to the use of atropine to treat intoxication by organophosphorus insecticides, which may cause cholinergic crises (such as an increase in secretion and bronchospasm) for days to weeks after the initial insult.[179–181]

The US military developed an inhaled form of atropine, called "medical aerosolized nerve agent antidote (MANAA)," which was approved by the FDA in 1990. It is not widely used but is still available in the national stockpile. The official doctrine for its use is as follows:

> MANAA is used mainly in medical treatment facilities by the individual casualty under medical supervision for symptomatic relief of nerve agent-induced secretions and muscle twitches. It is intended for use after the casualty has been decontaminated and evacuated to a clean environment where there is no need for MOPP, including the mask. The MANAA allows the patient to self-medicate on an "as needed" basis.[184]

MANAA has a limited role in patients recovering from nerve agent poisoning who still require some observation but who can self-medicate. It has not been stockpiled to any great extent in the civilian sector.

In hospital management of both vapor and liquid casualties, and, in many cases, in management en route to a hospital, such as in an ambulance, the preferred route of administration of atropine will be intravenous after the initial IM field doses. The clinical endpoint, that of patients breathing comfortably on their own without the complication of respiratory secretions, will be the same. A longer period of IV atropine administration should be expected in patients exposed through the skin than in vapor-exposed patients.

The management of patients exposed to nerve agent through open wounds will probably fall between that of vapor-exposed casualties and casualties exposed to nerve agent liquid on intact skin.

Oxime Therapy

Oximes are nucleophilic substances that reactivate the organophosphate-inhibited ChE (the phosphonylated enzyme) by removing the phosphyl moiety. Oximes may be considered a more physiologic method of treating nerve agent poisoning than atropine because they restore normal ChE enzyme function. However, several features limit their utility.

Mechanism of Action

After the organophosphorus compound attaches to the enzyme to inhibit it, one of the following two processes may occur:

1. The enzyme may be spontaneously reactivated by hydrolytic cleavage, which breaks the organophosphonyl–ChE bond, reactivating the enzyme.
2. The complex formed by the enzyme-ChE may lose a side group and become negatively charged, or "age," becoming resistant to reactivation by water or oxime.

Both of these processes are related to the size of the alkyl group attached to the oxygen of the organophosphorus compound, the group attached to the first carbon of this alkyl group, and other factors. Once the organophosphonyl–enzyme complex ages, it cannot be broken by an oxime.[14,15] Consequently, oxime therapy is not effective after aging occurs.

Because the nerve agents differ in structure, their rates of spontaneous reactivation and aging differ. For example, when complexed with VX, RBC-ChE spontaneously reactivates at a rate of roughly 0.5% to 1% per hour for about the first 48 hours. The VX–enzyme complex ages very little during this period.[44,47,113] The soman-enzyme complex does not spontaneously reactivate; the half-time for aging is about 2 minutes. The half-time for aging of the sarin-RBC-ChE complex is about 5 hours, and a small percentage (5%) of the enzyme undergoes spontaneous reactivation.[113] The half-time for aging of the tabun-enzyme complex is somewhat longer.

In the mid 1950s, Wilson and coworkers reported

that hydroxamine reactivated organophosphoryl-inhibited ChE faster than water did,[185] and later reported that an oxime (pyridine-2-aldoxime methiodide [2-PAM I]) was far more effective than hydroxamine in reactivating the enzyme.[186]

The oximes differ in their required doses, their toxicity, and their effectiveness. For example, TMB4 is more effective against tabun poisoning than is 2-PAM Cl. After thoroughly studying many of these compounds, 2-PAM Cl was chosen for use in the United States.[187] The choice was made because of research in both the civilian and military sectors experimentally demonstrated effectiveness as a reactivator and also because of the demonstrated clinical efficacy of 2-PAM Cl in treating organophosphorus insecticide poisoning.[188–194] At present, the only oxime approved by the FDA for use in the United States is 2-PAM Cl. The methanesulfonate salt of pralidoxime is the standard oxime in the United Kingdom, whereas TMB4 and toxogonin (obidoxime) are used in other European countries. Japan uses pralidoxime iodide. Other oximes, not yet approved, are of interest to several countries. HI-6 is advocated by some in Canada, while newer oximes are under study in the United States.

Because oximes reactivate the ChE inhibited by a nerve agent, they might be expected to completely reverse the effects caused by nerve agents. However, because it is possible that nerve agents produce biological activity by mechanisms other than inhibition of ChE, or because of reasons not understood, oximes are relatively ineffective in reversing effects in organs with muscarinic receptor sites. Oximes are also quaternary drugs and have limited penetration into the CNS. For these reasons, they are ineffective in reversing the central effects of nerve agent intoxication. They are much more effective in reversing nerve-agent–induced changes in organs with nicotinic receptor sites. In particular, when oximes are effective (ie, in the absence of aging), they decrease dysfunction in skeletal muscle, improving strength and decreasing fasciculations.

Dosage

The therapeutic dosage of 2-PAM Cl has not been established, but indirect evidence suggests that it is 15 to 25 mg/kg. The effective dose depends on the nerve agent, the time between poisoning and oxime administration, and other factors. An early study[195] showed that a plasma concentration of about 4 μg/mL in blood reversed the sarin-induced neuromuscular block in anesthetized cats; for years this concentration was generally accepted as being therapeutic for sarin. There is little data to support or disprove this contention. The 2-PAM Cl administered with the ComboPen or MARK 1 autoinjector (600 mg) produces a maximal plasma concentration of 6.5 μg/mL when injected intramuscularly in the average soldier (8.9 mg/kg in a 70-kg male).[178]

Different doses of 2-PAM Cl were administered (with atropine) in several studies. In sarin-poisoned rabbits, the protective ratio (PR; the ratio of the LD_{50} with treatment to the LD_{50} without treatment) increased from 25 to 90 when the IV dose of 2-PAM Cl increased from 5 to 10 mg/kg.[196] The PR increased from 1.6 to 4.2 when the IM dose of 2-PAM Cl increased from 30 to 120 mg/kg in sarin-poisoned rats,[160] and the PR increased from 1.9 to 3.1 when the IM dose of 2-PAM Cl increased from 11.2 to 22.5 mg/kg in VX-poisoned rabbits.[163] In the first two studies, the antidote was given immediately after the nerve agent. In the third, it was given at the onset of signs. No ventilatory support was used. When 2-PAM Cl was administered intravenously in humans 1 hour after sarin, a dose of 10 mg/kg reactivated 28% of the RBC-ChE, and doses of 15 or 20 mg/kg reactivated 58% of the enzyme. When given 3 hours after sarin, 5 mg/kg of 2-PAM Cl reactivated only 10% of the inhibited RBC-ChE, and 10 mg/kg or more reactivated more than 50%. When 2-PAM Cl was given at times from 0.5 to 24 hours after VX, doses of 2.5 to 25 mg/kg were found to reactivate 50% or more of the inhibited enzyme.[113]

For optimal therapy, 2-PAM Cl should be given intravenously, but usually this is not possible in the field. Even at small doses (2.5–5.0 mg/kg), the drug, when given intravenously in the absence of nerve agent poisoning, may cause transient effects, such as dizziness and blurred vision, which increase as the dose increases. Transient diplopia may occur at doses higher than 10 mg/kg. These effects, if they occur, are insignificant in a casualty poisoned with a ChE-inhibiting substance. Occasionally, nausea and vomiting may occur. The most serious side effect is hypertension, which is usually slight and transient at IV doses of 15 mg/kg or less, but may be marked and prolonged at higher doses.[197] 2-PAM Cl is commercially available as the cryodesiccated form (Protopam Chloride, manufactured by Wyeth-Ayerst Laboratories, Philadelphia, Pa) in vials containing 1 g, or about 14 mg/kg for a 70-kg person. Blood pressure elevations greater than 90 mm Hg systolic and 30 mm Hg diastolic may occur after administration of 45 mg/kg, and the elevations may persist for several hours.[197] Giving the oxime slowly (over 30–40 min) may minimize the hypertensive effect, and the hypertension can be quickly but transiently reversed by phentolamine 5 mg, administered intravenously (Figure 5-7).

2-PAM Cl is rapidly and almost completely excreted unchanged by the kidneys: 80% to 90% of an IM or IV

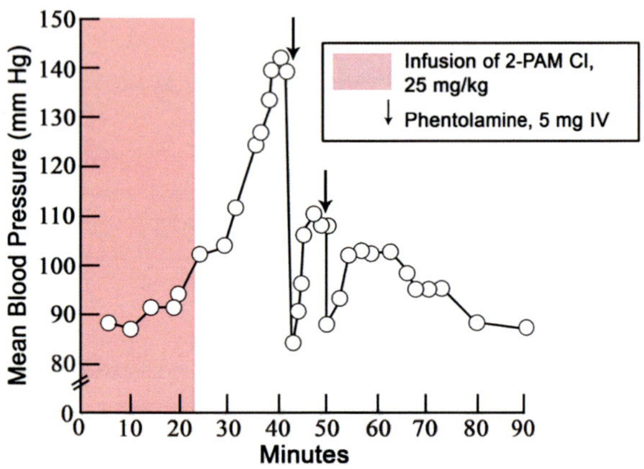

Fig. 5-7. An infusion of 25 mg/kg of 2-pyridine aldoxime methyl chloride (2-PAM Cl) over about 25 minutes produces marked hypertension, which is rapidly but transiently reversed by phentolamine (5 mg). The mean blood pressure is the diastolic plus one third of the difference between the systolic and the diastolic.

Reproduced with permission from: Sidell FR. Clinical considerations in nerve agent intoxication. In: Somani SM, ed. *Chemical Warfare Agents*. New York, NY: Academic Press; 1992: 181.

dose is excreted in 3 hours,[198] probably by an active tubular excretory mechanism (its renal clearance is close to that of p-aminohippurate[199]), with a half-time of about 90 minutes.[144] Both clearance and amount excreted are decreased by heat, exercise, or both.[200] Thiamine also decreases excretion (presumably by blocking tubular excretion), prolongs the plasma half-life, and increases the plasma concentration for the duration of thiamine activity.[198–202] Some[203] question the therapeutic benefit of thiamine.

An early clinical report[204] on the use of 2-PAM Cl in insecticide-poisoned people indicated that the oxime reversed the CNS effects of the poison (eg, patients regained consciousness and stopped convulsing shortly after the oxime was given). However, other early investigators found no oxime in the brains of animals[205,206] or the cerebrospinal fluid of humans[207] after experimental administration of 2-PAM Cl. Other investigators[74,208] found small amounts of 2-PAM Cl or reversal of the brain ChE inhibition in brains of animals poisoned with organophosphorus compounds.

Administration

An oxime should be initially administered with atropine. In cases of severe exposure, the contents of three Mark I kits or ATNAA should be administered; if these are not available, then oxime 1 to 1.5 g should be administered intravenously over a period of 20 to 30 minutes or longer. Additional atropine should be given to minimize secretions and to reduce ventilatory problems, thereby relieving the casualty's distress and discomfort.

Since an improvement in the skeletal muscle effects of the agent (ie, an increase or decrease in muscle tone and reduced fasciculations) may be seen after oxime administration, medical personnel may be tempted to repeat the oxime along with atropine. Because of side effects, however, no more than 2.5 g of oxime should be given within 1 to 1.5 hours. If the oxime is effective, it can be repeated once or twice at intervals of 60 to 90 minutes.

2-PAM Cl can be administered intravenously, intramuscularly, and orally. Soon after it became commercially available, 2-PAM Cl was administered orally both as therapy and as a pretreatment for those in constant contact with organophosphorus compounds (eg, crop dusters). At one time, the United Kingdom provided its military personnel with a supply of oxime tablets for pretreatment use, but it no longer does so. Enthusiasm for this practice waned for a number of reasons:

- erratic absorption of the drug from the gastrointestinal tract, leading to large differences (both between individuals and in the same person at different times) in plasma concentration;
- the large dose required (5 g to produce an average plasma concentration of 4 μg/mL);
- the unpopularity of the large, bitter 0.5-g or 1.0-g tablets; and
- the relatively slow absorption compared with that for administration by other routes.

In addition, the frequent administration (every 4–6 h) required by at-risk workers caused gastrointestinal irritation, including diarrhea. It is no longer common practice for crop workers to be given 2-PAM Cl as a pretreatment either, the rationale being that crop workers who take the medication might have a false sense of security and therefore might tend to be careless with safety measures.

Despite these drawbacks, 2-PAM Cl tablets may be the best alternative in certain cases, such as that of a depot worker exposed to a nerve agent who shows no effects except for an inhibition of RBC-ChE activity. An oxime might be given to restore the worker's RBC-ChE activity to 80% of the baseline value, which is necessary for return to work. (See Blood Cholinesterases section, above, for discussion of monitoring RBC-ChE activity.)

Oral administration may be considered preferable (although less reliable) to administration through a parenteral route because tablets can be self-administered and taking tablets avoids the pain of an injection.

IM administration of 2-PAM Cl with automatic injectors results in a plasma concentration of 4 μg/kg at 7 minutes, versus 10 minutes for conventional needle-and-syringe injection.[178] (A maximum plasma concentration of 6.9 μg/kg occurs at 19 min, versus 6.5 μg/kg at 22 min for the needle-and-syringe method.) About 80% to 90% of the intact drug is excreted unmetabolized in the urine; the half-life is about 90 minutes. When a 30% solution of 2-PAM Cl was injected intramuscularly at doses ranging from 2.5 to 30 mg/kg, the drug caused no change in heart rate or any signs or symptoms (except for pain at the injection site, as expected after an injection of 2 mL of a hypertonic solution).[198,199] When given intramuscularly, 30 mg/kg caused an elevation in blood pressure and minimal ECG changes, but no change in heart rate.[198]

Because of the rapid aging of the soman–AChE complex, oximes are often said to be ineffective in treating soman poisoning. Experimental studies in animals have shown that oximes are not as effective in treating soman intoxication as in sarin intoxication, but they do provide some therapeutic benefit (a 5%–10% reactivation of the inhibited enzyme).[209,210] Suggested reasons for this benefit are that an oxime acts as a cholinergic blocking drug at the nicotinic sites, analogous to atropine at the muscarinic sites,[209] or that it causes the circulation to improve, possibly by stimulating the release of catecholamines.[210]

Because of the hypertensive effect of 2-PAM Cl, US military doctrine states that no more than 2000 mg IV or three autoinjectors (600 mg each) should be given in 1 hour. If patients require additional treatment in the interim, atropine alone is used. Thus, as the ATNAA combined autoinjector replaces the MARK 1 set, atropine-only autoinjectors should also be available for use so that the 2-PAM Cl dosage limits are not exceeded during the treatment of a severe casualty.

Anticonvulsive Therapy

Convulsions occur after severe nerve agent exposure. In reports[20,66,104] of severe cases, convulsions (or what were described as "convulsive jerks" or "spasms") started within seconds after the casualty collapsed and lost consciousness, and persisted for several minutes until the individual became apneic and flaccid. The convulsions did not recur after atropine and oxime therapy and ventilatory support were administered. In these instances, no specific anticonvulsive therapy was needed nor given.

Laboratory studies indicate that the convulsive period lasts much longer (hours) in animals, even those given therapy, than in humans. The antidotes are given in a standard dose to experimental animals rather than titrated to a therapeutic effect as they are in human patients; this difference may account for the greater duration of convulsions in animal studies because the animals are protected from the immediate lethal effects of exposure but not the convulsant effects.

Diazepam, an anticonvulsant of the benzodiazepine family, has been shown to control nerve-agent–induced seizures/convulsions in rats, guinea pigs, rabbits, and monkeys.[128,211–215] It is commonly used to stop acute seizures (eg, status epilepticus) that may result from other etiologies,[141] including those produced by other anticholinesterases. Experimental studies also have shown that diazepam reduces or prevents nerve-agent–induced brain lesions due to this anticonvulsant activity.[128,129,131,132,135,211] Because of these properties and because diazepam is approved by the FDA for treatment of status epilepticus seizures by the IM route, diazepam was adopted by the US military as the drug for immediate anticonvulsant treatment of nerve agent casualties in the field.

During the Persian Gulf War, the US military issued an autoinjector containing 10 mg of diazepam (Convulsive Antidote, Nerve Agent, or CANA) to all military personnel (Figure 5-8). The Convulsive Antidote, Nerve Agent injector was not intended for self-use, but rather for use by a buddy when a soldier exhibited severe effects from a nerve agent. The

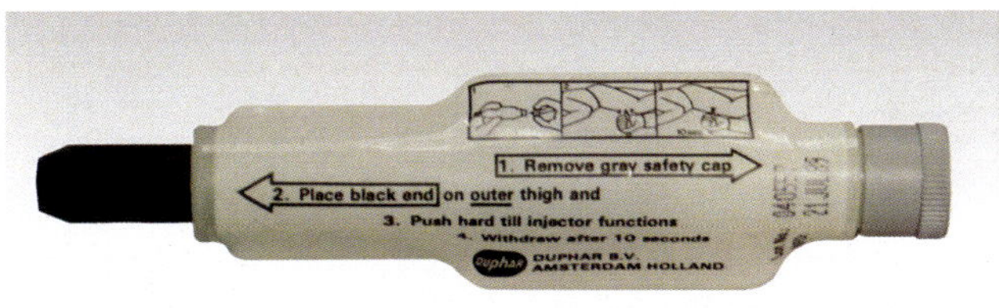

Fig. 5-8. The convulsive antidote nerve agent autoinjector (CANA) contains 10 mg of diazepam. The distinctive flared "wings" on each side make the shape of the injector unique and provide visual and tactual cues to indicate it is different from either the 2-pyridine aldoxime methyl chloride (2-PAM Cl) ComboPen or the antidote treatment nerve agent autoinjector (ATNAA).
Reproduced with permission from: Meridian Medical Technologies Inc, Bristol, Tenn.

buddy system was used because any soldier able to self-administer diazepam does not need it. Medics and unit lifesavers were issued additional diazepam autoinjectors and could administer two additional 10 mg doses at 10-minute intervals to a convulsing casualty. Current policy states that diazepam is given following the third Mark I or ATNAAs when the condition of the casualty warrants the administration of three Mark I kits or ATNAAs. The United Kingdom uses a drug similar to diazepam known as Avizafone.[132] Avizafone is a water-soluble, prodrug formulation of diazepam that is bioconverted to diazepam following injection.

If a convulsing or seizing casualty is being treated in a medical treatment facility, research has shown that other anticonvulsant benzodiazepines (eg, lorazepam [Ativan, Wyeth, Madison, New Jersey]), midazolam [Versed, Roche, Basel, Switzerland]) are just as effective in stopping nerve-agent–induced seizure as diazepam.[138] Experimental work has also shown that midazolam is twice as potent and twice as rapid in stopping nerve-agent–induced seizures compared to diazepam when the drugs are administered IM, the route of administration for immediate field treatment.[107,211] For these reasons, efforts are currently underway for FDA approval of midazolam as treatment of nerve-agent–induced seizures and the eventual replacement of diazepam by midazolam in the convulsive antidote nerve agent injectors.

Therapy for Cardiac Arrhythmias

Transient arrhythmias occur after nerve agent intoxication and after atropine administration in a normal individual. The irregularities generally terminate after the onset of atropine-induced sinus tachycardia (see discussion of cardiac effects above).

Experimental studies[156,215] have shown that when animals are poisoned with ChE inhibitors and then allowed to become cyanotic, rapid IV administration of atropine will cause ventricular fibrillation. This effect has not been reported in humans.

After severe intoxication from exposure to an organophosphate insecticide, a 20-year-old patient was stabilized with atropine and ventilatory support, but her ECG showed depression of the ST segment and flattening of the T wave, presumably because of persistent sinus tachycardia secondary to large doses of atropine (287 mg in 4 days; total of 830 mg). She was given a β-adrenergic blocking agent (propranolol), which slowed the heart rate to 107 beats per minute, normalizing the ST-T changes. The normal ECG pattern and heart rate of 107 beats per minute persisted, despite repeated doses of atropine. In effect, this produced a pharmacologically isolated heart, with both cholinergic and adrenergic blockade. The authors reporting on the case suggested that propranolol might be of value in protecting against the effects of atropine and organophosphorus intoxication.[216]

SPECIFIC TREATMENT BY EXPOSURE CATEGORY

The goals of medical therapy of any poisoning are, in most cases, straightforward: to minimize the patient's discomfort, to relieve distress, and to stop or reverse the abnormal process. These goals are the same in the treatment of a patient with nerve agent intoxication.

Therapy should be titrated against the complaints of dyspnea and objective manifestations, such as retching; administration of the contents of Mark I kits (or atropine alone) should be continued at intervals until relief is obtained. Seldom are more than two to three Mark I kits required to provide relief. Topical application of atropine or homatropine can effectively relieve eye or head pain not relieved by Mark I injections.

The signs of severe distress in a fellow soldier, such as twitching, convulsions, gasping for breath, and apnea, can be recognized by an untrained observer. A casualty's buddy will usually act appropriately, but because a buddy's resources are few, the level of assistance is limited: a buddy can administer three Mark I kits and diazepam and then seek medical assistance. In a more sophisticated setting, adequate ventilation is the highest priority, but even the best ventilators provide little improvement in the presence of copious secretions and high airway resistance. Atropine must be given until secretions (nose, mouth, airways) are decreased and resistance to assisted ventilation is minimal.

The goals of therapy must be realistic. Current medications will not immediately restore consciousness or respiration or completely reverse skeletal muscle abnormalities, nor will IM or IV drug therapy reverse miosis. Muscular fasciculations and small amounts of twitching may continue in a conscious patient long after adequate ventilation is restored and the patient is walking and talking.

Although in practice exposure categories are never clear-cut, different therapeutic measures are recommended for treating nerve agent casualties at different degrees of exposure severity. Treatment is based on the signs and symptoms caused by the particular exposure (Table 5-7). The following suggested exposure categories are based on the casualty presenting signs and symptoms.

TABLE 5-7

RECOMMENDED THERAPY FOR CASUALTIES OF NERVE AGENTS

Exposure Route	Exposure Category	Signs and Symptoms	Therapy
Inhalational (vapor)	Minimal	Miosis with or without rhinorrhea; reflex nausea and vomiting	< 5 min of exposure: 1 Mark I kit > 5 min of exposure*: observation
	Mild	Miosis; rhinorrhea; mild dyspnea; reflex nausea and vomiting	< 5 min of exposure: 2 Mark I kits > 5 min of exposure: 0 or 1 Mark I kit, depending on severity of dyspnea
	Moderate	Miosis; rhinorrhea; moderate to severe dyspnea; reflex nausea and vomiting	< 5 min of exposure: 3 Mark I kits and diazepam > 5 min of exposure: 1–2 Mark I kits
	Moderately severe	Severe dyspnea; gastrointestinal or neuromuscular signs	3 Mark I kits; standby ventilatory support; diazepam
	Severe	Loss of consciousness; convulsions; flaccid paralysis; apnea	3 Mark I kits; ventilatory support, suction; diazepam
Dermal (liquid on skin)	Mild	Localized sweating, fasciculations	1 Mark I kit
	Moderate	Gastrointestinal signs and symptoms	1 Mark I kit
	Moderately severe	Gastrointestinal signs plus respiratory or neuromuscular signs	3 Mark I kits; standby ventilatory support
	Severe	Same as for severe vapor exposure	3 Mark I kits; ventilatory support, suction; diazepam

*Casualty has been out of contaminated environment during this time.

Suspected Exposure

Suspected but unconfirmed exposure to a nerve agent sometimes occurs in an area where liquid agent was present. Workers without signs or symptoms may not be sure they are contaminated. In such cases, the suspected casualty should be thoroughly and completely decontaminated and kept under close medical observation for 18 hours. If a laboratory facility is available, blood should be drawn to measure RBC-ChE activity.

An individual working with nerve agent in an industrial or laboratory environment will have a baseline RBC-ChE activity value on record. If this value is still at baseline after a possible exposure, then no significant absorption has occurred and the new value provides confirmation of the baseline. (See Blood Cholinesterases section, above, on RBC-ChE activity monitoring.) If the activity is decreased, however, then absorption of the agent has occurred, but the decision to begin therapy should be based on signs or symptoms, not on the RBC-ChE activity (with one possible exception: an asymptomatic worker with decreased ChE activity; see Oxime Therapy section, above). The medical care provider must remember that the nadir of RBC-ChE activity may not occur for 18 to 24 hours, and if there has been no oxime therapy, then the final sample for analysis must be drawn during that time period.

Because the onset of effects caused by nerve agent exposure may occur as late as 18 hours after skin contact, prolonged observation is prudent. The longer the interval until the onset of signs and symptoms, the less severe they will be, but medical assistance will still be necessary. Since vapor (or inhaled aerosol) causes effects within seconds or minutes, it is extremely unlikely that a "suspected" asymptomatic casualty would be produced by this route.

Minimal Exposure

Miosis, with accompanying eye symptoms, and rhinorrhea are signs of a minimal exposure to a nerve agent, either vapor or vapor and liquid. This distinction is quite important in the management of this casualty. There are many situations in which one can be reasonably certain that exposure was by vapor alone (if the casualty was standing downwind from munitions or a container, for example, or standing across a laboratory or storeroom from a spilled agent or leaking container). On the other hand, if an unprotected individual is close to an agent splash or is walking in areas where liquid agent is present, exposure may be by both routes. Effects from vapor exposure occur quickly and are at their maximum within minutes, whereas effects from liquid agent on the skin may not occur until hours later.

Atropine (and oxime) should not be given systemically for miosis, if that is the only symptom, because it is ineffective in the usual doses (2 or 4 mg). If eye pain (or head pain) is severe, topical atropine or homatropine should be given. However, the visual blurring caused by atropine versus the relatively small amount of visual impairment caused by miosis must be considered. If the rhinorrhea is severe and troublesome, atropine (the 2 mg contained in one Mark I kit or one ATNAA) may provide some relief.

If liquid exposure can be excluded, there is no reason for prolonged observation.

Mild Exposure

An individual with mild or moderate dyspnea and possibly with miosis, rhinorrhea, or both can be classified as having a mild exposure to nerve agent. The symptoms indicate that the casualty has been exposed to a nerve agent vapor and may or may not have been contaminated by a liquid agent.

If an exposed person in this category is seen within several minutes after exposure, the contents of two Mark I kits or two ATNAA should be administered immediately. If 5 to 10 minutes have passed since exposure, the contents of only one kit should be given immediately. If no improvement occurs within 5 minutes under either circumstance, the casualty should receive the contents of another Mark I kit or ATNAA. The contents of an additional kit may be given if the casualty's condition worsens 5 to 10 minutes later, but it is unlikely that it will be needed. Only three oxime autoinjectors (Mark I kit) or three ATNAAs should be given; further therapy should be with atropine alone.

A person mildly exposed to a nerve agent should be thoroughly decontaminated (exposure to vapor alone does not require decontamination). The casualty should also have blood drawn to measure RBC-AChE activity prior to administering Mark I or ATTNA if facilities are available for the assay. Again, the MANAA inhaled atropine product may be helpful for patients under observation of a medic who can self-medicate.

Moderate Exposure

A casualty who has had moderate exposure to either a nerve agent vapor alone or to vapor and liquid will have severe dyspnea, with accompanying physical signs, and probably also miosis and rhinorrhea. The casualty should be thoroughly decontaminated, and blood should be drawn for assay of RBC-ChE activity if assay facilities are available. The contents of three Mark I kits or three ATNAAs and diazepam should be given if the casualty is seen within minutes of exposure. If seen later than 10 minutes after exposure, the casualty should receive the contents of two kits/ ATNAAs. Additional atropine should be given at 5-minute to 10-minute intervals until the dyspnea subsides. No more than three Mark I kits or ATNAAs should be used; however, additional atropine alone should be administered if the contents of three kits or ATNAAs do not relieve the dyspnea after 10 to 15 minutes. If there is reason to suspect liquid contamination, the patient should be kept under observation for 18 hours.

Nausea and vomiting are frequently the first effects of liquid contamination; the sooner after exposure they appear, the more ominous the outlook. Therapy should be more aggressive when these symptoms occur within an hour after exposure than when there is a longer delay in onset. If the onset is about an hour or less from the known time of liquid exposure, the contents of two Mark I kits or ATNAAs should be administered initially, and further therapy (the contents of a third Mark I kit or ATNAA to a total of three, then atropine alone) given at 5-minute to 10-minute intervals, with a maximum of three oxime injections. If the onset is several hours after the time of known exposure, the contents of one Mark I kit or ATNAA should be given initially, and additional Mark I kits or ATNAAs as needed to a total of three. Atropine alone should be used after the third Mark I or ATNAA. If the time of exposure is unknown, the contents of two Mark I kits or ATNAAs should be administered.

Nausea and vomiting that occur several hours after exposure have been treated successfully with 2 or 4 mg of atropine, and the symptoms did not recur. However, the exposure was single-site exposure (one drop at one place). It is not certain that this treatment will be successful if exposure is from a splash or from environmental contamination with multiple sites of exposure on the skin. Therefore, casualties with this degree of exposure should be observed closely for at least 18 hours after the onset of signs and symptoms.

Moderately Severe Exposure

In cases of moderately severe exposure, the casualty will be conscious and have one or more of the following signs and symptoms: severe respiratory distress (marked dyspnea and objective signs of pulmonary impairment such as wheezes and rales), marked secretions from the mouth and nose, nausea and vomiting (or retching), and muscular fasciculations and twitches. Miosis may be present if exposure was by vapor, but it is a relatively insignificant sign as a guideline for therapy in this context.

The contents of three Mark I kits or ATNAAs should be administered immediately. Preferably, if the means are available, 2 or 4 mg of atropine should be given intravenously, and the remainder of the total amount of 6 mg of atropine, along with the three oxime injections, should be given intramuscularly. Diazepam should always be given when the contents of three Mark I kits or ATNAAs are administered together. The casualty should be thoroughly decontaminated and have blood drawn for AChE assay before oxime is given.

Again, knowledge of the route of exposure is useful in planning further treatment. If the exposure was by vapor only and the casualty is seen in a vapor-free environment some minutes later, drug therapy should result in improvement. If the casualty has not lost consciousness, has not convulsed, and has not become apneic, improvement should be expected. If the exposure was the result of liquid agent or a combination of liquid and vapor, there may be a reservoir of unabsorbed agent in the skin; despite the initial therapy, the casualty's condition may worsen. In either case, medical care providers should be prepared to provide ventilatory assistance, including adequate suction, and additional drug therapy (atropine alone) if there is no improvement within 5 minutes after IV administration of atropine, or 5 to 10 minutes after IM administration of atropine.

The triad of consciousness, lack of convulsive activity, and spontaneous respiration is an indicator of a good outcome, provided adequate therapy is given early.

Severe Exposure

Casualties who are severely exposed to a nerve agent will be unconscious. They may be apneic or gasping for air with marked cyanosis, and may be convulsing or postictal. These casualties will have copious secretions from the mouth and nose and will have generalized fasciculations in addition to convulsive or large-muscle twitching movements. If they are postictal, or in nonconvulsive status epilepticus, they may be flaccid and apneic.

If the casualty shows no movement, including no signs of respiration, the initial response should be to determine if the heart is beating. This is not an easy task when the rescuer and the casualty are both in full mission-oriented, protective posture, level 4 gear, but it must be accomplished because a nonmoving, nonbreathing casualty without a heartbeat is not a candidate for further attention on the battlefield. A carotid pulse may be the easiest for the examiner to feel in mission-oriented, protective posture, level 4 gear. In a medical treatment facility, the medical personnel may be slightly more optimistic and proceed with aggressive therapy. After the Aum Shinrikyo sarin release in the Tokyo, Japan, subways, several casualties who were not breathing and who had no cardiac activity were taken to a hospital emergency department. Because of very vigorous and aggressive medical management, one or two of these casualties were able to walk out of the hospital several days later.

Despite the circumstances, self-protection from contamination via the patient is important. Since decontamination of the patient may not be the first priority, caregivers must wear appropriate protective equipment until they have an opportunity to decontaminate casualties and to remove them and themselves from the contaminated area.

The success of therapy under these circumstances is directly proportional to the viability of the casualty's cardiovascular system. If the heart rate is very slow or nonexistent, or if there is severe hypotension, the chances for success are poor, even in the best possible circumstances.

Medical personnel must first provide oxygenation and administer atropine by a technique that ensures it will be carried to the heart and lungs. If ventilatory assistance is not immediately available, the best treatment is to administer the contents of three Mark I kits or ATNAAs and diazepam. If ventilatory assistance will be forthcoming within minutes, the contents of the three Mark I kits or ATNAAs should be administered whether the circulation is intact or not. When there is no chance of rapid ventilatory assistance, little is gained by Mark I/ATNAA therapy, but an attempt at treatment should be made anyway.

In the case of a failed or failing cardiovascular system, routes of atropine administration other than IM should be considered. The IV route generally provides the fastest delivery of the drug throughout the body, but it is not without danger in an apneic and cyanotic patient. Whether or not concomitant ventilatory support can be provided, military medical personnel may consider administering atropine intratracheally by needle and syringe, if available, or with the atropine autoinjector (the AtroPen). Even if the casualty's systemic blood pressure is low, the peribronchial circulation may still have adequate blood flow to carry the drug to vital areas. If an endotracheal tube can be inserted, atropine could be injected into the tube either by needle and syringe or with the injector. In this case, because of the volume disparity, multiple atropine autoinjectors or ATNAAs are required to compensate for the volume of the tracheobronchial tree.

For severely exposed casualties, the initial dose of atropine should be at least the 6 mg from the three autoinjectors. An additional 2 mg or 4 mg should also be given intravenously if the capability is available and if the casualty is not hypoxic. Ventilatory support must be started before IV atropine is given. If additional atropine cannot be given intravenously, then the amount should be given intramuscularly. The total initial dose of atropine can be as much as 10 mg, but this dose should not be exceeded without allowing at least several minutes for a response. Further atropine administration depends on the response. If secretions decrease or if there are attempts at breathing, it may be prudent to wait even longer before administering additional atropine. All three injectors of 2-PAM Cl should be given with the initial 6 mg of atropine, but no more oxime should be given for an hour.

Possibly the most critical factor in the treatment of severely exposed casualties is restoration of oxygenation. Atropine alone might restore spontaneous breathing in a small number of apneic individuals. Ideally, an apparatus that delivers oxygen under positive pressure will be available. Even an RDIC or a mask-valve-bag apparatus used with ambient air will provide some assistance.

When the contents of three Mark I kits or ATNAAs are administered together to a severely poisoned casualty, diazepam should be administered with the contents of the third Mark I or ATNAA, whether or not there are indications of seizure activity. The risk of respiratory depression from this amount of diazepam given intramuscularly is negligible.

Hypotension need not be treated, at least initially. Generally the restoration of oxygenation and the increase in heart rate caused by atropine, aided perhaps by the hypertensive effects of 2-PAM Cl, will result in elevation of the blood pressure to an acceptable level.

Even with adequate oxygenation and large amounts of atropine, immediate reversal of all of the effects of the nerve agent will not occur. The casualty may remain unconscious, without spontaneous respiration, and with muscular flaccidity or twitching for hours. After respiration is at least partly spontaneous, secretions are minimized, and the casualty is partly alert, continued monitoring is necessary. Muscular fasciculations may continue for hours after the casualty is alert enough and has strength enough to get out of bed.

RETURN TO DUTY

Various factors should be considered before an individual who has been a nerve agent casualty is returned to duty. In an industrial setting (depot or laboratory), the criteria for reactivation are that the individual's RBC-ChE activity must have returned to greater than 90% of its baseline value and that the individual is otherwise symptom-free and sign-free.

In a military field setting, however, ChE activity measurements are not available, and the need to return the fighting soldier to duty may be more acute. The decision is largely a matter of judgment and should include the following considerations:

- If exposed to nerve agent again, will the soldier be in greater danger because of the previous exposure?
- How well can the soldier function?
- What is the military need for the soldier?

In the absence of blood ChE measurements, it is difficult to predict whether a soldier would be at greater risk from a second nerve agent exposure. Even an individual with rather mild effects (miosis and rhinorrhea) may have marked ChE inhibition. On the other hand, if an oxime (contained in the Mark I kit or ATNAA) was given and the agent was one susceptible to oxime therapy, then the enzyme activity may be restored. In a field setting, neither the identity of the agent nor the degree of ChE inhibition or restoration will be known. In any case, proper use of mission-oriented, protective posture, level 4 gear should protect against further exposure. The soldier should be returned to active duty if able and needed.

A soldier who has had signs of severe exposure with loss of consciousness, apnea, and convulsions, may have milder CNS effects for many weeks after recovery from the acute phase of intoxication. Except in dire circumstances, return to duty during this period should not be considered for such casualties. An individual with relatively mild effects (miosis, dyspnea, rhinorrhea) may be returned to duty within hours to several days following exposure, depending on the assignment and the military need. However, the soldier may experience visual problems in dim light and may have mental lapses for as long as 6 to 8 weeks,[18,45] and these factors must be considered before returning a soldier to duty. In one case, troops who were symptomatic (miosis, rhinorrhea, dyspnea) as a result of nerve agent exposure carried out maneuvers (including firing weapons) in a satisfactory, although suboptimal, manner. They did not do nearly as well at night because of visual problems.[88]

In another instance, workers in an industrial operation learned the effects of the agent after they had accidentally been exposed several times. They also learned that it was a bigger problem to seek medical aid (with the ensuing administrative processes) than to continue working in the presence of symptoms. They stopped going to the aid station if they noted the onset of only mild effects. These workers were generally not in positions requiring acute vision or complex decisions; it is not known how well they performed while symptomatic. However, they could continue to perform their jobs, and their supervisors apparently did not notice a decrement.[45]

The need for soldiers in a frontline military operation may require that every walking casualty be returned to duty. In an otherwise asymptomatic casualty, the primary limiting factors will be the soldier's visual acuity compared with the visual demands of the job, and the soldier's mental status compared with the intellectual demands of the job. Prolonged mental changes can be subtle and may require a careful examination to detect.

In the Iran-Iraq War, Foroutan[12] claims to have recommended to commanders that units who had come under nerve agent attack be held back from the front lines for a period of time until they had reconstituted their ChE. It is not clear whether the commanders followed his recommendation. This is the only instance known of a unit-level recommendation on a group of soldiers exposed to nerve agent. US doctrine is silent on this subject. In the planning for the 2003 invasion of Iraq, the authors were told that the theater surgeon responded to the issue, saying the commander on the ground would evaluate each situation as it presented itself.

TREATMENT GUIDELINES IN CHILDREN

Very little has been published on the treatment of nerve agent poisoning in the pediatric population. Rotenberg and Newmark have summarized the literature and extrapolated treatment guidelines based upon adult experience and animal data.[217]

In general, children are more susceptible to chemical agents than adults, based on the following: smaller mass and higher surface-to-volume ratio; immaturity of the respiratory system; immaturity of the stratum corneum in the skin of young children, which facilitates dermal absorption; and immaturity of the neurotransmitter systems, rendering children more likely to seize with an epileptogenic stimulus. In addition, the signs and symptoms of nerve agents in children may well differ from those seen in adults; miosis is less common in organophosphate poisonings in children than in adults, and children may present with less obvious convulsions/seizures than adults.

To treat children exposed to nerve agents, the authors recommend an atropine dose of at least 0.05 mg/kg IM or IV, with a higher dose of up to 0.1 mg/kg in a clear cholinergic crisis. Although technically off-label, the MARK 1 autoinjectors are probably safe to use in children who are large enough for the autoinjector needles. The FDA has approved 0.5 mg and 1 mg autoinjectors of atropine only, representing 25% and 50% of the adult (MARK 1/ATNAA) dose, with correspondingly shorter needles. For 2-PAM Cl, IV use is preferred in small children, and doses might not need to be repeated as frequently as in adults because the half-life of the drug in children appears to be twice that seen in adults. The treatment of seizures in children is similar to those in adults, with benzodiazepine dose adjusted for weight, as long as the caregiver remembers that status epilepticus may present differently in children than adults.

LESSONS FROM IRAN, JAPAN, AND IRAQ

With the exception of two soldiers exposed to sarin in Baghdad, Iraq in May 2004, the United States military has no experience with treating nerve agent casualties on the battlefield. Until then, the entire national experience had been with industrial accidents, many of which have already been described. In order to properly plan for either battlefield or terrorist incidents, it is crucial to learn from those who have dealt with these scenarios. The only appropriate experience comes from overseas, from the Iranian experience with battlefield nerve agent casualties in the Iran-Iraq War and from the Japanese experience with the 1994 and 1995 terrorist attacks.

Iran

From the 1930s until the 1981–1987 Iran-Iraq War, nerve agents were not used on the battlefield. Between 1984 and 1987, Iraq used tabun and sarin extensively against Iranian troops. Only in the last few years has good clinical data emerged from that experience. Foroutan, the first physician to run a chemical treatment station treating nerve agent battlefield casualties in world history, published his reminiscence of nerve agent and sulfur mustard casualty care in a series of articles in the Farsi-language *Kowsar Medical Journal* in the late 1990s.[218–227] The lessons Foroutan learned have been summarized in an English-language review paper.[12] Among the conclusions this analysis reached, Foroutan determined the differential diagnosis included cyanide poisoning, heat stroke, infectious diseases, fatigue, and psychiatric diagnoses, including combat s tress. At the time, the Iranians thought Iraq had also used cyanide, but that was never proven.

Foroutan used large amounts of atropine in his treatment protocols. This may have resulted from the lack of oxime therapy far forward; Iranian soldiers did not carry oxime with them, and even physicians had a very small supply to use. It may also have been due to Foroutan's inability to guarantee that atropine would be given during medical evacuation to the rear of his location. In a few cases, Foroutan actually gave 200 mg of atropine IV in a 10-minute to 15-minute period.

Although miosis is a poor guide to atropinization, due to the relative disconnection between the papillary muscle and the circulation, Foroutan noted that the disappearance of miosis or even the appearance of mydriasis was one indication to decrease atropine, "even if the patient's mouth has not completely dried."

Psychogenic casualties, whether those with actual psychiatric diagnoses or simply "worried well," were a major problem for Foroutan, just as they were in the civilian victims of the Tokyo subway attack. He stressed the need to identify them and remove them from the symptomatic patients requiring immediate attention. He also stressed the need to treat patients as quickly as possible in order to achieve optimal outcomes.

Foroutan's experience shows that a robust evacuation and triage system saves lives on the battlefield. In the Hosseiniyeh attack, the one which most overwhelmed his aid station, he received over 300 "severe" patients within 5 hours, along with 1,700 less severely affected patients. One aid station was not equipped to treat all of these patients. This illustrates the need to plan a robust and redundant system that can deal with mass casualties of nerve agent exposure.

Foroutan felt that the numbers of nerve agent casualties had been underestimated by the media and the government of Iran because, unlike sulfur mustard casualties, nerve agent casualties rapidly became well or died. As such, nerve agent survivors had no propaganda value, unlike the photogenic mustard casualties who were evacuated to Europe. He believed that there had been between 45,000 and 100,000 nerve agent casualties in the war, several times the United Nations estimate.

Japan

There is considerable literature on the medical aspects of the two terrorist attacks in Japan, in Matsumoto in 1994 and on the Tokyo subway system in 1995.[53,78,143,165,228–244] One of the major lessons from the Japanese attacks is that 80% of the patients who presented for medical attention were not found to have any signs or symptoms of sarin poisoning. This figure has become a major point in the teaching of mass casualty management of a future nerve agent attack. In Tokyo, for example, the combined figures show about 1,100 of the 5,500 people presenting to medical attention having signs and symptoms of sarin poisoning, ranging from extremely severe to extremely mild. The others could be considered the "worried well."[228] Even those patients who actually did have sarin poisoning symptoms tended to have mild symptoms. For example, at Saint Luke's International Hospital, which saw more patients than any other hospital (641), only 5 patients were deemed "critical."[165,229]

The physicians in the first attack, in the small city of Matsumoto, were able to make the diagnosis of organophosphate poisoning (cholinergic crisis) early by syndromic reasoning. In that part of central Japan insecticide poisoning is common, so the patients could be treated without knowing the specific organophosphate.[230] By contrast, in the later, larger Tokyo attack, diagnosis lagged considerably at many hospitals that were unaccustomed to seeing this condition.

In both the Matsumoto and the Tokyo subway attacks, miosis was the most common symptom.[53,165,229,231,232] Many of the patients had no demonstrated depression of ChE. This reinforces the principle that patients should be treated symptomatically, as laboratory values are not as effective a guide to their conditions as is the clinical examination. At Toranomon Hospital, ChE activity was also found to be a poor guide to the severity of poisoning, based on correlations with clinical picture and other values in 213 patients seen after the Tokyo attack.[233]

Four pregnant women, all with slightly decreased ChE levels, were among the patients evaluated at Saint Luke's International Hospital.[229] They were between 9 and 36 weeks' gestation at the time of poisoning. All delivered healthy infants on schedule and without complications. This may be the only series of pregnant exposed patients ever recorded.

The Japanese experience with acute nerve agent antidotal treatment is highly reassuring because even with delays of diagnosis, the standard protocols using atropine, oximes, and anticonvulsants saved many patients.[229,234,235] Those patients receiving 3 g or more of pralidoxime iodide recovered their ChE levels faster than those who did not. One peculiarity is that the Japanese oxime is 2-PAM iodide, not 2-PAM Cl, as in the United States. The reason for this is cultural. Japan has a high incidence of thyroid disease and often tries to develop drugs using iodide where possible.[237] Other than that, the Japanese hospital treatment protocols were essentially identical to those described in earlier sections of this chapter, and they were generally effective.

The value of acute therapy was validated in Tokyo. At Saint Luke's, of three patients who presented in full cardiopulmonary arrest, one patient was resuscitated and discharged on hospital day 6.[229] Although in a military situation, like the one described by Foroutan, or in an overwhelming civilian catastrophe, sufficient resources may not be available to give antidotal treatment, the Tokyo case demonstrates that even giving treatment to those who appear to be beyond saving is not necessarily futile.

One of the major lessons learned from the Japanese experience is that healthcare workers in an emergency room, even a well-ventilated one, are at high risk of secondary exposure when patients are neither stripped of their clothing nor decontaminated prior to entry.[236,238] At Keio University Hospital, 13 of 15 doctors in the emergency room reported dim vision, with severe miosis in 8, rhinorrhea in 8, chest tightness or dyspnea in 4, and cough in 2.[234] Six of the 13 received atropine, and one of the 13 received pralidoxime iodide. Despite that, all the doctors continued to practice throughout the day. At Saint Luke's, 23% of the staff reported mild physical disorders, including eye pain, headache, sore throat, dyspnea, nausea, dizziness, and nose pain (based upon a questionnaire in which only 45% of 1063 patients responded).[229]

Another major lesson from the Japanese experience is that, in contrast to many other chemical warfare agents, nerve agent casualties either die or improve in a relatively short period of time. At Saint Luke's, 105 patients were admitted overnight and 95% were discharged within 4 days,[228] indicating that nerve agent mass casualties create an acute, not chronic, problem for the health care system.

Among the most important lessons from the Japanese attacks is that there is the possibility of long-lasting clinical effects from sarin exposure.[236,238–244] Many of these effects overlap with or satisfy criteria for posttraumatic stress disorder and have been chronically disabling for some patients. In one questionnaire study, 60% of responders had symptoms 1, 3, and 6 months after exposure.[239] Many still met posttraumatic stress disorder criteria, and the reported symptoms varied widely, including fear of riding subways, depression, irritation, nightmares, insomnia, and flashbacks.[229] In 85 of 149 patients examined 1 and 2 years after the Matsumoto attack, six had been severely poisoned; of these six patients, four had persistent EEG abnormalities, one reported sensory neuropathies, and one had multifocal premature ventricular contractions. Of 27 moderately poisoned, one had persistent visual field defects.[244] In another series of 18 patients studied 6 to 8 months after exposure, at a time when they were clinically entirely normal, visually evoked responses (P[positive wave]100[milliseconds after the stimulaton]) and sensory evoked responses (P300) were prolonged, although brainstem auditory evoked responses were normal, and some of these patients also had posttraumatic stress disorder at the time.[239] An uncontrolled, 5-year, follow-up questionnaire of Saint Luke's patients suggests many may have developed posttraumatic stress disorder.[78] Within the survivor group, older patients seem to be more susceptible to insomnia.[243]

Iraq

In May 2004 two explosive ordnance soldiers in the US Army came in contact with an old sarin shell, presumably from the Iran-Iraq war, and experienced mild sarin poisoning. The soldiers made the syndromic diagnosis of possible nerve agent exposure themselves. This is noteworthy because no US soldiers had ever had documented nerve agent exposure before. The soldiers experienced miosis, dim vision, increased nasal and oral secretions, and mild dyspnea, and later reported some acute memory disturbances that were not well documented in their medical charts. Their ChEs were estimated by back-calculation to be 39% and 62% reduced from baseline.[245] One of the two soldiers appeared to recover fully but then developed memory difficulties several months later, which may or may not have been due to his documented sarin exposure.[246]

PYRIDOSTIGMINE BROMIDE AS A PRETREATMENT FOR NERVE AGENT POISONING

Aging half time places a significant limitation on oxime antidotal therapy for nerve agents, especially those agents that age rapidly. Aging is the reaction that takes place after ChE has bound to nerve agent, resulting in the loss of a side chain and placing a negative charge on the remaining ChE-agent complex. Oximes, such as 2-PAM Cl, cannot reactivate "aged" enzyme, and thus enzyme that has been bound to nerve agent and subsequently aged must be replaced by new synthesis of ChE by the body. Most nerve agents

TABLE 5-8

AGING HALF-TIME OF NERVE AGENTS

Nerve Agent	RBC-ChE Source	Aging Half-Time
GA (tabun)	Human (in vitro)	>14 h[1]
	Human (in vitro)	13.3 h[2]
GB (sarin)	Human (in vivo)	5 h[3]
	Human (in vitro)	3 h[1]
GD (soman)	Marmoset (in vivo)	1.0 min[4]
	Guinea pig (in vivo)	7.5 min[4]
	Rat (in vivo)	8.6 min[4]
	Human (in vitro)	2–6 min[1]
GF	Human (in vitro)	40 h[1]
	Human (in vitro)	7.5 h[5]
VX	Human (in vitro)	48 h[3]

RBC-ChE: red blood cell cholinesterase
(1) Mager PP. *Multidimensional Pharmacochemistry*. San Diego, Calif: Academic Press; 1984: 52–53. (2) Doctor BP, Blick DW, Caranto G, et al. Cholinesterases as scavengers for organophosphorus compounds: Protection of primate performance against soman toxicity. *Chem Biol Interact*. 1993;87:285–293. (3) Sidell FR, Groff WA. The reactivatibility of cholinesterase inhibited by VX and sarin in man. *Toxicol Appl Pharm*. 1974;27:241–252. (4) Talbot BG, Anderson DR, Harris LW, Yarbrough LW, Lennox WJ. A comparison of in vivo and in vitro rates of aging of soman-inhibited erythrocyte acetylcholinesterase in different animal species. *Drug Chem Toxicol*. 1988;11:289–305. (5) Hill DL, Thomas NC. *Reactivation by 2-PAM Cl of Human Red Blood Cell Cholinesterase Poisoned in vitro by Cyclohexylmethylphosphonofluoridate (GF)*. Edgewood Arsenal, Md: Medical Research Laboratory; 1969. Edgewood Arsenal Technical Report 43-13.

age slowly enough that this limitation is not crucial either tactically or clinically (Table 5-8). For example, although VX is extremely toxic, it ages so slowly that in any clinically relevant time frame, oxime will still be useful. The concern, however, has always centered upon rapid-aging nerve agents such as soman, whose aging half-time is on the order of minutes. Once several half-times have elapsed, oxime therapy is useless in a patient poisoned by such a nerve agent.

Due to the limitations of existing therapy, the US and other militaries turned to the carbamates. Pyridostigmine is one of the best known drugs of this class. Its chemical structure and that of a related carbamate, physostigmine, are shown in Figure 5-9. Physostigmine acts similarly, but because it crosses the blood-brain barrier, there is the possibility of behavioral side effects and it is therefore not used as a nerve agent pretreatment. Like the nerve agents, carbamates inhibit the enzymatic activity of AChE. As a quaternary amine, pyridostigmine is ionized under normal physiological conditions and penetrates poorly into the CNS. Pyridostigmine has been approved by the FDA since 1952 for the treatment of myasthenia gravis. In myasthenic patients, pyridostigmine prolongs the activity of ACh. Dosage of pyridostigmine for myasthenic patients in the United States starts at 60 mg by mouth every 8 hours and increases from there; patients receiving 480 mg per day are not unusual. Consequently, pyridostigmine has a long and favorable safety record in this patient population.

As an inhibitor of AChE, pyridostigmine in large doses mimics the peripheral toxic effects of the organophosphate nerve agents. It may seem paradoxical that carbamate compounds protect against nerve agent poisoning, but two critical characteristics of the carbamate-enzyme bond contribute to the usefulness of carbamates for this purpose. First, carbamoylation, the interaction between carbamates and the active site of AChE, is freely and spontaneously reversible, unlike the normally irreversible inhibition of AChE by the nerve agents. No oxime reactivators are needed to dissociate, or decarbamoylate, the enzyme from a carbamate compound. Carbamates do not undergo the aging reaction of nerve agents bound to AChE. The second characteristic is that carbamoylated AChE is fully protected from attack by nerve agents because the active site of the carbamoylated enzyme is not acces-

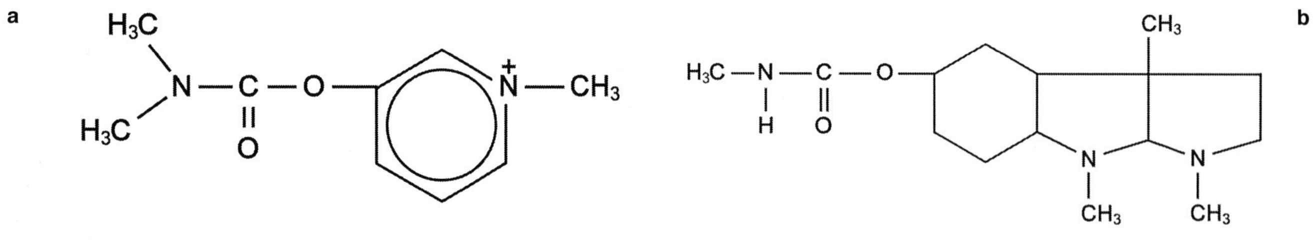

Fig. 5-9. The chemical structures of the carbamates **(a)** pyridostigmine and **(b)** physostigmine.

sible for binding nerve agent molecules. Functionally, sufficient excess AChE activity is normally present in synapses so that carbamoylation of 20% to 40% of the enzyme with pyridostigmine does not significantly impair neurotransmission.

Additionally, it must be recognized that the normal human carries excess ChE. Thus, temporary inhibition of a small portion of ChE is well tolerated by humans, with minimal side effect profiles, as detailed below.

When animals are challenged with a lethal dose of nerve agent, AChE activity normally decreases rapidly, becoming too low to measure. In pyridostigmine-pretreated animals with a sufficient quantity of protected, carbamoylated enzyme, spontaneous decarbamoylation of the enzyme regenerates enough AChE activity to sustain vital functions, such as neuromuscular transmission to support respiration. Prompt postexposure administration of atropine is still needed to antagonize ACh excess, and an oxime reactivator must also be administered if an excess of nerve agent remains to attack the newly uncovered AChE active sites that were protected by pyridostigmine.

Efficacy

Because it is impossible to test the rationale in humans exposed to nerve agents, the US military embarked upon a series of studies in animal models. Table 5-9 summarizes one study using male rhesus monkeys.[73] Pretreatment with orally administered, pyridostigmine-inhibited circulating red blood cell AChE (RBC-AChE) by 20% to 45%. (Inhibition of RBC-AChE by pyridostigmine is a useful index of its inhibition of AChE in peripheral synapses). Monkeys that had no pyridostigmine pretreatment were not well protected from soman by the prompt administration of atropine and 2-PAM Cl. The PR of 1.64 in these monkeys is typical of the most effective known postexposure antidote therapy in animals not given pretreatment to a soman challenge. In contrast to this low level of protection, however, the combination of pyridostigmine pretreatment and prompt postchallenge administration of atropine and 2-PAM Cl resulted in greatly improved protection (PR > 40 when compared with the control group; PR = 24 when compared with the group given atropine and 2-PAM Cl).

Because the number of animals available for soman challenge at extremely high doses was limited, accurate calculation of a PR was indeterminate in this experiment. The PR was well in excess of 40, clearly meeting the requirement for effectiveness of 5-fold improved protection. In a later study, four of five rhesus monkeys receiving pyridostigmine pretreatment

TABLE 5-9

EFFECT OF THERAPY ON MEDIAN LETHAL DOSE IN MONKEYS EXPOSED TO SOMAN

Group	Mean LD_{50} (μg/kg) [95% CL]	Mean Protective Ratio [95% CL]
Control (no treatment)	15.3 [13.7–17.1]	NA
Postexposure atropine + 2-PAM Cl	25.1 [22.0–28.8]	1.64 [1.38–19.5]
Pyridostigmine pretreatment + postexposure atropine + 2-PAM Cl	> 617	> 40*

*Indeterminate because of small number of subjects; PR relative to the atropine plus 2-PAM Cl group > 24 (617 ÷ 25.1)
2-PAM Cl: 2-pyridine aldoxime methyl chloride
CL: confidence limit (based on a separate slopes model)
LD_{50}: median lethal dose
NA: not applicable
PR: factor by which the LD_{50} of a nerve agent challenge is raised (in this experiment, the LD_{50} for group given therapy divided by the LD_{50} for control group)
Adapted from: Kluwe WM. Efficacy of pyridostigmine against soman intoxication in a primate model. In: *Proceedings of the Sixth Medical Chemical Defense Bioscience Review*. Aberdeen Proving Ground, Md: US Army Medical Research Institute of Chemical Defense; 1987: 233.

and postexposure therapy of atropine and 2-PAM Cl survived for 48 hours after being challenged with GF at a level 5-fold higher than its LD_{50}.[247]

Pyridostigmine pretreatment shows its strongest benefit, compared with atropine and oxime therapy alone, in animals challenged with soman and tabun, and provides little additional benefit against challenge by sarin or VX.[248–250] Table 5-10 shows the PRs obtained in animals given atropine and oxime therapy after challenge with the five nerve agents with and without pyridostigmine pretreatment. As shown, pyridostigmine pretreatment is essential for improved survival after soman and tabun challenge. With sarin or VX, depending on the animal system studied, pyridostigmine causes either no change or a minor decrease in PRs, which still indicate strong efficacy of atropine and oxime therapy for exposure to these agents. The data for GF show no benefit from pyridostigmine pretreatment for mice and a small benefit for guinea pigs. The only published data on protection of primates from GF show a PR of more than 5 with pyridostigmine pretreatment and atropine/oxime therapy, but a control group treated with atropine/oxime alone

TABLE 5-10

EFFECT OF THERAPY WITH AND WITHOUT PYRIDOSTIGMINE PRETREATMENT ON PROTECTIVE RATIOS IN ANIMALS EXPOSED TO NERVE AGENTS

		Protective Ratio	
Nerve Agent	**Animal Tested**	**Atropine + Oxime**	**Pyridostigmine + Atropine + Oxime**
GA (Tabun)	Rabbit[1]	2.4	3.9
	Mouse[2]	1.3	1.7/2.1*
	Guinea pig[2]	4.4	7.8/12.1*
	Rabbit[3]	4.2	> 8.5
GB (Sarin)	Mouse[2]	2.1	2.2/2.0*
	Guinea pig[2]	36.4	34.9/23.8*
GD (Soman)	Mouse[4]	1.1	2.5
	Rat[5]	1.2	1.4
	Guinea pig[6]	1.5	6.4/5.0*
	Guinea pig[7]	2.0	2.7/7.1*
	Guinea pig[8]	1.9	4.9
	Guinea pig[9]	1.7	6.8
	Rabbit[1]	1.4	1.5
	Rabbit[4]	2.2	3.1
	Rabbit[3]	1.9	2.8
	Rhesus monkey[10]	1.6	> 40
GF	Mouse[11]	1.4	1.4
	Guinea pig[11]	2.7	3.4
	Rhesus monkey[12]		> 5
VX	Mouse[2]	7.8	6.0/3.9*
	Rat[5]	2.5	2.1
	Guinea pig[2]	58.8	47.1/45.3*

*Two doses of pyridostigmine were used.

(1) Joiner RL, Dill GS, Hobson DW, et al. *Task 87-35: Evaluating the Efficacy of Antidote Drug Combinations Against Soman or Tabun Toxicity in the Rabbit.* Columbus, Oh: Battelle Memorial Institute; 1988. (2) Koplovitz I, Harris LW, Anderson DR, Lennox WJ, Stewart JR. Reduction by pyridostigmine pretreatment of the efficacy of atropine and 2-PAM treatment of sarin and VX poisoning in rodents. *Fundam Appl Toxicol.* 1992;18:102–106. (3) Koplovitz I, Stewart JR. A comparison of the efficacy of HI6 and 2-PAM against soman, tabun, sarin, and VX in the rabbit. *Toxicol Lett.* 1994;70:269–279. (4) Sultan WE, Lennox WJ. *Comparison of the Efficacy of Various Therapeutic Regimens, With and Without Pyridostigmine Prophylaxis, for Soman (GD) Poisoning in Mice and Rabbits.* Aberdeen Proving Ground, Md: US Army Chemical Systems Laboratory; 1983. ARCSL Technical Report 83103. (5) Anderson DR, Harris LW, Woodard CL, Lennox WJ. The effect of pyridostigmine pretreatment on oxime efficacy against intoxication by soman or VX in rats. *Drug Chem Toxicol.* 1992;15:285–294. (6) Jones DE, Carter WH Jr, Carchman RA. Assessing pyridostigmine efficacy by response surface modeling. *Fundam Appl Toxicol.* 1985;5:S242–S251. (7) Lennox WJ, Harris LW, Talbot BG, Anderson DR. Relationship between reversible acetylcholinesterase inhibition and efficacy against soman lethality. *Life Sci.* 1985;37:793–798. (8) Capacio BR, Koplovitz I, Rockwood GA, et al. *Drug Interaction Studies of Pyridostigmine with the 5HT3 Receptor Antagonists Ondansetron and Granisetron in Guinea Pigs.* Aberdeen Proving Ground, Md: US Army Medical Research Institute of Chemical Defense; 1995. USAMRICD Training Report 95-05. AD B204964. (9) Inns RH, Leadbeater L. The efficacy of bispyridinium derivatives in the treatment of organophosphate poisoning in the guinea pig. *J Pharm Pharmacol.* 1983;35:427–433. (10) Kluwe WM. Efficacy of pyridostigmine against soman intoxication in a primate model. In: *Proceedings of the 6th Medical Chemical Defense Bioscience Review.* Aberdeen Proving Ground, Md: USAMRICD; 1987: 227–234. (11) Stewart JR, Koplovitz I. The effect of pyridostigmine pretreatment on the efficacy of atropine and oxime treatment of cyclohexylmethylphosphonofluoridate (CMPF) poisoning in rodents. Aberdeen Proving Ground, Md: US Army Medical Research Institute of Chemical Defense; 1993. Unpublished manuscript. (12) Koplovitz I, Gresham VC, Dochterman LW, Kaminskis A, Stewart JR. Evaluation of the toxicity, pathology, and treatment of cyclohexylmethlyphosphonofluoridate (CMFF) poisoning in rhesus monkeys. *Arch Toxicol.* 1992;66:622–628.

for comparison was not included.[247] Clinical experts from all countries have concluded from these data that pyridostigmine isan essential pretreatment adjunct for nerve agent threats under combat conditions, where the identity of threat agents is uncertain.

The effectiveness of pyridostigmine pretreatment may not provide conclusive evidence of the importance of central mechanisms in respiratory arrest; it appears that there is at least partial permeability of the blood-brain barrier to polar compounds such as pyridostigmine, specifically in the regions of the fourth ventricle and brainstem, where respiratory centers are located. In addition, an increase in blood-brain barrier permeability occurs rapidly after soman administration.[251,252] The key observation remains that animals pretreated with pyridostigmine and promptly receive atropine and oxime therapy after an otherwise lethal soman exposure are able to maintain adequate respiration and survive.

Safety

Pyridostigmine maintains a good safety record following its administration to myasthenia gravis patients. Known adverse reactions have been limited to infrequent drug rashes after oral administration and the constellation of signs of peripheral cholinergic excess, which have been seen only when the dosage in patients with myasthenia gravis was increased to AChE inhibition levels well beyond the 20% to 40% range desired for nerve agent pretreatment. The recommended dose for nerve agent pretreatment, based upon non-human primate studies and human pharmacokinetic studies, is only half of the starting myasthenic dose of 60 mg orally every 8 hours, 30 mg orally every 8 hours. When this recommended adult dose regimen has been followed, no significant decrements have been found in the performance of a variety of military tasks. A review of British studies reported that pyridostigmine caused no changes in memory, manual dexterity, vigilance, day and night driving ability, or in psychological tests for cognitive and psychomotor skills.[253] No significant changes in sensory, motor, or cognitive functioning at ground level, at 800 ft, and at 13,000 ft were noted in 12 subjects in another study after their fourth 30-mg dose of pyridostigmine.[254]

The flight performance of subjects taking pyridostigmine in two studies was not affected,[255,256] and no impairment in neuromuscular function was noted in another study in which subjects took pyridostigmine for 8 days.[257] Cardiovascular and pulmonary function were normal at high altitudes in pyridostigmine-treated subjects in another study.[258] However, one study noted a slight decrement in performance in subjects taking pyridostigmine when they performed two tasks simultaneously; these subjects also had a slight decrement on a visual probability monitoring task.[259] Two studies found an increase in sweating and a decrease in skin blood flow in pyridostigmine-treated subjects subjected to heat/work stress.[260,261]

Although there has been wide experience with long-term administration of pyridostigmine to patients with myasthenia gravis, until recently, there was no comparable body of safety data in healthy young adults. Short-term pyridostigmine administration (on or two doses of 30 mg each) has been conducted in peacetime in some countries, including the United States, to screen critical personnel, such as aircrew, for unusual or idiosyncratic reactions, such as drug rash. The occurrence of such reactions has been well below the 0.1% level. Currently no military populations are routinely screened with administration of a test dose of pyridostigmine.

A limited number of animal studies of toxicological abnormalities and teratogenicity and mutagenicity in animals that were given pyridostigmine have had negative results (Hoffman-LaRoche, proprietary information).[262] In a study[263] in which pyridostigmine was administered to rats, either acutely or chronically, in doses sufficient to cause an average 60% AChE inhibition, ultrastructural alteration of a portion of the presynaptic mitochondria at the neuromuscular junction resulted, as well as alterations of nerve terminal branches, postsynaptic mitochondria, and sarcomeres. These morphological findings, which occurred at twice the AChE inhibition level desired in humans, have not been correlated with any evidence of functional impairment at lower doses, but they emphasize the need to limit enzyme inhibition to the target range of 20% to 40%. Pyridostigmine has been used by pregnant women with myasthenia gravis at higher doses and for much longer periods than it was used during the Persian Gulf War and has not been linked to fetal malformations.[264] Because safety in pregnancy has not been completely established, the FDA considers pyridostigmine a Class C drug (ie, the risk cannot be ruled out).

Several studies have sought information on pyridostigmine use under certain conditions: soldiers in combat who frequently take other medications; wounding and blood loss; and use while undergoing anesthesia. The possible interaction of pyridostigmine with other commonly used battlefield medications was reviewed by Keeler.[265] There appears to be no pharmacological basis for expecting adverse interactions between pyridostigmine and commonly used antibiotics, anesthetics, and analgesic agents. In a study[266] of pyridostigmine-treated swine, for example, the autonomic circulatory responses to hemorrhagic shock and resuscitation appeared normal. One potentially important effect of pyridostigmine deserves consideration by field anesthesiologists and anesthetists using muscle relaxants for anesthesia induction: depending on the duration of muscle-relaxant administration, there may be either up- or down-regulation of postsynaptic ACh receptors.[265] Clinical assessment of the status of neuromuscular transmission using a peripheral nerve stimulator should provide a basis for adjusting the dose of both depolarizing and nondepolarizing muscle relaxants to avoid an undesirable duration of muscle paralysis.

Wartime Use

Pyridostigmine was used to protect soldiers from an actual nerve agent threat in the Persian Gulf War. United States and Allied decisions to use pyridostigmine followed established doctrine, taking into account Iraqi capabilities and intentions. Iraq was known to have substantial stocks of sarin and VX, for which pyridostigmine pretreatment is unnecessary. However, Iraq was also known to be interested in acquiring any compounds that might defeat Allied protection, such as the rapidly aging nerve agent, soman. The security of Warsaw Pact stocks of soman, for example, was a growing concern in 1990.

It was also known in 1990 that Iraq had begun large-scale production of GF, a laboratory compound that had not earlier been manufactured in weapons quantity. International restrictions on the purchase of chemical precursors of the better-known nerve agents may have led Iraq to acquire cyclohexyl alcohol, which it was then able to use to produce GF. Very limited data on medical protection against GF were not reassuring. Although GF's aging time with AChE was reported to be relatively long (see Table 5-8), unpublished information from Allied countries suggested that postexposure atropine/oxime therapy in rodents exposed to GF did not protect against the effects of GF poisoning. As confirmed by the later studies shown in Table 5-10, atropine/oxime therapy only provided rodents with PRs in the range of 1.4 to 2.7. The only primate data available showed that rhesus monkeys given pyridostigmine pretreatment and atropine/oxime therapy uniformly survived a 5-LD_{50} challenge with GF.[246] Concern about Iraq's new GF capability, added to its known interest in acquiring soman, made Allied use of pyridostigmine a reasonable course of action.

Pyridostigmine bromide tablets, 30 mg, to be taken every 8 hours, are currently maintained in stocks of US combat units. The compound is packaged in a 21-tablet blister pack called the "nerve agent pyridostigmine pretreatment set," or NAPPS). One nerve agent pyridostigmine treatment set packet provides a week of pyridostigmine pretreatment for one soldier.[182,183]

The decision to begin pretreatment with pyridostigmine is made by commanders at Army division level or the equivalent, based on assessment of the nerve agent threat by their chemical, intelligence, and medical staff officers.[182,183,266] Because of the lack of data on long-term administration of pyridostigmine to healthy adults, current doctrine calls for a maximum pretreatment period of 21 days, with reassessment at frequent intervals of the need for continued pretreatment. A commander may extend the period once, but requires the approval of the first general or flag officer in the chain of command.

Pyridostigmine is poorly absorbed when taken orally; its bioavailability is 5% to 10%.[267] Ideally, two doses of pyridostigmine, taken 8 hours apart, should be administered prior to any risk of nerve agent exposure.[182,183,266] However, some benefit would be expected even if the first pyridostigmine dose is taken an hour before nerve agent exposure. Because excessive AChE inhibition can impair performance, no more than one 30-mg tablet should be taken every 8 hours. If a dose is forgotten or delayed, administration should simply be resumed on an 8-hour schedule as soon as possible, without making up missed doses.

In Operation Desert Storm in 1991, pyridostigmine was administered under combat conditions for the first time to US and Allied soldiers thought to be at risk for nerve agent exposure. Data on safety and possible adverse responses were collected from the unit medical officers caring for the 41,650 soldiers of the XVIII Airborne Corps, who took from 1 to 21 doses of pyridostigmine during January 1991.[268] Most major unit commanders continued the medication for 6 to 7 days, with over 34,000 soldiers taking it for that duration. They were able to perform their missions without any noticeable impairment, similar to findings with peacetime volunteers participating in studies.[253] However, they reported a higher-than- expected incidence of side effects, as noted in Table 5-11.

Gastrointestinal changes included flatus, loose stools, and abdominal cramps that were noticeable but not disabling. These side effects, together with urinary urgency, were of sufficient intensity for many soldiers to associate them with the medication. In most soldiers, these changes were noticed within hours of taking the first tablet. In many, the effects subsided after a day or two of administration, and in others they persisted as long as pyridostigmine was administered. Some units adopted a routine of taking pyridostigmine with meals, which was thought to minimize gastrointestinal symptoms.

Soldiers taking pyridostigmine during this period

TABLE 5-11

EFFECTS OF PYRIDOSTIGMINE PRETREATMENT* ON US SOLDIERS IN THE PERSIAN GULF WAR

Effect	Incidence (%) N=41,650
Gastrointestinal symptoms	≤50
Urinary urgency and frequency	5–30
Headaches, rhinorrhea, diaphoresis, tingling of extremities	< 5
Need for medical visit	< 1
Discontinuation on medical advice	< 0.1

*Dose was 30 mg pyridostigmine bromide, administered orally every 8 hours for 1 to 7 days.
Adapted with permission from: Keeler JR, Hurst CG, Dunn MA. Pyridostigmine used as a nerve agent pretreatment under wartime conditions. *JAMA*. 1991;266:694.

were also experiencing a wide range of other wartime-related stresses, such as repeatedly donning and removing their chemical protective suits and masks in response to alarms, sleep deprivation, and anticipation of actual combat. Because there was no comparable group of soldiers undergoing identical stresses but not administered pyridostigmine, it is not clear to what extent pyridostigmine itself was responsible for the symptoms noted above. The findings are thus a worst-case estimate for effects attributable to pyridostigmine use in wartime.

Among these soldiers, less than 1% sought medical attention for symptoms possibly related to pyridostigmine administration (483 clinic visits). Most of these had gastrointestinal or urinary disturbances. Two soldiers had drug rashes; one of them had urticaria and skin edema that responded to diphenhydramine. Three soldiers had exacerbations of bronchospasm that responded to bronchodilator therapy. Because the units of the XVIII Airborne Corps had been deployed to a desert environment for 5 months before pyridostigmine was used, most soldiers with significant reactive airways disease had already developed symptoms and had been evacuated earlier. The consensus among medical personnel more recently arrived was that they saw more pyridostigmine-related bronchospasm in their soldiers who had not been present in theater as long. Later, many soldiers said that they simply stopped taking the medication and did not report symptoms to their medical officers.[269]

Because of increased exposure to the work-of-breathing requirements of being masked, as well as inhaled dust, smoke, and particles, it was unclear whether pyridostigmine was a major causative factor in those who had bronchospasm at the onset of hostilities. Two soldiers from the XVIII Airborne Corps had significant blood pressure elevations, with diastolic pressures of 110 to 120 mm Hg, that manifested as epistaxis or persistent bleeding after a cut and subsided when pyridostigmine was stopped. Another soldier who took two pyridostigmine tablets together to make up a missed dose experienced mild cholinergic symptoms, self-administered an atropine autoinjector, and recovered fully after several hours. There were no hospitalizations or medical evacuations attributable to pyridostigmine among XVIII Airborne Corps soldiers. In other units, at least two female soldiers, both weighing approximately 45 to 50 kg, noted increased salivation, muscular twitching, severe abdominal cramps, and sweating that prompted medical observation. The symptoms subsided after pyridostigmine was stopped. This experience suggests that cholinergic symptoms may occur in a small number of individuals with relatively low body weight.

In a group of 213 soldiers in Israel who took pyridostigmine (30 mg every 8 h), 75% reported at least one symptom.[270] Included among these symptoms were excessive sweating (9%), nausea (22.1%), abdominal pain (20.4%), diarrhea (6.1%), and urinary frequency (11.3%). In a smaller group of 21 soldiers, pseudocholinesterase (also called butyrocholinesterase, which is discussed later in this chapter) activity was the same in the 12 who were symptomatic and the 9 who were not symptomatic.[40]

An Israeli soldier who developed cholinergic symptoms after taking pyridostigmine was reported to have a genetic variant of serum butyrlcholinesterase.[271] The variant enzyme has low binding affinity for pyridostigmine and other carbamates. The authors of the report suggested that people who are homozygous for the variant enzyme could therefore show exaggerated responses to anticholinesterase compounds. The soldier had a history of prolonged apnea after receiving succinylcholine premedication for surgery. People with similar histories of severe adverse responses to cholinergic medications should be carefully assessed concerning their potential deployability to combat, where they might face either a nerve agent threat or the potential need for resuscitative surgery involving emergency induction of anesthesia[265] using cholinergic medications.

Because pyridostigmine was used during the Persian Gulf War and troops were ordered to take it, and because some returning troops have reported unexplained medical symptoms, the possible role of pyridostigmine in the genesis of these problems has been questioned. A full discussion of this issue lies beyond the scope of this volume. Some studies performed since the Gulf War give reassurance that pyridostigmine used as called for in military doctrine does not by itself give rise to lasting neuromuscular problems such as fatigue, probably the most commonly related complaint. In one human study, a retrospective analysis showed that handgrip strength was not associated with pyridostigmine intake (P = 0.558).[272] In another study using animal muscle cells in culture, ultrastructural alterations seen by electron microscopy after 2 weeks of exposure to low-dose pyridostigmine were reversible following withdrawal of the drug.[273]

On the other hand, a more worrisome concern about pyridostigmine in a battlefield context is the situation in which a soldier who has been on the drug in accordance with pretreatment doctrine needs surgery acutely. Because pyridostigmine is a ChE inhibitor, one might expect that recovery from anesthesia using a neuromuscular blocking agent, such as succinylcholine, would be prolonged, and according to a prospective human study, such is the case.[274] This is of particular concern in those rare patients with mutant BuChE, as mentioned above.[271] Anesthesia providers in a combat zone must anticipate increased time to recovery of normal function, including that of the muscles of respiration, in troops on pyridostigmine, but the magnitude of the increase does not imply that this should affect the decision to go to surgery using these anesthetic agents.

It is now clear that pyridostigmine can be used effectively in large military populations under combat conditions without impairing mission performance. On the other hand, soldiers must have a clear understanding of the threat and the need for this medication. Otherwise, it seems unlikely that they will be willing to accept the associated gastrointestinal and urinary symptoms or to comply with an 8-hour dosage schedule.

Regulatory Status

Before the 1990 Persian Gulf War, the regulatory status of pyridostigmine for nerve agent pretreatment was as an off-label use of an approved medication. Additionally, the 30 mg dose was not approved, since the only on-label indication was for myasthenia gravis and the smallest adult dose was 60 mg. Because of the impending war, in 1991 the FDA waived informed consent for its use to make the best medical treatment available in a specific combat situation.[275,276] The FDA based this waiver on two factors. First, it relied on data from animal studies conducted in both the United States and other NATO countries that found that pyridostigmine increases survival when used as pretreatment against challenge by certain nerve agents (data on efficacy in humans challenged by nerve agents is not experimentally obtained). Second, it determined a long history of safety when the drug was used for approved indications at doses several-fold higher than the doses administered in the military.

The waiver of informed consent was withdrawn in 1992. From then until 2003, the status of pyridostigmine used for nerve agent pretreatment was that of an investigational new drug. This status resulted in the Department of Defense creating an informed consent protocol should the need again arise to order troops to take it. At no time was it illegal for a licensed physician to prescribe pyridostigmine to a patient, whether military or not, wishing to use the drug for this purpose.

In February 2003, on the eve of the invasion of Iraq, the FDA approved pyridostigmine as a nerve agent pretreatment for soman only. This was the first time the FDA applied the "animal rule" to approve a medication for use against chemical or biological warfare agents without Phase 2 and Phase 3 human clinical trial data. Technically, no other nerve agent is covered by this approval. Realistically, however, from a tactical standpoint, knowledge of the specific agent may not be available when a commander must decide whether or not to order troops to take it. Pyridostigmine is not suited for any population group not in imminent danger of exposure to a rapidly aging nerve agent. Despite increased concerns about chemical terrorism, no first-responder agency in the United States has seriously considered ordering responders to take pyridostigmine.

SUMMARY

Nerve agents are the most toxic chemical warfare agents known. They cause effects within seconds and death within minutes. These agents are in the military stockpiles of several countries, but have been used in only one war. They can be manufactured by terrorist groups and have been used in terrorist attacks.

Nerve agents cause biological effects by inhibiting the enzyme AChE, causing an excess of the neurotransmitter to accumulate. Hyperactivity in those organs innervated by cholinergic nerves results, with increased secretions from exocrine glands, hyperactivity of skeletal muscles leading to fatigue and paralysis, hyperactivity of smooth muscles with bronchoconstriction, and CNS changes, including seizure activity and apnea.

Therapy is based on the administration of atropine, which interferes with receptor binding of ACh at muscarinic but not nicotinic receptors, the oxime 2-PAM Cl, which breaks the agent-enzyme bond formed by most agents, and anticonvulsant treatment with diazepam or other benzodiazepines in cases of severe poisoning. Assisted ventilation and other supportive measures are also required in severe poisoning.

For proper protection, it may be necessary to pretreat those at high risk of exposure to a rapidly aging nerve agent, such as soman, with pyridostigmine, a carbamate that reversibly binds a fraction of the body's ChE. This medication now carries FDA approval against soman only.

REFERENCES

1. Koelle GB. Anticholinesterase agents. In: Goodman LS, Gilman A, eds. *The Pharmacological Basis of Therapeutics.* 5th ed. New York, NY: Macmillan; 1975: 445.
2. Davis W. *The Serpent and the Rainbow.* New York: Warner Books Inc; 1985: 36–37.
3. Fraser TR. On the characters, actions, and therapeutic use of the ordeal bean of Calabar. *Edinb Med J.* 1863;9:124–132.
4. Holmstedt B. Structure–activity relationships of the organophosphorus anticholinesterase agents. In: Koelle GB, ed. *Cholinesterases and Anticholinesterase Agents*. Berlin, Germany: Springer Verlag; 1963: 429.
5. Harris R, Paxman J. *A Higher Form of Killing*. New York, NY: Hill and Wang; 1982: 53.
6. Robinson JP. The rise of CB weapons. Vol 1. In: Stockholm International Peace Research Institute, ed. *The Problem of Chemical and Biological Warfare*. New York, NY: Humanities Press; 1971: 71.
7. Koelle GB. Organophosphate poisoning—an overview. *Fundam Appl Toxicol*. 1981;1:129–134.
8. Wilson Kenneth W. Research chemist, Directorate of Medical Research, Edgewood Arsenal, Md. Personal communication, interview, and lectures, 1976.
9. Wills JH, DeArmon IA. *A Statistical Study of the Adamek Report*. Army Chemical Center, Md: Medical Laboratories; 1954. Medical Laboratory Special Report 54.
10. Program Executive Officer, Program Manager for Chemical Demilitarization. *Chemical Stockpile Disposal Program: Final Programmatic Environmental Impact Statement.* Aberdeen Proving Ground, Md: Program Manager for Chemical Demilitarization; January 1988. Publication A3, vol 3.
11. Smith RJ. Army poison gas stockpile raises worries in Kentucky. *Washington Post.* January 22, 1989:A1.
12. Newmark J. The birth of nerve agent warfare: lessons from Syed Abbas Foroutan. *Neurology*. 2004;62:1590–1596.
13. Newark J. Neurologist, Washington, DC. Personal examination of one patient, 2005.
14. Koelle GB. Anticholinesterase agents. In: Goodman LS, Gilman A, eds. *The Pharmacological Basis of Therapeutics*. 4th ed. New York, NY: Macmillan; 1970: 446.
15. Taylor P. Anticholinesterase agents. In: Goodman LS, Gilman A, Hardman JG, Limbird LE, Gilman AG, eds. *Goodman and Gilman's The Pharmacological Basis of Therapeutics*. 10th ed. New York, NY: McGraw-Hill; 2001: 175–191.
16. Koelle GB. Protection of cholinesterase against irreversible inactivation by di-isopropyl fluorophosphate in vitro. *J Pharmacol Exp Ther*. 1946;88:232–237.
17. Koster R. Synergisms and antagonisms between physostigmine and di-isopropyl fluorophosphate in cats. *J Pharmacol Exp Ther.* 1946;88:39–46.

18. Freedman AM, Willis A, Himwich HE. Correlation between signs of toxicity and cholinesterase level of brain and blood during recovery from di-isopropyl fluorophosphate (DFP) poisoning. *Am J Physiol.* 1948;157:80–87.

19. Oberst FW, Christensen MK. Regeneration of erythrocyte and brain cholinesterase activity in rats after sublethal exposures to GB vapor. *J Pharmacol Exp Ther.* 1956;116:216–219.

20. Sidell FR. Soman and sarin: clinical manifestations and treatment of accidental poisoning by organophosphates. *Clin Toxicol.* 1974;7:1–17.

21. US Department of the Army, Office of the Assistant Secretary of the Army for Installations and Environment. *Implementation Guidance Policy for Revised Airborne Exposure Limits for GB, GA, GF, VX, H, HD, or HT.* Washington, DC: DA; June 2004.

22. Hayes WJ. Organic phosphorus pesticides. In: Hayes WJ, ed. *Pesticides Studied in Man.* Baltimore, Md: Williams & Wilkins; 1982: 284–435.

23. Adler M, Filbert MG. Role of butyrylcholinesterase in canine tracheal smooth muscle function. *FEBS Lett.* 1990;267:107–110.

24. Kent KM, Epstein SE, Cooper T, Jacobowitz DM. Cholinergic innervation of the canine and human ventricular conducting system. Anatomic and electrophysiologic correlations. *Circulation.* 1974:50:948–955.

25. Slavikova J, Vlk J, Hlavickova V. Acetylcholinesterase and butyrylcholinesterase activity in the atria of the heart of adult albino rats. *Physiol Bohemoslov.* 1982;31:407–414.

26. Kalow W, Genest K. A method for the detection of atypical forms of human serum cholinesterase; determination of dibucaine numbers. *Can J Biochem Physiol.* 1957;35:339–346.

27. Neitlich HW. Increased plasma cholinesterase activity and succinylcholine resistance: a genetic variant. *J Clin Invest.* 1966;45:380–387.

28. Johns RJ. Familial reduction in red cell cholinesterase. *N Engl J Med.* 1962;267:1344–1348.

29. Wetstone HJ, LaMotta RV. The clinical stability of serum cholinesterase activity. *Clin Chem.* 1965;11:653–663.

30. Sidell FR, Kaminskis A. Temporal intrapersonal physiological variability of cholinesterase activity in human plasma and erythrocytes. *Clin Chem.* 1975;21:1961–1963.

31. Shanor SP, van Hees GR, Baart N, Erdos EEG, Foldes FF. The influence of age and sex on human plasma and red cell cholinesterase. *Am J Med Sci.* 1961;242:357–361.

32. Sidell FR, Kaminskis A. Influence of age, sex, and oral contraceptives on human blood cholinesterase activity. *Clin Chem.* 1975;21:1393–1395.

33. Robertson GS. Serum protein and cholinesterase changes in association with contraceptive pills. *Lancet.* 1967;1:232–235.

34. Whittaker M, Charlier AR, Ramaswamy S. Changes in plasma cholinesterase isoenzyme due to oral contraceptives. *J Reprod Fertil.* 1971;26:373–375.

35. Callaway S, Davies DR, Rutland JP. Blood cholinesterase levels and range of personal variation in a healthy adult population. *Br Med J.* 1951;2:812–816.

36. Augustinsson K. The normal variation of human blood cholinesterase activity. *Acta Physiol Scand.* 1955;35:40–52.

37. Ketchum JS, Sidell FR, Crowell EB Jr, Aghajanian GK, Hayes AH Jr. Atropine, scopolamine, and ditran: comparative pharmacology and antagonists in man. *Psychopharmacologia.*1973;28:121–145.

38. Grob D, Lilienthal JL Jr, Harvey AM, Jones BF. The administration of di-isopropyl fluorophosphate (DFP) to man, I: Effect on plasma and erythrocyte cholinesterase; general systemic effects; use in study of hepatic function and erythropoieses; and some properties of plasma cholinesterase. *Bull Johns Hopkins Hosp.* 1947;81:217–244.

39. Rider JA, Moeller HC, Puletti EJ, Swader JI. Toxicity of parathion, systox, octamethyl pyrophosphoramide, and methyl parathion in man. *Toxicol Appl Pharmacol.* 1969;14:603–611.

40. Hayes GR Jr, Funckes AJ, Hartwell WV. Dermal exposure of human volunteers to parathion. *Arch Environ Health.* 1964;8:829–833.

41. Edson EF. No-effect levels of three organophosphates in the rat, pig, and man. *Food Cosmet Toxicol.* 1964;2:311–316.

42. Rider JA, Puletti EJ, Swader JI. The minimal oral toxicity level for mevinphos in man. *Toxicol Appl Pharmacol.* 1975;32:97–100.

43. Sidell FR, Groff WA. The reactivatibility of cholinesterase inhibited by VX and sarin in man. *Toxicol Appl Pharmacol.* 1974;27:241–252.

44. Sim VM. *Variability of Different Intact Human Skin Sites to the Penetration of VX.* Edgewood Arsenal, Md: Medical Research Laboratory; 1962. Chemical Research and Development Laboratory Report 3122.

45. Grob D, Harvey JC. Effects in man of the anticholinesterase compound sarin (isopropyl methyl phosphonofluoridate). *J Clin Invest.* 1958;37:350–368.

46. Grob D, Harvey AM. The effects and treatment of nerve gas poisoning. *Am J Med.* 1953;14:52–63.

47. Sim VM, Stubbs JL. *VX Percutaneous Studies in Man.* Edgewood Arsenal, Md: Medical Research Laboratory; 1960. Chemical Research and Development Laboratory Report 3015.

48. Craig FN, Cummings EG, Sim VM. Environmental temperature and the percutaneous absorption of a cholinesterase inhibitor, VX. *J Invest Dermatol.* 1977;68:357–361.

49. United Kingdom Ministry of Defence. *Cholinesterase as an Aid in the Early Diagnosis of Nerve Gas Poisoning. Part II: The Variation of Blood Cholinesterase in Man Before and After the Administration of Very Small Quantities of G Vapor by Inhalation.* London, England: Ministry of Defence. Unpublished report.

50. Harvey JC. *Clinical Observations on Volunteers Exposed to Concentrations of GB.* Edgewood Arsenal, Md: Medical Research Laboratory; 1952. Medical Laboratory Research Report 144.

51. Craig AB, Woodson GS. Observations on the effects of exposure to nerve gas. I. Clinical observations and cholinesterase depression. *Am J Med Sci.* 1959;238:13–17.

52. Sidell RF. Clinical considerations in nerve agent intoxication. In: Somani SM, ed. *Chemical Warfare Agents.* San Diego, Calif: Academic Press; 1992: 163.

53. Nohara M, Segawa K. Ocular symptoms due to organophosphorus gas (Sarin) poisoning in Matsumoto. *Br J Ophthalmol.* 1996;80:1023.

54. Namba T, Nolte CT, Jackrel J, Grob D. Poisoning due to organophosphate insecticides. *Am J Med.* 1971;50:475–492.

55. Rengstorff RH. Accidental exposure to sarin: vision effects. *Arch Toxicol.* 1985;56:201–203.

56. Johns RJ. *The Effects of Low Concentrations of GB on the Human Eye.* Edgewood Arsenal, Md: Medical Research Laboratory; 1952. Medical Laboratory Research Report 100.

57. Stewart WC, Madill HD, Dyer AM. Night vision in the miotic eye. *Can Med Assoc J.* 1968;99:1145–1148.

58. Craig AB Jr, Freeman G. *Clinical Observations on Workers Accidentally Exposed to "G" Agents*. Edgewood Arsenal, Md: Medical Research Laboratory; 1953. Medical Laboratory Research Report 154.

59. Rubin LS, Krop S, Goldberg MN. Effect of sarin on dark adaptation in man: mechanism of action. *J Appl Physiol.* 1957;11:445–449.

60. Rubin LS, Goldberg MN. Effect of tertiary and quaternary atropine salts on absolute scotopic threshold changes produced by an anticholinesterase (sarin). *J Appl Physiol.* 1958;12:305–310.

61. Trusov MS. The effect of eserine upon light sensitivity and dark adaptation of the eye [in Russian]. *Oftalmol Zh.* 1962;17:366–371.

62. Moylan-Jones RJ, Thomas DP. Cyclopentolate in treatment of sarin miosis. *Br J Pharmacol.* 1973;48:309–313.

63. United Kingdom Ministry of Defence. An evaluation of the functional changes produced by the inhalation of GB vapour. London, England: Ministry of Defence. Unpublished report.

64. United Kingdom Ministry of Defence. *Air-way Resistance Changes in Men Exposed to GB Vapour*. London, England: Ministry of Defence. Unpublished report.

65. Clements JA, Moore JC, Johnson RP, Lynott J. *Observations on Airway Resistance in Men Given Low Doses of GB by Chamber Exposure.* Edgewood Arsenal, Md: Medical Research Laboratory; 1952. Medical Laboratory Research Report 122.

66. Ward JR. Case report: Exposure to a nerve gas. In: Whittenberger JL, ed. *Artificial Respiration: Theory and Applications.* New York, NY: Harper & Row; 1962: 258–265.

67. De Candole CA, Douglas WW, Evans CL, et al. The failure of respiration in death by anticholinesterase poisoning. *Br J Pharmacol Chemother*. 1953;8:466–475.

68. United Kingdom Ministry of Defence. *The Predominantly Peripheral Effects of Acute GB Poisoning in Anaesthetized Animals.* London, England: Ministry of Defence. Unpublished report.

69. Johnson RP, Gold AJ, Freeman G. Comparative lung-airway resistance and cardiovascular effects in dogs and monkeys following parathion and sarin intoxication. *Am J Physiol.* 1958;192:581–584.

70. Fredriksson T, Hansson C, Holmstedt B. Effects of sarin in the anaesthetized and unanaesthetized dog following inhalation. Percutaneous absorption and intravenous infusion. *Arch Int Pharmacodyn Ther*. 1960;126:288–302.

71. Wright PG. An analysis of the central and peripheral components of respiratory failure produced by anticholinesterase poisoning in the rabbit. *J Physiol.* 1954;126:52–70.

72. Rickett DL, Glenn JF, Beers ET. Central respiratory effects versus neuromuscular actions of nerve agents. *Neurotoxicology*. 1986;7:225–236.

73. Kluwe WM, Chinn JC, Feder P, Olson C, Joiner R. Efficacy of pyridostigmine pretreatment against acute soman intoxication in a primate model. In: *Proceedings of the Sixth Medical Chemical Defense Bioscience Review*. Aberdeen Proving Ground, Md: US Army Medical Research Institute for Chemical Defense; 1987: 227–234. Report AD B121516.

74. Firemark H, Barlow CF, Roth LJ. The penetration of 2-PAM-C14 into brain and the effect of cholinesterase inhibitors on its transport. *J Pharmacol Exp Ther*. 1964;145:252–265.

75. Lipp JA. Cerebral electrical activity following soman administration. *Arch Int Pharmacodyn Ther*. 1968;175:161–169.

76. Carpentier P, Delamanche IS, LeBert M, Blanchet G, Bouchaud C. Seizure-related opening of the blood-brain barrier induced by soman: possible correlation with the acute neuropathology observed in poisoned rats. *Neurotoxicology.* 1990;11:493–508.

77. McDonough JH, Shih TM. Neuropharmacological mechanisms of nerve agent-induced seizure and neuropathology. *Neurosci Biobehav Rev.* 1997;21:559–579.

78. Kawana N, Ishimatsu S, Kanda K. Psycho-physiological effects of the terrorist sarin attack on the Tokyo subway system. *Mil Med.* 2001;166(12 suppl):23–26.

79. Romano JA, McDonough JH, Sheridan R, Sidell FR. Health effects of low-level exposure to nerve agents. In: Somani SM, Romano JA, eds. *Chemical Warfare Agents: Toxicity at Low Levels.* Boca Raton, Fla: CRC Press; 2001:1–24.

80. McDonough JH. Performance impacts of nerve agents and their pharmacological countermeasures. *Mil Psychol.* 2002;14(2):93-119.

81. Brown EC Jr. *Effects of G Agents on Man: Clinical Observations.* Edgewood Arsenal, Md: Medical Laboratory; 1948. Medical Division Report 158.

82. Craig AB Jr, Cornblath M. *Further Clinical Observations in Workers Accidentally Exposed to G Agents.* Edgewood Arsenal, Md: Medical Research Laboratory; 1953. Medical Laboratory Research Report 234.

83. Brody BB, Gammill JF. *Seventy-Five Cases of Accidental Nerve Gas Poisoning at Dugway Proving Ground.* Dugway Proving Ground, Utah: Medical Investigational Branch; 1954. Medical Investigational Branch Special Report 5.

84. Bowers MB, Goodman E, Sim VM. Some behavioral changes in man following anticholinesterase administration. *J Nerv Ment Dis.* 1964;138:383–389.

85. United Kingdom Ministry of Defence. Psychological effects of a G-agent on men. London, England: Ministry of Defence. Unpublished report.

86. United Kingdom Ministry of Defence. Psychological effects of a G-agent on men: 2nd report. London, England: Ministry of Defence. Unpublished report.

87. United Kingdom Ministry of Defence. The effects of a single exposure to GB (sarin) on human physical performance. London, England: Ministry of Defence. Unpublished report.

88. United Kingdom Ministry of Defence. The effects of a minor exposure to GB on military efficiency. London, England: Ministry of Defence. Unpublished report.

89. Brimblecombe RW, Buxton DA. Behavioural actions of anticholinergic drugs. *Prog Brain Res.* 1972;36:115–126.

90. Voytko ML. Cognitive functions of the basal forebrain cholinergic system in monkeys: memory or attention? *Behav Brain Res.* 1996;75:13–25.

91. Bartus RT, Dean RL 3rd, Beer B, Lippa AS. The cholinergic hypothesis of geriatric memory dysfunction. *Science.* 1982;217:408–417.

92. Davis KL, Berger PA, Hollister LE, Barchas JD. Cholinergic involvement in mental disorders. *Life Sci.* 1978;22:1865–1871.

93. Janowsky DS, Risch SC, Gillin JC. Adrenergic-cholinergic balance and the treatment of affective disorders. *Prog Neuropsychopharmacol Biol Psychiatry.* 1983;7:297–307.

94. Janowsky DS, Overstreet DH. Cholinergic dysfunction in depression. *Pharmacol Toxicol.* 1990;66(suppl 3):100–111.

95. Baghdoyan HA, Monaco AP, Rodrigo-Angulo ML, Assens F, McCarley RW, Hobson JA. Microinjection of neostigmine into the pontine reticular formation of cats enhances desynchronized sleep signs. *J Pharmacol Exp Ther.* 1984;231:173–180.

96. George R, Haslett WL, Jenden DJ. A cholinergic mechanism in the brainstem reticular formation: induction of paradoxical sleep. *Int J Neuropharmacol.* 1964;3:541–552.

97. Gnadt JW, Pegram GV. Cholinergic brainstem mechanisms of REM sleep in the rat. *Brain Res.* 1986;384:29–41.

98. Hobson JA. Sleep and dreaming: induction and mediation of REM sleep by cholinergic mechanisms. *Curr Opin Neurobiol.* 1992;2:759–763.

99. Gillin JC, Sitaram N, Mendelson WB, Wyatt RJ. Physostigmine alters onset but not duration of REM sleep in man. *Psychopharmacol (Berl).* 1978;58:111–114.

100. Gnadt JW, Atwood CW, Meighen GA, Pegram GV. Di-isopropyl-fluorophosphate (DFP): acute toxicity and sleep. *Neurotoxicology.* 1986;7:165–171.

101. Gnadt JW, Pegram GV, Baxter JF. The acetylcholinesterase inhibitor di-isopropyl-fluorophosphate increases REM sleep in rats. *Physiol Behav.* 1985;35:911–916.

102. Sitaram N, Wyatt RJ, Dawson S, Gillin JG. REM sleep induction by physostigmine infusion during sleep. *Science.* 1976;191:1281–1283.

103. Grob D, Harvey AM, Langworthy OR, Lilienthal JL Jr. The administration of di-isopropyl fluorophosphate (DFP) to man, III: effect on the central nervous system with special reference to the electrical activity of the brain. *Bull Johns Hopkins Hosp.* 1947;81:257–266.

104. Grob D. The manifestations and treatment of poisoning due to nerve gas and other organic phosphate anticholinesterase compounds. *AMA Arch Intern Med.* 1956;98:221–239.

105. Glenn JF, Hinman DJ, McMaster SB. Electroencephalographic correlates of nerve agent poisoning. In: Dun NJ, Perlman L, eds. *Neurobiology of Acetylcholine.* New York, NY: Plenum Press; 1987:503–534.

106. Koplovitz I, Skvorak JP. Electrocorticographic changes during generalized convulsive status epilepticus in soman intoxicated rats. *Epilepsy Res.* 1998;30:159–164.

107. Shih TM, Duniho SM, McDonough JH. Control of nerve agent-induced seizures is critical for neuroprotection and survival. *Toxicol Appl Pharmacol.* 2003;188:69–80.

108. Holmes JH, Gaon MD. Observations on acute and multiple exposure to anticholinesterase agents. *Trans Am Clin Climatol Assoc.* 1956;68:86–101.

109. Metcalf DR, Holmes JH. EEG, psychological, and neurological alterations in humans with organophosphorus exposure. *Ann N Y Acad Sci.* 1969;160:357–365.

110. Sekijima Y, Morita H, Shindo M, Okudera H, Shibata T. A case of severe sarin poisoning in the sarin attack at Matsumoto—one-year follow-up on the clinical findings and laboratory data [in Japanese]. *Rinsho Shinkeigaku [Clinical Neurology].* 1995;35:1241–1245.

111. Shih TM, Koviak TA, Capacio BR. Anticonvulsants for poisoning by the organophosphorus compound soman: pharmacological mechanisms. *Neurosci Biobehav Rev.* 1991;15:349–362.

112. Levin HS, Rodnitzky RL. Behavioral effects of organophosphate pesticides in man. *Clin Toxicol.* 1976;9:391–403.

113. Karczmar AG. Acute and long lasting central actions of organophosphorus agents. *Fundam Appl Toxicol.* 1984;4:S1–S17.

114. Duffy FH, Burchfiel JL, Bartels PH, Gaon M, Sim VM. Long-term effects of an organophosphate upon the human electroencephalogram. *Toxicol Appl Pharmacol.* 1979;47:161–176.

115. Petras JM. Soman neurotoxicity. *Fundam Appl Toxicol.* 1981;1:242.

116. Lemercier G, Carpentier P, Sentenac-Roumanou H, Morelis P. Histological and histochemical changes in the central nervous system of the rat poisoned by an irreversible anticholinesterase organophosphorus compound. *Acta Neuropathol (Berl).* 1983;61:123–129.

117. McLeod CG Jr, Singer AW, Harrington DG. Acute neuropathology in soman poisoned rats. *Neurotoxicology*. 1984;5:53–57.

118. Thornton KR, Fukuyama GS. *Morphological Changes in the Brain of* M. Mulatta *Treated for VX Poisoning with Atropine, Metaraminol and P2S.* Suffield Technical Paper No. 228; Canada: 1961.

119. Thornton KR, Brigden EG. *Morphological Changes in the Brains of Guinea Pigs Following VX Poisoning.* Suffield Technical Paper No. 230; Canada: 1962.

120. Petras JM. Neurology and neuropathology of soman-induced brain injury: an overview. *J Exp Anal Behav*. 1994;61:319–329.

121. McDonough JH Jr, Hackley BE Jr, Cross R, Samson F, Nelson S. Brain regional glucose use during soman-induced seizures. *Neurotoxicology*. 1983;4:203–210.

122. McDonough JH Jr, McLeod CG Jr, Nipwoda T. Direct microinjection of soman or VX into the amygdala produces repetitive limbic convulsions and neuropathology. *Brain Res*. 1987;435:123–137.

123. Deshpande SS, Smith CD, Filbert MG. Assessment of primary neuronal culture as a model for soman-induced neurotoxicity and effectiveness of memantine as a neuroprotective drug. *Arch Toxicol*. 1995;14:384–390.

124. Lallement G, Pernot-Marino I, Baubichon D, Burckhart MF, Carpentier P, Blanchet G. Modulation of soman-induced neuropathology with an anticonvulsant regimen. *Neuroreport*. 1994;5:2265–2268.

125. McDonough JH Jr, Dochterman LW, Smith CD, Shih TM. Protection against nerve agent-induced neuropathology, but not cardiac pathology, is associated with the anticonvulsant action of drug treatment. *Neurotoxicology*. 1995;15:123–132.

126. Lallement G, Clarencon D, Masqueliez C, Baubichon D, Galonnier M, Burckhart MF, Peoc'h M, Mestries JC. Nerve agent poisoning in primates: antilethal, anti-epileptic and neuroprotective effects of GK-11. *Arch Toxicol*. 1998;72:84–92.

127. Lallement G, Clarencon D, Galonnier M, Baubichon D, Burckhart MF, Peoc'h M. Acute soman poisoning in primates neither pretreated nor receiving immediate therapy: value of gacyclidine (GK-11) in delayed medical support. *Arch Toxicol*. 1999;73:115–122.

128. Martin LJ, Doebler JA, Shih TM, Anthony A. Protective effect of diazepam pretreatment on soman-induced brain lesion formation. *Brain Res*. 1985;325:287–289.

129. Hayward IJ, Wall HG, Jaax NK, Wade JV, Marlow DD, Nold JB. Decreased brain pathology in organophosphate-exposed rhesus monkeys following benzodiazepine therapy. *J Neurol Sci*. 1990;98:99–106.

130. Capacio BR, Shih TM. Anticonvulsant actions of anticholinergic drugs in soman poisoning. *Epilepsia*. 1991;32:604–615.

131. McDonough JH Jr, Jaax NK, Crowley RA, Mays MZ, Modrow HE. Atropine and/or diazepam therapy protects against soman-induced neural and cardiac pathology. *Fundam Appl Toxicol*. 1989;13:256–276.

132. Clement JG, Broxup B. Efficacy of diazepam and avizafone against soman-induced neuropathology in brain of rats. *Neurotoxicol*. 1993;14:485–504.

133. Anderson DR, Harris LW, Bowersox SL, Lennox WJ, Anders JC. Efficacy of injectable anticholinergic drugs against soman-induced convulsive/subconvulsive activity. *Drug Chem Toxicol*. 1994;17:139–148.

134. McDonough JH Jr, Shih TM. Pharmacological modulation of soman-induced seizures. *Neurosci Biobehav Rev*. 1993;17:203–215.

135. Philippens IH, Melchers BP, DeGroot DM, Wolthius OL. Behavioral performance, brain histology, and EEG sequela after immediate combined atropine/diazepam treatment of soman-intoxicated rats. *Pharmacol Biochem Behav*. 1992;42:711–719.

136. Raveh L, Weissman BA, Cohen G, Alkalay D, Rabinovitz I, Sonego H, Brandeis R. Caramiphen and scopolamine prevent soman-induced brain damage and cognitive dysfunction. *Neurotoxicol.* 2002;23:7–17.

137. Raveh L, Brandeis R, Gilat E, Cohen G, Alkalay D, Rabinovitz I, Sonego H, Weissman BA. Anticholinergic and antiglutamatergic agents protect against soman-induced brain damage and cognitive dysfunction. *Toxicol Sci.* 2003;75:108–116.

138. Raffaele K, Hughey D, Wenk G, Olton D, Modrow H, McDonough J. Long-term behavioral changes in rats following organophosphonate exposure. *Pharmacol Biochem Behav.* 1987;27:407–412.

139. McDonough JH Jr, Smith RF, Smith CD. Behavioral correlates of soman-induced neuropathology: deficits in DRL acquisition. *Neurobehav Toxicol Teratol.* 1986;8:179–187.

140. Modrow HE, Jaax NK. Effect of soman exposure on the acquisition of an operant alternation task. *Pharmacol Biochem Behav.* 1989;32:49–53.

141. Shorvon SD. *Status Epilepticus: Its Clinical Features and Treatment in Children and Adults.* Cambridge, England: Cambridge University Press; 1994: 195–213.

142. Nozaki H, Aikawa N, Fujishima S, et al. A case of VX poisoning and the difference from sarin. *Lancet.* 1995;346:698–699.

143. Himuro K, Murayama S, Nishiyama K, et al. Distal sensory axonopathy after sarin intoxication. *Neurology.* 1998;51:1195–1197.

144. Christensen MK, Cresthull P, Crook JW, Oberst FW, Ross RS, Umland CW 2nd. Resuscitation of dogs poisoned by inhalation of the nerve gas GB. *Mil Med.* 1956;119:377–386.

145. Pazdernik TL, Cross RS, Giesler M, Samson FE, Nelson SR. Changes in local cerebral glucose utilization induced by convulsants. *Neuroscience.* 1985;14:823–835.

146. Kiss Z, Fazekas T. Arrhythmias in organophosphate poisoning. *Acta Cardiol.* 1979;34:323–330.

147. Hassler CR, Moutvic RR, Hamlin RL. Studies of the action of chemical agents on the heart. In: *Proceedings of the Sixth Medical Chemical Defense Bioscience Review.* Aberdeen Proving Ground, Md: US Army Medical Research Institute for Chemical Defense; 1987: 551–554.

148. Hassler CR, Moutvic RR, Hobson DW, et al. Long-term arrhythmia analysis of primates pretreated with pyridostigmine, challenged with soman, and treated with atropine and 2-PAM. In: *Proceedings of the 1989 Medical Chemical Defense Bioscience Review.* Aberdeen Proving Ground, Md: US Army Medical Research Institute for Chemical Defense; 1989: 479–482.

149. Ludomirsky A, Klein HO, Sarelli P, et al. Q-T prolongation and polymorphous ("torsade de pointes") ventricular arrhythmias associated with organophosphorus insecticide poisoning. *Am J Cardiol.* 1982;49:1654–1658.

150. Allon N, Rabinovitz I, Manistersky E, Weissman BA, Grauer E. Acute and long-lasting cardiac changes following a single whole-body exposure to sarin vapor in rats. *Toxicol Sci.* 2005; 87:385–390.

151. Singer AW, Jaax NK, Graham JS, McLeod CG Jr. Cardiomyopathy in soman and sarin intoxicated rats. *Toxicol Lett.* 1987;36:243–249.

152. Baze WB. Soman-induced morphological changes: an overview in the non-human primate. *J Appl Toxicol.* 1993;13:173–177.

153. Britt JO Jr, Martin JL, Okerberg CV, Dick EJ Jr. Histopathologic changes in the brain, heart, and skeletal muscle of rhesus macaques, ten days after exposure to soman (an organophosphorus nerve agent). *Comp Med.* 2000;50:133–139.

154. Tryphonas l, Veinot JP, Clement JG. Early histopathologic and ultrastructural changes in the heart of Sprague-Dawley rats following administration of soman. *Toxicol Pathol*. 1996; 24:190–198.

155. Ludomirsky A, Klein HO, Sarelli P, et al. Q-T prolongation and polymorphous ("torsade de pointes") ventricular arrhythmias associated with organophosphorus insecticide poisoning. *Am J Cardiol*. 1982;49:1654–1658

156. Kunkel AM, O'Leary JF, Jones AH. *Atropine-Induced Ventricular Fibrillation During Cyanosis Caused by Organophosphorus Poisoning*. Edgewood Arsenal, Md: Medical Research Laboratory; 1973. Edgewood Arsenal Technical Report 4711.

157. Bellet S. *Clinical Disorders of the Heart Beat*. 2nd ed. Philadelphia, Pa: Lea & Febiger; 1963: 110.

158. Ganendran A. Organophosphate insecticide poisoning and its management. Anaesth Intensive Care. 1974;2:361–368.

159. Willems J, Vermeire P, Rolly G. Some observations on severe human poisonings with organophosphate pesticides. *Arch Toxicol*. 1971;28:182–191.

160. Davies DR, Green AL, Willey GL. 2-Hydroxyiminomethyl-N-methylpyridinium methanesulphonate and atropine in the treatment of severe organophosphate poisoning. *Br J Pharmacol Chemother*. 1959;14:5–8.

161. Sidell FR, Mershon MM, Savola RH, Schwartz HN, Wiles JS, McShane WP. *Treatment of Percutaneous VX Intoxication in Rabbits Under Conditions Simulating Self-Therapy in the Field*. Edgewood Arsenal, Md: Medical Research Laboratory. Technical Memorandum 114–22; 1968.

162. Ainsworth M, Shephard RJ. The intrabronchial distribution of soluble vapours at selected rates of gas flow. In: Davies CN, ed. *Inhaled Particles and Vapours*. New York, NY: Pergamon Press; 1961: 233–247.

163. Oberst FW. Factors affecting inhalation and retention of toxic vapors. In: Davies CN, ed. *Inhaled Particles and Vapours*. New York, NY: Pergamon Press; 1961: 249–265.

164. Oberst FW, Koon WS, Christensen MK, Crook JW, Cresthull P, Freeman G. Retention of inhaled sarin vapor and its effect on red blood cell cholinesterase activity in man. *Clin Pharmacol Ther*. 1968;9:421–427.

165. Okumura T, Takasu N, Ishimatsu S, et al. Report on 640 victims of the Tokyo subway attack. *Ann Emerg Med*.1996;28:129–135.

166. Fraser TR. An experimental research on the antagonism between the actions of physostigma and atropia. *Trans R Soc Edinb*. 1870;26:259–713.

167. Wills JH. Pharmacological antagonists of the anticholinesterase agents. In: Koelle GB, ed. *Cholinesterase and Anticholinesterase Agents*. Berlin, Germany: Springer Verlag; 1963: 897.

168. Vojvodic VB, Maksimovic M. Absorption and excretion of pralidoxime in man after intramuscular injection of PAM-2Cl and various cholinolytics. *Eur J Clin Pharmacol*. 1972;5:58-61.

169. Vojvodic V, Jovic R, Rosic N, Vojvodic M. Effect of a mixture of atropine, benactyzine, and pralidoxime mixture on the body and elements of fighting capability in volunteers [in Serbian]. *Vojnosanit Pregl*. 1972;29:103–107.

170. McDonough JH Jr, Zoeffel LD, McMonagle J, Copeland TL, Smith CD, Shih TM. Anticonvulsant treatment of nerve agent seizures: anticholinergics versus diazepam in soman-intoxicated guinea pigs. *Epilepsy Res*. 2000;38:1–14.

171. Jovic R, Milosevic M. Effective doses of some cholinolytics in the treatment of anticholinesterase poisoning. *Eur J Pharmacol*. 1970;12:85–93.

172. Bajgar J, Fusek J, Vachek J. Treatment and prophylaxis against nerve agent poisoning. *ASA Newsletter*. 1994;99;10–11.

173. Kassa J, Bajgar J. The influence of pharmacological pretreatment on efficacy of HI-6 oxime in combination with benactyzine in soman poisoning in rats. *Hum Exp Toxicol*. 1996;15;383–388.

174. Comstock CC, Krop S. German First Aid Kits for Treatment of Tabun (GA) Casualties. Edgewood Arsenal, Md: US Army Chemical Center; 1948. Medical Division Report No. 151.

175. Eddleston M, Buckley NA, Checketts H, et al. Speed of initial atropinisation in significant organophosphorus pesticide poisoning—a systematic comparison of recommended regimens. *J Toxicol Clin Toxicol*. 2004;42:865–875.

176. Eddleston M, Dawson A, Karalliedde L, et al. Early management after self-poisoning with an organophosphorus or carbamate pesticide—a treatment protocol for junior doctors. *Crit Care*. 2004;8:R391–R397.

177. Robinson S, Magenis TP, Minter DI, Harper H. The effects of varying doses of atropine on temperature regulation of men and dogs. In: Robinson S, ed. *The Physiological Effects of Atropine and Potential Atropine Substitutes*. Edgewood Arsenal, Md: Medical Research Laboratories; 1953. Medical Laboratory Contract Report 15.

178. Sidell FR, Markis JE, Groff W, Kaminskis A. Enhancement of drug absorption after administration by an automatic injector. *J Pharmacokinet Biopharm*. 1974;2:197–210.

179. Vale JA, Meredith TJ, Heath A. High dose atropine in organophosphorus poisoning. *Postgrad Med J*. 1990;66:878.

180. Chew LS, Chee KT, Yeeo JM, Jayaratnam FJ. Continuous atropine infusion in the management of organophosphorus insecticide poisoning. *Singapore Med J*. 1971;12:80–85.

181. LeBlanc FN, Benson BE, Gilg AD. A severe organophosphate poisoning requiring the use of an atropine drip. *J Toxicol Clin Toxicol*. 1986;24:69–76.

182. US Departments of the Army, the Navy, the Air Force, and Commandant, Marine Corps. *Field Manual: Treatment of Chemical Agent Casualties and Conventional Military Chemical Injuries*. Washington, DC: DA, DN, DAF, USMC; 1995. Field Manual 8-285, NAVMED P-5041, AFJMAN 44-149, Fleet Marine Force Manual 11-11.

183. Chemical Casualty Care Division, US Army Medical Research Institute of Chemical Defense. *Medical Management of Chemical Casualties Handbook*. 3rd ed. Aberdeen Proving Ground, Md: USAMRICD; 2000: 102–135.

184. Chemical-Biological Medical Systems, Joint Program Executive Office for Chemical-Biological Defense, Official Web site. Available at: http://www.jpeocbd.osd.mil. Accessed September 23, 2005.

185. Wilson IB. Acetylcholinesterase, XI. Reversibility of tetraethyl pyrophosphate. *J Biol Chem*. 1951;190:111–117.

186. Wilson IB, Ginsburg S. A powerful reactivator of alkyl phosphate-inhibited acetylcholinesterase. *Biochim Biophys Acta*. 1955;18:168–170.

187. Dawson RM. Review of oximes available for treatment of nerve agent poisoning. *J Appl Toxicol*.1994;14:317–331.

188. Quinby GE. Further therapeutic experience with pralidoximes in organic phosphorus poisoning. *JAMA*. 1964;187:202–206.

189. Quinby GE, Clappison GB. Parathion poisoning. A nearfatal pediatric case treated with 2-pyridine aldoxime methiodide (2-PAM). *Arch Environ Health*. 1961;3:538–542.

190. Quinby GE, Loomis TA, Brown HW. Oral occupational parathion poisoning treated with 2-PAM iodide (2-pyridine aldoxime methiodide). *N Engl J Med*. 1963;268:639–643.

191. Rosen FS. Toxic hazards: parathion. *N Engl J Med*. 1960;262:1243–1244.

192. Jacobziner H, Raybin HW. Parathion poisoning successfully treated with 2-PAM (pralidoxime chloride). *N Engl J Med*. 1961;265:436–437.

193. Funckes AJ. Treatment of severe parathion poisoning with 2-pyridine aldoxine methiodide (2-PAM); report of a case. *Arch Environ Health*. 1960;1:404–406.

194. Durham WF, Hayes WJ Jr. Organic phosphorus poisoning and its therapy. With special reference to modes of action and compounds that reactivate inhibited cholinesterase. *Arch Environ Health*. 1962;5:21–47.

195. Sundwall A. Minimum concentrations of N-methylpyridinium-2-aldoxime methane sulphonate (P2S) which reverse neuromuscular block. *Biochem Pharmacol*. 1961;8:413–417.

196. O'Leary JF, Kunkel AM, Jones AH. Efficacy and limitations of oxime-atropine treatment of organophosphorus anticholinesterase poisoning. *J Pharmacol Exp Ther*. 1961;132:50–57.

197. Calesnick B, Christensen, Richter M. Human toxicity of various oximes. 2-Pyridine aldoxime methyl chloride, its methane sulfonate salt, and 1,1'-trimethylenebis-(4-formylpyridinium chloride). *Arch Environ Health*. 1967;15:599–608.

198. Sidell FR, Groff WA. Intramuscular and intravenous administration of small doses of 2-pyridinium aldoxime methochloride to man. *J Pharm Sci*. 1971;60:1224–1228.

199. Swartz RD, Sidell FR. Renal tubular secretion of pralidoxime in man. *Proc Soc Exp Biol Med*. 1974;146:419–424.

200. Swartz RD, Sidell FR. Effects of heat and exercise on the elimination of pralidoxime in man. *J Clin Pharmacol Ther*. 1973;14:83–89.

201. Josselson J, Sidell FR. Effect of intravenous thiamine on pralidoxime kinetics. *Clin Pharmacol Ther*. 1978;24:95–100.

202. Josselson J, Sidell FR. *Dose-Response Effects of Intravenous Thiamine Hydrochloride on Pralidoxime Pharmacokinetics in Man*. Edgewood Arsenal, Md: Biomedical Laboratory; 1977. EB-TR 116117.

203. Jeevarathinam K, Ghosh AK, Srinivasan A, Das Gupta S. Pharmacokinetics of pralidoxime chloride and its correlation to therapeutic efficacy against diisopropyl fluorophosphate intoxication in rats. *Pharmazie*. 1988;43:114–115.

204. Quinby GE. Further therapeutic experience with pralidoximes in organic phosphorus poisoning. *JAMA*. 1964;187:202–206.

205. Kewitz H, Nachmansohn D. A specific antidote against lethal alkyl phosphate intoxication, IV. Effects in brain. *Arch Biochem Biophys*. 1957;66:271–283.

206. Loomis T. Distribution and excretion of pyridine-2-aldoxime methiodide (PAM), atropine and PAM in sarin poisoning. *Toxicol Appl Pharmacol*. 1963;5:489–499.

207. Jager BV, Stagg GN, Green N, Jager L. Studies on distribution and disappearance of pyridine-2-aldoxime methiodide (PAM) and of diacetyl monoxime (DAM) in man and in experimental animals. *Bull Johns Hopkins Hosp*. 1958;102:225–234.

208. De la Manche IS, Verge DE, Bouchard C, Coq H, Sentenac-Roumanou H. Penetration of oximes across the blood brain barrier. A histochemical study of the cerebral cholinesterase reactivation. *Experientia*. 1979;35:531–532.

209. Fleisher JH. Directorate of Medical Research, Biomedical Laboratory, Edgewood Arsenal, Md. Personal communication, 1970s.

210. Von Bredow J. Major, Medical Service Corps, US Army; Directorate of Medical Research, Biomedical Laboratory, Edgewood Arsenal, Md. Personal communication, 1970s.

211. McDonough JH Jr, McMonagle J, Copeland T, Zoeffel D, Shih TM. Comparative evaluation of benzodiazepines for control of soman-induced seizures. *Arch Toxicol*. 1999;73:473–478.

212. Lipp JA. Effect of benzodiazepine derivatives upon soma-induced seizure activity and convulsions in the monkey. *Acta Int Pharmacodyn Ther*. 1973;202:241–251.

213. Rump S, Grudzinska E, Edelwejn Z. Effects of diazepam on abnormalities of bioelectrical activity of the rabbit's brain due to fluostigmine. *Act Nerv Super (Praha)*. 1972;14:176–177.

214. Rump S, Grudzinska E, Edelwejn Z. Effects of diazepam on epileptiform patterns of bioelectrical activity of the rabbit's brain induced by fluostigmine. *Neuropharmacology*. 1973;12:813–817.

215. Wills JH, McNamara BP, Fine EA. Ventricular fibrillation in delayed treatment of TEPP poisoning. *Fed Proc*. 1950;9:136.

216. Valero A, Golan D. Accidental organic phosphorus poisoning: the use of propranolol to counteract vagolytic cardiac effects of atropine. *Isr J Med Sci*. 1967;3:582–584.

217. Rotenberg JS, Newmark J. Nerve agent attacks on children: diagnosis and management. *Pediatrics*. 2003;112:648–658.

218. Foroutan SA. Medical notes on chemical warfare, part I. *Kowsar Med J*. 1996;1:91–97.

219. Foroutan SA. Medical notes on chemical warfare, part II. *Kowsar Med J*. 1997;1:159–177.

220. Foroutan SA. Medical notes on chemical warfare, part III. *Kowsar Med J*. 1997;2:69–83.

221. Foroutan SA. Medical notes on chemical warfare, part IV. *Kowsar Med J*. 1997; 2:141–151.

222. Foroutan SA. Medical notes on chemical warfare, part V. *Kowsar Med J*. 1997;2:221–227.

223. Foroutan SA. Medical notes on chemical warfare, part VI. *Kowsar Med J*. 1998;2:289–301.

224. Foroutan SA. Medical notes on chemical warfare, part VII. *Kowsar Med J*. 1998;3:61–68.

225. Foroutan SA. Medical notes on chemical warfare, part IX. *Kowsar Med J*. 1998;2:211–221.

226. Foroutan SA. Medical notes on chemical warfare, part X. *Kowsar Med J*. 1999;3:278–290.

227. Foroutan SA. Medical notes on chemical warfare, part XI. *Kowsar Med J*. 1999;4:64–67.

228. Okumura T, Suzuki K, Fukuda A, et al. The Tokyo subway sarin attack: disaster management, part 2: hospital response. *Acad Emerg Med*. 1998; 5:618–624.

229. Ohbu S, Yamashina A, Takasu N, et al. Sarin poisoning on Tokyo subway. *Southern Med J*. 1997;90:587–593.

230. Okudera H, Morita H, Iwashita T, et al. Unexpected nerve gas exposure in the city of Matsumoto: report of rescue activity in the first sarin gas terrorism. *Am J Emerg Med*. 1997;15:527–528.

231. Kato T, Hamanaka T. Ocular signs and symptoms caused by exposure to sarin gas. *Am J Ophthalmol*. 1996;121:209–210.

232. Morita H, Yanagisawa N, Nakajima T, et al. Sarin poisoning in Matsumoto, Japan. *Lancet*. 1995;346:290–293.

233. Yokoyama K, Yamada A, Mimura N. Clinical profiles of patients with sarin poisoning after the Tokyo subway attack. *Am J Med*. 1996;100:586.

234. Suzuki J, Kohno T, Tsukagosi M, Furuhata T, Yamazaki K. Eighteen cases exposed to sarin in Matsumoto, Japan. *Internal Med*. 1997;36:466–470.

235. Suzuki T, Morita H, Ono K, Maekawa K, Nagai R, Yazaki Y. Sarin poisoning in Tokyo subway. *Lancet.* 1995;345:980.

236. Nozaki H, Aikawa N, Shinozawa Y, et al. Sarin poisoning in Tokyo subway. *Lancet*. 1995;345:980–981.

237. Takashima Y. Japanese Self-Defense Forces. Personal communication, 1996.

238. Nishiwaki Y, Maekawa K, Ogawa Y, Asukai N, Minami M, Omae K. Effects of sarin on the nervous system in rescue team staff members and police officers 3 years after the Tokyo subway sarin attack. *Environ Health Perspect*. 2001; 109:1169–1173

239. Murata K, Araki S, Yokoyama K, et al. Asymptomatic sequelae to acute sarin poisoning in the central and autonomic nervous system 6 months after the Tokyo subway attack. *J Neurol*. 1997;244:601–606.

240. Okudera H. Clinical features on nerve gas terrorism in Matsumoto. *J Clin Neurosci*. 2002;9:17–21.

241. Yokoyama K, Araki S, Murata K, et al. Chronic neurobehavioral and central and autonomic nervous system effects of Tokyo subway sarin poisoning. *J Physiol Paris*. 1998;92:317–323.

242. Nakajima T, Ohta S, Fukushima Y, Yanagisawa N. Sequelae of sarin toxicity at one and three years after exposure in Matsumoto, Japan. *J Epidemiol*. 1999; 9:337–343.

243. Kawada T, Katsumata M, Suzuki H, et al. Insomnia as a sequela of sarin toxicity several years after exposure in Tokyo subway trains. *Percept Mot Skills*. 2005;100:1121–1126.

244. Sekijima Y, Morita H, Yanagisawa N. Follow-up of sarin poisoning in Matsumoto. *Ann Intern Med*. 1997;127:1042.

245. Lefkowitz L. Biochemist, US Army Center for Health Promotion and Preventive Medicine. Personal communication, 1994.

246. Loh Y, Ingram V, Swanberg M, Newmark J. Long-term cognitive sequelae of sarin exposure. In preparation.

247. Koplovitz I, Gresham VC, Dochterman LW, Kaminskis A, Stewart JR. Evaluation of the toxicity, pathology, and treatment of cyclohexylmethlyphosphonofluoridate (CMPF) poisoning in rhesus monkeys. *Arch Toxicol*. 1992;66:622–628.

248. Leadbeater L. When all else fails. *Chem Br*. 1988;24:684–687.

249. Inns RH, Leadbeater L. The efficacy of bispyridinium derivatives in the treatment of organophosphate poisoning in the guinea-pig. *J Pharm Pharmacol*. 1983;35:427–433.

250. Koplovitz I, Harris LW, Anderson DR, Lennox WJ, Stewart JR. Reduction by pyridostigmine pretreatment of the efficacy of atropine and 2-PAM treatment of sarin and VX poisoning in rodents. *Fundam Appl Toxicol*. 1992;18:102–106.

251. Petrali JP, Maxwell DM, Lenz DE. A study on the effects of soman on rat blood–brain barrier. *Anat Rec*. 1985;211:351–352.

252. Petrali JP, Maxwell DM, Lenz DE, Mills KR. Effect of an anticholinesterase compound on the ultrastructure and function of the rat blood–brain barrier: a review and experiment. *J Submicrosc Cytol Pathol*. 1991;23:331–338.

253. Gall D. The use of therapeutic mixtures in the treatment of cholinesterase inhibition. *Fundam Appl Toxicol*. 1981;1:214–216.

254. Schiflett SG, Stranges SF, Slater T, Jackson MK. Interactive effects of pyridostigmine and altitude on performance. In: *Proceedings of the 6th Medical Chemical Defense Bioscience Review*. Aberdeen Proving Ground, Md: US Army Medical Research Institute of Chemical Defense; 1987:605–608.

255. Whinnery JE. Flight testing of pyridostigmine bromide in the tactical fighter aircraft operational environment. Kelly Air Force Base, Tex; 1993. Unpublished.

256. Schiflett SG, Miller JC, Gawron VJ. Pyridostigmine bromide effects of performance of tactical transport aircrews. In: *Proceedings of the 6th Medical Chemical Defense Bioscience Review*. Aberdeen Proving Ground, Md: US Army Medical Research Institute of Chemical Defense; 1987:609–611.

257. Glickson M, Achiron A, Ram Z, et al. The influence of pyridostigmine administration on human neuromuscular functions—studies in healthy human subjects. *Fundam Appl Toxicol*. 1991;16:288–298.

258. Krutz RW Jr, Burton RR, Schiflett S, Holden R, Fisher J. Interaction of pyridostigmine bromide with mild hypoxia and rapid decompression. In: *Proceedings of the 6th Medical Chemical Defense Bioscience Review*. Aberdeen Proving Ground, Md: US Army Medical Research Institute of Chemical Defense; 1987:601–604.

259. Graham C, Cook MR. *Effects of Pyridostigmine on Psychomotor and Visual Performance*. Wright-Patterson Air Force Base, Ohio; 1984. Final report, contract F33615-80-C-0606, MRI.

260. Stephenson LA, Kolka MA. Acetylcholinesterase inhibitor, pyridostigmine bromide, reduces skin blood flow in humans. *Am J Physiol*. 1990;258:R951–R957.

261. Kolka MA, Stephenson LA. Human temperature regulation during exercise after oral pyridostigmine administration. *Aviat Space Environ Med*. 1990;61:220–224.

262. Levine BS, Parker RM. Reproductive and developmental toxicity studies of pyridostigmine bromide in rats. *Toxicology*. 1991;69:291–300.

263. Hudson CS, Foster RE, Kahng MW. Neuromuscular toxicity of pyridostigmine bromide in the diaphragm, extensor digitorum longus and soleus muscles of the rat. *Fundam Appl Toxicol*. 1985;5:S260–S269.

264. Briggs GG, Freeman RK, Yaffe SJ. *Drugs in Pregnancy and Lactation*. Baltimore, Md: Williams & Wilkins; 1990: 543–544.

265. Keeler JR. Interactions between nerve agent pretreatment and drugs commonly used in combat anesthesia. *Milit Med*. 1990;155:527–533.

266. Wade CE, Waring PP, Trail DS, Gildengorin VL, Williams BF, Bonner GD. Effects of atropine, 2-PAM, or pyridostigmine in euvolemic or hemorrhagic conscious swine. *Milit Med*. 1988;153:470–476.

267. Aquilonius SM, Eckernas SA, Hartvig P, Lindstrom B, Osterman PO. Pharmacokinetics and oral bioavailability of pyridostigmine in man. *Eur J Clin Pharmacol*. 1980;18:423–428.

268. Keeler JR, Hurst CG, Dunn MA. Pyridostigmine used as a nerve agent pretreatment under wartime conditions. *JAMA*. 1991;266:693–695.

269. Dunn M, Commander, Fort Lewis, and Keeler J, Researcher, Army Medical Department Center and School. Personal communication, 2001.

270. Sharabi Y, Danon YL, Berkenstadt H, et al. Survey of symptoms following intake of pyridostigmine during the Persian Gulf war. *Isr J Med Sci*. 1991;27:656–658.

271. Loewenstein-Lichtenstein Y, Schwarz M, Glick D, Norgaard-Pedersen B, Zakut H, Soreq H. Genetic predisposition to adverse consequences of anti-cholinesterases in "atypical" BCHE carriers. *Nat Med*. 1995;1:1082–1085.

272. Kaiser KS, Hawksworth AW, Gray GC. Pyridostigmine bromide intake during the Persian Gulf War is not associated with postwar handgrip strength. *Mil Med*. 2000;165-168.

273. Drake-Baumann R, Seil FJ. Effects of exposure to low-dose pyridostigmine on neuromuscular junctions in vitro. *Muscle Nerve*. 1999;22:696–703.

274. Pellegrini JE, Baker AB, Fontenot DJ, Cardenas AF. The effect of oral pyridostigmine bromide nerve agent prophylaxis on return of twitch height in persons receiving succinylcholine. *Mil Med*. 2000;165:252–255.

275. Annas GJ. Changing the consent rules for Desert Storm. *N Engl J Med*. 1992;326:770–773.

276. Nightingale SL. Medicine and war. *N Engl J Med*. 1992;327:1097–1098.

Chapter 6

NEUROPROTECTION AS A TREATMENT FOR NERVE AGENT SURVIVORS

GERALD P.H. BALLOUGH, PhD*; JONATHAN NEWMARK, MD†; ERIC S. LEVINE, PhD‡; and MARGARET G. FILBERT, PhD§

*Professor of Biology, La Salle University, 1900 West Olney Avenue, Philadelphia, Pennsylvania 19141-1199
†Colonel, US Army, Deputy Joint Program Executive Officer, Joint Program Executive Office for Chemical/Biological Defense, Skyline #2, Suite 1609, 5203 Leesburg Pike, Falls Church, Virginia 22041-3203
‡Assistant Program Manager, Science Applications International Corporation, 3465 Boxhill Corporate Center Drive, MS 23, Abingdon, Maryland 21009
§Special Assistant to the Commander, US Army Medical Research Institute of Chemical Defense, 3100 Ricketts Point Road, Aberdeen Proving Ground, Maryland 21010-5400

Portions of this chapter appeared as: Filbert M, Levine E, Ballough G. Neuroprotection for nerve agent-induced brain damage by blocking delayed calcium overload: a review. *Journal of Medical, Chemical, Biological, and Radiological Defense*. 2005;3:1–21. Available at: http://jmedcbr.org/Issue_0301/Filbert/Filbert_1105.pdf. Accessed March 2007.

INTRODUCTION

Organophosphorus nerve agents are the principal chemical warfare agents known to produce brain injury. They block hydrolysis of the neurotransmitter acetylcholine by inhibiting the enzyme acetylcholinesterase, resulting in greatly increased postsynaptic acetylcholine levels. This causes a spectrum of effects, including miosis, excess secretions, nausea, vomiting, and muscle fasciculations. At moderate to high doses, nerve agents also cause seizures and associated convulsions. If left untreated, seizures rapidly progress to status epilepticus (SE) and cause irreversible seizure-related brain damage (SRBD).[1,2] The International Classification of Epileptic Seizures defines SE as any seizure lasting at least 30 minutes or intermittent seizures lasting longer than 30 minutes between which the patient does not regain consciousness.[3,4]

For over a decade acute therapy has effectively saved those poisoned by nerve agents on the battlefield,[5] after accidental exposures,[6] and in terrorist attacks, as in the Japan subway attacks in 1994 and 1995. One lesson learned from the 1995 Tokyo attack was that, lacking acute antidotal treatment, many survivors arrived at hospitals in convulsive SE. The Tokyo experience illustrates the necessity of acute antidotal therapy, such as the regimen adopted by the US military. This regimen is aimed primarily at treating cholinergic crisis with a postexposure anticholinergic (atropine sulfate) and an oxime reactivator (2-pralidoxime [2-PAM Cl]). In specific intelligence-driven situations, pyridostigmine bromide (PB) pretreatment is added. Although these medications greatly reduce morbidity and mortality, they do not always prevent seizures and brain damage in nerve agent casualties; therefore, the regimen now includes the anticonvulsant diazepam.[2]

Even with diazepam, however, the treatment regimen has limitations. The decision to include diazepam was based on animal data showing that it could terminate nerve-agent–induced seizures and convulsions and enhance survival when given in conjunction with the acute therapy described above.[7–11] However, the therapeutic window for arresting seizures and SE with diazepam is less than an hour following onset; after that, both are refractory to anticonvulsant therapy.[7,8,10–19]

Early use of an anticonvulsant does not guarantee that seizures, once stopped, will not return. The recurrence of seizures is often observed in animal studies in several species and is of concern in human exposures. Although neuropathology is reduced in diazepam-treated animals, the incidence and degree of protection afforded by diazepam is not complete.[9,20–23] Moreover, switching the fielded anticonvulsant to another benzodiazepine, such as midazolam or lorazepam, does not entirely solve the problem of refractory SE.

Seizures and SE are key causes of brain damage resulting from nerve agent poisoning, and their prevention or alleviation should be the primary objective.[24–26] However, because of the refractory nature of seizures and especially SE, prevention and alleviation become increasingly difficult as more time elapses before therapy begins. Also, there is high probability that seizures will return when anticonvulsants wear off. Therefore, it is reasonable to anticipate a high incidence of brain damage connected to the increased survival rate of nerve agent victims.

Casualties exhibiting seizures and SE can be anticipated not only from terrorist attacks but also from battlefield scenarios involving troops who were not in full protective ensemble at the time of the attack.[27] In the confusion following a terrorist attack or on the battlefield, prompt treatment of nerve agent casualties can be expected to be problematic, and some victims undergoing seizures may not receive anticonvulsants inside the antiseizure therapeutic window. It is also possible that some victims may undergo nonconvulsive SE, a state of continuous seizures without observable clinical movement.[28] For these victims, treatment might be inadvertently delayed beyond the therapeutic window. Under the Small Business Innovative Research Program, the US Army funds efforts to field a far-forward, simple seizure detector to identify these casualties.

This chapter presents a detailed overview of nerve-agent–induced neuropathology and explains the mechanisms of action of candidate neuroprotectants that have shown promise in various animal and human studies, especially those that have received US Food and Drug Administration (FDA) approval for other indications.

NEUROPATHOLOGY AND THE MECHANISM OF NERVE-AGENT–INDUCED DAMAGE

Although there is little neuropathological data from patients who have survived nerve agent attacks, abundant evidence is available from animal models, many of which involve persistent SE. The profound brain damage produced by nerve agents was first described by Petras[29]; Lemercier et al[30]; and McLeod et al.[31] Since then, numerous studies have greatly enhanced the understanding of neuropathology resulting from nerve agent intoxication.[23,32–38] These studies have established that prolonged seizures and SE resulting from nerve agent exposure are directly responsible for the vast majority, if not all, of the neuropathology produced by these agents. The associated damage is typically bilaterally symmetrical and most severe in temporal lobe structures (ie, piriform and entorhinal cortices, hippocampus, and amygdala) as well as in the thalamus.

Brain damage resulting from agent-induced seizures is the result of the complex, multiphasic response of individual neurons to numerous extracelluar and intracellular events. Following inhibition of acetylcholinesterase and accumulation of acetylcholine at cholinergic synapses, the hyperstimulation of cholinergic receptors on postsynaptic membranes triggers seizures.[10,39,40] Subsequently, recruitment and excessive activation of the glutamatergic neurotransmitter system occurs. Glutamate, the most abundant excitatory neurotransmitter in the brain, is responsible for sustaining soman-induced seizures and promoting the development of SE.[1,24,41–44] Large pathological elevations in the concentration of intracellular sodium and (especially) calcium are caused by excessive stimulation of ionotropic glutamate receptors, as is prolonged depolarization of postsynaptic membranes. This initiates a harmful cascade of pathological processes, most of which center around a prolonged increase in intracellular free calcium or delayed calcium overload, leading to excitotoxic cell death.[1,24,45–47]

Transient elevation in intracellular free calcium is a ubiquitous signaling mechanism and regulator of intracellular processes, from cell growth and metabolism to cell death.[48–50] Cytosolic free calcium is also a critical neuronal mediator of learning and memory.[51] However, when normal homeostatic control of intracellular calcium is lost and a sustained elevation occurs, the delayed calcium overload triggers neuronal cell death by necrosis or apoptosis (a form of programmed cell death).[52–56] In neurons, the majority of calcium influx occurs through *N*-methyl D-aspartate (NMDA) ionotropic glutamate receptors as well as voltage-gated calcium channels (eg, L-type). Calcium influx also occurs, though to a lesser extent, through the other two classes of ionotropic glutamate receptors (alpha-amino-3-hydroxy-5-methylisoxazole-4-proprionic acid and kainate receptors).[57] Excessive stimulation of NMDA receptors is the first step in glutamate excitotoxicity.[24,45]

The release of intracellular stores is also responsible for increased cytosolic free calcium. The endoplasmic reticulum (ER) releases calcium following binding of the second messenger, inositol triphosphate, to ionotropic receptors located on the ER membrane. Calcium is released from the ER via ryanodine receptors. These ionotropic receptors are also located on the ER membrane and open following binding of cytosolic calcium; thus, cytosolic free calcium augments its own concentration by stimulating calcium release from the ER.[49] The ER plays a critical role in normal calcium homeostasis. Excessive release or impaired uptake of calcium has been implicated in pathology resulting from calcium overload.[49,52] Brain mitochondria are important for calcium buffering as cytosolic concentrations rise, and their ability to sequester calcium is dependent on adenosine triphosphate (ATP).[58] However, when calcium overload occurs, mitochondria undergo a permeability transition characterized by loss of mitochondrial transmembrane potential, curtailment of ATP synthesis, mitochondrial swelling, release of stored calcium, and neuronal death by necrosis.[59–62]

The majority of soman-induced SRBD results from glutamate excitotoxicity and the delayed calcium overload that follows.[1,24,42,43] Delayed calcium overload in neurons initiates a pathological sequence characterized by activation of several potentially damaging enzymes. These include oxygenases, phospholipases, and nitric oxide synthase, which produce reactive oxygen species such as superoxide radical, hydrogen peroxide, hydroxyl radical, nitric oxide, and peroxynitrite. Neuronal injury induced by reactive oxygen species stems from direct damage to cell membranes, DNA, and intracellular proteins, and also induction of cytochrome C from mitochondria with subsequent caspase activation.[62] Release of cytochrome C, caspase activation, and DNA fragmentation are molecular hallmarks of apoptosis (Figure 6-1).[56,62,63]

Cysteine proteases called calpains are also activated by sustained elevations in intracellular free calcium. Calpains degrade various intracellular proteins, including those of the cytoskeleton, membrane channels, and metabolic enzymes, and cause neuronal death by necrosis.[56,62,63] (Necrosis produces localized inflammation, which exacerbates damage, while apoptosis is not associated with inflammation.) The culmination of these events may result in cell death hours or days after the initial insult.[53–55]

Necrosis and apoptosis are not an either/or phenomena, that is, they are not completely distinct forms of cell death with no overlap; a necrosis versus apoptosis dichotomy is a misleading over-simplification.[64,65] Martin and colleagues proposed an "apoptosis-necrosis continuum," reporting that dying neurons can exhibit intermediate forms between apoptosis and necrosis.[66] Recently, Baille and colleagues confirmed that neuronal injury, resulting from soman-induced seizures, exhibits a large variety of hybrid forms between necrosis and apoptosis, but that the majority show more necrotic features.[67] Whether soman-induced neuropathology is mostly necrotic, as it is in the piriform cortex of rats,[38] or contains elements of apoptosis as first proposed

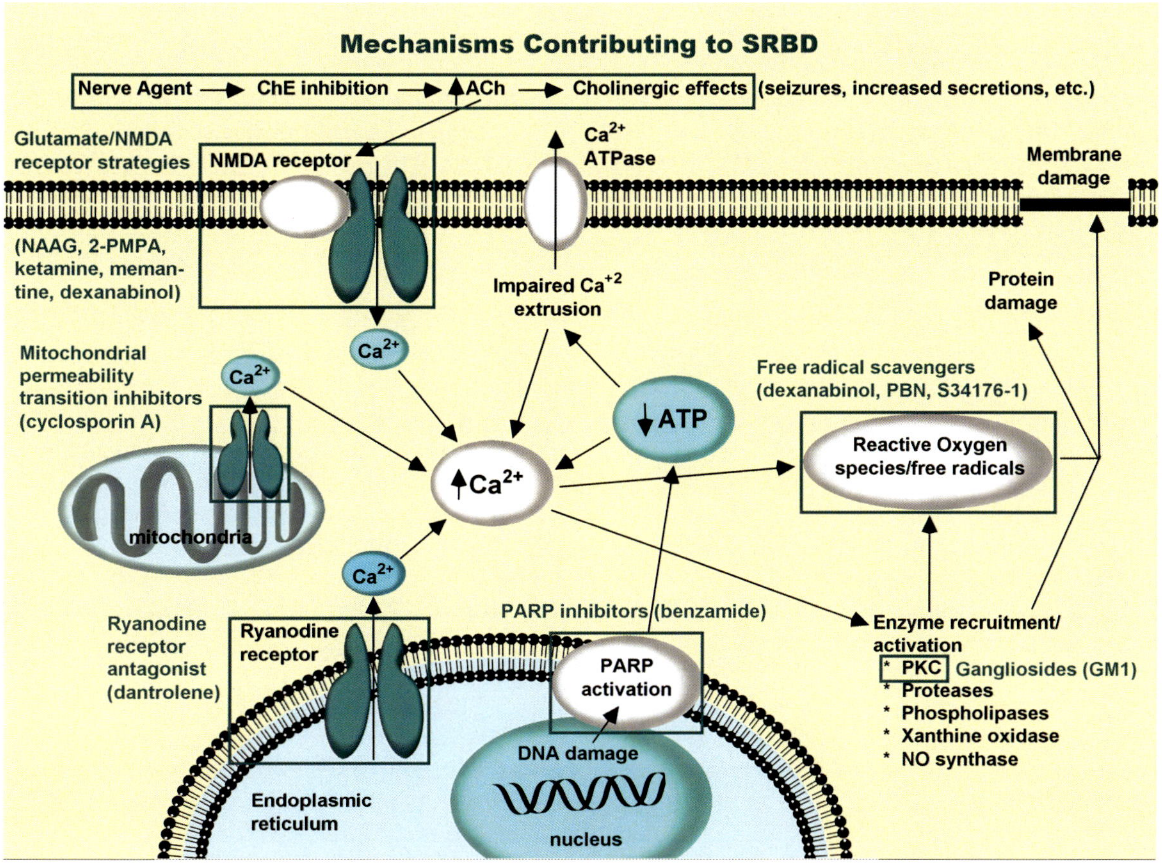

Fig. 6-1. Mechanisms contributing to nerve agent-induced SRBD. Calcium plays a pivotal role in glutamate excitotoxicity. A number of pharmacological approaches to neuroprotection have been investigated. Various sites in this pathway have been targeted. NMDA receptor antagonists block calcium entry through this glutamate ionotropic receptor. Gangliosides promote calcium extrusion indirectly by blocking PKC translocation (not indicated). PARP inhibitors enhance functionality of ion pumps and calcium extrusion by increasing ATP availability. Dantrolene blocks calcium release from intracellular stores. Free radical scavengers include free radical "traps" and endogenous free radical scavenging enzymes and small molecules prevent oxidative damage.

by Ballough et al in 1997 and definitively assessed by Baille et al is less important than the fact that both forms of neuronal cell death are triggered by nerve-agent–induced seizures.[38,67,68]

Candidate drugs may alter the relative proportions of neurons undergoing death by necrosis versus apoptosis. Studies have reported that insufficient ATP availability is an important determinant of whether a cell that has been triggered to undergo apoptosis is instead forced to die by necrosis.[55,69,70] Therefore, it is conceivable that a neuroprotectant candidate that enhances ATP availability (for example, poly(ADP-ribose) polymerase [PARP] inhibitors) could suppress necrosis while facilitating apoptosis. Neither possibility should be excluded during pathological evaluations of neuroprotectant candidates.

SPECIFIC RELEVANCE OF NEUROPROTECTION TO NERVE AGENT SURVIVORS

The term "neuroprotection" is defined as "pharmacological intervention that produces enduring benefits by favorably influencing underlying etiology or pathogenesis and thereby forestalling the onset of disease or clinical decline."[71,72] Within this broad definition, neuroprotection has acquired many different connotations. As a result, a search of the term "neuroprotection" on the National Library of Medicine's PubMed search page produces several thousand studies, mostly on disease states in which subsets of neurons are specifically vulnerable and die prematurely (as happens in Parkinson's disease, Huntington's disease, frontotemporal dementia, and a host of metabolic disorders) or accumulate neuropathology seen to a slight degree in normal brains but in an accelerated fashion in some diseases (such as Alzheimer's disease and trisomy 21). However, such interventions are unlikely to be relevant to the survivor of a single, brief nerve agent exposure that has already caused sustained seizures and SE. On the other hand, research on neuroprotection following stroke has provided valuable insights and clues that do apply to the nerve agent survivor.

In this chapter, the term "neuroprotection" specifically refers to a putative intervention given over a short period, ideally closely following the diagnosis of nerve agent exposure or before the acute toxic syndrome of exposure has been adequately treated. The best neuroprotectant would have the longest therapeutic window during which administration would be beneficial (even if the window is still only a matter of hours). At the same time, for logistical and doctrinal reasons, the neuroprotection initiative does not extend to prophylactic treatments administered to troops likely to experience nerve agent exposure (which would constitute a pretreatment, such as the bioscavenger initiative [see Chapter 7, Nerve Agent Bioscavenger: Development of a New Approach to Protect Against Organophosphorus Exposure]). Therefore, in this chapter, neuroprotection refers only to postexposure treatment.

There are similarities between brain damage resulting from nerve-agent–induced seizures and secondary neuronal injury resulting from stroke.[73,74] Although the immediate aspect of stroke-related neuronal injury is necrosis, which stems from anoxia or hypoxia, there is a secondary component to stroke damage that takes 48 to 72 hours to become manifest. This component accounts for approximately 50% of the total damage resulting from the ischemic episode. Secondary stroke injury involves brain tissue immediately surrounding the necrotic core of primary injury (the penumbra). For the most part, glutamate excitotoxicity and ionic destabilization, especially intracellular calcium, induce penumbral damage.[73–75] Thus, the similarities between secondary stroke damage and damage resulting from nerve-agent–induced seizures become apparent: they both involve glutamate excitotoxicity, hinge on intracellular calcium destabilization, and lead to necrotic or apoptotic neuronal death. This similarity raises the possibility that neuroprotectants being developed for stroke may be useful for nerve agent survivors. Neuroprotective interventions in stroke models have been shown to save neurons that otherwise would have died via necrosis or apoptosis. There is hope, then, that a treatment can be found that can be administered after agent exposure and that, although it may not have any immediately discernible clinical effect, will produce a significantly improved long-term neurological outcome. Any of the many classes of compounds that have been suggested as acute stroke neuroprotectant candidates could be tried. This list is extensive; the Internet Stroke Center (http://www.strokecenter.org), maintained by Washington University,[76] offers a continuously updated list of compounds that have been tried in clinical stroke trials.

The rationale for developing a protective agent, especially one based on dissimilar clinical situations that give rise to similar neuronal pathology, assumes that preventing neuronal loss will produce a superior clinical outcome. In the case of stroke, this assumption is probably warranted. In the case of nerve-agent–induced nerve cell damage, this assumption has never been tested directly, but it is consistent with a wide variety of animal data in multiple models and species. The assumption that preventing brain damage will produce superior behavioral outcome is even supported by Lashley and Hebb's studies in the early to mid 1900s.[77] A neuroprotectant in this restricted sense should demonstrate that neurons that might have been lost are now saved and that behavioral or neurological outcome is improved. An ideal database to document such neuroprotectants would include both neuropathological evidence of neuron survival and behavioral (in animals) or cognitive (in people) evidence that the neurologic outcome is superior compared to subjects that did not receive the neuroprotectant. Finally, the FDA must approve use of the agent if it is a medication. (In clinical medicine, any FDA-approved medication can be used off-label by licensed physicians, but in military doctrine, specific on-label FDA approval is mandatory.)

NEUROPROTECTANTS WITH PROVEN EFFICACY AGAINST NERVE-AGENT–INDUCED SIEZURE-RELATED BRAIN DAMAGE

This research comes from the consensus that nerve-agent–induced seizures and SE lead to the development of glutamate-mediated excitotoxicity, in which delayed calcium overload is the intracellular trigger of the final sequences leading to cell death.[1,24,42,43,47,49,56,78–81] Classes of drugs that have been tested for their abilities to ameliorate nerve-agent–induced SRBD by specifically mitigating delayed calcium overload include the following:

- NMDA receptor antagonists that block extracellular calcium influx;
- glycosphingolipids that reduce intracellular calcium by blocking the translocation of

protein kinase C (PKC), thus enhancing the sodium-calcium exchange;
- ryanodine receptor antagonists that prevent the release of calcium from the ER; and
- PARP inhibitors that indirectly lower intracellular calcium by preventing ATP depletion.[82–89]

Increased ATP availability facilitates calcium efflux by plasma membrane Ca2+ ATPase and calcium sequestration by the mitochondria, and indirectly enhances sodium-calcium exchange by maintaining sodium-potassium-ATPase functionality.[58]

Gangliosides

Medications that target events subsequent to calcium overload have been tested against soman-induced SRBD in an effort to circumvent neurotoxicity associated with NMDA receptor antagonism and mitigate established delayed calcium overload. Intracerebroventricular infusion of GM1 monosialoganglioside (5 mg/kg/day, for 5 days before and 27 h after soman exposure) in rats markedly reduced cross-sectional areas of soman-induced temporal lobe necrosis (there was an 85.9% lesion reduction in the piriform cortex and contiguous structures, compared with unprotected soman-positive controls).[90] In this study, all rats were pretreated with PB before soman exposure, and then treated with atropine methylnitrate (AMN) and 2-pralidoxime (2-PAM). Considerable neuroprotection was also obtained with the water-soluble GM1 monosialoganglioside derivative, WILD20. As an adjunct to HI-6 pretreatment and AMN posttreatment, WILD20 (2.5 mg/kg, intraperitoneal injection [IP]) reduced volumetric temporal lobe necrosis by 75.2%. Neuroprotection by these two compounds occurred, and neither seizure intensity nor duration (assessed via electroencephalography [EEG] monitoring) was diminished.

Gangliosides are sialic-acid–containing glycosphingolipids that are natural constituents of cell membranes and are particularly abundant in neurons.[91–93] The mechanism by which GM1 monosialoganglioside and WILD20 exert their neuroprotective effects involves inhibition of PKC translocation to the plasma membrane.[75, 82–86,94,95] PKC activation and translocation enhance glutamate excitotoxicity.[96,97] Furthermore, PKC's role in the excitotoxic process is to prolong NMDA receptor activation and possibly inhibit calcium extrusion mechanisms.[82,75,98] In addition, WILD20 is reported to reduce inflammation by its inhibitory effects on specific leukocytes (neutrophils).[99] Despite the promising results with gangliosides, further studies have been discontinued because of concerns of possible contamination by prions associated with bovine spongiform encephalopathy (mad cow disease).[90,100]

Poly(ADP-ribose) Polymerase Inhibitors

Recent studies indicate that PARP inhibition is neuroprotective following neuropathological insults involving excitotoxicity, such as cerebral ischemia and traumatic brain injury.[101–108] PARP is an abundant nuclear enzyme that is activated by DNA strand breaks induced by reactive oxygen species.[108,109] With moderate insults, it facilitates DNA repair by utilizing cellular nicotinamide adenine dinucleotide to form poly(ADP-ribose). Excessive PARP activation leads to nicotinamide adenine dinucleotide depletion, metabolic inhibition via glycolysis block, ATP insufficiency, and cell death by necrosis.[104,109,110] Neurons are especially vulnerable to metabolic insufficiency resulting from PARP over-activation because glucose is normally the only metabolic substrate and the dependency on glycolysis is exceptionally high.[108] In excitotoxic models, over-activation of PARP is closely linked to calcium-induced nitric oxide synthase activation, which leads to the production of nitric oxide; the detrimental effects of nitric oxide are mostly mediated through peroxynitrite, which forms when nitric oxide reacts with superoxide.[109,111,112]

In 1999 Meier et al[113] reported reduced lesion volumes and increased survival in soman-exposed rats that received the PARP inhibitor benzamide. Further investigation into the neuroprotective efficacy of PARP inhibition warrants consideration, and subsequent studies should include several new-generation PARP inhibitors that have shown increased usefulness, such as ONO-1924H, DR2313, and FR247304.[105,107,114]

Ryanodine Receptor Antagonist

Dantrolene is another drug that has shown neuroprotective efficacy against soman-induced SRBD.[88] A ryanodine receptor antagonist that prevents the release of calcium from the ER, dantrolene is FDA-approved for use in malignant hyperthermia. Although some neuroprotection is produced by diazepam alone (20 mg/kg, intramuscular injection [IM], 40 min after seizure onset), this protection is significantly augmented in the dorsal and lateral cortices of rats by coadministration of dantrolene (10 mg/kg, intravenous [IV]).[88] Administering the full dosage of dantrolene in a single injection is difficult because of insolubility problems associated with the medication. To overcome these problems and achieve the desired dantrolene dosage, four separate IV injections were performed between

40 minutes and 8 hours after seizure onset, with a total injection volume approximating 1 mL per rat. A unique formulation of dantrolene (Lyotropic Therapeutics, Inc, Ashland, Va) as a nanocrystal dispersion has also been used to obviate solubility problems. With this formulation, it is possible to administer a much higher dose of dantrolene in a much lower injection volume. This is critical because when dantrolene is administered by IP injection, liver enzymes lower the concentration of dantrolene reaching the brain. The nanocrystal formulation of dantrolene minimizes the effects of the liver enzymes.

Our results with the dantrolene nanocrystal formulation not only overcame the insolubility problems of our previous dantrolene study, but corroborated and extended the results of that study. The nanocrystal study was unable to demonstrate significant protection in the piriform cortex, the most severely damaged region, but in this study the nanocrystal dispersion of dantrolene (40 mg/kg, IP) plus diazepam (20 mg/kg, IM) reduced piriform cortical necrosis by 15.6% more than diazepam alone (unpublished study by US Army Medical Research Institute of Chemical Defense). In these experiments, all soman-exposed rats also received HI-6 (125 mg/kg, IP, 30 min after soman) and AMN (2 mg/kg, IM, < 1 min after soman) to protect against the peripheral effects of soman and ensure survival. Neuroprotection by dantrolene in the above experiments occurred without changes in seizure intensity or duration, and dantrolene produced no discernible effects on the electrocorticographic profiles of soman-exposed subjects. These findings are consistent with those of Frandsen and Schouosboe,[115] who reported that dantrolene prevented glutamate neurotoxicity by blocking release of calcium from intracellular stores. The results are also consistent with those of Niebauer and Gruenthal,[87] who examined the protective effects of dantrolene on hippocampal neuronal damage produced by SE in rats. In their study, dantrolene (10 mg/kg, IP) was administered either 30 or 140 minutes after the onset of SE. Niebauer and Gruenthal reported that early administration produced a significant reduction in neuronal injury in all hippocampal subregions. When dantrolene administration was delayed until 140 minutes after SE onset, some protection was still seen in hippocampal field CA3, but not the other subregions.[87] Protection against kainic-acid–induced apoptosis has also been reported.[116]

N-methyl-D-aspartate Receptor Antagonists

MK-801 (Dizocilpine)

The first NMDA receptor antagonist to show promise as a putative neuroprotectant was MK-801 (dizocilpine); however, it has been shown to have toxic effects. When given in conjunction with PB, AMN, and 2-PAM, noncompetitive MK-801 was reported to reduce nerve-agent–induced SRBD in the piriform cortex, amygdala, hippocampus, and thalamus.[43] As mentioned, these are among the most severely damaged brain regions in SRBD resulting from soman exposure.[29–32,35,37,38,90] In the Sparenborg study, MK-801 (0.5, 1.0, or 5 mg/kg, IP) reduced brain damage and diminished or arrested seizures in guinea pigs when administered as a pretreatment 30 minutes before soman, and the effects were dose-dependent. The anticonvulsant profile of MK-801 against soman-induced seizures was definitively characterized by Shih.[11] He showed that the anticonvulsant effect of MK-801 is four times greater than that of diazepam, but at doses of 1 mg/kg or higher, MK-801 potentiated the lethal effects of soman. Some concern arose about the use of NMDA antagonists when it was reported that MK-801 induces neuronal degeneration in the posterior cingulate, retrosplenial cortices, and other corticolimbic regions.[117,118] This damage evidently occurs by disinhibition of multiple converging excitatory pathways.[119] Specifically, excessive blockage of glutamatergic pathways leads to excessive stimulation of cholinergic function.[120] This explanation is supported by the findings that neurotoxicity by MK-801 is augmented when cholinergic receptors (ie, muscarinic) are activated.[121]

Memantine

Memantine is a noncompetitive NMDA receptor antagonist[122] that has also been tested for its anticonvulsant effects against soman-induced seizures. Studies have suggested that memantine's pharmacokinetics make it a safer candidate than MK-801.[123,124] McLean et al[125] reported that memantine alone (18 mg/kg, subcutaneous [SC]) blocked the onset of soman-induced seizures and was able to terminate seizures when administered 15 minutes after soman injection. These findings, however, are inconsistent with those of Shih et al[17] who reported that memantine by itself is completely ineffective as an anticonvulsant against soman-induced seizures. The latter authors pointed to a need for EEG monitoring when determining anticonvulsant efficacy and suggested that McLean et al may have mistaken diminished convulsive behavior as evidence of reduced seizure activity. Neither study addressed the possible neuroprotective effects of memantine (ie, reduced neuropathology independent of anticonvulsant activity). On the other hand, Koplovitz et al[126] observed a modest reduction in piriform cortical damage following soman in rats treated with atropine and memantine, compared to those that received atropine alone. There were no differences between the

EEG power spectra of the two groups. Regardless of the above discrepancies, the neuroprotective benefit of memantine in other models of excitotoxicity is widely accepted.[124,127] For example, in a rat model of stroke, memantine given 2 hours after the ischemic event reduced brain damage by approximately 50%.[128] In addition, memantine is well tolerated and does not produce neurotoxicity at therapeutic dosages. It was recently approved by the FDA for treating Alzheimer's disease.[124]

HU-211 (Dexanabinol)

The first real proof of concept of postexposure neuroprotection came from work with HU-211 (dexanabinol), a nonpsychotropic analogue of tetrahydrocannabinol, the active ingredient in marijuana. Filbert and colleagues[129] showed that in rats exposed to high doses of soman, dexanabinol protected neurons in the piriform cortex (Figure 6-2) when given as late as 40 minutes after the EEG-proven onset of seizures. The drug was not an anticonvulsant and had no effect upon the seizures, indicating that the results showed a true neuroprotective effect and not part of an anticonvulsant effect. HU-211 has been reported to inhibit NMDA receptors, act as an antioxidant and free radical scavenger, suppress nitrous oxide and tumor necrosis factor-α generation, and stabilize calcium levels.[130–132] HU-211 is generally well tolerated in humans.[133]

When HU-211 (25 mg/kg, IP) was administered 5 minutes after the onset of soman-induced seizures, in conjunction with HI-6 and AMN pretreatment and posttreatment, respectively, temporal lobe lesion volume/necrosis (assessed at 28 h after seizure onset) was reduced by 86%, compared with unprotected soman-positive controls (see Figure 6-2).[134,135] HU-211 had no effect on the strength or duration of seizure activity, as determined by quantitative EEG analysis. Significant neuroprotection was also observed when HU-211 administration was delayed 40 minutes after seizure onset. Neuroprotection by HU-211 was most evident in the piriform cortex and contiguous temporal lobe structures, such as the amygdala, entorhinal, and perirhinal cortices, but did not extend to the thalamus. Administration of HU-211 and diazepam 40 minutes after seizure onset did not augment the neuroprotection obtained with diazepam alone.

In analyzing the mechanisms of neuroprotection by HU-211 and diazepam, it is important to differentiate between protection obtained by anticonvulsant effects

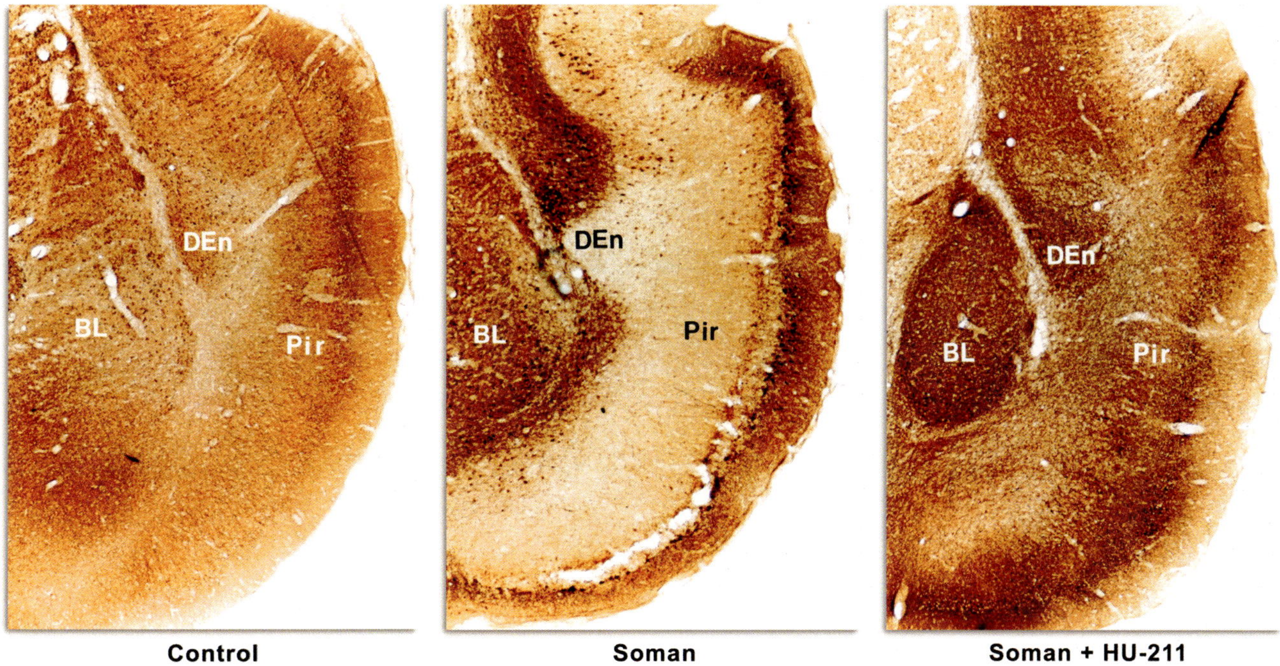

Fig. 6-2. Dexanabinol (HU-211) protects against soman-induced neurological damage. Microtubule-associated protein 2 (MAP-2) staining is neuron-specific. MAP-2 negative immunostaining indicates necrosis, except in areas of white matter.
BL: basolateral amygdaloid nuclear group
DEn: dorsal endopiriform nucleus
Pir: piriform cortex.

and that produced by interfering with delayed calcium overload. In the above studies, HU-211 was protective, despite the continued presence of undiminished seizures and SE, whereas diazepam attenuated (without stopping) seizure intensity and thereby reduced the initial insult. The anticonvulsant action of diazepam, via agonistic modulation of γ-aminobutyric A (GABA[A]) receptors, is well known. These mechanisms are nonoverlapping, and neuroprotective effects should be additive or synergistic. HU-211 is not approved for clinical use, and the company that owns the rights to it (Pharmos Ltd, Israel) is developing it as a possible adjunctive therapeutic for head trauma.

Gacyclidine

Gacyclidine (GK-11) is another NMDA receptor antagonist that has shown considerable neuroprotective efficacy. When GK-11 (0.01–0 .1 mg/kg, IV) was given to rats 10 minutes after soman exposure (in conjunction with PB pretreatment, and AS, 2-PAM, and diazepam posttreatments, 1 min after soman injections), it completely blocked SRBD when assessed 3 weeks after exposure.[136] In a more realistic battlefield scenario, GK-11 was administered 45 minutes after an exposure of 8 times the median lethal dose (LD_{50}) of soman in nonhuman primates. Animals also received PB pretreatment, followed by AS, 2-PAM, and diazepam posttreatments (1 min after soman exposure) equivalent to a single autoinjector of each in humans. When brain pathology was assessed 3 weeks after exposure, all three GK-11–treated primates showed little or no evidence of pathology in the frontal and entorhinal cortices, amygdala, caudate nucleus, hippocampus, thalamus, midbrain, pons, medulla, and cerebellum, compared with the only surviving soman-treated animal (1 of 3) that received AS, 2-PAM, and diazepam but not GK-11.[137] In a study that approximates casualty management following a terrorist attack, soman-intoxicated (2 times the LD_{50}) primates did not receive PB pretreatment and received delayed AS, 2-PAM, and diazepam treatments (one human-equivalent of each, as above) 30 minutes postexposure, followed by GK-11 (0.1 mg/kg, IV). In this study, the addition of GK-11 restored normal EEG activity and completely prevented neuropathology (assessed 5 weeks after exposure), compared with subjects that received AS, 2-PAM, or diazepam alone.[138] GK-11 has a binding affinity for NMDA receptors that is only one tenth that of MK-801. In addition, it binds to non-NMDA receptors when interaction with NMDA receptors is prevented. For these reasons, GK-11 is considered substantially less neurotoxic than MK-801.[139] It is currently being evaluated in human clinical trials for a different neuroprotective indication.[139,140]

Ketamine

Ketamine appears to be the most promising neuroprotectant candidate to date,[141,142] and it should be used in combination with a benzodiazepine, such as diazepam. Ketamine is an FDA-approved anesthetic that blocks neurotransmissions without depressing respiratory and circulatory functions. Its actions are mediated by low-affinity binding to NMDA receptor channels and prevention of calcium influx.[142–145] Ketamine is garnering considerable attention as a putative neuroprotectant against ischemic brain injury, damage resulting from seizures and SE, irrespective of etiology, and SRBD specifically resulting from nerve-agent–induced seizures.[144–149] Fujikawa[147] reported remarkable neuroprotection in 21 of 24 brain regions in rats when 100 mg/kg of ketamine was administered (IP) 15 minutes after lithium-pilocarpine-induced SE onset. Similarly, 100 mg/kg of ketamine (IP) prevented learning impairment in rats when administered immediately after lithium-pilocarpine-induced SE.[150] Borris et al[151] report that ketamine (58 mg/kg, the effective dose in 50% of those taking it [ED_{50}]) can control prolonged SE in rats when administered 1 hour after onset. Cumulative evidence for the beneficial effects of ketamine following SE onset has led to its recommended use in humans when SE cannot be alleviated by conventional anticonvulsant therapy.[148]

Based on its neuroprotective and anticonvulsant properties, Mion et al[145] recommend ketamine for victims of nerve agent exposure. More recently, Dorandeu et al[149] reported that ketamine proved effective in stopping seizures, highly reducing SRBD, and improving guinea pig survival when administered between 30 minutes and 2 hours after soman poisoning. Increasing dosages of ketamine (ie, 10–60 mg/kg, IM) were required as post-SE onset delay increased, and ketamine was always administered with atropine sulfate (2–10 mg/kg); in addition, guinea pigs received pyridostigmine (26 mg/kg, IM) 30 minutes prior to soman and AMN (4 mg/kg, IM) within 1 minute following the soman injection. Their study also provided compelling evidence of neuroprotection by ketamine at dosages that did not modify seizures (ie, 2–10 mg/kg), and suggested combining ketamine and benzodiazepine treatments when treatment is delayed 2 hours.

Results from the authors' laboratory corroborate reports of neuroprotection by ketamine following soman-induced SE. The authors observed that neuroprotection was greatly augmented by administering ketamine plus diazepam, compared to diazepam alone. When soman-exposed (1.6 times the LD_{50}) rats were administered 20 mg/kg diazepam (IM) and 25 mg/kg ketamine (IP), 40 minutes after seizure onset, the mean cross-sectional area of temporal lobe necrosis (ie, piriform cortex and surrounding structures) was reduced by 85.5% compared to soman-positive controls ($P = 0.018$). The mean reduction produced by diazepam alone was only 39.9% and was not significant. In the lateral dorsal thalamus and surrounding thalamic nuclei, diazepam plus ketamine reduced severe damage by 91.4% compared to soman controls ($P < 0.001$). The reduction in lateral dorsal thalamus damage by diazepam alone was only 27.4% and was not significant. Neuronal pathological assessments, using haematoxylin and eosin stain, confirmed these quantitative findings. It is likely that reduced seizure intensities contributed to the observed neuroprotection; however, this speculation is unconfirmed because EEGs were not obtained from these animals.

Taken together, the preponderance of evidence indicates that ketamine is a viable neuroprotectant candidate against nerve-agent–induced SRBD. However, ketamine is not FDA approved for this purpose. There have been no human or nonhuman primate studies to determine the optimal dose of ketamine to be used in combination with diazepam or other benzodiazepines to alleviate nerve-agent–induced SE. On the other hand, several case reports describe the effectiveness of ketamine, following benzodiazepine therapy, for refractory human SE from different causes. Therefore, off-label use of ketamine, as adjunct neuroprotective therapy following nerve agent intoxication, should be undertaken with caution and consideration of the best available evidence.

Because ketamine would be administered in conjunction with diazepam, and because of an increased risk of respiratory insufficiency by the combined treatments (see below), it is important to review treatment recommendations for diazepam. The autoinjector issued by the US military contains 10 mg diazepam. For a 70-kg (154-lb) individual, one autoinjector delivers a dose (0.14 mg/kg, IM) consistent with the diazepam loading dosage (0.15 mg/kg, IV) recommended by the recent Belgian Consensus on SE.[148] The autoinjector dose is also consistent with the diazepam dose (5–20 mg/70 kg) recommended by Durham[152] as initial treatment for SE, and is in agreement with the 20-mg diazepam dose (per rectum) recommended in "Treatment of Status Epilepticus in Adults: Columbia University Protocol," as first line therapy when IV access is not available.[153] The Belgian Consensus[148] further recommends 4 to 8 mg per hour IV maintenance dosing with diazepam. On the battlefield, medics and unit lifesavers are permitted to administer two additional 10-mg dosages of diazepam. Overall there is regularity in the recommended use of diazepam in the initial treatment of adult SE, regardless of cause. The main adverse effects of diazepam, and benzodiazepines in general, are respiratory depression, hypotension, and decreased consciousness.[148]

For intractable SE, the Belgian Consensus advocates an adult dosage of 50 to 100 mg ketamine as a follow up to diazepam for its "theoretical neuroprotective effects."[148] This dosage is consistent with Durham's[152] recommendation of 50 to 100 mg ketamine followed by 50 to 100 mg per hour, as a "second-line" treatment for refractory SE. Walker et al[154] report successfully treating an adult patient exhibiting "partial motor SE" with an anesthetic dosage of ketamine (ie, 100 mg/h). In a 13-year-old girl whose SE failed to respond to all standard treatments, control of clinical and electrographic SE was obtained within 90 seconds following a bolus injection (IV) of 2 mg/kg ketamine; control was maintained by continuous infusion of ketamine up to a maximum of 7.5 mg/kg per hour.[155]

Adverse effects of ketamine include a transient decrease in respiratory rate with bolus administration (ie, ≥ 2 mg/kg, IV), pulmonary secretions (controllable with atropine), transient cardiovascular stimulation and possible tachycardia, intracranial hypertension (making it contraindicated for closed head injury), and undesired psychic effects.[148,156] In field situations, ketamine is preferred above other anesthetics because it is relatively unlikely to cause respiratory depression. It is generally accepted that ketamine does not produce significant ventilatory depression in humans.[156]

Ketamine may also produce neurotoxicity typical of NMDA receptor antagonists. As mentioned above, NMDA receptor antagonists have been shown to cause neurotoxicity in the cingulate and retrosplenial cortices as well as cerebellar Purkinje cells.[117,118,157,158] A case of possible ketamine toxicity was seen in a 44-year-old man treated for refractory SE.[158] Control of his SE was achieved with an initial bolus injection of 2 mg/kg ketamine (IV, over 2 min), followed by a continuous infusion of 2 mg/kg per hour. Infusion dosages were progressively increased until achieving a final dose of 7.5 mg/kg per hour after 48 hours. Dosages were then titrated down over the next 72 hours. The patient exhibited diffuse cerebellar and cerebral atrophy consistent with animal models of NMDA antagonist-mediated neurotoxicity.[158] Studies have reported that the mechanism of this toxicity is indirectly mediated by excessive cholinergic stimulation,[119–121] and supplemental atropine could have an ameliorative effect. In addition, GABAergic stimulation is reportedly protective against this specific form of neurotoxicity.[119–121]

However, high dosages of both diazepam and ketamine could exacerbate respiratory distress already present in nerve agent casualties. Therefore, a conservative dose range for ketamine is advisable. In humans, a ketamine dose less than 1 mg/kg, IV, provides effective analgesia against acute and chronic pain.[146,156,159]

The anesthetic dose range in humans is 5 to 10 mg/kg, IV.[146,159] For a nerve agent victim on the battlefield, a ketamine dosage below 2 mg/kg, IV, should prove safe in combination with the high dosages of diazepam that are likely to be administered. While possibly not high enough to augment the anticonvulsant effects of diazepam and arrest SE, anesthetic or subanesthetic dosages of ketamine should provide considerable additional neuroprotection, compared to diazepam alone. Moreover, the ketamine dosage can be increased once patients reach a medical facility where intubation and ventilation can be provided.

ADDITIONAL NEUROPROTECTIVE APPROACHES

Free Radical Scavengers

Damage produced by reactive oxygen species or free radicals is a component of seizure and SE-related neurotoxicity,[47,160,161] including damage resulting from nerve agent poisoning.[160] The liberation of catalytic iron from extravasated hemoglobin may generate reactive oxygen species.[160,161] Reactive oxygen species could also be generated by xanthine oxidase or impaired mitochondrial electron transport,[161–163] offering the hope that nerve-agent–induced neurotoxicity could be mitigated by antioxidants or free radical scavengers.

Nitrone-based free radical traps, such as alpha-phenyl-N-tert-butylnitrone (PBN), which react with reactive oxygen species, have proven to be neuroprotective following cholinesterase inhibition. Pretreatment with PBN prevented seizures induced by diisofluorophosphate, an organophosphonate and nerve agent simulant.[164] Moreover, PBN (150 mg/kg, IP, 5 min after seizure onset) produced significant neuroprotection in the piriform cortices and other cortical areas of rats following lithium pilocarpine-induced SE.[165] Unfortunately (and reminiscent of the findings with HU-211 discussed above), thalamic damage was either exacerbated or not diminished by PBN in the latter study. Another report describes neuroprotective effects by PBN 12 hours after ischemic insult.[166] A pilot study of PBN did not show neuroprotection against soman-induced injury.[167] A new, centrally acting, nitrone-based free radical scavenger, S34176, has shown superior neuroprotective properties compared to PBN in stroke and other glutamate excitotoxicity models.[168] S34176 may prove useful against nerve-agent–induced injury.

Mitochondrial Permeability Transition Inhibitors

As mentioned above, damaging stimuli can induce neuronal mitochondria to undergo permeability transition, forming pores that allow the release of stored calcium into the neuronal cytoplasm. This is accompanied by curtailment of ATP synthesis, mitochondrial swelling, exacerbation of calcium overload, and neuronal death.[59–62] The assembly of mitochondrial transition pores can be blocked by cyclosporin A, an FDA -approved drug used in cancer chemotherapy. There is evidence that cyclosporin A and topiramate (another transition pore blocker) are neuroprotective in various models of excitotoxic brain injury.[169–174] Bauman and colleagues[169] found that cyclosporin A dramatically reduced brain injury in rats following seizures and SE induced by the organophosphate paraoxon. There is also evidence of neuroprotection by topiramate following pilocarpine-induced seizures and SE.[170]

Neuroprotective Hypothermia

Total-body cooling is an effective nonpharmacologic method of treating cerebrovascular disease. Several stroke experts have advanced this approach as holding great promise in reducing the amount of ischemic brain damage, and in 2004 the FDA approved a catheter for stroke and other specific uses that cools the blood in a penetrating artery. Less technologically complicated approaches to total-body cooling have been successful in limited numbers of animal studies.[175,176] Whether this approach would be practical in a battlefield situation, especially with mass casualties, is questionable, but it should be kept in mind as a possibility.

SUMMARY

A variety of neuroprotective compounds have proven useful in alleviating brain damage caused by nerve-agent–induced seizures and SE. Of these, ketamine, memantine, and dantrolene have received FDA approval for other indications, and several other compounds are in clinical trials. Based on the evidence, ketamine, in combination with diazepam, is the top candidate and most viable neuroprotectant for nerve agent survivors exhibiting seizures and SE. A dantrolene and diazepam combination is a viable possibility as well, though less efficacious. In addition, free radical scavengers (eg, S34176) and transition pore blockers (eg, cyclosporin A) show great promise. It is conceivable that the best possible neuroprotective approach will be a "cocktail" of two or more agents that affect, in a synergistic fashion, different legs of the excitotoxic pathway.[177]

REFERENCES

1. Solberg Y, Belkin M. The role of excitotoxicity in organophosphorous nerve agents central poisoning. *Trends Pharmacol Sci*. 1997;18:183–185.

2. Shih TM, Duniho SM, McDonough JH. Control of nerve agent-induced seizures is critical for neuroprotection and survival. *Toxicol Appl Pharm*. 2003;188:69–80.

3. DeLorenzo RJ. Management of status epilepticus. *Va Med Q*. 1996;123:103–111.

4. DeLorenzo RJ, Hauser WA, Towne AR, et al. A prospective, population-based epidemiologic study of status epilepticus in Richmond, Virginia. *Neurology*. 1996;46:1029–1035.

5. Newmark J. The birth of nerve agent warfare: lessons from Syed Abbas Foroutan. *Neurology*. 2004;62:1590–1596.

6. Sidell FR. Nerve Agents. In: Sidell FR, Takafuji ET, Franz DR, eds. *Medical Aspects of Chemical and Biological Warfare*. In: Zajtchuk R, Bellamy RF, eds. *Textbook of Military Medicine*. Washington, DC: Department of the Army, Office of The Surgeon General, Borden Institute; 1997: Chap 5.

7. Lipp JA. Effect of diazepam upon soman-induced seizure activity and convulsions. *Electroencephalogr Clin Neurophysiol*. 1972;32:557–560.

8. Lipp JA. Effect of benzodiazepine derivatives on soman-induced seizure activity and convulsions in the monkey. *Arch Int Pharmacodyn Ther*. 1973;202:244–251.

9. McDonough JH Jr, Jaax NK, Crowley RA, Mays MZ, Modrow HE. Atropine and/or diazepam therapy protects against soman-induced neural and cardiac pathology. *Fundam Appl Toxicol*. 1989;13:256–276.

10. McDonough JH Jr, Shih TM. Pharmacological modulation of soman-induced seizures. *Neurosci Biobehav Rev*. 1993;17:203–215.

11. Shih TM. Anticonvulsant effects of diazepam and MK-801 in soman poisoning. *Epilepsy Res*. 1990;7:105–116.

12. Shih TM, Koviak TA, Capacio BR. Anticonvulsants for poisoning by the organophosphorus compound soman: pharmacological mechanisms. *Neurosci Biobehav Rev*. 1991;15:349–362.

13. Capacio BR, Shih TM. Anticonvulsant actions of anticholinergic drugs in soman poisoning. *Epilepsia*. 1991;32:604–615.

14. Philippens IH, Melchers BP, de Groot DM, Wolthuis OL. Behavioral performance, brain histology, and EEG sequela after immediate combined atropine/diazepam treatment of soman-intoxicated rats. *Pharmacol Biochem Behav*. 1992;42:711–719.

15. Sparenborg S, Brennecke LH, Beers ET. Pharmacological dissociation of the motor and electrical aspects of convulsive status epilepticus induced by the cholinesterase inhibitor soman. *Epilepsy Res*. 1993;14:95–103.

16. Harris LW, Gennings C, Carter WH, Anderson DR, Lennox WJ, Bowersox SL, Solana RP. Efficacy comparison of scopolamine (SCP) and diazepam (DZ) against soman-induced lethality in guinea pigs. *Drug Chem Toxicol*. 1994;17:35–50.

17. Shih T, McDonough JH Jr, Koplovitz I. Anticonvulsants for soman-induced seizure activity. *J Biomed Sci*. 1999;6:86–96.

18. Lallement G, Renault F, Baubichon D, et al. Compared efficacy of diazepam or avizafone to prevent soman-induced electroencephalographic disturbances and neuropathology in primates: relationship to plasmatic benzodiazepine pharmacokinetics. *Arch Toxicol*. 2000;74:480–486.

19. McDonough JH Jr, Zoeffel LD, McMonagle J, Copeland TL, Smith CD, Shih TM. Anticonvulsant treatment of nerve agent seizures: anticholinergic versus diazepam in soman-intoxicated guinea pigs. *Epilepsy Res*. 2000;38:1–14.

20. Clement JG, Broxup B. Efficacy of diazepam and avizafone against soman-induced neuropathology in brain of rats. *Neurotoxicology*. 1993;14:485–504.

21. Hayward IJ, Wall HG, Jaax NK, Wade JV, Marlow DD, Nold JB. Decreased brain pathology in organophosphate-exposed rhesus monkeys following benzodiazepine therapy. *J Neurol Sci*. 1990;98:99–106.

22. McDonough JH Jr, Dochterman LW, Smith CD, Shih TM. Protection against nerve agent-induced neuropathology, but not cardiac pathology, is associated with the anticonvulsant action of drug treatment. *Neurotoxicology*. 1995;16:123–132.

23. Baze WB. Soman-induced morphological changes: an overview in the non-human primate. *J Appl Toxicol*. 1993;13:173–177.

24. Olney JW, de Gubareff T, Labruyere J. Seizure-related brain damage induced by cholinergic agents. *Nature*. 1983;301:520–522.

25. Sloviter RS. "Epileptic" brain damage in rats induced by sustained electrical stimulation of the perforant path. I. Acute electrophysiological and light microscopic studies. *Brain Res Bull*. 1983;10:675–697.

26. Meldrum BS. Concept of activity-induced cell death in epilepsy: historical and contemporary perspectives. *Progress Brain Res*. 2002;135:3–11.

27. Fanzone JF, Levine ES, Hursh SR. *Nerve Agent Bioscavenger Pretreatment Against Chemical Warfare Agents: Challenge, Casualty, and Intervention Modeling Support*. Aberdeen Proving Ground, Md: US Army Medical Research and Materiel Command. Interim Report. Contract No. DAMD17-98-D-0022; 2002.

28. DeLorenzo RJ, Waterhouse EJ, Towne AR, et al. Persistent nonconvulsive status epilepticus after the control of convulsive status epilepticus. *Epilepsia*. 1998;39:833–840.

29. Petras JM. Soman neurotoxicity. *Fundam Appl Toxicol*. 1981;1:242.

30. Lemercier G, Carpentier P, Sentenac-Roumanou H, Morelis P. Histological and histochemical changes in the central nervous system of the rat poisoned by an irreversible anticholinesterase organophosphorus compound. *Acta Neuropathol (Berl)*. 1983;61:123–129.

31. McLeod CG Jr, Singer AW, Harrington DG. Acute neuropathology in soman poisoned rats. *Neurotoxicology*. 1984;5:53–57.

32. Carpentier P, Delamanche IS, Le Bert M, Blanchet G, Bouchaud C. Seizure-related opening of the blood-brain barrier induced by soman: possible correlation with the acute neuropathology observed in poisoned rats. *Neurotoxicology*. 1990;11:493–508.

33. Kadar T, Cohen G, Sahar R, Alkalai D, Shapira S. Long-term study of brain lesions following soman, in comparison to DFP and metrazol poisoning. *Hum Exp Toxicol*. 1992; 11:517–523.

34. McDonough JH Jr, McLeod CG Jr, Nipwoda MT. Direct microinjection of soman or VX into the amygdala produces repetitive limbic convulsions and neuropathology. *Brain Res*. 1987;435:123–137.

35. Pazdernik TL, Cross R, Giesler M, Nelson S, Samson F, McDonough J Jr. Delayed effects of soman: brain glucose use and pathology. *Neurotoxicology*. 1985;6:61–70.

36. Petrali JP, Maxwell DM, Lenz DE, Mills KR. Effect of an anticholinesterase compound on the ultrastructure and function of the rat blood-brain barrier: a review and experiment. *J Submicrosc Cytol Pathol*. 1991;23:331–338.

37. Petras JM. Neurology and neuropathology of soman-induced brain injury: an overview. *J Exp Anal Behav*. 1994;61:319–329.

38. Ballough GP, Martin LJ, Cann FJ, et al. Microtubule-associated protein 2 (MAP-2): a sensitive marker of seizure-related brain damage. *J Neurosci Methods*. 1995;61:23–32.

39. Lallement G, Carpentier P, Collet A, Baubichon D, Pernot-Marino I, Blanchet G. Extracellular acetylcholine changes in rat limbic structures during soman-induced seizures. *Neurotoxicology*. 1992;13:557–567.

40. Tonduli LS, Testylier G, Marino IP, Lallement G. Triggering of soman-induced seizures in rats: multiparametric analysis with special correlation between enzymatic, neurochemical, and electrophysiological data. *J Neurosci Res*. 1999;58:464–473.

41. Wade JV, Samson FE, Nelson SR, Pazdernik TL. Changes in extracellular amino acids during soman- and kainic acid-induced seizures. *J Neurochem*. 1987;49:645–650.

42. Braitman DJ, Sparenborg S. MK-801 protects against seizures induced by the cholinesterase inhibitor soman. *Brain Res Bull*. 1989;23:145–148.

43. Sparenborg S, Brennecke LH, Jaax NK, Braitman DJ. Dizocilpine (MK-801) arrests status epilepticus and prevents brain damage induced by soman. *Neuropharmacology*. 1992;31:357–368.

44. Fosbraey P, Wetherell JR, French MC. Neurotransmitter changes in guinea-pig brain regions following soman intoxication. *J Neurochem*. 1990;54:72–79.

45. Choi DW. Calcium-mediated neurotoxicity: relationship to specific channel types and role in ischemic damage. *Trends Neurosci*. 1988;11:465–469.

46. Shih TM, Capacio BR, Cook LA. Effects of anticholinergic-antiparkinsonian drugs on striatal neurotransmitter levels of rats intoxicated with soman. *Pharmacol Biochem Behav*. 1993;44:615–622.

47. Fujikawa DG. Prolonged seizures and cellular injury: understanding the connection. *Epilepsy Behav*. 2005:7(suppl 3): S3–11.

48. Carafoli E. Calcium signaling: a tale for all seasons. *Proc Natl Acad Sci U S A*. 2002;99:1115–1122.

49. Verkhratsky A, Toescu EC. Endoplasmic reticulum Ca(2+) homeostasis and neuronal death. *J Cell Mol Med*. 2003;7:351–361.

50. Parekh AB. Store-operated Ca2+ entry: dynamic interplay between endoplasmic reticulum, mitochondria and plasma membrane. *J Physiol*. 2003;547(pt 2):333–348.

51. Bliss TV, Collingridge GL. A synaptic model of memory: long-term potentiation in the hippocampus. *Nature*. 1993;361:31–39.

52. Randall RD, Thayer SA. Glutamate-induced calcium transient triggers delayed calcium overload and neurotoxicity in rat hippocampal neurons. *J Neurosci*.1992;12:1882–1895.

53. Orrenius S, Burkitt MJ, Kass GE, Dypbukt JM, Nicotera P. Calcium ions and oxidative cell injury. *Ann Neurol*. 1992; 32(suppl):S33–42.

54. Orrenius S, Nicotera P. The calcium ion and cell death. *J Neural Transm Suppl*. 1994;43:1–11.

55. Nicotera P. Molecular switches deciding the death of injured neurons. *Toxicol Sci*. 2003;74:4–9.

56. Nicholls DG. Mitochondrial dysfunction and glutamate excitotoxicity studied in primary neuronal cultures. *Curr Mol Med*. 2004;4:149–177.

57. Jayakar SS, Dikshit M. AMPA receptor regulation mechanisms: future target for safer neuroprotective drugs. *Int J Neurosci*. 2004;114:695–734.

58. Kulak W, Sobaniec W, Wojtal K, Czuczwar SJ. Calcium modulation in epilepsy. *Pol J Pharmacol*. 2004;56:29–41.

59. Duchen MR. Mitochondria and calcium: from cell signaling to cell death. *J Physiology*. 2000;529:57–68.

60. Halestrap AP, McStay GP, Clarke SJ. The permeability transition pore complex: another view. *Biochimie*. 2002;84:153–166.

61. Chang LK, Putcha GV, Deshmukh M, Johnson EM Jr. Mitochondrial involvement in the point of no return in neuronal apoptosis. *Biochimie*. 2002;84:223–231.

62. Mattson MP. Excitotoxic and excitoprotective mechanisms: abundant targets for the prevention and treatment of neurodegenerative disorders. *Neuromolecular Med*. 2003;3:65–94.

63. Hou ST, MacManus JP. Molecular mechanisms of cerebral ischemia-induced neuronal death. *Intern Rev Cytol*. 2002;221:93–149.

64. Clarke PGH. Apoptosis versus necrosis--how valid a dichotomy for neurons: In: Koliatsos VE, Ratan RR, eds. *Cell Death and Diseases of the Nervous System*. Totowa, NJ: Humana Press Inc; 1999: 3–28.

65. Sloviter RS. Apoptosis: a guide for the perplexed. *Trends Pharmacol Sci* 2002;23:19–24.

66. Martin LJ, Al-Abdulla NA, Brambrink AM, Kirsch JR, Sieber FE, Portera-Cailliau C. Neurodegeneration in excitotoxicity, global cerebral ischemia, and target deprivation: a perspective on the contributions of apoptosis and necrosis. *Brain Res Bull*. 1998;46:281–309.

67. Baille V, Clarke PG, Brochier G, et al. Soman-induced convulsions: the neuropathology revisited. *Toxicology*. 2005;215:1–24.

68. Ballough GP, Forster JS, Makowski JP, Sordoni NC, Filbert MG. Soman-induced seizures produce neuronal apoptosis [abstract]. *Abstr Soc Neurosci*. 1997;23:1936.

69. Leist M, Single B, Castoldi AF, Kühnle S, Nicotera P. Intracellular adenosine triphosphate (ATP) concentration: a switch in the decision between apoptosis and necrosis. *J Exp Med*. 1997;185:1481–1486.

70. Nicotera P, Leist M, Ferrando-May E. Intracellular ATP, a switch in the decision between apoptosis and necrosis. *Toxicol Lett*. 1998;102–103:139–142.

71. Shoulson I. Experimental therapeutics of neurodegenerative disorders: unmet needs. *Science*. 1998;282:1072–1074.

72. Schulz, JB. Neurodegeneration. In: Bahr M, ed. *Neuroprotection: Models, Mechanisms, and Therapies*. Weinheim, Baden Württemberg, Germany: Wiley-VCH Verlag GmbH & Co; 2004: Chap 16.

73. Siesjo BK, Bengtsson F. Calcium fluxes, calcium antagonists, and calcium-related pathology in brain ischemia, hypoglycemia, and spreading depression: a unifying hypothesis. *J Cereb Blood Flow Metab*. 1989;9:127–140.

74. Silver B, Weber J, Fisher M. Medical therapy for ischemic stroke. *Clin Neuropharmacol*. 1996;19:101–128.

75. Costa E, Armstrong DM, Guidotti A, et al. Gangliosides in the protection against glutamate excitotoxicity. *Prog Brain Res*. 1994;101:357–373.

76. Washington University. The Internet Stroke Center. Available at: www.strokecenter.org. Accessed March 21, 2007.

77. Orbach J. *The Neuropsychological Theories of Lashley and Hebb: Contemporary Perspectives Fifty Years After Hebb's* The Organization of Behavior, *Vanuxem Lectures and Selected Theoretical Papers of Lashley*. Lanham, Md: University Press of America; 1998.

78. Choi DW. Ionic dependence of glutamate neurotoxicity. *J Neurosci*. 1987;7:369–379.

79. Lallement G, Carpentier P, Collet A, Pernot-Marino I, Baubichon D, Blanchet G. Effects of soman-induced seizures on different extracellular amino acid levels and on glutamate uptake in rat hippocampus. *Brain Res*. 1991;563:234–240.

80. Shih TM, McDonough JH Jr. Neurochemical mechanisms in soman-induced seizures. *J Appl Toxicol*. 1997;17:255–264.

81. McDonough JH Jr, Shih TM. Neuropharmacological mechanisms of nerve agent-induced seizure and neuropathology. *Neurosci Biobehav Rev.* 1997;21:559–579.

82. Manev H, Guidotti A, Costa E. Protection by gangliosides against glutamate excitotoxicity. *Adv Lipid Res.* 1993;25:269–288.

83. Tubaro E, Santiangeli C, Cavallo G, et al. Effect of a new de-N-acetyl-lysoglycosphingolipid on chemically-induced inflammatory bowel disease: possible mechanism of action. *Naunyn Schmiedebergs Arch Pharmacol.* 1993;348:670–678.

84. Otani S, Daniel H, Takita M, Crepel F. Long-term depression induced by postsynaptic group II metabotropic glutamate receptors linked to phospholipase C and intracellular calcium rises in rat prefrontal cortex. *J Neurosci.* 2002;22:3434–3444.

85. Monnet FP, Morin-Surun MP, Leger J, Combettes L. Protein kinase C-dependent potentiation of intracellular calcium influx by sigma1 receptor agonists in rat hippocampal neurons. *J Pharmacol Exp Ther.* 2003;307:705–312.

86. Chaban VV, Li J, Ennes HS, Nie J, Mayer EA, McRoberts JA. N-methyl-D-aspartate receptors enhance mechanical responses and voltage-dependent Ca2+ channels in rat dorsal root ganglia neurons through protein kinase C. *Neuroscience.* 2004;128:347–357.

87. Niebauer M, Gruenthal M. Neuroprotective effects of early vs. late administration of dantrolene in experimental status epilepticus. *Neuropharmacology.* 1999;38:1343–1348.

88. Ballough GPH, Filbert MG. *A Viable Neuroprotection Strategy Following Soman-Induced Status Epilepticus.* Aberdeen Proving Ground, Md: US Army Medical Research Institute of Chemical Defense; 2003. USAMRICD Technical Report 03-09, AD A443565.

89. Krause T, Gerbershagen MU, Fiege M, Weisshorn R, Wappler F. Dantrolene–a review of its pharmacology, therapeutic use, and new developments. *Anaesthesia.* 2004;59:364–373.

90. Ballough GP, Cann FJ, Smith CD, Forster JS, Kling CE, Filbert MG. GM1 monosialoganglioside pretreatment protects against soman-induced seizure-related brain damage. *Mol Chem Neuropathol.* 1998;34:1–23.

91. Ando S. Gangliosides in the nervous system. *Neurochem Int.* 1983;5:507–537.

92. Ledeen RW. Biology of gangliosides: neuritogenic and neuronotrophic properties. *J Neurosci Res.* 1984;12:147–159.

93. Yu RK, Goldenring JR, Kim JYH, DeLorenzo RJ. Gangliosides as differential modulators of membrane-bound protein kinase systems. In: Tettamanti G, Ledeen RW, Sandhoff K, Nagai Y, Toffano G, eds. *Fidia Research Series: Gangliosides and Neuronal Plasticity.* Vol 6. Padova, Italy: Liviana Press; 1986: 95–104.

94. Vaccarino F, Guidotti A, Costa E. Ganglioside inhibition of glutamate-mediated protein kinase C translocation in primary cultures of cerebellar neurons. *Proc Natl Acad Sci U S A.* 1987;84:8707–8711.

95. Manev H, Favaron M, Vicini S, Guidotti A. Ganglioside-mediated protection from glutamate-induced neuronal death. *Acta Neurobiol Exp (Wars).* 1990;50:475–488.

96. Wagey R, Hu J, Pelech SL, Raymond LA, Krieger C. Modulation of NMDA-mediated excitotoxicity by protein kinase C. *J Neurochem.* 2001;78:715–726.

97. Koponen S, Kurkinen K, Akerman KE, Mochly-Rosen D, Chan PH, Koistinaho J. Prevention of NMDA-induced death of cortical neurons by inhibition of protein kinase Czeta. *J Neurochem.* 2003;86:442–450.

98. Zhang L, Rzigalinski BA, Ellis EF, Satin LS. Reduction of voltage-dependent Mg2+ blockade of NMDA current in mechanically injured neurons. *Science.* 1996;274:1921–1923.

99. Tubaro E, Croce C, Cavallo G, Belogi L, Guida G, Santiangeli C, Cifone MG, Santoni A, Mainiero F. In vitro and in vivo impact of a new glycosphingolipid on neutrophils. *Agents Actions.* 1994;42:107–113.

100. Mattei V, Garofalo T, Misasi R, Gizzi C, Mascellino MT, Dolo V, Pontieri GM, Sorice M, Pavan A. Association of cellular prion protein with gangliosides in plasma membrane microdomains of neural and lymphocytic cells. *Neurochem Res.* 2002;27:743–749.

101. Eliasson MJ, Sampei K, Mandir AS, et al. Poly(ADP-ribose) polymerase gene disruption renders mice resistant to cerebral ischemia. *Nat Med.* 1997;3:1089–1095.

102. Mandir AS, Poitras MF, Berliner AR, et al. NMDA but not non-NMDA excitotoxicity is mediated by Poly(ADP-ribose) polymerase. *J Neurosci.* 2000;20:8005–8011.

103. Whalen MJ, Clark RS, Dixon CE, et al. Traumatic brain injury in mice deficient in poly-ADP(ribose) polymerase: a preliminary report. *Acta Neurochir Suppl.* 2000;76:61–64.

104. Abdelkarim GE, Gertz K, Harms C, et al. Protective effects of PJ34, a novel, potent inhibitor of poly(ADP-ribose) polymerase (PARP) in in vitro and in vivo models of stroke. *Int J Mol Med.* 2001;7:255–260.

105. Kamanaka Y, Kondo K, Ikeda Y, et al. Neuroprotective effects of ONO-1924H, an inhibitor of poly ADP-ribose polymerase (PARP), on cytotoxicity of PC12 cells and ischemic cerebral damage. *Life Sci.* 2004;76:151–162.

106. Sharma SS, Munusamy S, Thiyagarajan M, Kaul CL. Neuroprotective effect of peroxynitrite decomposition catalyst and poly(adenosine diphosphate-ribose) polymerase inhibitor alone and in combination in rats with focal cerebral ischemia. *J Neurosurg.* 2004;101:669–675.

107. Nakajima H, Kakui N, Ohkuma K, Ishikawa M, Hasegawa T. A newly synthesized poly(ADP-ribose) polymerase inhibitor, DR2313 [2-methyl-3,5,7,8-tetrahydrothiopyrano[4,3-d]-pyrimidine-4-one]: pharmacological profiles, neuroprotective effects, and therapeutic time window in cerebral ischemia in rats. *J Pharmacol Exp Ther.* 2005;312:472–481.

108. Ying W, Alano CC, Garnier P, Swanson RA. NAD+ as a metabolic link between DNA damage and cell death. *J Neurosci Res.* 2005;79:216–223.

109. Szabo C, Dawson VL. Role of poly(ADP-ribose) synthetase in inflammation and ischaemia-reperfusion. *Trends Pharmacol Sci.* 1998;19:287–298.

110. Virag L, Szabo C. The therapeutic potential of poly(ADP-ribose) polymerase inhibitors. *Pharmacol Rev.* 2002;54:375–429.

111. Park EM, Cho S, Frys K, et al. Interaction between inducible nitric oxide synthase and poly(ADP-ribose) polymerase in focal ischemic brain injury. *Stroke.* 2004;35:2896–2901.

112. Wang H, Yu SW, Koh DW, et al. Apoptosis-inducing factor substitutes for caspase executioners in NMDA-triggered excitotoxic neuronal death. *J Neurosci.* 2004;24:10963–10973.

113. Meier HL, Ballough GP, Forster JS, Filbert MG. Benzamide, a poly(ADP-ribose) polymerase inhibitor, is neuroprotective against soman-induced seizure-related brain damage. *Ann N Y Acad Sci.* 1999;890:330–335.

114. Iwashita A, Tojo N, Matsuura S, et al. A novel and potent poly(ADP-ribose) polymerase-1 inhibitor, FR247304 (5-chloro-2-[3-(4-phenyl-3,6-dihydro-1(2H)-pyridinyl)propyl]-4(3H)-quinazolinone), attenuates neuronal damage in vitro and in vivo models of cerebral ischemia. *J Pharmacol Exp Ther.* 2004;310:425–436.

115. Frandsen A, Schousboe A. Dantrolene prevents glutamate cytotoxicity and Ca2+ release from intracellular stores. *J Neurochem.* 1991;56:1075–1078.

116. Popescu BO, Oprica M, Sajin M, et al. Dantrolene protects neurons against kainic acid induced apoptosis in vitro and in vivo. *J Cell Mol Med.* 2002;6:555–569.

117. Olney JW, Labruyere J, Price MT. Pathological changes induced in cerebrocortical neurons by phencyclidine and related drugs. *Science.* 1989;244:1360–1362.

118. Fix AS, Horn JW, Wightman KA, et al. Neuronal vacuolization and necrosis induced by the noncompetitive N-methyl-D-aspartate (NMDA) antagonist MK(+)801 (dizocilpine maleate): a light and electron microscopic evaluation of the rat retrosplenial cortex. *Exp Neurol*. 1993;123:204–215.

119. Corso TD, Sesma MA, Tenkova TI, et al. Multifocal brain damage induced by phencyclidine is augmented by pilocarpine. *Brain Res*. 1997;752:1–14.

120. Olney JW, Labruyere J, Wang G, Wozniak DF, Price MT, Sesma MA. NMDA antagonist neurotoxicity: mechanism and prevention. *Science*. 1991;254:1515–1518.

121. Wozniak DF, Dikranian K, Ishimaru MJ, et al. Disseminated corticolimbic neuronal degeneration induced in rat brain by MK-801: potential relevance to Alzheimer's disease. *Neurobiol Dis*. 1998;5:305–322.

122. Bormann J. Memantine is a potent blocker of N-methyl-D-aspartate (NMDA) receptor channels. *Eur J Pharmacol*. 1989;166:591–592.

123. Chen HS, Pellegrini JW, Aggarwal SK, et al. Open-channel block of N-methyl-D-aspartate (NMDA) responses by memantine: therapeutic advantage against NMDA receptor-mediated neurotoxicity. *J Neurosci*. 1992;12:4427–4436.

124. Lipton SA. Excitotoxicity. In: Bahr M, ed. *Neuroprotection: Models, Mechanisms, and Therapies*. Weinheim, Baden Württemberg, Germany: Wiley-VCH Verlag GmbH & Co; 2004: Chap 14.

125. McLean MJ, Gupta RC, Dettbarn WD, Wamil AW. Prophylactic and therapeutic efficacy of memantine against seizures produced by soman in the rat. *Toxicol Appl Pharmacol*. 1992;112:95–103.

126. Koplovitz I, Schulz S, Shutz M, Railer R, Smith F, Okerberg C, Filbert M. Memantine effects on soman-induced seizures and seizure-related brain damage. *Toxicol Meth* 1997;7:227–239.[AQ2]

127. Parsons CG, Danysz W, Quack G. Memantine is a clinically well tolerated N-methyl-D-aspartate (NMDA) receptor antagonist--a review of preclinical data. *Neuropharmacology*. 1999;38:735–767.

128. Chen HS, Wang YF, Rayudu PV, et al. Neuroprotective concentrations of the N-methyl-D-aspartate open-channel blocker memantine are effective without cytoplasmic vacuolation following post-ischemic administration and do not block maze learning or long-term potentiation. *Neuroscience*. 1998;86:1121–1132.

129. Filbert MG, Forster JS, Smith CD, Ballough GP. Neuroprotective effects of HU-211 on brain damage resulting from soman-induced seizures. *Ann N Y Acad Sci*. 1999;890:505–514.

130. Shohami E, Novikov M, Mechoulam R. A nonpsychotropic cannabinoid, HU-211, has cerebroprotective effects after closed head injury in the rat. *J Neurotrauma*. 1993;10:109–119.

131. Biegon A, Joseph AB. Development of HU-211 as a neuroprotectant for ischemic brain damage. *Neurol Res*. 1995;17:275–280.

132. Lavie G, Teichner A, Shohami E, Ovadia H, Leker RR. Long term cerebroprotective effects of dexanabinol in a model of focal cerebral ischemia. *Brain Res*. 2001;901:195–201.

133. Darlington CL. Dexanabinol: a novel cannabinoid with neuroprotective properties. *IDrugs*. 2003;6:976–979.

134. Kitagawa K, Matsumoto M, Niinobe M, et al. Microtubule-associated protein 2 as a sensitive marker for cerebral ischemic damage—immunohistochemical investigation of dendritic damage. *Neurosci* 1989;31:401–411.

135. Gilland E, Bona E, Hagberg H. Temporal changes of regional glucose use, blood flow and microtubule-associated protein 2 immunostaining after hypoxia ischemia in the immature rat brain. *J Cereb Blood Flow Metab*. 1998:18:222–228.

136. Lallement G, Mestries JC, Privat A, et al. GK 11: promising additional neuroprotective therapy for organophosphate poisoning. *Neurotoxicology*. 1997;18:851–856.

137. Lallement G, Clarencon D, Masqueliez C, et al. Nerve agent poisoning in primates: antilethal, anti-epileptic, and neuroprotective effects of GK-11. *Arch Toxicol*. 1998;72:84–92.

138. Lallement G, Clarencon D, Galonnier M, Baubichon D, Burckhart MF, Peoc'h M. Acute soman poisoning in primates neither pretreated nor receiving immediate therapy: value of gacyclidine (GK-11) in delayed medical support. *Arch Toxicol*. 1999;73:115–122.

139. Hirbec H, Gaviria M, Vignon J. Gacyclidine: a new neuroprotective agent acting at the N-methyl-D-aspartate receptor. *CNS Drug Rev*. 2001;7:172–198.

140. Lepeintre JF, D'Arbigny P, Mathe JF, et al. Neuroprotective effect of gacyclidine. A multicenter double-blind pilot trial in patients with acute traumatic brain injury. *Neurochirurgie*. 2004;50(Part 1):83–95.

141. Lallement G. Centre de Recherches du Service de Sante des Armees, La Tronche, France. Personal communication with Ballough G, June 2005.

142. Dorandeu F. Centre de Recherches du Service de Sante des Armees, La Tronche, France. Personal communication with Ballough G, August 2006.

143. MacDonald JF, Nowak LM. Mechanisms of blockade of excitatory amino acid receptor channels. *Trends Pharmacol Sci*. 1990;11:167–172.

144. Werner C, Reeker W, Engelhard K, Lu H, Kochs E. Ketamine racemate and S-(+)-ketamine. Cerebrovascular effects and neuroprotection following focal ischemia. *Anaesthesist*. 1997;46(supp; 1):S55–S60.

145. Mion G, Tourtier JP, Petitjeans F, Dorandeu F, Lallement G, Ruttimann M. Neuroprotective and antiepileptic activities of ketamine in nerve agent poisoning. *Anesthesiology*. 2003;98:1517.

146. Ivani G, Vercellino C, Tonetti F. Ketamine: a new look to an old drug. *Minerva Anestesiol*. 2003;69:468–471.

147. Fujikawa DG. Neuroprotective effect of ketamine administration after status epilepticus onset. *Epilepsia*. 1995;36:186–195.

148. Van Rijckevorsel K, Boon P, Hauman H, et al. Standards of care for adults with convulsive status epilepticus: Belgian consensus recommendations. *Acta Neurol Belg*. 2005;105:111–118.

149. Dorandeu F, Carpentier P, Baubichon D, et al. Efficacy of the ketamine-atropine combination in the delayed treatment of soman-induced status epilepticus. *Brain Res*. 2005;1051:164–175.

150. Stewart LS, Persinger MA. Ketamine prevents learning impairment when administered immediately after status epilepticus onset. *Epilepsy Behav*. 2001;2:585–591.

151. Borris DJ, Bertram EH, Kapur J. Ketamine controls prolonged status epilepticus. *Epilepsy Res*. 2000;42:117–122.

152. Durham D. Management of status epilepticus. *Crit Care Resusc*. 1999;1:344–353.

153. Robakis TK, Hirsch LJ. Literature review, case report, and expert discussion of prolonged refractory status epilepticus. *Neurocrit Care*. 2006;4:35–46.

154. Walker MC, Howard RS, Smith SJ, Miller DH, Shorvon SD, Hirsch NP. Diagnosis and treatment of status epilepticus on a neurological intensive care unit. *QJM*. 1996;89:913–920.

155. Sheth RD, Gidal BE. Refractory status epilepticus: response to ketamine. *Neurology*. 1998;51:1765–1766.

156. Annetta MG, Iemma D, Garisto C, Tafani C, Proietti R. Ketamine: new indications for an old drug. *Curr Drug Targets*. 2005;6:789–794.

157. Nakki R, Koistinaho J, Sharp FR, Sagar SM. Cerebellar toxicity of phencyclidine. *J Neurosci*. 1995;15(pt 2):2097–2108.

158. Ubogu EE, Sagar SM, Lerner AJ, Maddux BN, Suarez JI, Werz MA. Ketamine for refractory status epilepticus: a case of possible ketamine-induced neurotoxicity. *Epilepsy Behav*. 2003;4:70–75.

159. Wolff K, Winstock AR. Ketamine: from medicine to misuse. *CNS Drugs*. 2006;20:199–218.

160. Pazdernik TL, Emerson MR, Cross R, Nelson SR, Samson FE. Soman-induced seizures: limbic activity, oxidative stress and neuroprotective proteins. *J Appl Toxicol*. 2001:21(suppl 1):S87–S94.

161. Pagni CA, Zenga F. Posttraumatic epilepsy with special emphasis on prophylaxis and prevention. *Acta Neurochir Suppl*. 2005;93:27–34.

162. Yokoi I, Toma J, Liu J, Kabuto H, Mori A. Adenosines scavenged hydroxyl radicals and prevented posttraumatic epilepsy. *Free Radic Biol Med*. 1995;19:473–479.

163. Davies KJ. Oxidative stress: the paradox of aerobic life. *Biochem Soc Symp*. 1995;61:1–31.

164. Zivin M, Milatovic D, Dettbarn WD. Nitrone spin trapping compound N-tert-butyl-alpha-phenylnitrone prevents seizures induced by anticholinesterases. *Brain Res*. 1999;850:63–72.

165. Peterson SL, Purvis RS, Griffith JW. Comparison of neuroprotective effects induced by alpha-phenyl-N-tert-butyl nitrone (PBN) and N-tert-butyl-alpha-(2 sulfophenyl) nitrone (S-PBN) in lithium-pilocarpine status epilepticus. *Neurotoxicology*. 2005;26:969–979.

166. Cao X, Phillis JW. Alpha-Phenyl-tert-butyl-nitrone reduces cortical infarct and edema in rats subjected to focal ischemia. *Brain Res*. 1994;644:267–272.

167. Meyerhoff JL. Division of Neurosciences, Walter Reed Army Institute of Research, Silver Spring, Md 20910-7500, USA. Personal communication with Newmark J, March 2006.

168. Lockhart B, Roger A, Bonhomme N, Goldstein S, Lestage P. In vivo neuroprotective effects of the novel imidazolyl nitrone free-radical scavenger (Z)-alpha-[2-thiazol-2-yl)imidazol-4-yl]-N-tert-butylnitrone (S34176). *Eur J Pharmacol*. 2005;511:127–136.

169. Bauman RA, Yourick DL, Wessner K, et al. A model for studying neuroprotection from seizure-induced brain injury resulting from exposure to organophosphate (OP) nerve agents. In: Proceedings of the NATO Task Group on Prophylaxis and Therapy Against Chemical Agents; May 23–27, 2005. Hradec Kralove, Czech Republic.

170. Kudin AP, Debska-Vielhaber G, Vielhaber S, Elger CE, Kunz WS. The mechanism of neuroprotection by topiramate in an animal model of epilepsy. *Epilepsia*. 2004;45:1478–1487.

171. Setkowicz Z, Ciarach M, Guzik R, Janeczko K. Different effects of neuroprotectants FK-506 and cyclosporin A on susceptibility to pilocarpine-induced seizures in rats with brain injured at different developmental stages. *Epilepsy Res*. 2004;61:63–72.

172. Santos JB, Schauwecker PE. Protection provided by cyclosporin A against excitotoxic neuronal death is genotype dependent. *Epilepsia*. 2003;44:995–1002

173. Okonkwo DO, Melon DE, Pellicane AJ, et al. Dose-response of cyclosporin A in attenuating traumatic axonal injury in rat. *Neuroreport*. 2003;14:463–466.

174. Friberg H, Wieloch T. Mitochondrial permeability transition in acute neurodegeneration. *Biochimie*. 2002;84:241–250.

175. De Keyser J, Uyttenboogaart M, Koch MW, et al. Neuroprotection in acute ischemic stroke. *Acta Neurol Belg*. 2005;105:144–148.

176. Li J, Luan X, Lai Q, et al. Long-term neuroprotection induced by regional brain cooling with saline infusion into ischemic territory in rats: a behavioral analysis. *Neurol Res*. 2004;26:677–683.

177. Filbert M, Levine E, Ballough G. Neuroprotection for nerve agent-induced brain damage by blocking delayed calcium overload: a review. *Journal of Medical Chemical Biological and Radiological Defense*. 2005;3:1–21. Available at http://jmedcbr.org/Issue_0301/Filbert/Filbert_1105.pdf.

Chapter 7

NERVE AGENT BIOSCAVENGER: DEVELOPMENT OF A NEW APPROACH TO PROTECT AGAINST ORGANO-PHOSPHORUS EXPOSURE

MICHELLE C. ROSS, DVM, PhD*; CLARENCE A. BROOMFIELD, PhD†; DOUGLAS M. CERASOLI, PhD‡; BHUPENDRA P. DOCTOR, PhD§; DAVID E. LENZ, PhD¥; DONALD M. MAXWELL, MS¶; AND ASHIMA SAXENA, PhD**

* *Colonel, US Army; Director of CBRN Medical Defense Policy, Office of the Assistant Secretary of Defense for Health Affairs, 5111 Leesburg Pike, Skyline 5, Falls Church, Virginia 22041*

† *Research Chemist, Research Division, Department of Pharmacology, US Army Medical Research Institute of Chemical Defense, 3100 Ricketts Point Road, Aberdeen Proving Ground, Maryland 21010*

‡ *Research Microbiologist, Research Division, Department of Physiology and Immunology, US Army Medical Research Institute of Chemical Defense, 3100 Ricketts Point Road, Aberdeen Proving Ground, Maryland 21010*

§ *Director, Division of Biochemistry, Walter Reed Army Institute of Research, 503 Robert Grant Avenue, Silver Spring, Maryland 20910*

¥ *Research Chemist, Research Division, US Army Medical Research Institute of Chemical Defense, 3100 Ricketts Point Road, Aberdeen Proving Ground, Maryland 21010*

¶ *Research Chemist, Research Division, Department of Pharmacology, US Army Medical Research Institute of Chemical Defense, 3100 Ricketts Point Road, Aberdeen Proving Ground, Maryland 21010*

** *Chief, Division of Biochemistry, Department of Molecular Pharmacology, Walter Reed Army Institute of Research, 503 Robert Grant Avenue, Silver Spring, Maryland 20910*

INTRODUCTION

Nerve agents are highly lethal chemical agent threats to the US population. Chemically, they belong to the organophosphorus (OP) compound group and are among the most toxic substances identified. OP compounds were originally developed for use as insecticides, but their extreme toxicity and rapid effects on higher vertebrates have led to their adoption as weapons of warfare. The OP compounds most commonly used as chemical weapons (referred to as "nerve agents") are O-ethyl N,N-dimethyl phosphoramidocyanidate (tabun; North Atlantic Treaty Organization [NATO] designation: GA), diisopropyl phosphonofluoridate (sarin; NATO designation: GB), pinacoloxymethyl-fluorophosphonate (soman; NATO designation: GD), cyclohexylmethyl phosphonofluoridate (cyclosarin; NATO designation: GF), and ethyl-S-diisopropylaminoethyl methylphosphonothiolate (VX). Newer, nontraditional nerve agents pose even greater dangers than these traditional ones.

Nerve agents in aerosol or liquid form can enter the body by inhalation or by absorption through the skin. Poisoning may also occur through the consumption of liquids or foods contaminated with nerve agents. Nerve agents are lethal at extremely low levels; exposure to a high concentration of nerve agent can result in death within minutes. Poisoning takes longer when the nerve agent is absorbed through the skin. The values for the median lethal dose (LD_{50}) in mammals, including estimates for humans, are in the μg/kg dose range for all routes of exposure except skin, in which LD_{50} values are in the mg/kg range.[1] Personnel may also be effected through secondary contact with contaminated victims. Survivors may have long-term central nervous system dysfunction following intoxication.[2]

The acute toxicity of OPs is attributed to their binding to and irreversible inhibition of acetylcholinesterase (AChE). The resulting increase in acetylcholine concentration manifests at the cholinergic synapses of both the peripheral and central nervous systems by over-stimulation at the neuromuscular junctions as well as alteration in the function of the respiratory center.[3–5] This precipitates a cholinergic crisis characterized by miosis, increased tracheobronchial and salivary secretions, bronchoconstriction, bradycardia, fasciculation, behavioral incapacitation, muscular weakness, and convulsions, culminating in death by respiratory failure.[3]

Nerve agents are stable, easily dispersed, and can be manufactured by readily available industrial chemical processes, including OP pesticide production facilities, which can easily be converted to produce nerve agents. Even the most dangerous forms of nerve agents are within the technical capability of sophisticated terrorist networks. Nerve agents possessed by rogue states and other potential US adversaries have long been known to pose a serious threat to US forces. Aum Shinrikyo's 1995 sarin attack in the Tokyo subway system demonstrated that nerve agents are also a real and potent terrorist threat to civilian populations. Nerve agents are attractive chemical weapons for terrorist use because small quantities are fast-acting and can cause death or harm by multiple routes. Some types of nerve agents are highly persistent, enabling terrorists to construct long-lasting hazards to target populations. For example, the administration of highly persistent nerve agents to frequently used public facilities, like subway trains, can effect mass disruption by causing citizens to fear using those facilities important to everyday life. The use of nerve agents in combination with other weapons may also make differentiating causalities challenging and place first responders and law enforcement personnel at risk when entering a contaminated area.

Current antidotal regimens for OP poisoning consist of a combination of pretreatment with a spontaneously reactivating AChE inhibitor, such as pyridostigmine bromide, and postexposure therapy with an anticholinergic drug, such as atropine sulfate, and an oxime, such as 2-pralidoxime chloride[6] and an anticonvulsant such as diazepam,[7] if needed. Although these antidotal regimens effectively prevent lethality and, in best cases, reverse toxicity following exposure, they do not prevent the exposed individual from becoming a casualty. Moreover, no current therapies for nerve agent exposure can provide sustained protection to an individual; they have to be readministered within minutes or hours and are therefore limited by practical and logistical issues. Treated patients often show signs of postexposure incapacitation, convulsions, and performance deficits or, in the case of recurring seizures, permanent brain damage.[8–10] Some nerve agents, such as soman, present an additional challenge because of the rapid dealkylation of soman-inhibited AChE that is resistant to therapeutic reversal by an oxime.

An urgent need exists for new medical countermeasures to nerve agent exposure that provide higher survival rates, eliminate or reduce enduring adverse effects to survivors, and significantly reduce or eliminate the need for repeated administration of therapeutic drugs. Ideally, medical treatment should be administered within approximately 1 minute after exposure and should be effective for all OP compounds. These challenges stimulated the development of enzyme bioscavengers as a pretreatment therapy to sequester highly toxic OPs in circulation before they reach their physiological targets.[11]

The use of enzymes as therapeutic agents is not unique; enzymes are used in wound healing, proteolysis, fibrinolysis, and depletion of metabolites in cancer. Enzymes have many advantages; they are specific, highly efficient, operate under physiological conditions, and cause essentially no deleterious side effects. However, there are certain requirements for an enzyme to be an effective therapy for OP toxicity in vivo: (*a*) it should react rapidly, specifically, and irreversibly with all OP nerve agents; (*b*) it should have a sustained half-life in circulation for it to be effective as a scavenger for long periods; (*c*) it should be readily available in sufficient quantities; and (*d*) it should not be immunogenic. The bioscavengers that have been explored to date for the detoxification of OPs fall into three categories: (1) those that stoichiometrically bind to OPs (ie, 1 mole of enzyme neutralizes 1 mole of OP, inactivating both), such as cholinesterase (ChE), carboxylesterase (CaE), and other related enzymes; (2) a group generally termed "pseudo catalytic," such as those combining AChE and an oxime so the catalytic activity of OP-inhibited AChE can rapidly and continuously be restored in the presence of oxime; and (3) those that can naturally catalytically hydrolyze OPs and thus render them nontoxic, such as OP hydrolase, OP anhydrase, and paraoxonase.

PLASMA-DERIVED STOICHIOMETRIC BIOSCAVENGERS

Candidate stoichiometric bioscavengers are naturally occurring human proteins that bind and react with nerve agents, including enzymes such as ChEs and CaEs. Each of these stoichiometric scavengers has the capacity to bind one molecule of nerve agent per molecule of protein scavenger.

Cholinesterases

Wolfe et al were the first to report the use of exogenously administered AChE as a bioscavenger.[12] They demonstrated that pretreatment of mice with fetal bovine serum (FBS) AChE afforded complete protection against VX, while providing a much lower level of protection against soman. However, FBS AChE pretreatment in conjunction with postexposure administration of atropine and 2-pralidoxime protected mice from both VX and soman. The authors also reported that animals displayed no detectable side effects in response to the administration of FBS AChE alone.

Maxwell et al conducted a similar set of experiments with rhesus monkeys.[13] Monkeys pretreated with FBS AChE that were challenged with either 1.5 or 2.5 times the LD_{50} of soman received total protection without decreased performance when assessed by a serial probe recognition task. Subsequently, Maxwell et al compared the relative protection afforded to mice against soman by three different treatment regimens: (1) pyridostigmine pretreatment with postexposure atropine therapy, (2) postexposure asoxime chloride with atropine therapy, and (3) FBS AChE pretreatment alone.[14] The researchers concluded that the FBS AChE pretreatment alone not only prevented the lethality of animals exposed to 8 to 10 times the LD_{50} of soman, but also protected against behavioral incapacitation.

Boomfield et al were the first to study the protection afforded by butyrylcholinesterase (BChE). They reported that a commercial preparation of equine serum (Eq) BChE afforded complete protection to rhesus monkeys against 2 times the LD_{50} challenge of soman, with no supporting therapy, and against 3 to 4 times the LD_{50} challenge of soman when combined with postexposure therapy with atropine.[15] Protection against a single LD_{50} of sarin without supporting therapy was also demonstrated. Furthermore, when animals were assessed for behavioral deficits using a serial probe recognition task, they all returned to baseline performance levels following soman exposure.

Raveh et al conducted the first study demonstrating the in vivo stoichiometry of OP neutralization by the bioscavenger.[16] They demonstrated that approximately 90% to 95% of FBS AChE that was administered by intravenous (IV) injection was found in the circulation of mice. Circulating enzyme concentrations rose to peak levels in 30 minutes to 1 hour and were maintained for up to 6 hours. This provided a window in which OP challenge of animals yielded a linear correlation between the moles of OP administered and the moles of enzyme neutralized. Ashani et al compared the OP scavenging properties of plasma-derived human (pHu) BChE with those of FBS AChE in mice, rats, and rhesus monkeys against several different nerve agents as well as other OPs.[17] They observed that in mice and rats, the same linear correlation existed between the concentration of pHu BChE in blood and the level of protection afforded against soman, sarin, or VX. They further noted that to be effective, a scavenger had to be present in circulation before OP exposure because the nerve agent had to be scavenged within one blood circulation time period. The window to determine stoichiometry of enzyme and OP became useful even when the enzyme was administered by intramuscular (IM) injection and the OP by subcutaneous injection.[18,19] Raveh et al reported that the same dose of enzyme could protect against 3.3 times the LD_{50} of soman or 2.1 times the LD_{50} of VX in rhesus monkeys.[19] They also reported substantial protection against soman-induced behavioral deficits using a spatial discrimination task.

Wolfe et al assessed the ability of FBS AChE or Eq BChE pretreatment to protect rhesus monkeys against multiple LD_{50} of soman.[20] Survival and the ability to perform the primate equilibrium platform behavioral task were concurrently assessed. Animals pretreated with FBS AChE were protected against a cumulative exposure of 5 times the LD_{50} of soman and showed no decrement in the primate equilibrium platform task. Two of the four monkeys that received purified Eq BChE showed a transient decrement in the primate equilibrium platform task performance when the cumulative dose of soman exceeded 4 times the LD_{50}. All experimental animals were observed for an additional 6 weeks and none displayed residual or delayed performance decrements, suggesting no residual adverse effects.

CaE is another enzyme with potential as a good anti-OP scavenger molecule. CaE can be distinguished from ChEs because while ChEs react with positively charged carboxylesters, such as acetylcholine and butyrylcholine, and are readily inhibited by carbamates, CaE does not react with positively charged substrates and is inhibited by carbamates only at high concentrations.[21] These differences in substrate specificity also extend to the reaction of CaE with OP compounds. Positively charged OP compounds, such as VX, react poorly with CaE, while neutral OP compounds such as soman, sarin, and paraoxon, react rapidly. CaE is synthesized in the liver and secreted into circulation.[22] The levels of circulating CaE vary between mammalian species, and animals that have high levels of plasma CaE require much larger doses of OP compounds to produce toxicity than do species with low levels of plasma CaE.[23] For example, the LD_{50} for soman in rats is 10-fold higher than the LD_{50} in nonhuman primates, which correlates with the differences in the plasma concentrations of CaE found in these species. Like nonhuman primates, humans do not express CaE in plasma.[24]

The primary evidence supporting the hypothesis that CaE can function as a stoichiometric scavenger against OPs (especially sarin and soman) but not for V agents was obtained by comparing LD_{50}s of OPs in animals possessing high endogenous plasma levels of CaE to LD_{50} in the same animal species following inhibition of plasma CaE with chemicals (Figure 7-1).[25] For example, inhibition of plasma CaE reduced the LD_{50} of soman in rats approximately 8-fold, suggesting that circulating CaE can be an effective bioscavenger against OPs. Furthermore, investigations of the reactivation of OP-inhibited CaE have suggested that it may be possible to increase its potential as an OP scavenger by exploiting its turnover of OPs. Maxwell et al observed that OP-inhibited CaE did not undergo aging that prevented oxime reactivation of OP-inhibited ChEs,[26] while Jokanovic et al found that OP-inhibited plasma CaE in rats underwent spontaneous reactivation with a half time of 1 to 2 hours.[27] Extensive investigations need to be carried out before considering using CaE as a bioscavenger for humans. Although human CaE has been cloned and expressed,[22] there is no commercial source of highly purified CaE for use in in-vivo testing of protective efficacy.

The absence of immunological or physiological side effects following transfusions of plasma in humans and the lack of adverse reaction to the administration of partially purified pHu BChE suggest that this enzyme would be the most promising prophylactic antidote for human use.[28,29] As an exogenously administered prophylactic, pHu BChE has several advantages for human use.[30] First, it reacts rapidly with all highly toxic OPs, offering a broad range of protection for nerve agents, including soman, sarin, tabun, and VX. Second, its retention time in human circulation is long

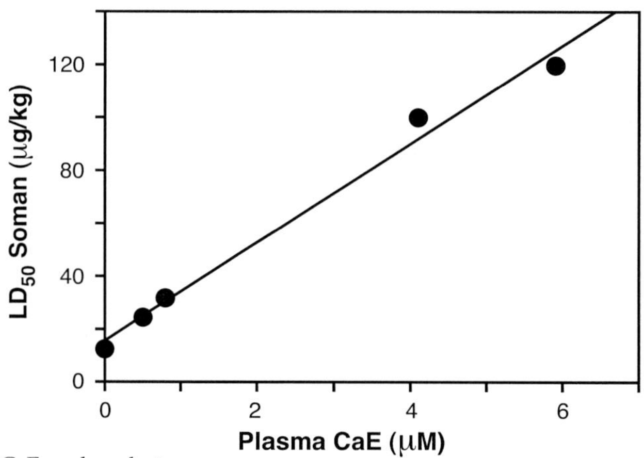

CaE: carboxylesterase
LD_{50}: median lethal dose

Fig. 7-1. Effect of plasma carboxylesterase concentration on soman median lethal dose (administered subcutaneously) in different species. Data points (from lower left to upper right of graph) for species were monkey, rabbit, guinea pig, rat, and mouse.

Reproduced with permission from: Maxwell DM, Wolfe AD, Ashani Y, Doctor BP. Cholinesterase and carboxylesterase as scavengers for organophosphorus agents, In: Massoulie J, Bacou F, Bernard E, Chatonnet A, Doctor BP, Quinn DM, eds. *Cholinesterases: Structure, Function, Mechanism, Genetics, and Cell Biology*. Washington, DC: American Chemical Society; 1991: 206.

and it is readily absorbed from injection sites. Third, because the enzyme is from a human source, it should not produce adverse immunological responses upon repeated administration to humans. Fourth, because the enzyme has no known physiological function in the body, it is unlikely to produce any physiological side effects. Because the biochemical mechanism underlying prophylaxis by exogenous pHu BChE was established and tested in several species, including nonhuman primates, results can be reliably extrapolated from animal experiments and applied to humans. A dose of 200 mg of pHu BChE is envisioned as prophylaxis for humans exposed to 2 to 5 times the LD_{50} of soman.

The foremost requirement to advance pHu BChE as a bioscavenger for human use was to obtain sufficient amounts of purified enzyme with which to conduct animal and clinical studies. Although a procedure for the purification of pHu BChE from human plasma, which contains ~ 2 mg of enzyme per liter of plasma, was described, this source is not suitable for producing gram quantities of pHu BChE.[31] Cohn Fraction IV-4 paste (a by-product of human plasma generated during the production of human blood proteins, such as γ-globulin and clotting factors), was identified as a rich source of pHu BChE. Cohn Fraction IV-4 paste contains ~ 150 mg of enzyme per kg, which is much higher than human plasma, and contains much lower quantities of other plasma proteins because of the fractionation steps employed in the production process. A procedure for the large-scale purification of pHu BChE from Cohn Fraction IV-4 paste was developed using batch procainamide affinity chromatography followed by anion exchange chromatography. Approximately 6 g of purified enzyme was obtained from 120 kg of Cohn fraction IV-4.[32]

Pharmacokinetics and the Safety of Plasma-Derived Human Butyrylcholinesterase

Purified pHu BChE displayed high bioavailability in the circulation of mice, guinea pigs, and nonhuman primates when administered by IV, IM, or intraperitoneal (IP) injections. The enzyme displayed a mean residence time (MRT) of about 48 hours in mice (IM, IP), 109 to 110 hours in guinea pigs (IM, IP) and 72 to 74 hours in rhesus (IV) or cynomolgus monkeys (IM).[32–34] The circulatory stability profiles were similar to those previously observed for enzyme purified from human plasma in rats and mice,[17–19] guinea pigs,[35] and rhesus monkeys.[19]

Because the major envisaged use of bioscavengers is prophylactic, it was important to demonstrate that pHu BChE was devoid of side effects of its own. Mice and guinea pigs with circulating levels of pHu BChE as high as 300 U/mL did not display any signs of clinical toxicity. Results of necropsy performed on animals, together with the examination of hematology and serum chemistry parameters, did not reveal any clinical signs of pathology following the administration of large doses of pHu BChE.[32,33]

In Vitro and In Vivo Stability of Plasma-Derived Human Butyrylcholinesterase

The thermal stability of purified pHu BChE stored at various temperatures has been evaluated.[32] Enzyme activity was stable when stored in lyophilized form at 4°, 25°, 37°, or 45°C for 2 years. The enzyme was also stable when stored in liquid form at 4° and 25°C for 1 year. The circulatory (in vivo) stability of enzyme stored in lyophilized form at −20°C was evaluated by measuring pharmacokinetic parameters in mice.[32] The pharmacokinetic properties of the enzyme were not affected upon storage at −20°C for 3 years.

Efficacy of Plasma-Derived Human Butyrylcholinesterase

The efficacy of pHu BChE was evaluated in guinea pigs and cynomolgus monkeys against multiple LD_{50} challenges of nerve agents.[34] Guinea pigs were protected against a cumulative dose of 5 times the LD_{50}s of either soman or VX, and there was a decrease in molar concentration of exogenously administered circulating pHu BChE equivalent to the amount of OP administered in a given time period.[36] For example, guinea pigs administered Hu BChE equivalent to 8 times the LD_{50} of soman attained peak blood BChE levels of approximately 300 U/mL. After challenge with 5.5 times the LD_{50} of soman, the enzyme level decreased to approximately 100 U/mL. This approximate 200 U/mL decrease in blood BChE level is equivalent to around 5 to 5.5 times the LD_{50} of soman. With VX challenge, proportionately less enzyme was administered because the LD_{50} of VX is smaller. No signs of poisoning were observed in the experimental animals during the efficacy studies. Animals were subjected to necropsy 7 or 14 days following nerve agent challenge and all tissues were normal upon light microscopic examination. In nonhuman primates, cynomolgus monkeys were protected against a cumulative challenge of 5.5 times the LD_{50} of soman. Of the six animals challenged, one died after the final challenge dose of soman (total 5.5 times the LD_{50} within 4 h) and one was euthanized 48 hours after the final dose of soman. The surviving animals displayed no signs of poisoning. Subsequent examination of these animals did not show any signs of delayed toxicity following examinations of blood chemistry and hematology parameters for less than 20 months.[37]

Most efficacy studies conducted to date have used IV or subcutaneous challenge of OPs. A study in which guinea pigs were administered soman by inhalation challenge following pretreatment with pHu BChE (IV or IM) showed that only 26% to 30% of enzyme was neutralized.[35] Because it is most likely that humans will be exposed to nerve agent through inhalation, more efficacy studies using inhalation are needed before the protective dose of enzyme can be established for humans.

Immunological Safety of Plasma-Derived Butyrylcholinesterase

A critical prerequisite for any potential bioscavenger is a prolonged circulatory residence time and the absence of antienzyme antibodies following repeated injections of the enzyme. Previously, it was demonstrated that multiple injections of Eq BChE into rabbits, rats, or rhesus monkeys resulted in an MRT spanning several days and the induction of antienzyme antibodies.[38–41] In these experiments, blood enzyme activity appeared to correlate negatively with anti-BChE immunogammaglobulin (IgG) levels. On the other hand, administering purified macaque BChE into macaques of the same species resulted in much longer MRT (225 ± 19 h) compared to that reported for heterologous Hu BChE (33.7 ± 2.9 h). A smaller second injection of macaque BChE given 4 weeks later attained predicted peak plasma levels of enzyme activity, although the four macaques showed wide variation in the MRT (54 to 357 h). No antibody response was detected in macaques following either injection of enzyme.[42]

More recently, the consequences of repeated injections of pHu BChE and plasma-derived mouse (pMo) BChE from CD-1 mice were examined in Balb/c[43] and CD-1[36] mice following two IM injections 4 weeks apart. The effects of two heterologous (pHu BChE) and homologous (pMo BChE) injections were monitored by following blood BChE activity and anti-BChE IgG levels. In Balb/c mice, the clearance of pMo BChE activity following the first injection occurred slowly (MRT = 91.8 h), compared to the heterologous pHu BChE injection (MRT = 56.7 h). As expected, the second injection of pHu BChE cleared much faster from the circulation of mice compared to the first injection. Surprisingly, the second injection of pMo BChE did not attain the predicted peak enzyme level, and a shorter MRT (61.6 h) was observed. No circulating anti-pHu BChE IgG was detected following the first pHu BChE injection, and significant levels of antibodies to pHu BChE could be detected 2 days after the second pHu BChE injection. As expected, no circulating anti-pMo BChE IgG was detected following the first pMo BChE injection. However, antibodies to pMo BChE, although 100-fold less than the levels observed with pHu BChE, were detected 5 days after the second Mo BChE injection. This could be due to differences in pBChEs from the two strains of mice and was subsequently resolved by repeating the study in CD-1 mice.

In CD-1 mice, the clearance of homologous pMo BChE activity following the first injection also occurred slowly (MRT = 73 h), compared to the heterologous Hu BChE injection (MRT = 48 h). As expected, the second injection of Hu BChE cleared much faster from the circulation of mice compared to the first injection (MRT = 26 h). The second injection of homologous Mo BchE, on the other hand, attained a peak enzyme level that was similar to that observed following the first injection and a similar MRT of 79 hours. As expected, circulating anti-Hu BChE IgG could be detected 5 days following the first pHu BChE injection, which increased dramatically after the second injection. No significant antibody response was detected following either of the two homologous pMo BChE injections. The absence of antibody responses following either injection in a homologous system are in agreement with the long retention times and the absence of significant adverse effects following administration of homologous macaque BChE into macaques. The observation that the second injection of pMo BChE resulted in a pharmacokinetic profile that was similar to that of the first injection is in agreement with the lack of a humoral response to the injected enzyme. The observed extended stability of exogenously administered pMo BChE into mice and macaque BChE into macaques suggests that even a single injection of homologous BChE is sufficient to maintain the enzyme at a long-lasting therapeutic level. The results of both studies with two injections of BChE have clearly demonstrated the utility of homologous BChE as an effective and safe scavenger, exhibiting high stability and low immunogenicity in recipient animals. With respect to the potential use of pHu BChE in humans, these results are consistent with a reported in-vivo half-life of 8 to 11 days and the absence of reported untoward immunological and physiological side effects following blood transfusions and IV injections of partially purified pHu BChE into humans.[28,29,44,45]

Behavioral Safety of Plasma-Derived Butyrylcholinesterase

Because the major use of bioscavengers is prophylactic, administered days or weeks prior to a potential exposure, it is essential that the enzyme be devoid of undesirable effects. Thus, several studies have evaluated the behavioral and physiological effects of pBChE administered alone as well as prior to nerve agent exposure.[46] For example, Genovese and Doctor evaluated the effects of highly purified Eq BChE on learned and unlearned behavior in rats.[47] Administration of 500 to 7500 U of Eq BChE (resulting in circulating BChE levels as high as ~ 55 U/mL) did not affect acquisition or retention of a passive avoidance task. Additionally, no disruption of performance of a food-maintained operant behavior task was observed. To evaluate unlearned performance, 24-hour spontaneous motor activity was evaluated before and after administration of Eq BChE. There was no disruption of either the total number of activity counts nor the circadian pattern of activity when monitored for 10 days following administration. Finally, the enzyme was shown to provide significant protection against performance degradation produced by 7-(methylethoxyphosphinyloxy)-1--methylquinolinium iodide (MEPQ), a peripherally active OP compound. The safety and efficacy of FBS AChE and Eq BChE was also evaluated in rhesus monkeys using a memory-intensive serial probe recognition task, in which subjects were required to recall a list of stimuli.[13,15,19] Repeated administration of a commercial preparation of Eq BChE that produced a 7- to 18-fold increase in circulating BChE levels did not systematically affect task performance,[41] and rhesus monkeys pretreated with 460 to 503 nmol of Eq BChE were protected against 2 or 3 times the LD_{50}s of soman or sarin.[15]

Similar studies were conducted to address the safety and efficacy of pHu BChE in mice,[17] rats,[48] guinea pigs,[35] and rhesus monkeys.[19] In all cases, doses of pHu BChE sufficient to protect against OP exposure were devoid of behavioral side effects. Brandeis et al demonstrated that pHu BChE was protective against soman and had no apparent effect on spatial memory as assessed by a Morris water-maze task.[48] Similarly, Raveh et al evaluated the safety of pHu BChE and its therapeutic efficacy against VX and soman toxicity using standardized observations and behavioral performance on a spatial discrimination task in rhesus monkeys.[19] For subjects in which the ratio of enzyme to OP was near or greater than 1, no or mild signs of toxicity were observed, largely with recovery by the next day. Regarding the safety of pHu BChE, three of four monkeys exposed to either 13 mg (10,400 U) or 34 mg (27,200 U) of pHu BChE did not show any observable deficits resulting from pHu BChE administration alone.[19] The transient behavioral effect observed in the fourth monkey was attributed to a nonspecific malaise induced by this enzyme preparation.

More recently, the behavioral safety of large doses of pHu BChE alone were evaluated in mice and rhesus monkeys. Clark et al showed that in mice, 2000 U of pHu BChE (the equivalent of 30 times the dose required for protecting humans from 2 times the LD_{50} of soman) did not significantly alter acoustic startle or prepulse inhibition behavior.[49] Similarly, administration of 30 mg/kg of pHu BChE was devoid of any adverse effects in rhesus monkeys when performance was assessed using a six-item serial probe recognition task.[50] Taken together, these studies demonstrate that pHu BChE pretreatment can provide protection against OP exposure while being devoid of adverse behavioral and physiological effects.

RECOMBINANT STOICHIOMETRIC BIOSCAVENGERS

Plasma-derived Hu BChE represents a first-generation biological scavenger. This material is obtained from outdated human plasma (Cohn Fraction IV-4 paste), and the overall availability is related to the quantity of fraction of the processed human plasma available at any given time. Sufficient amounts of Cohn Fraction IV-4 paste are generated in the United States by blood processing establishments to produce at least 100,000 doses of the bioscavenger product per year. Although this amount of material may be adequate for use by first responders in case of civilian exposure or deliberate, accidental, or limited combat engagement, it is not sufficient to protect the entire population or even the entire military. To identify a more reliable source of Hu BChE, recent research efforts focused on the development of Hu BChE from recombinant expression systems. If successful, such efforts will allow for a constant supply of material of reproducible purity and activity without dependence on the supply of outdated plasma. There are a variety of potential sources of recombinant Hu BChE (rHu BChE), including transgenic plants,[51] transgenic animals,[52] transfected insect larvae,[53] or algae.[54] In addition, rHu BChE can be expressed in cell lines.[55,56] The cell-derived rHu BChE was shown to be a mixture of monomers, dimers, and tetramers and contained incomplete glycan structures.[57] Similarly, goat-milk–derived rHu BChE is primarily a dimer, with some protein present as monomers and tetramers. In contrast, pHu BChE is predominantly tetrameric and possesses mostly biantennary complex and some high mannose glycan structures. Also, goat-milk–derived rHu BChE has a different glycosylation pattern than that of pHu BChE and contains a carbohydrate moiety that has been demonstrated to be immunogenic in humans.[58] Because of the lack of subunit assembly and complete glycan structures, rHu BChE has a much shorter circulatory half-life than pHu BChE.[57] To enhance its biological residence time, rHu BChE was modified to include polyethylene glycol adducts. The polyethylene glycolylated material had a pharmacokinetic profile similar to that of the pHu BChE,[55,59] suggesting that differences in pharmacokinetics between plasma-derived and recombinant enzymes can be addressed using in-vitro posttranslational modifications. Efficacy studies using rHu BChE from transgenic goat milk in guinea pigs against soman and VX have yielded results similar to those previously described that used pHu BChE.[59] These results suggest that effective recombinant stoichiometric bioscavengers can be developed, potentially providing a source for sufficient material for military members and civilians (such as first responders, emergency medical personnel, and agricultural workers) that may be occupationally exposed to OP pesticides.

CATALYTIC BIOSCAVENGERS

Although stoichiometric scavengers are able to afford good protection as long as the enzyme level in the body is higher than the amount of OP, they have a relatively high molecular weight; a comparatively large quantity is required to neutralize a small amount of nerve agent. A catalytic scavenger, even having the same high molecular weight, could be administered in smaller quantities and would potentially produce the same or greater extent of protection. It would also be advantageous because it would not be consumed in the process of detoxifying the nerve agent, making it available to protect against multiple OP exposures. Enzymes with intrinsic, catalytic, anti-OP activities come from a variety of sources, such as the OP hydrolase from *Pseudomonas diminuta*,[60] the OP anhydrase from A*lteromonas haloplanktis*,[61] and human paraoxonase 1 (Hu PON1).[62–66] Recombinant OP hydrolase from *Pseudomonas diminuta* was shown to protect mice against behavioral side effects and lethality caused by soman.[67] Similarly, pretreatment with only OP hydrolase purified from *Pseudomonas* species was shown to protect mice from lethality due to paraoxon, diethylfluorophosphate, and tabun.[68,69] Most of these enzymes possess short circulation times in vivo, and none has the ability to hydrolyze all known toxic OPs, nor do any have the high turnover required to dispose of the OPs from blood in one circulation time. In addition, these bacterial enzymes are likely to initiate potent immune responses in humans; therefore, they are not suitable for repeated use. Bacterial enzymes could conceivably be useful for skin protection as active components of topical skin protectants or covalently bound to the cornified layer of epidermis.[70] OPs can also be detoxified through enzymatic oxidation of their alkyl chains. In particular, breakdown of VX by horseradish peroxidase[71] or by *Caldariomyces fumago* chloroperoxidase[72] could be used in a polyfunctional active topical skin protectant and for skin decontamination.

Conversely, Hu PON1 can possibly afford protection without the potential complication of inducing an immune response. However, Hu PON1 does not possess the desired catalytic activity at a rate that is fast enough for use as a nerve agent pretreatment. Because agent must be cleared from the bloodstream within one circulation time (1 to 2 minutes) before it reaches critical targets,[15] a functional catalytic scavenger must have both a lower K_m (a measure of the strength of binding of a substrate to the enzyme) and a high turnover number (k_{cat}). Research efforts were directed toward creating such an enzyme by specific mutation of enzymes such as Hu BChE and Hu PON1. Hu BChE mutation designs were based on the fact that OP inhibitors are hemisubstrates for this enzyme. The acylation reaction is similar to that of normal substrates, but the subsequent reaction, equivalent to deacylation of the active site serine, cannot be affected because the amino acid group responsible for dephosphylation is not in the appropriate position.[73,74]

The perceived solution to this problem was to insert a second catalytic center into the active site specifically to carry out the dephosphylation step of the reaction.[74] Applying this rationale, wild-type Hu BChE was mutated in the oxyanion hole to create a mutated enzyme, G117H, with the ability to catalyze the hydrolysis of sarin, diisopropylfluorophosphate (DFP), paraoxon, VX, and other nonaging nerve agents.[74,75] Aging and reactivation are parallel first-order reactions in phosphylated enzymes. In the reactivation reaction, the phosphoryl group is removed from the active site serine residue (Ser198), restoring activity, whereas in the aging reaction one of the alkyl groups is removed from the phosphoryl group, rendering the inhibited enzyme nonreactivatable. To catalyze the hydrolysis of rapidly aging nerve agents such as soman, it is necessary to slow the rate of the aging reaction so that reactivation is faster. This was accomplished by replacing the carboxyl group Glu197 adjacent to the active site serine with an amide group.[76] Although these efforts were successful, the mutants have catalytic activities that are still too slow for practical use.

Hu PON1 is currently being subjected to mutation in efforts to generate faster catalytic antinerve agent enzymes. Because OPs are "accidental" substrates for paraoxonase,[62,64] it is likely that activity improvement can be realized through protein engineering. Two of the major difficulties in designing appropriate site-directed mutations in Hu PON1, the lack of knowledge on the residues at the active site and the enzyme's three-dimensional structure, were recently overcome by the work of Josse et al,[65,66] Harel et al,[77] Aharoni et al,[78] and Yeung et al.[79,80] Based on site-directed mutations of amino acids believed to be at or near the active site of Hu PON1 and on limited sequence homology with a DFPase, Josse et al had postulated that the molecule had the shape of a 6-fold beta propeller. Using a mouse-rat-rabbit-human chimera of paraoxonase 1 obtained through gene shuffling experiments and expressed in bacteria, Harel et al[77] and Aharoni et al[78] confirmed the postulated structure through X-ray crystallographic studies. Yeung et al have subsequently carried out site-directed mutation studies to identify and "map" amino acid residues critical for binding and involved in catalytic activity.[79,80] Further studies have revealed a degree of stereospecificity in the hydrolysis of soman by native Hu PON1, with the least toxic soman stereoisomer (C+P+) being hydrolyzed ~ 6 times more efficiently than the most toxic one (C–P–).[81] The observed stereospecificity is primarily due to preferential binding rather than to enhanced turnover of the (C+P+) stereoisomer by Hu PON1. All of these recent findings support the goal of designing a recombinant version of a naturally occurring human enzyme that can be developed as a catalytic biological scavenger to protect against nerve agent poisoning.

INTERAGENCY PARTNERSHIPS: PROJECT BIOSHIELD

Project BioShield was signed into law by President George W Bush on July 21, 2004. It grants the secretaries of the US Department of Health and Human Services and the US Department of Homeland Security authority to present the president and the director of the US Office of Management and Budget with recommendations for developing and procuring countermeasures to chemical, biological, radiological, and nuclear threats. Funding over 10 years was appropriated to the Department of Homeland Security for Project BioShield, establishing a new spending authority to spur development and procurement of "next generation" medical countermeasures (vaccines, therapeutics, and diagnostics) against chemical, biological, radiological, and nuclear agents. It also authorizes the National Institutes of Health to speed research and development in promising areas of medical countermeasures to these agents, grants increased flexibility and authority to award contracts and grants under expedited peer review procedures, and allows more rapid hiring of technical experts deemed necessary for research and development efforts. The Department of Defense is joining in this effort to leverage interagency resources. The objectives are to develop dual-use technologies and products that can be used to expand target populations (military and civilians) for US Food and Drug Administration licensure. Project BioShield legislation requires that products are manufactured under current Good Manufacturing Practices (practices recognized world-wide that ensure the safe manufacturing, management, testing, and control of goods, foods, and pharmaceuticals) and have completed a successful Phase I human clinical safety trial. Plasma-derived Hu BChE is currently being produced from human Cohn Fraction IV-4 and will be used for preclinical safety and toxicology testing with the intention of large-scale production and more extensive testing to be carried out leading to licensure. The bioscavenger countermeasure has been identified as a potential candidate for Project BioShield.

Collaborating in the BioShield process requires the Department of Defense to expand the concept of use to first responders, healthcare workers, and civilians. One way to protect those groups may be to stockpile sufficient amounts of pHu BChE, which could then be used in conjunction with extensive decontamination measures and personal protective equipment when indicated. In some settings, pHu BChE may replace the need for pyridostigmine bromide as a pretreatment medical countermeasure. Most studies tested the enzyme as a preventive countermeasure because once the nerve agent has reached the nerve synapse, pHu BChE becomes ineffective; at that point, intervention would include the traditional countermeasures (atropine, pralidoxime, and anticonvulsant). Although the majority of bioscavenger use will be in the preexposure setting, bioscavenger may also be useful in neutralizing on-going postexposure risks following skin absorption, which could lead to prolonged systemic exposure (ie, the "depot effect").

SUMMARY

OP nerve agents represent a very real threat not only to service members in the field but also to the public at large. Nerve agents have already been used by terrorist groups against civilians and, because of their low cost and relative ease of synthesis, are likely to be used again in the future. In addition, many commonly used pesticides and chemical manufacturing by-products can act as anticholinesterases and may be a low-dose exposure threat to workers in a variety of professions. Anticholinesterase pesticides may also be used against civilians in a terrorist context. Current therapeutic regimes for acute nerve agent exposure are generally effective in preventing fatalities if administered in an appropriate time period. For acute multi-LD_{50} levels of OP exposure, pyridostigmine pretreatment coupled with postexposure administration of an oxime, atropine, and an anticonvulsant does not prevent substantial behavioral incapacitation or, in some cases, permanent brain damage. It is therefore important from both military and domestic security perspectives to develop novel defenses against nerve agents, including the use of bioscavenger molecules, that avoid many of the difficulties associated with current treatments. While the use of nerve agents on the battlefield may be somewhat predictable, nerve agent use in a terrorist situation will be, in all probability, a surprise event. The potential to afford long-term protection to first-responders exposed to toxic or incapacitating concentrations of OPs is a notable advantage of biological scavengers.

Recent efforts have focused on identifying proteins that can act as biological scavengers of OP compounds and can remain stable in circulation for long periods of time. By prophylactically inactivating OPs before they inhibit central nervous system AChE, this approach avoids the side effects associated with current antidotes and the requirement for their rapid administration. Ideally, the scavenger should enjoy a long residence time in the blood stream (11–15 days), should be biologically inert in the absence of nerve agent, and should not present an antigenic challenge to the immune system. Taken together, pharmacological safety, toxicity, stability, and efficacy data strongly support pHu BChE as a safe pretreatment for chemical agent intoxication. Pharmacokinetic parameters of pHu BChE in mice, guinea pigs, and monkeys suggest that a single dose of enzyme can maintain blood BChE at a therapeutic concentration for at least 4 days. Safety and toxicity studies demonstrate that pHu BChE, even at a dose that is 30 times the therapeutic dose, is devoid of tissue toxicity and is safe for human use. Plasma Hu BChE has a long shelf life (2 years) in lyophilized

TABLE 7-1

PROTECTION BY HUMAN BUTYRYLCHOLINESTERASE AGAINST NERVE AGENT POISONING

Treatment	Test Species	Nerve Agent	Protection* (LD_{50})	Impairment	Recovery
pHu BChE	Rat	GD	1.5	None	Immediate
pHu BChE	Guinea pig	GD	5.5	None	Immediate
pHu BChE	Guinea Pig	VX	5.0	None	Immediate
pHu BChE	Rhesus monkey	GD	3.3	4 of 8	15 min to 2 h
pHu BChE	Rhesus monkey	VX	2.1	2 of 4	20 min to 20 h
pHu BChE	Cynomolgus monkey	GD	5.5	1 of 5	4 of 6†
rHu BChE	Guinea pig	GD	5.5	None	Immediate
rHu BChE	Guinea pig	VX	5.5		Immediate
ATR/2-PAM/DZP	Guinea pig	GD	1.5	4 of 4	2 of 4, days‡
ATR/2-PAM/DZP	Guinea pig	VX	1.5	10 of 10	10 of 10, days‡

*Values represent multiples of median lethal doses (LD_{50}s) of nerve agent survived after BChE administration.
†One animal died after the third dose of soman and one was impaired and later euthanized after 48 hours. The remaining four animals were normal, survived, and were held for long-term observations.
‡Two animals died in the first hour, while the other two remained impaired for 2 to 4 days.
2-PAM: 2-pyridine aldoxime methyl chloride
ATR: atropine
DZP: diazepam
Hu BChE: human butyrylcholinesterase
LD_{50}: median lethal dose
pHu BChE: plasma-derived human butyrylcholinesterase
rHu BChE: recombinant human butyrylcholinesterase
Data sources: (1) Genovese RF, Doctor BP. Behavioral and pharmacological assessment of butyrylcholinesterase in rats. *Pharmacol Biochem Behav.* 1995;51:647–654. (2) Lenz DE, Maxwell DM, Koplovitz I, et al. Protection against soman or VX poisoning by human butyrylcholinesterase in guinea pigs and cynomolgus monkeys. *Chem Biol Interact.* 2005;157–158:205–210. (3) Raveh L, Grauer E, Grunwald J, Cohen E, Ashani Y. The stoichiometry of protection against soman and VX toxicity in monkeys pretreated with human butyrylcholinesterase. *Toxicol Appl Pharmacol.* 1997;145:43–53. (4) Garcia GE, Moorad-Doctor D, Doctor BP, et al. Glycan structure comparison of native human plasma butyrylcholinesterase (Hu-BChE) and transgenic goat produced Hu-BChE. *FASEB J.* 2005;19:A867.

form at temperatures 4° to 25°C. Similarly, the pharmacokinetic properties of the enzyme were not affected upon storage at – 20°C for 3 years. Pretreatment with pHu BChE protected guinea pigs against a 5 times the LD_{50} of soman or VX. As expected, pHu BChE injection in mice or monkeys elicited the production of high levels of anti-BChE antibodies. No antibody response was detected following either of the two homologous mouse or monkey BChE injections. The observation that the second injection of homologous BChE resulted in a pharmacokinetic profile that was similar to that of the first injection is in agreement with the lack of a humoral response to the injected enzyme.

By nearly all criteria, the use of biological scavengers to protect against exposure to a lethal dose of a nerve agent offers numerous advantages over conventional treatment therapies (Table 7-1). Developing an effective prophylactic to nerve agent exposure will greatly reduce, if not eliminate, the need to know the precise length of exposure in a crisis situation. Successful prophylaxis will also preclude the need to repeatedly administer a host of pharmacologically active drugs with short durations of action. Also, the need to use personal protective equipment to protect against nerve agent exposure could be greatly reduced, which is particularly significant for first responders handling known casualties of nerve agent exposure. Finally, the appropriate scavenger would protect against all current nerve agent threats, including those that are refractory to treatment by atropine and oxime therapy. In cases of lower doses of nerve agents or in response to agents that potentially exert a time-release depot effect, pHu BChE could be used as a postexposure treatment to combat continued toxicity of the absorbed agent.

Several challenges must be met before bioscavengers can augment or replace the current therapeutic regimes for nerve agent intoxication. The immunogenicity and serum half-life of the scavenger must be determined in humans, and efforts may be required to minimize any immune consequences and maximize the residence time in circulation. Additionally, appropriate dosages of scavenger must be determined that will, based on animal models, protect against concentrations of nerve agents likely to be encountered in a wide range of scenarios. While research efforts to date have resulted in the successful transition to preclinical trials of stoichiometric scavengers, the use of either naturally or genetically engineered enzymes with catalytic activity to hydrolyze OPs holds the greatest theoretical promise for the development of a broad specificity, high efficacy, prophylactic scavenger. Current research efforts are focused on designing and expressing such enzymes and characterizing their in-vivo, antinerve agent efficacy in animal models acceptable to the Food and Drug Administration.

Acknowledgment

Special thanks to Dr Doug Cerasoli, US Army Medical Research Institute of Chemical Defense, for his contributions to sections of the chapter.

REFERENCES

1. Romano JA Jr, McDonough JH, Sheridan R, Sidell FR. Health effects of low-level exposure to nerve agents. In: Somani SM, Romano JA, Jr, eds. *Chemical Warfare Agents: Toxicity at Low Levels.* New York, NY: CRC Press; 2002: 1–18.

2. Yokoyama K, Araki S, Murata K, et al. Chronic neurobehavioral and central and autonomic nervous system effects of Tokyo subway sarin poisoning. *J Physiol Paris.* 1998;92:317–323.

3. De Candole CA, Douglas WW, Evans CL, et al. The failure of respiration in death by anticholinesterase poisoning. *Br J Pharmacol Chemother.* 1953;8:466–475.

4. Stewart WC, Anderson EA. Effect of a cholinesterase inhibitor when injected into the medulla of the rabbit. *J Pharmacol Exp Ther.* 1968;162:309–318.

5. Heffron PF, Hobbinger F. Relationship between inhibition of acetylcholinesterase and response of the rat phrenic nerve-diaphragm preparation to indirect stimulation at higher frequencies. *Br J Pharmacol.* 1979;66:323–329.

6. Gray AP. Design and structure-activity relationships of antidotes to organophosphorus anticholinesterase agents. *Drug Metab Rev.* 1984;15:557–589.

7. Lipp JA. Effect of diazepam upon soman-induced seizure activity and convulsions. *Electroencephalogr Clin Neurophysiol*. 1972;32:557–560.

8. Dirnhuber P, French MC, Green DM, Leadbeater L, Stratton JA. The protection of primates against soman poisoning by pretreatment with pyridostigmine. *J Pharm Pharmacol*. 1979;31:295–299.

9. McLeod CG Jr. Pathology of nerve agents: perspectives on medical management. *Fundam Appl Toxicol*. 1985;5:S10–S16.

10. Dunn MA, Sidell FR. Progress in medical defense against nerve agents. *JAMA*. 1989;262:649–652.

11. Doctor BP, Maxwell DM, Ashani Y, Saxena A, Gordon RK. New approaches to medical protection against chemical warfare nerve agents. In: Somani SM, Romano JA Jr, eds. *Chemical Warfare Agents: Toxicity at Low Levels*. New York, NY: CRC Press; 2002: 191–214.

12. Wolfe AD, Rush RS, Doctor BP, Koplovitz I, Jones D. Acetylcholinesterase prophylaxis against organophosphate toxicity. *Fundam Appl Toxicol*. 1987;9:266–270.

13. Maxwell DM, Castro CA, De La Hoz DM, et al. Protection of rhesus monkeys against soman and prevention of performance decrement by pretreatment with acetylcholinesterase. *Toxicol Appl Pharmacol*. 1992;115:44–49.

14. Maxwell DM, Brecht KM, Doctor BP, Wolfe AD. Comparison of antidote protection against soman by pyridostigmine, HI-6 and acetylcholinesterase. *J Pharmacol Exp Ther*. 1993;264:1085–1089.

15. Broomfield CA, Maxwell DM, Solana RP, Castro CA, Finger AV, Lenz DE. Protection by butyrylcholinesterase against organophosphorus poisoning in nonhuman primates. *J Pharmacol Exper Ther*. 1991;259:633–638.

16. Raveh L, Ashani Y, Levy D, De La Hoz D, Wolfe AD, Doctor BP. Acetylcholinesterase prophylaxis against organophosphate poisoning. Quantitative correlation between protection and blood-enzyme level in mice. *Biochem Pharmacol*. 1989;38:529–534.

17. Ashani Y, Shapira S, Levy D, Wolfe AD, Doctor BP, Raveh L. Butyrylcholinesterase and acetylcholinesterase prophylaxis against soman poisoning in mice. *Biochem Pharmacol*. 1991;41:37–41.

18. Raveh L, Grunwald J, Marcus D, Papier Y, Cohen E, Ashani Y. Human butyrylcholinesterase as a general prophylactic antidote for nerve agent toxicity. In vitro and in vivo quantitative characterization. *Biochem Pharmacol*. 1993;45:2465–2474.

19. Raveh L, Grauer E, Grunwald J, Cohen E, Ashani Y. The stoichiometry of protection against soman and VX toxicity in monkeys pretreated with human butyrylcholinesterase. *Toxicol Appl Pharmacol*. 1997;145:43–53.

20. Wolfe AD, Blick DW, Murphy MR, et al. Use of cholinesterases as pretreatment drugs for the protection of rhesus monkeys against soman toxicity. *Toxicol Appl Pharmacol*. 1992;117:189–193.

21. Augstinsson KB. Electrophoretic separation and classification of blood plasma esterases. *Nature*. 1958;151:1786–1789.

22. Scott DF, Chacko TL, Maxwell DM, Schlager JJ, Lanclos KD. Expression and partial purification of a recombinant secretory form of human liver carboxylesterase. *Protein Expr Purifi*. 1999;17:16–25.

23. Maxwell DM, Brecht KM, O'Neill BL. The effect of carboxylesterase inhibition on interspecies differences in soman toxicity. *Toxicol Lett*. 1987;39:35–42.

24. Li B, Sedlacek M, Manoharan I, et al. Butyrylcholinesterase, paraoxonase, and albumin esterase, but not carboxylesterase, are present in human plasma. *Biochem Pharmacol*. 2005;70:1673–1684.

25. Maxwell DM, Wolfe AD, Ashani Y, Doctor BP. Cholinesterase and carboxylesterase as scavengers for organophosphorus agents, In: Massoulie J, Bacou F, Bernard E, Chatonnet A, Doctor BP, Quinn DM, eds. *Cholinesterases: Structure, Function, Mechanism, Genetics, and Cell Biology*. Washington, DC: American Chemical Society; 1991: 206.

26. Maxwell DM, Lieske CN, Brecht KM. Oxime-induced reactivation of carboxylesterase inhibited by organophosphorous compounds. *Chem Res Toxicol.* 1994;7:428–433.

27. Jokanovic M, Kosanovic M, Maksimovic M. Interaction of organophosphorous compounds with carboxylesterases in the rat. *Arch Toxicol.* 1996;70:444–450.

28. Cascio C, Comite C, Ghiara M, Lanza G, Ponchione A. Use of serum cholinesterase in severe organophosphorus poisoning. Our experience. *Minerva Anesthesiol.* 1988;54:337–338.

29. Jenkins T, Balinsky D, Patient DW. Cholinesterase in plasma: first reported absence in the Bantu; half-life determination. *Science.* 1967;156:1748–1750.

30. Ashani Y. Prospective of human butyrylcholinesterase as a detoxifying antidote and potential regulator of controlled-release drugs. *Drug Dev Res.* 2000;50:298–308.

31. Grunwald J, Marcus D, Papier Y, Raveh L, Pittel Z, Ashani Y. Large-scale purification and long-term stability of human butyrylcholinesterase: a potential bioscavenger drug. *J Biochem Biophys Methods.* 1997;34:123–135.

32. Saxena A, Sun W, Luo C, Doctor BP. Human serum butyrylcholinesterase: in vitro and in vivo stability, pharmacokinetics, and safety in mice. *Chem Biol Interact.* 2005;157–158:199–203.

33. Sun W, Doctor BP, Saxena A. Safety and pharmacokinetics of human serum butyrylcholinesterase in guinea pigs. *Chem Bio Interact.* 2005;157–158:428–429.

34. Lenz DE, Maxwell DM, Koplovitz I, et al. Protection against soman or VX poisoning by human butyrylcholinesterase in guinea pigs and cynomolgus monkeys. *Chem Biol Interact.* 2005;157–158:205–210.

35. Allon N, Raveh L, Gilat E, Cohen E, Grunwald J, Ashani Y. Prophylaxis against soman inhalation toxicity in guinea pigs by pretreatment alone with human serum butyrylcholinesterase. *Toxicol Sci.* 1998;43:121–128.

36. Saxena A, Sun W, Luo C, et al. Development of human serum butyrylcholinesterase as a bioscavenger for medical protection against organophosphate chemical warfare agents. Paper presented at: *The 4th Singapore International Symposium on Protection Against Toxic Substances*; December, 2004; Singapore.

37. Sun 7W, Naik RS, Luo C, Lenz DE, Saxena A, Doctor BP. Long term effect of human butyrylcholinesterase pretreatment followed by acute soman challenge in cynomolgus monkeys. Paper presented at: *2005 Joint Service Science Conference on Chemical and Biological Defense Research*; November 14–16, 2005; Timonium, Md.

38. Genovese RF, Lu XCM, Gentry MK, Larrison R, Doctor BP. Evaluation of purified horse serum butyrylcholinesterase in rats. In: *Proceedings of the Medical Defense Bioscience Review.* Aberdeen Proving Ground, Md: US Army Medical Research Institute of Chemical Defense; 1993: 1035–1042. DTIC accession document no. AD A275669.

39. Gentry MK, Nuwayser ES, Doctor BP. Effects of repeated administration of butyrylcholinesterase on antibody induction in rabbits. In: *Proceedings of the Medical Defense Bioscience Review.* Aberdeen Proving Ground, Md: US Army Medical Research Institute of Chemical Defense; 1993: 1051–1056. DTIC accession document no. AD A275669.

40. Gentry MK, Nuwayser ES, Doctor BP. Immunological effect of repeated administration of cholinesterases in rabbits. In: *Proceedings of the Medical Defense Bioscience Review.* Aberdeen Proving Ground, Md: US Army Medical Research Institute of Chemical Defense; 1996: 183–191. DTIC accession document no. AD A321840

41. Matzke SM, Oubre JL, Caranto GR, Gentry MK, Galbicka G. Behavioral and immunological effects of exogenous butyrylcholinesterase in rhesus monkeys. *Pharmacol Biochem Behav.* 1999;62:523–530.

42. Rosenberg Y, Luo C, Ashani Y, et al. Pharmacokinetics and immunologic consequences of exposing macaques to purified homologous butyrylcholinesterase. *Life Sci.* 2002;72:125–134.

43. Sun W, Clark MG, Luo C, Bansal R, Doctor BP, Saxena A. Pharmacokinetics, stability, safety and toxicity of purified human serum butyrylcholinesterase in mice. Paper presented at: *NATO TG-004 Meeting*; September 29–October 3, 2003; Medicine Hat, Canada.

44. Stovner J, Stadskleiv K. Suxamethonium apnoea terminated with commercial serum cholinesterase. *Acta Anaesthesiol Scand.* 1976;20:211–215.

45. Ostergaard D, Viby-Mogensen J, Hanel HK, Skovgaard LT. Half-life of plasma cholinesterase. *Acta Anaesthesiol Scand.* 1988;32:266–269.

46. Lenz DE, Cerasoli DM. Nerve agent bioscavengers: protection with reduced behavioral effects. *Mil Psychol.* 2002;14:121–143.

47. Genovese RF, Doctor BP. Behavioral and pharmacological assessment of butyrylcholinesterase in rats. *Pharmacol Biochem Behav.* 1995;51:647–654.

48. Brandeis R, Raveh L, Grunwald J, Cohen E, Ashani Y. Prevention of soman-induced cognitive deficits by pretreatment with human butyrylcholinesterase in rats. *Pharmacol Biochem Behav.* 1993;46:889–896.

49. Clark MG, Sun W, Myers TM, Bansal R, Doctor BP, Saxena A. Effects of physostigmine and human butyrylcholinesterase on acoustic startle reflex and prepulse inhibition in C57BL/6J mice. *Pharmacol Biochem Behav.* 2005;81:497–505.

50. Myers TM, Sun W, Bansal R, Clark MG, Saxena A, Doctor BP. Safety evaluation of human serum butyrylcholinesterase in rhesus monkeys. In: *Proceedings of the Medical Defense Bioscience Review.* Aberdeen Proving Ground, Md: US Army Medical Research Institute of Chemical Defense; 2003: 1–8.

51. Mor TS, Sternfeld M, Soreq H, Arntzen CJ, Mason HS. Expression of recombinant human acetylcholinesterase in transgenic tomato plants. *Biotechnol Bioeng.* 2001;75:259–266.

52. Cerasoli DM, Griffiths EM, Doctor BP, et al. In vitro and in vivo characterization of recombinant human butyrylcholinesterase (Protexia) as a potential nerve agent bioscavenger. *Chem Biol Interact.* 2005;157–158:363–365.

53. Choudary PV, Kamita SG, Maeda S. Expression of foreign genes in *Bombyx mori* larvae using baculovirus vectors. *Methods Mol Biol.* 1995;39:243–264.

54. Siripornadulsil S, Traina S, Verma DP, Sayre RT. Molecular mechanisms of proline-mediated tolerance to toxic heavy metals in transgenic microalgae. *Plant Cell.* 2002;14:2837–2847.

55. Chilukuri N, Parikh K, Sun W, et al. Polyethylene glycosylation prolongs the circulatory stability of recombinant human butyrylcholinesterase. *Chem Biol Interact.* 2005;157–158:115–121.

56. Duysen EG, Bartels, CF, Lockridge O. Wild-type and A328W mutant human butyrylcholinesterase tetramers expressed in Chinese hamster ovary cells have a 16-hour half-life in the circulation and protect mice from cocaine toxicity. *J Pharmacol Exp Ther.* 2002;302:751–758.

57. Saxena A, Ashani Y, Raveh L, Stevenson D, Patel T, Doctor BP. Role of oligosaccharides in the pharmacokinetics of tissue-derived and genetically engineered cholinesterases. *Mol Phamacol.* 1998;53:112–122.

58. Garcia GE, Moorad-Doctor D, Doctor BP, et al. Glycan structure comparison of native human plasma butyrylcholinesterase (Hu-BChE) and transgenic goat produced Hu-BChE. *FASEB J.* 2005;19:A867.

59. Cerasoli DM, Robison CL, D'Ambrozio JA, et al. Pretreatment with pegylated protexia protects against exposure to the nerve agents VX and soman. *Society for Neuroscience.* 2005;31:337.

60. Serdar CM, Gibson DT. Enzymatic hydrolysis of organophosphates: cloning and expression of a parathion hydrolase gene from Pseudomonas diminuta. *Bio/Technology.* 1985;3:567.

61. Cheng T, Liu L, Wang B, et al. Nucleotide sequence of a gene encoding an organophosphorus nerve agent degrading enzyme from Alteromonas haloplanktis. *J Ind Microbiol Biotechnol.* 1997;18:49–55.

62. Masson P, Josse D, Lockridge O, Viguié N, Taupin C, Buhler C. Enzymes hydrolyzing organophosphates as potential catalytic scavengers against organophosphate poisoning. *J PhysiolParis.* 1998;92:357–362.

63. Gan KN, Smolen A, Eckerson HW, La Du BN. Purification of human serum paraoxonase/arylesterase. Evidence for one esterase catalyzing both activities. *Drug Metab Dispos.*1991;19:100–106.

64. Tuovinen K, Kalkiste-Korhonen E, Raushel FM, Hanninen O. Success of pyridostigmine, physostigmine, eptastigmine and phosphotriesterase treatments in acute sarin intoxication. *Toxicology.* 1999;134:169–178.

65. Josse D, Xie W, Renault F, et al. Identification of residues essential for human paraoxonase (PON1) arylesterase/organophosphatase activities. *Biochemistry.* 1999;38;2816–2825.

66. Josse D, Lockridge O, Xie W, Bartels CF, Schopfer LM, Masson P. The active site of human paraoxonase (PON1). *J Appl Toxicol.* 2001;21(suppl 1):7–11.

67. Broomfield CA. A purified recombinant organophosphorus acid anhydrase protects mice against soman. *Chem Biol Interact.* 1993;87:279–284.

68. Ashani Y, Rothschild N, Segall Y, Levanon D, Raveh L. Prophylaxis against organophosphate poisoning by an enzyme hydrolyzing organophosphorus compounds in mice. *Life Sci.* 1991;49:367–374.

69. Raveh L, Segall Y, Leader H, et al. Protection against tabun toxicity in mice by prophylaxis with an enzyme hydrolyzing organophosphate esters. *Biochem Pharmacol.* 1992;44:397–400.

70. Parsa R, Green H. Destruction of DFP by organophosphorus acid anhydrase covalently coupled to the cornified layer of human epidermis. Paper presented at: *The International Symposium on Applications of Enzymes in Chemical and Biological Defense*; May 14–18, 2001; Orlando, Fla.

71. Amitai G, Adani R, Rabinovitz I, Meshulam H. In vitro skin decontamination of VX by enzymatic peroxidation. Paper presented at: *Bioscience Review Meeting;* June 3–7, 2002; Hunt Valley, Md.

72. Amitai G, Adani R, Hershkovitz M, Bel P, Meshulam H, Rabinovitz R. Chloroperoxidase catalyzes the degradation of VX and sulfur mustard. In: Inestrosa NC, Campos EO, eds. *Cholinesterases in the Second Millenium: Biological and Pathological Aspects.* Pucon, Chile: Diseño e Impresiones J&J Ltda Press; 2002: 354.

73. Jarv S. Stereochemical aspects of cholinesterase catalysis. *Bioorg Chem.* 1984;12:259–278.

74. Millard CB, Lockridge O, Broomfield CA. Design and expression of organophosphorus acid anhydride hydrolase activity in human butyrylcholinesterase. *Biochemistry.* 1995;34:15925–15933.

75. Lockridge O, Blong RM, Masson P, Froment MT, Millard CB, Broomfield CA. A single amino acid substitution, Gly117His, confers phosphotriesterase (organophosphorus acid anhydride hydrolase) activity on human butyrylcholinesterase. *Biochemistry.* 1997;36:786–795.

76. Millard CB, Lockridge O, Broomfield CA. Organophosphorus acid anhydride hydrolase activity in human butyrylcholinesterase: synergy results in a somanase. *Biochemistry.* 1998;37:237–247.

77. Harel M, Aharoni A, Gaidukov L, et al. Structure and evolution of the serum paraoxonase family of detoxifying and anti-atherosclerotic enzymes. *Nat Struct Mol Biol.* 2004;11:412–419.

78. Aharoni A, Gaidukov L, Yagur S, Toker L, Silman I, Tawfik DS. Directed evolution of mammalian paraoxonases PON1 and PON3 for bacterial expression and catalytic specialization. *Proc Natl Acad Sci U S A.* 2004;101:482–487.

79. Yeung DT, Josse D, Nicholson JD, et al. Structure/function analyses of human serum paraoxonase (HuPON1) mutants designed from a DFPase-like homology model. *Biochim Biophys Acta.* 2004;1702:67–77.

80. Yeung DT, Lenz DE, Cerasoli DM. Analysis of active-site amino-acid residues of human serum paraoxonase using competitive substrates. *FEBS J.* 2005;272:2225–2230.

81. Yeung DT, Smith JR, Sweeny RE, Lenz DE, Cerasoli DM. Direct detection of stereospecific soman hydrolysis by wild-type human serum paraoxonase. *FEBS J.* 2007;274:1183–1191.

Chapter 8

VESICANTS

CHARLES G. HURST, MD*; JOHN P. PETRALI, PhD†; DAVID J. BARILLO, MD‡; JOHN S. GRAHAM, PhD§; WILLIAM J. SMITH, PhD¥; JOHN S. URBANETTI, MD¶; AND FREDERICK R. SIDELL, MD**

*Chief, Chemical Casualty Care Division, US Army Medical Research Institute of Chemical Defense, 3100 Ricketts Point Road, Aberdeen Proving Ground, Maryland 21010-5400

†Research Anatomist, Comparative Pathology Branch, Comparative Medicine Division, 3100 Ricketts Point Road, Building 3100, US Army Medical Research Institute of Chemical Defense, Aberdeen Proving Ground, Maryland 21010-5400

‡Colonel, Medical Corps, US Army; Surgical Intensivist and Chief, Burn Flight Team/Special Medical Augmentation Response Team—Burn (SMART-B), US Army Institute of Surgical Research, 3400 Rawley E. Chambers Avenue, Fort Sam Houston, Texas 78234-6315

§Research Biochemist, Medical Toxicology Branch, Analytical Toxicology Division, US Army Medical Research Institute of Chemical Defense, 3100 Ricketts Point Road, Aberdeen Proving Ground, Maryland 21010-5400

¥Chief, Cellular and Molecular Biology Branch, Research Division, US Army Medical Research Institute of Chemical Defense, 3100 Ricketts Point Road, Aberdeen Proving Ground, Maryland 21010-5400

¶Lecturer, Pulmonary Disease, Yale University School of Medicine, New Haven, Connecticut 06510

**Formerly, Chief, Chemical Casualty Care Office, and Director, Medical Management of Chemical Casualties Course, US Army Medical Research Institute of Chemical Defense, Aberdeen Proving Ground, Maryland 21010-5400; Deceased

INTRODUCTION

Vesicants are agents that produce chemical burns. Sulfur mustard, the first vesicant used as a chemical weapon, caused many injuries on the battlefields of World War I and is still considered a major chemical agent.[1-4] In the years since World War I, a number of recorded and suspected incidents of mustard use have occurred, culminating in the Iran-Iraq War in the 1980s. During this conflict, Iraq used mustard extensively against Iran. Graphic images of badly burned Iranian casualties in the media brought public attention to the horrors of chemical warfare. The possibility that Iraq would again use mustard caused major concern as the United States joined United Nations forces preparing to liberate Kuwait in fall 1990 (fortunately mustard was not used). Although mustard is the most important vesicant militarily, the vesicant category includes other agents such as lewisite and phosgene oxime (Table 8-1). The clinical differences among the vesicants discussed in this chapter are shown in Table 8-2.

There are two types of mustard: sulfur mustard and nitrogen mustard. Despretz probably synthesized poor quality sulfur mustard in 1822, but it was not identified. Riche, in 1854, and Guthrie, several years later, repeated Despretz's reaction to obtain the same product. Guthrie described the product as smelling like mustard, tasting like garlic, and causing blisters after contact with the skin. Niemann, in 1860, also synthesized the compound. In 1886 Meyer prepared higher quality mustard but discontinued his research because of the hazards involved. During World War I, Germany used Meyer's method of synthesis to manufacture mustard.[3]

Nitrogen mustard was first synthesized in the late 1930s. Although the properties of nitrogen mustard are similar to sulfur mustard, it was not found suitable for use as a weapon. One form of nitrogen mustard, HN2 (Mustargen, manufactured by Merck and Co, West Point, Pa) was found useful for chemotherapy of

TABLE 8-1

CHEMICAL, PHYSICAL, ENVIRONMENTAL, AND BIOLOGICAL PROPERTIES OF VESICATING AGENTS

Properties	Impure Sulfur Mustard (H)	Distilled Sulfur Mustard (HD)	Phosgene Oxime (CX)	Lewisite (L)
Chemical and Physical				
Boiling Point	Varies	227°C	128°C	190°C
Vapor Pressure	Depends on purity	0.072 mm Hg at 20°C	11.2 mm Hg at 25°C (solid) 13 mm Hg at 40°C (liquid)	0.39 mm Hg at 20°C
Density:				
Vapor	approx 5.5	5.4	<3.9	7.1
Liquid	approx 1.24 g/mL at 25°C	1.27 g/mL at 20°C	ND	1.89 g/mL at 20°C
Solid	NA	Crystal: 1.37 g/mL at 20°C	NA	NA
Volatility	approx 920 mg/m³ at 25°C	610 mg/m³ at 20°C	1,800 mg/m³ at 20°C	4,480 mg/m³ at 20°C
Appearance	Pale yellow to dark-brown liquid	Pale yellow to dark-brown liquid	Colorless, crystalline solid or a liquid	Pure: colorless, oily liquid As agent: amber to dark-brown liquid
Odor	Garlic or mustard	Garlic or mustard	Intense, irritating	Geranium
Solubility:				
In Water	0.092 g/100 g at 22°C	0.092 g/100 g at 22°C	70%	Slight
In Other Solvents	Complete in CCl_4, acetone, other organic solvents	Complete in CCl_4, acetone, other organic solvents	Very soluble in most organic solvents	Soluble in all common organic solvents

(Table 8-1 *continues***)**

certain neoplasms.[5-8] In the early years of chemotherapeutics, HN2 was a mainstay in cancer therapy.

A second group of vesicants is arsenicals. The major compound in this group is lewisite, which was synthesized, developed, and manufactured in the United States during the late stages of World War I.[1] A shipment of lewisite on its way to Europe when the war ended was destroyed at sea. There are no data on lewisite from battlefield use. As a weapon, lewisite has some advantages and disadvantages over mustard that will be discussed later in this chapter.

The third compound considered a vesicant by the US military is phosgene oxime. Phosgene oxime is not a true vesicant— unlike mustard and lewisite, it does not produce blisters; rather, it produces solid lesions resembling urticaria (hives). There are no verified battlefield uses of this compound, and it remains incompletely studied in the Western world. Both lewisite and phosgene oxime remain chemical weapons of concern because they were stockpiled by the former Soviet Union. Mixtures of agents such as mustard and lewisite also exist in these stockpiles.

MUSTARD

Although mustard ([bis-(2-chloroethyl)sulfide, also called 2,2′-dichlorodiethyl sulfide) was introduced late in World War I (July 1917), it caused more chemical casualties than chlorine, phosgene, and cyanide combined. Although lethality from mustard exposure was low, casualties filled the medical facilities. Considering the ease of its manufacture and extent of existing stockpiles, this fact is especially crucial.

Mustard allegedly received its name from its smell or taste (onion, garlic, mustard) or its color (which

Table 8-1 *continued*

Environmental and Biological				
Detection	Liquid: M8 paper Vapor: CAM	Liquid: M8 paper Vapor: CAM, M256A1 kit, ICAD	M256A1 ticket or card	Vapor, M256A1 ticket or card, ICAD
Persistence:				
In Soil	Persistent	2 wk–3 y	2 h	Days
On Materiel	Temperature-dependent; hours to days	Temperature-dependent; hours to days	Nonpersistent	Temperature-dependent; hours to days
Skin Decontamination	M2581 kit Dilute hypochlorite Water M291 kit	M258A1 kit Dilute hypochlorite Soap and water M291 kit	Water	Dilute hypochlorite M258A1 kit Water M291 kit
Biologically Effective Amount:				
Vapor ($mg \bullet min/m^3$)	LCt_{50}: 1,500	LCt_{50}: 1,500 (inhaled) 10,000 (masked)	Minimum effective Ct: approx 300; LCt_{50}: 3,200 (estimate)	Eye: <30 Skin: approx 200 LCt_{50}: 1,200–1,500 (inhaled) 100,000 (masked)
Liquid LD_{50}:	approx 100 mg/kg	LD_{50}: 100 mg/kg	No estimate	40–50 mg/kg

CAM: chemical agent monitor
CCl_4: carbon tetrachloride
ICAD: individual chemical agent detector
LD_{50}: dose that is lethal to 50% of the exposed population (liquid, solid)
LCt_{50}: (concentration • time of exposure) that is lethal to 50% of the exposed population (vapor, aerosol)
NA: not applicable
ND: not determined

TABLE 8-2

CLINICAL DIFFERENCES AMONG VESICANTS

		Onset	
Chemical Agent	**Blister**	**Pain**	**Tissue Damage**
Mustard	Fluid filled	Hours later	Immediate; onset of clinical effects is hours later
Lewisite	Fluid filled	Immediate	Seconds to minutes
Phosgene oxime	Solid wheal	Immediate	Seconds

varies from yellow, to light tan, to dark brown).[3,9] When Germany first used mustard, the Allies called it Hun Stoffe (German stuff), abbreviated as HS; later, it became known as H. Mustard manufactured by the Levinstein process is also known as H; it contains about 20% to 30% impurities (mostly sulfur). Distilled, or nearly pure, mustard is known as HD. Both forms of mustard, H and HD, can still be found today in munitions manufactured over 90 years ago. Sulfur mustard has also been called Lost or S-Lost (for the two German chemists who suggested its use as a chemical weapon, Lommell and Steinkopf); yellow cross (for its identifying mark on World War I shells); and yperite (for the site of its first use, Ypres, Belgium).

Nitrogen mustard has three forms: HN-1, HN-2, and HN-3. These agents are similar to sulfur mustard in many ways and seem to cause equally severe effects, particularly in the central nervous system (CNS). They regularly caused convulsions when administered intravenously to animals. However, the nitrogen mustards were not suitable as military agents for several reasons.[10] They will not be discussed further in this chapter because they have not been used militarily; unless stated otherwise the term "mustard" refers here to sulfur mustard.

Military Use

Mustard has been stockpiled in the arsenals of various countries since it was first used on July 12, 1917, when the Germans fired shells containing mustard at British troops entrenched near Ypres, Belgium.[1,2] Only a few months later, both sides were using mustard. Mustard caused at least 70% of the chemical casualties in World War I (when a single agent could be identified as the source of injury). The remaining 30% were caused by other agents, such as chlorine and phosgene (see Chapter 10, Toxic Inhalational Injury and Toxic Industrial Chemicals). The proportion of mustard injuries is remarkable considering there were 1.3 million chemical casualties in World War I (out of a total of 5 million chemical and conventional casualties) and that mustard was introduced only in the last year of the war. Of 180,983 chemical casualties among British soldiers; the injuries of 160,970 (88%) were caused solely by mustard, and 4,167 (2.6%) of these casualties died. Of 36,765 single-agent chemical casualties in the US military; the injuries of 27,711 (75%) were caused solely by mustard. Of all chemical casualties who reached a medical treatment facility (MTF), 599 (2.2%) died.[11] The conventional injury mortality rate for World War I was 7%. Although few mustard casualties died, the survivors required lengthy hospitalization averaging 42 days. The combination of long convalescent times and large numbers of casualties demonstrated the effectiveness of mustard.

Since World War I, mustard was reportedly used in a number of isolated incidents. In 1935, Italy probably used mustard against Abyssinia (now Ethiopia); Japan allegedly used mustard against the Chinese from 1937 to 1944; and Egypt was accused of using the agent against Yemen in the mid 1960s.[12]

Chemical agents were not used on the battlefield during World War II; one of several conjectures about why Germany did not use mustard was that Hitler had been a mustard victim during World War I and disdained its use. However, in December 1943, a German air raid destroyed the SS *John Harvey*, a US ship secretly carrying a large stockpile of mustard bombs, while it was docked with other Allied ships in Bari, Italy. There were 617 US mustard casualties (83 fatal) from exploded shells, burning mustard smoke, and oily mustard floating on the water surface. In addition, an unknown number of Italian civilians were casualties as a result of smoke.[13-15] The incident at Bari is discussed in greater detail in Chapter 2, History of Chemical Warfare.

During the Iran-Iraq War, one source estimated there were 45,000 mustard casualties.[16] In 1989 the journal *Annales Medicinae Militaris Belgicae* published a monograph by Jan L Willems that reported the western European experience treating a selected population of Iranian mustard casualties.[17] Willems reported that in March 1984, February 1985, and March 1986, Iranian casualties were sent to hospitals in Ghent, Belgium, and other western European cities for treatment. More casualties arrived in 1987. In an attempt to establish whether chemical warfare agents had been used, three United Nations missions (in 1984, 1986, and 1987) conducted field inspections, clinical examination of casualties, and laboratory analyses of chemical ammunition. The missions concluded that

- aerial bombs containing chemical weapons were used in some areas of Iran,
- sulfur mustard was the primary chemical agent, and
- there was some use of the nerve agent tabun.[17]

Since mustard's introduction, multiple accidental exposures have occurred. Several occurred in the North Sea, where fishermen were exposed after dredging up munitions that had been dumped after World War II.[18–21] Others occurred when children found and played with mustard shells. The children were injured when the shells exploded, and several died.[22,23] There have also been reported incidents of laboratory workers and, in one instance, of soldiers in their sleeping quarters who were accidentally exposed to mustard. In yet another incident, a souvenir collector unearthed a mustard shell.[24–26] Recently a US Air Force explosive ordinance disposal team was accidentally exposed to World War II munitions dredged from the Atlantic coast.

Properties

Mustard is an oily liquid generally regarded as a "persistent" chemical agent because of its low volatility, which usually allows the liquid to remain on surfaces longer than 24 hours. At higher temperatures, such as those in the Middle East during the hot season, 38° to 49°C (100° to 120°F), mustard vapor is a major hazard. The persistency of mustard in sand decreases from 100 hours to 7 hours as the temperature rises from 10° to 38°C (50° to 100°F).[27]

World War I data suggest that the warming of the air after sunrise caused significant evaporation of mustard from the ground.[28] Mustard attacks were frequently conducted at night, when the liquid agent did not readily evaporate in the cool night air; however, several hours after daybreak, the sun-warmed air caused the mustard to vaporize. At first, thinking the danger was over, soldiers removed their masks in the morning and fell victim to the evaporating mustard, but it soon became standard policy not to unmask for many hours after daybreak.

Mustard vapor has a 5.4-fold greater density than that of air, causing it to hug the ground and sink into trenches and gullies. Despite low volatility, more than 80% of the mustard casualties during World War I were caused by vapor, not the liquid form of mustard.[29]

The freezing/melting temperature for mustard is 57°F. This high freezing point makes mustard unsuitable for delivery by high-altitude aircraft or in the winter. To lower the freezing point, mustard must be mixed with another substance; during World War I it was mixed with chloropicrin, chlorobenzene, or carbon tetrachloride.[1] Mustard has also been mixed with lewisite to increase its volatility in colder weather. The mustard/lewisite combination has a freezing point close to 10°F.

Biochemical Mechanisms of Injury

Over the past few decades, scientists have made major advances in understanding the cellular and biochemical consequences of exposure to mustard and have put forth several hypotheses, two of which are discussed below, to explain mustard injury (Figure 8-1).[30–33] The mustards, both sulfur and nitrogen, are alkylating agents that act through cyclization of an ethylene group to form a highly reactive sulfonium or immonium electrophilic center. This reactive electrophile is capable of combining with any of the numerous nucleophilic sites present in the macromolecules of cells. The products of these reactions are stable adducts that can modify the normal function of the target macromolecule. Because nucleophilic areas exist in peptides, proteins, ribonucleic acid (RNA), deoxyribonucleic acid (DNA), and membrane components, researchers have tried to identify the most critical biomolecular reactions leading to mustard injury.

Because of the highly reactive nature of mustard, it is conceivable that the injury following tissue exposure may result from a combination of effects described in both hypotheses below, or injury may result from additional changes not yet described in a formal hypothesis. Whether the initiating event is alkylation of DNA or modification of other cellular macromolecules, these steps would disrupt the epidermal-dermal junction. Once the site of tissue injury is established, the pathogenic process leading to formation of fully developed blisters must involve an active inflammatory response and altered fluid dynamics in the affected tissue. Mustard also has cholinergic action, stimulating both muscarinic and nicotinic receptors.[34]

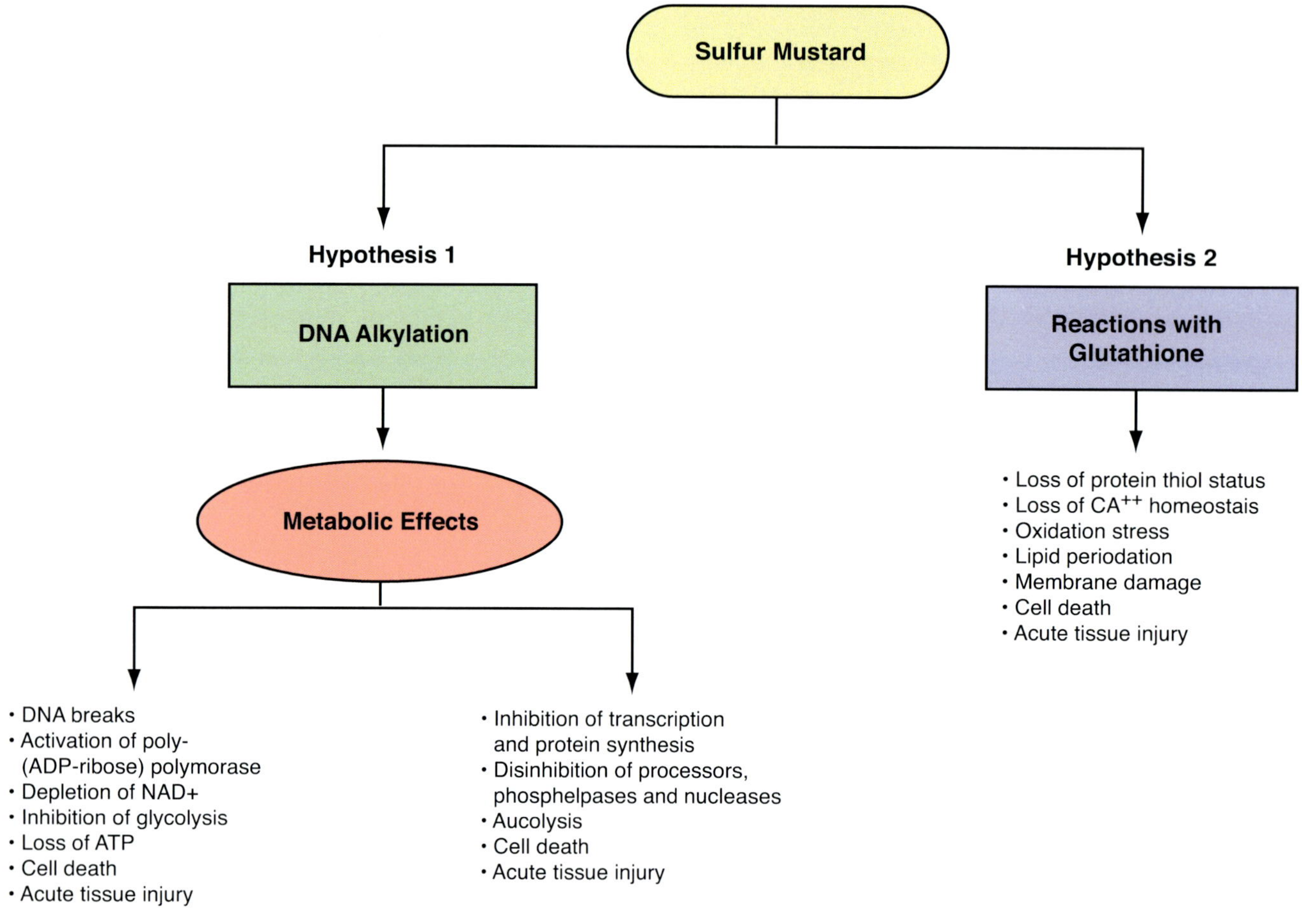

Fig. 8-1. The putative mechanisms by which sulfur mustard causes tissue damage.
ADP: adenosine 5′-diphosphate
ATP: adenosine triphosphate
Ca++: calcium ions
DNA: deoxyribonucleic acid
NAD+: nicotinamide adenine dinucleotide
Adapted from: US Army Medical Research Institute of Chemical Defense. A global picture of battlefield vesicants, I: a comparison of properties and effects. *Med Chem Def.* 1992;5(1):6.

Alkylation of Deoxyribonucleic Acid

The first proposed hypothesis about the mechanism of injury for mustard links alkylation of DNA with the cellular events of blister formation.[35] According to this proposal, alkylation of DNA by sulfur mustard results in strand breaks. The strand breaks trigger activation of a nuclear DNA repair enzyme, poly(adenosine diphosphate-ribose) polymerase (PADPRP). Excessive activity of this enzyme depletes cellular stores of nicotinamide adenine dinucleotide (NAD^+), a critical cofactor and substrate needed for glycolysis.[36-38] Inhibition of glycolysis would cause a buildup of glucose-6-phosphate, a substrate in the hexose monophosphate shunt.[39] Stimulation of the hexose monophosphate shunt results in activation of cellular proteases.[40] Since a principal target of mustard in the skin is the basal epidermal cell, protease from these cells could account for the cleavage of the adherent fibrils connecting the basal epidermal cell layer to the basement membrane.[41]

Thus far, data from animal and cellular systems are consistent with many aspects of this hypothesis, which considers DNA damage the initiating step and PADPRP activation a critical event. Studies with human skin grafts, epidermal keratinocytes, and leukocytes in culture, and with the euthymic hairless guinea pig, have shown decreases in cellular NAD^+ as a consequence of PADPRP activation following sulfur-mustard–induced DNA damage.[36,37,42,43] Niacinamide and other inhibitors of PADPRP can ameliorate the pathology developing in both living animal and cellular models.[36,37,43,44] Unfortunately, while niacinamide has some beneficial actions, the protection it affords is never complete and is limited in duration.[42,43] No evidence currently shows activation of the hexose monophosphate shunt following mustard exposure, but significant metabolic disruptions in human keratinocytes have been reported after mustard exposure.[45] Protease activity is increased in human cells exposed in vitro to mustard.[46–48]

Although many aspects of the PADPRP hypothesis have been verified, and there is good linkage between the proposed steps of this pathway and mustard-induced cytotoxicity, no direct correlation with the full range of tissue pathologies seen following mustard exposure has yet been established. Even though DNA is an important macromolecular target of mustard alkylation in the cell, several other hypotheses of mustard toxicity have been developed that are based on mustard's reaction with other cellular components. For a review of all such hypotheses, see *Medical Defense Against Mustard Gas: Toxic Mechanisms and Pharmacological Implications*; only those undergoing active investigation are discussed here.[31]

Reactions with Glutathione

The second major hypothesis to explain the effects of mustard proposes that the agent reacts with the intracellular free radical scavenger glutathione (GSH), thereby depleting it, resulting in a rapid inactivation of sulfhydryl groups and the consequent loss of protection against oxygen-derived free radicals, specifically those causing lipid peroxidation.[49] In 1987 Orrenius and Nicotera established that menadione-induced depletion of GSH resulted in loss of protein thiols and inactivation of sulfhydryl-containing enzymes.[50] Included in this class of thiol proteins are the calcium and magnesium adenosine triphosphatases, which regulate calcium homeostasis. With the inactivation of the enzymes that control thiol proteins, intracellular calcium levels would increase. High calcium levels within the cell trigger activation of protease, phospholipases, and endonucleases, which could give rise to the breakdown of membranes, cytoskeleton, and DNA that would result in cell death.

One report suggested that this mechanism could be activated by mustards and might be the mechanism of mustard injury.[51] While several aspects of the thiol-calcium hypothesis (eg, release of arachidonic acid and decrease in membrane fluidity) have been observed in cell cultures following sulfur mustard exposure, no definitive studies have drawn an association between calcium disruptions and mustard-induced pathology.[52]

Another proposed consequence of the assumed depletion of GSH following mustard exposure is lipid peroxidation.[53,54] According to this hypothesis, depletion of GSH allows the formation of oxygen-derived free radicals. The oxidizing compounds thus formed would react with membrane phospholipids to form lipid peroxides that could, in turn, lead to membrane alterations, changes in membrane fluidity, and eventual breakdown of cellular membranes.

As previously mentioned, studies have shown changes in membrane fluidity following sulfur mustard exposure.[52] In addition, in 1989 Elsayed and colleagues demonstrated the presence of lipid peroxidation indicators in the tissue of mice exposed to subcutaneous butyl mustard.[55] However, as with the thiol-calcium hypothesis, no studies have directly linked lipid peroxidation with mustard-induced injury.

Metabolism

As the first step in any of the mustard injury theories, mustard cyclizes to a sulfonium electrophilic center. This highly reactive moiety, in turn, combines with peptides, proteins, DNA, or other substances. After a few minutes in a biological milieu, intact mustard is no longer present; the reactive electrophile has attached to another molecule and is no longer reactive. The rapidity of this reaction also means that, within a few minutes, mustard has started to cause tissue damage. The clinical relevance is that intact mustard or its reactive metabolic product is not present in tissue or biological fluids, including blister fluid, a few minutes after the exposure; however, clothing, hair, and skin surfaces may still be contaminated hours later.

Several studies support the observation that intact or active mustard is not present in tissue or biological fluids after a few minutes.[31–33,56] Occluding the blood supply to areas of the intestinal tract or to selected bone marrow for a few minutes protected these organs from the effects of a lethal amount of intravenously administered mustard. Approximately 85% of S-labeled mustard disappeared from the blood of humans after several minutes, and the half-life for intravenously administered mustard to disappear from the blood of piglets was about 2 minutes.[37,57,58] Mustard blister fluid did not produce a reaction when instilled into the eyes of animals or humans or onto the skin of humans.[59,60] A continuing outbreak of smaller vesicles near a source of blister fluid is probably the result of these areas having received an additional exposure and not from contamination by the blister fluid.[59,61]

Clinical Effects

The organs most commonly affected by mustard are the skin, eyes, and airways (Table 8-3): the organs with which mustard comes into direct contact. After a significant amount of mustard has been absorbed through the skin or inhaled, the hemopoietic system, gastrointestinal tract, and CNS are also damaged. Mustard may also affect other organs, but rarely do these produce clinical effects.

During World War I, 80% to 90% of US mustard casualties had skin lesions, 86% had eye involvement, and 75% had airway damage; these percentages are not significantly different from those seen in Iranian casualties.[62] Of a group of 233 severely injured Iranian soldiers sent to western European hospitals by the Iranian government for treatment during the Iran-Iraq War, 95% had airway involvement, 92% had eye signs and symptoms, and 83% had skin lesions.[63] In a series of 535 Iranian casualties, including civilians, admitted to a dermatology ward, 92% had skin lesions and 85% had conjunctivitis; of the total number of patients, 79% had erythema and 55% had blisters. Casualties with more serious problems, including injury to the pulmonary tract, were admitted to other wards.[64]

The slightly higher percentage of airway and eye involvement in Iranian soldiers versus US World War I casualties is perhaps attributable to the higher ambient temperature in the area (compared with Europe), which caused more vaporization. The difference might also have resulted from the limited availability of Iranian protective equipment or poor mask seals with facial hair. In 1984, the year the first Iranian casualties were treated in Europe, protective clothing and gas masks were not commonly worn by Iranian soldiers.[17]

Mustard-related death occurs in about 3% of the casualties who reach an MTF; of those who die, most die 4 or more days after exposure. Table 8-4 illustrates the breakdown, in percentages, of British troops who died after exposure to mustard during World War I.[62] Of the casualties who died, 84% spent at least 4 days hospitalized. The causes of death from mustard exposure are pulmonary insufficiency from airway damage, superimposed infection, and sepsis. Rarely, the mustard exposure is overwhelming and causes death within 1 to 2 days; in these circumstances, death results from neurological factors or massive airway damage.[10,23] The Willems report on Iranian casualties treated in western European hospitals describes more recent treatment of mustard casualties. Clinical files of 65 of these casualties were studied in detail.[17] Eight patients died between 6 and 15 days after exposure. One patient died 185 days after exposure: he had received ventilatory support for an extended period because of severe bronchiolitis complicated by a series of loculate pneumothoraces. Most patients returned to Iran in fairly good condition after 2 to 10 weeks of treatment. The duration of hospitalization was determined

TABLE 8-3

INITIAL CLINICAL EFFECTS FROM MUSTARD EXPOSURE

Organ	Severity	Effects	Onset of First Effect
Eyes	Mild	Tearing Itching Burning Gritty feeling	4–12 h
	Moderate	Above effects, plus: Reddening Lid edema Moderate pain	3–6 h
	Severe	Marked lid edema Possible corneal damage Severe pain	1–2 h
Airways	Mild	Rhinorrhea Sneezing Epistaxis Hoarseness Hacking cough	6–24 h
	Severe	Above effects, plus: Productive cough Mild-to-severe dyspnea	2–6 h
Skin	Mild	Erythema	2–24 h
	Severe	Vesication	4–12 h

TABLE 8-4

DAY OF DEATH AFTER EXPOSURE IN WORLD WAR I FATAL MUSTARD CASUALTIES*

Day of Death (After Exposure)	Percentage of Deaths
≤1	1
2	2
3	5
4	8
5	22
≥6	62

*In 4,167 British troops who died from mustard exposure.
Data source: Gilchrist HL. *A Comparative Study of World War Casualties From Gas and Other Weapons*. Edgewood Arsenal, Md: US Chemical Warfare School; 1928: 14.

mainly by the time needed for healing of the deeper skin lesions. Despite medical advances since World War I, there was a 14% mortality rate among this group; this higher rate is because some of the most severely injured Iranian patients were sent to Europe.

Skin

The threshold amount of mustard vapor required to produce a skin lesion (erythema) is a *Ct* of about 200 mg•min/m^3. This amount varies greatly depending on a number of factors, including temperature, humidity, skin hydration, and body site. Warm, moist areas with thin skin, such as the perineum, external genitalia, axillae, antecubital fossae, and neck are much more sensitive than other areas of the body. A liquid droplet of about 10 μg will produce vesication. About 80% evaporates, and 10% enters the circulation, leaving about 10% on the skin surface to cause local topical injury. As little as 1 μg can cause simple vesicle formation. Evaporation of small droplets is rapid and nearly complete in 2 to 3 minutes; amounts larger than several hundred milligrams may take hours to evaporate.[65]

Mustard vapor rapidly penetrates the skin at the rates of 1.4 $\mu g/cm^2$/min at 70°F, and 2.7 $\mu g/cm^2$/min at 88°F.[27] Liquid mustard penetrates the skin at 2.2 $\mu g/cm^2$/min at 60°F and at 5.5 $\mu g/cm^2$/min at 102°F.[65]

The mildest and earliest form of visible skin injury is erythema, which resembles sunburn (Figure 8-2). Erythema begins to appear 1 to 24 hours after the skin is exposed to mustard, although onset can be later. Erythema is usually accompanied by pruritus (itching), burning, or stinging. After a small exposure, this might be the extent of the lesion. More commonly, small vesicles will develop within or on the periphery of the erythematous areas (like a string of pearls); these vesicles will later coalesce to form larger blisters (Figure 8-3). The effects from liquid mustard appear more rapidly than the effects from mustard vapor. Characteristically, the onset of erythema is about 4 to 8 hours after mustard exposure. Vesication begins about 2 to 18 hours later and may not be complete for several days.

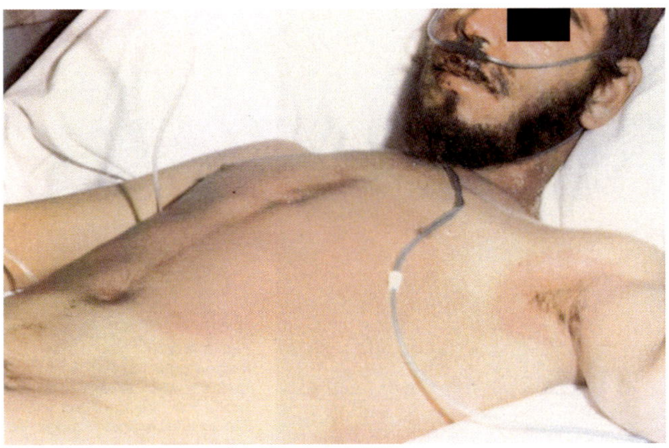

Fig. 8-2. Erythema of the chest of an Iranian casualty as it appeared 5 days after his exposure to mustard. He also had a pulmonary injury with an associated bronchopneumonia from infection with *Haemophilus influenzae.*
Reproduced with permission from: Willems JL. Clinical management of mustard gas casualties. *Ann Med Milit Belg.* 1989;3S:13.

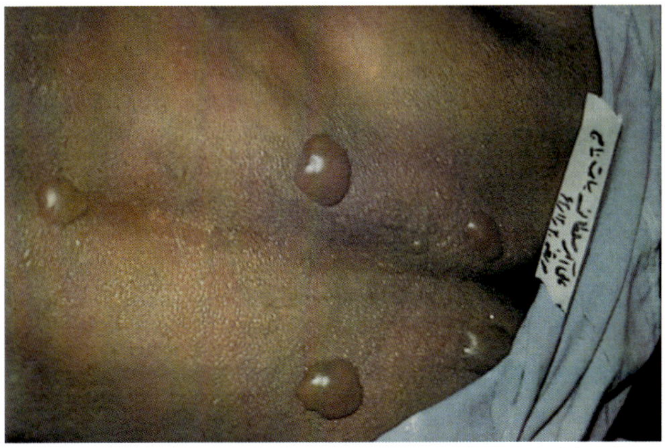

Fig. 8-3. The back of an Iranian casualty seen 16 hours after exposure to mustard. Note the large bullae that have resulted from coalescence of small vesicles.
Reproduced with permission from: Willems JL. Clinical management of mustard gas casualties. *Ann Med Milit Belg.* 1989;3S:8.

The typical bulla (large blister) is dome-shaped, thin-walled, superficial, translucent, yellowish, and surrounded by erythema; it can be 5 cm in diameter or larger (Figure 8-4). The blister fluid is initially thin and clear or slightly straw-colored; later it turns yellowish and tends to coagulate.[17,65,66] The blister fluid does not contain mustard and is not itself a vesicant. Thiodiglycol, a breakdown product of mustard, has been found in blister fluid and can be used to aid in diagnosis. Vapor injury is generally a first- or second-degree burn; liquid mustard may produce deeper damage comparable to a third-degree burn.

After exposure to extremely high doses, such as those resulting from contact with liquid mustard, lesions may be characterized by a central zone of coagulation necrosis, with blister formation at the periphery. These lesions are more severe, take longer to heal, and are more prone to secondary infection than lesions resulting from smaller doses.[29]

a

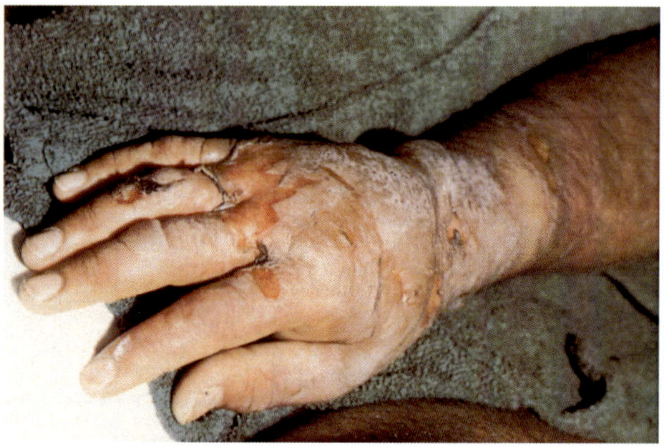

b

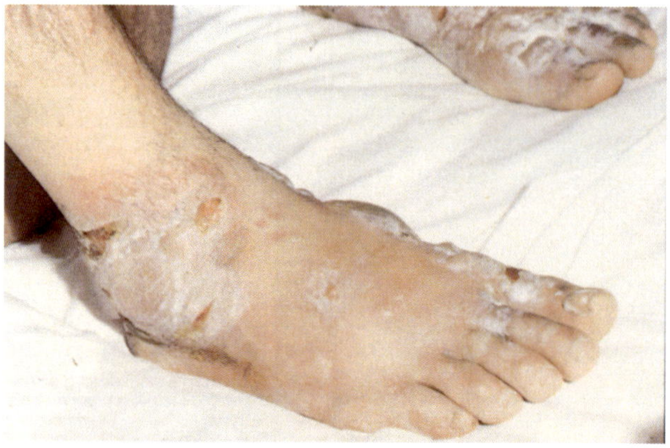

c

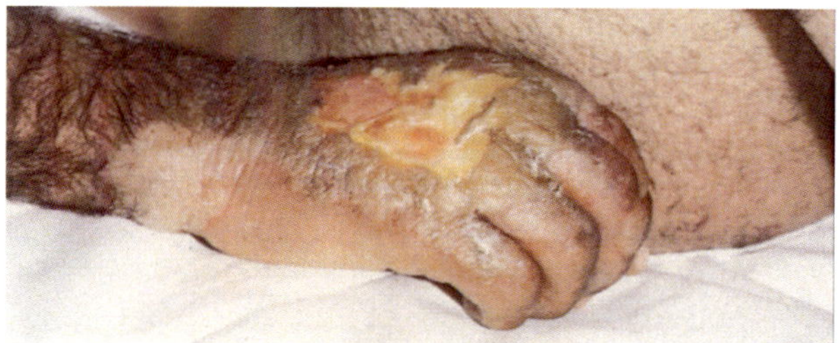

Fig. 8-4. Large and extensive bullae on **(a)** the hands and **(b)** the feet of Iranian casualties as they appeared 5 days after exposure to mustard. In **(c)**, also day 5, some of the bullae are disrupted and have a purulent base. Note the extensive edema of the surrounding skin. The whitish material is an antimicrobial salve.
Reproduced with permission from: Willems JL. Clinical management of mustard gas casualties. *Ann Med Milit Belg*. 1989;3S:14, 15.

The healing time for mustard skin lesions depends on the severity of the lesion. Erythema heals within several days, whereas severe lesions may require several weeks to several months to heal, depending on the anatomical site, the total area of skin surface affected, and the depth of the lesion (Figure 8-5).[17]

A characteristic of the cutaneous mustard injury that Willems reported in the Iranian casualties was transient blackening, or hyperpigmentation, of the affected skin (Figure 8-6).[17] When the hyperpigmented skin exfoliated, epithelium of normal color was exposed. Vesication was not necessary for hyperpigmentation to occur. The syndrome of hyperpigmentation and exfoliation was commonly recognized in World War I casualties, but less commonly in laboratory experiments using liquid mustard.[17] When the initial skin damage, inflammation, only stimulates the melanocyte (pigment cell), increased pigmentation (hyperpigmentation) can be seen. When the melanocyte is destroyed, hypopigmentation occurs, which lasts several months and occasionally becomes permanent. This blotchy hyperpigmentation and

a b

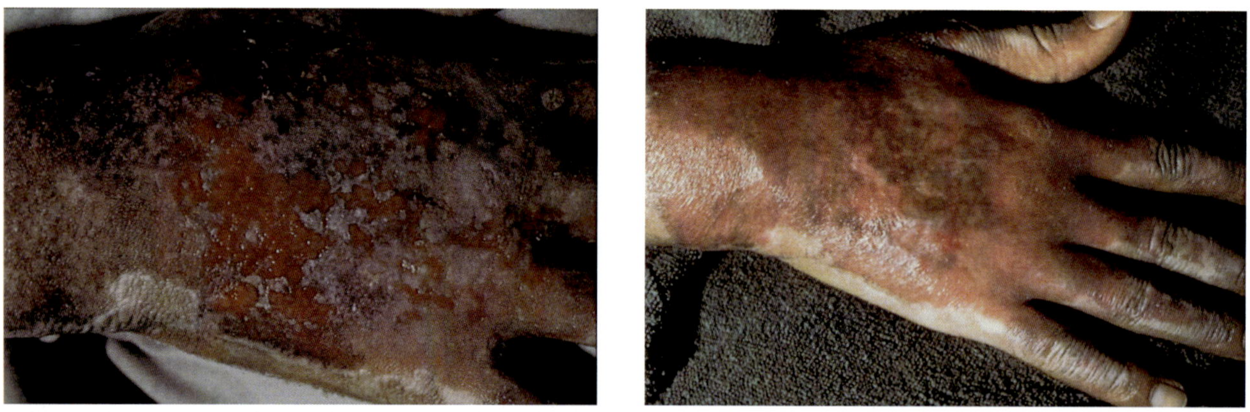

Fig. 8-5. Healing of a deep erosive mustard burn of the hand. **(a)** The appearance on day 49. Epithelialization occurred by ingrowth of cells from patches of less injured skin. **(b)** The appearance on day 66, when complete epithelialization had occurred. The thin and fragile nature of the new skin is clearly apparent.
Reproduced with permission from: Willems JL. Clinical management of mustard gas casualties. *Ann Med Milit Belg*. 1989;3S:36.

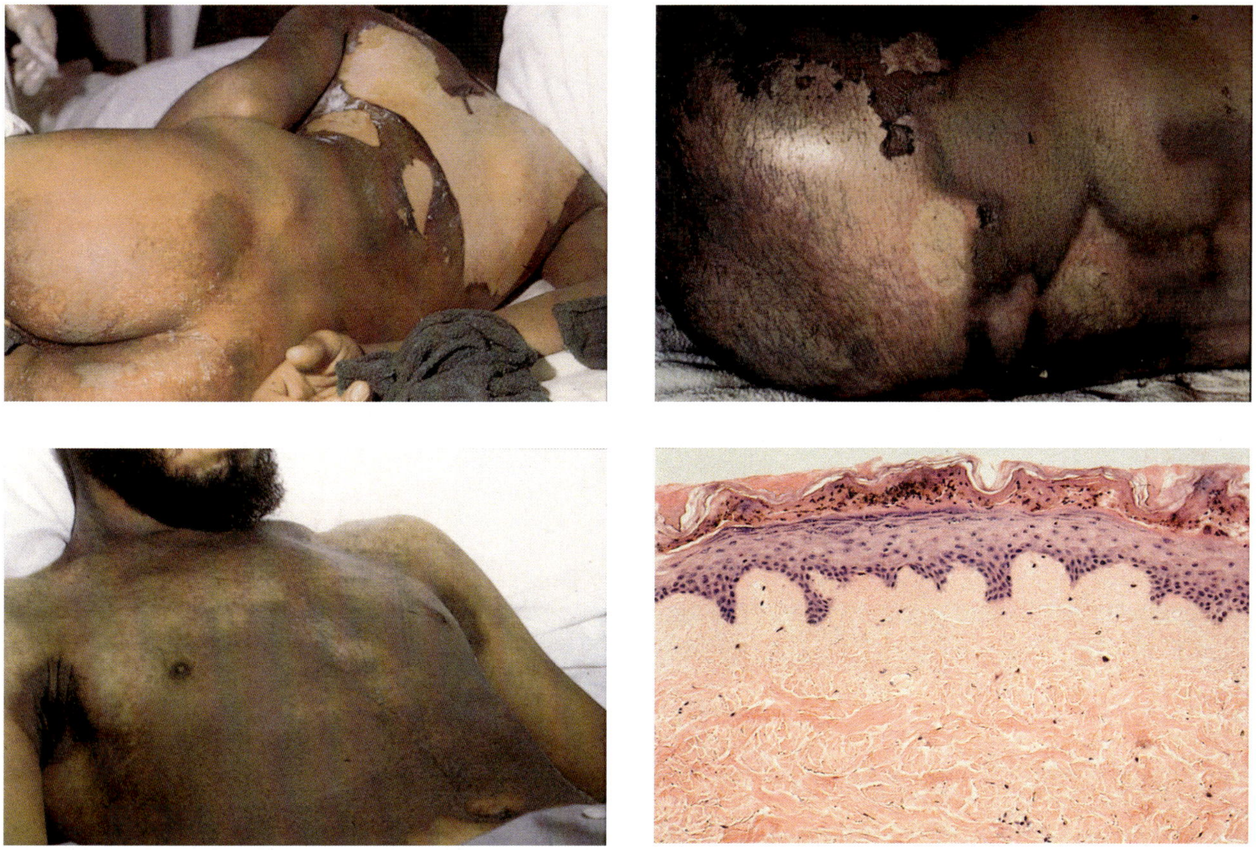

Fig. 8-6. Transient hyperpigmentation of the injured skin is frequently observed following mustard exposure. It is caused by the collection of melanin from dead melanocytes at the base of the soon-to-desquamate epidermis and resolves when the involved skin desquamates. Hyperpigmentation is not dependent on the formation of bullae. (**a**) An Iranian casualty is shown 5 days following exposure to mustard. Note the extensive desquamation of hyperpigmented skin on his back and the normal appearance of the underlying skin. This patient developed a profound leukopenia (400 cells per μL) and a bronchopneumonia of 10 days' duration. Resolution of these problems required a 5-week hospitalization. (**b**) A different Iranian casualty, seen 12 days after exposure to mustard, has darkening of the skin, desquamation, pink areas showing regeneration of the epidermis, and yellow-white areas of deeper necrosis. (**c**) Another casualty's blackening of the skin and beginning desquamation of the superficial layer of the epidermis is shown 15 days after mustard exposure. Note the prominence of these changes in the skin of the axilla. (**d**) The appearance on light microscopy of a hyperpigmented area. Note the melanin in the necrotic epidermal layer, under which is a layer of regenerating epidermis.
Reproduced with permission from: Willems JL. Clinical management of mustard gas casualties. *Ann Med Milit Belg*. 1989;3S:13, 18, 29, 30.

hypopigmentation can be extremely distressing to patients, because similar appearing skin changes are often associated with diseases such as leprosy and syphilis. Punctate repigmentation can be seen starting at and around hair follicles where the melanocytes were not destroyed (Figure 8-7).

Cytopathology. The major change at the dermal-epidermal junction, visualized by light microscopy, is liquefaction necrosis of epidermal basal cell keratinocytes (Figure 8-8). Nuclear swelling within basal cells starts as early as 3 to 6 hours after exposure, and progresses to pyknosis of nuclei and disintegration of cytoplasm.[31,67] The pathological process can be described as follows (Figure 8-9 further illustrates this process).

By a coalescence of neighboring cells undergoing the process of swelling, vacuolar degeneration, or hydropic degeneration ("liquefaction necrosis") and rupture, spaces of progressively increasing size are formed. This usually involves dissolution of cells of the basal layer, resulting in defects in the basal portion of the epidermis and separation of the upper layers of the epidermis from the corium. At first there are multiple focal areas of such microvesicle formation, with septa of as yet uninvolved epidermal cells.[68,69] Progressive dissolution of the cells of such septa follows, and although intact or partially degenerated basal cells may initially remain in the floor of the microvesicles, these

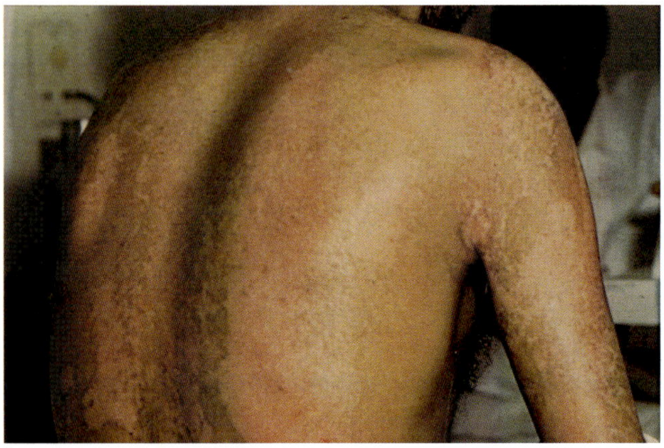

Fig. 8-7. By 32 days after exposure, this Iranian casualty has punctate hyperpigmentation in a healing deep mustard burn. This condition may be indicative of postinflammatory changes in the epidermis.
Reproduced with permission from: Willems JL. Clinical management of mustard gas casualties. *Ann Med Milit Belg.* 1989;3S:34.

also soon disintegrate as the vesicles enlarge.[70] An electron microscopy study of mustard lesions in human skin grafted onto nude mice confirmed that damage to the basal cells (nucleus, plasma membrane, anchoring filaments) resulted in the separation of epidermis from dermis and the formation of a subepidermal microblister.[71]

Models and histopathology. Morphopathological data at the light microscopy level gathered in controlled laboratory investigations are providing important clues about mechanisms of HD skin toxicity. Typically, mustard histopathology in animal skin is presented as occurring during a prevesication period and a vesication period.[72,73] In the prevesication period (the first 12 to 24 hours), beginning 4 to 6 hours postexposure, latent, lethal targeting of epidermal basal cells occurs; basal cell attachment mechanisms to the lamina densa of the skin basement membrane are disabled; and inflammatory cells within the dermal vasculature are recruited. Later, a progressive, inflammatory edema of the lamina lucida of the basement membrane zone contributes to the formation of lucidolytic microvesicles, which coalesce and persist as microblisters at the dermal-epidermal junction, leading to eventual subepidermal cleavage of the epidermis from the dermis (the vesication period).[74,75] Subepidermal vesication evident at 12 to 24 hours postexposure is the end stage of the pathology presented in laboratory animal models. Processes of healing and reepithelialization become evident during the resolution of microvesicles (see Figure 8-9). Leading contributions to this morphopathological data have been made through the use of in vivo models, such as human skin-grafted nude mice, hairless guinea pigs, domestic weanling pigs, and the mouse ear, and in vitro systems, such as cultured human skin equivalents

a

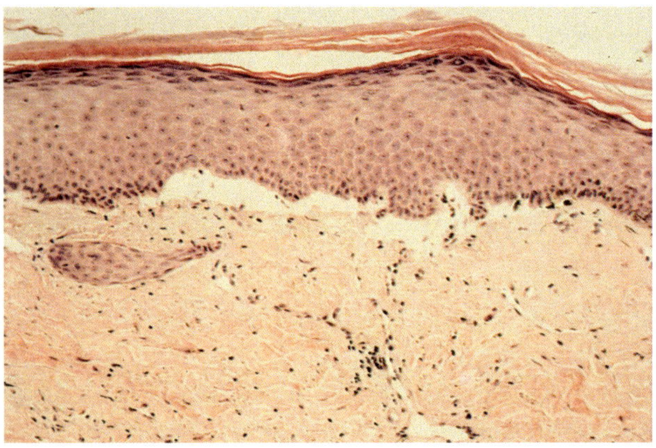

b

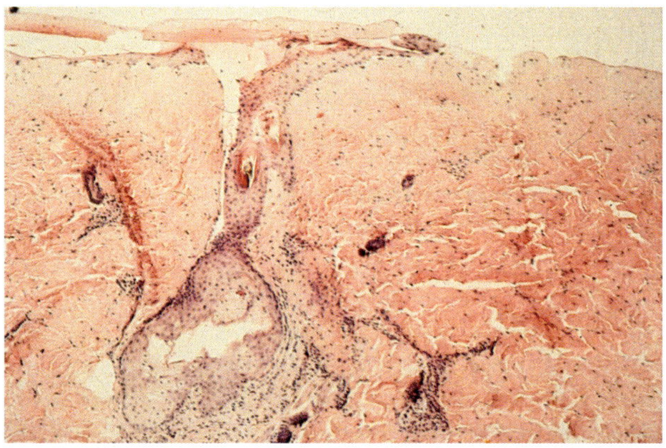

Fig. 8-8. The spectrum of cutaneous mustard injury as seen on light microscopy extends from superficially intact skin to sloughing of the epidermis. **(a)** A skin biopsy taken from an Iranian casualty on the 11th day following exposure to mustard. The gross appearance was of erythema. A cleavage plane is apparent between the dermis and epidermis, with edema extending into the stratum spinosum (note the enlarged spaces between individual cells). Changes in cells of the stratum germinativum are difficult to ascertain at this level of magnification, but nuclei of cells on the extreme right of the figure appear to be pyknotic (shrunken and dark). **(b)** This biopsy was taken at the site of an erosion. The epidermis has sloughed, and the superficial dermis is necrotic. White blood cells have infiltrated the deeper layers of the dermis. Part of an intact hair follicle is seen; the epidermis will ultimately regenerate from such structures.
Reproduced with permission from: Willems JL. Clinical management of mustard gas casualties. *Ann Med Milit Belg.* 1989;3S:19.

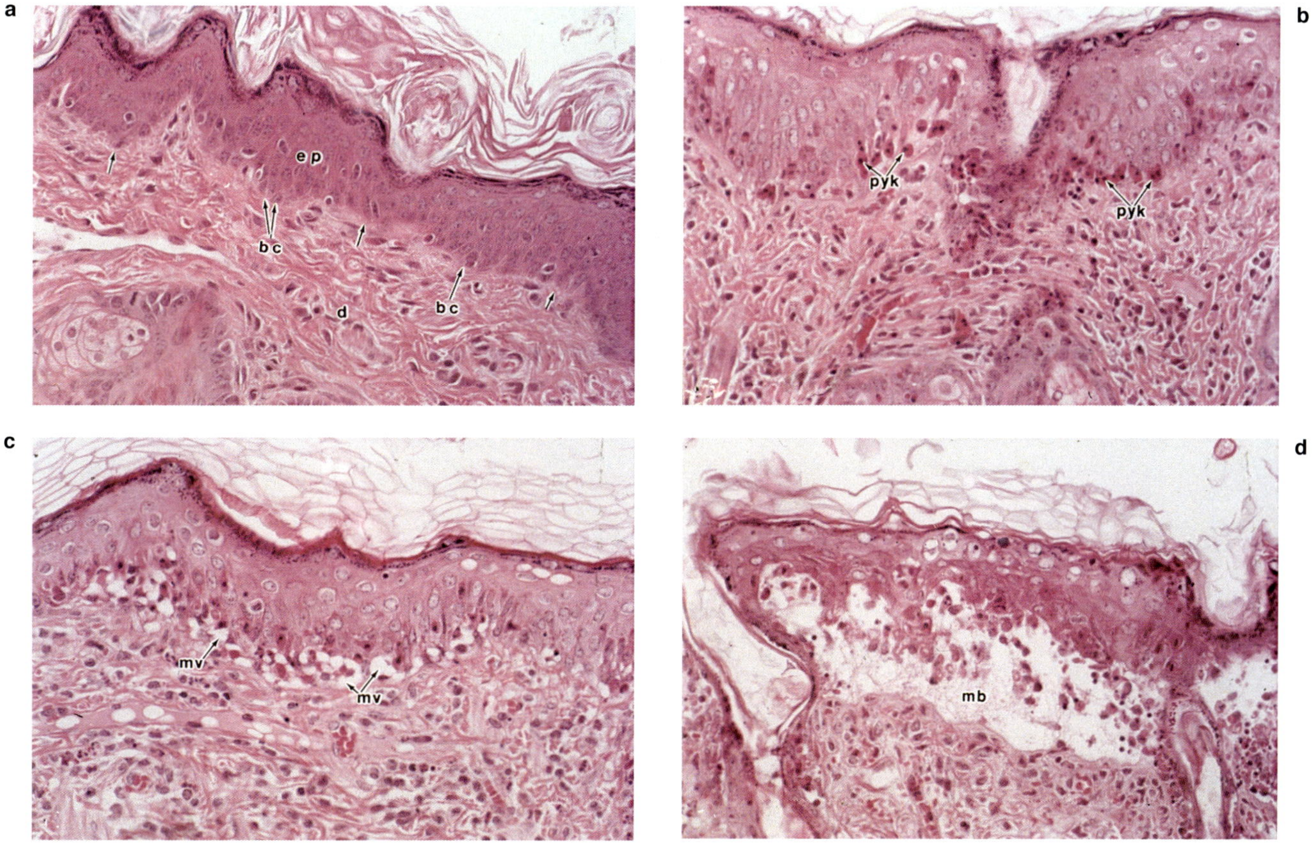

Fig 8-9. Light microscopic **(a, b)** and electron microscopic **(c, d)** presentations of hairless guinea pig skin exposed to sulfur mustard vapor reveal that the epithelial basal cell of the stratum germinativum is selectively affected to the exclusion of other epidermal cells. Following an apparent latency period of 4 to 6 hours, the basal cell pathology progresses to include extensive hydropic vacuolation, swollen endoplasmic reticulum, dilated mitochondria, coagulation of monofilaments, nuclear pyknosis, and cell death. At 12 to 24 hours, microvesicles/microblisters form at the dermal-epidermal junction, which cleave the epidermis from the dermis. The cavity formed within the lamina lucida of the basement membrane as a consequence of basal cell pathology, and perhaps as the result of disabling of basement membrane attachment proteins, is infiltrated with cellular debris, inflammatory cells, fibers, and tissue fluid. **(a)** Unexposed perilesional skin site serves as control, showing epidermis (ep), dermis (d), basement membrane (arrows), basal cells of the stratum germinativum (bc). **(b)** Affected skin 9 hours after exposure to HD vapor, showing degenerating basal cells with karyorrhectic and pyknotic nuclei (pyk). **(c)** Affected skin 12 hours after HD exposure, showing microvesicles (mv) forming at the basement membrane zone in association with the microenvironment of degenerating basal cells. **(d)** Affected skin 24 hours after HD exposure, showing microvesicles that have coalesced to form a characteristic microblister (mb) that separates the epidermis from the dermis. Original magnification × 220.

Photographs: Courtesy of John P Petrali, PhD, US Army Medical Research Institute of Chemical Defense, and Stephanie R Froberg, Graphics Department, US Army Medical Research Institute of Chemical Defense, Aberdeen Proving Ground, Md.

and isolated perfused porcine skin flaps.[74–80]

Ultrastructural pathology. Ultrastructural studies of in vivo models have expanded mustard investigations to elaborate important effects on subcellular entities of the basal cell and the basement membrane microenvironment.[73,74,81] During prevesication, models consistently present subcellular nuclear injury to basal cells to the exclusion of cells of other epidermal strata. These injuries, typically presenting at 6 hours postexposure, include nuclear chromatin condensations with margination, dilatations of the nuclear envelope, mitochondrial swelling, and tonofilament condensations.[75] These early basal cytopathologic changes were confirmed by immunohistochemistry to be associated with an HD-induced apoptosis. This finding suggests that HD-induced cell death involves early apoptosis and late necrosis, which temporarily overlap to produce a basal cell death pathway along an apoptotic-necrotic continuum (Figure 8-10).[82]

During vesication, in vivo models generate charac-

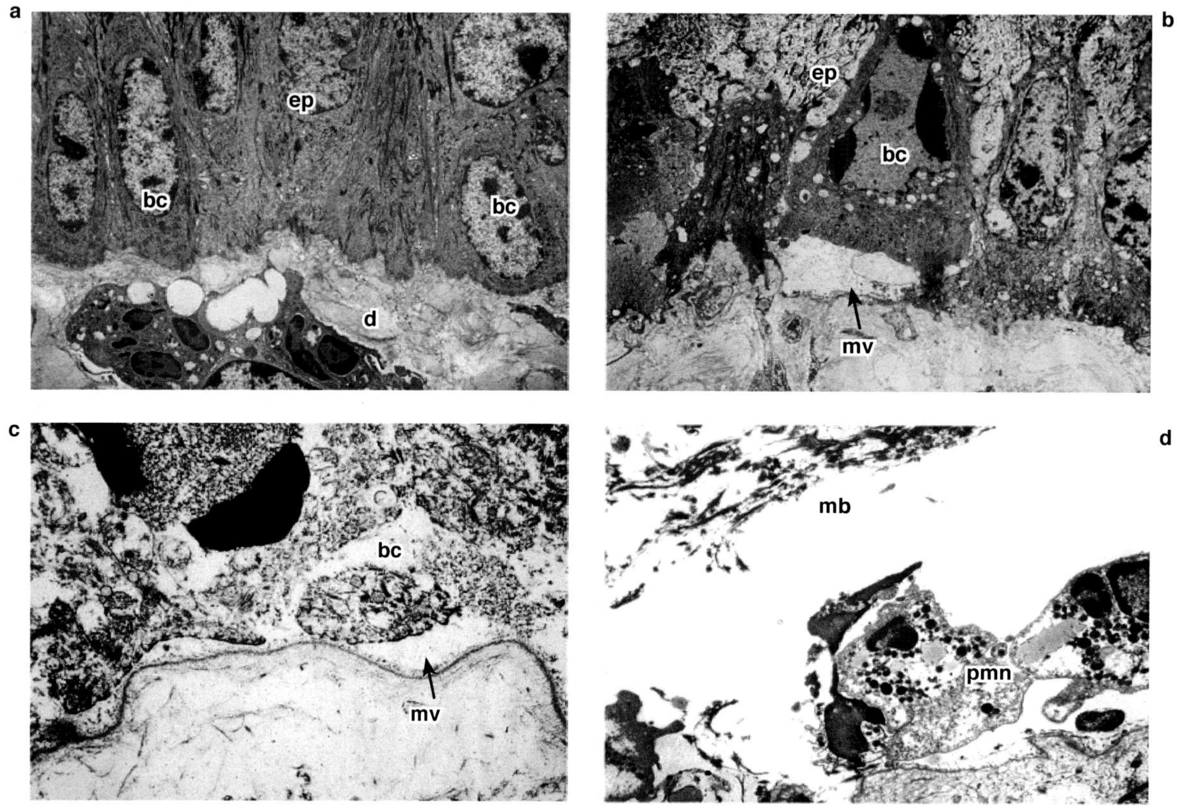

Fig 8-10. Transmission electron microscopy of hairless guinea pig skin. **(a)** Unexposed skin site at the level of the dermal-epidermal junction; epidermis (ep), basal cells of the stratum germinativum (bc), dermis (d). **(b)** Skin site exposed to sulfur mustard vapor 4–6 h postexposure; basal cell (bc) undergoing early apoptotic injury with marginal condensation of chromatin and formation of a microvesicle (mv) within the microenvironment of the basement membrane zone. **(c)** Skin site exposed to sulfur mustard vapor 24 h postexposure; disabling of hemidesmosomes (arrows) contributing to the formation of characteristic microvesicles (mv), basal cells undergoing advanced apoptotic injury and necrosis (bc). **(d)** The cavity of a large microblister (mb) infiltrated with polymorphonucleocytes (pmn).
Photographs (a, b, and d): Courtesy of John P Petrali, PhD, US Army Medical Research Institute of Chemical Defense, and Stephanie R Froberg, Graphics Department, US Army Medical Research Institute of Chemical Defense, Aberdeen Proving Ground, Md. Photograph (c) reproduced with permission from: Marlow DD, Mershon MM, Mitcheltree LW, Petrali JP, Jaax GP. Sulfur mustard-induced skin injury in hairless guinea pigs. *J Toxicol Cutan Ocular Toxicol.* 1990;9(3): 179–192.

teristic microvesicles within the lamina lucida of the basement membrane. The cavities of microvesicles formed as a consequence of basal cell pathology and the disabling of anchoring filaments of hemidesmosomes are bound by degenerating epidermal cells at the roof and by the lamina densa of the basement membrane at the floor. Microvesicles rapidly become infiltrated with inflammatory cells, phagocytic cells, degenerating cells, cellular debris, and tissue fluid, all exacerbating the lesion to form pervasive lucidolytic microblisters that later cleave the epidermis from the dermis (Figure 8-11).

Furthermore, investigative evidence shows that percutaneous carriers such as dimethyl sulfoxide can exacerbate mustard-gas–induced skin pathology.[83] Ultrastructural studies of monotypic human cells in culture, such as keratinocytes and lymphocytes, have added important subcellular information of HD temporal effects on nuclei, plasma membranes, and cytoplasmic organelles, perhaps reflecting predicted and expected biochemical lesions reported elsewhere in this chapter.

Skin proteins and immunohistopathology. Primary or secondary effects of HD toxicity on extracellular components of the basement membrane microenvironment are presently under investigation. Among these extracellular domains are structural adherent proteins known to be antigenically altered or lost to specific antisera in some clinical bullous diseases.[84] Although still the subject of study, proteins shown to be altered directly by the alkylating properties of HD or secondarily by released cellular proteases or by chemical mediators of the accompanying inflammatory response are bullous pemphigoid antigen, α-6 integrins, and laminin-5 (nicein).[80,85] Bullous pemphigoid antigen and α-6 integrins are recognized integral proteins of the hemidesmosome with complex molecular attachments to heads of anchoring filaments. Laminin-5 or nicein is the resident protein of anchoring filaments. Loss of immunospecificity of these proteins would indicate a pathogenesis associated with the disabling of anchoring filaments within the lamina lucida, a process (vida supra) documented by ultrastructural study of HD toxicity.

Histopathological and ultrastructural presentations of sulfur-mustard–induced toxicity—apparently irrespective of the model—demonstrate that epidermal/epithelial basal cells of the stratum germinativum layer are targeted early during the pathology to the exclusion of other epidermal/epithelial cells. Injured basal cells appearing approximately 4 to 6 hours after exposure present progressive signs of apoptosis and irreversible necrotic cell injury and death. Associated with basal cell injury is the apparent disabling of anchoring filaments of hemidesmosomes that leads to detachments within the subadjacent lamina lucida of the epidermal/epithelial basement membrane zone. Superimposed upon this cellular response is the effect on selected basement membrane adherent proteins that lose their immunospecificity to specific antisera

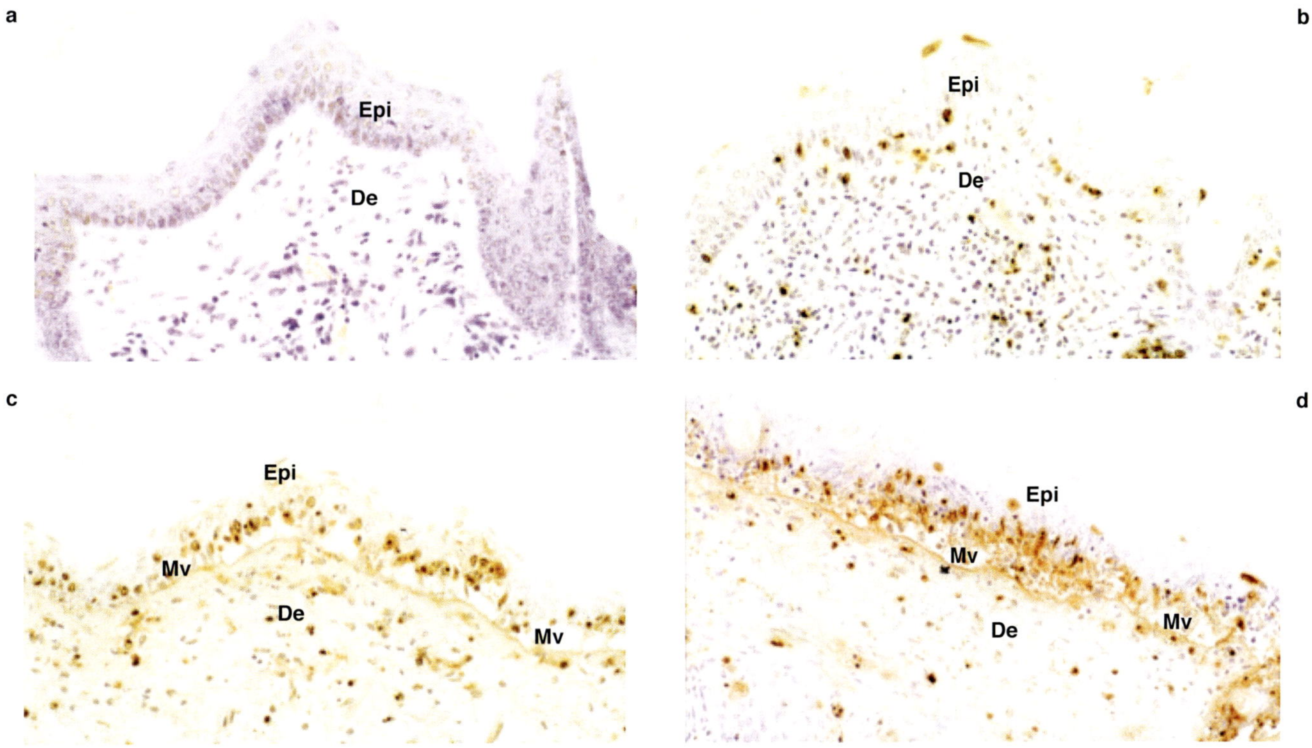

Fig. 8-11. ApopTag (Millipore Corp, Billerica, Mass) staining of paraffin-embedded skin sections demonstrating temporal progression of basal cell apoptotic profiles. **(a)** At 3 hr postexposure, no apoptotic basal cells were observed; only inflammatory cell infiltration was noted in papillary dermis (arrows). **(b)** At 6 hr postexposure, the occurrence of apoptotic basal cells is evident. ApopTag-positive cells exhibit typical characteristics of apoptosis, nuclear condensation, and margination (arrows). **(c)** At 12 hr postexposure, basal cells exhibiting apoptosis significantly increased at areas of microvesication (arrows). **(d)** At 24 hr postexposure, basal cell apoptosis progressed to necrosis, making identification of individual apoptotic cells among cellular debris difficult. Original magnification × 66.
Epi: epidermis
De: dermis
Mv: microvesication
Reproduced with permission from: Kan RK, Pleva CM, Hamilton TA, Anderson DR, Petrali JP. Sulfur mustard-induced apoptosis in hairless guinea pig skin. *Toxicol Pathol*. 2003;31(2): 185–190. Photographs: Courtesy of Stephanie R Froberg, Graphics Department, US Army Medical Research Institute of Chemical Defense, Aberdeen Proving Ground, Md.

and are predictive of attachment failures. Finally, the inflammatory response appears to exacerbate lesions, contributing to the formation of pervasive microvesicles that eventually cleave the epidermis/epithelium from their supporting, underlying structures, leading to epithelial/epidermal sloughing and denudation of basement membranes.

Eye

The eye is the external organ most sensitive to mustard. The latent period for eye damage is shorter than that for skin damage. Generally, the asymptomatic period varies with the concentration of mustard vapor and individual sensitivity. Eye irritation within minutes after exposure has been reported.[17,86] After a low *Ct* exposure, a slight irritation with reddening of the eye may be all that occurs (Figure 8-12). As the *Ct* increases, the spectrum of injury is characterized by progressively more severe conjunctivitis, blepharospasm, pain, and corneal damage.[31,66] Photophobia will appear, and even with mild exposures, may linger for weeks.

Corneal damage consists of edema with clouding, swelling, and infiltration of polymorphonuclear cells. Clinical improvement occurs after approximately 7 days, with subsiding edema. Corneal vascularization (pannus) with secondary edema may last for weeks. Vision will be lost if the pannus covers the visual axis. Severe effects from mustard exposure may be followed by scarring between the iris and the lens, which restricts pupillary movements and predisposes the individual to glaucoma.[31,87]

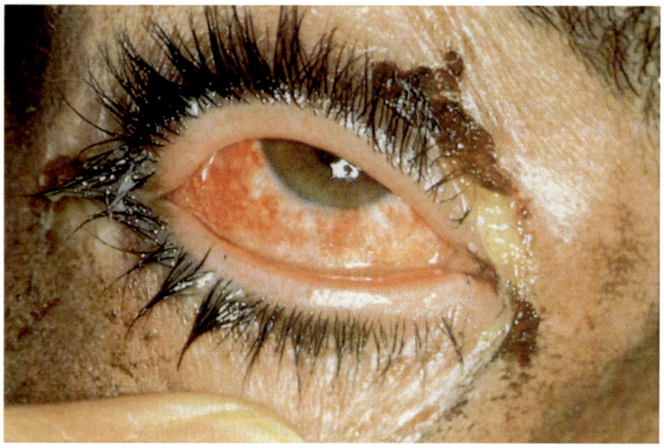

Fig. 8-12. An eye injury of lesser severity in an Iranian casualty (shown 7 d after exposure) caused by exposure to mustard. The characteristic findings were edema of the lid and conjunctival injection. Corneal ulcerations were found with more severe exposure.
Reproduced with permission from: Willems JL. Clinical management of mustard gas casualties. *Ann Med Milit Belg.* 1989;3S:12.

The most severe eye damage is caused by liquid mustard, which may be delivered by an airborne droplet or by self-contamination.[61] Symptoms may become evident within minutes after exposure.[66] Severe corneal damage with possible perforation of the cornea can occur after extensive eye exposure to liquid mustard. The patient may lose vision, or even the eye, from panophthalmitis, particularly if drainage of the infection is blocked, such as by adherent lids.[66] Miosis sometimes occurs, probably due to the cholinergic activity of mustard.

During World War I, mild conjunctivitis accounted for 75% of the eye injuries; complete recovery took 1 to 2 weeks. Severe conjunctivitis with minimal corneal involvement, blepharospasm, edema of the lids and conjunctivae, and orange-peel roughening of the cornea accounted for 15% of the cases; recovery from this condition occurred in 2 to 5 weeks. Mild corneal involvement with areas of corneal erosion, superficial corneal scarring, vascularization, and iritis accounted for 10% of the cases; convalescence took 2 to 3 months in these cases. Lastly, severe corneal involvement with ischemic necrosis of the conjunctivae, dense corneal opacification with deep ulceration, and vascularization accounted for about 0.1% of the injuries; convalescence from this condition lasted more than 3 months. Only one person out of 1,016 mustard casualties surveyed after World War I received disability payments for defective vision.[11]

Studies conducted on rabbit eyes indicate that mustard injury to the cornea is characterized by initial degeneration of the epithelial cells, with changes ranging from nuclear swelling and nuclear vacuolization, to pyknosis and nuclear fragmentation. Epithelial loosening and sloughing occurs either by separation of the basal cells from the basement membrane, or by shearing of the cell just above its attachment to the basement membrane.[88,89]

Mustard initially causes vasodilation and increased vascular permeability in the conjunctiva, which lead to progressive edema. Secretion of mucus occurs within minutes of exposure. Pyknosis of epithelial cells begins concurrently with or shortly after these changes, leading to desquamation of the epithelium. In the later stages, inflammatory infiltration of connective tissue and exudation are present.[88,89] Medical personnel have reported seeing delayed keratitis in humans from 8 months to 20 years after mustard exposure.[29,90] This delayed keratitis, in addition to the chronic inflammation, can lead to erosions and frank ulcerations.

Within approximately 5 minutes, liquid mustard

dropped into the eyes of rabbits was absorbed, had disappeared from the eye's surface, had passed through the cornea and the aqueous, and had produced hyperemia of the iris. Damage to other structures (eg, the Descemet membrane) also occurred within a similar length of time.[29] Because absorption and ocular damage occur so rapidly, decontamination must be performed immediately after liquid mustard contaminates the eye; after a few minutes, there will be no liquid remaining on the surface of the eye to decontaminate.

Descriptions of the pathology of ocular toxicity have been largely limited to gross and histological observations. Gross examination of human eye injury has been characterized at its peak as a progressive conjunctivitis with photophobia, blepharospasms, corneal stromal edema, and opacification. Histological examination of controlled animal eye injuries have presented dose- and time-dependent corneal epithelial degeneration and detachment.[91–94] Ultrastructural studies support progression of basal cell pathology, disabling of hemidesmosomes, and cleaving of the epithelium from the basement membrane, all appearing to be consistent with HD dermal exposure. At variance with dermal exposure is the absence of characteristic microblisters at the epidermal-stromal junction.[96,97] Lack of microblister formation may be directly attributable to the avascular anatomical organization of the cornea.[95]

Airways

Mustard produces dose-dependent damage to the mucosa of the respiratory tract, beginning with the upper airways, and descending to the lower airways as the amount of mustard increases. The inflammatory reaction, which varies from mild to severe, includes necrosis of the epithelium. When fully developed, the injury is characterized by an acute inflammation of the upper and lower airways, with discharge in the upper airway, inflammatory exudate, and pseudomembrane formation in the tracheobronchial tree. The injury develops slowly, intensifying over a period of days.

After a low-dose, single exposure, casualties might notice a variety of irritating symptoms accompanied by a dry cough; on examination, they might have pharyngeal and laryngeal erythema. Hoarseness is almost always present, and the patient often presents with a barking cough. Typically, this hoarseness may progress to a toneless voice, which appears to be particularly characteristic of mustard exposure. Patients characteristically note a sense of chest discomfort. All of these complaints typically commence approximately 4 to 6 hours after exposure, with sinus tenderness appearing hours later. Vapor concentrations sufficient to cause these symptoms typically produce reddened eyes, photophobia, lacrimation, and blepharospasm. There may be loss of taste and smell. Patients occasionally experience mild epistaxis and sore throat. Prominent wheezing and dyspnea (shortness of breath) may be present.[59]

Exposures to higher concentrations of vapor result in an earlier onset and greater severity of the above effects. Hoarseness rapidly progresses to aphonia. Severe tachypnea and early radiological infiltrates may appear. More severe respiratory exposures create necrotic changes in the respiratory epithelium that result in epithelial sloughing and pseudomembrane formation. There may be substantial airway occlusion from the inflammatory debris or from pseudomembranes, which can obstruct the upper airways as they form, or they can break off and obstruct lower airways.[17,59,61]

The initial bronchitis is nonbacterial. White blood cell elevation, fever, pulmonary infiltrates seen on radiograph, and colored secretions may all be present and mimic the changes of a bacterial process. This process is sterile during the first 3 to 4 days; bacterial superinfection occurs in about 4 to 6 days.[61]

Mustard has little effect on lung parenchyma. Its damage is usually confined to the airways and the tissue immediately surrounding the airways, except after an overwhelming exposure to mustard and as a terminal event.[96] The changes are most intense in the upper airways and decrease in the trachea, bronchi, and smaller bronchioles, presumably reflecting a differential disposition of vapor on the mucosal surface.[70,98] Pulmonary edema is not a usual feature, except in the case of hemorrhagic pulmonary edema with severe exposures, and it may occur in terminal stages.[61,96]

The lungs of animals exposed to mustard show alternating areas of atelectasis and emphysema. Atelectasis is thought to be caused by mucus clogging the bronchioles, and the emphysema is compensatory; these findings were confirmed when lungs resected at thoracotomy from Iranian casualties from the Iran-Iraq War showed similar effects.[17,97] As seen in Figure 8-13, the lungs showed bronchiectasis and severe chronic inflammation. The bronchiectasis was caused by full-thickness injury of the airways. In some casualties, this injury healed by scarring of such intensity that severe and unrelenting tracheobronchial stenosis developed.

Gastrointestinal Tract

Nausea and vomiting are common within the first few hours after mustard exposure, beginning at about the time the initial lesions become apparent. The early nausea and vomiting, which are generally transient

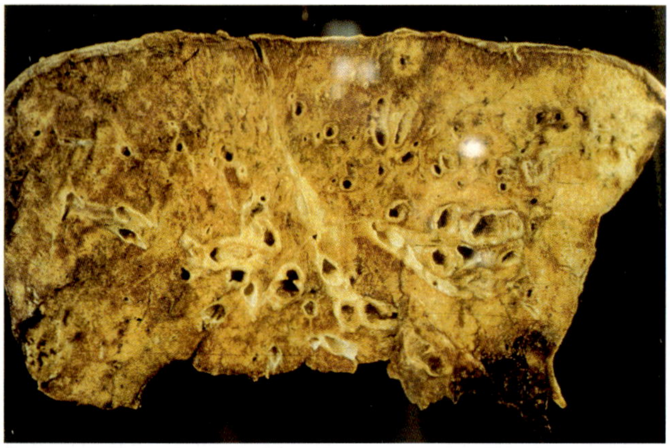

Fig. 8-13. A surgically excised lung from an Iranian mustard casualty showing bronchiectasis and severe chronic infection.
Reproduced with permission from: Freitag L, Firusian N, Stamatis G, Greschuchna D. The role of bronchoscopy in pulmonary complications due to mustard gas inhalation. *Chest*. 1991;100:1438.

and not severe, may be caused by the cholinergic activity of mustard, by a general reaction to injury, or because of the unpleasant odor.[9,33] Nausea and vomiting occurring 24 to 36 hours later results from the generalized cytotoxic activity of mustard and damage to the mucosa of the gastrointestinal tract.

Diarrhea is not common, and gastrointestinal bleeding seems to be even less common in humans. However, animals that were given potentially lethal doses of mustard administered either intravenously or subcutaneously had profuse diarrhea, which was frequently bloody; however, this was unusual when mustard was administered percutaneously or by inhalation.[61,98] Diarrhea in animals was more common after nitrogen mustard.[10] None of 107 autopsied human cases involved; and in the 57 cases in which the gastrointestinal tract was thoroughly examined, none had significant lesions.[99] In several reported series of Iranian casualties, totaling about 700 casualties, few had diarrhea and only a very few who died had bloody diarrhea.[17,63,100] Constipation was noted in casualties with mild exposure.[61]

Central Nervous System

Although the effects are not usually clinically prominent, mustard affects the CNS. Reports of World War I casualties described apathy, depression, intellectual dullness, and languor.[61] Approximately 83% of the 233 Iranian casualties sent to various European hospitals for medical care during the Iran-Iraq War had CNS complaints; most complaints, however, were mild and nonspecific.[63]

Large amounts of mustard administered to animals via the inhalational, intravenous, subcutaneous, or intramuscular routes caused hyperexcitability, abnormal muscular movements, convulsions, and other neurological manifestations.[61,101] Animals died a "neurological death" a few hours after receiving a lethal amount of mustard.[10] Autopsies of these animals disclosed few abnormalities.[101]

After three children were accidentally exposed to a large amount of mustard, two of them presented with abnormal muscular activity, and the third alternated between coma and agitation. The first two children died 3 to 4 hours after exposure, possibly from neurological mechanisms.[23] It is unknown whether these CNS manifestations are from a cholinergic activity of mustard or from other mechanisms.

Death

Most casualties die of pulmonary damage complicated by infection bronchopneumonia, immunosuppression, and sepsis. When exposure is not by inhalation, the mechanism of death is less clear. In studies with animals in which mustard was administered via routes other than inhalational, the animals died 3 to 7 days after the exposure; they had no signs of pulmonary damage and often had no signs of sepsis. The mechanism of death was not clear, but autopsy findings resembled those seen after radiation.[102] Mustard is considered radiomimetic because of the delayed onset of signs and symptoms and the accompanying immunosuppression with potentially lethal doses.

Diagnosis

The differential diagnosis of mustard casualties on the battlefield after a known chemical attack is not difficult. The history of a chemical attack is useful, particularly if the chemical agent is known. Simply questioning the casualty about when the pain started, whether it started immediately after the exposure or hours later, is very helpful. Pain from lewisite (the other vesicant that causes blistering) begins seconds to minutes after exposure; pain from mustard does not begin until the lesion begins to develop hours later.

Blisters appearing simultaneously in a large number of people, in the absence of a known chemical attack, should alert medical personnel to search the area with a chemical agent detector. The appearance of one or more blisters in an individual does not alone make a diagnosis. Friction, plants, insects, and other diseases also cause blisters.

Laboratory Tests

No "routine" laboratory test for mustard exposure exists. Investigational studies have demonstrated the presence of significant amounts of thiodiglycol, a major metabolite of mustard, in the urine of mustard casualties (except for being a breakdown product from sulfur mustard, thiodiglycol is harmless). In two studies, Iranian casualties had higher amounts of thiodiglycol in their urine than did control subjects.[103,104] In a third study, the urinary thiodiglycol secreted by a laboratory worker accidentally exposed to mustard was quantitatively measured for a 2-week period (his postrecovery urine was used as a control); the half-life of thiodiglycol was 1.18 days.[24] In a more recent accident, thiodiglycol was also found in the patient's blister fluid. The procedure for analysis of thiodiglycol is described in the US Army's Technical Bulletin Medical 296, *Assay Techniques for Detection of Exposure to Sulfur Mustard, Cholinesterase Inhibitors, Sarin, Soman, GF, and Cyanide*.[105] The procedure for handling urine samples of suspected victims is on USAMRICD's Web site (http://ccc.apgea.army.mil). See also Chapter 22, Medical Diagnostics.

Patient Management

Decontamination within 1 or 2 minutes after exposure is the only established, effective means of preventing or decreasing tissue damage from mustard. This decontamination is not done by medical personnel; it must be performed by the soldier immediately after the exposure. Generally, a soldier will not seek medical help until the lesions develop hours later. By that time, skin decontamination will not help. Mustard fixes to the skin within minutes, and tissue damage will already have occurred.[65]

If any mustard remains on the skin, thorough decontamination later will prevent further spreading to other areas. After several hours, spreading will have occurred, because oily substances flow on warm skin. Decontamination at that time, however, will prevent mustard from spreading to personnel who handle the casualty and possible contamination of the MTF. By the time skin lesions develop, most mustard will have been absorbed and fixed to tissue. Unless the site was occluded, the remaining unabsorbed agent will have evaporated.

Mustard droplets disappear from the surface of the eye very quickly. The eye should still be flushed as soon as possible. All mustard casualties must be thoroughly decontaminated before they enter a clean MTF. This should be done with the realization that by the time a contaminated soldier reaches an MTF, this decontamination will rarely help the casualty; it does, however, prevent exposure to medical personnel.

Mustard casualties generally fall into three categories. Individuals in the first category may be returned to duty. These individuals have a small area of erythema or one or more small blisters on noncritical areas of their skin; eye irritation or mild conjunctivitis; and/or late-onset, mild upper respiratory symptoms, such as hoarseness or throat irritation and a hacking cough. If these casualties are seen 48 to 72 hours after exposure, there is good reason to believe that the lesion will not progress significantly, and they can be given symptomatic therapy and returned to duty.

The second category includes casualties who appear to have non-life–threatening injuries, but who are unable to return to duty. Casualties with the following conditions must be hospitalized for further care:

- a large area of erythema (with or without blisters);
- an extremely painful eye lesion or an eye lesion that hinders vision; or
- a respiratory injury with moderate symptoms that include a productive cough and dyspnea.

Some of these conditions may develop into life-threatening injuries. For example, an area of erythema caused by liquid mustard that covers 50% or more of the body surface area suggests that the individual was exposed to a potentially lethal dose. Likewise, dyspnea occurring within 4 to 6 hours after the exposure suggests inhalation of a potentially lethal amount of mustard.

The third category comprises those casualties who appear to have life-threatening injuries when they first present at an MTF. Life-threatening injuries include large skin burns caused by liquid mustard and early onset of moderate to severe pulmonary symptoms. Some of the casualties in this category will die from their injuries. Because conditions listed in category two may become life-threatening (category three), the categories should be used only to assess a casualty's presenting condition.

Many mustard casualties will fall into the first category, the majority will fall into the second category, and only a very small percentage of casualties will fall into the third category. Data from World War I, in which only 3% of mustard injuries were lethal despite the unsophisticated medical care at that time (eg, no antibiotics, intravenous fluids, or electrolytes), suggest that most mustard casualties are not severely injured and most will survive.

Most casualties of mustard exposure will, however,

require some form of medical care—from a few days to many weeks. Eye care and airway care will promote healing within weeks; skin lesions take the longest to heal and may necessitate hospitalization for months.[17] Casualties with mild to moderate mustard damage need supportive care. Pain control is extremely important. Fluids and electrolytes should be carefully monitored. Although there is not as great a fluid loss from mustard burns (compared with thermal burns), patients will probably be dehydrated when they enter the MTF. Parenteral fluid supplements and vitamins are of benefit. Patients who have lost their eyesight because of mustard exposure should be reassured that they will recover their vision. Casualties who do become critically ill from their exposure to mustard present with large areas of burns, major pulmonary damage, and immunosuppression. Some may die from sepsis or from overwhelming damage to the airways and lungs.

There are no controlled human studies comparing different treatments for mustard exposure; nor have uniform standards of care been developed. However, suggestions for the care required for each organ system is described in the section below. Recommendations for skin care are based on research and experience with thermal burns. Most casualties have more than one system involved, and many of these casualties will be dehydrated and have other injuries as well.

Skin

Current treatments. Significant cutaneous HD injuries can take several months to heal, necessitate lengthy hospitalizations, and result in significant cosmetic and/or functional deficits. There are currently no standardized or optimized methods of casualty management and no specific US Food and Drug Administration (FDA) approved treatment regimens for HD injury. Historically, blister aspiration and/or unroofing (epidermal removal), physical debridement, irrigation, topical antibiotics, and sterile dressings have been the main courses of action in the medical management of cutaneous HD injuries.[106–110] Current treatment strategy consists of symptomatic management and is designed to relieve symptoms, prevent infection, and promote healing.

Decisions regarding appropriate treatment methods must consider the number of casualties involved and the exposure setting. The management of a small number of workers exposed to liquid HD in a laboratory setting or while handling munitions would be different from the treatment of hundreds of soldiers with vapor exposure in a far-forward environment. Before commencement of any treatment, patient clothing should be carefully removed and treated as potentially contaminated, and the patient thoroughly decontaminated. For a general overview of decontamination procedures, see Chapter 16, Decontaminationof Chemical Casualites.

Skin injury from HD can be considered a chemical burn. Within military medical facilities, chemical burn injuries would meet the criteria established by the American Burn Association for referral to a burn center.[111] The similarity between HD skin injury and toxic epidermal necrosis (TEN), and between HD lung injury and smoke inhalation injury further support burn center referral, where the requisite expertise to treat these conditions is available. Within the military medical system, the designated center for the treatment of major HD burns and other chemical burn injuries is the US Army Institute of Surgical Research/Army Burn Center located at Brooke Army Medical Center in San Antonio, Texas.[112] In the civilian sector, there are 132 burn centers located in the United States. Locations and contact information for these centers is available through the American Burn Association at 1-800-548-BURN or online at www.ameriburn.org.

The appearance of a superficial to moderate HD skin injury mimics that of a first- or second-degree burn, and the appearance of a deep HD injury resulting from direct liquid contact or secondary infection mimics that of a full thickness or third-degree burn. On this basis, many burn care practitioners erroneously conclude that thermal and HD injuries are the same. However, direct comparisons in the literature between HD and thermal burns are scarce. Papirmeister et al noted that disintegration of the basal cell layer caused by thermal burns has been shown to produce an intraepidermal blister that contains fragments of the basal cell layer attached to the basal lamina, unlike the almost totally denuded basement membrane in HD lesions.[31] Also, mustard injuries take considerably longer to heal compared to similar-sized thermal or chemical burns. A major argument against the adage "a burn is a burn" is that HD initially targets a specific cell type (epithelial basal cells), unlike a thermal burn, in which damage occurs first at the stratum corneum and then progresses downward.

Since the stratum corneum is the structure largely responsible for barrier function, water loss rates are very high immediately after a thermal burn (140–180 $g/m^2/h$ in humans).[113] After a cutaneous HD injury, the stratum corneum remains intact for 2 to 3 days, after which barrier function becomes compromised by loss of sloughing epidermis or unroofing of the blister. Thus, the systemic fluid derangements and nutritional requirements seen in cutaneous HD injury are less than is seen with thermal burns.[17] The recommended infusion rates and formulas (Parkland, Modified Brooke) used to calculate total volume requirements for thermal burn patients, based on body weight and total body surface area (TBSA) will overestimate fluid needs of HD casualties and should not be routinely applied in HD casualty management.[114] Iatrogenic hypervolemia and pulmonary edema documented in HD casualties during the Iran-Iraq War showed that fluid requirements appear to have been relatively independent of TBSA.[17,108] Fluids and electrolytes should be closely monitored for HD casualties because fluids may be lost to edematous areas, with resultant dehydration. The exact fluid replacement requirements for cutaneous HD injuries should be based on individual patient hemodynamic status and electrolyte balance. Monitoring of heart rate and urine output are simple and reliable field guides to the adequacy of resuscitation. In hospitalized patients, serum sodium levels also accurately reflect water status. The fluids used in replacement fluid therapy for non-HD burns, which would likely be appropriate for use in HD injuries if fluid replacement is required, are described by Settle, Brisebois, and Thomas et al.[114–116] The requirements of casualties with both HD exposure and multiple traumatic injury will likely follow the resuscitation requirements of the associated traumatic injury.

In some respects, superficial to moderate HD injuries exhibit similarities to exfoliative diseases such as TEN. Although the nomenclature of exfoliative diseases is both controversial and confusing to the nonspecialist, the term TEN type II can be used (on basis of biopsy) to include classic TEN, Lyell disease, erythema multiforme majus or exudativum, acute disseminated epidermal necrosis, and Stevens-Johnson syndrome.[117–119] Both HD injury and TEN type II patients have skin lesions with a cleavage plane at the dermal-epidermal junction; a decrease in white blood cell count which may become life-threatening; involvement of mucosal surfaces (gastrointestinal and trachea); and intravenous fluid needs greater than maintenance but less than expected for a correspondingly sized thermal burn. There is ample evidence in both the burn and dermatology literature that mortality decreases and outcomes improve when patients with TEN are managed in a burn center.[117, 119–124] Given the similarities between TEN and HD injury, burn center referral, when available, is advocated.

HD casualties should be kept comfortable and their lesions regularly cleansed to prevent infection. Limbs may need to be immobilized, because movement of joints can aggravate existing lesions. Blisters arising on the trunk require protective dressings to avoid or minimize damage from friction with clothing or bedding.

Current treatment of cutaneous HD injury depends upon the level and extent of skin involvement. The earliest and most superficial manifestation is erythema, which usually has an onset of 4 to 8 hours (range 1–24 h) after exposure. The erythema has the appearance of a sunburn and is usually accompanied by pruritis, burning, or stinging. This level of injury may or may not progress to vesicle formation. If blisters or vesicles do not form and the skin remains intact, management consists of protecting the skin from further damage, and the application of antipruritic creams or lotions (calamine lotion, 0.25% camphor, menthol). Systemic analgesics and antipruritics may be indicated, depending on the discomfort level of the patient. There is some evidence that topical steroid creams may prevent progression or speed healing of superficial injury. Topical steroids should not be applied to open wounds, vesicles, or large body surfaces. Resolution of erythema generally requires several days.

Deeper or more prolonged exposure results in vesicle formation, which typically begins 2 to 18 hours after vapor exposure and continues for several days. The vesicles may start as a "string of pearls" within or at the periphery of sites of erythema. Small vesicles may coalesce to form bulla or blisters, typically 0.5 to 5 cm in diameter. The fluid contained in vesicles or blisters does not contain active agent, does not cause further vesication, and does not pose any hazard to health care providers beyond that of normal body fluids. Blisters less than 1 cm in diameter should be left intact. The area surrounding the blister should be irrigated at least once per day, followed by application of a topical antibiotic. A petrolatum gauze bandage can be put in place over these unbroken blisters, if desired. Any such dressings should be changed every 3 to 4 days.

There is no consensus on whether larger, intact blisters should be unroofed. Blister fluid from intact blisters provides a sterile wound covering, but the blisters are fragile and easily ruptured. For this reason, military medical manuals generally recommend that blisters greater than 1 cm in diameter be unroofed or debrided, irrigating the underlying area two to four times per day with saline, sterile water, clean soapy water, or Dakin solution.[125–127] For patients presenting with intact frank blisters, it may be beneficial to aspirate the blister fluid with a sterile needle and syringe, allowing the roof of the blister to act as a sterile dressing until a physician can remove it. Blister roofs have been reattached via epidermal grafting using the tops of suction blisters in the treatment of vitiligo, as well as in experimental suction blisters in humans following aspiration of blister fluid.[128–130] (A suction blister is iatrogenically induced by applying suction to the skin to separate the epidermis from the dermis for the purpose of harvesting the epidermis for autotransplantation.) The roofs of HD blisters, however, are not expected to reattach to the blister floor because of HD-induced damage to basal cells and basement membrane zone (BMZ) components. Sloughing will eventually occur. Weak attachment of the neoepidermis to the underlying dermis (fragile skin) has been noted in human HD casualties and experimentally exposed weanling pigs.[131] Once the lesions have fully reepithelialized, protective dressings may initially be needed to avoid or minimize damage from friction with clothing or bedding.

For patients presenting with ruptured HD-induced blisters, careful removal of the blister roof with scissors, application of an antibiotic ointment, and placement of a sterile dressing is warranted. For both of these scenarios, more complete debridement is necessary for large lesions.

In hospital settings, vesicles that have coalesced or become confluent, as well as larger intact blisters can be unroofed and cleansed by gently rubbing the affected areas with a saline soaked course mesh gauze or laparotomy pad under general anesthesia or conscious sedation. Alternately, sharp scissor debridement can be carried out. In field settings, sharp debridement may be more practical. Following debridement or unroofing, the wounds will require protection from infection and desiccation. Options include various topical antimicrobials, or the use of biologic or synthetic dressings.

Intact vesicles or blisters that are debrided in clean hospital settings may benefit from the application of biologic dressings, such as porcine heterograft (pigskin); collagen-laminated nylon dressings such as Biobrane (Dow Hickam Pharmaceuticals Inc, Sugar Land, Tex); or silver-containing dressings such as Acticoat (Smith and Nephew, Largo, Fla); Silverlon (Argentum, Lakemont, Ga); or Silvasorb (Medline Industries, Mundelein Ill).[131–137] These dressings create a moist healing environment, decrease pain, and obviate the need for daily dressing changes. Biobrane has the added advantage of flexibility, facilitating movement. If adherent, pigskin and Biobrane may be left in place until reepithelialization occurs. Silver-containing dressings need to be changed every few days, following manufacturers' recommendations. Biologic, synthetic, or silver dressings that are not adhered to the wound bed should be promptly removed, followed by wound cleansing and application of an appropriate topical antibiotic. Fluid could build up underneath dressings that do not remain in complete contact with the wound bed, resulting in masceration. Dressings should also be removed if infection or cellulitis develops. Field application of these dressings is usually impractical because the appropriate level of cleanliness cannot be maintained.

Wounds that are not freshly debrided, are dirty or contaminated, or contain blisters already broken should be unroofed or debrided and cleansed with soap and water or appropriate surgical detergents, such as chlorhexidine gluconate solution. Extrapolating from burn experience, iodine-containing surgical detergents or prep solutions have poor coverage against *Pseudomonas* species and should be avoided. Following cleansing, the area should be liberally covered with a topical antibiotic (eg, 1% silver sulfadiazine cream, aqueous 5% mafenide acetate solution, Dakin solution, 0.5% silver nitrate solution, bacitracin antibiotic ointment, or Neosporin ointment [Pfizer Inc, New York, NY]), and a sterile dressing should then be applied. Biologic or synthetic dressings should not be used in this setting. The choice of antibiotic is largely a matter of personal experience and hospital or battlefield availability, for there is little scientific data in actual HD injuries to strongly advocate one agent over another. The use of bacitracin and Neosporin ointments should be limited to small wounds (less than 1% TBSA) and employed for very brief periods (3–5 days) because of their high capacity to provoke allergic cutaneous reactions.[138] Bacitracin is only effective against Gram-positive bacteria, but Neosporin has a broader antimicrobial spectrum. The use of 11.1% mafenide acetate cream should be avoided because of the severe pain it causes when applied to partial-thickness wounds and the possibility of metabolic acidosis. Mafenide acetate cream would be appropriate over insensate full thickness injuries caused by liquid HD exposure; over superficial (partial thickness) injuries that become infected and convert to full thickness; or over wounds that are visibly infected (see below). Following application of any topical antibiotic, a sterile dressing should be put in place.

Several antimicrobials are available in liquid form, facilitating wound debridement and inspection. These include 0.5% silver nitrate solution, Dakin solution (0.25%–0.5% sodium hypochlorite), and 5% mafenide acetate solution.[140] Silver nitrate 0.5% solution is inexpensive, readily available, and has bacteriostatic coverage against a broad spectrum of Gram-positive and Gram-negative bacteria and yeast-like organisms. Silver nitrate solution is a primary topical therapy for toxic epidermal necrosis; silver sulfadiazene is a poor choice because sulfa drugs are often the inciting agent. Silver nitrate solution does not penetrate deep wounds and works best on minimally colonized, debrided, or superficial injury.[139] It has the disadvantages of staining instruments, clothing, and bed linens and causes hypochloremia, hypocalcemia, and hyponatremia with prolonged use. Dakin solution is likewise inexpensive and readily available, with bacteriocidal activity against a broad spectrum of Gram-positive and Gram-negative organisms.[139] Dakin solution must be freshly compounded to be effective. Aqueous mafenide 5% solution (acetate or hydrochloride) is bacteriostatic against a broad spectrum of Gram-positive and Gram-negative bacteria and has strong coverage against pathogens commonly encountered in gunshot wounds, blast injuries, open fractures, necrotizing fascitis, and Fournier gangrene.[140,141] The drug is particularly active against *Pseudomonas* and *Clostridia* species.[142] The acetate salt is commercially available as Sulfamylon (Bertek Pharmaceuticals, Morgantown, WV). An isoosmolar solution is produced by 50 g of powder mixed in 1 L of sterile water; if mixed in sterile saline, the solution is hyperosmolar and painful on application. Mendelson points out that aqueous mafenide is an excellent battlefield or mass casualty drug, because 5 lb of powder mixed with local water sources can supply sufficient solution to provide a patient with a 50% TBSA burn with 455 dressing changes of 10% solution or 910 dressing changes of a 5% solution.[140,143] In austere conditions, where gloves and dressing supplies are unavailable, 5% or 10% mafenide solution has been applied with spray bottles to wounds that are then left uncovered.[140,144,145]

Deep skin injury may be produced by exposure to liquid HD, causing coagulation necrosis. Delayed treatment may allow progression of superficial injury to deeper levels. Concurrent trauma or wound contamination may predispose the wound to infection. Infection complicating superficial HD wounds may convert a partial thickness injury to full thickness. Deep HD skin injuries should be washed twice daily with a surgical detergent (chlorhexidine gluconate solution), rinsed with saline or water, and covered with silver sulfadiazine cream followed by protective gauze dressings. Wounds that are obviously full thickness benefit from "alternating agents," application of 11% mafenide acetate cream during the day followed by application of silver sulfadiazine cream at night. The combination of these agents provides a broader antimicrobial spectrum, limits emergence of resistant organisms, and has fewer side effects (neutropenia and metabolic acidosis) than when either agent is used alone.[139] Mafenide acetate cream alone may be applied twice daily on wounds that are very deep, heavily contaminated, or infected. Mafenide acetate cream has the best eschar penetration of any topical agent; it is useful in situations where injuries are deep and battlefield conditions preclude proper wound debridement or excision. Full thickness or infected injuries will also require surgical debridement or excision. Following excision, split-thickness autografting will shorten wound healing time.

Wounds should be inspected periodically for signs of infection. The risk of secondary infection of HD wounds is at least as high as in thermal injury. Infection is a significant factor in causing delayed healing of cutaneous HD injuries, although even uninfected HD burns exhibit delayed wound healing. Infected wounds require surgical debridement or excision. Any biologic or synthetic dressings should be removed when cellulitis is present, the wounds should be debrided of any nonviable tissue, and penicillin should be administered orally. Intravenous antibiotics may be indicated for cellulitis that does not respond to oral antibiotics. There is no indication for the routine administration of systemic antibiotics to patients with HD injury.

The decision to evacuate and hospitalize an HD casualty is based upon the magnitude and type of exposure (vapor versus liquid); systemic, ocular, and pulmonary manifestations; and the extent and severity of skin lesions, in consideration with other injuries that may be present (eg, respiratory, ocular). For patients experiencing only cutaneous HD injuries, erythema covering more than 5% of TBSA in noncritical areas requires hospitalization. Erythema covering less than 5% TBSA may require hospitalization, depending upon the site of the injury (eg, face, inguinal area) and level of impairment (eg, limitation of limb movement due to pain, edema). Multiple or large areas of vesication also require hospitalization. Since blister formation may initially be slight, the patient should be watched for a progression in the size and number of blisters. Topical antibacterial creams such as silver sulfadiazine can be prescribed to patients who do not require close medical monitoring, with instructions to apply a thin layer to the affected area twice, four times a day. Following application of the cream, the area should be covered with a loose gauze dressing such as a petrolatum gauze bandage.

Development of improved therapies. Treatment strategies for improved and rapid healing of cutaneous HD injuries recently formulated by a working group of US and UK researchers and physicians are summarized below.[138] Research is underway to experimentally support these strategies and determine which medical devices, supplies, and pharmaceuticals are most efficacious. The ultimate goal is to determine the most efficacious treatment regimen to be applied in the clinical management of HD casualties. The ideal regimen should return damaged skin to optimal appearance and normal function in the shortest time. Improved treatment will result in a better cosmetic and functional outcome for patients and enable them to return to normal activities sooner.

Immediate treatment. For those patients who are

beginning to present with erythema or those who are in the latent period and suspect an exposure may have occurred, systemic administration of an antiinflammatory agent will likely help decrease the amount of damage ultimately induced. HD-induced inflammatory responses themselves likely contribute to the severity of the pathology, and numerous animal studies have shown the benefits of prophylactic or therapeutic use of antiinflammatory agents.[32,146–148] It remains to be determined which nonsteroidal antiinflammatory drug (NSAID) or combination of drugs, route of administration, length of administration, and dosing regimen is the most efficacious in preventing or ameliorating the effects of HD on skin. It is likely that an NSAID will need to be administered for 2 to 5 days. Topically delivered intracellular scavengers such as 4-methyl-2-mercaptopyridine-1-oxide and dimercaprol have proven effective in animal experiments in reducing the severity of HD-induced cutaneous injuries, and concurrent use of one of these agents with an NSAID may yield the best results.[49,148] Corticosteroid antiinflammatory agents, such as hydrocortisone (given systemically or topically for cutaneous HD injuries) and dexamethasone (tested in vitro on primary alveolar macrophages and given topically for ocular HD injuries), also appear to be promising therapeutic agents.[147–150] Other topical, steroidal, antiinflammatory agents of much greater potency that would likely be very efficacious if used early in the lesion development stage, such as betamethasone dipropionate, clobetasol propionate, and diflorasone diacetate. Superpotent (class 1), potent (class 2) and upper midstrength (class 3) topical corticosteroids should be tested for their efficacy in ameliorating HD-induced cutaneous injury.

Depletion of GSH and accumulation of endogenous oxidants and ultimate formation of potent oxidizing species (eg, toxic lipid peroxides) may be contributory factors in HD-induced cytotoxicity.[31] Topically applied HD has been shown to negatively affect antioxidant enzymes in blood cells and body tissues of rats.[151] Several antioxidants have been shown to protect liver and lung from oxidative damage following inhalation or percutaneous exposure to HD in a mouse model.[152] It has been suggested that administration of antioxidants may be protective and useful.[153] Thus, initial antioxidant treatment aimed at affecting the progression of lesions that is instituted during the erythema phase may prove to be of benefit. The effectiveness and role of the interruption of the inflammatory cascade by the inclusion of topical and systemic antioxidant agents as well as a determination of the optimal timing for such therapy are important and intriguing avenues for investigation.[138]

Placement of an occlusive or semiocclusive dressing will likely prove helpful in promoting autolytic debridement and preventing desiccation. Debridement plays a central role in improving the healing of cutaneous HD lesions, and beginning the process early may be beneficial. How soon following exposure these dressings can be applied remains to be determined. Although maintaining a moist environment has long been known to facilitate wound healing, caution needs to be observed because very early occlusion that increases moisture levels in the skin will exacerbate the lesion.[154–157] Additionally, there is a period following exposure to sulfur mustard during which off-gassing of unbound HD occurs in weanling pigs and African green monkeys.[131,158] These studies have suggested that off-gassing after a large exposure can continue for 24 to 36 hours. Limiting the escape of this unbound HD by occlusive dressings may worsen the lesion, so delayed placement of occlusive dressings for at least 24 hours following exposure should be considered. Keeping clothing off of the exposed area to prevent vapor build-up may also be of benefit.

Injury assessment. Before HD injuries can be appropriately treated, assessment of the injuries must occur. TBSA of the injuries should be established and depth of injury determined. TBSA can be determined using Wallace's rule of nines and the Lund and Browder chart for estimating burn severity.[159,160] Determination of injury depth is a more challenging task; however, accurate depth assessment is important because it dictates how aggressive treatment must be to minimize or prevent cosmetic and functional deficits.

In thermal burns, depth of injury is typically assessed by physical examination, with a goal of wound healing by day 14. Surface appearance, assessment of intact sensation, the pinprick test to assess pain, the blanch-capillary return test to evaluate microcirculation, and surface temperature difference between burned and unburned skin are often utilized.[161] Using these methods, diagnosing very superficial burns (which will heal nonoperatively) and very deep burns (which will require immediate excision and grafting) is relatively easy for the experienced burn surgeon. Burns of intermediate depth are more often problematic. At present, no technology reliably predicts which intermediate-depth burns will require grafting and which will heal nonoperatively, a decision best left to the experienced burn surgeon. Determining depth of HD injuries is even more challenging. First, the full extent of cutaneous injury can take several days to manifest. Secondly, superficial appearances do not accurately predict depth of injury nor need for grafting. The presence of blisters in thermal burns is generally associated with superficial dermal injuries, but blistering in HD injuries can occur in deep dermal/full-thickness injuries because of the unique nature of the agent and the unique progression of the injury.

Noninvasively examining cutaneous blood flow can greatly assist the physician in making depth of injury determinations. Laser Doppler perfusion imaging (LDPI) and indocyanine green (ICG) fluorescence imaging may prove to be very valuable tools in prognosticating optimal wound healing of cutaneous HD injuries.[138]

Laser Doppler flowmetry and LDPI have been used for prolonged, noninvasive monitoring of tissue viability and wound healing, and for the assessment of peripheral vascular disease, inflammation, ischemia, reperfusion, skin graft acceptance (take), and burn depth. Brown et al found that laser Doppler perfusion images of vesicant vapor burns on the backs of swine correlated well with histopathological findings (thrombosis and necrosis of subepidermal capillaries) between 1 hour and 7 days postexposure and suggested that clinical management decision making on how to treat early vesicant burns could be aided by LDPI.[162] Chilcott et al used several noninvasive bioengineering methods to monitor wound healing in a large white pig model for 7 days following exposure to HD and lewisite vapors.[163] They found LDPI to be a promising prognostic tool.

ICG fluorescence imaging is a minimally invasive procedure that requires the placement of an intravenous line. The fluorescence of intravenous ICG has been shown to estimate burn depth in small animals.[164] In contrast to fluorescein fluorescence, ICG fluorescence is capable of distinguishing superficial and deep partial-thickness burns from full-thickness burns.[165] The fluorescence intensity of ICG decreases exponentially with burn depth for burns of similar age.[166] ICG fluorescence was successfully used to estimate burn depth in a porcine model.[167] An imaging system with a diagnostic algorithm was developed at the Wellman Laboratories of Photomedicine (Boston, Mass); the system accurately diagnosed burns that healed within 21 days with minimal scarring from those that took longer to heal by secondary means. The algorithm was shown to be dependent on the age of the burn and independent of the location of the burn. This technology showed promise in plastic surgical applications and accurate determination of thermal burn depth in humans.[168–170] ICG fluorescence imaging also shows promise in diagnosing depth of HD injury.[171] Unlike LDPI, multiple images over large areas can be captured in a relatively short period of time. Images are typically collected 5 to 10 minutes after ICG injection to allow uptake and distribution. The dye is then excited (eg, 780 nm), and the resultant fluorescence emission (eg, 810 nm) immediately captured and saved by a computer and analyzed for burn/normal skin fluorescence ratio. ICG binds strongly to plasma globulins, limiting both extravasation within burn-injured vascular epithelia and extravascular transport to areas nearby.[166] Large signals are thought to be the result of vasodilation and hyperemia, and smaller signals are thought to be attributable to vascular occlusion and edema.[164,166]

Treatment of deep injuries. Previous animal studies have shown that surgically aggressive approaches are needed to prevent or minimize significant cosmetic and functional deficits that result from deep HD injury. For the best outcome, deep dermal/full-thickness cutaneous HD injuries require full-thickness debridement followed by autologous split-thickness skin grafting.[172,173] To be successful, the skin grafts must be placed on a hemostatically secure wound bed, devoid of blood clots, debris, or necrotic tissue. The recipient bed must have an adequate blood supply to nourish the skin grafts, and the grafts must be protected from shearing forces, motion, and mechanical disruption. A variety of modalities are available for achieving initial graft adherence and subsequent acceptance ("take"). These include sutures, surgical staples, fibrin glue, tie-over bolsters, compression dressings, and a variety of antishear dressing techniques. The choice of fixation and dressing technique is determined by the size and location of the wounds, and the experience and preferences of the surgeon.[138]

In thermal burn management, deep burns are grafted to promote timely wound closure and improve outcome with minimal cosmetic and functional deficits. The decision to graft is based upon depth of injury, and deep HD injuries will require surgically aggressive approaches. As with thermal burns, depth of HD injury should be accurately assessed before treatment begins. Reported long-term effects such as fragile skin and scarring likely indicate that injury depth was not accurately diagnosed and treatment was not sufficiently aggressive.

Treatment of partial-thickness injuries. Epidermal and superficial dermal HD injuries may have greater clinical relevance on the battlefield than deep injuries. Partial thickness injuries need debridement, but not grafting. The standard treatment, after assessing the injury and deroofing frank blisters, is to perform adequate debridement of partial-thickness injuries, then treat the lesions like chronic cutaneous ulcers or partial-thickness thermal burns using contemporary medical approaches. Debridement is followed by one or more treatment adjuncts. Examples of adjuncts under consideration are dressings, growth factors, skin substitutes, and Vacuum-Assisted Closure (VAC) Therapy (KCI, San Antonio, Tex).

Debridement. Experimental approaches to vesicant

wound debridement have included powered dermabrasion, sharp surgical excision, laser debridement, and enzymatic debridement.[172–180] Powered dermabrasion has been shown to speed up the reepithelialization process of cutaneous HD injuries. Kjellstrom et al found sharp surgical excision with primary suturing of the skin defect to be effective in decreasing healing time of HD vapor lesions in guinea pigs.[174, 175,177] Powered dermabrasion, pulsed CO_2 laser ablation and erbium: yttrium-aluminium-garnet (Er:YAG) laser ablation have been shown to accelerate the rate of healing of full-thickness cutaneous lewisite vapor burns in swine without the need for split-thickness skin grafting.[176,178] Eldad et al found that excimer laser ablation and Debridase (Biotechnology General Ltd, Kiryat Malchi, Israel) enzymatic debridement were efficacious in improving the healing of partial-thickness nitrogen mustard burns in a guinea pig model.[179]

Laser debridement of cutaneous vesicant wounds has proven to be an effective method of improving the rate of wound healing in pig models. Graham et al showed that viability, thickness, and organization of the epidermis were all significantly improved by partial-thickness pulsed CO_2 laser debridement of small, mild to moderately severe cutaneous HD vapor injuries.[180] Laser debridement followed by skin grafting was as efficacious in improving the wound healing of deep HD burns as sharp surgical tangential excision followed by grafting (the "gold standard" in human deep dermal/full-thickness thermal burns medicine).[172,173] Middermal debridement by sharp excision or laser ablation without grafting produced less desirable results but was better than no treatment.[172,173] A 4-fold improvement in reepithelialization of lewisite injuries was achieved at 1 week following laser dermabrasion, with almost 100% reepithelialization by 3 weeks.[178] It is not apparent why these full-thickness lewisite injuries (10 cm^2) did not require grafting, as did HD injuries (12.6 cm^2) or as would a full-thickness thermal burn.[172,173] There are differences in biochemical action and rates of spontaneous reepithelialization between lewisite and HD.[178] Further studies must be conducted to fully examine the comparative healing of deep lewisite, HD, and thermal injuries.

Laser debridement offers additional benefits, including hemostatic control during surgery, minimal risk of exposure to aerosolized pathogens, and time efficiency. Another major advantage to the use of lasers is the ability to control the amount of normal perilesional skin that is removed. Eldad et al noted that controlling the amount of tissue removed by surgical tangential excision is technically difficult, and laser ablation of nitrogen mustard burns in a guinea pig model enabled control of the amount of tissue removed with minimal blood loss.[179] Minimizing the amount of tissue removed is a cosmetic benefit to the patient.

A number of lasers manufactured in the United States, Canada, and Europe may be considered for routine debridement of vesicant injuries. Acland and Barlow have reviewed the current uses of lasers in dermatological practice and list the types of lasers used for specific procedures.[181] They list CO_2 and Er: YAG lasers as the most appropriate for cutaneous resurfacing. Er:YAG lasers have been used for a wide variety of procedures, ranging from facial resurfacing to burn debridement.[181–185] They have been shown to be particularly useful in the debridement of partial-thickness burns and the management of deep lewisite injuries.[179,186] Unlike the Gaussian beam profiles created by CO_2 lasers, Er:YAG laser beams tend to be uniform and produce uniform depths of ablation.[185] (These techniques require trained and skilled personnel taking all necessary precautions including eye protection.)

Another alternative under consideration for debridement of HD injuries is enzymatic debridement. The enzymes, categorized as proteolytics, fibrinolytics, and collagenases, are designed to dissolve necrotic tissue from wounds, and they are often used to debride chronic wounds (eg, decubitus ulcers, venous stasis ulcers, arterial insufficiency ulcers, diabetic foot ulcers).[186] Many have been found to be safe and effective in removing devitalized tissue and accelerating healing in burns.[187–194] Any burn eschar present is typically surgically cross-hatched to allow the agent to penetrate into the wound. Other agents, such as the bacterial proteolytic enzymes streptokinase and streptodornase, have given disappointing results in deep burns because they do not break down the collagen that separates vital from nonvital tissue.[195] Use of fibrinolytics may impair wound healing of HD lesions, because fibrin is an early matrix protein essential for wound healing. Fibrinolysin is typically combined with deoxyribonuclease, and this combination also digests DNA in the dividing fibroblasts that play a role in healing.[186] Some effective enzymes have produced better results than others, with enzyme concentration, skin moisture level, and the presence of certain antibacterial agents affecting results. Secondary dressings are needed to keep the wound moist and to allow these agents to work.[186] Klasen offers an excellent review of the use of enzymatic debridement agents in burns.[195] The most popular and effective agents on the market today are collagenases and papain/urea combinations. A promising proteolytic enzyme extracted from the stem of the pineapple plant is in US and European clinical trials for the treatment of deep partial- and full-thickness burns. Enzymatic debridement of HD injuries is a promising and cheaper alternative to laser debridement, albeit more time consuming. However, burn wound sepsis and bacteremias have been noted in burn patients undergoing enzymatic debridement.[186,195] Concomitant use of a topical antibiotic that does not interfere with the action of the enzyme under study may be warranted as a preventative measure. Research is underway for determining which enzymatic debridement product is most efficacious in debriding partial-thickness HD injuries.

In addition to vesication and death of epidermal keratinocytes, HD exposure results in sublethal damage to keratinocytes along the periphery of the gross lesion. Damage to the BMZ and underlying collagen in the papillary dermis has also been noted. Unroofing frank blisters followed by timely removal of this adjacent and subjacent damage will likely improve the rate of reepithelialization. Nonlethal damage is clearly noted at the periphery of cutaneous HD lesions and has been reported previously.[196–198] Nikolsky sign, characterized by separation and loss of the epidermis from the dermis when the skin is pressed with a sliding or twisting motion, has been demonstrated in weanling pig skin following HD vapor exposure.[196,198,199] Nikolsky sign is also a clinical hallmark of TEN, reinforcing the similarity between this disease and HD injury.[117] These weakened areas of the dermal-epidermal junction occur along the periphery of gross lesions and are indicative of sublethally damaged basal cells and/or altered proteins of extracellular matrices of the BMZ. Sublethally injured cells at the periphery of an HD lesion and in hair follicles and other adnexal structures may be partly responsible for the slow rate of reepithelialization seen in these injuries. Rice et al suggested that the level of damage to cellular DNA at the margins of HD lesions may be sufficient to delay or prevent effective replication of those keratinocytes.[175] Removal of these sublethally damaged keratinocytes at the margins of the lesions by debridement beyond the visible borders of the lesion will likely speed up the reepithelialization process.

HD induces damage to the BMZ at the level of the lamina lucida.[200,201] The floor of the blister retains portions of the damaged BMZ and needs to be removed to provide an adequate scaffold over which keratinocytes feeding the reepithelialization process can migrate. Thus, at minimum, debridement needs to proceed down into the papillary dermis after removal of the blister roof. Beyond the BMZ, dermal collagen itself is affected by HD exposure and can impede the wound healing process.[175,202,203] Brown and Rice reported coagulation and hypereosinophilia of the papillary dermis in Yucatan minipig skin 12 to 24 hours following saturated HD vapor exposure, with the deeper reticular dermis unaffected.[203] Rice et al[175] and Lindsay and Rice[202] suggested that following exposure to HD, papillary dermal collagen is altered and may no longer function normally as a healthy scaffold over which epidermal cells can migrate.

The question of how deep to debride must be addressed. Ablative lasers that create less than 160 ± 60 µm of residual thermal damage permit optimal skin graft take and healing.[204] Domankevitz and Nishioka concluded that lasers that induce residual thermal damage zones of less than 200 µm are useful for cutaneous surgery and burn wound debridement prior to skin grafting.[205] Lam et al were able to improve wound healing of full-thickness cutaneous lewisite injuries in pigs by partial-thickness laser debridement.[178] Graham et al were also able to improve wound healing of deep cutaneous HD injuries in pigs by partial-thickness debridement without grafting, albeit not to the extent attained by full-thickness debridement followed by grafting.[172] These studies indicate that retaining some amount of damaged dermal tissue does not significantly impede wound healing. Complete debridement of partial-thickness injury, therefore, will likely not be required. Debridement of partial-thickness HD injury into the papillary dermis or upper reticular dermis will likely be adequate.

Dressings. Following wound debridement of HD injuries, an appropriate dressing will be needed to promote moist wound healing. Beneficial effects of such dressings include prevention of tissue dehydration and cell death, accelerating angiogenesis, increased breakdown of dead tissue and fibrin (eg, pericapillary fibrin cuffs), significant reduction in pain, and potentiation of growth factor and target cell interaction.[157] Helfman et al[154] and Singhal et al[186] have provided overviews of various types of occlusive and semiocclusive dressings. Hydrocolloids, hydrogels, foam dressings, alginates, and transparent film dressings are commercially available from a large number of manufacturers. Silver impregnated dressing materials may be of great potential benefit in treating these wounds because of their antimicrobial efficacy and demonstrated ability to enhance rates of reepithelialization.[132,206–209] A number of these dressing materials are currently employed in burn and chronic wound care; other more advanced silver dressings are in various stages of development. Application of silver impregnated dressings following Er:YAG laser debridement has shown great promise in improving HD wound healing in a weanling pig model.[131]

Growth factors. During cutaneous wound healing, growth factors play dominant roles in regulating cell proliferation, differentiation, and synthesis of the extracellular matrix.[210] Epidermal growth factor, transforming growth factor-beta, platelet-derived growth factor, insulin-like growth factor, keratinocyte growth factor, hepatocyte growth factor, granulocyte-macrophage colony-stimulating factor, and fibroblast growth factors play important and critical roles in the healing of cutaneous wounds.

Platelet-derived growth factor and keratinocyte growth factor have been shown to improve the healing of burns and skin grafted lesions.[211–213] A recombinant human platelet-derived growth factor BB has been approved for human use by the FDA and is commercially available. Keratinocyte growth factor is in several ongoing US clinical trials to test its ability to prevent mucositis in patients undergoing chemotherapy with bone marrow transplantation, and for the treatment of venous ulcers and ulcerative colitis. These products may prove useful in improving the healing of cutaneous HD injuries. Concomitant use of protease inhibitors or a dressing designed to bind or inactivate matrix metalloproteases and protect growth factors (eg, Promogran Matrix Wound Dressing, Johnson and Johnson Wound Management Worldwide, Somerville, NJ) will likely be necessary until HD-induced inflammatory responses have subsided.

Skin substitutes. Skin substitutes may provide an excellent temporary wound dressing for debrided HD injuries. Permanent wound closure can only be achieved by spontaneous reepithelialization or by the provision of autologous skin by means of skin grafting. The use of skin substitutes to temporarily restore the multiple functions of normal skin may be of substantial benefit in the management of cutaneous HD injuries.[138]

The selection of the most suitable and effective temporary skin substitute will require a critical assessment of the products attributes when applied to HD wounds, as well as cost, ease of use, availability, and consistency of results.[138] Skin substitutes are widely used in human thermal burns management and can be (*a*) temporary or permanent, (*b*) epidermal, dermal, or composite, and (*c*) biologic or synthetic.[133,214–218] They have also been shown to be effective in reducing time to closure of chronic leg and foot ulcers, surgical excision sites, and partial-thickness donor sites. They may be a source of growth factors and are generally semiocclusive in nature. Generally flexible and pliable, skin substitutes can provide barrier function; add tensile strength to the wound; markedly reduce pain, inflammation, and drainage; and provide a moist wound healing environment. A number of skin substitutes are available on the market and should be tested for their efficacy in improving wound healing of cutaneous HD injuries. Several marketed products are currently under consideration: (*a*) living bilayered skin substitutes, (*b*) bilayered composites consisting of a synthetic epidermal analog and a biologic (collagen-based) dermal analog, (*c*) complex weaves of biopolymers that produce a thin protective membrane, and (*d*) acellular dermal matrices. Permanent skin substitute products that are designed for treating deep injuries and require application of a thin epithelial autograft will likely be inappropriate for use in treating partial-thickness HD injuries.

Cultured epithelial allografts and autografts have been used for about 2 decades as a treatment for chronic ulcers and thermal burns. Keratinocytes can be harvested from skin biopsies and grown to confluence by the method originally described by Rheinwald and Green.[219,220] Large amounts of stratifying epidermis can thus be grown in the laboratory in short periods of time and used to restore defects in the epidermis.[221] Such grafts can be used immediately or cryopreserved for use at a later date. In addition to their usefulness in improving the healing of deep ulcers and burns, these grafts have shown efficacy in improving the rate of reepithelialization of partial-thickness burns and split-thickness skin graft donor sites. Cultured keratinocyte allografts speed healing by providing cover and producing growth factors and extracellular matrix proteins.[222] Because these coverings can be produced in large quantities and would thus be more readily available than cadaver skin, their application in the treatment of debrided partial-thickness HD injuries should be considered. Cultured epidermal autografts (CEAs) would be safer to use from the perspective of disease transmission and would not require donor-screening procedures. They do, however, require lenticular surgical small-punch biopsies collected from the patient and a lag time of about 2 weeks to grow the graft material. Several US laboratories perform this service for their local burn centers. Commercially produced CEAs are also available. Durability has been increased by placing the CEA on a scaffolding of widely meshed autograft.[223] Alternatively, CEAs placed over deepithelialized allograft (ie, engrafted allodermis) have also proved successful.[224]

Finally, application of keratinocytes in suspension has been shown to improve epidermal wound healing in pig and mouse models.[225–228] Keratinocyte suspension technology does not require the length of time necessary to produce cultured epidermal sheets, and it has proven efficacious in treating thermal burns in humans.[229] After a small biopsy is collected, the cells are cultured and expanded in a clinical laboratory, then placed into a syringe-like spraying mechanism and sprayed onto the wound 2 to 5 days following biopsy. Products are commercially available for use in the treatment of partial- to full-thickness burns, donor sites, scars, chronic ulcers, and pigment loss, and for cosmetic skin rejuvenation following laser resurfacing, dermabrasion, and chemical peels. An innovative medical device currently available (ReCell, Clinical Cell Culture, Coral Springs, Fla) allows rapid harvesting of cells from a thin split-thickness biopsy followed by spray application onto small wounds (up to 2% TBSA) within 30 minutes of collecting the biopsy, without the need of culturing the keratinocytes in a clinical laboratory.

Vacuum-Assisted Closure Therapy. Application of topical negative pressure in the management of chronic wounds and burns has gained popularity in the last 5 years. Also known as VAC, the procedure involves placing an sterile open cell foam into the wound bed (cut to conform to the shape of the wound), sealing it with an adhesive drape, and applying subatmospheric pressure (125 mm Hg below ambient) that is transmitted via an evacuation tube by a vacuum pump.[230,231] The procedure is becoming widely used for the closure of chronic wounds such as stage III and IV pressure ulcers; venous, arterial, and neuropathic ulcers; and subacute and acute wounds such as dehisced incisions, split-thickness meshed skin grafts, and muscle flaps.[232,233] This methodology increases local blood perfusion and nutrient delivery to the wound, accelerates the rate of granulation tissue formation, and decreases wound tissue bacterial levels.[230,231] Before VAC application wounds must be debrided of all necrotic tissue. Contraindications to VAC placement include the presence of fistulas, osteomyelitis, exposed organs, exposed blood vessels or malignancy in or around the wound. The dressings are typically changed every 1 to 4 days until wound closure. VAC has been shown to be effective in preventing progression of partial-thickness burns to a deeper injury in a swine model, likely the result of increased delivery of oxygen and nutrients to the zone of stasis.[232] The method has also been shown to increase the rate of skin graft donor site reepithelialization in pigs and humans, and it is a safe and effective method for securing split-thickness skin grafts, providing improved graft survival.[233,234] Following debridement of partial-thickness HD injuries, VAC may prove efficacious in significantly speeding the reepithelialization process. Recently the FDA approved the use of VAC in treating partial-thickness burns. Several VAC systems are commercially available, including a lightweight, portable system for ambulatory care.

Eye

The basic principles of eye care are to prevent infection and scarring. Although mustard is unlikely to remain in the eye by the time the casualty is seen, the eye should be irrigated to remove any chemical agent that might be on the lashes and any inflammatory debris that might be on the surface of the eye. Mild lesions (eg, conjunctivitis) can be treated three to four times daily with a soothing eye solution.

Casualties with more severe eye lesions should be hospitalized. Care for these patients should consist of at least one daily irrigation, preferably more, to remove inflammatory debris; administration of a topical antibiotic three to four times daily; and administration of a topical mydriatic (atropine or homatropine) as needed to keep the pupil dilated to prevent later synechiae formation. Vaseline or a similar material should be applied to the lid edges to prevent them from adhering to each other; this reduces later scarring and also keeps a path open for possible infection to drain. When animals' eyes were kept tightly closed, a small infection could not drain, and a panophthalmitis developed that perforated and structurally destroyed the eyes.[66]

Topical analgesics may be used for the initial examination; however, they should rarely be used routinely because they can cause accidental corneal damage. Pain should be controlled with systemic analgesics. The benefit of topical steroids is not established in humans (see experimental animal data discussed below); however, most ophthalmologists feel that topical steroids may be helpful if used within the first 48 hours after exposure.[235] In any case, an ophthalmologist must be consulted as early as possible. Keeping the casualty in a dim room or providing sunglasses reduces discomfort from photophobia.

The transient loss of vision is usually the result of edema of the lids and other structures rather than corneal damage. Medical personnel should assure the patient that vision will return. Recovery may be within days for milder injuries, although those with severe damage will take approximately a month or longer to recover.

Airways

The therapeutic goal for mild airway symptoms (eg, irritation of the throat, nonproductive cough) is to keep the patient comfortable. In a casualty with severe problems, the goal is to maintain adequate oxygenation.

Hypoxia is secondary to abnormalities in ventilation caused by inflammatory bronchitis. Bronchial mucosal sloughing (pseudomembrane formation) further complicates this abnormality. Bronchospasm is easily triggered, requiring therapy with bronchodilators. Casualties with bronchospasm not responding to bronchodilators may benefit from steroid treatment, with careful attention to increased risk of infection. Oxygen supplementation may be necessary for prolonged periods. Ventilatory support may be necessary to assist oxygenation and adequate carbon dioxide clearance. The use of certain antibiotic skin creams (such as mafenide acetate) to treat skin lesions may complicate the acid–base status of the individual by inducing a metabolic acidosis.

Initially, bronchitis resulting from mustard exposure is nonbacterial. White blood cell elevation, fever, pulmonary infiltrates on chest radiograph, and colored sputum may all be present. Careful assessment of sputum by Gram stain and culture demonstrates that bacterial superinfection typically is not present during the first 3 to 4 days. Antibiotic therapy should be withheld until the identity of a specific organism becomes available. Of particular importance is the patient's immune status, which may be compromised by a progressive leukopenia beginning about day 4 or 5. The development of leukopenia signals severe immune system dysfunction; intensive medical support may become necessary for these patients. In these instances, sepsis typically becomes a complicating factor.

Casualties with evidence of deteriorating pulmonary status should be intubated early, before laryngeal spasm makes it difficult or impossible. Intubation assists in ventilation and also allows suction of necrotic and inflammatory debris. Bronchoscopy may be necessary to remove intact pseudomembranes or fragments of pseudomembranes (one of the Iranian casualties treated in western European hospitals during the Iran-Iraq War died of tracheal obstruction by a pseudomembrane, as did World War I casualties). Early use of positive end-expiratory pressure or continuous positive airway pressure may be beneficial. The need for continuous ventilatory support suggests a poor prognosis; of the Iranian casualties treated in European hospitals who required assisted ventilation, 87% died.[17]

An especially devastating pulmonary complication, severe and progressive stenosis of the tracheobronchial tree (Figure 8-14), developed in about 10% of the Iranian casualties treated in European hospitals. With the Iranian casualties, bronchoscopy was of value when used both for diagnosis and for therapeutic dilation.[236] (This complication was possibly not recognized in World War I mustard casualties because the degree of exposure required to cause severe tracheobronchial injury resulted in early death from pneumonia.)

Gastrointestinal Tract

Initial nausea and vomiting are rarely severe and can usually be relieved with atropine or common antiemetics. Prolonged vomiting and diarrhea beyond 24 hours are usually indicative of systemic toxicity requiring intensive care.

Bone Marrow

Suppression of hemopoietic elements cannot be predicted from the extent of skin lesions (eg, the lesions might be from vapor and therefore superficial, but significant amounts of mustard may have been absorbed through inhalation). Frequent counts of the formed blood elements must be performed on casualties with significant skin lesions or airway damage. Mustard destroys the precursor cells, and cell elements in the blood are depressed. Because white blood cells have the shortest life span, their numbers decrease first; red blood cells and thrombocytes soon follow. Typically, leukopenia begins at day 3 through day 5 after exposure, and reaches a nadir in 7 to 21 days. Leukopenia with a cell count lower than 200 cells/mm^3 usually signifies a poor prognosis, as does a rapid drop in the cell count; for example, from 30,000 to 15,000 cells/mm^3 in a day.[17,61]

Medical personnel should institute therapy with nonabsorbable antibiotics that sterilize the gut at the onset of leukopenia.[17] Cellular replacement may also be successful (see also the comments on granulocyte colony stimulating factor below).

Eye. Research at USAMRICD with rabbits exposed to sulfur mustard showed remarkable results using steroids and antibiotic eye combinations. In the study, the treatments were given both by injection and topically in the form of solutions and ointments. Eyes that would have been nearly destroyed appeared almost normal when these combinations were applied early and frequently. Based on this research, USAMRICD recommended that commercially available ophthalmologic steroid/antibiotic solutions or ointments be added to field medical sets. Recommended use is as soon as possible for even the mildest mustard eye injury. Frequency of use is every 1 to 2 hours until the full extent of the developing mustard injury becomes known. Treatment should then be modified accordingly, with consultation and examination by an ophthalmologist. This initial treatment would be applied only in the absence of a penetrating injury to the eye or in the case of obvious secondary bacterial infection. Eye pain can be severe enough to require narcotic analgesia.[237]

Lung. No specific antidotes for the mustard injury to the lung exist. However, a tremendous amount of supportive care is available for all pulmonary injuries. Mustard lung injuries in the trachea and bronchi have a high rate of secondary bacterial infection starting as early as 3 days and developing as late as 2 to 3 weeks

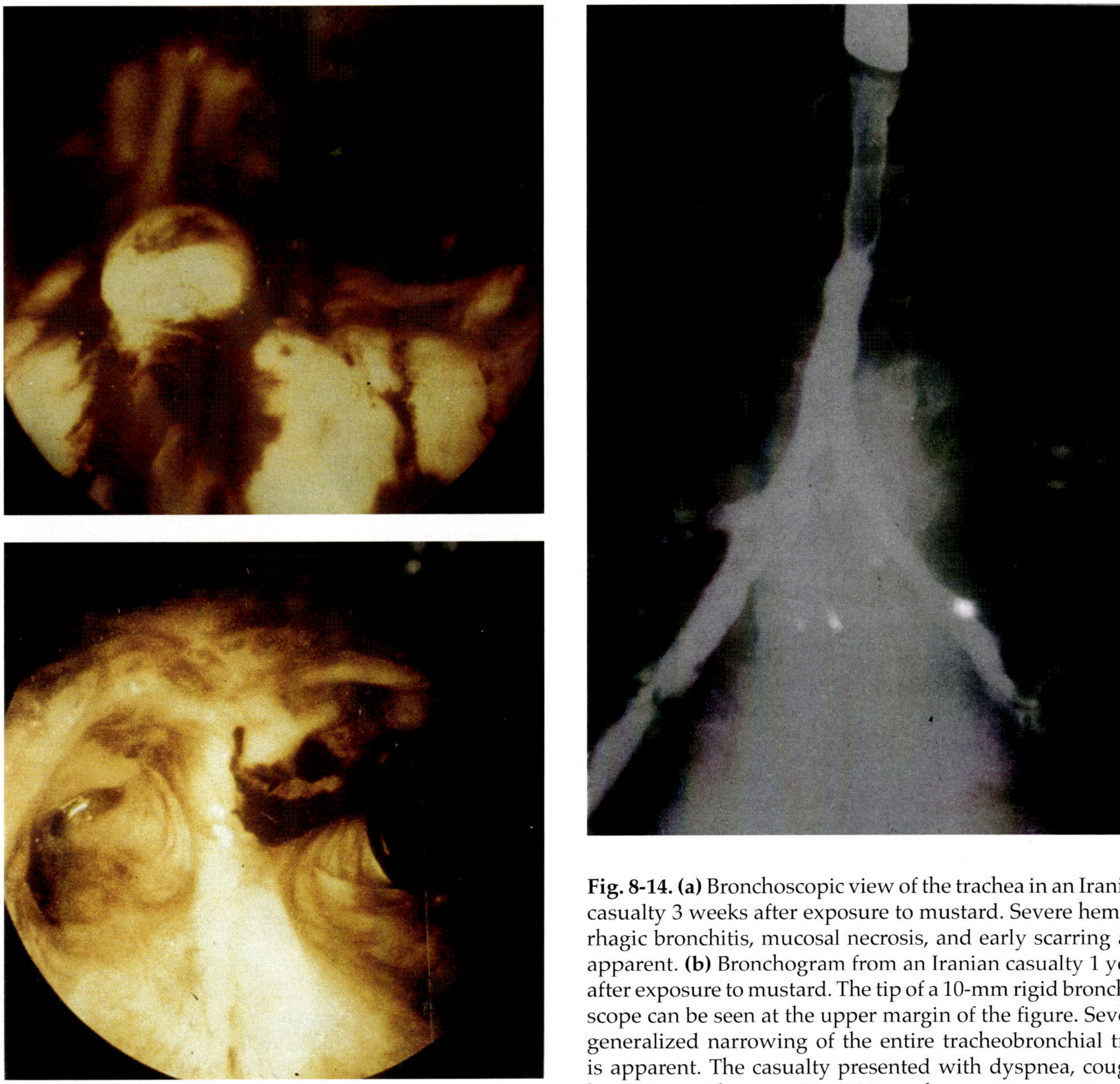

Fig. 8-14. (a) Bronchoscopic view of the trachea in an Iranian casualty 3 weeks after exposure to mustard. Severe hemorrhagic bronchitis, mucosal necrosis, and early scarring are apparent. **(b)** Bronchogram from an Iranian casualty 1 year after exposure to mustard. The tip of a 10-mm rigid bronchoscope can be seen at the upper margin of the figure. Severe generalized narrowing of the entire tracheobronchial tree is apparent. The casualty presented with dyspnea, cough, hypoxia, and hypercarbia. **(c)** Bronchoscopic appearance of the carina of an Iranian casualty who had been exposed to mustard several years before. There is nearly total occlusion of the left main-stem bronchus.
Reproduced with permission from: Freitag L, Firusian N, Stamatis G, Greschuchna D. The role of bronchoscopy in pulmonary complications due to mustard gas inhalation. *Chest*. 1991;100:1437–1438.

after exposure. The late development is especially frequent with exposures leading to significant bone marrow depression. Prophylactic administration of antibiotics is contraindicated and leads to the selection of resistant bacterial infections. Medical personnel should vigilantly watch for early signs and symptoms of infection, using Gram stains, and culture and sensitivity testing to select the most appropriate antibiotic.

Treatment for sloughing of the necrotic bronchial mucosa is rigorous percussion, postural drainage, and provision of humidified air with supplemental moisturized air or oxygen. Fiberoptic bronchoscopy may be needed to remove blockage. Bronchospasm with asthma-like symptoms can be a frequent complication of mustard lung injury. Medications used for bronchospasm are the same as in asthma: beta adrenergic dilators, steroids, and theophylline-type drugs. Although steroid antiinflammatory agents have yet to be shown beneficial in preventing human mustard lung injury, steroids may help relieve bronchospasm if beta-adrenergic bronchodilators do not provide complete relief. Caution is warranted in the use of steroids because of the likelihood of secondary bacterial infection.

With significant irritation to the larynx, acute closure caused by laryngospasm is possible and can result in death if a patent airway is not maintained. Pulmonary edema is not a normal feature of mustard lung injury, except in the case of very large exposures, when hemorrhagic pulmonary edema may be seen. Mounting circumstantial evidence suggests the possibility of chronic bronchial disease developing after significant pulmonary exposure.

Mustard is a proven carcinogen, but no cases of cancer have been documented with acute exposures. However, some factory workers chronically exposed to low doses of sulfur mustard in World War I developed cancers of the respiratory tract (nasopharynx, larynx, and lung). A small amount of laboratory data in rats and mice points to reproductive abnormalities. Anecdotal stories now emerging from Iran and Iraq will take years to substantiate with epidemiological studies. The possibility of a causal link between mustard exposure and late onset or chronic health effects should always be investigated in patients with a documented or suspected history of exposure.

Skin. In general, mustard skin burns are more superficial than thermal burns, but the services of an intensive care unit or surgical burn unit are often needed. Mustard can cause tremendous inflammation in skin wounds, and wounds can easily develop secondary bacterial cellulitis. These two conditions can be easily confused. Infection surveillance and specialty consultation may be necessary. Infection requires the use of appropriate systemic antibiotics. Mustard casualties with skin injury may require narcotics for analgesia. Recent studies in the US (USAMRICD) and England (Chemical and Biological Defence Establishment) have shown that appropriate debridement of deeper mustard burns leads to more usual healing times and return to normal skin architecture.

Bone marrow. Sulfur mustard, like nitrogen mustard and certain chemotherapeutic compounds, is an alkylating agent. Systemic absorption of sulfur mustard above 25% of a lethal dosage can lead to significant bone marrow depression. This systemic effect of sulfur mustard has sometimes been described as radiomimetic. The earliest indicator of a significant systemic exposure is nausea and vomiting persisting longer than the first hour or 2 after exposure. Nausea and vomiting 24 hours later is definitely a warning sign. The next most sensitive indicator is a fall in the lymphocyte count; this lymphopenia may occur as early as the first 24 hours. The polymorphonuclear cell count may actually rise in the first 24 hours. Other cellular components of blood may show a significant decline as early as 3 days after exposure, and patients develop profound marrow suppression by 1 to 3 weeks following exposure. The complication of sepsis or septic pneumonia can be fatal. Treatment may include transfusions, isolation techniques, hormonal stimulation of the marrow, and appropriate antibiotics.

Granulocyte colony stimulating factor is a commercially available product for use in chemotherapy; however, it causes undesirable levels of marrow suppression. Studies in nonhuman primates by the Navy using nitrogen mustard and by the Army with sulfur mustard showed an improved bone marrow recovery time using this product.[238,239]

Gastrointestinal tract. Severe hemorrhagic diarrhea may be caused either by direct ingestion of sulfur mustard or by systemic absorption following exposure by other routes. High doses of sulfur mustard can induce a necrosis and sloughing of the gastrointestinal mucosa. The most important aspect of treatment is intravenous fluids and electrolytes. Anticholinergics to control bowel spasm and possibly narcotic analgesia are indicated if an acute surgical abdomen is not a complication. Hemorrhage could be severe enough to require transfusion.

Central nervous system. In the first few hours of exposure to sulfur mustard, patients can experience mood swings ranging from depression to euphoria. The mechanism for these mood changes is not understood; supportive care is indicated. A few individuals in World War I who received massive exposures to sulfur mustard experienced seizures and died rapidly. This same phenomenon has been observed in animals.

Guidelines for Return to Duty

Because of the slow healing properties of sulfur mustard injuries, any casualty with significant injury to the eyes, respiratory tract, skin, gastrointestinal tract, or CNS should not return to duty for weeks to months.

Eye. Patients with only the mildest eye irritations to sulfur mustard, those requiring only soothing eye drops, will be able to return to duty. Even the mildest form of conjunctivitis causes a functional blindness from pain, photophobia, and spasm of the eyelid muscles; this conjunctivitis resolves in an average of 2 weeks. As the severity of the injury increases, so does the time for healing. Moderate conjunctivitis may require a 2-month recovery before return to duty is possible. In a few rare instances, blindness may result from severe exposures.

Lung. Only those individuals experiencing irritation without significant tissue injury will be able to return to duty. Determining the level of injury requires observation for 3 to 7 days. Anyone with documented mustard lung injury producing bronchial pneumonia or pseudomembrane formation will be unable to return to duty for several months. Those with severe cases may never return to duty.

Skin. Only patients with small TBSA injuries (less than 5%) in noncritical areas will be able to return to duty following treatment with topical antibiotic, dressings, and oral analgesics. Burns to the hands, feet, face, axillae, and groin are all potentially disabling. (A recent accident victim required hospitalization in a burn center for burns on the arm and leg amounting to 6% to 7% TBSA, sustaining serious disability from a relatively small surface area injury.) For all but the mildest of injuries return to duty will require weeks to months.

Burns by liquid on the skin and in the eye cause the most severe injury. It is possible, however, to receive a nearly total body burn with mustard vapor with effects no more severe than those from a second-degree sunburn. Such a mild vapor burn would take 48 or more hours to develop. However, a vapor burn developing in only a few hours could be as severe as a liquid burn. Severity of a mustard burn is dependent upon the total absorbed dose of vapor and liquid.

Long-Term Effects

Mustard burns may leave areas of hypopigmentation or hyperpigmentation, sometimes with scarring. Individuals who survive an acute, single mustard exposure with few or no systemic or infectious complications appear to recover fully. Previous cardiopulmonary disorders, severe or inadequately treated bronchitis or pneumonitis, a prior history of smoking, and advanced age all appear to contribute to long-term chronic bronchitis; there is no definitive way to determine whether these conditions are the result of aging, smoking, or a previous mustard exposure. Casualties with severe airway lesions may later have postrecovery scarring and stenosis, which predispose the individual to bronchiectasis and recurrent pneumonia.[59]

An important late sequela of mustard inhalation is a tracheal/bronchial stenosis that necessitates bronchoscopy and possible dilatation, isotonic saline lavages, laser surgery, or silicone stents.[235] Mustard has been reported to create a long-term sensitivity to smoke, dust, and similar airborne particles, probably as a result of clinically inapparent bronchospasm.[59,240]

The relationship between mustard exposure and subsequent cancer has been the subject of much study. It seems clear that individuals who were exposed to mustard daily for long periods (eg, workers in mustard production plants) have a slightly higher incidence of cancer of the airways, primarily the upper airways.[241–243] According to two separate reports, the association of one or two exposures on the battlefield with subsequent cancer is not clear; in a third report, the relation between mustard exposure and subsequent cancer is equivocal.[244–246] Watson and associates reviewed the mustard exposure–cancer incidence relation in 1989, concluding that the maximum estimates of lifetime cancer risks with sulfur mustard are not great, but neither are they entirely negligible.[247]

In 1991 the National Academy of Sciences appointed a committee to survey the health effects of mustard and lewisite.[246] Veterans of World War II who had been exposed to mustard and lewisite as subjects in test programs were presenting at Veterans Administration hospitals with complaints of illnesses they believed to be associated with the exposures. The committee was requested to survey the literature to assess the strength of association between these chemical agents and the development of specific diseases. The committee reported finding a causal relationship between exposure and various cancers and chronic diseases of the respiratory system; cancer and certain other problems of the skin; certain chronic eye conditions; psychological disorders; and sexual dysfunction. They found insufficient evidence for a causal relationship between exposure and gastrointestinal diseases, hematological diseases, neurological diseases, and cardiovascular diseases (except those resulting from infection following exposure). Some of these conclusions were not well supported. For example, there were no cases of skin cancer reported, and the alleged psychological disorders were from the trauma of exposure, not from the agent (see Chapter 9, Long-Term Health Effects of Chemical Threat Agents).

LEWISITE

Lewisite (b-chlorovinyldichloroarsine), an arsenical vesicant, is of secondary importance in the vesicant group of agents. It was synthesized in the early 20th century and has seen little or no battlefield use.[248] Lewisite is similar to mustard in that it damages the skin, eyes, and airways; however, it differs from mustard because its clinical effects appear within seconds of exposure. An antidote, British antilewisite (BAL [dimercaprol]), can ameliorate the effects of lewisite if used soon after exposure. For use as a chemical warfare agent, lewisite has some advantages over mustard but also some disadvantages.

Military Use

A research team headed by US Army Captain WL Lewis is generally credited with the synthesis of lewisite in 1918, although German scientists had studied this material earlier.[1,59,248–250] The United States manufactured a large quantity for battlefield use and sent a shipload to Europe; however, World War I ended while the shipment was at sea, and the vessel was sunk.[1,250]

No battlefield use of lewisite has been verified, although Japan may have used it against China between 1937 and 1944.[246] Lewisite is probably in the chemical warfare stockpile of several countries. Lewisite is sometimes mixed with mustard to lower the freezing point of mustard; Russia has stores of this mixture.[251]

Properties

Pure lewisite is an oily, colorless liquid, and impure lewisite is amber to black. It has a characteristic odor of geraniums. Lewisite is much more volatile and persistent in colder climates than mustard. Lewisite remains fluid at lower temperatures, which makes it perfect for winter dispersal. Lewisite hydrolyzes rapidly, and, on a humid day, maintaining a biologically active concentration of vapor may be difficult.[252]

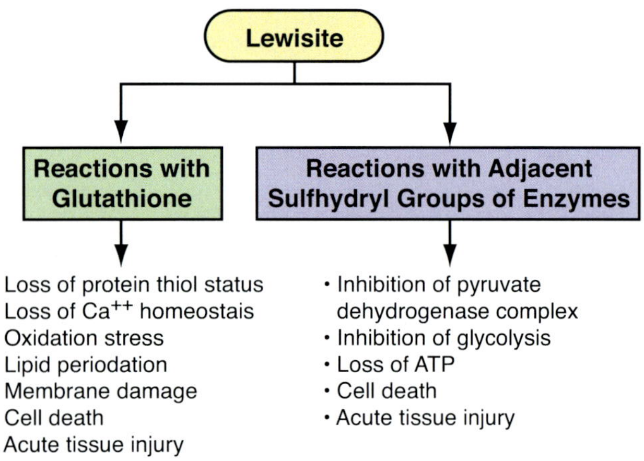

Fig. 8-15. The putative mechanisms by which lewisite causes tissue damage.
ATP: adenosine triphosphate
Ca++: calcium ions
Adapted from: US Army Medical Research Institute of Chemical Defense. A global picture of battlefield vesicants, I: a comparison of properties and effects. *Med Chem Def.* 1992;5(1):6.

Toxicity

The toxicity of lewisite vapor is very similar to that of mustard vapor. Vesication is caused by 14 μg of liquid.[98,250] Blister fluid from a lewisite-caused blister is nonirritating; however, it does contain 0.8 to 1.3 mg/mL of arsenic. In some instances intact lewisite or equally damaging breakdown products have been found in blister fluid.[59,250]

Biochemical Mechanisms of Injury

Lewisite shares many biochemical mechanisms of injury with the other arsenical compounds. It inhibits many enzymes, in particular, those with thiol groups such as pyruvic oxidase, alcohol dehydrogenase, succinic oxidase, hexokinase, and succinic dehydrogenase (Figure 8-15). As is true with mustard, the exact mechanism by which lewisite damages cells has not been completely defined. Inactivation of carbohydrate metabolism, primarily because of inhibition of the pyruvate dehydrogenase complex, is thought to be a key factor.[250]

Clinical Effects

Lewisite damages skin, eyes, and airways by direct contact and has systemic effects after absorption. Unlike mustard, it does not cause immunosuppression. Data on human exposure are few. Lewisite was applied to human skin in a few studies; however, most information on its clinical effects is based on animal studies.[59,253–255]

Skin

Lewisite liquid or vapor produces pain or irritation within seconds to minutes after contact. Pain caused by a lewisite lesion is much less severe than that caused by mustard lesions, and it diminishes after blisters form.[59] Erythema is evident within 15 to 30 minutes after exposure to liquid lewisite, and blisters start within several hours; these times are somewhat longer after vapor exposure. Lewisite is absorbed by the skin within 3 to 5 minutes (compared with 20 to 30 minutes for an equal amount of mustard) and spreads over a wider area than the same amount of mustard. The lewisite blister begins as a small blister in the center of the erythematous area and expands to include the entire inflamed area, whereas vesication from mustard begins as a "string of pearls" at the periphery of the lesion, and the small blisters eventually merge.[59] Other differences between the lesions produced by these two chemical agents are as follows:

- the inflammatory reaction from lewisite generally occurs much faster;
- the lesions from lewisite heal much faster;
- secondary infection is less common after lewisite exposure; and
- subsequent hyperpigmentation or hypopigmentation is likewise less common.[59]

Goldman and Dacre provide a further review of lewisite and its toxicology.[256]

Eye

A person is less likely to receive severe eye injury from lewisite vapor than from mustard vapor because the immediate irritation and pain caused by lewisite will produce blepharospasm, effectively preventing further exposure. A small droplet of lewisite (0.001 mL) can cause perforation and loss of an eye.[257]

In tests performed on rabbits, lewisite caused almost immediate edema of the lids, conjunctiva, and cornea, as well as early and severe involvement of the iris and ciliary body, followed by gradual depigmentation and shrinkage of the iris stroma.[257] Miosis appeared early. In this same study, miosis was not noted after mustard exposure. No long-term effects of lewisite were noted, such as the delayed keratitis seen after mustard exposure.

Airways

Lewisite vapor is extremely irritating to the nose and lower airways, causing exposed individuals to seek immediate protection, thus limiting further exposure. The airway lesion of lewisite is very similar to the lesion caused by mustard exposure except that lewisite vapor is extremely irritating to the mucous membranes. This results in sneezing, coughing, choking, and eventual necrosis of the epithelial surface. In large amounts, lewisite causes pulmonary edema.

After exposure to lewisite, dogs exhibited massive nasal secretions, lacrimation, retching, vomiting, and labored respiration. These symptoms worsened until death occurred. On autopsy, the lungs were edematous, and a pseudomembrane often extended from the nostrils to the bronchi. Tracheal and bronchial mucosa was destroyed, and the submucosa was congested and edematous. Bronchopneumonia was commonly mixed with edema.[61]

Other Effects

"Lewisite shock" is seen after exposure to large amounts of lewisite. This condition is the result of protein and plasma leakage from the capillaries and subsequent hemoconcentration and hypotension. A small amount of lewisite on the skin causes local edema because of its effects on local capillaries. With a large amount of lewisite, the pulmonary capillaries are also affected; there is edema at the site of exposure and pulmonary edema. With even larger amounts of lewisite, all capillaries are affected, and proteins and plasma leak from the circulation into the periphery. Even after small amounts of lewisite, the fluid loss can be sufficient to cause diminution of renal function and hypotension.[256] Arsines are known to cause hemolytic anemia, but there is little mention of this in reports on lewisite exposure. A "true or hemolytic anemia" has been noted with lewisite shock.[256]

Diagnosis

Lewisite exposure can be distinguished from mustard exposure by the history of pain on contact with the agent. Phosgene oxime also causes pain on contact, but phosgene oxime does not produce a liquid-filled blister. If a single individual has an isolated blister, other plant or animal causes of vesication should be sought. See also Chapter 22, Medical Diagnostics.

Laboratory Tests

No specific laboratory test exists for lewisite. Urinary arsenic excretion might be helpful. Hemolytic anemia may be seen in lewisite-exposed patients.

Patient Management

Medical personnel should follow the same principles for managing lewisite skin, eye, and airway lesions that they follow for managing mustard lesions. BAL prevents or greatly decreases the severity of skin and eye lesions if applied topically within minutes after the exposure and decontamination (however, preparations of BAL for use in the eyes and on the skin are no longer available). Given intramuscularly, BAL reduces the severity of systemic effects. BAL binds to the arsenic of lewisite more strongly than do tissue enzymes, thereby displacing lewisite from the cellular receptor sites.[250,256] BAL reduced mortality in dogs when it was given within 100 minutes after they had inhaled a lethal amount of lewisite.[258] Burns of the eyes from lewisite can be prevented if BAL is applied within 2 to 5 minutes of exposure; when it was applied within an hour after exposure, BAL prevented vesication in humans.[256,259] BAL has some unpleasant side effects, including hypertension and tachycardia; the user should read the package insert.

Long-Term Effects

There are no data on human exposure from which to predict the long-term effects from lewisite. No substantial evidence exists to suggest that lewisite is carcinogenic, teratogenic, or mutagenic.[256] The National Academy of Sciences committee reported a causal relationship between lewisite exposure and chronic respiratory diseases, and also that acute, severe injuries to the eye from lewisite will persist.[246]

PHOSGENE OXIME

Phosgene oxime is not a true vesicant because it does not produce vesicles. Instead, phosgene oxime is an urticant or nettle agent: it causes erythema, wheals, and urticaria (hives). Its lesions have been compared with those caused by nettle stings. Because it causes extensive tissue damage, phosgene oxime has been called a corrosive agent. Phosgene oxime is not known to have been used on a battlefield, and there is very little information regarding its effects on humans. This compound must be distinguished from phosgene, which exerts effects on the alveolar-capillary membrane. Phosgene oxime is made from phosgene, hence the name.

Military Use

German scientists first synthesized phosgene oxime in 1929, and Russia and Germany had developed it before World War II. Both countries may have had weapons that contained the agent.[260,261] The United States also studied phosgene oxime before World War II but rejected it as a possible chemical agent because of its biological effects, or lack thereof, and its instability.[107] The apparent lack of biological effects was later found to result from the low concentrations (1%–2%) used in the pre–World War II studies. Later studies indicated that concentrations below 8% cause no or inconsistent effects.[261,262]

Phosgene oxime is of military interest because it

- penetrates garments and rubber much more quickly than do other chemical agents and
- produces a rapid onset of severe and prolonged effects.

When mixed with another chemical agent (eg, VX), the rapid skin damage caused by phosgene oxime renders the skin more susceptible to the second agent. Also, if unmasked soldiers were exposed to phosgene oxime before donning a mask, the pain caused by the exposure would prompt them to unmask again.

Properties

Pure phosgene oxime (dichloroformoxime) is a colorless, crystalline solid; the munitions grade compound is a yellowish-brown liquid. Its melting point is 35° to 40°C (95° to 104°F). The solid material produces enough vapor to cause symptoms.[252]

Biochemical Mechanisms of Injury

Phosgene oxime is the least well studied of the chemical agents discussed in this volume, and its mechanism of action is unknown. It might produce biological damage because of the necrotizing effects of the chlorine, because of the direct effect of the oxime, or because of the carbonyl group (Figure 8-16). The skin lesions, in particular, are similar to those caused by a strong acid. The agent seems to cause its greatest systemic effects in the first capillary bed it encounters. For example, cutaneous application or intravenous injection of phosgene oxime causes pulmonary edema; injection into the portal vein produces hepatic necrosis but not pulmonary edema.[262]

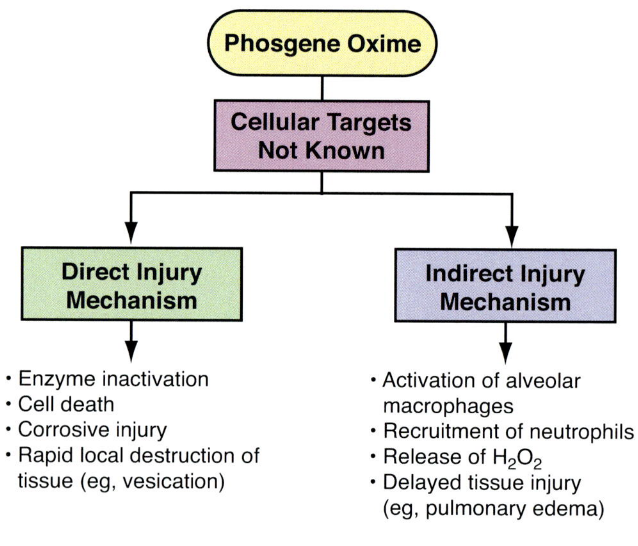

Fig. 8-16. The putative mechanisms by which phosgene oxime causes tissue damage.
H202: hydrogen peroxide
Adapted from: US Army Medical Research Institute of Chemical Defense. A global picture of battlefield vesicants, I: a comparison of properties and effects. *Med Chem Def.* 1992;5(1):6.

Clinical Effects

Phosgene oxime affects the skin, eyes, and lungs. The effects are almost instantaneous, and it causes more severe tissue damage than other vesicants. A characteristic of phosgene oxime is the immediate pain or irritation it produces on the skin, in the eyes, and in the airways. No other chemical agent produces such an immediately painful onset followed by rapid tissue necrosis.

Skin

Pain occurs immediately on contact with the liquid or solid form of this agent. Approximately 5 to 20 seconds after solutions containing 8% to 70% phosgene oxime were applied, pain and blanching occurred at the application site. Following the initial exposure, the site became grayish, with a border of erythema. Within 5 to 30 minutes after the exposure, edema formed around the edges of the tissue; the tissue later became necrotic. During the next 30 minutes, a wheal formed but disappeared overnight. The edema regressed over the following 24 hours and the original blanched area became pigmented. A dark eschar formed over the following 7 days; this gradually healed from below by granulation. The lesion extended into the underlying panniculus and muscle and was surrounded by an inflammatory reaction. In some subjects, healing was incomplete 4 to 6 months after exposure.[262] In both animal and human subjects, the skin had completely absorbed the phosgene oxime within seconds—by the time pallor appeared.[262]

Eye

Eye lesions from phosgene oxime are similar to those caused by lewisite; these lesions result in immediate pain, conjunctivitis, and keratitis.[261–263] An exact description of these effects, however, is not available.

Airways

The main lesion of phosgene oxime in the lungs is pulmonary edema. This effect occurs after either inhalation or systemic absorption of the agent. The pulmonary edema may be accompanied by necrotizing bronchiolitis and thrombosis of pulmonary venules. A large amount of phosgene oxime on the skin may produce pulmonary edema after a several-hour delay; pulmonary thromboses are prominent.[262]

Patient Management

There is no antidote for phosgene oxime, nor is there a recommended therapeutic regimen. Medical personnel should treat necrotic areas of the skin the same way other necrotic lesions are treated, by keeping them clean and preventing infection. The eye lesions require the same care as would be done for damage from a corrosive substance. The pulmonary lesion, noncardiac pulmonary edema, should be managed as suggested in Chapter 10, Toxic Inhalational Injury and Toxic Industrial Chemicals. Decontamination, or self-aid, must be accomplished immediately after contact because the agent is absorbed from the skin within seconds.

SUMMARY

The US military has considered vesicants to be major chemical warfare agents since 1917. Mustard, however, is the only vesicant known to have been used on the battlefield. Mustard and lewisite (in much smaller amounts), are known to be in the stockpiles of other countries.

Mustard was used on a large scale in World War I, causing a great number of casualties; it was also used during the Iran-Iraq War. Data from World War I indicate that more than 95% of mustard casualties survived but most required lengthy hospitalizations; data from the Iran-Iraq War are not as complete. If mustard is ever used again, military medical personnel must be prepared to accept and care for large numbers of casualties, who will require long-term care.

REFERENCES

1. Prentiss AM. *Chemicals in War: A Treatise on Chemical War.* New York, NY: McGraw-Hill; 1937.

2. Heller CE. *Chemical Warfare in World War I: The American Experience, 1917-1918.* Fort Leavenworth, Kan: US Army Command and General Staff College, Combat Studies Institute; 1984. Leavenworth Papers No. 10.

3. Medema J. Mustard gas: the science of H. *Nucl Biol Chem Defense Technol Int.* 1986;1:66–71.

4. Dacre JC, Goldman M. Toxicology and pharmacology of the chemical warfare agent sulfur mustard. *Pharmacol Rev.* 1996;48:289–326.

5. Jacobson LO, Spurr C, Barron ESG, Smith T, Lushbaugh C, Dick GF. Nitrogen mustard therapy. *JAMA.* 1946;32:263–271.

6. Gilman A. The initial clinical trial of nitrogen mustard. *Am J Surg.* 1963;105:574–578.

7. Goodman LS, Wintrobe MM, Dameshek W, Goodman MJ, Gilman A, McLennan MT. Nitrogen mustard therapy. *JAMA.* 1946;132:126–132.

8. Rhoads CP. Nitrogen mustards in the treatment of neoplastic disease: official statement. *JAMA.* 1946;131:656–658.

9. Fries AA, West CJ. Dichloroethylsulfide: mustard gas. In: Fries AA, West CJ, eds. *Chemical Warfare.* New York, NY: McGraw Hill; 1921:150–179.

10. Graef I, Karnofsky DA, Jager VB, Krichesky B, Smith HW. The clinical and pathologic effects of nitrogen and sulfur mustards in laboratory animals. *Am J Pathol.* 1948;24:1–47.

11. Gilchrist HL. Statistical consideration of gas casualties, I: Gas casualties. In: Weed FW, ed. *Medical Aspects of Gas Warfare.* Vol 14. In: *The Medical Department of the United States Army in the World War.* Washington, DC: Government Printing Office; 1926: 273–279.

12. Balali-Mood M, Farhoodi M, Panjvani FK. Report of three fatal cases of war gas poisoning. In: *Proceedings of the 2nd World Congress on New Compounds in Biological and Chemical Warfare, 24–27 August 1986.* Ghent, Belgium: International Association of Forensic Toxicologists; 1986. Abstract.

13. Alexander SF. Medical report of the Bari Harbor mustard casualties. *Mil Surg.* 1947;101:1–17.

14. Infield G. *Disaster at Bari.* New York, NY: Bantam; 1988.

15. Deeter DP, Gaydos JC, eds. *Occupational Health: The Soldier and the Industrial Base.* Part 3, Vol 2. In: Zajtchuk R, Bellamy RF, eds. *Textbooks of Military Medicine.* Washington, DC: US Department of the Army, Office of The Surgeon General, and Borden Institute; 1993.

16. Carus WS. *Chemical Weapons in the Middle East.* Washington, DC: The Washington Institute for Near East Policy; 1988. Research Memorandum 9.

17. Willems JL. Clinical management of mustard gas casualties. *Ann Med Milit Belg.* 1989;3S:1–61.

18. Aasted A, Darre MD, Wulf HC. Mustard gas: clinical, toxicological, and mutagenic aspects based on modern experience. *Ann Plast Surg.* 1987;19:330–333.

19. Aasted A, Wulf HC, Darre E, Niebuhr E. Fishermen exposed to mustard gas: clinical experiences and cancer risk evaluation. *Ugeskr Laeger.* 1985;147:2213–2216.

20. Jorgensen BS, Olesen B, Berntsen O. Mustard gas accidents near Bornholm. *Ugeskr Laeger.* 1985;147:2251–2254.

21. Wulf HC, Aasted A, Darre E, Neibuhr E. Sister chromatid exchanges in fishermen exposed to leaking mustard gas shells. *Lancet.* 1985;1:690–691.

22. Hobbs FB. A fatal case of mustard gas poisoning. *Br Med J.* 1944;2:306–307.

23. Heully F, Gruninger M. Collective intoxication caused by the explosion of a mustard gas shell. *Ann Med Legal.* 1956;36:195–204.

24. Jakubowski EM, Sidell FR, Evans RA, et al. Quantification of thiodiglycol in human urine after an accidental sulfur mustard exposure. *Toxicol Methods.* 2000;10:143–150.

25. Aitken RS. Effects of accidental exposure to mustard-gas vapor. *Lancet.* 1943;245:602–603.

26. Ruhl CM, Park DJ, Danisa O, et al. A serious skin sulfur mustard burn from artillery shell. *J Emerg Med.* 1994;12(2):159–166.

27. Chemical Research and Development Engineering Command. *Persistency Times of Chemical Agents on CARC Painted Vehicles and Sand*. Aberdeen Proving Ground, Md: CRDEC; 1990. CRDEC SMCCR-OPA.

28. Blewett WK. *Defense Against Mustard: A P2NBC2 Review and Analysis*. Aberdeen Proving Ground, Md: Physical Protection Directorate; 1992. Chemical Research and Development Engineering Command Technical Report 3270.

29. Mann I, Pullinger BD. A study of mustard-gas lesions of the eyes of rabbits and men. *Am J Ophthalmol.* 1944;26:1253–1277.

30. Marshall EK Jr, Lynch V, Smith HW. On dichlorethylsulphide (mustard gas), II: Variations in susceptibility of the skin to dichlorethylsulphide. *J Pharm Exp Therap.* 1919;12:291–301.

31. Papirmeister B, Feister AJ, Robinson SI, Ford RD. *Medical Defense Against Mustard Gas: Toxic Mechanisms and Pharmacological Implications.* Boca Raton, Fla: CRC Press; 1991.

32. Smith WJ, Dunn MA. Medical defense against blistering chemical warfare agents. *Arch Dermatol.* 1991;127:1207–1213.

33. Somani SM, Babu SR. Toxicodynamics of sulfur mustard. *Int J Clin Pharm Therap Toxicol.* 1989;9:419–435.

34. Anslow WP, Houck CR. Systemic pharmacology and pathology of sulfur and nitrogen mustards. In: *Chemical Warfare Agents, and Related Chemical Problems.* Parts 3–6. Washington, DC: Office of Scientific Research and Development, National Defense Research Committee, Div 9; 1946:440–478.

35. Papirmeister B, Gross CL, Meier HL, Petrali JP, Johnson JB. Molecular basis for mustard-induced vesication. *Fundam Appl Toxicol.* 1985;5:S134–S149.

36. Gross CL, Meier HL, Papirmeister B, Brinkley FB, Johnson JB. Sulfur mustard lowers nicotinamide dinucleotide concentrations in human skin grafted to athymic nude mice. *Toxicol Appl Pharmacol.* 1985;81:85–90.

37. Meier HL, Gross CL, Papirmeister B. 2,2'-dichlorodiethyl sulfide (sulfur mustard) decreases NAD^+ levels in human leukocytes. *Toxicol Lett.* 1987;39:109–122.

38. Mol MAE, van de Ruit AMBC, Kluivers AW. NAD^+ levels and glucose uptake of cultured human epidermal cells exposed to sulfur mustard. *Toxicol Appl Pharmacol.* 1989;98:159–165.

39. Dixon M, Needham DM. Biochemical research on chemical warfare agents. *Nature.* 1946;158:432–438.

40. Schnyder J, Bagglionoi M. Induction of plasminogen activator secretion in macrophages by electrochemical stimulation of the hexose monophosphate shunt by methylene blue. *Proc Natl Acad Sci USA.* 1980;77:414–417.

41. Papirmeister B, Gross CL, Petrali JP, Hixson CL. Pathology produced by sulfur mustard in human skin grafts on athymic nude mice, I: Gross and light microscopic changes. *J Toxicol Cutan Ocular Toxicol.* 1984;3:371–391.

42. Smith WJ, Gross CL, Chan P, Meier HL. The use of human epidermal keratinocytes in culture as a model for studying sulfur mustard toxicity. *Cell Biol Toxicol.* 1990;6:285–291.

43. Yourick JJ, Clark CR, Mitcheltree LW. Niacinamide pretreatment reduces microvesicle formation in hairless guinea pigs cutaneously exposed to sulfur mustard. *Fund Appl Toxicol.* 1991;17:533–542.

44. Petrali JP, Oglesby SB, Meier HL. Ultrastructural correlates of the protection afforded by niacinamide against sulfur mustard–induced cytotoxicology of human lymphocytes in vitro. *Ultrastructural Pathol.* 1990;14:253–262.

45. Martens ME, Smith WJ. Mechanisms of sulfur mustard induced metabolic injury. In: *Proceedings of the 1993 Medical Chemical Defense Bioscience Review, Baltimore, Md, 10–13 May 1993.* Aberdeen Proving Ground, Md: US Army Medical Research Institute of Chemical Defense; 1993: 257–363. Defense Technical Information Center A275667.

46. Cowan FM, Broomfield CA, Smith WJ. Effect of sulfur mustard exposure on protease activity in human peripheral blood lymphocytes. *Cell Biol Toxicol.* 1991;7:239–248.

47. Cowan FM, Broomfield CA, Smith WJ. Inhibition of sulfur mustard-increased protease activity by niacinamide, n-acetyl cysteine or dexamethasone. *Cell Biol Toxicol.* 1992;8:129–138.

48. Smith WJ, Cowan FM, Broomfield CA. Increased proteolytic activity in human epithelial cells following exposure to sulfur mustard. *FASEB J.* 1991;5:A828.

49. Gentilhomme E, Neveux Y, Hua A, Thiriot C, Faure M, Thivolet J. Action of bis(betachloroethyl)sulphide (BCES) on human epidermis reconstituted in culture: morphological alterations and biochemical depletion of glutathione. *Toxicol in Vitro.* 1992;6:139–147.

50. Orrenius S, Nicotera P. On the role of calcium in chemical toxicity. *Arch Toxicol Suppl.* 1987;11:S11–S19.

51. Ministry of Defence. A literature review upon the toxicology, mechanism of action, and treatment of sulphur and nitrogen mustard poisoning. United Kingdom: Ministry of Defence; nd. Unpublished report.

52. Ray R, Legere RH, Broomfield CA, Petrali JP. Mechanism of action of alkylating agents: Membrane effects. In: *Proceedings of the 1991 Medical Defense Bioscience Review, Aberdeen Proving Ground, Md, 7–8 August 1991.* Aberdeen Proving Ground, Md: US Army Medical Research Institute of Chemical Defense; 1991: 139–142. AD B158588.

53. Miccadei S, Kyle ME, Gilfor D, Farber JL. Toxic consequences of the abrupt depletion of glutathione in cultured rat hepatocytes. *Arch Biochem Biophys.* 1988;265:311–320.

54. Paulet G. Metabolisme cellulaire et action cutanée du sulfure d'ethyle dichlore (yperite): Role devolu au potentiel d'oxydation cellulaire [in French]. *CR Séances Soc Bio.* 1952;146:925–928.

55. Elsayed NM, Omaye ST, Klain GJ, et al. Response of mouse brain to a single subcutaneous injection of the monofunctional sulfur mustard, butyl 2-chloroethyl sulfide (BCS). *Toxicol.* 1989;58:11–20.

56. Karnofsky DA, Graef I, Smith HW. Studies on the mechanism of action of the nitrogen and sulfur mustards in vivo. *Am J Pathol.* 1948;24:275–291.

57. Davison C, Rozman RS, Smith PK. Metabolism of bis-beta-chloroethyl sulfide (sulfur mustard gas). *Biochem Pharmacol.* 1961;7:65–74.

58. Zhang B, Wu Y. Toxicokinetics of sulfur mustard. *Chinese J Pharm Toxicol.* 1987;1:188–194.

59. Buscher H. *Green and Yellow Cross.* Conway N, trans. Cincinnati, Ohio: Kettering Laboratory of Applied Physiology, University of Cincinnati; 1944.

60. Keeler JR. Lieutenant Colonel, US Army Nurse Corps. Personal communication, 1990.

61. Vedder EB. Vesicants. In: Vedder EB, ed. *The Medical Aspects of Chemical Warfare.* Baltimore, Md: Williams & Wilkins; 1925: 125–166.

62. Gilchrist HL. *A Comparative Study of World War Casualties From Gas and Other Weapons.* Edgewood Arsenal, Md: US Chemical Warfare School; 1928: 1–51.

63. Balali-Mood M, Navaeian A. Clinical and paraclinical findings in 233 patients with sulfur mustard poisoning. In: *Proceedings of the 2nd World Congress on New Compounds in Biological and Chemical Warfare, 24–27 August 1986.* Ghent, Belgium: International Association of Forensic Toxicologists; 1986: 464–473.

64. Momeni A, Enshaeih S, Meghdadi M, Amindjavaheri M. Skin manifestations of mustard gas. *Arch Dermatol.* 1992;128:775–780.

65. Renshaw B. Mechanisms in production of cutaneous injuries by sulfur and nitrogen mustards. In: *Chemical Warfare Agents, and Related Chemical Problems.* Parts 3–6. Washington, DC: Office of Scientific Research and Development, National Defense Research Committee, Div 9; 1946: 478–520.

66. Warthin AS. Pathologic action of mustard gas (dichlorethylsulphide). In: Weed FW, ed. *Medical Aspects of Gas Warfare.* Vol. 14. In: *The Medical Department of the United States Army in the World War.* Washington, DC: Government Printing Office; 1926: 512–661.

67. Henriques FC Jr, Moritz AR, Breyfogle HS, Paterson LA. The mechanism of cutaneous injury by mustard gas: an experimental study using mustard prepared with radioactive sulfur. In: *Chemical Warfare Agents, and Related Chemical Problems.* Parts 3–6. Washington, DC: Office of Scientific Research and Development, National Defense Research Committee, Div 9; 1946.

68. Marzulli FN, Maibach HI, eds. *Dermatotoxicology*. 5th ed. Washington, DC: Taylor & Francis; 1996: chapter 5.

69. Sidell FR, Takafuji ET, Franz DR, eds. *Medical Aspects of Chemical and Biological Warfare.* In: Zajtchuk R, Bellamy RF, eds. *Textbooks of Military Medicine.* Washington, DC: Department of the Army, Office of The Surgeon General, Borden Institute; 1997.

70. Ginzler AM, Davis MIJ. *The Pathology of Mustard Burns of Human Skin*. Edgewood Arsenal, Md: US Army Medical Research Laboratory; 1943.

71. Petrali JP, Oglesby SB, Mills KR. Ultrastructural correlates of sulfur mustard toxicity. *J Toxicol Cutan Ocular Toxicol.* 1990;9:193–204.

72. Petrali JP, Oglesby SB, Hamilton, TA, Mills KR. Comparative morphology of sulfur mustard effects in the hairless guinea pig and a human skin equivalent. *J Submicrosc Cytol Pathol.* 1993;25:113–118.

73. Petrali JP, Oglesby-Megee S. Toxicity of mustard gas skin lesions. *Microsc Res Tech.* 1997;37:221–228.

74. Petrali JP, Oglesby SB, Mills KR. Ultrastructural correlates of sulfur mustard toxicity. *J Toxicol Cutan Ocular Toxicol.* 1990;9:193–214.

75. Petrali JP, Oglesby SB, Justus TA. Morphological effects of sulfur mustard on a human skin equivalent. *J Toxicol Cutan Ocular Toxicol.* 1991;10:315–324.

76. King JR, Monteiro-Riviere NA. Cutaneous toxicity of 2-chloroethyl methyl sulfide in isolated perfused porcine skin. *Toxicol Appl Pharmacol.* 1990;104:167–179.

77. Mershon MM, Mitcheltree LW, Petrali JP, Braue EH, Wade JV. Hairless guinea pig bioassay model for vesicant vapor exposure. *Fundam Appl Toxicol.* 1990;15:622–630.

78. Papirmeister B, Gross CL, Petrali JP, Hixson CJ. Pathology produced by sulfur mustard in human skin grafts on athymic nude mice. *J Toxicol Cutan Ocul Toxicol.* 1984;3:371–408.

79. Petrali JP, Oglesby SB, Meier HL. Ultrastructural correlates of the protection afforded by niacinamide against sulfur mustard-induced cytotoxicity of human lymphocytes in vitro. *Ultrastruct Pathol.* 1990;14:253–262.

80. Petrali JP, Oglesby SB, Hamilton TA. Mustard gas skin lesion and bullous pemphigoid antigen. In: Bailey GW, Garratt-Reed, eds. *Proceedings of the 52nd Annual Meeting of the Microscopy Society of America, New Orleans, La, August 1994.* San Francisco, Calif: San Francisco Press, Inc; 1994: 254–255.

81. Moore KG, Schofield BH, Higuchi K, et al. Two sensitive in vitro monitors of chemical toxicity to human and animal skin (in short term organ culture). I. Paranuclear vacuolization in glycol metharylate tissue sections. II. Interface with 14-c-leucine incorporation. *J Toxicol Cutan Ocul Toxicol.* 1986; 5:285–302.

82. Kan RK, Pleva CM, Hamilton TA, Anderson DR, Petrali JP. Sulfur mustard-induced apoptosis in hairless guinea pig skin. *Toxicol Pathol.* 2003;31(3):185–190.

83. Petrali JP, Hamilton TA, Benton B, et al. Dimethyl sulfoxide accelerates mustard gas-induced skin pathology. *J Med Chem Biol Rad Defense* [serial online]. April 29, 2005. Available at http://www.jmedcbr.org/Issue_0301/Petrali/Petrali_0405.html. Accessed May 21, 2007.

84. Fine J. Altered skin basement membrane antigenicity in epidermolysis bullosa. *Curr Probl Dermatol.* 1987;17:111–126.

85. Kan RK, Pleva CM, Backof DR, Hamilton TA, Petrali JP. Free-floating cryostat sections for immunoelectron microscopy: bridging the gap form light to electron microscopy. *Microsc Res Tech.* 2001;54:246–253.

86. Reed CI. The minimum concentration of dichlorethylsulphide (mustard gas) effective for the eyes of man. *J Pharm Exp Therap.* 1920;15:77–80.

87. Geeraets WJ, Abedi S, Blanke RV. Acute corneal injury by mustard gas. *South Med J.* 1977;70:348–350.

88. Warthin AS, Weller CV. *The Medical Aspects of Mustard Gas Poisoning.* St Louis, Mo: CV Mosby; 1919.

89. Maumenee AE, Scholz RO. The histopathology of the ocular lesions produced by the sulfur and nitrogen mustards. *Bull Johns Hopkins Hosp.* 1948;82:121–147.

90. Atkinson WS. Delayed keratitis due to mustard gas (dichlorodiethyl sulfide) burns. *Arch Ophthalmol.* 1948;40:291–301.

91. Petrali JP, Miskena FJ, Hamilton TA, Finger AS, Janny SJ. Sulfur mustard toxicity of the rabbit eye: an ultrastructural study. *J Toxicol Cutan Ocul Toxicol.* 1997;16(4):227–237.

92. Petrali JP, Henein M, Ali AH, Devamanoharan PS, Hamilton TA, Varma SD. Morphological correlates of the protection afforded by varma mixture in rat cornea exposed to half mustard (CEES): a proposed new treatment for sulfur mustard toxicity. *Proceedings Microscopy and Microanalysis, Microscopy Society of America 57th Annual Meeting, Portland, Ore, 3–7 August 1999.* Portland, Ore: Microscopy Society of America; 1999: 1178–1179.

93. Varma SD, Devamanoharan PS, Ali AH, et al. Corneal damage by half mustard (2-chloroethyl ethyl sulfide, CEES) in vitro preventive studies: a histologic and electron microscopic revaluation. *J Ocul Pharmacol Ther.* 1998;14(5):413–421.

94. Varma SD, Devamanoharan PS, Ali AH, et al. Half mustard (CEES) induced damage to rabbit cornea: attenuating effect of taurine-pyruvate-alpha-ketoglutarate-pantothenate mixture. *J Ocul Pharmacol Ther.* 1998;14(5):423–428.

95. Petrali JP, Dick EJ, Brozetti JJ, Hamilton TA, Finger AV. Acute ocular effects of mustard gas: ultrastructural pathology and immunohistopathology of exposed rabbit cornea. *J Appl Toxicol.* 2000; 20:S173–S175.

96. Gilchrist HL. Symptoms and treatment. In: Weed FW, ed. *Medical Aspects of Gas Warfare.* Vol 14. In: *The Medical Department of the United States Army in the World War.* Washington, DC: Government Printing Office; 1926: 250–272.

97. Winternitz MC, Finney WP Jr. The pathology of mustard poisoning. In: *Collected Studies on the Pathology of War Gas Poisoning.* New Haven, Conn: Yale University Press; 1920: 99–114.

98. Houck CR, Crawford B, Bannon JH, Smith HW. Studies on the mechanism of death in dogs after systemic intoxication by the intravenous injection of methyl-bis(beta-chloroethyl)amine or tris(beta-chloroethyl)amine. *J Pharm Exp Therap.* 1947;90:277–292.

99. Pappenheimer AM. Pathological action of war gases. In: Weed, FW, ed. *Medical Aspects of Gas Warfare.* Vol 14. In: *The Medical Department of the United States Army in the World War.* Washington, DC: Government Printing Office; 1926: 87–249.

100. Sohrabpour H. Clinical manifestations of chemical agents on Iranian combatants during the Iran–Iraq conflict. In: Heyndrickx A, ed. *Proceedings of the 1st World Congress on New Compounds in Biological and Chemical Warfare: Toxicological Evaluation, May 21–23, 1984.* Ghent, Belgium: Rijksuniversiteit; 1984: 291–297.

101. Marshall EK Jr. Physiological action of dichlorethyl sulphide (mustard gas). In: Weed FW, ed. *Medical Aspects of Gas Warfare*. Vol 14. In: *The Medical Department of the United States Army in the World War.* Washington, DC: Government Printing Office; 1926: 369–406.

102. Philips FS. Recent contributions to the pharmacology of bis(2-haloethyl) amines and sulfides. *Pharmacol Rev.* 1950; 2:281–323.

103. Wils ERJ, Hulst AG, de John AL, Verweij A, Boter HL. Analysis of thiodiglycol in urine of victims of an alleged attack with mustard gas. *J Anal Toxicol.* 1985;9:254–257.

104. Wils ER, Hulst AG, van Laar J. Analysis of thiodiglycol in urine of victims of an alleged attack with mustard gas, II. *J Anal Toxicol.* 1988;12:15–19.

105. US Department of the Army. *Assay Techniques for Detection of Exposure to Sulfur Mustard, Cholinesterase Inhibitors, Sarin, Soman, GF, and Cyanide*. Washington, DC: Headquarters, DA; May 1996. Technical Bulletin Medical 296.

106. Mellor SG, Rice P, Cooper GJ. Vesicant burns. *Br J Plast Surg.* 1991; 44(6):434–437.

107. Borak J, Sidell FR. Agents of chemical warfare: sulfur mustard. *Ann Emerg Med.* 1992; 21(3):303–308.

108. Sidell FR, Urbanetti JS, Smith WJ, Hurst CG. Vesicants. In: Sidell FR, Takafuji ET, Franz DR, eds. *Medical Aspects of Chemical and Biological Warfare.* In: Zajtchuk R, Bellamy RF, eds. *Textbooks of Military Medicine.* Washington, DC: Department of the Army, Office of The Surgeon General, Borden Institute, 1997: 197–228.

109. Ruhl CM, Park SJ, Danisa O, et al. A serious skin sulfur mustard burn from an artillery shell. *J Emerg Med.* 1994;12(2):159–166.

110. Kadivar H, Adams SC. Treatment of chemical and biological warfare injuries: insights derived from the 1984 Iraqi attack on Majnoon Island. *Mil Med.* 1991;156(4):171–177.

111. Barillo DJ, Cancio LC, Goodwin CW. Treatment of white phosphorus and other chemical burn injuries at one burn center over a 51 year period. *Burns.* 2004;30:448–452.

112. Cancio LC, Horvath EE, Barillo DJ, et al. Burn support for Operation Iraqi Freedom and related operations, 2003–2004. *J Burn Care Rehabil.* 2005;26:151–161.

113. Arturson G. Local effects. In: Settle JAD, ed. *Principles and Practice of Burns Management.* New York, NY: Churchill Livingstone, 1996: 83–94.

114. Settle JAD. Principals of replacement fluid therapy. In: Settle JAD, ed. *Principles and Practice of Burns Management.* New York, NY: Churchill Livingstone; 1996: 217–222.

115. Brisebois RJ. Fluid resuscitation in the Canadian Forces. *J Trauma.* 2003;54(5Suppl):S36–S38.

116. Thomas SJ, Kramer GC, Herndon DN. Burns: military options and tactical solutions. *J Trauma.* 2003;54(5Suppl):S207–S218.

117. Winfree J, Barillo DJ. Burn management. Nonthermal injuries. *Nurs Clin North Am.* 1997;32:275–296.

118. Barillo DJ, Goodwin CW. Dermatologists and the burn center. *Dermatol Clin.* 1999;17:61–75.

119. Ducic I, Shalom A, Rising W, Nagamoto K, Munster AM. Outcome of patients with toxic epidermal necrolysis syndrome revisited. *Plast Reconstr Surg.* 2002;110:768–773.

120. Halebian PH, Corder VJ, Madden MR, Finklestein JL, Shires GT. Improved burn center survival of patients with toxic epidermal necrolysis managed without corticosteroids. *Ann Surg.* 1986;204:503–512.

121. Heimbach DM, Engrav LH, Marvin JA, Harnar TJ, Grube BJ. Toxic epidermal necrolysis: a step forward in treatment. *JAMA*. 1987;257:2171–2175.

122. Keleman JJ 3rd, Cioffi WG, McManus WF, Mason AD Jr, Pruitt BA Jr. Burn center care for patients with toxic epidermal necrolysis. *J Am Coll Surg*. 1995;80:273–278.

123. Palmieri TL, Greenhalgh DG, Saffle JR, et al. A multicenter review of toxic epidermal necrolysis treated in US burn centers at the end of the twentieth century. *J Burn Care Rehabil*. 2002;23:87–96.

124. McGee T, Munster A. Toxic epidermal necrolysis syndrome:mortality rate reduced with early referral to regional burn center. *Plast Reconstr Surg*. 1998;102:1018–1022.

125. *Field Management of Chemical Casualties Handbook*. 2nd ed. Aberdeen Proving Ground, Md: US Army Medical Research Institute of Chemical Defense; 2000. Available at https://ccc.apgea.army.mil/products/info/products.htm. Accessed May 21, 2007.

126. *Medical Management of Chemical Casualties Handbook*. 3rd ed. Aberdeen Proving Ground, Md: US Army Medical Research Institute of Chemical Defense, 2000. Available at https://ccc.apgea.army.mil/products/info/products.htm. Accessed May 21, 2007.

127. US Department of the Army. NATO handbook on the medical aspects of NBC defensive operations, AmedP-6(B). Study draft 1, 2001. Army Field Manual 8-9, Part III, Chap 3.

128. Koga M. Epidermal grafting using the tops of suction blisters in the treatment of vitiligo. *Arch Dermatol*. 1988;124:1656–1658.

129. Tang WY, Chan LY, Lo KK. Treatment of vitiligo with autologous epidermal transplantation using the roofs of suction blisters. *Hong Kong Med J*. 1998;4(2):219–224.

130. Kiistala U, Mustakallio KK. In-vivo separation of epidermis by production of suction blisters. *Lancet*. 1964;1:1444–1445.

131. Graham JS, Stevenson RS, Hamilton TA, et al, unpublished research, 2005.

132. Yin HQ, Langford R, Burrell RE. Comparative evaluation of the antimicrobial activity of ACTICOAT antimicrobial barrier dressing. *J Burn Care Rehabil*. 1999;20(3):195–200.

133. Sheridan RL, Tompkins RG. Skin substitutes in burns. *Burns*. 1999;25(2):97–103.

134. Tredget EE, Shankowsky HA, Groeneveld A, Burrell R. A matched pair-randomized study evaluating the efficacy and safety of acticoat silver-coated dressings for the treatment of burn wounds. *J Burn Care Rehabil*. 1998;19:531–537.

135. Heggers J, Goodheart RE, Washington J, et al. Thereapeutic efficacy of three silver dressings in an infected animal model. *J Burn Care Rehabil*. 2005;26:53–56.

136. Kucan JO. Use of Biobrane in the treatment of toxic epidermal necrolysis. *J Burn Care Rehabil*. 1995;16:324–327.

137. Smith DJ Jr. Use of Biobrane in wound management. *J Burn Care Rehabil*. 1995;16:317–320.

138. Graham JS, Chilcott RP, Rice P, Milner SM, Hurst CG, Maliner BI. Wound healing of cutaneous sulfur mustard injuries: strategies for the development of improved therapies. *J Burns Wounds* [serial online]. 2005;4(1)1–45. Available at http://www.journalofburnsandwounds.com/volume04/jobw04e1.pdf. Accessed May 21, 2007.

139. Barillo DJ, McManus AT. Infection in burn patients. In: Cohen J, Powderly WG, eds: *Infectious Diseases*. 2nd ed. London, England: Mosby International; 2003.

140. Barillo DJ. Using mafenide acetate in acute and chronic wounds. *Ostomy Wound Manage*. 2002(Suppl):5–10.

141. Barillo DJ, McManus AT, Cancio LC, Sofer A, Goodwin CW. Burn center management of necrotizing fasciitis. *J Burn Care Rehabil.* 2003;24:127–132.

142. Mendelson JA, Lindsey D. Sulfamylon (mafenide) and penicillin as expedient treatment of experimental massive open wounds with *C. perfringens* infection. *J Trauma.* 1962;2:239–261.

143. Mendelson JA. Topical mafenide hydrochloride aqueous spray in initial management of massive contaminated wounds with devitalized tissue. *Prehospital Disaster Med.* 2001;16:172–174.

144. Mendelson JA. The management of burns under conditions of limited resources using topical aqueous sulfamylon (mafenide) hydrochloride spray. *J Burn Care Rehabil.* 1997;18:238–244.

145. Mendelson JA, Pratt HJ, Amato JJ, et al. Mafenide hydrochloride and mafenide acetate in spray and ointment forms as topical therapy C Perfringins contaminated massive wounds: experimental study. *J Trauma.* 1970;10:1132–1144.

146. Smith WJ, Babin MC, Kiser RC, Casillas RP. Development of medical countermeasures to sulfur mustard vesication. In: Salem H, Katz SA, eds. *Alternative Toxicological Methods.* Boca Raton, Fla: CRC Press; 2003: 323–328.

147. Babin MC, Ricketts K, Skvorak JP, Gazaway M, Mitcheltree LW, Casillas RP. Systemic administration of candidate antivesicants to protect against topically applied sulfur mustard in the mouse ear vesicant model (MEVM). *J Appl Toxicol.* 2000;20:S141–S144.

148. Casillas RP, Kiser RC, Truxall JA, et al. Therapeutic approaches to dermatotoxicity by sulfur mustard. I. Modulation of sulfur mustard-induced cutaneous injury in the mouse ear vesicant model. *J Appl Toxicol.* 2000;20:S145–S151.

149. Amir A, Chapman S, Kadar T, Gozes Y, Sahar R, Allon N. Sulfur mustard toxicity in macrophages: effect of dexamethasone. *J Appl Toxicol.* 2000;20:S51–S58.

150. Amir A, Turetz J, Chapman S, et al. Beneficial effects of topical anti-inflammatory drugs against sulfur-mustard-induced ocular lesions in rabbits. *J Appl Toxicol.* 2000;20:S109–S114.

151. Husain K, Dube SN, Sugendran K, Singh R, Das Gupta S, Somani HD. Effect of topically applied sulphur mustard on antioxidant enzymes in blood cells and body tissues of rats. *J Appl Toxicol.* 1996;16(3):245–248.

152. Kumar O, Sugendran K, Vijayaraghavan R. Protective effect of various antioxidants on the toxicity of sulphur mustard administered to mice by inhalation or percutaneous routes. *Chem Biol Interact.* 2001;134(1):1–12.

153. Naghii MR. Sulfur mustard intoxication, oxidative stress and antioxidants. *Mil Med.* 2002;167(7):573–575.

154. Helfman T, Ovington L, Falanga V. Occlusive dressings and wound healing. *Clin Dermatol.* 1994;12(1):121–127.

155. Chang H, Wind S, Kerstein MD. Moist wound healing. *Dermatol Nurs.* 1996;8(3):174–176.

156. Kerstein MD. Moist wound healing: the clinical perspective. *Ostomy Wound Manage.* 1995;41(7A Suppl):37S–44S.

157. Field CK, Kerstein MD. Overview of wound healing in a moist environment. *Am J Surg.* 1994;167(1A):2S–6S.

158. Logan TP, Graham JS, Martin JL, Zallnick JE, Jakubowski EM, Braue EH. Detection and measurement of sulfur mustard (HD) offgassing from the weanling pig following exposure to saturated sulfur mustard vapor. *J Appl Toxicol.* 2000;20:S199–204.

159. Marsden AK. Accident department. In: Settle JAD, ed. *Principles and Practice of Burns Management.* New York, NY: Churchill Livingstone, 1996: 209–215.

160. Johnson RM, Richard R. Partial-thickness burns: identification and management. *Adv Skin Wound Care.* 2003;6(4):178–189.

161. Arturson G. Mechanism of injury. In: Settle JAD, ed. *Principles and Practice of Burns Management.* New York, NY: Churchill Livingstone, 1996: 61–82.

162. Brown RFR, Rice P, Bennett NJ. The use of laser Doppler imaging as an aid in clinical management decision making in the treatment of vesicant burns. *Burns.* 1998; 24(8):692–698.

163. Chilcott RP, Brown RFR, Rice P. Non-invasive quantification of skin injury resulting from exposure to sulphur mustard and Lewisite vapours. *Burns.* 2000;26(3):245–250.

164. Green HA, Bua D, Anderson RR, Nishioka NS. Burn depth estimation using indocyanine green fluorescence. *Arch Dermatol.* 1992;128:43–49.

165. Black KS, Hewitt CW, Miller DM, et al. Burn depth evaluation with fluorometry: is it really definitive? *J Burn Care Rehabil.* 1986;7(4):313–317.

166. Schomacker KT, Torri A, Sandison DR, Sheridan RL, Nishioka NS. Biodistribution of indocyanine green in a porcine burn model: light and fluorescence microscopy. *J Trauma.* 1997;43:813–819.

167. Jerath MR, Schomacker KT, Sheridan RL, Nishioka NS. Burn wound assessment in porcine skin using indocyanine green fluorescence. *J Trauma.* 1999;46(6):1085–1088.

168. Holm C, Mayr M, Tegeler J, Becker A, Pfeiffer U, Muhlbauer W. Laser-induced fluorescence of indocyanine green: plastic surgical applications. *Eur J Plast Surg.* 2003;26:19–25.

169. Holm C, Mayr M, Hofter E, Becker A, Pfeiffer UJ, Muhlbauer W. Intraoperative evaluation of skin-flap viability using laser-induced fluorescence of indocyanine green. *Br J Plast Surg.* 2002;55(8):635–644.

170. Sheridan RL, Schomacker KT, Lucchina LC, et al. Burn depth estimation by use of indocyanine green fluorescence: initial human trial. *J Burn Care Rehabil.* 1995;16(6):602–604.

171. Braue EH, Graham JS, Doxzon BF, et al. Non-invasive methods for determining lesion depth from vesicant exposure. *J Burn Care Res.* 2007;28(2):275–285.

172. Graham JS, Schomacker KT, Glatter RD, Briscoe CM, Braue EH, Squibb KS. Efficacy of laser debridement with autologous split-thickness skin grafting in promoting improved healing of deep cutaneous sulfur mustard burns. *Burns.* 2002;28(8):719–730.

173. Graham JS, Schomacker KT, Glatter RD, Briscoe CM, Braue EH Jr, Squibb KS. Bioengineering methods employed in the study of wound healing of sulfur mustard burns. *Skin Res Technol.* 2002;8(1):57–69.

174. Rice P. The use of dermabrasion to accelerate the naturally slow rate of epidermal healing mustard injuries in pigs. In: *Proceedings of the 1995 NATO Research Study Group 3 Meeting on Prophylaxis and Therapy Against Chemical Agents, Porton Down, Salisbury, England, 18–21 September 1995.* Porton Down, Salisbury, England: Chemical and Biological Defence Establishment, 1995. CTIC No. AD-B209142.

175. Rice P, Brown RFR, Lam DGK, Chilcott RP, Bennett NJ. Dermabrasion—a novel concept in the surgical management of sulphur mustard injuries. *Burns.* 2000;26(1):34–40.

176. Rice P, Bennett NJ, Lam DGK, Brown RFR. The role of dermabrasion in Lewisite-induced skin injury. In: *Proceedings of the 2000 Medical Defense Bioscience Review, Hunt Valley, Md, 4–9 June 2000.* Aberdeen Proving Ground, Md: US Army Medical Research Institute of Chemical Defense; 2000: 1179–1186.

177. Kjellstrom BT, Persson JK, Runn P. Surgical treatment of skin lesions induced by sulfur mustard ("mustard gas")—an experimental study in the guinea pig. *Ann Acad Med Singapore.* 1997;26(1):30–36.

178. Lam DG, Rice P, Brown RF. The treatment of Lewisite burns with laser debridement—'lasablation.' *Burns.* 2002;28(1):19–25.

179. Eldad A, Weinberg A, Breiterman S, Chaouat M, Palanker D, Ben-Bassat H. Early nonsurgical removal of chemically injured tissue enhances wound healing in partial-thickness burns. *Burns.* 1998;24(2):166–172.

180. Graham JS, Smith KJ, Braue EH, et al. Improved healing of sulfur mustard-induced cutaneous lesions in the weanling pig by pulsed CO_2 laser debridement. *J Toxicol Cutan Ocul Toxicol.* 1997;16(4):275–295.

181. Acland KM, Barlow RJ. Lasers for the dermatologist. *Br J Dermatol.* 2000;143(2):244–255.

182. Tanzi EL, Alster TS. Side effects and complications of variable-pulsed erbium:yttrium-aluminum-garnet laser skin resurfacing: extended experience with 50 patients. *Plast Reconstr Surg.* 2003;111(4):1524–1529.

183. Tanzi EL, Alster TS. Single-pass carbon dioxide versus multiple-pass Er:YAG laser skin resurfacing: a comparison of postoperative wound healing and side-effect rates. *Dermatol Surg.* 2003;29(1):80–84.

184. Jeong JT, Park JH, Kye YC. Resurfacing of pitted facial acne scars using Er:YAG laser with ablation and coagulation mode. *Aesthetic Plast Surg.* 2003;27:130–134.

185. Reynolds N, Cawrse N, Burge T, Kenealy J. Debridement of a mixed partial and full-thickness burn with an erbium:YAG laser. *Burns.* 2003;29(2):183–188.

186. Singhal A, Reis ED, Kerstein MD. Options for nonsurgical debridement of necrotic wounds. *Adv Skin Wound Care.* 2001;14(2):96–103.

187. Ozcan C, Ergun O, Celik A, Corduk N, Ozok G. Enzymatic debridement of burn wound with collagenase in children with partial-thickness burns. *Burns.* 2002;28(8):791–794.

188. Orgill DP, Liu PY, Ritterbush LS, Skrabut EM, Samuels JA, Shames SL. Debridement of porcine burns with a highly purified, ananain-based cysteine protease preparation. *J Burn Care Rehabil.* 1996;17(4):311–322.

189. Hansbrough JF, Achauer B, Dawson J, et al. Wound healing in partial-thickness burn wounds treated with collagenase ointment versus silver sulfadiazine cream. *J Burn Care Rehabil.* 1995;16:241–247.

190. Soroff HS, Sasvary DH. Collagenase ointment and polymyxin B sulfate/bacitracin spray versus silver sulfadiazine cream in partial-thickness burns: a pilot study. *J Burn Care Rehabil.* 1994;15:13–17.

191. Ahle NW, Hamlet MP. Enzymatic frostbite eschar debridement by bromelain. *Ann Emerg Med.* 1987;16(9):1063–1065.

192. Houck JC, Chang CM, Klein G. Isolation of an effective debriding agent from the stems of pineapple plants. *Int J Tissue React.* 1983;5(2):125–134.

193. Levenson HD, Gruber DK, Gruber C, Lent R, Seifter E. Chemical debridement of burns: mercaptans. *J Trauma.* 1981;21(8):632–644.

194. Gant TD. The early enzymatic debridement and grafting of deep dermal burns to the hand. *Plast Reconstr Surg.* 1980;66(2):185–190.

195. Klasen HJ. A review on the nonoperative removal of necrotic tissue from burn wounds. *Burns.* 2000;26(3):207–222.

196. Graham JS, Martin JL, Zallnick JE, et al. Assessment of cutaneous sulfur mustard injury in the weanling pig. *Skin Res Technol.* 1999;5(1):56–67.

197. Reid FM, Graham JS, Niemuth NA, Singer AW, Janny SJ. Sulfur mustard-induced skin burns in weanling swine evaluated clinically and histopathologically. *J Appl Toxicol.* 2000;20:S153–S160.

198. Braue EH, Nalls CR, Way RA, Zallnick JE, Reider RG, Mitcheltree LW. Nikolsky's sign: a novel way to evaluate damage at the dermal-epidermal junction. *Skin Res Technol.* 1997;3(4):245–251.

199. Goodman H. Nikolsky sign. *Arch Dermatol Syphilol.* 1953;68:334–335.

200. Petrali JP, Oglesby SB, Hamilton TA, Mills KR. Ultrastructural pathology and immunohistochemistry of mustard gas lesion. In: *Proceedings of the 1993 Medical Chemical Defense Bioscience Review, Baltimore, Md, 10–13 May 1993.* Aberdeen Proving Ground, Md: US Army Medical Research Institute of Chemical Defense; 1993: 15–20. AD A275667.

201. Petrali JP, Oglesby SB, Hamilton TA, Mills KR. Ultrastructural pathology and immunohistochemistry of mustard gas lesion. In: Bailey GW, Bentley J, Small JA, eds. *Proceedings of the 50th Annual Meeting of the Electron Microscopy Society of America, 16–21 August 1992, Boston, Mass*. San Francisco, Calif: San Francisco Press, Inc; 1992.

202. Lindsay CD, Rice P. Changes in connective tissue macromolecular components of Yucatan mini-pig skin following application of sulphur mustard vapor. *Hum Exp Toxicol.* 1995;14:341–348.

203. Brown RFR, Rice P. Histopathological changes in Yukatan minipig skin following challenge with sulfur mustard. A sequential study of the first 24 hours following challenge. *Int J Exp Path.* 1997;78:9–20.

204. Green HA, Burd EE, Nishioka NS, Compton CC. Skin graft take and healing following 193-nm excimer, continuous-wave carbon dioxide (CO_2), pulsed CO_2, or pulsed holmium:YAG laser ablation of the graft bed. *Arch Dermatol.* 1993;129:979–988.

205. Domankevitz Y, Nishioka NS. Effects of a rapidly scanned carbon dioxide laser on porcine dermis. *J Burn Care Rehabil.* 1997;18(3):206–209.

206. Thomas S, McCubbin P. A comparison of the antimicrobial effects of four silver-containing dressings on three organisms. *J Wound Care.* 2003;12(3):101–107.

207. O'Neill MA, Vine GJ, Beezer AE, et al. Antimicrobial properties of silver-containing wound dressings: a microcalorimetric study. *Int J Pharm.* 2003;263(1–2):61–68.

208. Olson ME, Wright JB, Lam K, Burrell RE. Healing of porcine donor sites covered with silver-coated dressings. *Eur J Surg.* 2000;166(6):486–489.

209. Demling RH, DeSanti MDL. The rate of re-epithelialization across meshed skin grafts is increased with exposure to silver. *Burns.* 2002;28(3):264–266.

210. Paddock HN, Schultz GS, Mast BA. Methods in reepithelialization. In: DiPietro LA, Burns AL, eds. *Wound Healing*. Totowa, NJ: Humana Press, 2003:17–36.

211. Danilenko DM, Ring BD, Tarpley JE, et al. Growth factors in porcine full and partial-thickness burn repair. Differing targets and effects of keratinocyte growth factor, platelet-derived growth factor-BB, epidermal growth factor and neu differentiation factor. *Am J Pathol.* 1995;147(5):1261–1277.

212. Wang HJ, Wan HL, Yang DS, Chen TM, Chang DM. Acceleration of skin graft healing by growth factors. *Burns.* 1996;22(1):10–14.

213. Smith PD, Polo M, Soler PM, et al. Efficacy of growth factors in the accelerated closure of interstices in explanted meshed human skin grafts. *J Burn Care Rehabil.* 2000;21:5–9.

214. Sheridan RL, Moreno C. Skin substitutes in burns. *Burns.* 2001;27(1):92.

215. Shakespeare P. Burn wound healing and skin substitutes. *Burns.* 2001;27(5):517–522.

216. Balasubramani M, Kumar TR, Babu M. Skin substitutes: a review. *Burns.* 2001;27(5): 534–544.

217. Hansen SL, Voigt DW, Wiebelhaus P, Paul CN. Using skin replacement products to treat burns and wounds. *Adv Wound Care.* 2001;14(1):37–44.

218. Supp DM, Boyce ST. Engineered skin substitutes: practices and potentials. *Clin Dermatol*. 2005;23(4):403–412.

219. Rheinwald JG, Green H. Serial cultivation of strains of human epidermal keratinocytes: the formation of keratinizing colonies from single cells. *Cell.* 1975;6(3):331–343.

220. Randolph RK, Simon M. Characterization of retinol metabolism in cultured human epidermal keratinocytes. *J Biol Chem.* 1993;268(13):9198–9205.

221. Green H, Kehinde O, Thomas J. Growth of cultured human epidermal cells into multiple epithelia suitable for grafting. *Proc Natl Acad Sci USA.* 1979;76(11):5665–5668.

222. Fratianne R, Papay F, Housini I, Lang C, Schafer IA. Keratinocyte allografts accelerate healing of split-thickness donor sites: applications for improved treatment of burns. *J Burn Care Rehabil.* 1993;14:148–154.

223. Braye F, Oddou L, Bertin-Maghit M, et al. Widely meshed autograft associated with cultured autologous epithelium for the treatment of major burns in children: report of 12 cases. *Eur J Pediatr Surg.* 2000;10(1):35–40.

224. Hickerson WL, Compton C, Fletchall S, Smith LR. Cultured epidermal allografts and allodermis combination for permanent burn wound coverage. *Burns.* 1994;20(suppl 1):S52–S55.

225. Svensjo T, Yao F, Pomahac B, Eriksson E. Autologous keratinocyte suspensions accelerate epidermal wound healing in pigs. *J Surg Res.* 2001;99(2):211–221.

226. Navarro FA, Stoner ML, Park CS, et al. Sprayed keratinocyte suspensions accelerate epidermal coverage in a porcine microwound model. *J Burn Care Rehabil.* 2000; 1(6):513–518.

227. Voigt M, Schauer M, Schaefer DJ, Andree C, Horch R, Stark GB. Cultured epidermal keratinocytes on a microspherical transport system are feasible to reconstitute the epidermis in full-thickness wounds. *Tissue Eng.* 1999;5(6):563–572.

228. Horch RE, Bannasch H, Kopp J, Andree C, Stark GB. Single-cell suspensions of cultured human keratinocytes in fibrin-glue reconstitute the epidermis. *Cell Transplant.* 1998;7(3):309–317.

229. Wood F. Clinical potential of autologous epithelial suspension. *Wounds.* 2003;15(1):16–22.

230. Mendez-Eastman S. Negative pressure wound therapy. *Plast Surg Nurs.* 1998;18(1):27–29, 33–37.

231. Morykwas MJ, Argenta LC, Shelton-Brown EI, McGuirt W. Vacuum-assisted closure: a new method for wound control and treatment: animal studies and basic foundation. *Ann Plast Surg.* 1997;38(6):553–562.

232. Morykwas MJ, David LR, Schneider AM, et al. Use of subatmospheric pressure to prevent progression of partial-thickness burns in a swine model. *J Burn Care Rehabil.* 1999;20(1):15–21.

233. Genecov DG, Schneider AM, Morykwas MJ, Parker D, White WL, Argenta LC. A controlled subatmospheric pressure dressing increases the rate of skin graft donor site reepithelialization. *Ann Plast Surg.* 1998;40:219–225.

234. Scherer LA, Shiver S, Chang M, Meredith JW, Owings JT. The vacuum assisted closure device: a method of securing skin grafts and improving graft survival. *Arch Surg.* 2002;137(8):930–934.

235. Personal communications with ophthalmologists at US Army Medical Research Institute of Chemical Defense Medical Management of Chemical and Biological Casualties course training, 1995.

236. Freitag L, Firusian N, Stamatis G, Greschuchna D. The role of bronchoscopy in pulmonary complications due to mustard gas inhalation. *Chest.* 1991;100:1436–1441.

237. Hurst CG. Unpublished document on managing mustard casualties, 2003–2004.

238. Anderson DR, Holmes WW, Lee RB, et al. Sulfur mustard-induced neutropenia: treatment with granulocyte colony-stimulating factor. *Mil Med.* 2006;171(5):448–453.

239. Meisenberg BR, Melaragno AJ, Monroy RL. Granulocyte colony stimulating factor (G-CSF) for mustard-induced bone marrow suppression. *Mil Med.* 1993;158:470–474.

240. Morgenstern P, Koss FR, Alexander WW. Residual mustard gas bronchitis: effects of prolonged exposure to low concentrations of mustard gas. *Ann Intern Med.* 1947;26:27–40.

241. Tokuoka S, Hayashi Y, Inai K, et al. Early cancer and related lesions in the bronchial epithelium in former workers of a mustard gas factory. *Acta Pathol Jpn.* 1986;36:533–542.

242. Wada S, Miyanishi M, Nishimoto Y, Kambe S, Miller RW. Mustard gas as a cause of respiratory neoplasia in man. *Lancet.* 1968;1:1161–1163.

243. Manning KP, Skegg DCG, Stell PM, Doll R. Cancer of the larynx and other occupational hazards of mustard gas workers. *Clin Otolaryngol.* 1981;6:165–170.

244. Norman JE. Lung cancer mortality in World War I veterans with mustard-gas injury: 1919–1965. *J Natl Cancer Inst.* 1975;54:311–317.

245. Beebe GW. Lung cancer in World War I veterans: possible relation to mustard-gas injury and 1918 influenza epidemic. *J Natl Cancer Inst.* 1960;25:1231–1252.

246. Pechura CM, Rall DP, eds. *Veterans at Risk.* Washington, DC: National Academy Press; 1993.

247. Watson AP, Jones TD, Griffin GD. Sulfur mustard as a carcinogen: application of relative potency analysis to the chemical warfare agents H, HD, and HT. *Regul Toxicol Pharmacol.* 1989;10:1–25.

248. Lewis WL, Stiegler HW. The beta-chlorovinyl-arsines and their derivatives. *Am Chem Soc.* 1925;47:2546–2555.

249. Harris R, Paxman J. *A Higher Form of Killing.* New York, NY: Hill and Wang; 1982.

250. Trammel GL. Toxicodynamics of organoarsenic chemical warfare agents. In: Somani SM, ed. *Chemical Warfare Agents.* San Diego, Calif: Academic Press; 1992:255–270.

251. Madsen J. Major, Medical Corps, US Army. Personal communication, 1995.

252. US Department of Defense. *Potential Military Chemical/Biological Agents and Compounds.* Washington, DC: Headquarters, Departments of the Army, Navy, and Air Force; 1990. Field Manual 3-9, Air Force Manual 355-7, Navy Publication P-467.

253. Rovida G. Lewisite, III: Action on the human skin. *Sperimentale.* 1929;83:115–120.

254. Wardell EL. *Lewisite (M-1): Summary of Physiologic and Toxicologic Data.* Edgewood Arsenal, Md: Chemical Warfare Service; 1940. Edgewood Arsenal Technical Report 285.

255. Dailey LE, Clark JW, Stolp BN, Conner JC Jr. *A Controlled Laboratory Experiment to Compare Lesions Resulting From Application of Mustard, Lewisite and Nitrogen Mustards to the Skin of the Forearms of Humans.* Washington, DC: Naval Research Laboratory; 1941. NRL Report P-2364.

256. Goldman M, Dacre JC. Lewisite: its chemistry, toxicology, and biological effects. *Rev Environ Contam Toxicol.* 1989;110:75–115.

257. Mann I, Pirie A, Pullinger BD. A study of Lewisite lesions of the eyes of rabbits. *Am J Ophthalmol.* 1946;29:1215–1227.

258. Harrison HE, Ordway HK, Durlacher SH, Albrink WS, Bunting H. Poisoning from inhalation of the vapors of Lewisite and phenyldichlorarsine: its pathology in the dog and treatment with 2,3-dimercaptopropanol (BAL). *J Pharm Exp Therap.* 1946;87:76–80.

259. Peters RA, Stocken LA, Thompson RHS. British anti-Lewisite (BAL). *Nature.* 1945;156:616–619.

260. Prandtl W, Sennewald K. Trichloronitrosomethane, dichloroformoxime (phosgene oxime) and some of their derivatives. *Berichte.* 1929;62B:1754–1768.

261. Joffe MH, Barry MC, Marzulli FN. *Effects of Aqueous Solutions of Cutaneously Applied Phosgene Oxime on Humans.* Edgewood Arsenal, Md: Army Chemical Center; 1954. Medical Laboratories Research Report 288.

262. McAdams AJ Jr, Joffe MH. *A Toxico-pathologic Study of Phosgene Oxime.* Army Chemical Center, Md; 1955. Medical Laboratories Research Report 381.

263. Augerson WS, Cadigan FC Jr, Goyer MM, Sivak A. *Chemical Casualty Treatment Protocol.* Cambridge, Mass: Arthur D Little, Inc; 1987: Chap 3.

Chapter 9

LONG-TERM HEALTH EFFECTS OF CHEMICAL THREAT AGENTS

WILLIAM J. SMITH, PhD*; MATTHEW G. CLARK, PhD†; THOMAS B. TALBOT, MD, MS‡; PATRICIA ANN CAPLE, RN§; FREDERICK R. SIDELL, MD¥; AND CHARLES G. HURST, MD¶

*Chief, Cellular and Molecular Biology Branch, Research Division, US Army Medical Research Institute of Chemical Defense, 3100 Ricketts Point Road, Aberdeen Proving Ground, Maryland 21010-5400

†Major, Medical Service Corps, US Army; Chief, Neurobehavioral Toxicology Branch, Analytical Toxicology Division, US Army Medical Research Institute of Chemical Defense, 3100 Ricketts Point Road, Aberdeen Proving Ground, Maryland 21010-5400

‡Major, Medical Corps, US Army; Chief of Operations Branch, Chemical Casualty Care Division, US Army Medical Research Institute of Chemical Defense, 3100 Ricketts Point Road, Aberdeen Proving Ground, Maryland 21010-5400

§Lieutenant Colonel, Nurse Corps, US Air Force; Chemical Casualty Care Division, US Army Medical Research Institute of Chemical Defense, 3100 Ricketts Point Road, Aberdeen Proving Ground, Maryland 21010-5400

¥Formerly, Chief, Chemical Casualty Care Office, and Director, Medical Management of Chemical Casualties Course, US Army Medical Research Institute of Chemical Defense, Aberdeen Proving Ground, Maryland 21010-5400; Deceased

¶Chief, Chemical Casualty Care Division, US Army Medical Research Institute of Chemical Defense, 3100 Ricketts Point Road, Aberdeen Proving Ground, Maryland 21010-5400

INTRODUCTION

Chemical warfare agents were used extensively in World War I (the United States had approximately 70,000 chemical casualties[1]) and have been employed or allegedly employed in about a dozen conflicts since then.[2] The most recent large-scale use of these weapons was by Iraq in its war with Iran in the late 1980s. During that conflict, Iraq used nerve agents and the vesicant mustard[3]; after the war it maintained stockpiles of the two agents and the capability to manufacture them. Before coalition forces liberated Kuwait early in 1991 during the Persian Gulf War, Iraq was expected to use these agents when attacked. No reports of the use of chemical weapons during that conflict were made, however, despite the vigilance of the press corps and military medical personnel, who were trained to report, investigate, and care for chemical casualties.[4,5] One US soldier developed skin blisters 8 hours after exploring an underground bunker.[4] His clinical findings and mass spectroscopy readings (performed by a chemical detection team) from his clothing and the bunker supported a diagnosis of accidental mustard exposure, which was mild. The exposure was not confirmed by later testing of clothing samples, from which trace amounts of the agent may have dissipated.

Although the acute effects of the nerve agents and of mustard agent are well known,[6,7] the long-term effects after a single exposure or multiple exposures are less well recognized. The nerve agents are the subject of Chapter 5, Nerve Agents, and mustard is discussed in Chapter 8, Vesicants. This chapter focuses on the long-term effects of exposure to these agents.

MUSTARD

Two well-known forms of mustard exist. Sulfur mustard (designated by the military as H or HD) was first synthesized in the early 1800s, has been used in warfare on several occasions, and is a major chemical warfare agent.[6] Nitrogen mustard is of more recent origin, has not been used in warfare, and is a cancer chemotherapeutic agent. In this chapter, the word "mustard" will refer to sulfur mustard.

Mustard is best known as a skin vesicant, but in a series of Iranian patients exposed to mustard, 95% had airway effects, 92% had eye injuries, and 83% had skin lesions.[8] After absorption, mustard, an extremely potent alkylating agent, has the potential to damage all cells and all organs.[6] Absorption and systemic distribution of a significant amount of mustard damages the bone marrow, where it destroys the precursor cells, resulting in pancytopenia.[6] Less commonly, clinical effects are seen in the gastrointestinal tract (usually as a terminal event)[9,10] and in the central nervous system (CNS), with ill-defined symptoms such as lethargy and apathy.[8,11]

On the skin, a *Ct* (the concentration [C] of agent vapor or aerosol in air, as mg/m^3, multiplied by the time [*t*] of exposure, in minutes) of 50 $mg{\bullet}min/m^3$ or a droplet of 10 μg of mustard is adequate to produce vesication.[6] (One study[12] indicates that 8 of the 10 μg evaporate and 1 μg enters the systemic circulation, leaving 1 μg to produce the skin lesion.) Eye lesions can be produced by a *Ct* of 10 $mg{\bullet}min/m^3$.[13] Airway injury occurs at a *Ct* of 100 $mg{\bullet}min/m^3$ or higher.[6]

The mode of biological activity of mustard is less well defined than that of the nerve agents. The initial event is felt to be a reaction of mustard and deoxyribonucleic acid (DNA) with subsequent damage to the DNA. A series of intracellular events then occur, leading to cellular damage accompanied by inflammation and cellular death. Cellular damage begins within 1 to 2 minutes of contact of mustard to skin or mucous membranes.[6] The onset of clinical effects following exposure to mustard occurs hours after the exposure.[6] The delay usually ranges from 2 to 24 hours, is inversely proportional to the amount of mustard, and depends on other factors as well. No specific therapy for mustard exposure exists.[6] Decontamination within a minute or two will prevent or diminish the lesion, and later care consists of symptomatic management of the lesion.

Studies have established that the chemical agent mustard has long-term sequelae. Both Morgenstern et al[14] and Buscher[15] emphasize that chronic low-dose exposure over months to years in occupationally exposed workers leads to chronic bronchitis, bronchial asthma, hoarseness, aphonia, and hypersensitivity to smoke, dust, and fumes. Affected individuals typically show persistent disability, with increased susceptibility to respiratory tract infections and evidence of bronchitis and bronchiectasis.[6,14,15] Laboratory animal studies[16–18] have found that mustard is mutagenic and carcinogenic, and it is reported to be carcinogenic in humans.[19]

A 1993 study[19] sponsored by the Veterans Administration and conducted by the Institute of Medicine reported that a causal relationship exists between mustard exposure and the following conditions:

- chronic respiratory diseases (asthma, chronic bronchitis, emphysema, chronic obstructive pulmonary disease, chronic laryngitis);
- respiratory cancers (nasopharyngeal, laryngeal, and lung);
- pigmentation abnormalities of the skin;
- chronic skin ulceration and scar formation;
- skin cancer;
- chronic conjunctivitis;
- recurrent corneal ulcerative disease;
- delayed recurrent keratitis;
- leukemia (nitrogen mustard);
- bone marrow depression and (resulting) immunosuppression;
- psychological disorders (mood disorders, anxiety disorders, and traumatic stress disorders); and
- sexual dysfunction as a result of scrotal and penile scarring.

Although laboratory evidence suggests that all of these *might* occur, there is no data in humans to indicate that all *have* occurred. The study report recognized this by stating, "It is also possible that skin cancers did not occur in the studied populations..."[19] and "...underrepresented in human studies is information on chronic or delayed effects [on the bone marrow and immune system]."[19] The report also pointed out that the psychological disorders were from the stress of the exposure and not from the agent, and there seemed to be no data on sexual dysfunction. Moreover, it is not clear from the report whether these effects follow one or multiple mustard exposures.

All human studies dealing with chronic mustard disease processes are retrospective and fraught with the problems inherent in retrospective studies. These problems include bias in the sampling populations; lack of epidemiological controls for the effects of smoking, lifestyle, race, gender, age, or exposure to other chemicals; differential quality of available health care; and incorrect diagnosis.[6] These limitations make absolute interpretation of the studies difficult.

Over the past several years, Iranian investigators have provided a number of papers that study the late toxic effects of mustard exposure in patients 16 to 20 years after the Iran-Iraq conflicts of the 1980s.[20–26] Balali-Mood and Hefazi[27] have summarized most of these data in a comparative review of early and late toxic effects of mustard.

Carcinogenesis

Mustard is an alkylating agent similar to drugs that have been used in cancer chemotherapy, such as nitrogen mustard, Cytoxan (Bristol-Myers Squibb Oncology Division, Princeton, NJ), and methotrexate. Since DNA is one of mustard's most sensitive targets, it is not surprising that carcinogenesis and radiomimetic effects are seen.

In studies[18,28,29] conducted from 1949 through 1953 by WE Heston with mustard and strain-A mice (immunocompromised), the occurrence of pulmonary tumors was easily demonstrated. Studies conducted at Edgewood Arsenal, Maryland, examined the carcinogenic effects on rats in whole-body chamber exposures. Mustard readily produced skin malignancies in rats, but no excess tumors at other sites.[30] Subcutaneous injections totaling about 6 mg/kg of mustard produced sarcomas and other malignancies at injection sites in C3H, C3Hf, and strain-A mice, but did not result in an increase of malignancies at other sites.[29]

Human data on the carcinogenicity of mustard are from *(a)* battlefield exposures, *(b)* accidents, and *(c)* workers in chemical factories. Both British and American studies have investigated the increased incidence of pulmonary carcinoma arising from World War I battlefield exposure. All are difficult to interpret, owing to the lack of controls for age, chronic pulmonary disease, cigarette smoking, and other factors that might have affected the outcome.[31–33]

In contrast to battlefield exposures, studies of factory workers involved in the production of mustard have shown a definite link between prolonged exposure to low doses of mustard and cancer.[6] Several studies[17,34–38] have provided evidence of an increased risk of respiratory tract cancers in factory workers. Easton et al[35] found a 45% increase in deaths due to lung cancer, a 170% increase in death from cancer of the larynx, and a 450% increase in deaths from cancer of the pharynx, compared with expected deaths in the general population. The risks for cancer of the pharynx and lung were significantly related to the duration of employment at the factory. For reasons analyzed more fully elsewhere,[39] the association between a single exposure to mustard and airway cancer is not as well established.

Japanese studies suggest a greater potential risk of cancer from mustard than do the British studies. Easton et al[35] and Manning et al[17] suggest that the difference is related to the design of the Japanese studies and to the lower industrial hygiene standards in Japan at the time of the studies.[6] The weight of the evidence—cellular, epidemiological, and toxicological—indicates a causal association between mustard exposure and the occurrence of excess respiratory cancer, skin cancer, and possibly leukemia. Inadequate exposure information limits accurate estimation of the cancer excesses that may be expected.[19]

The Iranian data suggest that surviving victims of mustard exposure during the Iran-Iraq War are exhibiting carcinoma of the nasopharynx, bronchogenic carcinoma, and adenocarcinoma of the stomach, as well as acute myeloblastic and lymphoblastic leukemia.[27] Definitive studies of the nature and types of cancers seen in this patient population have yet to be published.

Chronic Pulmonary Disease

Inhalation of mustard vapor primarily affects the laryngeal and tracheobronchial mucosa.[6] Evidence suggests that mustard inhalation causes sustained respiratory difficulties even after the acute lesions have healed. Clinical follow-ups on 200 Iranian soldiers who were severely injured by mustard during the Iran–Iraq War indicate that about one third had experienced persistent respiratory effects 2 years after initial exposure. Reported problems included chronic bronchitis, asthma, rhinopharyngitis, tracheobronchitis, laryngitis, recurrent pneumonia, bronchiectasis, and in some cases, severe, unrelenting tracheobronchial stenosis.[22,40–43]

Of the British soldiers exposed to mustard in World War I, 12% were awarded disability compensation for respiratory disorders that were believed to be from mustard exposures during combat.[44] Bronchitis was the major complaint; emphysema and asthma were also reported. However, epidemiological studies of the relationship between agent exposure and subsequent respiratory disability were severely limited for several reasons. Often, individuals had experienced multiple combined exposures to mustard and other chemical agents. Also, influenza and other respiratory ailments frequently made diagnosis of the mustard vapor injury difficult.[6] Finally, no epidemiological controls for smoking or for postexposure environmental and occupational histories were included in the studies.[45]

Wada et al[34] suggest a causal relationship between mustard exposure and subsequent bronchitis, tuberculosis, and pneumonia in factory workers involved in the production of mustard. Again, Morgenstern et al[14] and Buscher[15] emphasize that chronic low-dose exposure over prolonged periods (presumably months to years) leads to lingering bronchitis, bronchial asthma, hoarseness, aphonia, and hypersensitivity to smoke, dust, and fumes. Affected individuals typically show persistent disability, with increased susceptibility to respiratory tract infections and evidence of bronchitis and bronchiectasis.[6]

Little contemporary information regarding the pathogenesis of the respiratory lesions is available, and few data from people or animals exposed to nonlethal concentrations of mustard vapor exist. Even fewer studies investigate the histopathology of the recovery process in animals exposed to mustard.[19] However, two studies[9,46] conducted during World War I suggest that low-level exposure or survivable exposures in dogs and rabbits may produce scar tissue following small ulcerations in the trachea and larynx, causing contractions of these areas. The more severe respiratory tract lesions described in animals exposed to mustard vapor appear to be similar in type and location to those described in humans.[6]

The Iranian database shows that in the 3-year postexposure time frame the most severely affected patients demonstrated restrictive pulmonary disease patterns. By 16 years postexposure, these patterns had become obstructive in nature.[27] Sixteen to twenty years after exposure, the main respiratory complications were chronic obstructive pulmonary disease, bronchiectasis, asthma, large airway narrowing, and pulmonary fibrosis.[27]

Chronic Eye Disease

Individuals who sustain acute ocular injury from high-dose mustard exposure may experience difficulties even after the initial effects of the injury have subsided.[47–50] Recurrent or persistent corneal ulceration can occur after latent periods of 10 to 25 years. This delayed keratopathy[49,51] may be accompanied by chronic conjunctivitis and corneal clouding. Anecdotal accounts suggest that low-dose exposure also causes increased sensitivity to later exposures to mustard,[52] although the existence of increased sensitivity is difficult to substantiate with available scientific evidence.[6] About 10% of those with eye injury in World War I had severely affected eyes, with both the cornea and the conjunctiva being involved. Members of this group developed the "delayed keratitis" noted above 8 to 25 years later.[48]

The 1993 Institute of Medicine study[19] of the effects of mustard and lewisite exposure on the health of veterans concluded that acute, severe injury of the eye from mustard might result in recurrent corneal ulcerative disease for the remainder of the patient's life, with a maximum incidence occurring 15 to 20 years after the injury. Based on extensive data, the study concluded that a causal relationship between severe exposure to mustard and the development of delayed recurrent keratitis exists.[47] The study also found a causal relationship between exposure to mustard and the development of prolonged, intractable conjunctivitis.

Scarring of Epithelial Surfaces

Residual cutaneous lesions most often take the form of scars that result from uncontrolled fibroblastic activity and overgrowth of connective tissue during the process of wound repair. Even wounds that are well cared for on joints and sites that are not easily immobilized, such as shoulders, knees, elbows, and male genitalia, often heal with severe residual scar formation. Pigmentation is often altered (either increased or decreased) at these sites, although the degree of alteration does not differ from that observed in injuries caused by burns and other forms of physical and chemical insult. In the absence of melanocyte destruction, hyperpigmentation predominates. If melanocytes are locally destroyed, and inward migration from destroyed adnexal structures does not occur, depigmentation predominates. In a prospective study of delayed toxic effects from mustard exposure, Balali-Mood[22] followed a group of Iranian solders exposed to mustard gas during the Iran–Iraq War. After 2 years, 41% of the exposed victims were experiencing pigmentary disorders. Any previously injured sites have been described as being "sensitive" to subsequent mechanical injury. These sites may show recurrent blisters after mild injury.[19] Renshaw[12] reported on the development of contact sensitivity in humans following localized exposure to liquid mustard. Cutaneous sensitivity may be seen within 8 days following the first application, and a more pronounced effect is seen after 4 weeks. The incidence of hypersensitivity varies between 30% and 65% of exposed individuals. Sensitivity may be immediate hives or delayed dermatitis and appears to last a lifetime. Sensitivity may also take the form of flares of old, healed mustard injury sites after a fresh application of mustard to normal, unaffected skin.[12] The occurrence of skin cancers at the site of old scar formation is an acknowledged biological phenomenon.[53,54] Cutaneous cancers resulting from acute mustard exposure usually localize in scars, whereas those caused by chronic exposure can occur on any exposed site.[55]

In its study of mustard and lewisite effects,[19] the Institute of Medicine concluded that the evidence indicates a causal relation between acute, severe exposure to mustard agents and increased pigmentation and depigmentation in human skin; acute and severe exposure can lead to chronic skin ulceration, scar formation, and the development of cutaneous cancer (but see the caveat in the previous discussion of this report's conclusions); and chronic exposure to minimally toxic and even subtoxic doses can lead to skin pigmentation abnormalities and cutaneous cancer. Among the Iranian victims at 16 to 20 years after exposure, the most common skin lesions, by order of occurrence, were hyperpigmentation, erythematous popular rash, dry skin, multiple cherry angioma, atrophy, and hyperpigmentation.[27]

Central Nervous System

Excitation of the CNS after mustard exposure, resulting in convulsions and followed by CNS depression, has been reported.[56] Convulsions and cardiac irregularities appear to occur only after extremely acute, high doses,[57] which are probably attainable only in laboratory settings.[6] Mustard casualties of the Iran–Iraq War did not display severe CNS or cardiac abnormalities.[40]

Acute neuropsychiatric symptoms, including severe depression and changes in mentation, are common after high-dose exposures to mustard agents. These symptoms are produced both directly by the chemical and secondarily to other physiological changes.[19] Follow-up of workers in German chemical warfare plants showed a high prevalence of various neurological disorders, including impaired concentration, diminished libido, and sensory hypersensitivity.[58] To what extent mustard agents were responsible is not clear because multiple exposures to other agents, including nerve agents, were known to have occurred.

Balali-Mood et al[23] conducted studies on peripheral neuropathic processes in victims exhibiting severe late manifestations of mustard poisoning using electromyography and nerve conduction velocity. Seventy percent of the patients demonstrated disturbances in the peripheral nervous system. Nerve conduction abnormalities were more common in sensory nerves and more prevalent in lower extremities than in upper extremities. Forty percent of the patients exhibited incomplete interference patterns in electromyographic studies.

Mutagenesis, Teratogenesis, and Reproductive Toxicity

Mustard causes cross-linking of DNA and is known to alkylate DNA at the O^6 position of guanine. Some authors[59,60] suggest that intrastrand DNA cross-links, rather than interstrand cross-links,[61,62] are the lesions primarily responsible for producing chromosomal aberrations. Mustard causes chromosomal breakage and induces sister chromatid exchanges in a wide variety of cells including mammalian cells.[63] The International Agency for Research on Cancer in Lyon, France (an agency of the World Health Organization), has classified mustard as a human carcinogen based on the findings of epidemiological studies. Taken together, these observations highlight the potential of this compound to induce genetic damage and become a long-term health hazard. The agency also suggests that mustard could be a reproductive toxin.[19]

The 1993 Institute of Medicine report[19] noted that the quality of human data on the reproductive toxicity of mustard is quite poor. Follow-up of the occupational or battlefield cohorts to determine the nature of any reproductive toxicity or teratogenic effects attributable to these exposures has been insufficient. The evidence suggests a causal relationship between mustard exposure and reproductive toxicity in laboratory animals, but the database is far too small and unreliable to allow a clear understanding of human reproductive risk from exposure to mustard. Mustard can cause genetic alterations in the sperm of male rats after inhalation or gastric exposure, but rodent studies[64] showed that mustards are not detectable teratogens in animals. The human data are insufficient for reliable interpretation.[19]

NERVE AGENTS

Nerve agents are esters of phosphonic acid and are extremely potent chemicals. Their military designations are GA (tabun), GB (sarin), GD (soman), GF (cyclosarin), and VX. The agent VX has no common name. In contrast to the information available on both short- and long-term effects of mustard in humans from its battlefield use in World War I and the Iran–Iraq War, and from experimental studies during the World War I and World War II periods,[19] limited data from the battlefield use of nerve agents are available.

The toxic effects of nerve agents are caused primarily by their inhibition of acetylcholinesterase (AChE) and the resulting accumulation of acetylcholine.[65] Other biological activities of these agents have been described, but the relation of these activities to clinical effects has not been recognized. For example, some nerve agents affect ionic channels,[66] and all affect structures other than AChE.[67] Several milligrams of VX, the least volatile nerve agent, absorbed through the skin causes clinical signs and symptoms.[68,69] A *Ct* of 2 to 3 mg•min/m^3 of sarin produces miosis and rhinorrhea in humans.[70] This *Ct* can be attained with exposure to a concentration of 2 mg/m^3 for 1 minute or a concentration of 0.05 mg/m^3 for 40 minutes. The initial signs of exposure to small quantities of agent vapor are miosis, rhinorrhea, and airway constriction.[7,71] Larger amounts cause loss of consciousness, seizure activity,[71] cessation of respiration[72] and cardiac activity, and death, unless there is medical intervention. Effects occur within minutes of exposure,[71,72] and after a large exposure (*Ct* of 10–200 mg•min/m^3, depending on the agent[73]), death occurs in 10 to 15 minutes. After exposure to a sublethal amount on the skin (1–3 mg), the onset time for clinical effects may be hours.[68,69] The initial effect is usually vomiting, which may be followed by muscular weakness. A lethal amount of VX on the skin causes effects within several minutes,[71] and death occurs shortly afterwards.

Treatment consists of the administration of atropine, a drug that blocks the effects of the excess acetylcholine at muscarinic cholinergic receptor sites, and of 2-pyridine aldoxime methyl chloride (2-PAM Cl, also called 2-pralidoxime chloride), an oxime that removes the agent from AChE, thereby reactivating the enzyme after poisoning by some agents.[74] 2-PAM Cl, however, is ineffective against soman intoxication[71] because of soman's rapid aging. (Aging is the process by which one of the nerve agent's alkyl groups leaves the molecule after binding to AChE. After dealkylation, an AChE-bound nerve agent molecule can no longer be removed from the enzyme by an oxime. The aging half-time of soman is about 2 min.) Ventilatory support is necessary when breathing has stopped or is inadequate,[71,72] and the anticonvulsant diazepam may need to be administered.

Information on the effects of nerve agents in humans comes from the accidental exposure of hundreds of people mildly or moderately exposed while working with nerve agents and from a handful of workers who had severe exposures. Investigational studies carried out in hundreds of people also provide information. More recently, terrorists used sarin in two separate attacks in Matsumoto and Tokyo, Japan, in 1994 and 1995. These attacks have provided a great deal of information on both the short- and long-term impact of organophosphorus nerve agents in humans. Information on the effects of organophosphorus insecticides is also included so that medical officers can compare and contrast the two. Because both nerve agents and insecticides are organophosphorus compounds, people often tend to extrapolate the biological effects of one to the other, but in fact there are many differences between the two. The authors of some reports did not recognize the differences and grouped them together.[75,76]

Although the organophosphate insecticides are similar to nerve agents in inhibiting cholinesterase, they differ in other characteristics. For example, the cholinergic crisis caused by acute, severe intoxication with the insecticides is generally much longer than that caused by nerve agents (days to weeks for insecticides[77–79] vs hours for nerve agents[71,72]). Not only do insecticides differ from nerve agents, but they also differ among themselves in some of their biological effects; for example, some cause polyneuropathy, and others do not.[79] Because of these differences, all of which have probably not been defined, the similarity between the effects of insecticides in humans and the effects of nerve agents in humans cannot be assumed. (As stated earlier, insecticides are included here only so that the similarities and differences can be noted; readers should be careful not to confuse the two.)

Polyneuropathy

Insecticides

Organophosphorus ester–induced delayed neurotoxicity (OPIDN) has been recognized as a clinical syndrome in humans and animals for over 50 years. After exposure to certain organophosphates, incoordination, ataxia, spasticity, and flaccid paralysis develop over the following 1 to 3 weeks; the paralysis begins distally in the lower limbs and eventually spreads to the upper limbs. Part or all of the lesion may be reversible, but in its most severe form it can cause lifetime quadriplegia. Structural changes begin at the distal, nonmyelinated portion of the nerve, followed by progressive demyelination associated with degeneration of more proximal nerve segments.[79] This syndrome was initially associated with ingestion of triorthocresyl phosphate rather than an insecticide. After organophosphate insecticides became available, the syndrome was seen after exposure to some, but not all, of them.[79]

The best animal model for studying the effects of exposure to organophosphates is the chicken.[80,81] Extensive studies have been performed to elucidate the mechanism of action that causes OPIDN and to screen new organophosphate insecticides for this effect.[79,80] The exact mechanism of action is still unknown, but much evidence suggests that the inhibition of neurotoxic esterase in nerve tissue is involved.[81] Administration of oximes and atropine has no effect on the production of this neurotoxicity.[82]

OPIDN is not seen with all insecticides.[79,80] Generally, insecticides that have been shown to cause polyneuropathy have been removed from the market; only those that have been demonstrated not to cause this effect in animal models are available.

Nerve Agents

Nerve agents have caused polyneuropathy in animals only at doses many fold greater than the LD^{50} (the dose [D] that is lethal [L] to 50% of the exposed population)—doses that require massive pretreatment and therapy to ensure survival of the animals. Davies et al[83] produced polyneuropathy in chickens with sarin only at 60 or more times the LD^{50}. (The animals were protected with atropine and oxime to permit survival.) Neuropathy was not detected at 8 times the LD^{50} of soman. Davies's group also detected no polyneuropathy at doses of VX of 45 µmol/kg.[84]

In another study,[85] polyneuropathy was found in hens after 30 to 60 times the LD^{50} for sarin was administered, but not at 38 times the LD^{50} for soman or 82 times the LD^{50} for tabun. VX was not examined in this study because its ability to inhibit neurotoxic esterase is negligible. At 120 times the acute LD^{50} in hens, soman and tabun caused polyneuropathy in some surviving animals.[86] Cyclosarin is a stronger inhibitor of neurotoxic esterase in vitro than the other nerve agents.[87] However, cyclosarin, in addition to tabun, soman, and VX, did not cause polyneuropathy at very high doses.[88]

Polyneuropathy has not been noted in the handful of humans severely exposed to nerve agents or in the hundreds of humans with mild-to-moderate effects from nerve agents. However, one report details a case study in which a patient who survived for 15 months following the Tokyo sarin terrorist attack showed distal sensory axonopathy on postmortem analysis.[89] The patient survived the initial attack, but was maintained on mechanical ventilation and total parenteral nutrition until he died of pneumonia. He initially showed signs of tremor and decerebrate rigidity, which changed to flaccid quadriparesis 6 months following the sarin intoxication. He then developed distal-dominant, severe muscle atrophy with clawhand and foot drop deformity. The postmortem analysis confirmed the distal axonopathy as well as severe hypoxic-ischemic CNS damage. Obvious limitations of this report include the fact that the patient was maintained for an extended period with life support and was largely immobile, and there is no information regarding the total sarin exposure the man received. Nevertheless, the case report is one of the first to show temporally delayed distal neuropathy in humans. Studies using smaller doses of tabun, sarin, and soman are described in the toxicology section later in this chapter.

Muscle Necrosis

Insecticides

Necrosis of rat skeletal muscle in the region of the motor endplate has been noted after administration of cholinesterase-inhibiting compounds in amounts sufficient to cause signs.[90] Swelling, eosinophilia, and loss of striations of myofibers can be observed by light microscopy in the motor endplate regions as early as 2 hours after administration of the organophosphate, and the lesion is fully developed in 12 to 24 hours. In affected fibers, the sarcolemma remains intact and is the focus of later repair of the fiber. Recovery begins in 2 days and is complete by 2 weeks. The lesion can be prevented or lessened by denervation or by administration of atropine and oxime within the first 2 hours; the lesion is more severe in muscles of high activity, such as the diaphragm, and in type II fast-twitch muscle fibers.[90]

Muscle necrosis was seen in the diaphragm of a man who died after drinking parathion. No cholinesterase could be demonstrated in the myoneural junctions of any muscle, but necrosis was limited to the diaphragm. Each focus involved one to four sarcomeres of both types of myofibers, varying from acute swelling to vacuolar disintegration of the fibers. The nerve endings in the segmental necrotic zones were degenerated.[91]

Nerve Agents

The circumscribed muscular necrosis seen with insecticides has also been seen after sarin[92,93] and tabun[94] administration to experimental animals. Soman produced necrosis in one study,[95] but not in another.[94] On stimulation of the nerve, the muscle was unable to sustain a tetanic contraction at frequencies of 100 and 200 Hz.[93]

Intermediate Syndrome

Insecticides

A second type of delayed neurological manifestation of organophosphate insecticide poisoning is the "intermediate syndrome." In a series of 200 consecutive cases of organophosphate insecticide poisoning, 36 patients developed a weakness of the proximal muscles of the limbs, cranial nerve weaknesses, bilateral pyramidal tract signs, and areflexia.[96] This disturbance began 12 to 84 hours after hospital admission. In most cases, the cholinergic crisis had resolved, and the 21 patients who survived recovered completely by 96 hours. The lesion was unresponsive to large amounts of atropine; 2-PAM Cl was not available. The authors of the report[96] divided the signs of organophosphate intoxication into two groups, which they called type I and type II. According to these authors, type I signs were muscarinic in nature and were amenable to atropine therapy, whereas type II signs were nicotinic in nature, appeared 12 to 48 hours after exposure, and were resistant to atropine therapy.

Ten additional cases were later described.[97] These patients received atropine (up to 40 mg every 24 h) and 2-PAM Cl (1 g every 12 hour for 24 to 48 h) during the cholinergic-crisis phase. About 24 to 96 hours after poisoning, the 10 patients developed a syndrome that included palsies of cranial nerves III, IV, VI, VII, and X; weakness of the respiratory muscles (four patients required immediate intubation and assisted ventilation at the onset of the syndrome); weakness of the proximal limb muscles; and pyramidal tract signs. Recovery occurred in 5 to 18 days. Electromyography in limb muscles and nerve conduction were normal. Tetanic stimulation of the abductor pollicis brevis showed a marked fade with no posttetanic facilitation. The authors of the report[45] called this condition the "intermediate syndrome," meaning that it is intermediate between the acute cholinergic effects and the later, well-recognized delayed polyneuropathy. Consequently, the term intermediate syndrome, rather than type II signs, has been adopted.

Two additional cases of this syndrome were reported several years later; both patients required ventilatory support during the paralytic phase.[98] In another series, 29 of 90 patients with organophosphate poisoning had the intermediate syndrome.[99] Tetanic fade with no posttetanic facilitation was maximal between days 4 and 6, and the response to electrical stimulation had returned to normal by 8 to 10 days. The author suggested that a neuromuscular junction defect was responsible for the lesion. Other cases have since been reported[100–103] and in some, the weakness or paralysis lasted for days to weeks. Lack of early oxime therapy had been thought to contribute to the development of the syndrome,[104] but it has occurred with adequate amounts of oxime.[100,101,105] The cause of this neuromuscular dysfunction has not been elucidated, nor has an animal model been described. Intermediate syndrome may be related to the myopathy seen at the neuromuscular junction.

Nerve Agents

The occurrence of the intermediate syndrome following nerve agent exposure is not well characterized.[106] In one experiment, single fiber electromyography was used to examine the syndrome in volunteers exposed to a low level of sarin.[107] Significant, albeit small, changes in single fiber electromyography were observed at 3 hours and at 3 days following exposure. However, the electromyographic changes did not accompany clinical neuromuscular symptoms. The small changes observed were resolved when the volunteers were evaluated 2 years later.

Another study examined the delayed neurotoxic effects of repeated sarin inhalation in mice.[108] Female

Swiss mice received repeated whole-body exposure to 5 mg/m^3, 20 minutes daily for 10 days. The mice were evaluated daily for changes in gross behavior, and 4 days following the last exposure, the mice were examined histopathologically. The sarin-exposed mice exhibited muscular weakness in the limbs, twitching, and slight ataxis on the 14th day (4 days after the final exposure), despite clear anti-AChE signs. The histopathology results showed depressed neurotoxic esterase activity in the CNS and platelets, and axonal degeneration was observed in the spinal cord. The time frame of onset of the observed results is consistent with the intermediate syndrome, but could potentially have been OPIDN. The report did not follow mice past the 4th day postexposure, so it is unclear whether the symptoms would have resolved. Overall, there is limited information regarding the occurrence of the intermediate syndrome following nerve agent exposure.

Neuropsychiatric Effects

Many neuropsychiatric problems have been associated with single and repeated exposures to insecticides and nerve agents. In many cases these symptoms were studied shortly after the patients were exposed, and the duration of the problems was not noted. However, several studies examined the effects long after the acute insult. These effects include disturbances in memory, sleep, and vigilance; depression; posttraumatic stress disorder (PTSD); anxiety and irritability; and problems with information processing. In cases of exposure to nerve agents, the traumatic impact of experiencing a chemical warfare attack potentially confounds the evaluation of the long-term health effects of nerve agent exposure alone. Thus, whether caused by the direct effects of the chemical compound or by the event itself, the neuropsychological effects presented will still require attention by the attending clinician.

Insecticides

In 1961 Gershon and Shaw[109] described 16 patients with psychiatric problems who had been exposed to pesticides repeatedly over a 1.5- to 10-year period. Five were schizophrenic, seven were severely depressed, one was in a state of fugue, and all had impairment of memory and concentration. These conditions followed multiple symptomatic exposures to organophosphate insecticides, and the patients recovered within 6 to 12 months after the onset of their signs and symptoms. Because neuropsychiatric sequelae of organophosphate insecticides had not been widely recognized, the authors suggested that these sequelae might be more common than generally thought.

Gershon and Shaw's report was criticized[110,111] because no information on the exposure history was included; because few objective measures, either of mental status or of blood cholinesterase, were used; and because the conditions reported had not been reported in much larger series of patients exposed to organophosphate insecticides. Later studies failed to find evidence of thought disorders after pesticide exposure,[112,113] although diisopropyl fluorophosphate administration aggravated psychosis.[114] Less severe neuropsychiatric manifestations of organophosphate insecticide exposure, occurring either acutely or as sequelae, have been subsequently reported.

Durham et al[115] examined 187 individuals who were routinely involved in pesticide work (eg, crop dusting) for mental alertness. The groups were people with varying degrees of exposure to organic phosphorus pesticides and the control group were persons with no known previous exposure to these materials. The subjects were studied, using a complex reaction time, (*a*) at the time of maximal work with insecticides and (*b*) during "nonexposure" periods. Control subjects were studied at similar times. Both groups, subjects and controls, did better on tests during nonexposure periods, and both groups scored poorer during the higher risk periods. The performance of the exposed subjects improved during and after convalescence. The authors emphasized repeatedly that mental effects were not seen in the absence of clinical signs of poisoning. Problems with memory after insecticide exposure were reported by Gershon and Shaw[109] (the problems resolved 6 to 12 months after the acute exposure) and by Metcalf and Holmes[113] (the patients were studied more than a year after exposure). In the latter study, testing was performed to corroborate the report of memory deficit. Other reports have mentioned memory problems, but they provide few data.

Steenland et al[116] examined 128 agricultural workers who had been previously poisoned with at least one organophosphate pesticide between 1982 and 1990. Subjects were evaluated using a neurological test battery that included assessments of mood, motor speed, sustained visual attention, hand-eye coordination, simple reaction time, coding speed, visual memory, serial digit learning and memory, dexterity, and pursuit aiming. Total results showed consistent and significant impairments in mood scale, sustained visual attention, and coding speed. The researchers further performed a nerve conduction and vibrotactile sensitivity assessment of the same population, observing that nerve conductions were normal, but vibrotactile sensitivity was reduced. Together the results indicated that central and peripheral neurological damage related to organophosphorus pesticide poisoning likely occurred.

Anxiety, irritability, giddiness, tension, and restlessness persisting for months after exposure to insecticides were reported by Namba et al[117] and by Gershon and Shaw.[109] Both studies emphasized that these effects occurred only in patients who had demonstrated symptoms of exposure. Metcalf and Holmes[113] reported similar effects, but did not indicate their duration or the time after exposure that they occurred. Depression has been reported[117] from insecticide exposure immediately following the acute symptomatic exposure, but it did not persist. More prolonged (6 to 12 months) depression has been reported[109] after insecticide exposure. In contrast, Levin et al[112] found no evidence of depression using a structured interview and a depression inventory in asymptomatic workers with histories of chronic exposure. Sleep disturbances, such as excessive dreaming, nightmares, and insomnia, generally of relatively short duration (days to weeks), after insecticide exposure have also been reported.[113,117]

Psychomotor performance has been evaluated after exposure to insecticides. Rowntree et al[114] found that daily administration of an organophosphate compound caused slowness in thought and decreased performance speed. Metcalf and Holmes[113] noted slowed thinking and calculation in patients who had been exposed to insecticides more than a year previously. Difficulties in concentration and vigilance have been reported after insecticide exposure,[109,113,115,117,118] although some of the studies indicate marginal decreases, and others lack objective data (eg, Gershon and Shaw[109]). In all of the cases, the impairment occurred after an episode in which the patient had exhibited symptoms of exposure to the compound.

Tabershaw and Cooper[119] evaluated 87 patients who had been exposed to an organophosphate insecticide more than 3 years previously and who had had persistent complaints for over a 6-month period. The symptoms involved the visual, gastrointestinal, cardiorespiratory, and neuropsychiatric systems. In each instance, the complaint could be attributed to other problems; for example, several cases of visual blurring were due to presbyopia, a case of chronic abdominal pain was due to a peptic ulcer, and in one case, nervousness and tremors were due to chronic alcoholism.

In a more recent study, Rosenstock et al[120] examined 38 patients more than a year after their hospitalization for organophosphate insecticide exposure. Control subjects had also worked with organophosphate insecticides but had not had a symptomatic exposure. The poisoned group did significantly less well than the control group on tests assessing a wide variety of neuropsychological functions, including auditory attention, visual memory, visuomotor speed, sequencing and problem solving, and motor steadiness, reaction, and dexterity.

Nerve Agents

Bowers et al[68] reported that subjects had difficulty with memory for 24 hours after they were given VX, but had no evidence of major thought disorders. Other investigators[65] noted depression acutely after nerve agent exposure, but the depression did not persist. Sleep disturbances were also short-lived.[68,121,122] After exposure to VX, subjects had decreased performance on an arithmetic test, decreased reading comprehension, and decreased ability to play chess.[68] In some instances these performance decrements occurred before other signs of intoxication or in the absence of other signs. Impaired concentration and vigilance have been reported after nerve agent exposure.[121] These effects can persist for several weeks after symptomatic exposure to nerve agents.[123]

A report[122] of 297 cases of accidental exposure to nerve agent among manufacturing workers indicated that about 20% of the individuals had neuropsychiatric effects such as disturbed sleep, disturbance in mood, irritability, nervousness, disturbance in ability to think clearly, absentmindedness, fatigability, and lightheadedness. The duration of these effects was not indicated, but the report noted that supervisors and coworkers detected these effects when the casualties returned to work prematurely.

A single subject, a biochemist exposed to soman, was evaluated at 2 weeks, 4 months, and 6 months after exposure, using a psychiatric interview and a battery of psychological tests.[71] The person had been severely exposed, requiring ventilatory support for about 30 minutes. On initial testing, he had high scores on the hypochondriasis and hysteria scales on the Minnesota Multiphasic Personality Inventory; these improved on later testing. On the initial testing he did poorly on a visual retention task, word association proverbs, and an ink blot test. While taking the tests, he used delaying tactics, had difficulty generating verbal associations, and failed the harder proverbs. Results on the later tests were much improved and indicated full use of his intellectual faculties. In another case, a physician was exposed to sarin and required ventilatory support for more than 3 hours. Although psychiatric and psychological studies were not performed, he returned to work after recovery with no apparent problems.[72]

Although few data on the duration of these neuropsychiatric effects in people exist, evidence suggests that they are relatively short-lived (days or weeks). Because of the nature of their work, people handling nerve agents in manufacturing plants, at depots, or in research and development facilities were relatively few in number, tended to remain in the same job for a long period, and comprised closely knit groups. Most were thoroughly familiar with the effects of nerve agents, and most knew their coworkers very well. If a worker did not seem "right," his coworker or supervisor recognized it.[122] A medical facility dedicated to the treatment of nerve agent casualties, with a staff experienced in this type of injury, was always available; workers were encouraged to use it, and supervisors were instructed to send employees who were not "normal" to the medical facility for evaluation.

One neuropsychiatric disorder that has been reported to persist following the Tokyo incident is PTSD. Soon after the events in the Tokyo subway in 1995, one hospital reported that as many as 60% of patients exhibited symptomatic PTSD up to 6 months after the initial event.[124] Furthermore, 32% of the victims were still feeling fear, 29% displayed insomnia, and 16% had flashbacks of their experience. Still others displayed depression (16%), irritability (16%), and persistent nightmares (10%). A 5-year follow-up of 34 patients involved in the Tokyo incident[125,126] examined serum cholesterol, uric acid, cholinesterase, and PTSD. From this group, eight patients (23%) developed PTSD following the event, and two were diagnosed with the disorder at the time of the assessment. Comorbidity of PTSD with other mental illness, including anxiety, agoraphobia, panic disorders, and severe depression, was also observed in the group that developed the disorder. Although no relationship of PTSD with cholesterol or uric acid was apparent, the disorder had a surprising relationship to serum cholinesterase. Relative to patients who did not develop PTSD, the patients who developed PTSD had lower serum cholinesterase both within 3 days of the attack and 5 years following the event. However, both groups had significantly reduced cholinesterase immediately following the attack versus the 5-year assessment; thus, the relationship of reduced cholinesterase and PTSD is not readily apparent.

Other studies show the development of PTSD with related neuropsychiatric symptoms in sarin-exposed patients following the Tokyo subway incident, but not all showed persistent decreased cholinesterase. A group of 18 male and female sarin patients were neurobehaviorally assessed 6 to 8 months following the terrorist incident.[127] Relative to matched controls, the sarin patients presented with significantly depressed cholinesterase activity at the time of hospital admission that had recovered by the time of the assessment. At the follow-up assessment the sarin patients showed significantly more psychiatric symptoms; fatigue; impaired Wechslar Adult Intelligence Scale digit symbol performance (a measure of motor persistence, sustained attention, response speed, and visuomotor coordination); and extended latencies for P300 auditory event-related and P100 visual brain-evoked potentials related to PTSD. The P300 evoked potential serves as a neural marker of the ability to allocate and sustain attention, and the P100 visual evoked potential is a marker for the conduction time from the retina to the visual cortex.

In summary, studies intended to examine the neuropsychiatric effects of organophosphate compounds vary in their adequacy, and in some instances the results are contradictory. Most studies agree, however, that acute neuropsychiatric effects result from exposure to both insecticides and nerve agents. These effects include inability to concentrate, memory problems, sleep disturbances, anxiety, irritability, depression, problems with information processing and psychomotor tasks, and potentially PTSD. With pesticides, these effects do not occur in the absence of the conventional signs of poisoning. The duration of these effects is less well studied. Some studies suggest that after exposure to insecticides, problems might persist for a year or longer, but supporting data are not always provided. The two reports of patients exposed to nerve agents and personal observation suggest that these effects are of shorter duration in this class of compounds.

Electroencephalographic Abnormalities

Insecticides and Other Organophosphates

Electroencephalographic abnormalities were reported in subjects given daily doses of diisopropyl fluorophosphate for 2 to 7 days.[128] These abnormalities consisted of faster frequencies, higher voltages, and occasional bursts of slow waves of high voltage at 3 to 6 Hz. Their severity was directly related to the degree of initial cholinesterase inhibition. The changes persisted for 3 to 4 weeks. Changes were noted in the electroencephalograms (EEGs) of 50 industrial and agricultural workers within 72 hours of accidental exposure to insecticides (both organophosphate and chlorinated hydrocarbons, on separate occasions), although the relationship to work history, blood cholinesterase, and exposure type, duration, and severity were not mentioned.[113]

Nerve Agents

In a patient severely intoxicated with sarin, an EEG (taken after the loss of consciousness but before the onset of convulsions) showed marked slowing, with bursts of high-voltage slow waves at 5 Hz in the temporofrontal leads. These abnormalities persisted for 6 days, after which no residual effects were noted.[121]

Because of the reports on insecticides and concern for employees working with or in the vicinity of nerve agents, the US government sponsored a series of studies[129–132] on the long-term effects of sarin exposure as seen in EEG examinations. In the first study, monkeys were dosed with sarin in one of two dose schedules: (1) a single large dose that produced convulsions or (2) a series of 10 weekly doses that caused no clinical effects. In the second study, workers who had had at least one documented exposure to sarin (signs, cholinesterase depression) more than a year before the study were evaluated. Control subjects were coworkers who had no possibility of organophosphate exposure.

In the nonhuman primates, animals from both dose schedules had increases in high-frequency beta activity a year after exposure. Spectral analysis of the EEGs of the humans showed increased beta activity in the sarin-exposed population compared to the control population. Visual reading of the records suggested decreased amounts of alpha and increased amounts of slow delta and theta activity in the exposed group. Increased amounts of rapid-eye movement sleep in the exposed group were also found. Individual records could not be categorized. The investigators noted that the relationship between these changes and alterations in brain function was not known.

Toxicological Studies on Nerve Agents

The effects of exposure to nerve agents on a chronic or subchronic basis were reported in two studies on animals. In a two-part, 90-day study[133,134] of subchronic exposure, rats were given one of three doses of tabun or soman 5 days per week by gavage. At the end of the study, no abnormalities were found on gross or histological examination of tissue. In a study[135] of chronic exposure to sarin, dogs received a C*t* of 10 mg•min/m^3 of sarin over a 6-month period. Some animals were dosed 5 days per week, and some were dosed 7 days per week. No tissue abnormalities that could be attributed to the agent were noted on gross or microscopic examination. Several of the male animals were bred after the exposure and the pups were normal. In studies[136–139] in which tabun, sarin, and soman were given to hens in single or multiple doses, in amounts maximally tolerated with the coadministration of atropine, no evidence of polyneuropathy was noted clinically or on microscopic examination.

Sarin and soman were deemed not mutagenic after they were studied using Ames *Salmonella*, mouse lymphoma, and Chinese hamster ovary cell systems.[140] Tabun was found to be weakly mutagenic in the mouse lymphoma cell test,[141] Chinese hamster ovary system,[142] and Ames bacterial system.[143]

CYANIDE

Cyanide is a lethal poison that can produce death within 10 minutes. Cyanide compounds are used extensively in industry and are present in the environment from many sources. Humans can be exposed to cyanide by ingestion, inhalation, or injection. However, humans produce minute quantities of cyanide for normal metabolic processes and also possess a limited capability to detoxify ingested or inhaled cyanide. This review of cyanide long-term effects differentiates the long-term outcomes of a high-level acute exposure as compared to a long-term exposure.

Physiology

Cyanide is a potent inhibitor of aerobic metabolism through interruption of oxygen binding within mitochondrial cytochrome oxidase. Tissues that depend greatly on aerobic respiration, such as cardiac muscle and nerve tissue, are most affected. Besides these effects and those on many other enzymes, cyanide is also cardiotoxic and neurotoxic.[144] Much of the CNS toxicity of cyanide appears to be related to direct toxicity on neurons with glutamic acid receptors. Cyanide-induced striatal degeneration is mediated by short-term, high-level exposures affecting *N*-methyl D-aspartate glutamate receptors.[145] Neuronal degeneration based upon long-term exposure to cyanide and its metabolites appears to be mediated through α-amino-3-hydroxy-5-methyl-isoxazole-4-propionic acid glutamate receptors.[146]

Cyanide detoxification is extensively reviewed in Chapter 11, Cyanide Poisoning, though it is important to note that the primary biological means of detoxification is the conversion of cyanide to thiocyanate through a sulphurtransferase reaction followed by urinary excretion.

Long-Term Effects of an Acute Insult

Outcomes of severe cyanide intoxications are highly variable. Many victims of moderate to severe exposures who recover have no sequelae. For others, the outcome often is a factor of timely diagnosis and effective treatment.

A chemical company that produces large quantities of cyanide for plastic manufacturing reported the results of eleven cyanide inhalations and two cutaneous exposures. The cases varied in severity of symptoms from headache and dizziness to death (although only one person died, and this individual was in extremis when found). All individuals in the report who had vital signs at the time of discovery recovered. Most of the victims inhaled cyanide fumes for 30 to 90 seconds and became unconscious with irregular respirations or apnea. All these patients received supportive care of bagged oxygen and amyl nitrite within 5 minutes. One surviving patient required intravenous antidotes as well as amyl nitrite, and the rest recovered with amyl nitrite and artificial ventilation alone. Nearly all the patients recovered quickly, and some were even sent back to work after a few hours of observation. No long-term effects were reported. These cases demonstrate the efficacy of simple field treatment if implemented within a few minutes of exposure. It is noteworthy that patients who remained conscious after inhalation of cyanide recovered with supplemental oxygen and no antidotes.[147]

Medical reports from severe ingestions include various outcomes. Many patients responded to treatment and experienced complete recovery. Other outcomes were difficult to discern because the patients may have developed global deficits from prolonged hypoxia. In some severe casualties, a distinct pattern of neurological impairment occurred. The basal ganglia appeared to be particularly vulnerable to insult from cyanide, with frequent involvement of the globus pallidus and putamen.[148] Symptoms reported were parkinsonian, with bradykinesia, shuffling gait, rigidity, and other symptoms resembling a generalized dystonia. Cognitive function sometimes remained intact.[149] In all cases with long term sequelae, the patients experienced significant delays of 30 minutes to hours before antidote administration. (There are several excellent case examples in Chapter 11, Cyanide Poisoning.)

Long-Term Exposure

Long-term exposure to cyanide contributes to a number of conditions, although the different diseases usually have several features in common. First, they are primarily neurological diseases. Second, they involved prolonged exposures to cyanide-containing food or medication. Third, those affected tend to subsist on a monotonous diet with insufficient protein.

The most common dietary exposure is bitter cassava root, *Manihot esculenta* Crantz, which is widely consumed in the tropics and sub-Saharan Africa, where it ranks fourth in nutritional importance after rice, wheat, and maize. Cassava is a staple during times of famine because it can grow in poor soil and climate conditions. Cassava's cyanogenicity confers immunity to pests. Procedures such as prolonged soaking, smashing, or boiling are necessary to remove cyanogenic compounds such as linamarin. Fresh cassava roots can contain up to 1,500 mg hydrogen cyanide equivalent per kilogram.[145] Acute intoxications, even death, have resulted from consumption of raw cassava, though long-term exposures from incompletely processed cassava are more likely.

Konzo ("tied legs") is a form of spastic paraparesis found among poor rural populations of central and east Africa who primarily consume cassava. It affects individuals of all ages. Konzo is symmetrical, isolated, and permanent. It is associated with sensations of heaviness and weakness in legs that can cause the inability to stand. It is often present in entire families and varies in severity from a mild toe-scissor gait, to requiring a walking stick, and to the point where walking is not possible. Those at risk for konzo have ankle clonus and lower extremity hyperreflexia.[150] Konzo is also associated with optic neuropathy.[151] Individuals with konzo are noted to have very high levels of urinary thiocyanate. They are also protein deficient, with a great deal of ingested amino acid sulphur diverting to cyanide detoxification.[152] Linamarin has been identified as a specific toxic factor in this disease. It is also thought that overwhelmed detoxification mechanisms and an abrupt increase in metabolites over their chronic levels lead to the sudden clinical presentation of konzo.[153]

Tropical ataxic neuropathy is a distinct cyanide-related disease with several other names that is classically associated with prisoners of war or middle-aged and elderly persons in southwestern Nigeria. It is a polyneuropathy associated with bilateral optic atrophy, bilateral neurosensory deafness, and sensory gait ataxia. This condition was widespread in Nigeria until an improved diet resulting from the 1970s oil boom relegated this condition to rural areas.[154] Tropical ataxic neuropathy is a gradual onset, permanent condition associated thiocyanate, cyanate, and a monotonous cassava diet.[155]

Smokers are known to have blood cyanide levels significantly higher than the nonsmoking population.[156] Tobacco amblyopia is caused by chronic cyanide levels sometimes coupled with malnutrition and alcoholism. Symptoms are loss of color perception and decreased vision, which is often recoverable after discontinuation of smoking or even administration of cyanide antidotes. This once-common syndrome has become rare in the United States.[157]

Another cyanide-related disorder is Leber hereditary optic neuropathy (LHON). LHON, first described in 1871, is a maternally inherited disease of highly variable penetrance that impairs oxidative phosphorylation. LHON is the model disease for mutations of the mitrochondrial genome. The disease is heteroplasmic, usually requiring more than 60% mutant genes for symptoms to present. Patients with LHON are normal until the sudden onset of blindness between the ages of 15 and 35.[158] The stressor leading to cell death of the highly aerobic optic nerve is the elevated blood cyanide level associated with smoking and the associated blood cyanide level.[159]

Given the likely acute high-level exposure expected in a military environment, it is reasonable to ask whether cyanide exposure can lead to blindness in some individuals. This is theoretically possible in the small fragment of the population with LHON mutations, although no cases have been reported. There is only one case of blindness from acute cyanide poisoning in the literature, a temporary case caused by a sodium nitroprusside overdose.[160]

Cyanide can also be responsible for some cases of goiter. Elevated levels of thiocyanate as well as thyroid abnormalities have been documented in individuals on cyanogenic food diets and those in industries with chronic exposures such as electroplating.[161] Thiocyanate prevents uptake of iodine into the thyroid gland.[162]

Patients with chronic renal failure who smoke have been known to develop a condition known as uremic neuropathy, a result of the accumulation of thiocyanate, the major detoxification metabolite of cyanide. In these patients, thiocyanate cannot be removed from the body, even with dialysis. Treatment involves administration of hydroxocobalamin antidote, which uses a different chemical pathway.[163]

Several conditions were previously thought to be associated with cyanide, including lathyrism, a neurological disorder associated with grass pea ingestion. Subacute combined degeneration of the spinal cord, attributed to cyanide in the past, is now well known to be related to vitamin B12 metabolism.

In summary, the long-term effects of cyanide exposure are highly variable. Severe exposures and cases with delayed treatment may manifest in a Parkinsonian akinetic syndrome. Long-term exposure to cyanide is likely in areas where cassava is the staple food and represents a likely risk to future prisoners of war in these areas. Long-term cyanide exposure combined with poor protein intake leads to neuromotor and neurosensory disorders. Smoking represents a chronic cyanide exposure that may lead to permanent blindness in rare individuals. Most importantly, the majority of cyanide-exposed individuals who receive prompt treatment may expect no long-term sequelae following an acute cyanide exposure. This fact emphasizes the importance of prompt casualty care.

TOXIC INHALATION INJURY

The pulmonary agents are absorbed almost exclusively by inhalation. They readily penetrate to the level of the respiratory bronchioles and alveoli, that is, to the peripheral compartment of the respiratory tree. However, most of these agents are essentially consumed by reactions occurring at the alveolar-capillary membrane, or more proximally in the respiratory tract, and are not systemically distributed to a clinically significant extent.

Inhalation of selected organohalides, oxides of nitrogen, and other compounds can result in varying degrees of pulmonary edema, usually after a symptom-free period that varies in duration with the amount inhaled. Chemically induced acute lung injury by these agents involves a permeability defect in the blood–air barrier (the alveolar-capillary membrane); however, the precise mechanisms of toxicity remain an enigma. The United States produces over a billion pounds of phosgene per year for industrial uses; however, it is not stockpiled for military use.

Perfluoroisobutylene (PFIB) is a toxic pyrolysis product of tetrafluoroethylene polymers encountered in military materiel (eg, Teflon [DuPont, Wilmington, Del] found in the interior of many military vehicles). The oxides of nitrogen are components of blast weapons or may be toxic decomposition products. Smokes (eg, HC) contain toxic compounds that cause the same effects as phosgene.[164] The long-term health effects of phosgene exposure also apply to casualties from agents such as PFIB and oxides of nitrogen.[165]

Phosgene

Phosgene produces pulmonary edema following a clinical latent period of variable length that depends primarily on the intensity of exposure (ie, the C*t*), but also partly on the physical activity of the exposed individual. After the latent period, the patient experiences worsening respiratory distress that at first is unaccompanied by objectively verifiable signs of pulmonary damage, but may progress relentlessly to pulmonary edema and death.

During the time preceding the appearance of shortness of breath, individuals exposed to particularly high concentrations of organohalides may report symptoms associated with mucous membrane irritation. Exposure to large quantities of phosgene may irritate moist mucous membranes, presumably because of the generation of hydrochloric acid from the hydrolysis of phosgene. Transient burning sensation in the eyes with lacrimation and chemical conjunctivitis may coexist with mild, early onset cough and a substernal ache with a sensation of pressure. Irritation of the larynx by very large concentrations of the agent may lead to sudden laryngeal spasm and death.

A clinical latent period during which the patient is asymptomatic may follow low C*t* exposure or the transient irritation associated with substantial phosgene exposure. This asymptomatic period may persist up to 24 hours after organohalide inhalation. The duration of the latent period is shorter following a high dose and is shortened by physical exertion following exposure.

The most prominent symptom following the clinical latent period is dyspnea, perceived as shortness of breath, with or without chest tightness. These sensations reflect hypoxemia, increased ventilatory drive, and decreased lung compliance, all of which result from the accumulation of fluid in the pulmonary interstitial and peripheral airways. Fine crackles can be heard at the lung bases, but these may not be clearly audible unless auscultation is conducted after a forced expiration. Later, auscultation reveals coarse crackles and rales in all lung fields, and increasing quantities of thin, watery secretions are noted. The buildup of fluid in the lungs has two clinically pertinent effects. First, developing pulmonary edema interferes with oxygen delivery to alveolar capillaries and may lead to hypoxemia, and if a sufficient percentage of hemoglobin is unoxygenated, cyanosis will become apparent. Second, the sequestration of plasma-derived fluid (up to 1 L per hour) in the lungs may lead to hypovolemia and hypotension, interfering with oxygen delivery to the brain, kidneys, and other crucial organs. Death results from respiratory failure, hypoxemia, hypovolemia, or a combination of these factors. Hypoxia and hypotension may progress particularly rapidly, which suggests a poor prognosis. The development of symptoms and signs of pulmonary edema within 4 hours of exposure is an especially accurate indicator of a poor prognosis; in the absence of immediately available intensive medical support, such patients are at high risk of death. Complications include infection of damaged lungs and delayed deaths following such respiratory infections.[164] Several studies sponsored by the Veterans Administration using animals and humans reported that after phosgene exposure pulmonary edema appeared very early.[166]

In July 1920, Winternitz's[167] report on experimental work with dogs revealed acute changes in the cardiorespiratory system following exposure to lethal concentrations of phosgene. The upper portion of the respiratory tract was not affected, but the alveoli of the lungs and the finer bronchi gave evidence of congestion, inflammation, and edema. The inflammatory reaction following phosgene exposure resulted in congestion of the bronchial and spread into the surrounding air cells, indicative of an early bronchopneumonia with a marked edema of the lungs. Dilatation, reflex bronchiolar spasm, and plugging of the bronchiols with exudates led to patches of atelectasis and emphysema. A substantial amount of fibrin on alveolar walls, crossing and obstructing the capillaries, led to resistance in the pulmonary circulation, with a consequent dilatation of the right heart. In the dogs, damage occurred principally in the respiratory tract, and lesions varied according to the length of survival after the exposure. Initial pulmonary edema associated with congestion reached a maximum intensity toward the end of the first 24 hours and gradually disappeared in animals surviving 10 days or longer. With the edema, there was an associated inflammatory exudation of fibrin and leucocytes. This cellular exudate was found especially in the finer bronchioles and extended into the alveolar tissue. It was suggestive of a lobular pneumonia. The pneumonia was frequently complicated by necrotization of the walls of the bronchioles, which also involved the adjacent alveoli and resulted in abscess formation. In some cases, although the inflammatory process was succesesfully overcome, an obliterative bronchiolitis resulted.

In the exposed dogs, the pathology was localized to the trachea and bronchi. The epithelium of the trachea and larger bronchi was damaged, while the smaller bronchi and bronchioles were the most seriously affected. In addition to changes in the mucosa, there were contractions, distortions of the bronchioles, and more or less obliteration of the lumina. All this led to mechanical disturbance in the air sacs, with resting atelectasis and emphysema.

The Veterans Administration conducted a study reviewing the histories of 10 veterans who had been gassed with phosgene and showed evidence of physical effects a number of years later.[166] This historical study revealed that chronic bronchitis was the most frequent long-term effect noted. Emphysema was noted in three of the veterans, pulmonary fibrosis was noted in two, chronic-active pulmonary tuberculosis was found in one case, and bronchial asthma was found in another. This study also revealed that the symptoms of the pulmonary disabilities were observed immediately after the phosgene gas exposure and continued to be the causative factor the long-term pulmonary effects at the time of the study.[166]

According to the Veterans Administration, the following pathological changes were noted in soldiers who died following phosgene gas exposure[166]:

- Pulmonary edema, usually very marked, occurred. The pleural cavities generally contained an excess of fluid.
- The lungs, upon removal from the thorax, were voluminous, heavy, and bluish-red in color; occasionally, petechial hemorrhages and alternating patches of emphysema and collapsed lung tissue were noted.
- Section of lungs showed an exudation of frothy fluid from the cut surface.
- Irregular, alternating areas of edema and acute emphysema were noted.
- The trachea, bronchi, and bronchiole were generally filled with thin, yellowish, serosanguineous fluid.
- There was little or no inflammatory change in the larynx, trachea, and bronchi.
- The veins were engorged.
- The heart, especially on the right side, was dilated.
- Petechial hemorrhages were often found beneath the endocardium.
- The pericardial fluid increased in amount.
- The abdominal viscera showed the presence of generalized venous engorgement and congestion.
- The meninges of the brain were congested.

Methyl Isocyanate

In December 1984, in Bhopal, India, a massive leak of methyl isocyanate resulted from operational and equipment malfunctions in a pesticide plant. Many thousands of residents of the city, most in proximity to the plant, suffered sublethal and lethal respiratory injuries, the expected consequences of high-level exposure to this type of potent irritant chemical vapor. Animal toxicological information was limited prior to the accident, but has since confirmed that the lung is the major target of these lethal injuries, invariably with pulmonary edema. Early concerns about acute cyanide intoxication were not supported by subsequent scientific inquiry. Superficial corneal erosions did not result in permanent eye injury. The primary unresolved (and perhaps irresolvable) medical issue is the incidence and determinants of long-term respiratory injury in the survivors. Limited available evidence suggests that chronic damage, when present, is or resembles fibrosing bronchiolitis obliterans, the expected consequence when permanent injury results from acute, high-level irritant gas exposure. Definition of the follow-up population is uncertain, and exposure information is lacking. Dose-response relationships are not likely to emerge from follow-up studies.[168]

Perfluoroisobutylene

PFIB primarily affects the peripheral compartment of the pulmonary system. Although animal studies occasionally report disseminated intravascular coagulation and other organ involvement, these effects only occur with substantial pulmonary injury to the peripheral compartment of the pulmonary system, suggesting that systemic hypoxia is a major factor.[169] No human studies have reported organ involvement other than the respiratory system. Pathological data on acute human exposure to PFIB are not available; however, pathological data on animals show both histological and ultramicroscopic changes occurring within 5 minutes of exposure.[170] Interstitial edema with alveolar fibrin deposition progresses rapidly over 24 hours, and then gradually subsides until the patient is fully recovered. At 72 hours, a type II pneumocyte hyperplasia is seen (interpreted as consistent with known reparative processes). Some long-term pathological changes in animals have been noted but most animal studies do not identify such long-term effects.[171] Human long-term pathological data are available for only one reported case: a 50-year-old woman who experienced approximately 40 episodes of polymer fume fever—typically occurring from smoking contaminated cigarettes. Eighteen months after her last episode, progressive exercise dyspnea was noted. A cardiopulmonary physical examination, chest radiograph, and arterial blood gas were all normal. Pulmonary function testing supported a provisional diagnosis of alveolar capillary block syndrome (decreased diffusion capacity of carbon monoxide, increased exercise alveolar-arterial oxygen gradient, and minimal airway disease). Death occurred from an unrelated cause. The autopsy provided histological evidence of moderate interstitial fibrosis with minimal chronic inflammatory cell infiltrate.[172] Only two human deaths from pyrolysis products of polymerized organofluorides have been reported.[173,174]

Oxides of Nitrogen

Inhalation of nitric oxide causes the formation of methemoglobin. Inhalation of nitrogen dioxide results in the formation of nitrite, which leads to a fall in blood pressure, production of methemoglobin, and cellular hypoxia, which causes rapid onset pulmonary edema.

The clinical response to oxides of nitrogen exposure is essentially triphasic. In phase 1, symptoms appear more or less quickly, depending on the intensity of exposure. With a low dose, initial eye irritation, throat tightness, chest tightness, cough, and mild nausea may appear. Once the casualty is removed from the source of exposure, these symptoms disappear spontaneously over the next 24 hours. However, at 24 to 36 hours postexposure, a particularly severe respiratory symptom complex may appear suddenly; exertion seems to be a prominent precipitating factor. There may be severe cough, dyspnea, and rapid onset of pulmonary edema. If the patient survives this stage, spontaneous remission occurs within 48 to 72 hours postexposure. More intense exposures produce a relatively rapid onset of acute bronchiolitis with severe cough, dyspnea, and weakness, without the above-mentioned latent period. Again, spontaneous remission occurs at approximately 3 to 4 days postexposure.[175]

Phase 2 is a relatively asymptomatic period lasting approximately 2 to 5 weeks. A mild residual cough with malaise and perhaps minimal shortness of breath may occur, as well as a sense of weakness that may progress. The chest radiograph, however, typically is clear. In phase 3, symptoms may recur 3 to 6 weeks after the initial exposure. Severe cough, fever, chills, dyspnea, and cyanosis may develop. Crackles are identified on physical examination of the lung. The polymorphonuclear white blood cell count is elevated, and the partial pressure of carbon dioxide may be elevated as well.[176] The chest radiograph demonstrates diffuse, scattered, fluffy nodules of various sizes, which may become confluent progressively, with a butterfly pulmonary edema pattern and a prominent acinar component. At this point, pathological study demonstrates classic bronchiolitis fibrosis obliterans, which may clear spontaneously or may progress to severe, occasionally lethal respiratory failure. The fluffy nodular changes noted in the chest radiograph typically show no clinical improvement. Pulmonary function testing may show long-term persistence of airways obstruction.[177–179]

Zinc Oxide

Hexachloroethane (HC) smoke, a mixture of equal amounts of HC and zinc oxide with additional ingredients, is a toxic military smoke and obscurant. HC's toxicity is attributed to the irritating effects of zinc chloride. Most likely, carbon monoxide, phosgene, hexachloroethane, and other products contribute to the observed respiratory effects. The damage to the pulmonary system is confined largely to the upper respiratory tract, where zinc chloride acts much like a corrosive irritant. Studies reveal that HC exposure can produce a gradual decrease in total lung capacity, vital capacity, and diffusion capacity of carbon monoxide. HC is associated with the presence of pulmonary edema, increased airway resistance, and decreased compliance. When HC smoke exposure is discontinued, the pulmonary changes are reversible in all but 10% to 20% of those effected, who could develop pulmonary fibrotic changes.[180]

In a study by Conner et al[181] performed with guinea pigs, exposure to ultrafine HC particles (0.05 μm) in increasing degrees was associated with a dose-response elevation in protein, neutrophils, and angiotensin-converting enzyme found in lavage fluid. A direct relationship also was observed with alkaline phosphatase, acid phosphatase, and lactate dehydrogenase in lavage fluid. Centriacinar inflammation was seen histologically, indicating evidence of pulmonary damage. A study by Marrs et al[182] involving mice, rats, and guinea pigs demonstrated a positive association of alveologenic carcinoma in a dose-response trend to HC smoke, as well as a variety of inflammatory changes. The article states that hexachloroethane and zinc, as well as carbon tetrachloride (which may be present in HC smoke), may be animal carcinogens in certain circumstances. This raises the suspicion of HC as a potential carcinogen.

Metal fume fever is a well-documented acute disease induced by intense inhalation of metal oxides, especially zinc oxide. The exact pathology is not understood, but the clinical syndrome is well described and has been studied at length. A study by Kuschner et al[183] on human volunteers showed that pulmonary cytokines such as tumor necrosis factor, interleukin 6, and interleukin 8 may play important initial roles in mediating metal fume fever. Prolonged exposures or exposures to very high doses of HC may result in sudden early collapse and death, possible as a result of laryngeal edema or glottal spasm. If severe exposure does not kill the individual immediately, hemorrhagic ulceration of the upper airway may occur, with paroxysmal cough and bloody secretions. Death may occur within hours secondary to an acute tracheobronchitis.

Most individuals with HC inhalation injuries progress to complete recovery. Of exposed individuals, 10% to 20% develop fibrotic pulmonary changes. Distinguishing between those who will recover and those who will not is difficult, because both groups make an early clinical recovery.

SUMMARY

A wide variety of chemical agents and industrial products are associated with long-term health consequences after an acute insult. Others are known to be harmful with prolonged low-level exposure. The linkage between these associations is sometimes tenuous given the limitations of retrospective studies and case reports up to 90 years old. Research laboratory efforts and future case reports will continue to strengthen the understanding of these effects. In the meantime, the existing knowledge base provides clinicians sufficient reason to monitor for these possible outcomes and apply proactive surveillance to individuals working with these chemicals on a daily basis.

REFERENCES

1. Prentiss AM. *Chemicals in War: A Treatise on Chemical Warfare*. New York, NY: McGraw-Hill; 1937: 653.

2. Robinson JP. *The Rise of CB Weapons*. Vol 1. In: *The Problem of Chemical and Biological Warfare*. New York, NY: Humanities Press; 1971.

3. United Nations Security Council. *Report of Specialists Appointed by the Secretary General to Investigate Allegations by the Islamic Republic of Iran Concerning the Use of Chemical Weapons*. New York, NY: United Nations; 1984. UN Report S/16433.

4. Wade JV, Gum RM, Dunn MA. Medical chemical defense in Operations Desert Shield and Desert Storm. *J US Army Med Dept*. 1992;1/2:34–36.

5. Sidell FR. The medical management of chemical casualty course in CONUS and Europe during Desert Storm. *J US Army Med Dept*. 1992;3/4:10–12.

6. Papirmeister B, Feister AJ, Robinson SI, Ford RD. *Medical Defense Against Mustard Gas: Toxic Mechanisms and Pharmacological Implications*. Boca Raton, Fla: CRC Press; 1991.

7. Sidell FR. Clinical considerations in nerve agent intoxication. In: Somani SM, ed. *Chemical Warfare Agents*. San Diego, Calif: Academic Press; 1992: 156–194.

8. Balali-Mood M, Navaeian A. Clinical and paraclinical findings in 233 patients with sulfur mustard poisoning. In: *Proceedings of the 2nd World Congress on New Compounds in Biological and Chemical Warfare: Toxicological Evaluation, Industrial Chemical Disasters, Civil Protection and Treatment, 24–27 August 1986*. Ghent, Belgium: International Association of Forensic Toxicologists; 1986: 464–473.

9. Warthin AS, Weller CV. The lesions of the respiratory and gastrointestinal tract produced by mustard gas (dichlorethyl sulphide). *J Lab Clin Med*. 1919;4:229–264.

10. Sohrabpour H. Clinical manifestations of chemical agents on Iranian combatants during the Iran–Iraq conflict. In: Heyndrickx A, ed. *Proceedings of the 1st World Congress on New Compounds in Biological and Chemical Warfare: Toxicological Evaluation, 21–23 May 1984*. Ghent, Belgium: State University of Ghent; 1984: 291–297.

11. Vedder EB, ed. *The Medical Aspects of Chemical Warfare*. Baltimore, Md: Williams & Wilkins; 1925.

12. Renshaw B. Mechanisms in production of cutaneous injuries by sulfur and nitrogen mustards. In: *Chemical Warfare Agents and Related Chemical Problems*. Parts 3–6. Washington, DC: Office of Scientific Research and Development, National Defense Research Committee, Div 9; 1946: 478–520.

13. Reed CI. The minimum concentration of dichlorethylsulphide (mustard gas) effective for the eyes of man. *J Pharmacol Exp Ther*. 1920;15:77–80.

14. Morgenstern P, Koss FR, Alexander WW. Residual mustard gas bronchitis: effects of prolonged exposure to low concentrations of mustard gas. *Ann Intern Med*. 1947;26:27–40.

15. Buscher H. *Green and Yellow Cross*. Conway N, trans. Cincinnati, Ohio: Kettering Laboratory of Applied Physiology, University of Cincinnati; 1944.

16. Prokes J, Svovoda V, Hynie I, Proksova M, Keel K. The influence of x-radiation and mustard gas on methionin-35S incorporation in erythrocytes. *Neoplasma*. 1968;15:393–398.

17. Manning KP, Skegg DC, Stell PM, Doll R. Cancer of the larynx and other occupational hazards of mustard gas workers. *Clin Otolaryngol Allied Sci*. 1981;6:165–170.

18. Heston WE. Induction of pulmonary tumors in strain A mice with methyl-bis (beta-chloroethyl)amine hydrochloride. *J Natl Cancer Inst*. 1949;10:125–130.

19. Pechura CM, Rall DP, eds. *Veterans at Risk: The Health Effects of Mustard Gas and Lewisite*. Washington, DC: National Academy Press; 1993.

20. Afshinniaz F, Ghanei M. *Relationship of the Chronic Respiratory Symptoms With Spirometric and Laboratory Parameters* [dissertation]. Isfahan, Iran: Isfahan University of Medical Sciences; 1996.

21. Balali M. The evaluation of late toxic effects of sulfur mustard poisoning in 1428 Iranian veterans. In: *Proceedings of the Seminar on Late Complications of Chemical Warfare Agents in Iranian Veterans.* Tehran, Iran: Veteran Foundation; 1992: 15–37.

22. Balali-Mood M. First report of delayed toxic effect of Yperite poisoning in Iranian fighters. In: *Proceedings of the 2nd World Congress on New Compounds in Biological and Chemical Warfare: Toxicological Evaluation, Industrial Chemical Disasters, Civil Protection and Treatment, 24–27 August 1986*. Ghent, Belgium: International Association of Forensic Toxicologists; 1986: 489–495.

23. Balali-Mood M, Hefazi M, Mahmoudi M, et al. Long term complications of sulfur mustard poisoning in severely intoxicated Iranian veterans. *Fundam Clin. Pharmacol.* 2005;19:713–721.

24. Ghanei M, Vosoghi AA. An epidemiologic study to screen for chronic myelocytic leukemia in war victims exposed to mustard gas. *Environ Health Prespect.* 2002;110:519–521.

25. Hefazi M, Attaran D, Mahmoudi M, Balali-Mood M. Late respiratory complications of mustard gas poisoning in Iranian veterans. *Inhal Toxicol.* 2005;17:587–592.

26. Khateri S, Ghanei M, Soroush M, Haines D. Incidence of lung, eye and skin lesions as late complications in 34,000 Iranians with wartime exposure to mustard agent. *J Occ Environ Med.* 2003; 452:1136–1143.

27. Balali-Mood M, Hefazi M. Comparison of early and late toxic effects of sulfur mustard in Iranian veterans. *Basic Clin Parma Toxicol.* 2006;99:273–282.

28. Heston WE. Carcinogenic action of the mustards. *J Natl Cancer Inst*. 1950;11:415–423.

29. Heston WE. Occurrence of tumors in mice injected subcutaneously with sulfur mustard and nitrogen mustard. *J Natl Cancer Inst*. 1953;14:131–140.

30. McNamara BP, Owens EJ, Christensen MK, Vocci FJ, Ford DF, Rozimarek H. *Toxicological Basis for Controlling Levels of Mustard in the Environment*. Aberdeen Proving Ground, Md: Edgewood Arsenal Biomedical Laboratory; 1975. EB-SP-74030.

31. Case RAM, Lea AJ. Mustard gas poisoning, chronic bronchitis, and lung cancer: an investigation into the possibility that poisoning by mustard gas in the 1914–1918 war might be a factor in the production of neoplasia. *Br J Prev Soc Med*. 1955;9:62–72.

32. Norman JR Jr. Lung cancer mortality in World War I veterans with mustard-gas injury: 1919–1965. *J Natl Cancer Inst*. 1975;54:311–317.

33. Fletcher C, Peto R, Tinker C, Speizer FE. *The Natural History of Chronic Bronchitis and Emphysema*. Oxford, England: Oxford University Press; 1976.

34. Wada S, Miyanishi M, Nashimoto Y, Kambe S, Miller RW. Mustard gas as a cause of respiratory neoplasia in man. *Lancet*. 1968;1:1161–1163.

35. Easton DF, Peto J, Doll R. Cancers of the respiratory tract in mustard gas workers. *Br J Ind Med*. 1988;45:652–659.

36. Minoue R, Shizushiri S. Occupationally-related lung cancer—cancer of the respiratory tract as sequentia from poison gas plants. *Jpn J Thorac Dis*. 1980;18:845–859.

37. Albro PW, Fishbein L. Gas chromatography of sulfur mustard and its analogs. *J Chromatogr*. 1970;46:202–203.

38. Yanagida J, Hozawa S, Ishioka S, et al. Somatic mutation in peripheral lymphocytes of former workers at the Okunojima poison gas factory. *Jpn J Cancer Res*. 1988;79:1276–1283.

39. Watson AP, Jones TD, Grinnin GD. Sulfur mustard as a carcinogen: application of relative potency analysis to the chemical warfare agents H, HD, and HT. *Regul Toxicol Pharmacol*. 1989;10:1–25.

40. Willems JL. Clinical management of mustard gas casualties. *Ann Med Milit Belg*. 1989;3(suppl):1–61.

41. Urbanetti JS. Battlefield chemical inhalation injury. In: Loke J, ed. *Pathophysiology and Treatment of Inhalation Injuries*. New York, NY: Marcel Dekker; 1988.

42. Balali M. Clinical and laboratory findings in Iranian fighters with chemical gas poisoning. In: Heyndrickx B, ed. *Proceedings of the 1st World Congress on New Compounds in Biological and Chemical Warfare: Toxicological Evaluation, 21–23 May 1984*. Ghent, Belgium: State University of Ghent; 1984: 254–259.

43. Freitag L, Firusian N, Stamatis G, Greschuchna D. The role of bronchoscopy in pulmonary complications due to mustard gas inhalation. *Chest*. 1991;100:1436–1441.

44. Gilchrist HL. *A Comparative Study of World War Casualties From Gas and Other Weapons*. Edgewood Arsenal, Md: US Chemical Warfare School; 1928.

45. Beebe GW. Lung cancer in World War I veterans: possible relation to mustard-gas injury and 1918 influenza epidemic. *J Natl Cancer Inst*. 1960;25:1231–1252.

46. Winternitz MC. Anatomical changes in the respiratory tract initiated by irritating gases. *Milit Surg*. 1919;44:476–493.

47. Rimm WR, Bahn CF. Vesicant injury to the eye. In: *Proceedings of the Vesicant Workshop, February 1987*. Aberdeen Proving Ground, Md: US Army Medical Research Institute of Chemical Defense; 1987.

48. Hughes WF Jr. Mustard gas injuries to the eyes. *Arch Ophthalmol*. 1942;27:582–601.

49. Blodi FC. Mustard gas keratopathy. *Int Ophthalmol Clin*. 1971;2:1–13.

50. Duke-Elder S, MacFaul PA. Chemical injuries. In: Duke-Elder S, MacFaul PA, eds. *Injuries*. Vol 14. In: Duke-Elder S, MacFaul PA, eds, *System of Ophthalmology*. St. Louis, Mo: CV Mosby; 1972.

51. Duke-Elder WS, MacFaul PA, eds. *System of Ophthalmology*. St. Louis, Mo: CV Mosby; 1958–1976.

52. Otto CE. *A Preliminary Report on the Ocular Action of Dichlorethyl Sulfide (Mustard Gas) in Man as Seen at Edgewood Arsenal*, Edgewood, Maryland. Edgewood Arsenal, Md: Chemical Warfare Service; 1946. EAL 539.

53. Novick M, Gard DH, Hardy SB, Spira M. Burn scar carcinoma: a review and analysis of 46 cases. *J Trauma*. 1977;17:809–817.

54. Treves N, Pack GT. Development of cancer in burn scars: analysis and report of 34 cases. *Surg Gynecol Obstet*. 1930;51:749–782.

55. Inada S, Hiragun K, Seo K, Yamura T. Multiple Bowen's disease observed in former workers of a poison gas factory in Japan with special reference to mustard gas exposure. *J Dermatol*. 1978;5:49–60.

56. US Army, US Navy, and US Air Force. Vesicants (blister agents). Section I—Mustard and nitrogen mustard. In: *NATO Handbook on the Medical Aspects of NBC Defensive Operations*. Washington, DC: US Army, US Navy, US Air Force; 1973. AMedP-6.

57. Anslow WP, Houch CR. Systemic pharmacology and pathology of sulfur and nitrogen mustards. In: *Chemical Warfare Agents and Related Chemical Problems*. Washington, DC: Office of Scientific Research and Development; 1946.

58. Lohs K. *Delayed Toxic Effects of Chemical Warfare Agents*. Stockholm, Sweden: Almqvist & Wilksell; 1979. SIPRI monograph.

59. Lawley PD, Lethbridge JH, Edwards PA, Shooter KV. Inactivation of bacteriophage T7 by mono- and difunctional sulphur mustards in relation to crosslinking and depurination of bacteriophage DNA. *J Mol Biol*. 1969;39:181–198.

60. Flamm WG, Bernheim NJ, Fishbein L. On the existence of intrastrand crosslinks in DNA alkylated with sulfur mustard. *Biochim Biophys Acta*. 1970;224:657–659.

61. Fox M, Scott D. The genetic toxicology of nitrogen and sulphur mustard. *Mutat Res*. 1980;75:131–168.

62. Scott D, Fox M, Fox BW. The relationship between chromosomal aberrations, survival and DNA repair in tumor cell lines of differential sensitivity to X-rays and sulphur mustard. *Mutat Res*. 1974;22:207–221.

63. Wulf HC, Aasted A, Darre E, Neibuhr E. Sister chromatid exchanges in fishermen exposed to leaking mustard gas shells. *Lancet*. 1985;1:690–691.

64. Sasser LB, Miller RA, Kalkwarf DR, Buschbom RL, Cushing JA. *Toxicology Studies on Lewisite and Sulfur Mustard Agents: Two-Generation Reproduction Study of Sulfur Mustard (HD) in Rats*. Richland, Wash: Pacific Northwest Laboratory; 1989.

65. Taylor P. Anticholinesterase agents. In: Hardman JG, Limbird LE, Gilman AG, eds. *The Pharmacological Basis of Therapeutics*. New York, NY: Pergamon Press; 2001: 175–193.

66. Albuquerque EX, Akaike A, Shaw KP, Rickett DL. The interaction of anticholinesterase agents with the acetylcholine receptor–ionic channel complex. *Fundam Appl Toxicol*. 1984;4:S27–S33.

67. O'Neill JJ. Non-cholinesterase effects of anticholinesterases. *Fundam Appl Toxicol*. 1981;1:154–169.

68. Bowers MB, Goodman E, Sim VM. Some behavioral changes in man following anticholinesterase administration. *J Nerv Ment Dis*. 1964;138:383–389.

69. Craig FN, Cummings EG, Sim VM. Environmental temperature and the percutaneous absorption of a cholinesterase inhibitor, VX. *J Invest Dermatol*. 1977;68:357–361.

70. Johns RJ. *The Effects of Low Concentrations of GB on the Human Eye*. Edgewood Arsenal, Md: Medical Research Laboratory; 1952. MRL Report 100.

71. Sidell FR. Soman and sarin: clinical manifestations and treatment of accidental poisoning by organophosphates. *Clin Toxicol*. 1974;7:1–17.

72. Ward JR. Exposure to a nerve gas. In: Whittenberger JL, ed. *Artificial Respiration: Theory and Applications*. New York, NY: Harper & Row; 1962: 258–265.

73. Program Executive Officer–Program Manager of Chemical Demilitarization. *Chemical Stockpile Disposal Program Final Programmatic Environmental Impact Statement*. Aberdeen Proving Ground, Md: Program Executive Officer–Program Manager of Chemical Demilitarization; 1988: B-23–B-25.

74. Sidell FR, Groff WA. The reactivatibility of cholinesterase inhibited by VX and sarin in man. *Toxicol Appl Pharmacol*. 1974;27:241–252.

75. Boskovic B, Kusic R. Long-term effects of acute exposure to nerve gases upon human health. In: *Chemical Weapons: Destruction and Conversion*. New York, NY: Crane, Russak; 1980: 113–116.

76. Fullerton CS, Ursano RJ. Behavioral and psychological responses to chemical and biological warfare. *Mil Med*. 1990;155:54–59.

77. Chew LS, Chee KT, Yeeo JM, Jayaratnam FJ. Continuous atropine infusion in the management of organophosphorus insecticide poisoning. *Singapore Med J.* 1971;12:80–85.

78. LeBlanc FN, Benson BE, Gilg AD. A severe organophosphate poisoning requiring the use of an atropine drip. *Clin Toxicol.* 1986;24:69–76.

79. Metcalf RL. Historical perspective of organophosphorus ester-induced delayed neurotoxicity. In: Cranmer JM, Hixson EJ, eds. *Delayed Neurotoxicity.* Little Rock, Ark: Intox Press; 1984: 7–23.

80. Takade DY. Delayed neurotoxicity in perspective: summary and objectives of the workshop. In: Cranmer JM, Hixson EJ, eds. *Delayed Neurotoxicity.* Little Rock, Ark: Intox Press; 1984: 2–6.

81. Johnson MK. Organophosphorus esters causing delayed neurotoxic effects. *Arch Toxicol.* 1975;34:259–288.

82. Davies DR, Holland P. Effect of oximes and atropine upon the development of delayed neurotoxic signs in chickens following poisoning by DFP and sarin. *Biochem Pharmacol.* 1972;21:3145–3151.

83. Davies DR, Holland P, Rumens MJ. The relationship between the chemical structure and neurotoxicity of alkyl organophosphorus compounds. *Brit J Pharmacol.* 1960;15:271–278.

84. Davies, et al Cited in: Gordon JJ, Inns RH, Johnson MK, et al. The delayed neuropathic effects of nerve agents and some other organophosphorus compounds. *Arch Toxicol.* 1983;52(3):71–81.

85. Gordon JJ, Inns RH, Johnson MK, et al. The delayed neuropathic effects of nerve agents and some other organophosphorus compounds. *Arch Toxicol.* 1983;52(3):71–81.

86. Willems JL, Nicaise M, De Bisschop HC. Delayed neuropathy by the organophosphorus nerve agents soman and tabun. *Arch Toxicol.* 1984;55:76–77.

87. Vranken MA, DeBisschop HC, Willems JL. "In vitro" inhibition of neurotoxic esterase by organophosphorus nerve agents. *Arch Int Pharmacodyn.* 1982;260:316–318.

88. Willems JL, Palate BM, Vranken MA, DeBisschop HC. Delayed neuropathy by organophosphorus nerve agents. In: *Proceedings of the International Symposium on Protection Against Chemical Warfare Agents, Stockholm, Sweden, 6–9 June 1983.* Umea, Sweden: National Defence Research Institute; 1983.

89. Himuro K, Murayama S, Nishiyama K, et al. Distal sensory axonopathy after sarin intoxication. *Neurology.* 1998;51(4):1195–1197.

90. Hayes WJ Jr. Organic phosphorus pesticides. In: *Pesticides Studied in Man.* Baltimore, Md: Williams & Wilkins; 1982: 294.

91. DeReuck J, Willems J. Acute parathion poisoning: myopathic changes in the diaphragm. *J Neurol.* 1975;208:309–314.

92. Meshul CK, Boyne AF, Deshpande SS, Albuquerque EX. Comparison of the ultrastructural myopathy induced by anticholinesterase agents at the end plates of rat soleus and extensor muscles. *Exp Neurol.* 1985;89:96–114.

93. Kawabuchi M, Boyne AF, Deshpande SS, Albuquerque EX. The reversible carbamate (–) physostigmine reduced the size of synaptic end plate lesions induced by sarin, an irreversible organophosphate. *Toxicol Appl Pharmacol.* 1989;97:98–106.

94. Ariens AT, Meeter E, Wolthuis OL, van Benthem RMJ. Reversible necrosis at the end-plate region in striated muscles of the rat poisoned with cholinesterase inhibitors. *Experientia.* 1969;25:57–59.

95. Dettbarn W. Pesticide induced muscle necrosis: mechanisms and prevention. *Fundam Appl Toxicol.* 1984;4:S18–S26.

96. Wadia RS, Sadagopan C, Amin RB, Sardesai HV. Neurological manifestations of organophosphorous insecticide poisoning. *J Neurol Neurosurg Psychiatry.* 1974;37:841–847.

97. Senanayake N, Karalliedde L. Neurotoxic effects of organophosphorus insecticides. *N Engl J Med*. 1987;316:761–763.

98. Karademir M, Erturk F, Kocak R. Two cases of organophosphate poisoning with development of intermediate syndrome. *Hum Exp Toxicol*. 1990;9:187–189.

99. Nadarajah B. Intermediate syndrome of organophosphorus insecticide poisoning: a neurophysiological study. *Neurology*. 1991;41(suppl 1):251.

100. DeBleecker J, Willems J, Neucker KVD, DeReuck J, Vogelaers D. Prolonged toxicity with intermediate syndrome after combined parathion and methyl parathion poisoning. *Clin Toxicol*. 1992;30:333–345.

101. DeBleecker J, Neucker KVD, Willems J. The intermediate syndrome in organophosphate poisoning: presentation of a case and review of the literature. *Clin Toxicol*. 1992;30:321–329.

102. Perron R, Johnson BB. Insecticide poisoning. *N Engl J Med*. 1969; 281:274–275.

103. Gadoth N, Fisher A. Late onset of neuromuscular block in organophosphorus poisoning. *Ann Intern Med*. 1978;88:654–655.

104. Benson B. Is the intermediate syndrome in organophosphate poisoning the result of insufficient oxime therapy? *Clin Toxicol*. 1992;30:347–349.

105. Haddad LM. Organophosphate poisoning—intermediate syndrome? *Clin Toxicol*. 1992;30:331–332.

106. Brown M, Brix K. Review of health consequences from high-, intermediate- and low-level exposure to organophosphorus nerve agents. *J Appl Toxicol*. 1998;18,393–408.

107. Baker DJ, Segwick EM. Single fibre electromyographic changes in man after organophosphate exposure. *Hum Exp Toxicol*. 1996;15:369–375.

108. Husain K, Vijayaraghavan R, Pant SC, Raza SK, Pandey KS. Delayed neurotoxic effect of sarin in mice after repeated inhalation exposure. *J Appl Toxicol*. 1993;13(2):143–145.

109. Gershon S, Shaw FH. Psychiatric sequelae of chronic exposure to organophosphorus insecticides. *Lancet*. 1961;1:1371–1374.

110. Bidstrup PL. Psychiatric sequelae of chronic exposure to organophosphorus insecticides. *Lancet*. 1961;2:103. Letter.

111. Biskind MS. Psychiatric manifestations from insecticide exposure. *JAMA*. 1972;220:1248. Letter.

112. Levin HS, Rodnitzky RL, Mick DL. Anxiety associated with exposure to organophosphate compounds. *Arch Gen Psychiatry*. 1976;33:225–228.

113. Metcalf DR, Holmes JH. EEG, psychological, and neurological alterations in humans with organophosphorus exposure. *Ann N Y Acad Sci*. 1969;160:357–365.

114. Rowntree DW, Nevin S, Wilson A. The effects of diisopropylfluorophosphate in schizophrenic and manic depressive psychosis. *J Neurol Neurosurg Psychiatry*. 1950;13:47–62.

115. Durham WF, Wolfe HR, Quinby GE. Organophosphorus insecticides and mental alertness. *Arch Environ Health*. 1965;10:55–66.

116. Steenland K, Jenkins B, Ames RG, O'Malley M, Chrislip D, Russo J. Chronic neurological sequelae to organophosphate pesticide poisoning. *Am J Public Health*. 1994;84:731–736.

117. Namba T, Nolte CT, Jackrel J, Grob D. Poisoning due to organophosphate insecticides. *Am J Med*. 1971;50:475.

118. Dille JR, Smith PW. Central nervous system effects of chronic exposure to organophosphate insecticides. *Aerospace Med*. 1964;35:475–478.

119. Tabershaw IR, Cooper WC. Sequelae of acute organic phosphate poisoning. *J Occup Med*. 1966;8:5–20.

120. Rosenstock L, Keifer M, Daniell WE, McConnell R, Claypoole K. Chronic central nervous system effects of acute organophosphate pesticide intoxication. *Lancet*. 1991;338:223–227.

121. Grob D. The manifestations and treatment of poisoning due to nerve gas and other organic phosphate anticholinesterase compounds. *Arch Intern Med*. 1956;98:221–239.

122. Gaon MD, Werne J. *Report of a Study of Mild Exposures to GB at Rocky Mountain Arsenal*. Rocky Mountain Arsenal, Colo: US Army Medical Department; nd.

123. Sidell FR. Formerly, Chief, Chemical Casualty Care Office, US Army Medical Research Institute of Chemical Disease. Personal observations, 1994

124. Ohbu S, Yamashina A, Takasu N, et al. Sarin poisoning on Tokyo subway. *South Med J*. 1997;90(6);587–593.

125. Tochigi M, Umekage T, Otani T, et al. Serum cholesterol, uric acid and cholinesterase in victims of the Tokyo subway sarin poisoning: a relation with post-traumatic stress disorder. *Neurosci Res*. 2002;44: 267–272.

126. Tochigi M, Otani T, Yamasue H, et al. Support for relationship between serum cholinesterase and post-traumatic stress disorder; 5-year follow-ups of victims of the Toyko subway sarin poisoning. *Neurosci Res*. 2005;52:129–131.

127. Yokoyama K, Araki S, Murata K, et al. Chronic neurobehavioral effects of Tokyo subway sarin poisoning in relation to posttraumatic stress disorder. *Arch Environ Health*. 1998;53:249–256.

128. Grob D, Harvey AM, Langworthy OR, Lillienthal JL. The administration of di-isopropyl fluorophosphate (DFP) to man. *Bull Johns Hopkins Hosp*. 1947; 31:257.

129. Duffy FH, Burchfiel JL. Long term effects of the organophosphate sarin on EEGs in monkeys and humans. *Neurotoxicol*. 1980;1:667–689.

130. Duffy FH, Burchfiel JL, Bartels PH, Gaon M, Sim VM. Long-term effects of an organophosphate upon the human electroencephalogram. *Toxicol Appl Pharmacol*. 1979;47:161–176.

131. Burchfiel JL, Duffy FH. Organophosphate neurotoxicity: chronic effects of sarin on the electroencephalogram of monkey and man. *Neurobehav Toxicol Teratol*. 1982;4:767–778.

132. Burchfiel JL, Duffy FH, Sim V. Persistent effect of sarin and dieldrin upon the primate electroencephalogram. *Toxicol Appl Pharmacol*. 1976;35:365–379.

133. Bucci TJ, Parker RM, Crowell JA, Thurman JD, Gosnell PA. *Toxicity Studies on Agent GA (Phase II): 90 Day Subchronic Study of GA (Tabun) in CD Rats*. Jefferson, Ark: National Center for Toxicological Research; 1992.

134. Bucci TJ, Parker RM, Gosnell PA. *Toxicity Studies on Agents GB and GD (Phase II): 90-Day Subchronic Study of GD (Soman) in CD-Rats*. Jefferson, Ark: National Center for Toxicological Research; 1992.

135. Jacobson KH, Christensen MK, DeArmon IA, Oberst FW. Studies of chronic exposures of dogs to GB (isopropyl methylphosphono-fluoridate) vapor. *Arch Indust Health*. 1959;19:5–10.

136. Bucci TJ, Parker RM, Cosnell PA. *Toxicity Studies on Agents GB and GD (Phase II): Delayed Neuropathy Study of Sarin, Type I, in SPF White Leghorn Chickens*. Jefferson, Ark: National Center for Toxicological Research; 1992.

137. Bucci TJ, Parker RM, Gosnell PA. *Toxicity Studies on Agents GB and GD (Phase II): Delayed Neuropathy Study of Sarin, Type II, in SPF White Leghorn Chickens*. Jefferson, Ark: National Center for Toxicological Research; 1992.

138. Henderson JD, Higgins RJ, Rosenblatt L, Wilson BW. *Toxicity Studies on Agent GA: Delayed Neurotoxicity—Acute and Repeated Exposures of GA (Tabun)*. Davis, Calif: University of California Davis Lab for Energy; 1989.

139. Bucci TJ, Parker RM, Gosnell PA. *Toxicity Studies on Agents GB and GD.* Jefferson, Ark: National Center for Toxiological Research; 1992.

140. Goldman M, Klein AK, Kawakami TG, Rosenblatt LS. *Toxicity Studies on Agents GB and GD.* Davis, Calif: University of California Davis Laboratory for Energy; 1987.

141. Kawakami TG, Goldman M, Rosenblatt L, Wilson BW. *Toxicity Studies in Agent GA: Mutagenicity of Agent GA (Tabun) in the Mouse Lymphoma Assay.* Davis, Calif: University of California Davis Laboratory for Energy; 1989.

142. Nasr M, Cone N, Kawakami TG, Goldman M, Rosenblatt L. *Toxicity Studies on Agent GA: Mutagenicity of Agent GA (Tabun) in the In Vitro Cytogenetic Sister Chromatid Exchange Test Phase I.* Davis, Calif: University of California Davis Laboratory for Energy; 1988.

143. Goldman M, Nasr M, Cone N, Rosenblatt LS, Wilson BW. *Toxicity Studies on Agent GA: Mutagenicity of Tabun (GA) in the Ames Mutagenicity Assay.* Davis, Calif: University of California Davis Laboratory for Energy; 1989.

144. Baskin SI. Cardiac effects of cyanide. In: Ballantyne B, Marrs TC, eds. *Clinical and Experimental Toxicology of Cyanide.* Bristol, United Kingdom: Wright; 1987:138–155.

145. Patel MN, Tim GK, Isom GE. N-methyl-D-aspartate receptors mediate cyanide-induced cytotoxicity in hippocampal cultures. *Neurotoxicology.* 1983;14:35–40.

146. Spencer PS. Food toxins, AMPA receptors and motor neuron diseases. *Drug Metab Rev.* 1999;31(3):561–587.

147. Wurzburg H. Treatment of cyanide poisoning in an industrial setting. *Vet Hum Toxicol.* 1996;38(1):44–47.

148. Rachinger J, Fellner FA, Stieglbauer K, Trenkler J. MR changes after acute cyanide ingestion. *AJNR Am J Neuroradiol.* 2002;23:1398–1401.

149. Borgohain R, Singh AK, Radhakrishna H, Rao VC, Mohandas S. Delayed onset generalized dystonia after cyanide poisoning. *Clin Neurol Neurosurg.* 1995;97:213–215.

150. Cliff J, Nicala D, Saute F, et al. Ankle clonus and thiocyanate, linamarin, and inorganic sulphate excretion in school children in communities with Konzo, Mozambique. *J Trop Pediatr.* 1999; 45(3):139–142.

151. Mwanza JC, Tshala-Katumbay D, Kayembe DL, Eeg-Olofsson KE, Tylleskar T. Neuro-opthalmologic findings in konzo, an upper motor neuron disorder in Africa. *EurJ Ophthalmol.* 2003;13(4):383–389.

152. Tylleskar T, Banea M, Bikangi N, Cooke RD, Poulter NH, Rosling H. Cassava cyanogens and konzo, an upper motoneuron disease found in Africa. *Lancet.* 1992;339(8787):208–211.

153. Banea-Mayambu JP, Tylleskar T, Gitebo N, Matadi N, Gebre-Medhin M, Rosling H. Geographical and seasonal association between linamarin and cyanide exposure from cassava and the upper motor neurone disease konzo in former Zaire. *Trop Med Int Health.* 1997;2(12):1143–1151.

154. Oluwole OS, Onabolu A O, Link H, Rosling H. Persistence of tropical ataxic neuropathy in a Nigerian community. *J Neurol Neurosurg Psychiatry.* 2000;69:96–101.

155. Tor-Agbidye J, Palmer VS, Lasarev MR, et al. Bioactivation of cyanide to cyanate in sulfur amino acid deficiency: relevance to neurological disease in humans subsisting on cassava. *Toxicol Sci.* 1999;50:228–235.

156. Lundquist P, Rosling H, Sorbo B, Tibbling L. Cyanide concentrations in blood after cigarette smoking, as determined by a sensitive fluorimetric method. *Clin Chem.* 1987;33(7): 1228–1230.

157. Mackey D, Howell N. Tobacco amblyopia. *Am J Ophthalmol.* 1994;117(6):817–819.

158. Brown MD, Voljavec AS, allot MT, MacDonald I, Wallace DC. Leber's hereditary optic neuropathy: a model for mitochondrial neurodegenerative diseases. *FASEB J.* 1992;6:2791–2799.

159. Tsao K, Aitken P, Johns DR. Smoking as an aetiological factor in the pedigree with Leber's hereditary optic neuropathy. *Br J Ophthalmol.* 1999;83:577–581.

160. Olgunturk R, Yener A, Tunaoglu FS, Gokgoz L, Aslamci S. Temporary blindness due to sodium nitroprusside overdosage in a postoperative patient: an unusual adverse effect. *Clin Pediatr (Phila).* 1992; 31(6):380–381.

161. El-Ghawabi SH, Gaafar Ma, El-Saharti AA, Ahmed SH, Malash KK, Fares R. Chronic cyanide exposure: a clinical, radioisotope, and laboratory study. *Br J Ind Med.*1975;32(3):215–219.

162. Erdogan MF. Thiocyanate overload and thyroid disease. *BioFactors* 2003;19:107–111.

163. Koyama K, Yoshida A, Takeda A, Morozumi K, Fujinami T, Tanaka N. Abnormal cyanide metabolism in uraemic patients. *Nephro Dial Transplant.* 1997;12:1622–1628.

164. US Army Medical Research Institute of Chemical Defense, Chemical Casualty Care Office. *Medical Management of Chemical Casualties Handbook.* 2nd ed. Aberdeen Proving Ground, Md: USAMRICD; 1995.

165. US Army Medical Research Institute of Chemical Defense, Chemical Casualty Care Office. *Medical Management of Chemical Casualties Handbook.* 3rd ed. Aberdeen Proving Ground, Md: USAMRICD; 2000.

166. Gilchrist HL, Matz PB. The residual effects of warfare gases: the use of phosgene gas, with report of cases. *Med Bull Veterans Admin.* 1933;10:1–37.

167. Winternitz MC. *Pathology of War Gas Poisoning*. Yale University Press, New Haven, 1920.

168. Weill H. Disaster at Bhopal: the accident, early findings and respiratory health outlook in those injured. *Bull Eur Physiopathol Respir.* 1987;23:587–590.

169. Akbar-Khanzadeh F. Short-term respiratory function changes in relation to work shift welding fumes exposures. *Int Arch Occup Environ Health.* 1993;64:393–397.

170. Nold JB, Petrali JP, Wall HG, Moore DH. Progressive pulmonary pathology of two organofluorine compounds in rats. *Inhalation Toxicol*. 1991;3:12

171. Karpov BD. Establishment of upper and lower toxicity parameters of perfluroisobutylene toxicity. *Tr Lenig Sanit-Gig Med Inst*. 1977;111:30–33.

172. Williams N, Atkinson W, Patchefsky AS. Polymer-fume fever: not so benign. *J Occup Med*. 1974;16:519–522.

173. Auclair F, Baudot P, Beiler D, Limasset JC. Minor and fatal complications due to treating polytetrafluoroethylene in an industrial environment: clinical observations and physiochemical measurement of the polluted atmosphere [in French]. *Toxicol Eur Res*. 1983;5(1):43–48.

174. Makulova ID. Clinical picture of acute poisoning with perflurosebutylene. *Gig Tr Prof Zabol*. 1965;9:20–23.

175. Ramirez RJ. The first death from nitrogen dioxide fumes. *JAMA*. 1974;229:1181–1182.

176. Lowry T, Schuman LM. Silo-filler's disease. *JAMA*. 1956;162:153–155.

177. Ramirez RJ, Dowell AR. Silo-filler's disease: nitrogen dioxide–induced lung injury. *Ann Intern Med*. 1971;74:569–576.

178. Becklake MR, Goldman HI, Bosman AR, Freed CC. The long-term effects of exposure to nitrous fumes. *Am Rev Tuberc*. 1957;76:398–409.

179. Jones GR, Proudfoot AT, Hall JT. Pulmonary effects of acute exposure to nitrous fumes. *Thorax*. 1973;28:61–65.

180. National Research Council, Committee on Toxicology, Commission on Life Sciences. *Toxicity of Military Smokes and Obscurants*. Vol 1. Washington DC: National Academy Press; 1997.

181. Conner MW, Flood WH, Rogers AE, Amdur MP. Lung injury in guinea pigs caused by multiple exposures to ultrafine zinc oxide: changes in pulmonary lavage fluid. *J Toxicol Environ Health.* 1988; 25(1):57–69.

182. Marrs TC, Colgrave HF, Edginton JA, Brown RF, Cross NL. The repeated dose toxicity of a zinc oxide / hexachloroethane smoke. *Arch Toxicol.* 1988; 62(2-3):123–132.

183. Kuschner WG, D'Alessandro A, Wong H, Blanc PD. Early pulmonary cytokine responses to zinc oxide fume inhalation. *Environ Res.* 1997;75(1):7–11.

Chapter 10

TOXIC INHALATIONAL INJURY AND TOXIC INDUSTRIAL CHEMICALS

SHIRLEY D. TUORINSKY, MSN,* AND ALFRED M. SCIUTO, PHD†

*Lieutenant Colonel, AN, US Army; Executive Officer, Combat Casualty Care Division, US Army Medical Research Institute of Chemical Defense, 3100 Ricketts Point Road, Aberdeen Proving Ground, Maryland 21010-5400

†Research Physiologist, Analytical Toxicology Division, Medical Toxicology Branch, US Army Medical Research Institute of Chemical Defense, 3100 Ricketts Point Road, Aberdeen Proving Ground, Maryland 21010-5400

INTRODUCTION

Toxic industrial chemicals (TICs) are a wide variety of lung-damaging chemical agents used in manufacturing. TICs are commonly found in communities of industrialized nations that manufacture petroleum, textiles, plastics, fertilizers, paper, pesticides, and many other products. These extensively used chemicals are inexpensive; easily acquired; and transported by ship, train, pipeline, and truck, making them an obvious choice for terrorists. The list of these chemicals is extremely long. According to the North Atlantic Treaty Organization, TICs are chemicals at least as poisonous as ammonia that are produced in large quantities. By this definition, TICs could be released in sufficient quantities to produce mass casualties on or off the battlefield.

The toxicity of TICs varies greatly: some are acutely toxic, whereas others have little toxicity. They come in liquid, vapor, and solid form (Table 10-1); the liquid and vapor forms generally lead to the greatest intensity of exposure. A crucial aspect of the medical management of acute toxic inhalational casualties is determining the respiratory system compartment or compartments affected, then treating the compartmental damage, rather than adhering to a specific treatment protocol for each agent. Knowing the identity of the specific TIC released is helpful but not necessary in the medical evaluation of the pulmonary agent casualty, which should concentrate on the location of lung compartment damage. Clinical recognition of damage to the central compartment or the peripheral compartment or both should be enough to guide medical management in the absence of identification of specific chemicals.

Determining the damaged compartment is done on the basis of the chemical's aqueous solubility, chemical reactivity, and dose received. Lung-damaging TICs can cause damage to central or peripheral compartments of the respiratory system. The central compartment of the respiratory system consists of the conducting airways, larynx, trachea, and bronchi. The peripheral compartment consists of the smaller airway, in which gas exchange takes place. Effects of agents that act on the peripheral airway are found in the bronchioles to the alveoli of the respiratory system. Centrally acting TICs normally form strong acids or bases (alkali) with the water in the central airway tissues, which leads to the destruction of these tissues. The damaged tissue swells and may slough into the airway, restricting breathing. Ammonia and sulfur mustard are examples of centrally acting TICs. Peripherally acting chemicals cause life-threatening pulmonary edema. However, both centrally and peripherally acting TICs cause damage in the lungs by inhalation. TICs do not affect the lungs when they are absorbed through the skin, injected, or orally ingested. This chapter will be restricted to those chemical agents with acute local pulmonary effects.

TABLE 10-1

DEFINITIONS OF AIRBORNE TOXIC MATERIAL

Gas	The molecular form of a substance, in which molecules are dispersed widely enough to have little physical effect (attraction) on each other; therefore, there is no definite shape or volume to gas.
Vapor	A term used somewhat interchangeably with gas, vapor specifically refers to the gaseous state of a substance that at normal temperature and pressure would be liquid or solid (mustard vapor or water vapor compared with oxygen gas). Vaporized substances often reliquefy and hence may have a combined inhalational and topical effect.
Mist	The particulate form of a liquid (droplets) suspended in air, often as a result of an explosion or mechanical generation of particles (by a spinning disk generator or sprayer). Particle size is a primary factor in determining the airborne persistence of a mist and the level of its deposition in the respiratory tract.
Fumes, Smokes, and Dusts	Solid particles of various sizes that are suspended in air. The particles may be formed by explosion or mechanical generation or as a by-product of chemical reaction or combustion. Fumes, smokes, and dusts may themselves be toxic or may carry, adsorbed to their surfaces, any of a variety of toxic gaseous substances. As these particles and surfaces collide, adsorbed gases may be liberated and produce local or even systemic toxic injury.
Aerosol	Particles, either liquid or solid, suspended in air. Mists, fumes, smokes, and dusts are all aerosols.

The potential for accidental or deliberate exposure to lung-damaging TICs exists for the military and civilian populations. These industrial chemicals provide effective and readily accessible materials to develop improvised explosives, incendiaries, and poisons.[1] On April 30, 2007, newspapers around the world reported an incident in Ramadi, Iraq, in which insurgents exploded a tanker loaded with chlorine gas, causing many civilian deaths and injuries. This chapter will help to prepare the military medical community to recognize the symptoms of lung-damaging TICs and provide treatment.

HISTORY AND USE

Military Uses

The use of chemical or even biological warfare agents goes back to antiquity. Early agents of choice were smokes, which could be generated from a combustible source and serve as a formidable offensive weapon in favorable wind conditions. The Greeks were known to expose their enemies to concoctions of smoke and flame mixed with sulfur.[2] In 1456 arsenical smokes were used defensively in Belgrade against the Turks.[3] During World War I chemical agents such as phosgene, chlorine, sulfur mustard, diphosgene (trichloromethylchlorformate), diphenylarsine, chloropicrin, and diphenylchloroarsine were used offensively by both the Allies and the Axis to produce mass casualties.

These agents were largely used in some combination for ease of use and to maintain the persistence of the gas on the battlefield to attain the greatest exposure effects. For example, phosgene, the principal nonpersistent gas, had to be cooled in salt brine during the mixing process because of its low boiling point (8°C), so it was combined with either chlorine or diphosgene for more efficient weaponization.[4] Phosgene was the gas of choice because of its well-known toxicity and capacity to produce the most casualties. Battlefield exposure to gas mixtures such as chlorine-phosgene was responsible for approximately 71,000 casualties or about 33% of all casualties entering the hospital; however, phosgene was reportedly directly responsible for only 6,834 casualties and 66 deaths[4] (this contradicts some reports that suggest phosgene alone was responsible for nearly 80% of all gas casualty deaths during 1914–1918[5]). Although the number of fatalities was low, phosgene gassing during the war caused men to lose 311,000 days to hospitalization, equal to 852 person-years.[4] Because chemical warfare agents are used not solely to exterminate the opposition, but also to take soldiers off the battlefield, phosgene was an effective agent. France first weaponized phosgene in 1916, and Germany quickly followed, choosing to combine phosgene with diphosgene because its higher boiling point (128°C) made the concoction easier to pour into shells. Also, diphosgene was believed to break down to phosgene under proper conditions, especially when it reached the lung.[6]

During the latter course of the war, thousands of chemical agent shells were fired by both sides. The largest number of American casualties from one artillery attack occurred at the Battle of the Marne on June 14–15, 1918, when 1,559 soldiers were gassed.[6] Later that year, on August 2, the Germans fired 20,000 shells, which produced 349 casualties, and on August 7 and 8, they used 8,000 to 10,000 gas-filled shells, producing over 800 casualties and 47 deaths.[6] Table 10-2 gives an overview of the chronological use of chemical warfare agents in World War I.

Because of the massive battlefield casualties and the long-term postwar health effects from the chemical weapons in World War I, the Geneva Protocol was established to ban the use of offensive chemicals in war. The ban was neither generally accepted nor adhered to by all countries, and it was not ratified by the United States until 1975. Egypt reportedly used chemical agents in Yemen between 1963 and 1967, and evidence cites the use of CS (tear gas [2-chlorobenzylidene malonitrile]) and Agent Orange (a plant defoliant) by US forces in Vietnam in the late 1960s and early 1970s.[7]

Nonmilitary Uses

The chemical agents discussed above, used as incapacitating agents or weapons of mass casualty, also have important uses as industrial chemical intermediates or are the end products of nonweapons manufacturing processes. The large number of potentially toxic gases described below and listed in Table 10-3 are limited to those that have been studied under experimental conditions and have an associated human exposure/treatment database.[8]

Ammonia, a naturally occurring soluble alkaline gas, is a colorless irritant with a sharp odor. It is widely used in industrial processes, including oil refining as well as the production of explosives, refrigerants, fertilizers, and plastics. Ammonia is also used as a fixative in photographic, blueprinting, and duplicating processes. It is a particularly significant airborne environmental hazard in swine and poultry confinement areas. Another source of exposure can be from well-known ammonium-based cleaning agents. Ammonia is transported daily by rail and road across the

TABLE 10-2

CHEMICAL AGENTS USED IN WORLD WAR I (IN CHRONOLOGICAL ORDER)

Agent	Type	First Use	Agent	Type	First Use
Ethyl bromoacetate	I	Aug 1914	Trichloromethyl chloroformate	R	May 1916
o-Dianisidine chlorosulfonate	I	Oct 1914	Hydrogen cyanide	R	Jul 1916
Chloroacetone	I	Nov 1914	Hydrogen sulfide	R	Jul 1916
Xylyl bromide	I	Jan 1915	Chloropicrin	R	Aug 1916
Xylylene bromide	I	Jan 1915	Cyanogen bromide	R	Sept 1916
Benzyl bromide	I	Mar 1915	Cyanogen chloride	R	Oct 1916
Chlorine	R	Apr 1915	Phenylcarbylamine chloride	—	May 1917
Bromine	R	May 1915	Diphenylchlorarsine	I	Jul 1917
Methyl chlorosulfonate	I	Jun 1915	Bis(2-chloroethyl) sulfide	S	Jul 1917
Ethyl chlorosulfonate	I	Jun 1915	Phenyldichloroarsine	I	Sept 1917
Chloromethyl chloroformate	I	Jun 1915	Bis(chloromethyl) ether	R	Jan 1918
Dichloromethyl chloroformate	I	Jun 1915	Bis(bromomethyl) ether	R	Jan 1918
Bromoacetone	I	Jun 1915	Thiophosgene	I	Mar 1918
Bromomethylethylketone	I	Jul 1915	Ethyldichloroarsine	S	Mar 1918
Iodoacetone	I	Aug 1915	Methyldichloroarsine	S	Mar 1918
Dimethyl sulfate	I	Aug 1915	Diphenylcyanoarsine	I	May 1918
Perchloromethyl mercaptan	R	Sep 1915	*N*-ethylcarbazole	I	Jul 1918
Ethyl iodoacetate	I	Sep 1915	α-Bromobenzylcyanide	I	Jul 1918
Benzyl iodide	I	Nov 1915	10-Chloro-5,10-dihydro-phenarsazine	I	Sep 1918
Phosgene	R	Dec 1915	Phenyldibromoarsine	I	Sep 1918
o-Nitrobenzyl chloride	I	1915	Ethyldibromoarsine	S	Sep 1918
Benzyl chloride	I	1915	Cyanoformate esters	—	1918
Acrolein	I	Jan 1916			

I: primary irritant; R: lethal via respiratory route; S: mainly skin effects; —: no data.
Data source: Beswick FW. Chemical agents used in riot control and warfare. *Hum Toxicol*. 1983;2:247-256.

country. Industrial exposure of approximately 1,700 parts per million (ppm) of ammonia has been shown to cause severe airway obstruction.[9]

Chlorine, a greenish to yellowish compound, is another irritant gas. Chlorine was used as a chemical warfare agent during World War I because of its heavier-than-air capacity to occupy low-lying areas such as trenches. Chlorine is widely used in the paper and pulp mill production industries; over 10 million tons of chlorine are manufactured in the United States and Europe each year.[10] Accidental exposure to chlorine can occur in the household or anywhere bleach is mixed with acidic cleansers in an unventilated room. Other common sources of exposure are swimming pools, where an imbalance in mixing or dilution can result in increased release of chlorine gas. Since World War I over 200 major incidents involving mild to toxic chlorine exposure have occurred worldwide.[11]

Intentional exposures are not limited to the battlefield. Irritating, poorly water-soluble smokes such as CS, CN (chloroacetophenone), and CR (dibenz[b,f]-1,4-oxazepine), commonly referred to as riot control agents or tear gas, have been used for many years to quell social disturbances. CS was first introduced in Britain by Corson and Stoughton in 1958 to replace CN for riot control because it was safer and more effective.[12] These gases effect the sensory nerves of the skin and mucosa in the nose, eyes, and mouth, causing uncomfortable irritation at the sites of exposures. The overall effects of CS and CN inhalation are respiratory and ventilatory depression. CS has also been linked to reactive airways dysfunction syndrome (RADS) resulting from a single intentional exposure.[13] These agents have no practical use in the chemical and manufacturing industries. Olajos and Salem have provided a review of the tear gases.[14]

Hydrogen cyanide (HCN) is one of the gases most toxic to humans. It may be encountered in industrial processes as sodium or potassium cyanate or as acrylonitrile. Exposures to the salts may occur during the extraction of gold, in electroplating, or in photographic processes. HCN can be manufactured as a byproduct during the synthesis of acrylonitrile, which is a more common industrial hazard used in the production of synthetic rubber and as a fumigant. Mixtures of sodium cyanide, magnesium carbonate, and magnesium

TABLE 10-3

US ARMY CENTER FOR HEALTH PROMOTION AND PREVENTIVE MEDICINE TOXIC INDUSTRIAL CHEMICALS

Chemical	Rate of Onset	Persists in Environment	Toxicity Threshold ppm/hr impairment fatality	Odor	Related hazards / Source Use	Symptoms (from inhalation & dermal Contact)	Decontamination & Treatment
Allyl alcohol (colorless liquid)	Immediate	Days-weeks +	7.7 22	mustard-like	Rapidly absorbed through skin highly flammable with caustic fumes; used as contact pesticide. plastic/perfume manufacture	General Mild Health Effects Nausea, dizziness, headaches chills, coughing, choking throat irritation Specific and More Severe Effects Eyes: Irritation; tearing/watering pain; intolerance to light (eg from hydrogen sulfide) Skin: (particularly if liquid contact): Irritation; burning; blisters (eg with hydrogen fluoride; vesiculation (nitric and sufuric acid) dermatitis; and frostbite (e.g. Acryonitrite) Respiratory Tract/Lungs: Breathing difficulty, respiratory distress; laryngeal spasm (e.g. from hydrogen chloride, or hydrogen bromide); pulmonary edema. Chest/Heart: chest pain; tachardia (rapid heart beat) Systemic; Blood: Cyanotic (blue skin from lack of Oxygen to blood) (e.g. from SO_2, SO_3, NO_2, ethylene oxide Convulsions/seizures hemolytic anemia;kidney damage (Arsine) Additional Chemical Specific Symptoms: pink froth/sputum: Ammonia mucoid frothy sputum: SO_2, SO_3, NO_2 Peculiar taste: Ethylene oxide asphyxia and metal taste: Acrylonitrite garlic breath: Hydrogen Selenide	Decontamination: Flush (15min) eyes & skin with water; Soap optional after initial water rinse Treatment & Diagnostic procedures/options: Eye injuries Saline wash Antibiotic ointments Skin burns/blisters/irritation topical corticosteroids and/or antihistamines inject $MgSO_4$at affected site (hydrogen fluoride) Breathing/respiratory distress: Oxygen and ventilation Prophylactic antibiotics X-rays Pulse Ox/ blood gas NOTE: avoid mouth to mouth to protect against cross contamination Bronchospasm/Pulmonary Edema: Inhale corticosterioids Beta2 agonist Endotracheal Intubation Hemolysis (e.g. Arsine): IV transfusion Seizures: Diazepam
Acrolein (colorless-yellow liq)	Immediate	Minutes-hour	0.1 1.4	1ppm-sharp acrid, sweet	Toxic and corrosive fumes: Herbicide		
Acrylonitrile (clear/pale yellow liq)	Immediate	Minutes to Hours	35 75	17ppm-unpleasant sweet(peach)	Flammable gas; used in plastics, coatings, adhesives idhesives industries; dyes, pharmaceuticals		
Ammonia (colorless gas)	Immediate	Minutes	110 1100	17ppm-sharp suffocating dry urine	Explosives manufacture; pesticides; detergents industry		
Arsine (colorless gas)	Immediate to 24 hours	Minutes to Hours	0.2 0.5	0.5ppm garlic like	reacts with H_20 (don't use H_20 in fires); Used in electronics industry		
Chlorine (greenish-yellow gas)	Immediate to hours	Minutes to Hours	3 22	3.5ppm-pungent(bleach) suffocating	Irritating corr fumes; heavier than air; Cleaner/disinfectant in many industries; water treatment; WWI war gas		
Diborane (colorless gas)	Immediate	Minutes to Hours	>1 15	2.5ppm-sickly sweet	Very Flammable; Intermediate chemical manufacturing		
Ethylene oxide (colorless gas/liq)	Immediate	Minutes to Hours	45 200	425ppm-sweet ether-like	Very Flammable Rocket propellant; fumigant sterilization in health care industry		
Formaldehyde (clear-white gas/liq)	Immediate	Hours	10 25	1ppm-pungent suffocating	Flammable; Disinfection/germicide; fungicide; textile; health care (tissue fixing)		
Hydrogen bromide (pale yellow liq)	Immediate	Minutes to Hours	3 30	2ppm-sharp stinging	Chemical Manufacturing industry; very corrosive		
Hydrogen chloride (hydrochloric acid) (pale yellow-colorless liq)	Immediate	Minutes to Hours	22 104	0.77ppm pungent ittitation	Corrosive Liquid; Ore, other metal refining/cleaning; food/pickling; petroleum		
Hydrogen Cyanide (colorless-white-pale) (blue gas; liq <75 F)	Immediate	Minutes	7 15-50	1-5ppm-bitter/ sweet almond-like	Weak acide except in Water or mucous membranes-then corrosive/ irritating; used as War gas, pesticide herbicide; other industries		
Hydrogen fluoride (colorless gas/fuming liq)	Immediate & Delayed	Minutes to Hours	24 44	0.4ppm-strong irritating	Corrosive liquid, Aluminum & other metal industries, insecticide manufacturing		
Hydrogen selenide (colorless gas)	Immediate	Minutes-hour	0.2 1.5+	0.3ppm-decayed horseradish	Highly flammable/explosive; can cause burns/frostbite; decomposes rapidly to form elemental selenium metals & semiconductor prep	→	

(**Table 10-3** *continues*)

sulfate are used as rodenticides. Exposure to cyanide can result from the release of HCN gas when the solid mixture comes into contact with water. Exposure to HCN gas, which is lighter than air, can also result from fires because many organic compounds release HCN during combustion or pyrolysis processes.[15] Cyanide, a metabolic poison that smells like almonds, is a potent inhibitor of cytochrome-*c*-oxidase, the terminal enzyme in the mitochondrial electron transport chain required for cellular respiration.[16] Chapter 11, Cyanide Posoning, contains more details on HCN.

Hydrogen sulfide (H_2S), or sour gas, has a well-known pungent and irritating odor that smells like rotten eggs. A heavier-than-air and colorless gas, H_2S

Table 10-3 *continued*

Chemical	Rate of Onset	Persists in Environment	Toxicity Thresholds ppm/hr impairment fatality	Odor	Related hazards/Source Use	Symptoms (from inhalation & dermal contact)	Decontamination & Treatment
Hydrogen Sulfide (colorless gas)	Immediate & Delayed	Minutes to Hours	30 100	0.1 ppm- rotten egg	Disinfectant lubrcat/oils; Interm for HC manfacture; deadens sense of smell	General Mild Health Effects Nausia, dizziness, headaches, chills, coughing, choking, throat irritation Specific and More Severe Effects Eyes: Irritation; tearing/watering; pain;intolerance to light (eg from hydrogen sulfide) Skin: (particularly if liquid contact): Irritation; burning; blisters (eg with hydrogen fluoride; vesiculation (nitric & sulfuric acid) dermatitis & frostbite (e.g. Acryonitrite) Respiratory Tract/Lungs: Breathing difficulty, respiratory distress; laryngeal spasm (e.g. from hydrogen chloride, or hydrogen bromide); pulmonary edma Chest/Heart: chest pain; tachardia (rapid heartbeat) Systemic Blood: Cyanotic (blue skin from lack of Oxygen to blood) (e.g. from SO_2, SO_3, NO_2, ethylene oxide) Convulsions/seizures; hemolytic anemia; kidney damage (Arsine sulfuric acid, hydrazine) Additional Chemical Specific Symptoms: pink froth/sputum: Ammonia mucoid frothy sputum: SO_2, SO_3, NO_2 Peculiar taste: Ethylene oxide asphyxia & metal taste: Acrylonitrile garlic breath: Hydrogen Selenide Miosis, Sweating,↓AchE: Parathion Coffe ground vomit- Sulfuric acid	Decontamination Flush (15 min) eyes & skin with water; Soap oprional after initial water use Treatment & Diagnostic procedures/options: Eye injuries: Saline wash Antibiotic ointments Skin burns/blisters/irritation: topical corticosteroids and/or antihistamines inject $MgSO_4$ at affected site (hydrogen fluoride) Breathing/respiratory distress: Oxygen & ventilation Prophylactic antibiotics X-rays Pulse Ox/ blood gas NOTE: avoid mouth to mouth to protect against cross contamination Bronchospasm/Pulmonary Edema: inhale corticosteroids Beta2 agonist Endotracheal intubation Hemolysis (e.g Arsie): IV transfusion Seizures: Diazepam
Methyle Hydrazine	Immediate & Delayed (lungs)	Hours-Days	1 3	1-1-ppm- ammonia like	Irritating vapors; Flammable- Once ignited continues to burn; Used as solvent; rocket fuel		
Hydrazine colorless, oil (fuming) liq/waxy solid or crystals	Immediate & Delayed (lungs)	Hours-Days	13 35	3-4 ppm- ammonia like	Flammable- Once ignited continues to burn; irritating vapors; used as solvent; rocket fuel		
Methyle isocyanate (colorless liquid)	Immediate	Minutes-Hours	0.5 5	2.1ppm- sharp pungent	intermediate in manufacturing reacts with H2O (don't use in fire)		
Methyle mercaptan (colorless gas;liquid <43°F)	Immediate	Minutes-Hours	5 23	0,002ppm-rotten cabbage (1ppm odor fatigue)	From decayed organic matter- pulp mills, oil refineries; highly flammable liquid burns/frostbite		
Nitrogen dioxide (colorless gas/pale liq)	Delayed (24-72 hours	Minutes-Hours	12 20	1ppm- ?	Intermediate for manufacture of nitric acid & sulfuric acid; explosives/rocket propellant		
Nitric acid (colorless, yellow, or red fuming liquid)	Immediate	Hours-Days +	4 22+	~1ppm- choking, sweet-acrid	Used in many industries; Very corrosive to skin/mucous membranes as well as metals & other materials		
Parathion (pale yellow to brown liq)	Immediate but often Delayed (weeks)	Days-Weeks	0.2 0.8	0.04ppm	Organophosphate (insecticide); similar symptoms (and thus treatment) as nerve gases;penetrates leather/ canvas & plastic/rubber coatings		
Phosgene (colorless-light yellow gas)	Immediate & Delayed (lungs)	Minutes-Hours	0.3 0.8 -5	0.5ppm-musty hay	Dye, pesticide & other industries; Histpry as a war gas; corrosive/ irritating		
Phosphine (colorless gas)	Immediate & Delayed (lungs)	Minutes-Hours	0.3 1.1 -30	0.9ppm-rotten fish, garlic	Insecticide; used in the manufacture of flame retardants & incendiaries		
Sulfuric Acid (clear colorless-brown oily liquid)	Immediate	Hours, Days	2.5 7.5	Oderless (acrid taste)	Toxic fumes when heated Battery/dyes/paper/glue/metals industries; volcanic gas		
Sulfur dioxide/trioxide (from sulfuric acide colorless gas)	Immediate & Delayed	Minutes-Hours	>3 15-100	1ppm-pungent (metalic taste)	Disinfectant & preserving in breweries & food/canning textile industry; batteries		
Toluene diisocyanate (2.4) (water-white to pale yellow liq, or crystals)	Immediate	Hours-Weeks	0.08 0.51	0.4-2ppm-sharp pungent	Skin irritant Polyurethane (wood coatings, foam), nylon industries		

Reproduced from: US Army Center for Health Promotion and Preventive Medicine. *Industrial Chemical Prioritization and Determination of Critical Hazards of Concern.* Aberdeen Proving Ground, Md: USACHPPM; 2003: Appendix B. USACHPPM Report 47-EM-6154-03.

may occur in industrial processes associated with mining, crude oil refining, tanning, farming, paper pulp mills, sewage treatment, and rubber production. It is also a component of natural gas, a major component of volcanic eruptions, and a major airborne hazard in animal confinement areas. H_2S is nearly as toxic as HCN and acts almost as rapidly. It is responsible for more deaths than any other gas.[17] Case reports indicate that exposure can cause neurological symptoms, with focal necrosis of the brain implicated in a fatal outcome.[18] Environmental release of H_2S can cause breathlessness and eye and nasopharyngeal irritation.[19] Reiffenstein et al[20] have provided an early review of H_2S reporting that the typical "rotten-egg" odor is inadequate warning of short-term exposures to high levels, which can cause an inability to smell the gas (olfactory paralysis), among other adverse health effects.

Oxides of nitrogen come in four stable forms: (1) nitrogen oxide (N_2O), an anesthetic compound, and (2) nitric oxide (NO), an important byproduct of intracellular biochemical nitrogen metabolism, which also forms (3) nitrogen dioxide (NO_2) and (4) nitrogen tetroxide (N_2O_4) when oxidized in air. Oxides of nitrogen are important reactive end products of air pollution. The reactive dioxide form is a pulmonary irritant that can be found in fresh silage from agricultural processes preserving green crops such as alfalfa and corn (silo-filler's disease), in unventilated areas with high temperature arc welding, and the production and transport of nitric acid. N_2O may also be produced in the dipping of aluminum, brass, and copper and in combustion and pyrolysis processes.[21]

Polytetrafluoroethylene (Teflon [Dupont, Wilmington, Del]) can form toxic gases when heated to temperatures above 400°C. Combustion and pyrolysis byproducts of Teflon, which have been known for some time, have been implicated in pulmonary injury and even deaths following a single exposure.[22] Illnesses caused by the inhalation of combustion byproducts have been given the label "polymer fume fever." One of the more common byproducts is perfluoroisobutylene (PFIB), which is reportedly 10 times more toxic than phosgene.[23]

Phosgene has been used extensively for the past 60 years in the production of pharmaceuticals, aniline dyes, polyfoam rubber, isocyanates, and plastic products in the United States and worldwide. In 1998 the United States used 4.3 million pounds of phosgene in manufacturing processes.[24] Phosgene is used in a "phosgenation" reaction to help supply chlorine groups to reaction products. Babad and Zeiler[25] have reviewed phosgene chemical reactions, finding that phosgene rapidly reacts with water to form carbon dioxide and hydrochloric acid, and it also reacts with macromolecules containing sulfhydryl, amine, and hydroxyl groups in aqueous solutions. Phosgene can be formed by the thermal decomposition of chlorinated hydrocarbons and poses a threat for welders, refrigeration mechanics, and automobile mechanics.[26] Commonly used industrial degreasers contain chlorinated hydrocarbons, such as perchloroethylene, which can form phosgene when heated. Therefore, industrial workers, fire fighters, military personnel, and others are at risk for accidental or occupational exposure to phosgene. In Poland, for example, because of heavy industrialization in proximity to densely populated areas, phosgene, along with chlorine, ammonia, and sulfur dioxide, has been identified as one of the most significant threats to the environment.[27]

Smoke is a general classification of a complex mixture of particulate/gaseous emissions. Smokes are products of the combustion process of burning or smoldering. The major cause of death from fire-related events is smoke inhalation. Smoke can include many of the chemicals mentioned earlier. Particulate matter such as carbon soot particles can make up a significant proportion of toxic smoke, as can carbon monoxide, HCN, phosgene, aldehydes such as formaldehyde, ammonia, and PFIB.

Sulfur dioxide is a major air pollutant and a principal source of photochemical smog and acid rain. A colorless, water-soluble gas 2.26 times heavier than water, sulfur dioxide is used in a number of industrial processes such as the smelting production of copper, iron, lead, and zinc ores. When it comes into contact with moist surfaces, sulfur dioxide is hydrolyzed and oxidized to form sulfuric acid. It is extremely corrosive to the nasopharynx region, eyes, and upper airways. Inhalation exposure may progress to acute respiratory distress syndrome (ARDS) and has been implicated in causing RADS.[28] Prolonged exposure causes inflammation of the airways and impairs the immune system and lung resistance.[29] Table 10-4 provides a very limited overview of some well-known gaseous irritants.

MECHANISMS OF TOXICITY

Numerous studies have been undertaken to determine the mechanisms of toxicity and the basis for lung injury from exposure to toxic gases. These investigations have historically involved animal models. As early as 1919 the progression and intensity of exposure to agents such as phosgene was demonstrated in dogs. In later decades, animal models included mice, rats, guinea pigs, swine, and monkeys to more accurately predict the temporal effects of injury progression and scope in humans. Many of these models involved the use of inhalation techniques, focused essentially on the establishment of a fundamental relationship: lethal concentration (C), in ppm, times the duration (T), in minutes, of exposure (also known as Haber's law).[30] The product of C × T corresponds to a standard response measure describing a biological endpoint of edema formation, death, or any other consistent physiological parameter. Conceptually, this product simply meant that the same biological endpoint would occur whether the animals were exposed to 100 ppm of gas for 10 minutes, 50 ppm for 20 minutes, or 20 ppm for 50 minutes (all resulting in a C × T of 1,000 ppm•min). However, later experiments showed that for a gas such as phosgene and other irritants, Haber's law was applicable only over short exposure times.[31,32] It is now generally agreed that concentration rather than duration of exposure determines the gas's effect.

As implied by this discussion of Haber's law, the use of such a general quantitative assessment for exposure-response effects includes inherent problems. Many fundamental physiological, toxicological, histopathological, and biochemical effects are lost in such an evaluation, especially when death is the endpoint. As shown in Table 10–4, many of these compounds have varying solubility ranges, resulting in a range of effects within the pulmonary tree. For example,

TABLE 10-4

MECHANISMS OF LUNG INJURY OF GASEOUS RESPIRATORY IRRITANTS

Irritant Gas	Mechanism of Injury
Ammonia (NH_2) Source: Agriculture, rain, plastic, explosives	Alkali burns
Hydrogen chloride (HCl) Source: Dyes, fertilizers, textiles, rubber, thermal degradation of polyvinyl chloride	Acid burns
Sulfur dioxide (SO_2) Source: Smelting, combustion of coal/oil, paper manufacturing, food preparation	Acid burns
Chlorine (Cl_2) Source: Paper, textile manufacturing, sewage treatment	Acid burns, free radical formation
Oxides of nitrogen (NO, NO_2, N_2O_4) Source: Agriculture, mining, welding, manufacturing of dyes/lacquers	Acid burns, free radical formation
Phosgene ($COCl_2$) Source: Firefighters, welders, paint strippers, chemical intermediates (isocyanate, pesticides, dyes, pharmaceuticals)	Acid burns

Colors indicate water solubility. Red: high; yellow: intermediate; green: low.
Data source: Schwartz DA. Acute inhalational injury. *Occup Med*. 1987;2:298.

inhalation of compounds that have limited solubility results in lower lung injury, whereas compounds that are miscible in water affect the upper regions of the respiratory tree. Compounds discussed earlier, such as phosgene, chlorine, oxides of nitrogen, and PFIB, are considered lower airway (peripheral compartment) irritants based on their solubility characteristics. Gases such as ammonia, sulfur dioxide, and hydrochloric acid are generally considered upper airway (central compartment) irritants but can affect the lower lung regions if exposure concentration and duration are sufficient. Carbon monoxide, H_2S, and HCN are classified as systemic chemical asphyxiants.

Rational and effective medical countermeasures against the inhalational injury caused by gases, smokes, fumes, and mists depend on mechanistic evidence of exposure responses at the tissue and cellular levels. The investigation required to determine the correct treatment route, therapeutic window, and dosing levels is costly and time consuming. Study of representative compounds from a class of gases can provide general insight into the mechanisms responsible for tissue and cellular injury and the subsequent repair processes. In recent years extensive data on the mechanisms of phosgene, chlorine, H_2S, and oxides of nitrogen gas exposure have been published.[32–34] These studies evaluated the following range of effects over time and at various exposures:

- histopathology of exposed lung tissue;
- biochemical pathway assessment of lung tissue markers of exposure such as a simple determination of wet/dry weight ratio for pulmonary edema estimates;
- inflammation pathways;
- metabolic markers of exposure such as arachidonate mediators;
- physiological assessment of blood gas and hemodynamic status;
- cell differential counts;
- pulmonary function as measured by plethysmography;
- tissue and bronchoalveolar lavage fluid redox and antioxidant status;
- behavioral effects;
- genomic expression markers;
- immunosuppression effects; and
- mortality as determined by survival rate studies.

Mechanistic Effects of Inhaled Pulmonary Agents

Exposure to inhaled agents can compromise the entire pulmonary tree through a range of altered physiological, biochemical, and pathophysiological processes. The general mechanisms of toxic gas exposure are shown in Figure 10-1. Researchers have used animal models to examine these dysfunctional pathways in many ways. In an obligate nose-breathing experimental animal like the rodent, the basic mammalian life processes are extrapolated to humans, allowing for reasonable estimates of potential human exposure responses. This chapter will cover studies of prominent pathways through which

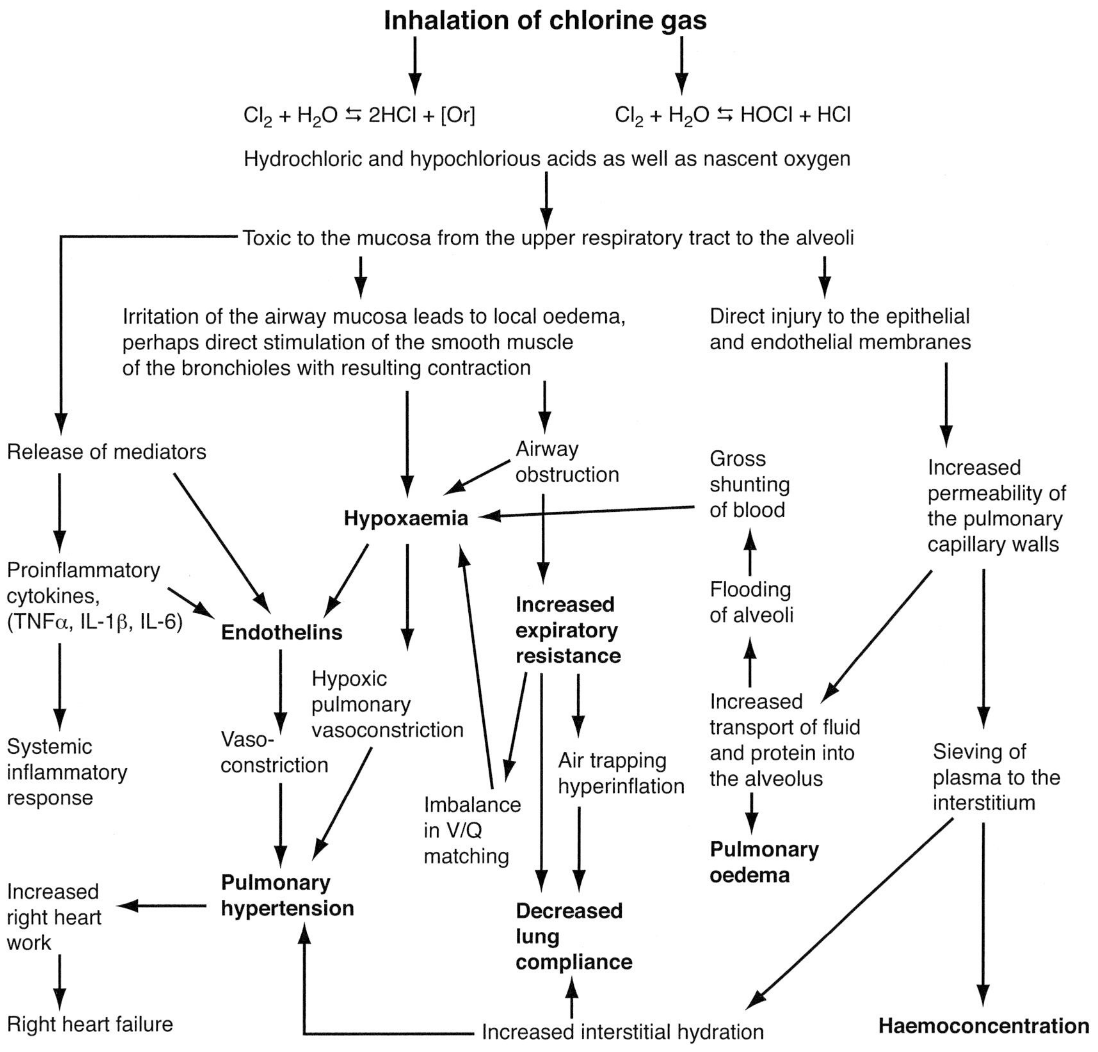

Fig. 10–1. General mechanisms of toxic gas exposure.
IL: interleukin
TNF: tumor necrosis factor
V/Q: ventilation profusion ratio
Reproduced with permission from: Wang J. *Pathophysiology and Treatment of Chlorine Gas-Induced Lung Injury: An Experimental Study in Pigs* [dissertation]. Linköping, Sweden: Linköping University; 2004: 36.

inhaled compounds affect basic life processes.

It should be kept in mind that the effects of an inhalational event are related to the chemical reactivity of the toxicant, its concentration, and the duration of exposure. In accidental exposure scenarios, there is generally poor quantifiable information on concentration and exposure duration; in some cases the identity of the agent may be uncertain. Also, the possibility of multiple simultaneous chemical exposures, which can occur in a chemical plant explosion, must be considered. In Bhopal, India, an accidental release of methylisocyanate used in the production of the pesticide carbaryl was responsible for over 60,000 casualties and nearly 5,000 deaths in December 1984.[35] Inhalation of the toxic gas resulted in a range of pulmonary symptoms that included irritation and coughing. Pulmonary edema and atelectasis were the eventual causes of death. Long-term survivors were diagnosed with lung inflammation, fibrosis, and compromised lung function. Survivors continue to have health issues related to catastrophe event after nearly 25 years.[36]

Physiological Responses

Many studies have shown that the adverse effects

of toxic gas inhalation can easily be assessed by measuring basic pulmonary function. Several irritants such as phosgene, chlorine, and PFIB initiate reactions that result in problems with physiological breathing processes. Cranial nerve input in the nasopharyngeal region is mainly responsible for initiating changes in respiratory function, as evidenced by altered breathing mechanics. Experiments in mice exposed to phosgene show that minute ventilation is increased following exposure,[37] caused by an increase in respiratory rate in response to local irritation from the gas. Inspiratory and expiratory flow rates are also compromised by local sensory irritation because of formation of hydrochloric acid in the mucous membranes in the upper airway of the central airway compartment. Several studies found decreased dynamic compliance and increases in both airway resistance and tracheal pressure to be predictable patterns of response following irritant gas exposure.[38–41] Phosgene exerts much of its toxic effect in the peripheral compartment of the lung, and histopathologic specimens show a significant alteration of the acinar type I and II epithelial cell layers of the air–blood barrier. Exposure causes significant pulmonary edema and respiratory acidosis through increased P_{CO_2} saturation, decreased Pa_{O_2}saturation, and decreased arterial pH.[42–44] Similar responses have been observed in animal models using chlorine, PFIB, and ammonia. Studies involving PFIB have demonstrated that rats made to exercise following exposure exhibited an enhancement of transcellular transport of blood proteins to the alveolar surface.[45,46] These data suggest that although the lung may be injured and edematous, fleeing from the site of exposure may not in itself contribute to the edematous effect.

Decreased body weight is a useful indicator of exposure and systemic toxicity. Pulmonary edema formation can be estimated by the lung wet weight to dry weight ratio, which increases over time as the injury progresses . Although the wet/dry weight ratio is an important measure of edema, it may not show subtle effects that preexist fulminant alveolar edema. A valuable indicator of what is actually occurring in the deep lung environment is bronchoalveolar lavage fluid (BALF). BALF tests provide a wealth of information. Lavage fluid protein levels give a good indication of subtle changes in the integrity of the air–blood barrier. Increased protein levels can be measured in some cases hours prior to gross alveolar edema formation. This may indicate that interstitial edema is occurring. Much use has been made of the electrolyte homeostatic responses to toxic gas exposure. Sciuto et al have shown that phosgene exposure can produce a possibly deleterious effect on lung homeostatic process by altering ionized Ca^{++}, Na^{+}, and K^{+} levels indirectly, thus indicating possible compromised Na^{+}, K^{+}, or Ca^{++}-adenosine triphosphatase pump function.[47] Inhalation of irritants such as phosgene is known to eventually result in immunosuppression, which may increase mortality via infection in the compromised lung.[48,49]

Genomic studies have provided insight into the effects of toxic gas exposure on gene expression levels. In phosgene-exposed mice, it was demonstrated that the earliest changes (occurring within 1 to 4 hours) in lung tissue involved increased expression levels of antioxidant enzymes of the glutathione redox cycle.[50] These data strongly suggest that free-radical–mediated injury processes are active well before gross pathophysiologic changes become manifest. It has been shown that in vitro exposure of epithelial cells to nitrogen dioxide can cause a range of problems in the entire length of the respiratory tract. Many of these detrimental effects are the result of activated reactive nitrogen species free radicals such as the peroxy radical $OONO^-$ or the nitrogen dioxide radical $\bullet NO_2$ itself.[51]

Riot control agents, also called incapacitants, can cause ocular and cutaneous as well as acute pulmonary responses during exposure. Although generally nonlethal, incapacitants may have magnified contact problems if exposure occurs within a confined space. Symptoms resulting from a single exposure can last for years.[8]

Pathophysiological Effects of Exposure

Examination of histopathological effects on chemically exposed lung tissue provides critical information on the effects of a C × T response. The mechanisms of lung injury and repair are summarized in Figure 10-2.[52] Evaluation of phosgene-induced pulmonary injury to the peripheral compartment revealed characteristic temporal acute toxicity lesions. Early lesions of a toxic gas exposure can be characterized by leakage of edema, fibrin, and erythrocytes from the pulmonary microvasculature into the alveolar spaces and interstitial tissues. In general, alveolar and interstitial edema can characterize the earliest and most significant pulmonary changes. Epithelial damage in the terminal bronchioles and alveoli as well as mild inflammatory cell infiltrates can accompany increasing pulmonary edema. The repair and regeneration of epithelial damage centered on the terminal bronchioles may complement the resolution of edema.[53] In this study early indicators of phosgene-induced pulmonary injury were identified by comparing acute pulmonary histopathologic changes to bronchoalveolar lavage and lung wet-weight gravimetric measurements. Of the BALF parameters studied, lactate dehydrogenase and

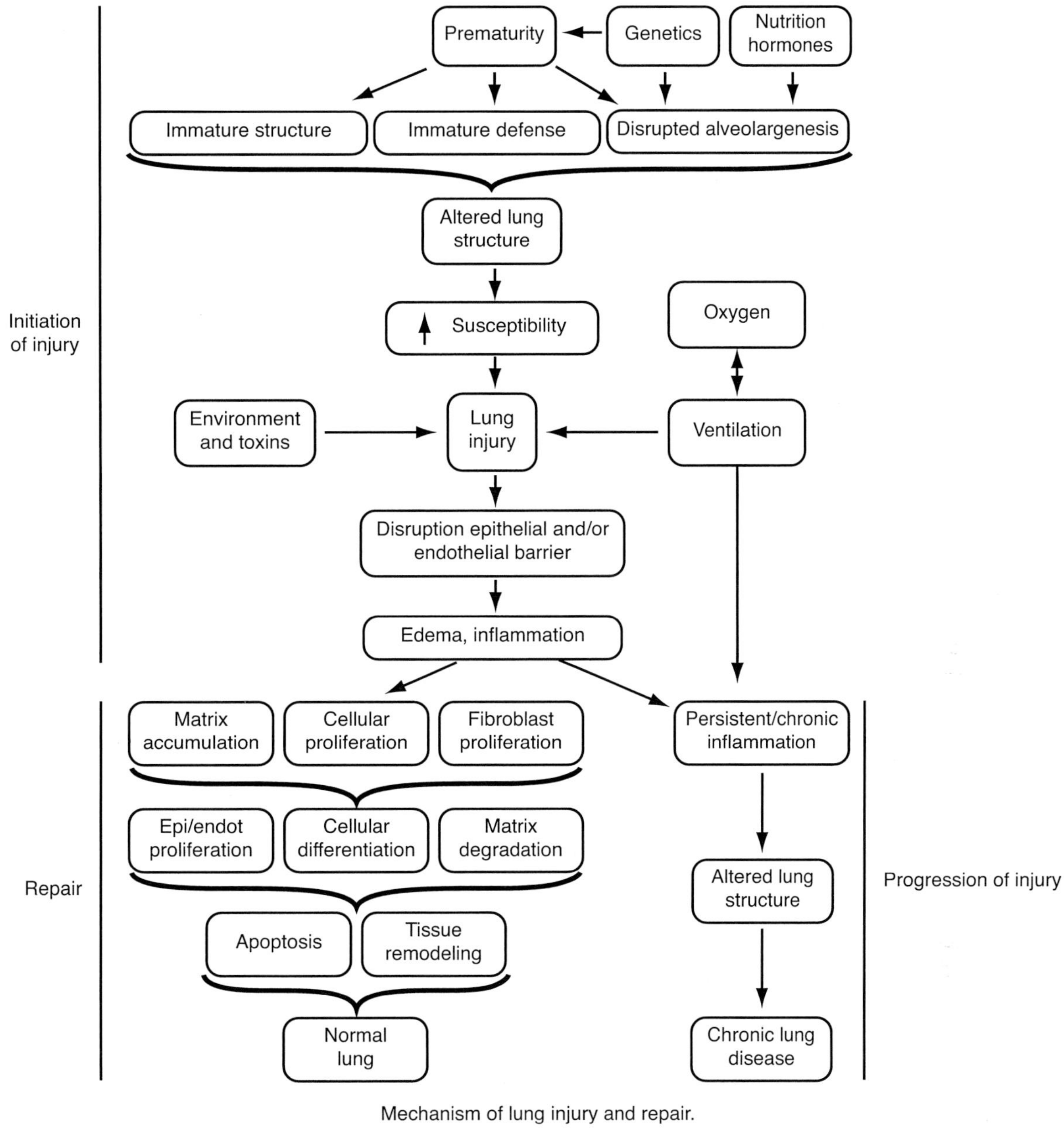

Fig. 10-2. Pathophysiology of toxic gas inhalation.
Epi/Endot: epithelial and/or endothelial
Adapted with permission from: Copland I, Tanswell K, Post M. Principals of lung development, growth, and repair. In: Notter RH, Finkelstein JN, Holm BA, eds. *Lung Injury: Mechanisms, Pathophysiology, and Therapy.* Boca Raton, Fla: Taylor & Francis Group; 2005: 19–66.

protein levels were the most sensitive early indicators of pulmonary edema. In experiments in rats exposed to PFIB, as the mass exposure concentration increased, the earlier tissue injury occurred. Epithelial and endothelial cell blebbing occurred, which progressed over time to endothelial swelling and fenestrations of the epithelial barrier, denudement of the alveolar surface, and interstitial edema.[45] PFIB and phosgene exposure also caused alteration of the production of specific surfactant phospholipids, which can have important implications for reduced lung compliance and the subsequent treatment of this injury.[54] In rats exposed to the pyrolysis products of Teflon at 450°C, ultrastructural changes in the lung consisted of pulmonary edema, hemorrhage, and necrotic tracheobronchial epithelium, accompanied by pneumocyte bleb formation, denudation, and fragmentation.[55]

Lung tissue and cellular responses to inhalation exposure can also be manifested in the form of cell membrane destruction. This can be measured to some degree by determining the extent of lipid peroxidation, an indicator of oxidative stress caused by the abundance of free radicals. Lipid peroxidation is a process whereby the rigid lipid bilayer of the membrane becomes more fluid, resulting in the activation of intracellular metabolic pathways regulated by altered enzyme function. One of the more important pathways is the arachidonic acid (AA) pathway, which leads to the production of mediators of inflammation and edema such as the leukotrienes. The other metabolic arm of the AA pathway leads to vasoactive compounds such as prostaglandins, which are in part responsible for vascular tone. Both leukotrienes and prostaglandins have been implicated in toxic-gas–induced acute lung injury.[56–59] Adenlyate cyclase is yet another injury-activated enzyme system responsible for the cleavage of adenosine triphosphate to form adenosine 3′,5′-cyclic monophosphate (cAMP), which is required for endothelial and epithelial tight-junction formation. The initial step in this process is damage to membrane surface β-adrenergic receptors, which aid in the regulation of cAMP formation. With the deactivation of cAMP formation, tight junctions become more permeable and allow the passage of fluid or water into intracellular and extracellular spaces. Decreased cAMP production and the resultant pulmonary edema have been implicated in toxic-gas–induced acute lung injury.[39]

Acute exposure to nitrogen dioxide causes a range of pathological effects characterized by increased epithelial permeability and the proliferation of Clara and type II epithelial cells.[60] Chronic exposure induces bronchiolitis, alveolar bronchiolarization, ciliated cysts, and emphysema. Exposure effects may be more pronounced in those with preexisting compromised lung function such as asthma. In experiments in an asthmatic population exposed to 1 ppm nitrogen dioxide, increased levels of mediators of inflammation and vasoactive compounds were measured in the BALF.[61] Metabolites of the cyclooxygenase pathway of the AA cascade, such as 6-keto-prostaglandin F_1-α (responsible for bronchodilation) were decreased; however, both prostaglandin D_2 and thromboxane B_2 (responsible for bronchoconstriction) were increased. Elevated levels of leukotrienes such as C_4, D_4, and E_4, which are products of the lipoxygenase pathway of the AA cascade related to bronchial hyperresponsiveness, were also involved in the inflammatory response.

Exposure to smoke has been shown to cause sufficiently severe acute lung injury to ultimately result in death. In human smoke-related fatalities, the lungs were shown to exhibit soot staining in the tracheobronchial mucosa, and they were heavy (edematous) and hyperemic. Light microscopy indicated pulmonary congestion, and electron microscopy revealed carbon particles as well as interstitial and intraalveolar edema.[62]

Inflammatory Pathways

Inflammation is a critical result of toxic-gas–inhalation injury. Many studies have demonstrated a decrease in the number of macrophages, which are important in clearance mechanisms, and an increase in neutrophils, which aid in detoxification of toxic mediators and metabolites. These shifts in cell populations generally occur over time and are usually a function of the gas involved, the depth of inhalation, the concentration, and the duration of exposure. In the case of some inhaled gases, the chemical reaction in the tissue can produce deleterious amounts of free radicals. These radicals in turn can damage migrating cells such as neutrophils, causing them to dump their toxic proteases, proinflammatory cytokines and chemokines, and additional toxic free radicals such as the hydroxyl species •OH and superoxide anion O_2^- into the intracellular environment, causing greater damage. This additive effect may account for some of the latent injury responses seen following inhalation of gases such as phosgene and possibly other irritants, some of which have well-described latency (1–24 hours) effects.

Markers of inflammation and the timing of their release after exposure can provide useful information about the potential therapeutic window for eventual and successful treatment. Many studies have focused on cytokines, which are produced by a variety of white cells, fibroblasts, and epithelial and endothelial cells, to assess the inflammatory response. Cytokines can have a wide range of proinflammatory and antiinflammatory effects in tissue injury responses. These compounds serve as important mediators of tissue and injury repair processes and as such represent suitable markers of inflammation injury and signal transduction pathways (Table 10-5).[63]

For example, in phosgene-exposed mice, BALF cytokine and chemokine analysis over 72 hours clearly demonstrated that the cytokine interleukin-6 and the chemokine macrophage inflammatory protein-2, the analog in mice for human interleukin-8, were both significantly increased within 4 to 8 hours of exposure.[64] Both interleukin-1β and tumor necrosis factor-α were significantly increased 24 to 72 hours after exposure. The data support the postulation that tumor necrosis

TABLE 10-5

MAIN INFLAMMATORY AGENTS INVOLVED IN ACUTE LUNG INJURY, THEIR SOURCE AND ACTION

Agent	Source	Actions
	Cytokines (Proteins)	
IL-1	In response to infection/injury from activated macrophage. Induced by TNF from mononuclear and endothelial cells.	Regulates systemic inflammatory response, causes increase in blood neutrophils; causes fever. Induces other cytokines. Stimulates NO production, produces PLA_2, PAF, releases histamine.
IL-6	Induced by IL-1 from epithelial cells.	Creates pyrogen, activates stromal bone marrow to produce CSF.
IL-8	Secreted by macrophages, endothelial cells, T cells and fibroblasts in response to LPS, IL-1 or TNF stimulation.	Chemotactic for neutrophils and activates macrophages.
TNF-α	Large amounts from endotoxin-stimulated macrophages.	Induces arachidonic metabolites and synthesis of cytokines. Chemotactic for neutrophils and macrophages. Synergistic with IL-1. Causes fever.
	Lipids (Arachidonic Acid Metabolites)	
Leukotrienes (B_4, C_4, D_4, E_4)	Enzymatic pathway from membrane phospholipid.	Causes vasoconstriction, bronchoconstriction, enhancement of capillary leakage.
Prostaglandin E_2	Enzymatic pathway from membrane phospholipid.	A vasodilator, has proinflammaotry and antiinflammatory potential.
Thromboxane A_2	Enzymatic pathway from membrane phospholipid.	Potent vasodilator, causes platelet sequestration.
PAF	Epithelial cells via the arachidonic acid pathway, also neutrophils, basophils and platelets.	Causes platelet aggregation. Recruits eosinophils, causes vasodilation, increases vascular permeability, causes degranulation of neutrophils. Spasmogenic on bronchial smooth muscle.
	Reduced Oxygen Species (Free Radicals)	
OH, H_2O_2, superoxide anion	LPS stimulated macrophage/monocyte cell.	Very reactive, responsible for lung tissue injury. Interacts with arachidonic acid pathway to increase levels of eicosanoids.

CSF: colony-stimulating factor
H_2O_2: hydrogen peroxide
IL: interleukin
LPS: lipopolysaccharide
NO: nitric oxide
OH: hydroxyl radical
PAF: platelet-aggregating factor
PLA_2: phospholypase A2
TNF: tumor necrosis factor

factor-α may aid in fluid clearance in this injury model. The nature of lung injury in response to an inhalational event can be extremely complex. Figure 10-3 provides a visual representation of the alveolar region of the peripheral lung compartment following exposure to toxic gas. The difficulty in treating an injury with a large array of metabolic chaos is that many of these pathways are activated and on-going simultaneously.

Biochemical Responses

Understanding the biochemical responses to inha-

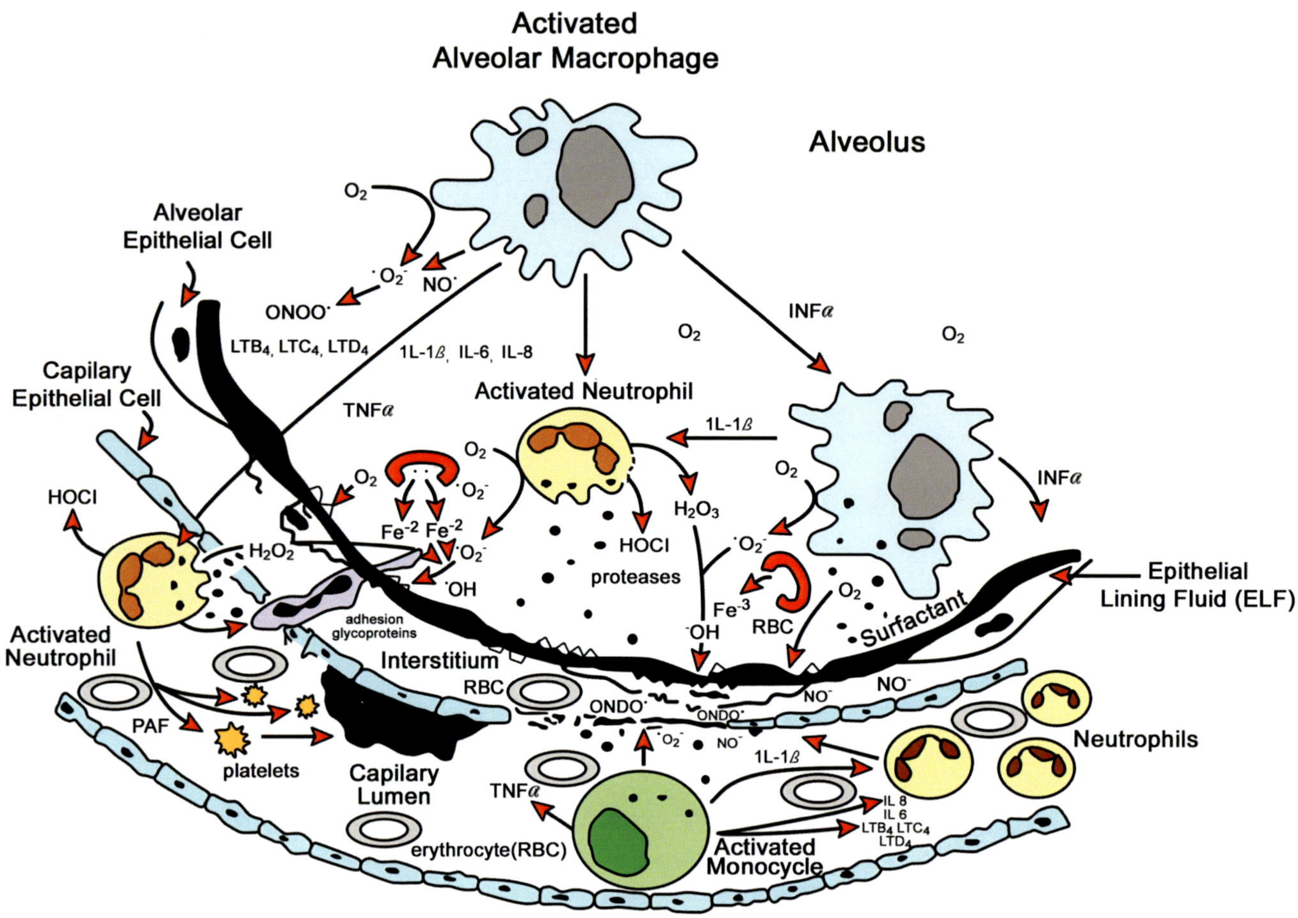

Fig. 10–3. General schema for the study of acute and chronic lung injury.
HOCl: hypochlorous acid
INF: interferon
H_2O_2: hydrogen peroxide
H_2O_3: dihydrogen trioxide
IL: interleukin
LT: leukotriene
PAF: platelet-aggregating factor
RBC: red blood cell
TNF: tumor necrosis factor
Courtesy of: US Army Medical Research Institute of Chemical Defense, Aberdeen Proving Ground, Md.

lation exposure can provide a wealth of information about pathways that may lead to successful treatment strategies. One of the most important pathways is the glutathione (GSH) cycle. GSH is an important and ubiquitous intracellular antioxidant. The GSH redox cycle is activated in response to free-radical–mediated tissue and cellular injury. GSH also aids in maintaining the proper balance between naturally occurring free radical metabolism processes and antioxidant detoxification. Basically, it helps to create equilibrium in the antioxidant/oxidant ratio. Exposure to inhaled chemical toxins can elicit a response that favors the liberation of extremely toxic free radicals. Exposure to phosgene has been demonstrated to cause a significant decrease in lung tissue GSH across a range of species.[65] Concurrent with decreased GSH protection in the lung tissue, BALF shows a marked increase in GSH levels.[65] Increased BALF GSH is believed to be a response of damaged lung tissue for the purpose of transporting GSH to critical areas in the alveolar regions. This occurs to protect the surfactant and epithelial integrity of the gas-exchanging units in response to free radical activity. This same response mechanism has been demonstrated in smokers.[66] It is well established that the toxic effect of smoking is largely a free radical-mediated process.

SPECIFIC INHALED TOXIC-GAS–INDUCED EFFECTS AND THEIR TREATMENTS

Defining treatment strategies and clinical medical management for toxic gas exposure is problematic. In most cases the chemical inhalant is unknown. In other cases there may be multiple chemical exposure, patients may be too confused to accurately recall the duration of inhalation, and the patient's health and age may affect the outcome. Many chemicals can cause hyposmia or even anosmia following inhalation, making the assessment of duration and type of chemical agent inhaled all the more difficult. Some individuals are known to be much more chemically sensitized than others, especially if, for example, asthma, smoking, or an acquired sensitivity is present. Many of the chemicals discussed thus far are listed as causing RADS or occupationally-induced asthma.[67,68] Currently, most doctrines describe management, including ventilation support, pulmonary function tests, chest radiographs, supportive fluid replacement, and antiinflammatory treatment. The mechanisms of toxicity in acute lung injury processes are largely consistent from chemical to chemical, and injuries detected early will respond more readily to supportive or specialized treatment. Several compounds for which experimental or even clinical supportive therapy has been successfully used are detailed below.

Ammonia

Inhalation exposure to ammonia, generally considered a central airway compartment irritant, can cause damage to the airway epithelium and the alveolar-capillary membrane. Acute signs and symptoms of inhalation, typical of irritant gases, include coughing, bronchospasm, difficulty in breathing, pulmonary edema, hypoxemia, and respiratory failure.[69] At death, hemorrhagic pulmonary edema can be a hallmark of exposure. Interstitial fibrosis has been observed in patients following accidental exposure to ammonia.[70]

In rabbits exposed to nebulized ammonia at an estimated accidental exposure level (35,000–39,000 ppm over 4 minutes), acute and severe lung injury occurred. Decreased Pao_2 and increases in airway pressure and $Paco_2$ were evident from 1 to 6 hours after exposure.[69] In this experimental model, the use of inhaled corticosteroids such as budesonide administered 30 minutes after exposure was not effective in improving gas exchange or reducing elevated airway pressure. Corticosteroids are controversial for therapy following ammonia inhalation and ingestion exposure in humans.

Chlorine

Affecting both the central and peripheral airway compartments, chlorine inhalation leads to abrupt bronchoconstriction, increased airway resistance, and decreased compliance. In humans who have died from chlorine poisoning, severe pulmonary edema, pneumonia, and ulcerative tracheobronchitis have been seen.[71] Recently, epithelial cell necrosis, small airway dilation, and microvascular permeability have been found.[44] Efficacious therapeutic treatments have been tested in experimental models using large swine. Aerosolized terbutaline or the corticosteroid budesonide reduced acute lung injury when administered 30 minutes after a 400 ppm × 20-minute exposure.[72] Lung function was improved even more when both compounds were administered in combination. The effect of terbutaline or budesonide corroborates the biochemical response mentioned earlier: terbutaline helps increase cAMP levels through the stimulation of β-adrenergic signaling pathways and adenylate cyclase, thereby increasing tight junction strength and the integrity of the air–blood barrier, which reduces fluid transport through compromised basement membranes. Budesonide can work by reducing proinflammatory cytokines and by stabilizing membranes by limiting the effects of membrane lipid peroxidative processes and the subsequent release of reactive mediators.

Hydrogen Cyanide

As a metabolic poison, HCN presents a challenge for effective postexposure treatment. It is also considered to be a cardiotoxin. Acute exposure to HCN rarely causes specific changes in histopathological or pathological changes.[73] Many people believe that the slightest contact with HCN means instant death, but studies of experimental animals have disproven this belief. Sublethal concentrations can produce incapacitation, with dizziness and nausea reported in some exposed people.[74] However, treatment should always be provided as rapidly as possible. Supportive and antidote treatments against HCN include the use of sodium thiosulfate, which hastens the detoxification of CN; sodium nitrite, a methemoglobin former; and rhodanese, an enzyme currently used in experimental trials. In some instances 100% oxygen supportive therapy in conjunction with sodium thiosulfate and sodium nitrite may be synergistically beneficial. Treatment with sodium bicarbonate can be used to reverse lactate acidosis. Ballantyne and Salem[75] provide an in-depth review of HCN exposure effects, mechanisms of action, antidotes, and sources of exposure, and Chapter 11, Cyanide Poisoning, provides additional information.

Perfluoroisobutylene

A significant exposure hazard from fires and chemical industrial accidents, PFIB causes severe pulmonary edema in the peripheral airway compartment. In mice PFIB exposure caused a significant reduction in protective sulfhydryl concentrations and myeloperoxidase activity, as well as enhancement of the influx of polymorphonuclear leukocytes into the lung.[76] Exposure can disrupt the air–blood barrier, cause hemorrhagic pulmonary edema, and increase BALF protein leak. Treatment with cholinolytic 3-quinuclidinyl benzilate 30 minutes before or 10 hours after exposure resulted in reduced indices of acute lung injury as measured by lung wet weight to body weight ratio, reduced blood viscosity and reduced mortality.

Phosgene

Because of phosgene's extensive industrial use and extreme toxicity, a great deal of experimental model development, mechanistic toxicology, and therapeutic testing has taken place over the past 25 years. Phosgene is very chemically reactive, especially with important cellular components of biomolecules, such as sulfhydryl, amine, and hydroxyl groups.[25] This chemical reactivity occurs primarily in the distal lung peripheral airway compartment, and exposure has been found to directly affect type I pneumocytes,[77,78] increase lavage polymorphonuclear phagocytes,[79] decrease both cytochrome-*c*-oxidase and adenosine triphosphatase activity,[80] and significantly reduce lung adenosine triphosphate concentrations.[81] Some limited and questionable evidence suggests that phosgene inhalation may be involved in toxic encephalopathy in humans[82]; however, this study involved long-term exposure to many chemical solvents in an industrial environment, which may have confounded the role of phosgene as a single causative agent of neurotoxicity.

Recent experimental work with phosgene in animals has shown that bronchoconstriction, enhanced pulmonary edema formation, elevated leukotriene production, increased lipid peroxidation byproducts, and decreases in both dynamic compliance and lung tissue cAMP are several of the major responses of the lung to phosgene inhalation.[59,83,84] Phosgene has been found to be toxic through normal metabolic detoxification mechanisms unrelated to direct inhalation exposure. In hepatocytes, phosgene binds with phospholipids such as phosphatidylcholine and ethanolamine under hypoxic or normoxic conditions.[85–87] These bonds could be mechanistically important during the injury process because alveolar surfactant is largely phospholipid in content and alveolar edema causes a locally hypoxic environment. Experimental evidence has shown that phosgene exposure has a significant effect on lung surfactant levels.[88]

Based on these detrimental effects, postexposure therapeutic efforts have succeeded in reducing lung injury in exposed animals. Studies involving rodents and rabbits have shown that the effects of increased pulmonary edema, airway pressure, and pulmonary artery pressure, as well as the inhibition of the release of reactive metabolites (such as the permeability-enhancing leukotrienes, vasoactive prostaglandins, and free radicals) can all be reduced following treatment after exposure. Compounds approved by the US Food and Drug Administration such as isoproterenol, ibuprofen, aminophylline, and N-acetylcysteine can protect the lung from further damage.[33,83,89,90] In some cases, treatment can enhance survival rates.[89] No data supports the use of steroids to treat human exposure. However, medical management guidelines from the Centers for Disease Control and Prevention recommend starting intravenous corticosteroids in cases of severe exposure even if the patient is asymptomatic. Steroids administrated intravenously seem to be more beneficial when administered before exposure,[59] although this finding has yet to be tested clinically on a large scale. Not all effective treatment against phosgene-induced lung injury involves the use of drugs. In large swine exposed to phosgene, effective therapy involved the modification of ventilation parameters after exposure. Lower tidal volume, decreased ventilation rates, and decreased positive end-expiratory pressure, in addition to intravenous saline and glucose support, reduced cardiovascular effects, lung damage (reduced edema formation), and the histopathological response of the lung tissue.[40]

In addition to producing acute lung injury to the central and peripheral compartments, phosgene, chlorine, riot control agents, smokes, and ammonia can have long-term effects. Fibrosis, bronchiolitis obliterans, chronic obstructive pulmonary disease, RADS, pulmonary function abnormalities, alveolitis, and bronchiectasis are some of the sequela of exposure. The exposure could have been a one-time event, chronic exposure over years, or a multiple chemical exposure. In addition, gases such as PFIB, phosgene, and chlorine may give rise to ARDS in the days to weeks after exposure, especially if the exposure requires intensive care intervention. Both long-term effects and the potential for developing an ARDS-like response must be taken into account in the administration of therapeutic countermeasures.

CLINICAL PRESENTATION AND DIAGNOSIS

This section considers only TICs that pose a potential threat to military personnel. Although this list is not complete, casualties from other lung-damaging agents are managed in the same way as these examples. In low doses, highly reactive TICs have a greater effect on the central airway; some TICs act on both the central and peripheral airways; and still others that are not as reactive in the central airway can defuse deeper into the respiratory tract and destroy the tissues of the alveoli-capillary membrane in the peripheral airways, leading to noncardiac pulmonary edema. Any large inhaled dose of a TIC causes both central and peripheral airway damage (Figure 10-4).

Centrally Acting Toxic Industrial Chemicals

Centrally acting chemicals affect the respiratory system from the nasopharynx to the bronchioles. Centrally acting TICs normally form strong acids or bases (alkali) with the water in the central airway tissues, which leads to the destruction of these tissues. The damaged tissue swells, causing sloughing of the epithelium lining into the airway and reactive smooth muscle contraction, causing restriction of breathing.

Levels of exposure to toxic gases are defined by the short-term exposure limit (STEL), time-weighted average (TWA), and concentrations at which toxic gasses are immediately dangerous to life or health (IDLH). STEL is the concentration of exposure that after 15 minutes may cause immediate or chronic compromise to health. TWA is the concentration for an 8-hour workday of a 40-hour workweek that most workers can be exposed to without adverse effects.[91]

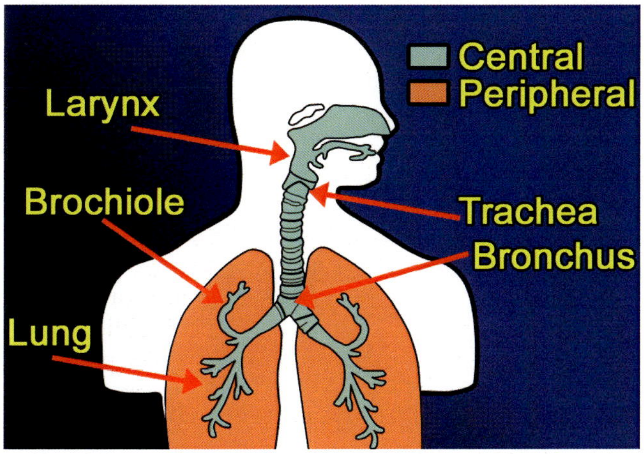

Fig. 10-4. Airway compartments: central and peripheral. Courtesy of: US Army Medical Research Institute of Chemical Defense, Aberdeen Proving Ground, Md.

Ammonia

This highly caustic and reactive gas has not been used in warfare but may be encountered in industrial accidents. Ammonia has a TWA of 25 ppm, an STEL of 35 ppm and an IDLH of 500 ppm. Most injuries from ammonia are caused by inhalation. In low doses it is primarily a centrally acting TIC (Table 10-6). Ammonia gas usually causes damage when it contacts the moist, watery tissues of the central airway, which results in the formation of a strongly alkaline solution. This reaction is exothermic—capable of causing significant thermal burns and destruction to tissues —which could lead to the victims presenting with a laryngospasm and airway collapse.

In 1941 Caplin classified accidental ammonia inhalation as mild, moderate, and severe. Casualties with mild exposure present with pain and conjunctival and upper respiratory inflammation but no signs of respi-

TABLE 10-6

GASEOUS AMMONIA EFFECTS AT VARIOUS CONCENTRATIONS

Amount (ppm)	Effects
25–50	Detectable odor; adverse effects unlikely
50–100	Mild eye, nose, and throat irritation
140	Moderate eye irritation
400	Moderate throat irritation
700	Immediate eye injury
1,000	Directly caustic to airway
1,700	Laryngospasm
2,500	Fatal (after half-hour exposure)
2,500–6,500	Sloughing and necrosis of airway mucosa, chest pain, pulmonary edema and bronchospasm
5,000	Rapidly fatal

Data source: Issley S. Toxicity, ammonia. eMedicine from WebMD. Available at: http://www.emedicine.com/EMERG/topic846.htm. Accessed August 6, 2007.

ratory distress. Casualties with moderate exposure present with the same signs but more exaggerated symptoms. Casualties with a severe exposure present with frank respiratory distress, productive cough, pulmonary edema, and dysphagia. After a brief exposure damage is usually limited to the upper airway mucosa. However, a brief exposure at a very high concentration can be overwhelming to the victim and the entire respiratory system.

Ammonia inhalation injuries also lead to pain of the oroharyngeal and retrosternal areas. Symptoms of dyspnea, hemoptysis, hoarseness, and loss of consciousness could be noted. Tissues of the airway become swollen, and, longer term, scar tissue may form along the airway. Frequently, damaged tissue in the airway will die, slough off, and lead to obstruction. Individuals with reactive airway disease are particularly sensitive to ammonia inhalation.

Ammonia can also be absorbed by dust particles that travel to the small airways. Respiratory symptoms can develop after the ingestion of ammonia products if aspiration pneumonia or pneumonitis complicates ingestion. Most casualties who survive the first 24 hours will recover. Patients show improvement within 48 to 72 hours, and patients with mild exposure could recover fully in this time. For patients with more severe respiratory symptoms, recovery can be expected within several weeks to months.[91]

Sulfur Mustards

Produced solely for warfare, sulfur mustards are vesicants and alkylating agents that act on the central airway if inhaled. Sulfur mustards cause a dose-dependent inflammatory reaction in the upper and lower airways that develops several hours after exposure and progresses. Burning of the nasal pathway results in pain, epistaxis, larynigitis, loss of taste and smell, coughing, wheezing, and possible dyspnea. Necrosis of the respiratory epithelium causes tissue to slough off in large sheets, known as pseudomembranes, causing local airway obstruction.[92] Prolonged or repeated acute exposure to sulfur mustards could lead to chronic respiratory disease. Repeated exposures result in cumulative effects because mustards are not detoxified naturally in the body.[93] Chapter 8, Vesicants, provides more information on the medical management of sulfur mustards agents.

Peripherally Acting Toxic Industrial Chemicals

Air moves in the peripheral compartment of the airways only by diffusion. When peripherally acting lung-damaging TICs are inhaled, they travel to the smallest segments of the respiratory system, the terminal and respiratory bronchioles, the alveolar ducts, the alveolar sacs, and the alveoli. These agents also cause inflammation and necrosis to the thin membrane that separates the capillaries from the alveoli by reacting with the proteins and enzymes in the membranes. The function of these membranes is to separate the blood in the capillaries from the air in the alveoli, but when the membranes become damaged, this process cannot occur. When the normal elimination of plasma serum from the respiratory system is interrupted because of this damage, the plasma leaks into the alveolar septa, causing the air sacs to fill with fluid, blocking oxygen exchange. The casualty then suffers oxygen deprivation leading to hypoxia and apnea. The pulmonary tissue fills with massive amounts of fluid (up

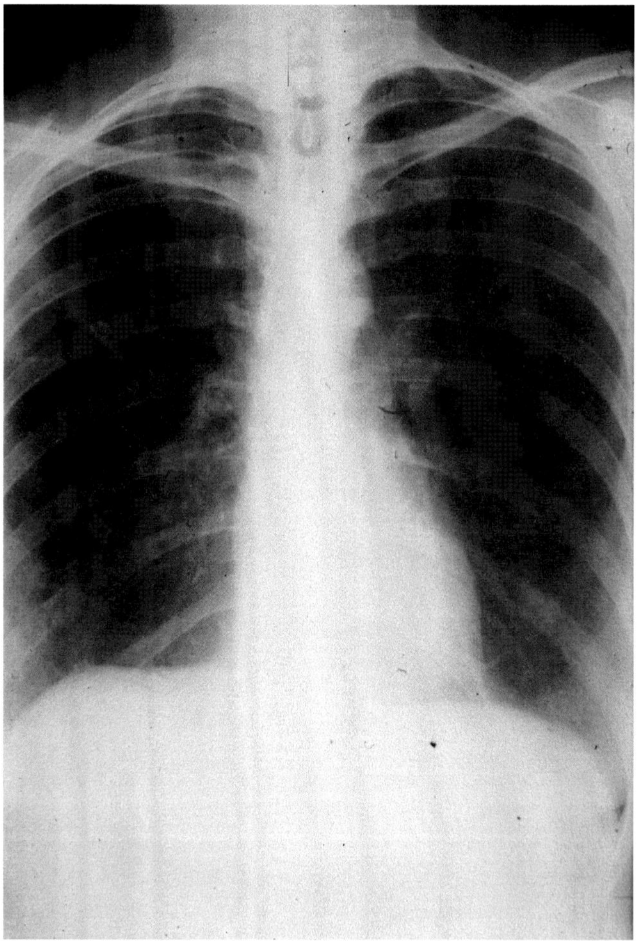

Fig. 10–5. The chest radiograph of a male chemical worker 2 hours postexposure to phosgene with mild resting dyspnea for the 2nd hour. His physical examination was normal with a Po_2 of 88 mm Hg breathing room air. The radiograph is normal.

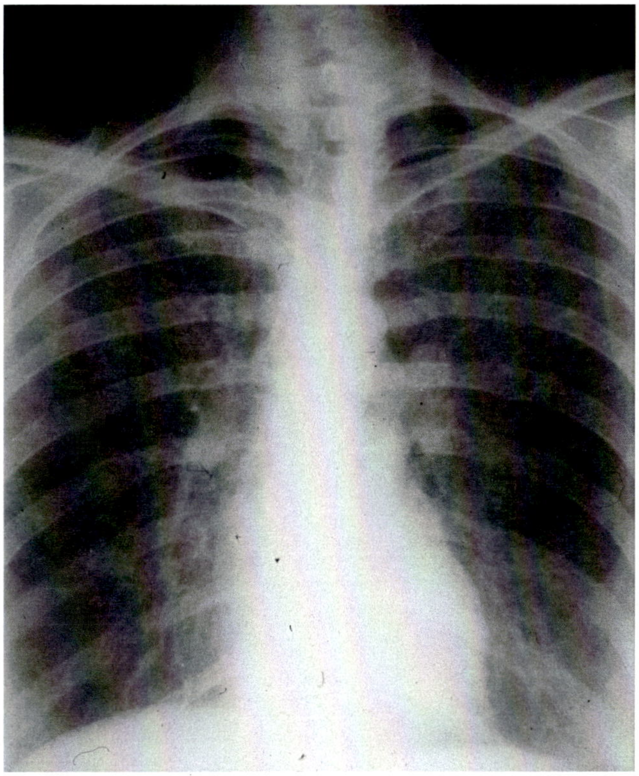

Fig. 10-6. The same patient seen in Figure 10-5 now 7 hours postexposure to phosgene with moderate resting dyspnea, a few crackles on auscultation, and a Po_2 of 64 mm Hg breathing room air. The radiograph shows mild interstitial edema.

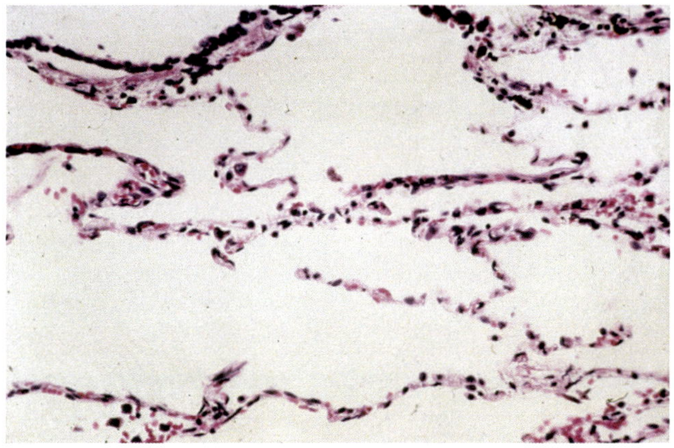

Fig. 10–7. A lung section from the patient whose chest radiographs are shown in Figures 10-5 and 10-6. This section shows normal lung tissues without evidence of interstitial fibrosis or inflammation. Hematoxylin and eosin stain; original magnification × 400.

to 1 L/h), which leads to noncardiogenic pulmonary edema (Figures 10-5 – 10-8). For this reason, peripherally acting TIC poisoning is sometimes referred to as "dry land drowning." The damage following acute exposure to peripherally acting lung-damaging TICs is proportionate to the product of the concentration and duration of exposure (Haber's law); however, with chronic exposure Haber's law does not apply.[1]

Perfluoroisobutylene

Produced as a common by-product in the fluoropolymer industry, PFIB is used for long-term protection against high temperatures and corrosive chemicals in automobiles, jet aircraft, and other products. Teflon's lubricity, high dielectric constant, and chemical inertness make it a desirable component for the interior of many military vehicles, such as tanks and aircraft. PFIB smoke is given off when Teflon burns at temperatures above 400°C, such as in a vehicle fire. Closed-space fires in military vehicles have prompted research on the toxicity of exposure to the by-products

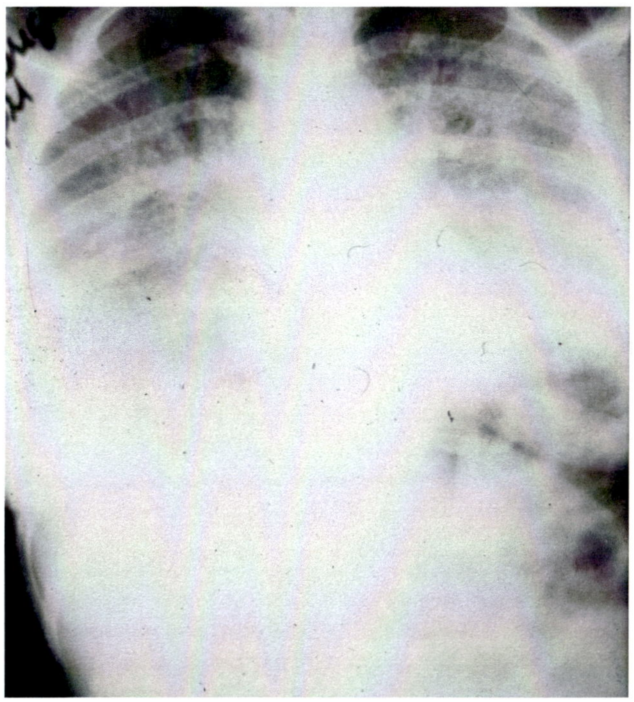

Fig. 10–8. The chest radiograph of a female chemical worker 2 hours postexposure to phosgene. Dyspnea progressed rapidly over the 2nd hour; Po_2 was 40 mm Hg breathing room air. This radiograph shows bilateral perihilar, fluffy, and diffuse interstitial infiltrates. The patient died 6 hours postexposure.

created from incinerated organofluorines released by PFIB. The pyrolysis of PFIB produces a particulate smoke, which produces symptoms termed "polymer fume fever" when inhaled. Polymer fume fever is an influnza-like, self-limited symptom complex with a latent period of some hours followed by fever, chills, and myalgias (which could lead to the misdiagnosis of an acute viral illness). Typically, polymer fume fever episodes resolve within 24 hours; however, some cases have been reported to last longer. Only supportive care including antipyretics and hydration is recommended. If wheezing or other obstructive respiratory changes occur, inhaled bronchodilators are indicated. With bronchospasms or productive cough, inhaled steroids may be indicated. Patients with polymer fume fever should be observed for at least 24 to 48 hours for other lung consolidation changes such as chemical pneumonitis or noncardiogenic pulmonary edema. Oxygen therapy including intubation with positive end-expiratory pressure may be necessary if respiratory distress is severe. Use of antibiotic and systemic steroids should be considered, depending on the patient's condition. Survivors of vehicle fires who are short of breath should be questioned carefully about smoke exposure and should be observed over a period of time.[94]

Oxides of Nitrogen

Oxides of nitrogen, or NOx, are components of photochemical smog, which can be produced by the detonation of nitrate-based explosives or by electric or arc welding. Significant quantities of nitrogen dioxide are found in the exhaust of diesel engines. These dangerous nitrous fumes can build to high concentrations on the battlefield where artillery is fired and in enclosed spaces with inadequate ventilation, such as gun pits, ship magazines, armored vehicles, and turrets, as well as in mining and tunneling operations. Inhalation of NOx leads to the formation of nitrite, the production of methemoglobin, and cellular hypoxia. Inhalation of high concentrations could cause rapid death without the formation of pulmonary edema; however, a severe exposure may result in death with the production of yellow frothy fluid in the nasal passages, mouth, and trachea, as well as with marked pulmonary edema. Symptoms following inhalation of NOx are mostly due to nitrogen dioxide. The diagnosis is made from the history, from symptoms described by the patient, and possibly by the yellowish discoloration of the exposed membranes. NOx exposure should be suspected in soldiers who experience shortness of breath after heavy artillery firing in an enclosed space (tanks, ships).[95]

Hexachloroethane Smoke

Hexachloroethane (HC) smoke, a mixture of equal amounts of HC and zinc oxide with approximately 7% grained aluminum or aluminum powder, is used in the military for obscuration. HC smoke is probably the most acutely toxic of the military smokes and obscurants. Its toxicity is due mainly to the irritating effects of the zinc chloride. The more humid the air, the denser HC smoke will be. HC smoke is dispersed by grenades, candles, pots, artillery shells, and special air bombs.[95]

Zinc oxide cause upper respiratory tract (central compartment) damage from its irritant and corrosive action. In severe exposures, chemical pneumonia with pulmonary edema can appear. A chest radiograph of a 60-year-old sailor 8 hours after exposure to HC while in an enclosed space onboard ship shows diffuse dense peripheral pulmonary infiltrates (Figure 10-9). He had symptoms of moderately severe resting dyspnea during the 7th and 8th hours, with diffuse coarse crackles noted on auscultation.[96] Metal fume fever, which has been documented with an intense inhalation of metal oxides such as zinc oxide, has a delayed onset of 4 to 48 hours after exposure, with symptoms including dryness of the throat, coughing, substernal chest pain or tightness, and fever. Respiratory symptoms generally resolve in 1 to 4 days with supportive care. Most individuals with HC inhalation injuries progress to complete recovery; however, 10% to 20% develop fi-

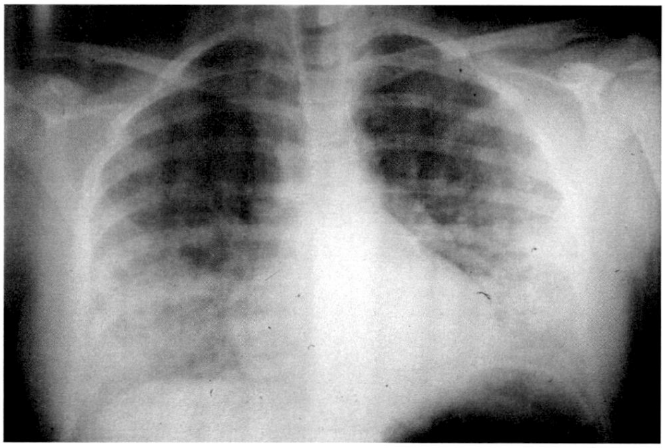

Fig. 10-9. Chest radiograph taken 8 hours postexposure of a 60-year-old male sailor who inhaled zinc oxide in an enclosed space. He showed symptoms of moderately severe resting dyspnea during the 7th and 8th hours, diffuse coarse crackles on auscultation, and a Po_2 of 41 mm Hg breathing room air. The radiograph confirms diffuse dense peripheral pulmonary infiltrates.

brotic pulmonary changes. Appropriate precautions, such as wearing protective masks, must be taken when HC smoke is used.[95]

Chemicals That Act on Both the Central and Peripheral Airways

Chlorine

Chlorine is a good example of a combination agent, one that acts on both airway compartments in low doses because of its intermediate water solubility. Chlorine's effectiveness as a warfare agent was greatly reduced once protective masks became widely available in World War I, but it continues to be seen in industrial accidents. The Occupational Safety and Health Administration's permissible exposure level of chlorine is 1 ppm. The National Institute for Occupational Safety and Health has determined that the IDLH concentration is 25 ppm. Chlorine turns to hydrochloric acid when it contacts the moisture of the airway; the hydrochloric acid then causes tissue burns to the epithelia of the conjunctivae and upper respiratory mucus membranes.[97] Chlorine produces signs and symptoms similar to those associated with exposure to both centrally and peripherally acting agents. A chest radiograph of a chemical worker 2 hours after exposure to chlorine shows diffuse pulmonary edema without considerable cardiomegaly (Figure 10-10). This person also experienced severe resting dyspnea and diffuse crackles on auscultation. Although the central lung damage of chlorine injury may seem to be the primary concern in some patients (ie, they are coughing and wheezing), the healthcare provider must anticipate treatment for potential development of peripheral symptoms and take seriously any patient complaints about chest tightness or breathing difficulty.[96]

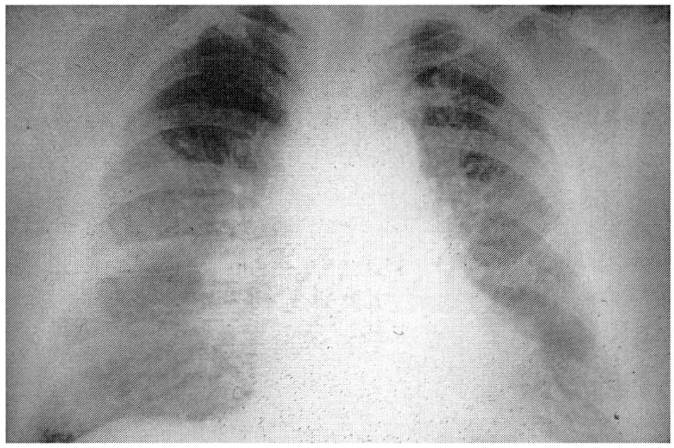

Fig. 10-10. The chest radiograph of a female chemical worker 2 hours postexposure to chlorine inhalant. On medical examination she had severe resting dyspnea during the 2nd hour, diffuse crackles/rhonchi on auscultation, and a Po_2 of 32 mm Hg breathing room air. The radiograph shows diffuse pulmonary edema without significant cardiomegaly.

Clinical Effects

Centrally Acting Agents

Almost immediately after exposure to these gasses or vapors, the casualty can develop a laryngospasm, which could cause sudden death. As the airways are irritated and damaged, the individual may experience a wide variety of symptoms including sneezing; development of rhinorrhea; tachypea; pain in the nasopharynx, indicating early inflammation; dysphagia from the pain of swallowing; oropharyngeal inflammation; hoarseness; a feeling of choking; noise with exhalation caused by laryngeal edema (the hallmark sign of centrally acting agents); chest pain or retrosternal burning; coughing, which could be violent at times; wheezing during breathing from the trachea and bronchi inflammation; and edema. If the exposure is severe enough and the TIC has penetrated into the peripheral airway, the casualty may experience peripheral effects. Later, scarring of the central airway can cause permanent airway narrowing, depending on the agent involved and the dose received.

Peripherally Acting Agents

Peripherally acting agents exert a direct toxic effect on the peripheral compartment of the respiratory tract, leading to damage of the alveolar-capillary membrane and the hallmark clinical effect—dyspnea. The time to onset of clinical effects from peripherally acting agents depends on dose, duration, and concentration. Shortly after low concentration exposure to phosgene or other agents affecting the peripheral airway, the casualties are typically asymptomatic for 30 minutes to 72 hours (although they may notice irritation of the eyes, nose, and throat). However, symptoms may progress to complaints of coughing and dyspnea on exertion. The major effects do not occur until hours later. More significant exposures have a latency period of less than 24 hours. Chlorine, which can affect both compartments but primarily affects the central compartment of the respiratory tract, can also exhibit delayed effects in the peripheral compartment.

Approximately 2 to 24 hours after exposure, the casualty with peripheral damage will notice shortness of breath and tightness in the chest, which are symptoms of the development of noncardiogenic pulmonary edema. These symptoms may initially be mild, but as the damage progresses, dyspnea on exertion will become resting dyspnea. Coughing is at first nonproductive with chest tightness or discomfort described as retrosternal burning, but if the damage is severe, the casualty will start producing clear to yellow frothy sputum. This is caused by necrosis and inflammation of the lower airway and alveolar tissue and subsequent leakage of serum into the alveolar septa.

The eventual severity of dyspnea is related to dose, concentration, and duration of the exposure. A casualty with a very mild exposure will develop dyspnea 6 to 24 hours after exposure, first noticed after heavy exertion. Later, however, the casualty becomes short of breath after any activity. With proper care, complete recovery is expected. A casualty with a severe exposure will notice shortness of breath within 4 to 6 hours after exposure. Dyspnea, even at rest, results from inability of the pulmonary lymph system to eliminate the large amount of fluid produced from the necrosis of the alveolar-capillary membrane. This leads to the clinical presentation of noncardiogenic pulmonary edema, causing hypoxia and apnea. These casualties, even with intensive pulmonary care, may not survive.

Many of the casualties exposed to lung-damaging agents are between these two extreme situations. When the onset of dyspnea is more than 6 hours after exposure, there may be progression to dyspnea at rest. However, with good pulmonary care beginning early after the onset of effects, the casualty should recover completely. Failure to consider the asymptomatic period and delayed onset of peripherally acting lung-damaging agents may lead to early discharge from the emergency room, without an adequate period of observation, and possibly to a poor outcome.[1]

Diagnostic Tests

No commonly available laboratory tests exist for the specific identification or quantification of exposure to lung-damaging agents; however, an increase in the hematocrit may reflect the hemoconcentration induced by transudation of fluid into the pulmonary parenchyma from the peripherally acting agents. Arterial blood gases may show a low PaO_2 or $PaCO_2$, which is an early, nonspecific warning of increased interstitial fluid in the lung. Peak expiratory flow rate may decrease early after a massive exposure to peripherally acting agents. This nonspecific test helps assess the degree of airway damage and the effect of bronchodilator therapy. Decreased lung compliance and carbon monoxide diffusing capacity are particularly sensitive indicators of interstitial fluid volume in the lung, but because of their complexity, these tests are usually performed only in hospitals.

Chest Radiograph

Initial findings on a chest radiograph may be normal; as the disease process progresses, the radiograph may demonstrate bilateral diffuse interstitial infiltrates. The early finding on a chest radiograph is hyperinflation, which suggests toxic injury of the smaller airway that results in air being diffusely trapped in the alveoli. The appearance of "batwing" infiltrates is caused by pulmonary edema secondary to the alveolar capillary membrane damage. Pulmonary edema develops later and without cardiovascular changes of redistribution or cardiomegaly. Radiological changes from centrally acting lung-damaging agents may occur for hours to days, so the use of a chest radiograph may be of limited value.

Arterial Blood Gases

Measuring carboxyhemoglobin and methemoglobin levels can help determine whether the casualties have been exposed to methylene chloride or confirm suspected carbon monoxide exposure; methemoglobinemia may suggest other causes. Serial arterial blood gases in cases of significant respiratory distress demonstrate the degree of hypoxemia. Hypoxia is often the result of exposure to both centrally and peripherally acting lung-damaging agents. The measurement of the partial pressure of oxygen (PO_2) can give insight into the treatment of hypoxia, but it is a nonspecific tool in the diagnosis of exposure to a lung-damaging agent.[1]

Pulmonary Function Tests

A variety of airway and pulmonary parenchymal function measures can be performed in rear-medical treatment facilities. Initial and follow-up measurements of the flow-volume loop, lung volumes, and lung diffusing capacity for carbon monoxide are particularly useful in assessing and managing long-term effects of a lung-damaging TIC exposure. Although such laboratory studies are of minimal value in an acute-care setting, flow-volume loop measures may document a previously unrecognized degree of airway obstruction. A degree of reversibility may also be demonstrated if bronchodilators are tested at the same time. Substantial airway obstruction may be present with little clinical evidence. In all cases of unexplained dyspnea, regardless of clinical findings, careful pulmonary function measurements should be undertaken. Ideally, these studies should be performed in an established pulmonary function laboratory and would include lung diffusing capacity for carbon monoxide and arterial blood gas measurements. These studies should also be performed during exertion if the patient has dyspnea on exertion that cannot otherwise be explained by pulmonary function studies performed at rest.[1]

Bronchoalveolar Lavage

Bronchoalveolar lavage is a diagnostic procedure that involves washing a sample of cells and secretions from the alveolar and bronchial airspaces. An inflammatory response can be detected by polymorphonuclear leukocytes and an increase in protein content in the lung washings. Cell death or membrane damage can be indicated by the release of cytoplasmic enzymes and lactate dehydrogenase into the acellular portion of the lavage fluid. Animals chronically exposed to insoluble particles show a large increase in some lysosomal enzymes found in the bronchoalveolar lavage fluid. Also, angiotensin-converting enzymes have been found to be elevated with endothelial cell damage in the pulmonary capillaries. Although bronchoalveolar lavage has been used to validate the presence of acute lung injury from TICs, the method is limited by the large range of normal values for each parameter.[53]

Other Tests

- Pulmonary capillary wedge pressure should be monitored in cases of severe pulmonary edema or ARDS.
- Ventilation/perfusion scans can show abnormal air trapping in the setting of lower airway obstruction and may be useful to help gauge severity or progress of respiratory disease; however, these findings are unlikely to change acute medical management.
- Carbon dioxide levels should be monitored in patients with prior lung disease such as asthma and chronic obstructive pulmonary disease; these patients may be affected more severely and are at greater risk of retaining carbon dioxide.

MEDICAL MANAGEMENT

Lung-damaging TIC casualties may have minimal signs and symptoms during the acute phase, and the prognosis should be guarded. Ongoing reassessment is an essential component of the early medical management of these casualties, for they could rapidly develop severe noncardigenic pulmonary edema. However, many of the casualties who survive for more than 48 hours recover without sequelae. A complete medical history is one of the most important aspects in the medical management of these casualties. In contrast to most occupational inhalational exposures, lung-damaging chemical warfare agents need specific immediate treatment in addition to the usual supportive care (the suspicion of exposure to lung-damaging chemical warfare agents is of course higher in times of war or terrorist activity).

Patient History

Collecting historical data from the casualty is a critical aspect of assessing and treating individuals exposed to lung-damaging agents. No specific statement can determine the correct diagnosis and ultimate treatment, but careful questioning of an exposed individual will often greatly simplify the diagnosis and medical therapy. Different approaches to collecting a history may be needed depending on the circumstances of the events involved (see Exhibit 10-1 for a list of example questions). If a casualty is unable to provide a history of the incident, an observation of the scene can be helpful in determining treatment, the amount of time needed for observation, and the likely prognosis. Other personnel on the scene of the incident, who may have conducted reconnaissance or any atmospheric monitoring, may be able to assist in the clinical decision making.

Physical Examination

Physical examination may be particularly difficult in the event of combined lung-damaging TICs and conventional injuries; therefore, it is essential that medical personnel note the patient's physical condition (specific conditions to look for are listed in Exhibit 10-2). Symptoms of lung-damaging TIC inhalation injuries can be delayed in onset, but some conditions that may precede the onset of delayed symptoms include facial burns, inflamed nares, wheezing, altered mental status, and productive cough. Coughing will more than likely be the first symptom noted (although an occasional

EXHIBIT 10–1

HISTORY ASSESSMENT FOR CASUALTIES EXPOSED TO LUNG-DAMAGING AGENTS

- **Environment**: Were the explosions observed? Was there obvious smoke? If so, what color was it? Was the smoke heavier than air or close to the ground? What was the weather condition (temperature, rain, wind, daylight, fog)? Were there pools of liquid or a thickened substance in evidence?
- **Protective posture:** What was the level of mission-oriented protective posture (MOPP)? Was there face mask or suit damage? Did the face mask fit adequately? When was the filter last changed? How well trained was the indivual in using the appropriate protective posture? Were other factors present (eg, consumption of alcoholic beverages, exposure to other chemicals, psychiatric status)?
- **Prior exposure:** Was there prior exposure to other chemical agents? Is the individual a cigarette smoker? (For how many years? How recently did he or she last smoke? How many cigarettes smoked a day?)
- **Pulmonary history:** Is there a prior history of chest trauma, hay fever, asthma, pneumonia, tuberculosis, exposure to tuberculosis, recurrent bronchitis, chronic cough or sputum production, or shortness of breath on exertion?
- **Cardiac and endocrine history:** Is there a history of cardiac or endocrine disorder?
- **Acute exposure history:** What were the initial signs and symptoms?
  - **Eyes:** Is there burning, itching, tearing, or pain? How long after exposure did symptoms occur: minutes, hours, days?
  - **Nose and sinuses:** Was a gas odor detected? Is there rhinorrhea, epistaxis, or pain? How long after exposure did symptoms occur: minutes, hours, days?
  - **Mouth and throat:** Is there pain, choking, or cough? How long after exposure did symptoms occur: minutes, hours, days?
  - **Pharynx and larynx:** Are there swallowing difficulties, cough, stridor, hoarseness, or aphonia? How long after exposure did symptoms occur: minutes, hours, days?
  - **Trachea and mainstem bronchi:** Is there coughing, wheezing, substernal burning, pain, or dyspnea? How long after exposure did symptoms occur: minutes, hours, days?
  - **Peripheral airways and parenchyma:** Is there dyspnea or chest tightness? How long after exposure did symptoms occur: minutes, hours, days?
  - **Cardiac:** Are there palpitations, angina, or syncope? How long after exposure did symptoms occur: minutes, hours, days?
  - **Central nervous system:** Is there diffuse or focal neurological dysfunction?

Data source: Bickley LS, Szilagyi PG. *Bates' Guide to Physical Examination and History Taking*. 9th ed. Philadelpha: Lippincott-Raven; 2005.

cough may be a symptom of asthma).

Acute Medical Management

Exposure to lung-damaging agents can be limited by removing casualties from the environment in which the toxicant is present. Careful decontamination serves to limit reexposure to the toxicant from body surfaces or clothing, as well as reducing the risk of secondary exposure of healthcare personnel. Listed below are important steps in the acute management of lung-damaging agents. See Exhibit 10-3 for triage procedures.

Terminate Exposure and Decontaminate

The first vital measure is to physically remove the casualty from the contaminated environment or properly fit the person with a protective mask. Decontamination starts with the staff and decontamination team in the appropriate protective gear. Decontamination of any liquid agent on skin and removal of clothing (where agent vapors could be trapped) will fully terminate the exposure from these sources. Removal of the casualty's clothing, if it has been contaminated with liquid agent, prevents cross contamination of any unprotected staff or casualty. If eye involvement is reported, remove contact lenses, if present, and irrigate with copious amounts of water or saline. If the skin exposure is significant, wash with copious amounts of water and mild soap.[97]

Implement ABCs

Establishing an airway is especially crucial in a patient exhibiting hoarseness or stridor; such individuals may face impending laryngeal spasm. Establishing a

EXHIBIT 10-2

PHYSICAL ASSESSMENT FOR CASUALTIES OF LUNG-DAMAGING CHEMICAL AGENTS

- **Reliability:** Is the casualty alert and oriented?
- **Appearance**: Is the casualty anxious or tachypneic?
- **Vital Signs:** What are the casuality's weight, blood pressure, pulse, temperature and pulse oximetry?
- **Trauma:** Is there a head injury? Are there burns in the region of the eyes, nose, or mouth?
- **Skin**: Are there signs of burns, erythema, cyanosis, sweating, or dryness? Are there facial or oral burns and ulceration?
- **Eyes**: Is there conjunctivitis, corneal burns or abrasion, lacrimation, miosis, or mydriasis?
- **Nose**: Is there erythema, rhinorrhea, or epistaxis?
- **Oropharynx**: Is there evidence of perioral burns or erythema?
- **Neck**: Is there hoarseness, stridor, or subcutaneous emphysema?
- **Chest**: Is there superficial chest wall trauma, tenderness, crepitation, dullness, or hyperresonance? Palpitatons? Angina?
- **Respiration**: Is tachypnea present? What is the oxygen saturation? Is the a productive cough (with phosgene, cough is initially nonproductive, later frothy white to yellow sputum) Hemoptysis? Are inspiratory crackles, wheezes, rhonchi present?
- **Central nervous system:** Is there loss of consciousness? Headache (thought to be secondary to hypoxemia and the inflammatory response initiated in the pulmonary parenchyma)?

Data source: Bickley LS, Szilagyi PG. *Bates' Guide to Physical Examination and History Taking*. 9th ed. Philadelpha: Lippincott-Raven; 2005.

clear airway also aids in interpretation of auscultatory findings. Steps to minimize the work of breathing must be taken. Because of the always present danger of hypotension induced by pulmonary edema or positive airway pressure, accurate determination of the casualty's circulatory status is vital not only initially, but also at regularly repeated intervals and whenever indicated by the clinical situation.

Implement Rest

Even minimal physical exertion may shorten the clinical latent period and increase the severity of respiratory symptoms and signs in a lung-damaging agent casualty. Physical activity in a symptomatic patient may precipitate acute clinical deterioration and even death. Strict limitation of activity (eg, forced bed rest) and litter evacuation are mandatory for patients suspected of having inhaled any of the edematogenic agents. This is true whether or not the patient has respiratory symptoms and whether or not objective evidence of noncardiogenic pulmonary edema is present.

Manage Airway Secretions; Prevent and Treat Bronchospasm

Unless superinfection is present, secretions present in the airways of lung-damaging agent casualties are usually copious and watery. Secretions may serve as an index to the degree of noncardiogenic pulmonary edema and do not require specific therapy apart from suctioning and drainage. Antibiotics should be reserved for patients with an infectious process documented by sputum Gram staining and culture. Bronchospasm may occur in individuals with reactive airways and should be treated with theophylline or beta-adrenergic bronchodilators. Steroid therapy is also indicated for bronchospasm but must be parenterally administered; inhaled therapy may result in inadequate distribution to damaged airways. Methylprednisolone, 700 to 1,000 mg, or its equivalent may be given intravenously in divided doses during the first day and then tapered during the duration of the clinical illness. The increased susceptibility to bacterial infection during steroid therapy mandates careful surveillance of the patient. There is some support in the literature for steroid use in those exposed to HC smoke (zinc/zinc oxide) and oxides of nitrogen, because steroids can theoretically reduce autoimmune reactions that foster scar development and subsequent bronchiolitis obliterans. In the case of phosgene exposure, the literature suggests that corticosteroid administration in the first 15 minutes postexposure reduces the degree of noncardiogenic pulmonary edema.[98] The literature does not give strong support for the use of steroids in the treatment of other toxic inhalants because steroids reduce lung bacterial clear-

EXHIBIT 10-3

TRIAGE FOR CASUALTIES OF LUNG-DAMAGING TOXIC INDUSTRIAL CHEMICALS

Patients Seen Within 12 Hours of Exposure

- **Immediate**: Patients with pulmonary edema only, and if intensive pulmonary care is immediately available. In general, a shorter latent period portends a more serious illness.
- **Delayed:** Patients who are dyspneic without objective signs should be observed closely and retriaged hourly if not sooner.
- **Minimal**: Asymptomatic patients with known exposure, these patients must be observed and retriaged every 2 hours. If a patient remains asymptomatic 24 hours after exposure, the patient could be discharged. If exposure is doubtful and the patient remains asymptomatic 12 hours following putative exposure, consider discharge.
- **Expectant:** Patients who present with pulmonary edema, cyanosis, and hypotension are classified as expectant. A casualty who presents with these signs within 6 hours of exposure generally will not survive; a casualty with the onset of these signs 6 hours or longer after exposure may possibly survive with immediate, intensive medical care. If ventilatory support is not available, but adequate evacuation assets are, these patients should have priority for urgent evacuation to a facility where adequate ventilatory support is available.[1]

Patients Seen More Than 12 Hours After Exposure

- **Immediate:** Patients who present with pulmonary edema, if they can receive intensive care treatment within several hours.
- **Delayed:** Patients who are dyspneic should be observed closely and retriaged at least every 2 hours. Patients who are recovering from the exposure could be discharged 24 hours after exposure.
- **Minimal:** Patients who are asymptomatic or have resolving dyspnea are classified as minimal. Patients who are asymptomatic 24 hours after exposure may be discharged.
- **Expectant:** Patients who present with persistent hypotension despite intensive medical care interventions. If cyanosis and hypotension are present with pulmonary edema, triage the patient as expectant.

Examples: Patients with only eye or upper airway irritation who are otherwise asymptomatic and with normal physical examination 12 hours later may be returned to duty. If the patient's original complaint was dyspnea only and on physical examination the chest radiograph and arterial blood gases are all normal at 24 hours, he or she may be returned to duty. Patients who presented with symptoms of an abnormal physical examination, chest radiograph, or arterial blood gas require close supervision; however, if physical examination, chest radiograph, and arterial blood gases are all normal at 48 hours, they can be returned to duty.

(1) US Army Medical Research Institute of Chemical Defense. *Medical Management of Chemical Casualties Handbook.* 4th ed. Aberdeen Proving Ground, Md: USAMRICD; 2007.

ance and increase the potential for bacterial pneumonia as a late complication of inhalation injuries, which outweighs any potential antiinflammatory effects. Thus, steroids are not recommended in individuals without evidence of overt or latent reactive airway disease.[99]

Prevent and Treat Pulmonary Edema

Positive airway pressure provides some control over the clinical complications of pulmonary edema. Early use of a positive pressure mask may be beneficial. Positive airway pressure may exacerbate hypotension by decreasing thoracic venous return, necessitating intravenous fluid administration and perhaps judicious use of a pneumatic antishock garment.

Prevent and Treat Hypoxia

Oxygen therapy is definitely indicated and may require supplemental positive airway pressure administered via one of several available devices for generating intermittent or continuous positive pressure. Intubation, with or without ventilatory assistance, may be required, and positive pressure may need to be applied during at least the end-expiratory phase of the ventilator cycle. Humidified oxygen supplementation may be needed.

Prevent and Treat Hypotension

Sequestration of plasma-derived fluid in the lungs

may cause hypotension that may be exacerbated by positive airway pressure. Due to fluid shifts, urgent intravenous administration of either crystalloid or colloid solution (which in this situation appear equally effective) and the use of a pulmonary artery catheter monitor (to avoid excessive fluid administration) may be required to maintain appropriate fluid balance while treating hypotension. The use of vasopressors is a temporary measure until fluids can be replaced.

Clinical Care

Acute lung injury is one of the causes of noncardiogenic pulmonary edema, which causes an increase in lung vascular permeability, leading to accumulation of protein-rich edema in the interstitial and air spaces. Cardiogenic or high-pressure pulmonary edema is caused by elevated pulmonary venous pressure from left ventricular dysfunction, valvular disease, or intravascular volume overload. In addition to ARDS, noncardiogenic pulmonary edema is referred to as "clinical acute lung injury." The care of these patients requires careful attention to the underlying causes such as a treatable pulmonary infection. The modes of mechanical ventilation and hemodynamic management in ARDS patients have been controversial for years, although the National Institutes of Health and other institutions have established a protocol for ARDS patients on mechanical ventilation. Discussion of this protocol and any other strategies is beyond the scope of this chapter; however, one certainty is that ARDS management demands quick recognition and intensive care protocols.[100,101]

Patient Transport

Lung-damaging TIC casualties may need to be evacuated to a higher level of care if the receiving facility does not have an intensive care setting. When a casualty is transferred to a higher level of care, supplemental oxygen and appropriate evaluation monitors must be provided.

Long-Term Effects

The replacement of damaged airway epithelium with granular tissue is one of the major etiologies of chronic lung disease following centrally acting chemical agents such as ammonia.[91] See Chapter 9, Long-Term Health Effects of Chemical Threat Agents, for more detail.

SUMMARY

The respiratory system, both the central and peripheral compartments, can efficiently absorb inhaled lung-damaging agents, leading to airway and pulmonary injury. Few specific antidotes exist for treating inhaled toxicants. Common pathophysiologic pathways link the syndrome of acute inhalation injury to preferential methods of clinical treatment. Understanding the mechanisms of inhalation injury can simplify the decision-making process for treating a casualty with a potential lung-damaging TIC inhalation exposure.

Acknowledgment

The authors wish to thank the following individuals for their efforts: Jennifer L Collins, biologist (USAMRICD), for reviewing the manuscript, and Peter Hurst, graphic designer (USAMRICD), for artwork.

REFERENCES

1. US Army Medical Research Institute of Chemical Defense. *Medical Management of Chemical Casualties Handbook*. 4th ed. Aberdeen Proving Ground, Md: USAMRICD, Chemical Casualty Care Division; 2007.

2. Beswick FW. Chemical agents used in riot control and warfare. *Hum Toxicol*. 1983;2:247–256.

3. Stockholm International Peace Research Institute. *Chemical/Biological Weapons and Biological Warfare.* Vol 1 in: *The Problem of Chemical and Biological Warfare*. New York, NY: Humanities Press, 1971.

4. Jackson KE. Phosgene. *J Chem Educ*. 1933;622–626.

5. Elsayed NM, Salem H. Chemical warfare agents and nuclear weapons. In: Salem H, Katz SA, eds. *Inhalation Toxicology*. 2nd ed. Boca Raton, Fla: CRC/Taylor & Francis; 2006: Chap 22.

6. Gilchrist H. The residual effects of warfare gases: the use of phosgene gas, with report of cases. *Med Bull Vet Admin*. 1933;10:1–36.

7. Department of the Army. *Employment of Riot Control Agent CS*. San Francisco, Calif: HQ, 25th Infantry Division; 1970. DA Letter of Instructions 23–70.

8. US Army Center for Health Promotion and Preventive Medicine. *Industrial Chemical Prioritization and Determination of Critical Hazards of Concern*. Aberdeen Proving Ground, Md: USACHPPM; 2003: Appendix B. USACHPPM Report 47-EM-6154-03.

9. Walton M. Industrial ammonia gassing. *Br J Ind Med*. 1973;30:78–86.

10. Das R, Blanc PD. Chlorine gas exposure and the lung: a review. *Toxicol Ind Health*. 1993;9:439–455.

11. Baxter PJ, Davies PC, Murray V. Medical planning for toxic releases into the community: the example of chlorine gas. *Br J Ind Med*. 1989;46:277–285.

12. Ballantyne B, Callaway S. Inhalation toxicology and pathology of animals exposed to o-chlorobenzylidene malononitrile (CS). *Med Sci Law*. 1972;12:43–65.

13. Hu H, Christiani D. Reactive airways dysfunction after exposure to teargas. *Lancet*. 1992;339:1535.

14. Olajos EJ, Salem H. Riot control agents: pharmacology, toxicology, biochemistry and chemistry. *J Appl Toxicol*. 2001;21:355–391.

15. Norris JC, Ballantyne B. Toxicology and implications of the products of combustion. In: Ballantyne B, Marrs TC, Syversen T, eds. *General and Applied Toxicology*. 2nd ed. London, England: Macmillan; 1999: 1915–1933.

16. Isom GE, Way JL. Effects of oxygen on the antagonism of cyanide intoxication: cytochrome oxidase, in vitro. *Toxicol Appl Pharmacol*. 1984;74:57–62.

17. Oehme FW, Rumbeiha WK. Veterinary toxicology. In: Ballantyne B, Marrs TC, Syversen T, eds. *General and Applied Toxicology*. 2nd ed. London, England: Macmillan; 1999: Chap 69.

18. Burnett WW, King EG, Grace M, Hall WF. Hydrogen sulfide poisoning: review of 5 years' experience. *Can Med Assoc J*. 1977;117:1277–1280.

19. Haahtela T, Marttila O, Vilkka V, Jäppinen P, Jaakkola JJ. The South Karelia Air Pollution Study: acute health effects of malodorous sulfur air pollutants released by a pulp mill. *Am J Public Health*. 1992;82:603–605.

20. Reiffenstein RJ, Hulbert WC, Roth SH. Toxicology of hydrogen sulfide. *Annu Rev Pharmacol Toxicol*. 1992;32:109–134.

21. Morgan WKC, Seaton A. Toxic gases and fumes. In: Morgan WKC, Seaton A, eds. *Occupational Lung Diseases*. 2nd ed. Philadelphia, Pa: WB Saunders Company; 1984: Chap 20.

22. Karpov BD. Establishment of upper and lower toxicity parameters of perfluoroisobutylene toxicity. *Tr Lenig Sanit-Gig Med Inst*. 1977;III:30–33.

23. Oberdorster G, Gelein RM, Ferin J, Weiss B. Association of particulate air pollution and acute mortality: involvement of ultrafine particles? *Inhal Toxicol*. 1995;7:111–124.

24. Chemical profile for phosgene. *Chemical Market Reporter*. June 21, 1999:1–4.

25. Babad H, Zeiler AG. The chemistry of phosgene. *Chem Rev*. 1973;73:75–91.

26. Brown JE, Birky MM. Phosgene in the thermal decomposition products of poly (vinyl chloride) Generation, detection, and measurement. *J Anal Toxicol*. 1980;4:166–174.

27. Krajewski JA. Chemical accidents and catastrophes as a source of the greatest hazard to the environment and human health in Poland. *Med Pr*. 1997;48:93–103.

28. Charan NB, Myers CG, Lakshminarayan S, Spencer TM. Pulmonary injuries associated with acute sulfur dioxide inhalation. *Am Rev Respir Dis*. 1979;119:555–560.

29. Meng Z, Liu Y, Wu D. Effects of sulfur dioxide inhalation on cytokine levels in lungs and serum of mice. *Inhal Toxicol*. 2005;17:303–307.

30. Haber FR. Zur geschichte des gaskrieges [On the history of the gas war]. In: *Fuenf Vortraege aus den Jahren 1920–23* (Five lectures from the years 1920–1923). Berlin, Germany: Verlag von Julius Springer; 1924: 76–92.

31. Rhinehart WE, Hatch T. Concentration-time product (CT) as an expression of dose in sublethal exposures to phosgene. *Am Ind Hyg Assoc J*. 1964;25:545–553.

32. Gelzleichter TR, Witschi H, Last JA. Concentration-response relationships of rat lung to exposure to oxidant air pollutants: a critical test of Haber's Law for ozone and nitrogen dioxide. *Toxicol Appl Pharmacol*. 1998;112:73–80.

33. Sciuto AM, Hurt HH. Therapeutic treatments of phosgene-induced lung injury. *Inhal Toxicol*.2004; 16: 565–580.

34. Jiang XZ, Buckley LA, Morgan KT. Pathology of toxic responses to the RD50 concentration of chlorine gas in the nasal passages of rats and mice. *Toxicol Appl Pharmacol*. 1983;71:225–236.

35. Bucher JR. Methyl isocyanate: a review of health effects research since Bhopal. *Fundam Appl Toxicol*. 1987;9:367–379.

36. Andersson N, Kerr Muir M, Mehra V, Salmon AG. Exposure and response to methyl isocyanate: results of a community based survey in Bhopal. *Br J Ind Med*. 1988;45:469–475.

37. Sciuto AM, Lee RB, Forster JS, Cascio MB, Clapp DL, Moran TS. Temporal changes in respiratory dynamics in mice exposed to phosgene. *Inhal Toxicol*. 2002;14: 487–501.

38. Stavert DM, Lehnert BE. Potentiation of expression of nitrogen dioxide-induced lung injury by post-exposure exercise. *Environ Res*. 1989;48:87–99.

39. Sciuto AM, Strickland PT, Kennedy TP, Guo YL, Gurtner GH. Intratracheal administration of Dibutyryl Camp attenuates edema formation in acute phosgene-induced lung injury. *J Appl Physiol*. 1996;80:149–157.

40. Brown RF, Jugg BJ, Harban FM, Platt J, Rice P. Pathological improvement following protective ventilation strategy in an inhalationally induced lung injury model. *Am J Resp Crit Care Med*. 2003;16:A775.

41. Wang J, Zhang L, Walther SM. Inhaled budesonide in experimental chlorine gas lung injury: influence of time interval between injury and treatment. *Intensive Care Med*. 2002;28:352–357.

42. Sciuto AM, Moran TS, Narula A, Forster JS. Disruption of gas exchange in mice following exposure to the chemical threat agent phosgene. *Mil Med*. 2001;166:809–814.

43. Wang J. *Pathophysiology and Treatment of Chlorine Gas-Induced Lung Injury: An Experimental Study in Pigs* [dissertation]. Linköping, Sweden: Linköping University; 2004: 7–53.

44. Wang J, Walther SM. Chlorine gas inhalation: mechanisms of injury and treatment. *Int J Disast Med*. 2004;2:75–81.

45. Lehnert BE, Archuleta D, Behr MJ, Stavert DM. Lung injury after acute inhalation of perfluoroisobutylene: exposure concentration-response relationships. *Inhal Toxicol*. 1993;5:1–32.

46. Lehnert BE, Archuleta D, Gurley LR, et al. Exercise potentiation of lung injury following inhalation of a pneumoedematogenic gas: perfluoroisobutylene. *Exp Lung Res*. 1995;21:331–350.

47. Sciuto AM, Carpin LB, Moran TS, Forster JS. Chronological changes in electrolyte levels in arterial blood and broncheoalveoler lavage fluid in mice after exposure to an edemagenic gas. *Inhal Toxicol*. 2003;15:663–674.

48. Burleson GR, Keyes LL. Natural killer activity in Fischer-344 rat lungs as a method to assess pulmonary immunocompetence: immunosuppression by phosgene inhalation. *Immunopharmacol Immunotoxicol*. 1989;11:421–443.

49. Selgrade MK, Starnes DM, Illing JW, Daniels MJ, Graham JA. Effects of phosgene exposure on bacterial, viral, and neoplastic lung disease susceptibility in mice. *Inhal Toxicol*. 1989;1:243–259.

50. Sciuto AM, Phillips CS, Orzolek LD, Hege AI, Moran TS, Dillman JF. Genomic analysis of murine pulmonary tissue following carbonyl chloride inhalation. *Chem Res Toxciol*. 2005;18:1654–1660.

51 Persinger RL, Poynter ME, Ckless K, Janssen-Heininger YM. Molecular mechanisms of nitrogen dioxide induced epithelial injury in the lung. *Mol Cell Biochem*. 2002;234–235:71–80.

52. Copland I, Tanswell K, Post M. Principals of lung development, growth, and repair. In: Notter RH, Finkelstein JN, Holm BA, eds. *Lung Injury: Mechanisms, Pathophysiology, and Therapy*. Boca Raton, Fla: Taylor & Francis; 2005: 19–66.

53. Duniho SM, Martin J, Forster JS, et al. Acute changes in lung histopathology and bronchoalveolar lavage parameters in mice exposed to the choking agent gas phosgene. *Toxicol Pathol*. 2002;30:339–349.

54. Jugg B, Jenner J, Rice P. The effect of perfluoroisobutene and phosgene on rat lung fluid surfactant phoslipids. *Human Exp Toxicol*. 1999;18:93–102.

55. Lee KP, Zapp JA, Sarver JW. Ultrastructural alterations of rat lung exposed to pyrolysis products of polytetrafluoroethylene (PTFE, Teflon). *Lab Invest*. 1976;35:152–160.

56. Sciuto AM, Strickland PT, Kennedy TP, Gurtner GH. Postexposure treatment with aminophylline protects against phosgene-induced acute lung injury. *Exp Lung Res*. 1997;23:317–332.

57. Sciuto AM, Strickland PT, Gurtner GH. Post-exposure treatment with isoproterenol attenuates pulmonary edema in phosgene-exposed rabbits. *J Appl Toxicol*. 1998;18:321–329.

58. Madden MC, Freidman M, Keyes LK, Koren S, Burleson GR. Effects of phosgene on lung arachidonic acid metabolism. *Inhal Toxicol*. 1991;3:73–90.

59. Guo YL, Kennedy TP, Michael JR, et al. Mechanisms of phosgene-induced toxicity: role of arachidonate mediators. *J Appl Physiol*. 1990;69:1615–1622.

60. Warheit DB. Interspecies comparisons of lung responses to inhaled particles and gases. *Crit Rev Toxicol*. 1989;20:1–29.

61. Jörres R, Nowak D, Grimminger F, Seeger W, Oldigs M, Magnussen H. The effect of 1 ppm nitrogen dioxide on bronchoalveolar lavage cells and inflammatory mediators in normal and asthmatic subjects. *Eur Respir J*. 1995;8:416–424.

62. Burns TR, Greenberg SD, Cartwright J, Jachimczyk JA. Smoke inhalation: an ultrastructural study of reaction to injury in the human alveolar wall. *Environ Res*. 1986;41:447–457.

63. Lane SR, Nicholls PJ, Sewell RDE. The pharmacology and toxicology of inhaled dusts, endotoxins, and glucans. In: Salem H, Katz SA, eds. *Inhalation Toxicology*. 2nd ed. Baco Raton, Fla: CRC/Taylor & Francis; 2006: Chap 31.

64. Sciuto AM, Clapp DL, Hess ZA, Moran TS. The temporal profile of cytokines in the bronchoalveolar lavage fluid in mice exposed to the industrial gas phosgene. *Inhal Toxicol*. 2003;15:687–700.

65. Sciuto AM. Assessment of early acute lung injury in rodents exposed to phosgene. *Arch Toxicol*. 1998;72:283–288.

66. Cantin AM, North SL, Hubbard RC, Crystal RG. Normal alveolar epithelial lining fluid contains high levels of glutathione. *J Appl Physiol*. 1987;63:152–157.

67. Tarlo SM, Broder I. Irritant-induced occupational asthma. *Chest*. 1989;96:297–300.

68. Alberts WM, do Pico GA. Reactive airways dysfunction syndrome. *Chest*. 1996;109:1618–1626.

69. Sjöblom E, Höjer J, Kulling PE, Stauffer K, Suneson A, Ludwigs U. A placebo-controlled experimental study of steroid inhalation therapy in ammonia-induced lung injury. *J Toxicol Clin Toxicol*. 1999;37:59–67.

70. Brautbar N, Wu MP, Richter ED. Chronic ammonia inhalation and interstitial pulmonary fibrosis: a case report and review of the literature. *Arch Environ Health*. 2003;58:592–596.

71. Adelson L, Kaufman J. Fatal chlorine poisoning: report of two cases with clinicopathologic correlation. *Am J Clin Pathol*. 1971;56:430–442.

72. Wang J, Zhang L, Walther SM. Administration of aerosolized terbutaline and budesonide reduces chlorine gas –induced acute lung injury. *J Trauma*. 2004;56:850–862.

73. Ballantyne B. Autopsy findings following death by intramuscular hydrogen cyanide: an experimental study. *Med Sci Law*. 1970;10:171–174.

74. Maynard RL. Toxicology of chemical warfare agents. In: Ballantyne B, Marrs TC, Syversen T, eds. *General and Applied Toxicology*. 2nd ed. London, England: Macmillan; 1999: Chap 98.

75. Ballantyne B, Salem H. Experimental, clinical, occupational toxicology, and forensic aspects of hydrogen cyanide with particular reference to vapor exposure. In: Salem H, Katz SA, eds. *Inhalation Toxicology*. 2nd ed. Boca Raton, Fla: CRC/Taylor & Francis; 2006: Chap 30.

76. Zhang T, Zhang X, Shoa Z, et al. The prophylactic and therapeutic effects of cholinolytics on perfluoroisobutylene inhalation induced acute lung injury. *J Occup Health*. 2005;47:277–285.

77. Diller WF, Bruch J, Dehnen W. Pulmonary changes in the rat following low phosgene exposure. *Arch Toxicol*. 1985;57:184–190.

78. Pawlowski R, Frosolono MF. Effect of phosgene on rat lung after a single high-level exposure. II. Ultrastructural alterations. *Arch Environ Health*. 1977;32:278–283.

79. Currie WD, Hatch GE, Frosolono MF. Pulmonary alterations in rats due to phosgene inhalation. *Fundam Appl Toxicol*. 1987;8:107–114.

80. Frosolono MF, Pawlowski R. Effect of phosgene on rat lungs after single high-level exposure. *Arch Environ Health*. 1977;32:271–277.

81. Currie WD, Hatch GE, Frosolono MF. Changes in lung ATP concentration in the rat after low-level phosgene exposure. *J Biochem Toxicol*. 1987;2:105–114.

82. Callender TJ, Morrow L, Subramanian K, Duhon D, Ristovv M. Three-dimensional brain metabolic imaging in patients with toxic encephalopathy. *Environ Res*. 1993;60:295–319.

83. Kennedy TP, Michael JR, Hoidal JR, et al. Dibutyryl cAMP, aminophylline, and betaadrenergic agonists protect against pulmonary edema caused by phosgene. *J Appl Physiol*. 1989;67:2542–2552.

84. Sciuto AM, Stotts RR, Chittenden V, Choung E, Heflin M. Changes in absorbance at 413 nm in plasma from three rodent species exposed to phosgene. *Biochem Biophys Res Commun*. 1996;226:906–911.

85. De Curtis V, Gemma S, Sbraccia M, Testai E, Vittozzi L. The contribution of electrophilic and radicalic intermediates to phospholipid adducts formed by halomethanes in vivo. *J Biochem Toxicol*. 1994;9:305–310.

86. Guastadisegni C, Balduzzi M, Vittozzi L. Preliminary characterization of phospholipid adducts by [14C]-CHCl3 reactive intermediates in hepatocyte suspensions. *J Biochem Toxicol*. 1996;11:21–25.

87. Guastadisegni C, Guidoni L, Balduzzi M, Viti V, DiConsiglio E, Vittozzi L. Characterization of a phospholipid adduct formed in Sprague Dawley rats by chloroform metabolism: NMR studies. *J Biochem Mol Toxicol*. 1998;12:93–102.

88. Wang Z, Holm BA, Matalon S, Notter RH. Surfactant activity and dysfunction in lung injury. In: Notter RH, Finkelstein JN, Holm BA, eds. *Lung Injury: Mechanisms, Pathophysiology, and Therapy*. Boca Raton, Fla: Taylor & Francis; 2005: Chap 9.

89. Sciuto AM. Ibuprofen treatment enhances the survival of mice following exposure to phosgene. *Inhal Toxicol*. 1997;9:389–403.

90. Sciuto AM, Stotts RR, Hurt HH. Efficacy of ibuprofen and pentoxifylline in the treatment of phosgene-induced acute lung injury. *J Appl Toxicol*. 1996;16:381–384.

91. Issley S. Toxicity, ammonia. eMedicine from WebMD. Available at: http://www.emedicine.com/EMERG/topic846.htm. Accessed August 6, 2007.

92. Willems JL. Clinical management of mustard gas casualties. *Ann Med Milit Belg*. 1989;3:1.

93. Khateri S, Ghanei M, Keshavarz S, Souoush M, Haines D. Incidence of lung, eye, and skin lesions as late complication in 34,000 Iranians with wartime exposure to mustard agent. *J Occup Envron Med*. 2003;45(11):1136–1143.

94. Shusterman DJ. Polymer fume fever and other fluorocarbon pyrolysis-related syndromes. *Occup Med*. 1993;8:519–531.

95. Smith DT, Dupont AM. CBRNE—lung damaging agents. eMedicine from WebMD. http://www.emedicine.com. Accessed: November 2004.

96. Urbanetti JS. Toxic inhalational injury. In: Sidell FR, Takafuji ET, Franz DR, eds: *Medical Aspects of Chemical and Biological Warfare*. In: Zajtchuk R, Bellamy RF, eds. *Textbook of Military Medicine*. Washington, DC: Department of the Army, Office of The Surgeon General, Borden Institute; 1997: Chap 9.

97. Segal E, Lang E. Toxicity, chlorine gas. eMedicine from WebMD. Available at: http://www.emedicine.com/EMERG/topic851.htm. Accessed August 6, 2007.

98. Noltkamper D, Burgher SW. Toxicity, phosgene. eMedicine from WebMD. Available at: http://www.emedicine.com/emerg/topic849.htm. Accessed August 6, 2007.

99. Miller K, Chang A. Acute inhalation injury. *Emerg Med Clin North Am*. 2003;21:533–557.

100. Matthay MA, Uchida T, Fang X. Clinical acute lung injury and acute respiratory distress syndrome. *Curr Treat Options Cardiovaxc Med*. 2002;4:139–149.

101. Fulkerson WJ, MacIntyre N, Stamler J, Crapo JD. Pathogenesis and treatment of the adult respiratory distress syndrome. *Arch Intern Med*. 1996;156:29–38.

Chapter 11

CYANIDE POISONING

STEVEN I. BASKIN, PhD*; JAMES B. KELLY†; BEVERLY I. MALINER, DO, MPH‡; GARY A. ROCKWOOD, PhD§; AND CSABA K. ZOLTANI, PhD¥

* *Deputy Research Coordinator, Cyanide Medical Countermeasures, Analytical Toxicology Division, US Army Medical Research Institute of Chemical Defense, 3100 Ricketts Point Road, Aberdeen Proving Ground, Maryland 21010-5400*

† *Research Chemist, US Army Medical Research Institute of Chemical Defense, 3100 Ricketts Point Road, Room 92, Aberdeen Proving Ground, Maryland 21010-5400*

‡ *Colonel, Medical Corps, US Army; Director, Department of Occupational and Environmental Medicine, US Army Center for Health Promotion and Preventive Medicine, 5158 Blackhawk Road, Building E1930, Aberdeen Proving Ground, Maryland 21010-5403*

§ *Research Coordinator, Cyanide Medical Countermeasures, Analytical Toxicology Division, US Army Medical Research Institute of Chemical Defense, 3100 Ricketts Point Road, Aberdeen Proving Ground, Maryland 21010-5400*

¥ *Research Physicist, Army Research Laboratory, Building 394, Aberdeen Proving Ground, Maryland 21005*

INTRODUCTION

Cyanide has been used as a poison for thousands of years. In World War I, however, possibly because of inefficient delivery, cyanide was not highly successful as a chemical warfare agent. The effects of high-dose cyanide are quick, and death occurs within minutes. Antidotes are effective if administered in time (although antidotes are unlikely to be available in time with high-dose exposures).

Cyanide is ubiquitous. It is present in some foods and in the products of combustion of synthetic materials, and it is widely used in industry. The cyanides of military interest are the volatile liquids hydrocyanic acid (or hydrogen cyanide [HCN], North Atlantic Treaty Organization [NATO] designation: AC) and cyanogen chloride (NATO designation: CK); however, a great number of cyanide compounds actually release active cyanide. Cyanides are stored and used in either liquid form or as solid salts (Table 11-1).

HISTORICAL USE

Discovery and Ancient Use of Cyanide

Since the time of ancient Egypt, plants containing cyanide derivatives, such as bitter almonds, cherry laurel leaves, peach pits, and cassava, have been used as lethal poisons.[1,2] Peach pits used in judicial executions by the ancient Egyptians are on display in the Louvre Museum, Paris, and an Egyptian papyrus refers to the "penalty of the peach."[2] The Romans used cherry laurel leaves as a method of execution (also known

TABLE 11-1

CHEMICAL, PHYSICAL, ENVIRONMENTAL, AND BIOLOGICAL PROPERTIES OF CYANIDES

Properties	Hydrogen Cyanide (AC)	Cyanogen Chloride (CK)
Chemical and Physical		
Boiling Point	25.7°C	12.9°C
Vapor Pressure	740 mm Hg	1,000 mg Hg
Density		
Vapor	0.99 at 20°C	2.1
Liquid	0.68 g/mL at 25°C	1.18 g/mL at 20°C
Solid	NA	Crystal: 0.93 g/mL at –40°C
Volatility	1.1×10^6 mg/m^3 at 25°C	2.6×10^6 mg/m^3 at 12.9°C
Appearance and Odor	Gas: Odor of bitter almonds or peach kernals	Bitter almonds scent; colorless gas or liquid; irritating to upper airway, eyes
Solubility		
In water	Complete at 25°C	6.9 g/100 mL at 20°C
In other solvents	Completely miscible in almost all organic solvents	Most organic solvents (mixtures are unstable)
Environmental and Biological		
Detection	ICAD; M254A1 kit	M256A1 kit
Persistency		
In soil	< 1 h	Nonpersistent
On material	Low	Nonpersistent
Skin Decontamination	Water; soap and water	Water; soap and water
Biologically Effective Amount		
Vapor (mg•min/m^3)	LCt_{50}: 2,500–5,000 (time-dependent)	LCt_{50}: 11,000
Liquid (mg/kg)	LD_{50}(skin): 100	LD_{50}(skin): 100

ICAD: individual chemical agent detector
LCt_{50}: the vapor or aerosol exposure (concentration • time) lethal to 50% of the exposed population
LD_{50}: the dose lethal to 50% of the exposed population
NA: not applicable

as "the cherry death"), and the Roman emperor Nero used cherry laurel water to poison members of his family and others who displeased him. Dioscorides, a Greek physician who served in Nero's army, compiled information on more than 600 species of plants with medicinal value in the five books titled *De Materia Medica,* recognizing the poisonous properties of bitter almonds. Napoleon III proposed the use of cyanides to enhance the effectiveness of his soldiers' bayonets during the Franco–Prussian War; it has also been suggested that Napoleon died from cyanide.[3]

The first description of cyanide poisoning, by Wepfer in 1679, dealt with the effects of extract of bitter almond administration.[2] In 1731 Maddern demonstrated that cherry laurel water given orally, into the rectum, or by injection, rapidly killed dogs.[4] Although substances containing cyanide have been used for centuries as poisons, cyanide was not identified until 1782, when Swedish pharmacist and chemist Carl Wilhelm Scheele[2] isolated cyanide by heating the dye Prussian Blue with dilute sulfuric acid, obtaining a flammable gas (hydrogen cyanide) that was water soluble and acidic. Scheele called this new acid Berlin blue acid, which later became known as prussic acid and today is known as cyanide (from the Greek word "kyanos," meaning "blue"). Scheele's discovery may have cost him his life several years later, from either engaging in unsafe experimental practices such as taste testing and smelling HCN, or accidentally breaking a vial of the poison. A better understanding of the cyanides was achieved in 1815 by the French chemist Joseph Louis Gay-Lussac.[2] Gay-Lussac identified a colorless, poisonous gas called cyanogen, which had an almond-like flavor and considerable thermal stability. His work on acids, including HCN, led to the realization that acids do not need to contain oxygen, and that the cyanogen moiety could be shifted from compound to compound without separating the individual carbon and nitrogen atoms.

Terrorist and Military Uses

Although ancient civilizations used plants containing cyanides to kill, it was not until World War I, in late 1915 and early 1916, that cyanide was produced expressly for the purpose of killing. France started the large-scale use of cyanide as a chemical weapon, producing approximately 8 million pounds of HCN by distilling a concentrated solution of potassium cyanide (KCN) with dilute sulfuric acid. Even though HCN had quick-kill properties and was not readily absorbed on charcoal (allowing penetration through enemy gas masks), its use provided no tactical advantage. This was due, in part, to small payload munitions and the high volatility of cyanide with no cumulative effects (cyanide is lighter than air, persisting for only a few minutes in the open air). Concentrations sufficient to incapacitate or kill were not achieved. In addition, Germany learned of its use and equipped its troops with masks capable of filtering out the gas.

In September 1916, France tried another cyanide-based poison, cyanogen chloride, which is heavier and less volatile than HCN and had a cumulative effect on its victims. Cyanogen chloride was produced by chlorinating a saturated solution of KCN at 0°C (32°F). Its toxicity was similar to that of HCN, but cyanogen chloride was more effective at low concentrations because it irritated the eyes and lungs. Cyanogen chloride also had a delayed toxic effect similar to lung irritants such as chlorine and phosgene. At the same time that France launched cyanogen chloride, Austria introduced a poisonous gas derived from KCN and bromine. The resulting cyanogen bromide was still highly volatile, yet it had only a quarter of the volatility of HCN and was less toxic. Cyanogen bromide had a strong irritating effect on the conjunctiva and the mucous membranes of the respiratory system; however, because it corroded metals and was unstable in storage (gradually polymerizing into a toxicologically inert substance), the Austrians abandoned its use.[5]

During World War II, the Nazis employed HCN adsorbed onto a dispersible pharmaceutical base (Zyklon B) to exterminate millions of civilians and enemy soldiers in the death camps. Cyanide was detected in the walls of crematoria almost 50 years later.[6,7] Zyklon B was also used as a fumigant and rodenticide to rid ships of rodents by the United States and other countries. Japan allegedly used cyanide against China before and during the war.

In the late 1980s, reports indicated that cyanide-like agents may have been used against the inhabitants of the Syrian city of Hama,[8] the Kurdish city of Halabja, Iraq,[9] and possibly Shahabad, Iran, during the Iran-Iraq War.[10] In addition to military operations, cyanide has been used by individuals and terrorist organizations. One notorious incident was the poisoning of Tylenol (acetaminophen, manufactured by McNeill Consumer Products Co, Fort Washington, Pa) in the Chicago area in 1982, which killed seven people.[11] An acid and a cyanide salt were found in several subway restrooms in Tokyo, Japan, in the weeks following the release of nerve agents in the city in March 1995.[12]

Executions and Suicides

Cyanide has been the typical agent used in "gas chambers," in which a cyanide salt is dropped into an acid to produce HCN. Gas chambers used in some states to judicially execute murderers provide information on the effect of HCN. In US gas chambers HCN was usually released by dropping a bag of sodium cyanide into sulfuric acid. Unconsciousness was thought to be instant, with death following in 5 to 10 minutes. In 1994 District Judge Marilyn Hall Patel ruled that the gas chamber was an inhumane method of punishment and outlawed its practice in California. Two years later the 9th US Ciruit Court of Appeals supported Patel's decision and ruled that gas chambers violated the Eighth Amendment to the Constitution because of the horrible pain observed for several minutes. However, in several states, death row inmates still have the right to choose the gas chamber over lethal injection, as Walter LeGrand did in Arizona in 1999.

Cyanide has often been used by individuals and groups to commit suicide.[13] One of the most notorious of such events happened in 1978 near Port Kaituma, Guyana, when the followers of Jim Jones drank a grape-flavored drink laced with cyanide, resulting in the deaths of more than 900 children and adults.[14]

Cyanide Sources and Accidental Poisoning

Although there are many chemical forms of cyanide, HCN (or the cyanide anion CN^-) is the primary toxic agent, regardless of its origin. Military personnel and civilians may be exposed to common natural and anthropogenic sources of cyanide through edible and nonedible plants, industrial operations, fires, and cigarette smoke. Ongoing low-level cyanide exposures are managed by the body through reaction pathways that detoxify amounts in excess of biological tolerances. Much of the medical information on cyanide poisoning has come from civilian experiences of poisoning, fires, and industrial accidents.

HCN is released into the atmosphere from volcanoes, plants, bacteria, and fungi.[15–21] However, the primary natural source of cyanide poisoning in humans and animals is from plants. Over 2,000 plant species, including edible fruits and vegetables, contain cyanogenic glycosides, which can release cyanide when ingested.[18,22,23] Rapid hydrolysis of cyanogenic glycosides and release of HCN occurs when the plant cell structure is disrupted. Thus consumption of improperly processed plants with cyanogen-containing glycosides will release HCN and may result in illness or death. Some common cyanogenic edible plants reported to cause cyanide poisoning include cassava, sorghum, sweet potatoes, yams, maize, millet, bamboo, sugarcane, peas, lima beans, soybeans, almond kernels, lemons, limes, apples, pears, peach, chokecherries, apricots, prunes, and plums.[18,22–30] Cassava (manioc) and sorghum are staple foods for hundreds of millions of people in many tropical countries and are blamed in part for the high incidence of central and peripheral neuropathies in those areas.[31] Known cyanogenic glycosides in plants include amygdalin, linamarin, prunasin, dhurrin, lotaustralin, and taxiphyllin.

Worldwide manufacturing of cyanide to support industrial and agricultural demand is in the range of 2.5 million US tons annually. In industries using cyanide, occupational exposures occur primarily by the dermal and inhalation routes. Nonindustrial accidental exposures of clinical significance are typically associated with commercial fires involving the burning of plastics.[32,33]

Inhalation of tobacco smoke, another source of cyanide, has been associated with tobacco amblyopia, a syndrome of visual failure occurring in association with the use of tobacco, thought to result from nutritional or idiopathic deficiencies in certain detoxification mechanisms, particularly those that target the cyanide component of tobacco smoke.[34] Cyanide levels in smokers versus nonsmokers are often used as a sensitivity test in analytical methods for determination of cyanide or its metabolites in biological fluids.[35] HCN concentrations in inhaled smoke from US-manufactured cigarettes range from 10 to 400 μg per cigarette. In non–US-manufactured cigarettes, cyanide concentrations range from 280 to 550 μg per cigarette in inhaled smoke and from 53 to 111 μg per cigarette in second-hand smoke.[15,36–38] Cyanide has also been found to be a metabolic product of certain pharmacological preparations such as laetrile, nitroprusside, and succinonitrile. Some of these formulations have caused cyanide poisoning, in some cases resulting in death.[21, 39–43]

BIOCHEMICAL BASIS FOR POISONING

Cyanide is known to bind and inactivate several enzymes, particularly those containing iron in the ferric (Fe^{3+}) state and cobalt. It is thought to exert its ultimate lethal effect of histotoxic anoxia by binding to the active site of cytochrome *c* oxidase, the terminal protein in the electron transport chain located within mitochondrial membranes (Figure 11-1). By this means, cyanide prevents the transfer of electrons to molecular oxygen. Thus, despite the presence of oxygen in the blood, it cannot be utilized toward adenosine triphosphate (ATP) generation, thereby stopping aerobic cell metabolism.[44,45] Initially cells attempt to replenish the ATP energy source through glycolysis, but the replenishment is short lived, particularly in the metabolically

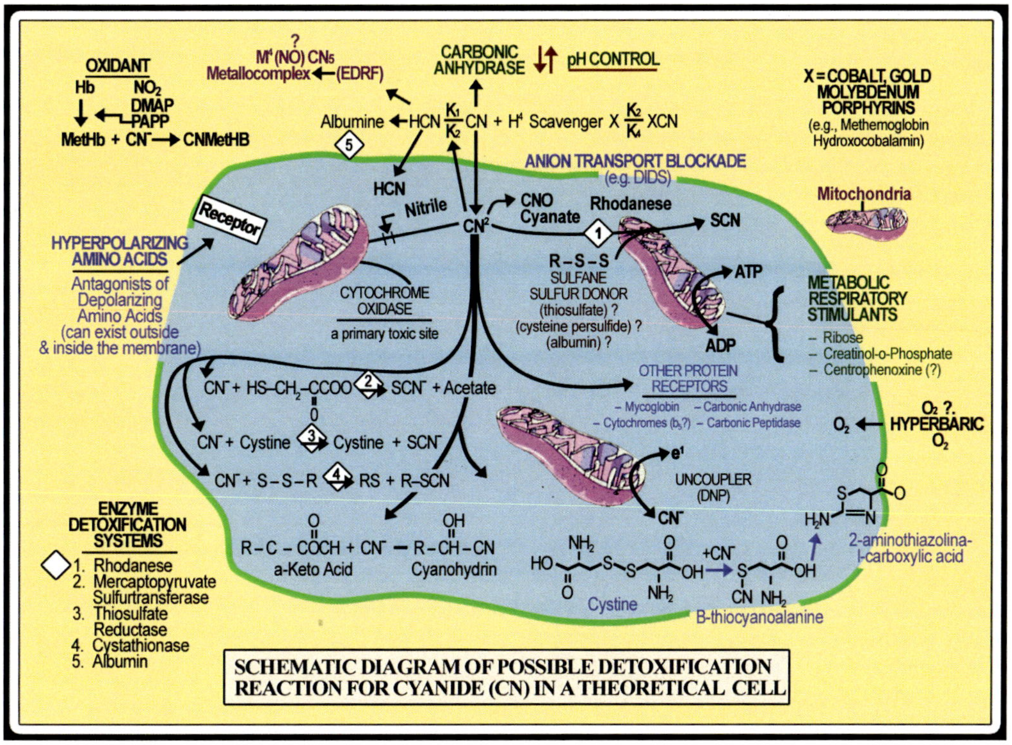

Fig. 11-1. Likely detoxification reactions for cyanide are shown for this hypothetical cell. The enzyme detoxification systems are as follows:

1. Rhodanese: an intramitochondrial liver enzyme that catalyzes the transfer of sulfur from a donor molecule to cyanide to form thiocyanate. Rhodanese is the major pathway for cyanide detoxification.
2. Mercaptopyruvate sulfurtransferases: a group of enzymes widely distributed in the body that catalyze the transfer of a sulfane sulfur atom from a donor molecule to a thiophilic acceptor substrate for the limitation of cyanide.
3. Thiosulfate reductase: enzymes found in the liver, kidney, heart, brain, intestine, and testis that use electrons from thiols, which in vivo probably use electrons from glutathione, to reduce the sulfane sulfur atoms of inorganic thiosulfate and organic thiosulfonate anions to the sulfide level. Sulfide production from these thiol-dependent reductases is thought to be used in the synthesis of Fe-S proteins.
4. Cystathionase: enzymes widely distributed in the body that can transfer sulfur from one cysteine to another, generating thiocysteine and pyruvate. Transamination of cysteine leads to the production of thiosulfate and the limitation of cyanide.
5. Albumin: molecules that act like an enzyme in the detoxification of cyanide. Albumin molecules contain sulfur sites that bind to and limit cyanide.

ADP: adenosine diphosphate
ATP: adenosine triphosphate
ATCA: 2-aminothiazoline-4-carboxylic acid
CN^-: cyanide ion
CNMetHb: cyanomethemoglobin
CNO: cyanate
DIDS: 4,4′-diisothiocyano-2,2′-disulfonic stilbene
DMAP: dimethylaminophenol
DNP: deoxyribonucleoprotein
EDERF: endothelium-derived relaxing factor
Hb: hemoglobin
MedHb: methemoglobin
PAPP: p-aminopropiophenone
R: reduction factor
S: substrate
Drawing: Courtesy of Steven I Baskin, PhD, and Fred Sidell, PhD, US Army Research Institute of Chemical Defense, Aberdeen Proving Ground, Md.

active heart and brain. Binding to the cytochrome oxidase can occur in minutes.[46] A more rapid effect appears to occur on neuronal transmission. Cyanide is known to inhibit carbonic anhydrase,[47] and this enzyme interaction may prove to be an important contributor to the well-documented metabolic acidosis resulting from clinically significant cyanide intoxication.

Cyanide can be removed by several processes before it can enter cells. Cyanide may form a complex with endothelial-derived relaxing factor (thought to be nitric oxide). Heavy metals (eg, gold, molybdenum, or cobalt salts) or organic compounds with metal centers (eg, hydroxocobalamin) may scavenge cyanide, effectively removing it before it can enter the cell. Finally, albumin can exhibit enzyme-like behavior and use bound elemental sulfur[48] to detoxify cyanide.

Cyanide can be removed by several processes within cells. Perhaps of greatest importance is the formation of cyanomethemoglobin in red blood cells, which is produced when cyanide reacts with methemoglobin. At least four intracellular enzymes may be involved in cyanide detoxification. The generalized reactions of rhodanese, mercaptopyruvate sulfurtransferase, thiosulfate reductase, and cystathionase in the cell are shown in Figure 11-1. Cyanide also reacts with cystine to form 2-aminothiazoline-4-carboxylic acid (ATCA). Oxygen supplementation enhances recovery from cyanide intoxication, although the mechanism by which this happens is uncertain.[49]

Cyanide is readily diffusible through epithelium. This property contributes to its lethality after inhalation of HCN gas, ingestion of cyanide salts or cyanogens, or percutaneous absorption of cyanide from high-concentration solutions. Because cyanides are present at low concentrations in several naturally occurring environmental sources, it is not surprising that animals have intrinsic biochemical pathways for detoxification of the cyanide ion.

The most important route of cyanide excretion is by formation of thiocyanate (SCN^-), which is subsequently excreted in the urine.[31] Thiocyanate possesses a less inherent toxicological hazard than cyanide, cyanate (CNO^-), or isocyanate. Thiocyanate formation is catalyzed directly by the enzyme rhodanese(EC 2.8.1.1) and indirectly via a spontaneous reaction between cyanide and the persulfide sulfur products of the enzymes 3-mercaptopyruvate sulfurtransferase (EC 2.8.1.2)[50] and thiosulfate reductase (EC 2.8.1.3) (see Figure 11-1). The mechanisms of all three enzymes[51] as well as the pharmacokinetics of thiocyanate formation[52,53] have been studied. The enzymatic routes are efficient but constrained in situations of overwhelming acute overdose by insufficient sulfur donor substrate. The mitochondrial sulfurtransferase reactions are exploited by the administration of sodium thiosulfate (used in therapy and discussed later in this chapter) in the treatment of acute poisonings.

The interaction of cystine and cyanide to form ATCA and its tautomer account for approximately 20% of cyanide metabolism.[54] This percentage increases with toxic doses of cyanide.[55] A minor route of metabolism, the exact extent of which is unknown, is the conversion of cyanide to cyanate.

Combined, these metabolic routes detoxify 0.017 mg of cyanide per kilogram of body weight per minute in the average human (1.19 mg/min in a 70-kg person).[56,57] Cyanide is one of the few chemical agents that does not follow Haber's law, which states that the Ct (the product of concentration and time) necessary to cause a given biological effect is constant over a range of concentrations and times; for this reason, the LCt_{50} (the vapor or aerosol exposure that is lethal to 50% of the exposed population) for a short exposure to a high concentration is different from a long exposure to a low concentration.

Cyanide Pharmacokinetics and Pharmacodynamics

Cyanide appears to display first-order kinetics during the period of initial toxicity.[52] The volume of distribution for cyanide appears to change as the blood levels of the chemical change,[58] but these alterations probably reflect the marked intracellular sequestration of the molecule. Animal studies[59,60] show a differential disposition of inhaled HCN, with the highest tissue levels found in the lung, heart, and brain. These data seem to corroborate the evidence from other animal studies and from clinical reports that emphasize the importance of these organs in cyanide toxicity. Ingestion of cyanide results in much higher levels in the liver than does inhalation exposure; this is a useful differential point in forensic investigations. Cyanide also has wide-ranging cardiovascular effects, including a poorly understood increase in vascular resistance in the early phases of poisoning[61] and a marked increase in cerebral blood flow in dogs.[62]

Data from rodent studies suggest that a single, acute administration of a cyanide salt can result in death or complete recovery. Data from HCN inhalational studies in dogs, rabbits, monkeys, and humans suggest that death may be delayed for up to 8 days.[63,64] The neurological sequelae of cyanide intoxication may be delayed for up to a year.[2] These delayed changes in regional sensitivities of the brain are thought to be caused by hypoxic stress and are analogous to those seen following sublethal carbon monoxide poisoning.

Toxicity

Although generally considered to be very toxic substances when compared with other lethal chemical warfare agents, cyanides are among the least toxic. The LCt_{50} for HCN is generally stated to be 2,500 to 5,000 mg•min/m^3; for cyanogen chloride, about 11,000 mg•min/m^3. (Comparable values for the nerve agents are 10–200 mg•min/m^3; for sulfur mustard, 1,500 mg•min/m^3; and for phosgene, 3,000 mg•min/m^3.)[65] The estimated intravenous dose of HCN for humans that is lethal to 50% of the exposed population (LD_{50}) is approximately 1.0 mg/kg, and the estimated LD_{50} for liquid on the skin is about 100 mg/kg.

DETECTION OF CYANIDE AND CYANIDE METABOLITES

The determination of cyanide, or its metabolites thiocyanate and ATCA, in biological fluids is often needed for forensics, clinical, research, or veterinary purposes. Although the detection of cyanide and cyanide compounds in other matrices is important to industrial, environmental, and research applications, it is not discussed in this chapter. This chapter will briefly discuss the available techniques and identify problems in cyanide analysis. Analytical methods for direct determination of cyanide and cyanide metabolites in biological samples have been reviewed.[15,54,66,67] Methods of analysis include spectrochemical absorption or luminescence methods,[21,35,68–104] electrochemical methods,[68–76] capillary electrophoresis,[77,78] and gas[105–126] or liquid chromatography techniques[127–149] coupled to a variety of detection techniques. The number of literature references (more than 200) that examine the detection of cyanide and cyanide metabolites in biological fluids can add to the difficulty in choosing a method. In addition, the numerous uncertainties and discrepancies in the literature have made comparison and selection of a method complicated for the novice. Obviously the first decision will be whether to choose cyanide, one of its metabolites, or both as the substance or substances to look for. Factors that influence this choice are cellular absorption and detoxification kinetics, sampling and analysis time, sample storage time and conditions, sample matrix, interferences, detection limits, available equipment and expertise, and budget allowances.

The analytical determination of cyanide and/or cyanide metabolites before antidotal treatment provides a more accurate assessment of the severity of poisoning and insight into antidote dose levels (especially because high doses of antidotes can also be toxic).[19,79,80] However, no available method is simple, accurate, and fast enough to justify waiting for test results before antidotal treatment is administered (ie, cyanide can kill faster than the analysis can be performed). Measurement of cyanide and its metabolites may have diagnostic or therapeutic value when sublethal; minimally or moderately symptomatic exposure is part of the differential diagnosis. In addition, biological samples should be assessed for confirmation or refutation of a putative diagnosis of cyanide intoxication.

Blood has been the biological sample of choice when determining cyanide concentrations. However, cyanide is rapidly removed from blood by detoxification processes, binding to proteins and enzymes that contain metal centers or heme moieties, or sequestering in other favorable cellular entities.[21,40,67,81–92] Cyanide characteristics[93,94] suggest that a biological sample should be collected quickly, and analysis should be performed as soon as possible. If analysis of cyanide cannot be performed quickly, then the sampling and storage of biological samples for later testing should consider the following:

- **Cyanide resides mainly in erythrocytes rather than plasma**. Cyanide in blood primarily resides in erythrocytes (red blood cells)[40,82,89–92,95] by binding to methemoglobin, forming cyanomethemoglobin, but may also be present in plasma, especially if cyanide concentrations exceed erythrocyte concentrations.[40,82,89] Test results are improved by working with whole blood that is not coagulated. Heparinized vials should be used in the collection of the blood sample for determination of cyanide concentration. Containers that contain anticoagulants such as heparin and ethylenediaminetetraacetate (EDTA) help prevent clotting and also ensure efficient harvesting of plasma after the blood has been centrifuged. Lundquist et al demonstrated that the cyanide binding capacity of erythrocytes due to methemoglobin increased from 89,000 nM to 517,000 nM upon addition of sodium nitrite.[82]
- **Cyanide may evaporate because of HCN volatility at the physiological pH, and cyanide nucleophilic action should be reduced**. The next considerations should be reducing the evaporation and loss of cyanide from biological samples and preventing nucleophilic reactions. Using tightly sealed vials,

TABLE 11-2

ANALYTICAL METHODS TO IDENTIFY CYANIDE AND ITS METABOLITES IN BIOLOGICAL FLUIDS*

Analyte	Matrix Studied	Analytical Method	Detection Limit†		Estimated Time	Study
			nM	ng/mL		
		Gas Chromatography				
HCN	Human blood (whole)	Headspace analysis GC-MS (internal standard: $K^{13}C^{15}N$)	300	8	~20	1
HCN	Human blood (whole)	Headspace analysis GC with NPD (also used SPME); calibration curve	519	14	~ 17 min	2
HCN	Human blood (whole)	Headspace analysis GC with NPD and cryogenic oven (internal standard: propionitrile)	74	2	~ 35 min	3
HCN	Human blood (whole)	HPLC-MS after derivatization (internal standard: $K^{13}C^{15}N$)	185	5	~ 45 min	4
HCN	Cow serum, rumen, liver	GCMS after derivatization (internal standard: bromocyclohexane in ethyl acetate)	700	18	~ 55 min	5
HCN, SCN^-	Human blood (whole)	For HCN: GC-EC after derivatization; for SCN^-: GC-EC after derivatization; (internal standard: 1,3,5 tribromo-benzene in ethyl acetate)	10,000 3,000	270 174	~55 min	6
ATCA	Blood plasma, urine	GC-MS; (internal standard: ATCA-d_2)	171.2	25	> 1 h	7
		Electrochemical				
HCN	Human blood (whole)	Voltammetry with Ag RDE following trapping of HCN gas	1,000	27	> 50 min	8
SCN^-	Human urine and saliva	Thiocyanate selective polymeric membrane electrode (electrode conditioning requires 24 h; pH range 5–10)	48	2.8	15 or 120 s for conditioned electrode	9
		Liquid Chromatography				
HCN	Human blood (whole)	HPLC with fluorometric detection after derivatization	74	2	> 2 h	10
HCN, SCN^-	Human blood (whole)	For HCN: IC with F detection after derivatization; for SCN^-: IC with UV detection	3.8 86	0.10 5	~ 45 min	11
SCN^-	Human urine	Ion interaction LC with UV detection	1,720	100	~ 10 min	12
SCN^-	Human urine	IC with electrochemical detection	500	29	~ 15 min	13
SCN^-	Human blood (whole)	HPLC with fluorometric detection after derivatization	0.165	0.0096	> 1 h	14
SCN^-	Human plasma and urine	IC with spectrophotometric detection following chlorination	930	54	~ 25 min	15
ATCA	Human urine	HPLC with fluorometric detection after derivatization	300	44	> 3 h	16

(**Table 11-2** *continues*)

Table 11-2 *continued*

		Spectrochemical Absorption or Luminescence				
HCN	Human blood (whole)	Fluorometric	2,000	52	~ 17 min	17
HCN	Equine blood	Spectrophotometry following trapping of HCN gas	74	2	~ 16 h	18
HCN	Human blood (whole)	Spectrophotometry	1,000	27	~ 45 min	19
SCN^-	Human blood serum, urine, saliva	Flame atomic absorption spectrometry; calibration	69	4	~ 20 min	20

*This table is meant to give a general overview of analytical methods in this area and their detection limits. It is not meant to be all-inclusive. The 2004 US Department of Health and Human Services Agency for Toxic Substances and Disease Registry toxicology profile for cyanide also includes biological analytical methods not mentioned above and environmental analytical methods, including the US Environmental Protection Agency and National Institute for Occupational Safety and Health standard methods.[21]

†Conversion of units; figures are multiplied by the molecular weight of HCN, 27 g/mol.

EC: electron capture; GC: gas chromatography; GCMS: gas chromatography mass spectrometry; HCN: hydrogen cyanide; HPLC: high-performance liquid chromatography; IC: ion chromatography; LC: liquid chromatography; LCMS: liquid chromatography mass spectrometry; NPD: nitrogen phosphorous detector; RDE: rotating disk electrode; SPME: solid phase microextraction; SCN^-: thiocyanate; UV: ultraviolet

Data sources: (1) Dumas P, Gingras G, LeBlanc A. Isotope dilution-mass spectrometry determination of blood cyanide by headspace gas chromatography. *J Anal Toxicol.* 2005;29:71–75. (2) Calafat AM, Stanfill SB. Rapid quantitation of cyanide in whole blood by automated headspace gas chromatography. *J Chromatogr B Analyt Technol Biomed Life Sci.* 2002; 772:131–137. (3) Ishii A, Seno H, Watanabe-Suzuki K, Suzuki O, Kumazawa T. Determination of cyanide in whole blood by capillary gas chromatography with cryogenic oven trapping. *Anal Chem.* 1998;70:4873–4876. (4) Tracqui A, Raul JS, Geraut A, Berthelon L, Ludes B. Determination of blood cyanide by HPLC-MS. *J Anal Toxicol.* 2002;26:144–148. (5) Meiser H, Hagedorn HW, Schultz R. Development of a method for determination of cyanide concentrations in serum and rumen fluid of cattle. *Am J Vet Res.* 2000;61:658–664. (6) Kage S, Nagata T, Kudo K. Determination of cyanide and thiocyanate in blood by gas chromatography and gas chromatography-mass spectrometry. *J Chromatogr B Biomed Appl.* 1996;675:27–32. (7) Logue BA, Kirschten NP, Petrikovics I, Moser MA, Rockwood GA, Baskin SI. Determination of the cyanide metabolite 2-aminothiazoline-4-carboxylic acid in urine and plasma by gas chromatography-mass spectrometry. *J Chromatogr B Analyt Technol Biomed Life Sci.* 2005;819:237–244. (8) Westley AM, Westley J. Voltammetric determination of cyanide and thiocyanate in small biological samples. *Anal Biochem.* 1989;181:190–194. (9) Ganjali MR, Yousefi M, Javanbakht MJ, et al. Determination of SCN^- in urine and saliva of smokers and non-smokers by SCN(-)- selective polymeric membrane containing a nickel(II)-azamacrocycle complex coated on a graphite electrode. *Anal Sci.* 2002;18:887–892. (10) Felscher D, Wulfmeyer M. A new specific method to detect cyanide in body fluids, especially whole blood, by fluorimetry. *J Anal Toxicol.* 1998;22:363–366. (11) Chinaka S, Takayama N, Michigami Y, Ueda K. Simultaneous determination of cyanide and thiocyanate in blood by ion chromatography with fluorescence and ultraviolet detection. *J Chromatogr B Biomed Sci Appl.* 1998;713:353–359. (12) Connolly D, Barron L, Paull B. Determination of urinary thiocyanate and nitrate using fast ion-interaction chromatography. *J Chromatogr B Analyt Technol Biomed Life Sci.* 2002;767:175–180. (13) Casella IG, Guascito MR, De Benedetto GE. Electrooxidation of thiocyanate on the copper-modified gold electrode and its amperometric determination by ion chromatography. *Analyst.* 1998;123:1359–1363. (14) Chen SH, Yang ZY, Wu HL, Kou HS, Lin SJ. Determination of thiocyanate anion by high-performance liquid chromatography with fluorimetric detection. *J Anal Toxicol.* 1996;20:38–42. (15) Lundquist P, Kagedal B, Nilsson L. An improved method for determination of thiocyanate in plasma and urine. *Eur J Clin Chem Clin Biochem.* 1995;33:343–349. (16) Lundquist P, Kagedal B, Nilsson L, Rosling H. Analysis of the cyanide metabolite 2-aminothiazoline-4-carboxylic acid in urine by high-performance liquid chromatography. *Anal Biochem.* 1995;228:27–34. (17) Groff WA, Stemler FW, Kaminskis A, Froehlich HL, Johnson RP. Plasma free cyanide and blood total cyanide: a rapid completely automated microdistillation assay. *J Toxicol Clin Toxicol.* 1985;23:133–163. (18) Hughes C, Lehner F, Dirikolu L, et al. A simple and highly sensitive spectrophotometric method for the determination of cyanide in equine blood. *Toxicol Mech Methods.* 2003;13:1–10. (19) Lundquist P, Sörbo B. Rapid determination of toxic cyanide concentrations in blood. *Clin Chem.* 1989;35:617–619. (20) Chattaraj S, Das AK. Indirect determination of thiocyanate in biological fluids using atomic absorption spectrometry. *Spectrochica Acta.* 1992;47:675–680. (21) *Toxicological Profile for Cyanide.* Atlanta, Ga: US Department

low temperature, and preserving agents are common procedures used to prevent loss of cyanide. Rubber stoppers have been shown to adsorb or dissolve HCN when in contact with the gas, so use of rubber stoppers to seal vials should be avoided.[95] Storing samples at low temperatures to slow chemical reactions has been tested, and temperature studies for biological samples containing cyanide have been performed. However, there are many temperature discrepancies in the literature.[69,81,83,96,97] The temperature study performed by Lundquist et al resulted in the following four determinations[82]: (1) cyanide in whole blood is reasonably stable at −20°C, and this stability decreased at the higher temperatures of 4°C and room temperature; (2) the addition of silver ions (silver sulfate) immediately after collection appeared to stabilize cyanide at the higher temperatures; (3) the addition of the silver sulfate immediately after collection increased storage time of biological samples at 4°C for at least 2 weeks; and (4) the addition of silver sulfate also appeared to quench the reaction of cyanide and bovine serum albumin to form iminothiazolidine and cysteine residues in blood plasma. Forming other stable cyanide complexes, for example, by adding sodium nitrite to form methemoglobin or by adding hydroxocobalamin, has also been performed successfully.[87,98]

- **Cyanide may form during storage**. Artifactual formation of cyanide may also occur in biological samples depending on storage conditions.[91,97,99–101] It has been suggested that oxyhemoglobin,[100] thiocyanate oxidase,[91,101] and granulocytes (white blood cells)[99] may oxidize thiocyanate to cyanide and that these reactions are dependent on the temperature and pH of the sample. Lundquist's temperature dependence analysis was found to be different from earlier studies[69,96,97] and his use of silver ions may also improve thiocyanate stability.[82] Microorganisms are also responsible for cyanide production,[101] and low temperature storage helps to eliminate their growth.

These considerations, common to all the analytical methods, are a major source for the vast discrepancies in cyanide and cyanide metabolite levels reported from casualties. Because of the detoxification processes and cyanide's physical and nucleophilic properties, direct analysis of cyanide is not normally done with urine or saliva samples, although traces have been found in urine, saliva, and expired air. The cyanide metabolites thiocyanate and ATCA may be determined in urine, saliva, and blood plasma. Correlation of their concentrations to cyanide exposure have been examined.[96,102–104,150–153] Advantages to measuring thiocyanate are that appreciable concentrations may be found immediately after exposure, and that it is considered to be more stable than cyanide. However, the true concentration may also be difficult to determine because of its conversion back to cyanide during storage.[153] ATCA is stable in biological samples for months at freezing and ambient temperatures.[154] Based on determination of pK_a values (carboxylic acid: 2.03; amine: 8.48) and nuclear magnetic resonance studies,[154] ATCA forms a bipolar ion in solution and is therefore not volatile. It has been suggested that ATCA has lower initial concentrations than thiocyanate, but its stability and applicability to sensitive analytical techniques may prove more beneficial. Disadvantages for both ATCA and thiocyanate, as with cyanide, include naturally occurring background levels that are different for each person, making it difficult to quantify low-level cyanide exposure without establishing baseline levels for an individual prior to exposure.[96,155] In addition, cyanide distribution and concentrations in organs differ depending on the route of administration and primate species type. Organ cyanide concentrations have also been used for blood cyanide intoxication levels in forensic cases; however, the postmortem production and transformation of cyanide must be considered in interpreting the results.[85,86,92,156–159]

The analytical determination of cyanide is not an easy task because of its volatility, nucleophilic properties, and lack of color. Although numerous methods have been developed, each must be used with precautions because of interferences and instrumentation capabilities. However, all the methods have helped in some way or another to provide insight into the detection of cyanide in biological fluids. When selecting an analytical method, several factors in addition to the detection limit and length of time needed (Table 11-2) must be considered:

- Does the method include consideration of preserving cyanide and its metabolites during storage?
- Does the method include correct storage of stock solutions[95] or use fresh preparations daily?
- Does the method include consideration of typical interferences found in blood?
- Does the method test for cyanide with and without clinically used antidotes present?
- Does the method include analysis procedures (eg, pH, heating, and acidification) that could result in the loss of cyanide? Are rubber stoppers or septums used?
- Are the chemicals used in the determination toxic or carcinogenic?
- Is the method precise, accurate, inexpensive, and practical?

The literature displays a great deal of inconsistency in reporting on how cyanide or thiocyanate analytical methods faired during storage, the validation of the method in the presence of antidotes, and timing of sample collection. Several authors strongly emphasize the importance of collection and storage of cyanide-contaminated biological samples.[82,87,105–109,158–160] Because no simple, fast, lightweight, sensitive, and accurate methods are currently available for detection of cyanide in biological fluids, none are appropriate for diagnostic

TABLE 11-3

ENDOGENOUS CYANIDE CONCENTRATIONS FOR SMOKERS AND NONSMOKERS*

	Cyanide							
	Nonsmokers				**Smokers**			
Subsample Size in Study	**Whole Blood (ng/mL)**	**Erythrocytes (ng/mL)**	**Plasma (ng/mL)**	**Saliva (ng/mL)**	**Whole Blood (ng/mL)**	**Erythrocytes (ng/mL)**	**Plasma (ng/mL)**	**Saliva (ng/mL)**
n=20[1]	4.4 ± 1.0			9.9 ± 6.8	7.0 ± 1.8			17.1 ± 13.5
n=5 smokers; n=10 nonsmokers[2]	3.5 ± 2.1	6.5 ± 5.9	0.54 ± 0.54		8.9 ± 3.2	18.0 ± 5.4	0.81 ± 0.54	
n=10 nonsmokers[3]	51.3 ± 17.3							
	Thiocyanate							
	Whole Blood (ng/mL)	**Plasma (ng/mL)**	**Urine (ng/mL)**	**Saliva (ng/mL)**	**Whole Blood (ng/mL)**	**Plasma (ng/mL)**	**Urine (ng/mL)**	**Saliva (ng/mL)**
n=20[1]		1.94 ± 1.47		31.4 ± 23.5		6.54 ± 5.34		96.0 ± 48.8
	2-Aminothiazoline-4-carboxylic Acid							
	Whole Blood (ng/mL)	**Plasma (ng/mL)**	**Urine (ng/mL)**	**Saliva (ng/mL)**	**Whole Blood (ng/mL)**	**Plasma (ng/mL)**	**Urine (ng/mL)**	**Saliva (ng/mL)**
n=19 smokers; n=21 nonsmokers[4]			85 ± 47				233 ± 237	
n=27 smokers; n=27 nonsmokers[5]		11.8 ± 4.7				17.2 ± 5.2		

*The nonsmoker averages 0.06 μg/mL of cyanide in blood, whereas the smoker averages 0.17 μg/ mL.
Data sources: (1) Seto Y. False cyanide detection. *Anal Chem.* 2002;74:134A–141A. (2) Lundquist P, Rosling H, Sorbo B. Determination of cyanide in whole blood, erythrocytes and plasma. *Clin Chem.* 1985;31:591–595. (3) Lundquist P, Sörbo B. Rapid determination of toxic cyanide concentrations in blood. *Clin Chem.* 1989;35:617–619. (4) Logue BA, Kirschten NP, Petrikovics I, Moser MA, Rockwood GA, Baskin SI. Determination of the cyanide metabolite 2-aminothiazoline-4-carboxylic acid in urine and plasma by gas chromatography-mass spectrometry. *J Chromatogr B Analyt Technol Biomed Life Sci.* 2005;819:237–244. (5) Maserek WK, Rockwood GA, Platoff GE, Baskin SI, Logue BA. Feasibility of using the cyanide metabolite 2-amino-2-thiazoline-4-carboxylic acid as a retrospective marker of cyanide exposure. *Toxicol Sci.* 2006;abstract 1918:392. (6) Clark CJ, Campbell D, Reid WH. Blood carboxyhaemoglobin and cyanide levels in fire survivors. *Lancet.* 1981;1:1332–1335.

use by first responders. Emergency personnel have to rely initially on the history and physical symptoms of the patient, rather than wait for laboratory results, recognizing that cyanide poisoning can have symptoms similar to other poisonings.[101,110] Blood and urine samples should be collected and analyzed as soon as possible for confirmation or refutation. Table 11-2 is a method list, and Table 11-3 contains baseline concentrations (neither are intended to be all-inclusive). In addition, some of the methods listed have not been thoroughly examined against suggestions 1 through 5 above. When testing cannot be performed immediately, procedures such as those in Exhibit 11-1 should be used to collect and store samples for later analysis.

CLINICAL PRESENTATION AND MANAGEMENT OF CASUALTIES

Principles of Therapy

The effects of cyanide poisoning are those of progressive tissue hypoxia (Figure 11-2). Many cyanide compounds exist, but this chapter deals only with the toxicities of HCN. Additional signs and symptoms may occur as a result of the parent compound. For example, cyanogen chloride also produces irritation of the eyes and mucous membranes similar to that produced by chlorine.

Lesser degrees of poisoning are survivable even in the absence of specific antidotal therapies. Acute, severe cyanide intoxication, however, is a life-threatening emergency. It is survivable with aggressive acute care

EXHIBIT 11-1

PROCEDURES FOR COLLECTING AND STORING BLOOD SAMPLES FOR DELAYED CYANIDE ANALYSIS

Procedure 1

Step 1. Collect a blood sample in a blood collection tube containing an anticoagulant (eg, EDTA, heparin, sodium citrate).

Step 2. Add 0.05 mL of 0.05 mol/L sodium nitrite per 1 mL of blood, cover, and let stand for 2 minutes.

Step 3. Store at -20 °C until analysis can be performed.[1]

Procedure 2

Step 1. Prepare blood collection tubes containing the anticoagulant sodium citrate (~ 17 mg). Add 20 μL of 50% aqueous solution of sodium nitrite (~10 mg), and dry in vacuo over anhydrous calcium chloride.

Step 2. Collect a 5-mL blood sample.

Step 3. Store at 5°C.[2]

Procedure 3

Step 1. Collect a blood sample in a blood collection tube containing an anticoagulant (EDTA or heparin). Ensure that the top is not made of rubber.

Step 2. Add 1 mL of whole blood to 10 mL of the acid silver sulfate reagent (20 mmol in 0.5 mmol H_2SO_4).

Step 3. Store at -20°C until analysis can be performed.[3]

(1) Lundquist P, Sörbo B. Rapid determination of toxic cyanide concentrations in blood. *Clin Chem.* 1989;35:617–619. (2) Vesey CJ, Langford RM. Stabilization of blood cyanide. *J Anal Toxicol.* 1998; 22:176–178. (3) Lundquist P, Rosling H, Sorbo B. Determination of cyanide in whole blood, erythrocytes and plasma. *Clin Chem.* 1985;31:591–595.

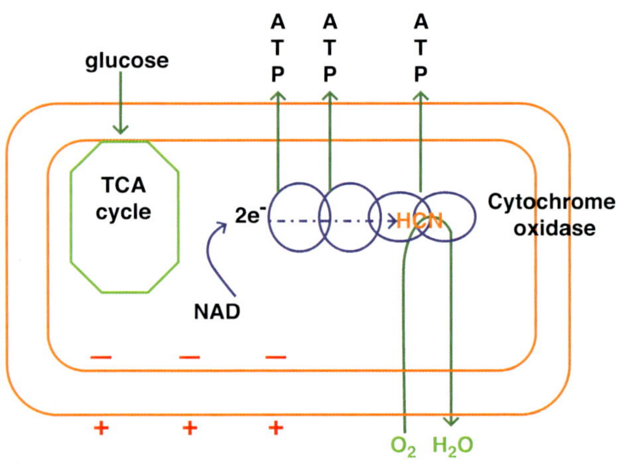

Fig. 11-2. Cyanide binds the terminal enzyme of the cytochrome oxidase enzyme system. The enzyme system is located within the inner lamina of the mitochondria. The blockade interrupts the electron flow through the cytochrome oxidase system, thereby disrupting ATP production and both mitochondrial and cytoplasmic ionic balance.
ATP: adenosine triphosphate
HCN: cyanide
NADH: nicotinamide adenine dinucleotide
TCA: tricarboxylic acid cycle
$2e^-$: two electrons

and support during recovery. Often, but not always, recovery is complete. In addition to medical therapeutics, it may be necessary for rescuers and providers to protect themselves from cyanide in the environment, on the casualty, or in exhaled air and vomitus. Once successful medical care begins, providers will need to support the casualty through neurological crisis including coma, seizures, and respiratory failure. They will need to manage cardiorespiratory crisis, including pulmonary edema, and they may need to manage other organ effects, such as toxic hepatitis and renal failure. After acute recovery, they need to prepare for psychiatric care and possible delayed neuropathology.

Cyanide is known to inhibit some 40 enzymes, including several metalloenzymes containing iron, copper, or molybdenum.[125] These reactions may well contribute to cyanide toxicity. The dominant effects of acute, high-dose exposure, however, result from cyanide's primary effect of inhibiting cytochrome *c* oxidase. This action impairs oxygen uptake and utilization, resulting over time in partial or complete cessation of oxidative metabolism, termed histotoxic anoxia. In massive cyanide poisoning, the mechanisms of toxicity appear to be more complex. In particular, cyanide may cause both pulmonary arteriolar and/or coronary artery vasoconstriction, resulting in decreased cardiac output—a shock state unrelated to inhibition of the cytochrome-*c*-oxidase system.[126] Given its high dependency on oxidative metabolism and limited anaerobic capacity, central nervous system impairments unsurprisingly dominate the clinical picture of significantly exposed persons. Unless relieved, neuronal progression to cellular death occurs. The clinical record demonstrates that the single most important factor driving successful conversion of a potentially lethal exposure into full recovery is timeliness of rescue.

Cyanide is a rapidly acting poison with a steep dose-effect curve. A lethal dose of cyanide salts is generally considered to be approximately 300 mg or more.[126,127] Whole blood cyanide levels above 2.7 mg/L are potentially lethal.[128] Dysfunction of the central nervous system dominates the clinical picture. A severe, gapped metabolic acidosis, with a large anion gap is common due to overwhelming lactic acidosis. Cardiovascular instability is typical as the clinical course progresses. Differential diagnosis includes all other causes of rapid loss of consciousness and all other causes of lactic acidosis with anion gap. Chen and coworkers describe the usual findings (based on some 600 cyanide poisonings) as follows:

> Clinically, the odor of bitter almond oil in breath is highly suggestive of cyanide poisoning. On the other hand, its absence does not rule out the possibility of cyanide poisoning. Other signs, while not specific or pathognomonic, consist of rapid respiration, later slow and gasping, accelerated pulse, vomiting, and convulsions which are followed by coma and cyanosis.[129]

Common themes in case presentations (acute, severe) include rapid onset of coma; mydriasis with variable pupil reactivity; burnt/bitter/pungent almond scent; tachycardia; metabolic acidosis, often extreme; cyanosis of mucous membranes and/or flushed skin; absence of cyanosis despite respiratory failure; ECG showing the T wave originating high on the R (most severe); absence of focal neurological signs; distant heart sounds; an irregular pulse; and similar oxygen tension in both arterioles and venules (Figure 11-3). In a few cases of massive poisoning, pulmonary edema has been reported, likely a result of myocardial injury from the cyanide leading to temporary left heart failure and increased central venous pressure.[130–132] Another uncommonly reported acute complication is rhabdomyolysis.[133] Although patients in some reported cases received treatment with hemodialysis either to remove unknown toxins or to treat complications of treatment, acute renal failure secondary to cyanide poisoning is not reported. Similarly, toxic hepatitis is not reported, presumably because few cyanide patients survive longer than the 6 hours of postcyanide shock usually necessary to induce toxic hepatitis.[134]

General supportive measures in the setting of acute reaction to moderate or high dose cyanide focus on assuring an airway, administering 100% oxygen, establishing intravenous (IV) access, ablating seizures, and monitoring vital signs and electrocardiograms (EKGs). Blood should be drawn (while noting its color) for a complete blood count, pH, Po_2, Pco_2, electrolytes, glucose, and whole-blood cyanide. Additional studies may be indicated, particularly if the cause of illness is unknown. Subsequent interventions depend on clinical presentation, and the treatment team must be prepared to adjust therapies. Common adjuncts include pressor support; IV hydration; benzodiazapines; insulin; mannitol for pulmonary edema; antiarrhythmics; gastrointestinal clearance (lavage, activated charcoal, diarrheals); and sodium bicarbonate. In general, patients recovering from cyanide intoxication need 24 to 48 hours' observation to support early intervention in the event of acute complications and/or recurring intoxication from incompletely cleared cyanide.

Antidotal enhancement of cyanide excretion is a two-step process, represented in Figure 11-4. The first simplistically uses "scavengers" to restore aerobic energy production. The second prepares cyanide through sulfation for renal clearance from the body. The second step is required to eliminate the threat of reintoxication. Nitrites and sodium thiosulfate have been used worldwide for many decades to treat cyanide intoxication. Thiosulfate, a sulfane donor, is the rate-limiting substrate for the sulfur transferase rhodanese. Rhodanese is the dominant system for clearing cyanide, working by converting cyanide into the renally excretable thiocyanate. Rhodanese is widely distributed, although most concentrated in the liver, and is intramitochondrial. Physiological reserves of thiosulfate are low, thereby limiting endogenous rhodanese activity. Excess thiosulfate is cleared through the kidneys. Experimental data indicate that thiosulfate and rhodanese effectively remove free HCN, resulting in restored cytochrome oxidase activity.[135] Although unrecorded as the sole therapeutic drug in human case history, sodium thiosulfate is likely a sufficient antidote for moderately severe poisonings, but insufficient for greater exposures.[136] Given its large safety margin, sodium thiosulfate may have particular value when clinicians are reluctant to apply more toxic or more complicated antidotes.

Nitrites available in the United States are amyl nitrite and sodium nitrite. Amyl nitrite (0.35 mL/crushable capsule) is considered a first aid inhalable form.

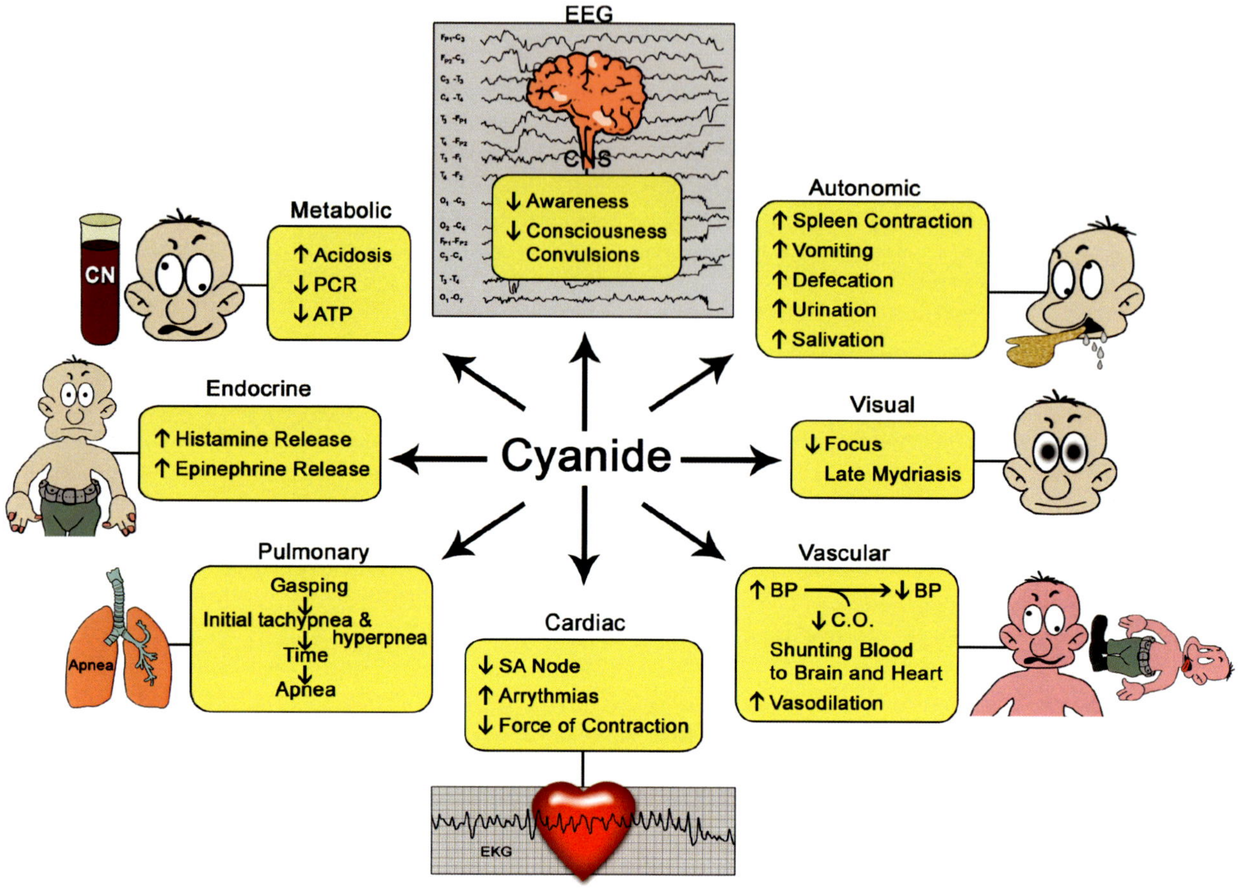

Fig. 11-3. Cyanide can affect the function of vascular, visual, pulmonary, central nervous, cardiac, autonomic, endocrine, and metabolic systems. The toxicodynamic effects can vary depending on the dose, route and speed of administration, chemical form (liquid, gas, solid) of the cyanide, and other factors, including the gender, age, weight, stress level, and general physical condition of the recipient. Proceeding clockwise from the top of the diagram: *Vascular* effects of cyanide can include an initial transient increase, followed by a decrease, in cardiac output. Blood pressure falls as the cardiac inotropic effect decreases and as vasodilation occurs. *Visual* effects can include decreased capacity to focus, with late-onset mydriasis secondary to hypoxia. One of the first *pulmonary* effects from cyanide is a respiratory gasp, caused by stimulation of chemoreceptor bodies near the aortic bifurcation. Hyperventilation follows this response. Over time (the response is dose-dependent, occurring in seconds to minutes), the frequency and depth of breathing diminish. *Central nervous system* effects initially manifest as decreased awareness and increased release of enkephalins, followed by loss of consciousness and convulsions. *Cardiac* effects include an increase in heart rate, then a decrease; both are accompanied by arrhythmias and negative inotropy. Cyanide produces a number of *autonomic nervous system* effects, based on the route and dose of the agent. Cyanide can also produce multiple *endocrine* effects, including epinephrine and histamine release, and *metabolic* actions that decrease energy production by the inhibition of the use of cytochrome *c* oxidase.
ATP: adenosine triphosphate
CNS: central nervous system
CO: cardiac output
EEG: electroencephalogram
EKG: electrocardiogram
PCr: phosphocreatine

Sodium nitrite is the intravenous, definitive treatment form. Nitrite delivery increases endogenous methemoglobin, which binds cyanide but does not clear it from the body. Treatment with nitrites must be accompanied by treatment with sodium thiosulfate. Both amyl and sodium nitrite are potent vasodilators, which may afford additional therapeutic advantage.[137] The value of combined intravenous sodium nitrite and sodium thiosulfate was recognized early and was summarized (as follows) by Chen et al:

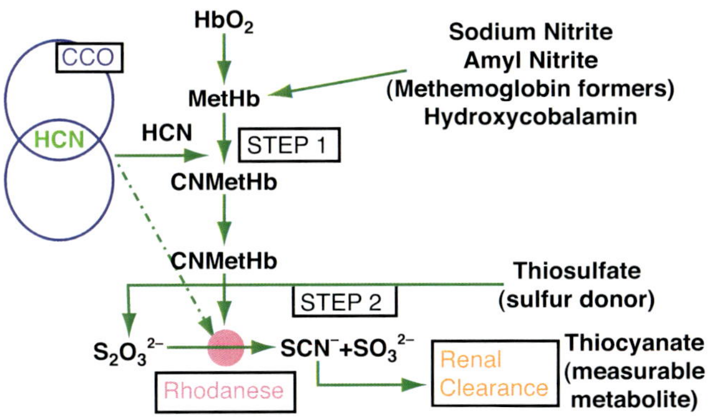

Fig. 11-4. Fundamentals of cyanide antidote therapy. Clearance of excess cyanide is essentially a two-step process. The first step restores mitochondrial aerobic energy production by accelerating cyanide removal from cytochrome *c* oxidase. The second step enhances conversion of cyanide into a form suitable for renal clearance. It should be noted that the clearance process crosses multiple compartments and organ systems, and it works efficiently in the presence of adequate substrate and intact hepatic and renal function.
CCO: cytochrome *c* oxidase
HCN: cyanide
MetHb: methemoglobin
CNMetHb: cyanomethemoglobin
$S_2O_3^{2-}$: thiosulfate ion
SO_3^{2-}: sulfite
SCN^-: thiocyanate

> The two substances intravenously injected, one after the other, namely, the nitrite followed by the thiosulfate, are capable of detoxifying approximately twenty lethal doses of sodium cyanide in dogs, and are effective even after respiration has stopped. As long as the heart is still beating, the chances of recovery by this method of treatment are very good. Since dogs are more susceptible to the poison than man, these observations are especially significant. When sodium nitrite is used alone, about four lethal doses of the cyanide are detoxified. Sodium thiosulfate, when injected alone, nullifies about three lethal doses of the cyanide. Thus, there is not only a summation but a definite potentiation of action when the nitrite and the thiosulfate are administered together . . . . Another nitrite, namely amyl nitrite, by inhalation has the same detoxifying value as sodium nitrite by intravenous injection.[129]

More recent case experience confirms early reports.[137]

Because nitrite formers elevate methemoglobin levels and are powerful hypotensive agents, both methemoglobin levels and hypotension must be monitored during the course of therapy and nitrites withheld if necessary until recovery of acceptable blood pressure and treatment of methemoglobinemia. Therapeutic levels of methemoglobin are usually well under 10% when measured, often 3% to 5%. Induced cyanomethemoglobin levels are usually unknown; available oxygen carrying capacity is always less than methemoglobin levels alone predict.

The two chief formations of cobalt antidotes are hydroxocobalamin and dicobalt edetate. Although cobalt EDTA is quite toxic, hydroxocobalamin appears to have a safety profile preferable to the nitrites, particularly in settings in which induction of methemoglobin is undesirable. No efficacy studies compare performance of nitrites against that of cobalts.

Oxygen is an important medicament for cyanide intoxication. It significantly enhances the antidotal value of nitrite plus thiosulfates, increasing the LD_{50} dose 6-fold (drugs alone) to over 8-fold.[49] Oxygen's mechanisms of action are uncertain. The additional gain afforded by hyperbaric oxygen is uncertain, with some patients responding well and other attempts unsuccessful unless carbon monoxide intoxication coexists.[138] Patients should receive 100% humidified oxygen. If a mask is used, it should be a nonrebreathing mask to prevent rebreathing of exhaled cyanide.

Several case reports have been published in which full recovery occurred in the absence of specific antidotal therapy. In each case, indicated general supportive measures were otherwise provided.[126,133,139,140] Blood levels of cyanide in these individuals ranged from 2.14 to 7.7 mg/L. Levels exceeding 3 mg/L are usually considered potentially lethal, and levels exceeding 2 mg/L severe. These cases do not, however, justify withholding specific antidotal therapies if antidotes are available.[56] These survivors likely were more tolerant of the exposures than is typical. In addition, their postacute recovery statuses are not reported. Yen et al report the only published English language epidemiological case comparison between severe cyanide intoxications receiving nitrite/thiosulfate antidotes and those receiving supportive care alone.[137] In the absence of anoxic encephalopathy, administration of specific antidotes offered clear survival advantage.

Full treatment, including antidotes, should be administered to pregnant women who are seriously impaired by cyanide. Fetal effects other than methemoglobin induction have not been reported. Risks to the fetus from maternal incapacitation override concerns from possible fetal methemoglobin induction. In addition, the evidence suggesting the teratogenic risk of antidotes during pregnancy is very limited.[141] In a life-saving situation, therapies should not be modified as a consequence of pregnancy.

In summary, the fundamental principles of toxicologic therapies apply to treatment of cyanide-injured casualties. The first is to recognize the situation and to protect those responding. The second is to rapidly intervene to avoid unnecessary complications. The third is to provide supportive measures according to the extent of injury. And the fourth is to provide specific antidotes even in the absence of confirmatory laboratory testing while controlling for undesirable side effects (Table 11-4). If these principles are followed, most persons arriving for medical care will recover within hours to days. Once discharged, all seriously affected persons should receive periodic follow-up to ensure that any underlying psychiatric problems or delayed neurological and other consequences are detected and managed (see below).

Triage, Decontamination and Patient Transport (Evacuation)

Triage is necessitated by the presence of overwhelming demands on the available medical system. It provides for a methodical and orderly approach to casualties. Triage, decontamination, and timely transport to prepared medical receivers depend on a trained, prepared, and well-integrated organizational system. A coordinated system is at least as critical to casualty survival as are specific antidotes.[142] The remainder of this discussion will assume reader awareness of general principles of casualty rescue: protection of workers from exposure; reduction of contamination by evacuation from the contamination source, undressing, and removal of obvious liquid cyanide; provision of general life support including seizure ablation; and, finally, medical decontamination and definitive medical care.

Triage of a cyanide mass casualty event focuses on identifying casualties who require emergent care to survive with the least possible consequence to later function, including neurological function. Casualties absent of heart rate are termed expectant or black. Comatose, seizing, hypotensive, or hypopneic casualties are classified immediate or red. These patients must receive immediate respiratory support, oxygen, circulatory support, and antiseizure medications in addition to having obvious cyanide removed. As soon as possible, specific cyanide antidotes must be administered. Thiosulfate may be the preferred antidote in mass casualty situations because of its favorable safety profile. If personnel are available to monitor for nitrite-induced hypotension and to adjust the rate of administration, then the addition of nitrites will enhance recovery. Because their condition can be expected to deteriorate rapidly, persons who have ingested cyanide or who have liquid contamination should be considered for early intravenous access with possible initiation of thiosulfate infusion *even before overt signs develop.*

Remaining casualties are removed from further exposure and sorted into delayed (yellow) and minimal (green) categories. Minimal (green) is assigned to mildly affected, vapor-exposed persons. These casualities experience nausea and dizziness, and may be agitated or hyperventilating. They require only removal from exposure, a calming environment, and reassurance. Once recovered, they may be asked to provide assistance to the response effort, because they will sustain no injury from their exposure and may benefit from early return to useful activity. Delayed (yellow) casualties are those who have received initial treatment and are under observation during recovery. Casualties who are alive at the time of first medical contact should be expected to survive given full care.

Cyanide decontamination is straightforward. If

TABLE 11-4

US APPROACH TO CYANIDE ANTIDOTES

Mechanism	Natural Process of Elimination	Treatment
Unload cyanide from cellular cytochrome oxidase	Use methemoglobin 1%–2% (Fe^{3+})	Amyl nitrite ampules (inhaled), sodium nitrite (300 mg IV), or hydroxocobalamin (5 g, diluted, IV)
Transfer CN^- from stable, time-release depot to excretable molecule	Rhodanese conjugates CN^- with thiocyanate ion → SCN + sulfite	Sodium thiosulfate (50 mL of 25% solution, IV)
Remove from body	Renal excretion	Renal excretion
Potentiate effects of nitrite and thiosulfate	None	Supplemental oxygen (100% humidified)
Reduce burden of ingested cyanide	Vomit	Gastric lavage

CN^-: cyanide anion
SCN^-: thiocyanate

cyanide has been ingested the gut should be decontaminated through gastric lavage and the administration of activated carbon. All cutaneous cyanide can be removed by washing with water or soap and water. Water temperature should be comfortably warm if possible, but decontamination should not be delayed while water is heated. Early decontamination definitely reduces the extent of illness by decreasing total body burden. Decontamination also protects emergency responders and healthcare personnel. Personnel conducting decontamination and any predecontamination care require appropriate personal protective equipment so that they themselves do not become casualties. Personnel conducting autopsy examinations on persons recently deceased from cyanide poisoning should also apply safety precautions. At the least, these include adequate ventilation to the outside, frequent breaks in uncontaminated spaces, and containment of heavily contaminated organs. Any personnel who become symptomatic should refrain from continued exposure. Documentation of postexposure blood cyanide levels can be considered.[143]

Transport of cyanide-intoxicated casualties to definitive care facilities should be done as rapidly as possible unless general supportive care and antidotes can be delivered by emergency responders. In the event of a suicide attempt, this could be at the home or workplace or in the ambulance en route to the hospital. In the event of an urban release, initial stabilization could occur in the warm zone (decontamination corridor). In the event of a military situation, initial stabilization would probably occur in the dirty side of the patient decontamination station. In any case, stabilization of critically ill casualties must be done before complete decontamination. Transport vehicles and personnel should be prepared to provide oxygen (100% if possible), intravenous lines, cardiopulmonary rescusitation, and antiseizure medications. Ideally they will also be equipped to initiate specific antidotal therapy, particularly with amyl nitrite and thiosulfate. Because of its side-effect profile, sodium nitrite should not be administered unless the care providers are equipped to monitor blood pressure closely and to adjust rates of administration.

Laboratory Findings

Serious cyanide toxicity is characterized by obstruction of aerobic metabolism and forced anaerobic metabolism. These conditions cause lactic acidosis, manifesting as metabolic acidosis with anion gap and lactic acidemia, and reduced arteriovenous oxygen content difference. A lactate level measurement refines the more general impression of metabolic acidosis; depending on the results, renal insufficiency would be a less likely cause of anion gapped metabolic acidosis. In the setting of severe and potentially fatal cyanide poisoning, pulse oximetry correctly demonstrates the high blood oxygen content. It will not, however, correctly reflect deficient oxygen delivery and uptake at tissue level.

As therapy proceeds and cellular respiration resumes, venous oxygen levels will drop, lactic acid levels will return to normal, and pH will move towards neutral.[144–148] Estimation of oxygen saturation by pulse oximetry will remain misleading, however, because of the presence of methemoglobin as a consequence of nitrite therapy.[149] Hemoximetry (in vitro multiwavelength cooximetry) can quantify the deficit in functional saturation resulting from methemoglobin and carboxyhemoglobin but does not account for additional, and likely significant, decrements caused by cyanomethemoglobin (unless newer machines capable of directly measuring cyanomethemoglobin are used).[161] Measured methemoglobin levels after administration of a 300-mg ampule of sodium nitrite will likely not exceed 7% to 10% and may be lower; the remaining oxygen carrying capacity will be something less than 90% to 93%, depending on the degree of dyshemoglobinemia present.

Interpretation of cyanide levels for clinical management is unreliable. Cyanide is continually eliminated from the body as long as the person remains alive. Cyanide can be measured in either plasma or whole blood. Whole blood levels more accurately reflect the total body burden because most cyanide is rapidly bound into red blood cells, but plasma levels may more correctly predict cellular exposure.[144] Blood cyanide levels do not reliably predict severity of illness. In addition, most centers are unable to receive test results quickly enough to support diagnostic use. Therefore, blood or plasma cyanide levels currently have limited value in the acute care setting outside of research hospitals. They remain valuable for confirmatory testing and forensic purposes. In the near future, the cyanide metabolite ATCA may prove to be a useful additional biomarker of excessive cyanide exposure because of its stability over time.[151]

Long-Term Effects

Comparatively few persons survive acute, high-dose exposures to cyanide. Survivors typically either receive early aggressive medical support or represent the subpopulation with increased resistance to the poison. One other subgroup is those with gastric anacidity. They tolerate large amounts of cyanide salts, apart from local erosions.[162] The understanding of the health impacts of survival of otherwise lethal cyanide intoxications is necessarily framed by the few published case reports that follow survivors over time.[127,162–170] These reports indicate that the major system resulting in clinically relevant pathology is the central nervous system, particularly the brain, but also to some extent the spinal cord.[171]

Cyanide does not uniformly affect all brain cells. For example, CA1 neurons in the hippocampus are more susceptible than CA3 cells to metabolic inhibition by cyanide.[172] Nearly all long-term neurological sequelae of acute high-dose exposure result from damage to the basal ganglia and sensorimotor cortex, with additional defects referencing cerebellar Purkinje neurons. Cell death occurs slowly after brief ischemia. Current theory favors cellular apoptosis as the mechanism of demise as opposed to necrotic death.[163,167] Casualties with long-term effects manifest parkinsonian-like conditions and akinetic rigid syndromes, typically after intervals of weeks to months. Usually lacking are tremor, pathological reflexes, disorders of sensitivity, or intellectual deficits. Occasionally, the clinical picture partially improves over time. Some patients demonstrate partial improvement with medication. The following eight case synopses address the neuroanatomical pathology of survivors of large cyanide doses, with brief summaries of overall presentation and radiological/histopathologic features. (Note that advancing technologies allow gradually improved understanding of functional as well as anatomical consequences of survival from potentially lethal cyanide intoxications.)

Case Study 11-1. An 18-year-old male survived a 975- to 1,300-mg KCN ingestion.[176] He developed parkinsonian syndrome, characterized primarily by akinesia and rigidity, and died 19 months later. The autopsy revealed major destructive changes in the globus pallidus and putamin. The substantia nigra was intact.

Case Study 11-2. A 29-year-old male survived a 500-mg KCN ingestion.[162] Within 3 weeks he developed slowed and cumbersome speech and impaired swallowing. Within 4 weeks he overshot his trunk movements with postural change and had stiff gait, flat facies, hypokinesia, unmodulated speech, dyscoordination of speech, cogwheel phenomenon, severe bradydiadochokinesia, brisk monosynaptic reflexes, and absence of pathologic reflexes. T2-weighted magnetic resonance imaging (MRI) showed symmetrical signal elevation in both putamina. By 5 months, his clinical status was improved, although slow speech and pronounced bradydiadochokinesia of upper limbs persisted. The putamina were hypodense on MRI.

Case Study 11-3. A 46-year-old male survived a 1,500-mg KCN ingestion.[167] Within 3 days he had mild difficulty with tandem gait and halting speech. Examination 3 weeks after recovery revealed marked bradykinesia; masked facies; slow, shuffling gait; mild rigidity; and weak dysphonic voice. Little tremor was present. MRI 12 months after ingestion revealed multiple, bilaterally symmetrical areas of high-signal intensity in the globus pallidus and posterior putamen on T2-weighted images. A 6-fluorodopa positron emission tomography revealed diffuse decreased activity in fluoridopa in the basal ganglia and markedly decreased activity in the posterior regions of the basal ganglia, similar to patients with parkinsonism.

Case Study 11-4. A 28-year-old male survived a 800-mg KCN ingestion.[164] Within several weeks he developed extrapyramidal signs including marked drooling, profound micrographia, masked facies, mild intention tremor, and cogwheel rigidity. MRI 3 months after poisoning demonstrated wedge-shaped areas of increased signal intensity in the T2-weighted images, particularly in the globus pallidi. Repeat scanning 12 months later disclosed no change in the extent of basal ganglial abnormality but showed the development of mild cerebellar atrophy.

Case Study 11-5. A 31-year-old male with epilepsy recovered fully after ingesting 20 to 40 gm KCN dissolved in milk.[166] As long as 1.5 years after the poisoning, he showed no signs or symptoms. His temporal lobe epilepsy was unchanged. Memory and intelligence were unaffected. T1-weighted images on MRI at day 51 demonstrated bilaterally symmetrical high-signal intensity in both putamina. Both regions became isointense to white matter by day 146 and remained so by day 286.

Case Study 11-6. A 27-year-old female survived a 300-mg KCN ingestion.[165] Over the next 2 months she developed gradually progressive stiffness and weakness of all four limbs, along with unclear speech, severe hyperkinetic dysarthria due to dystonia, mild left facial weakness, generalized lead pipe rigidity, and bradykinesia. She also demonstrated hemiplegic dystonia with bilateral involvement characterized by flexed upper limbs, extended lower limbs, and normal deep tendon reflexes with flexor plantar responses. Her upper limbs were flexed and supinated, with fingers tightly flexed and thumb strongly opposed. Her neck and spine were rigidly extended. She showed no tendency to spontaneous improvement. Cranial computed tomography scan showed bilateral putaminal hypodensities, which were seen to be hyperintense on MRI T2-weighted images. Multimodal evoked potentials were normal.

Case Study 11-7. A 19-year-old female survived inhalational exposure of a large dose (the exact amount was unknown) as an intended victim of homicide.[173] During trial proceedings 8 months after the poisoning, she was noted to be fully recovered with the exception of a mild dragging of one leg. No imaging studies were reported.

Case Study 11-8. A 35-year-old female survived a usually lethal ingestion of KCN.[163] By day 5 she displayed agitation and choreoathetotic movements of all four extremities and the trunk, which was suppressed while she was communicating. Deep tendon reflexes were brisk, and both plantar responses were positive. By week 3, the choreoathetotic movements abated to a state of akinetic mutism with loss of power, resembling generalized dystonia. She was dysarthric and had limited swallowing. An electroencephalogram (EEG) revealed diffuse, abnormal beta activity, more pronounced in frontal and front-temporal regions, but no focal epileptic activity. Serial evoked potentials testing revealed central axonal auditory and somatosensory propagation damage. MRI revealed acute and subacute damage to the caudate nucleus and globus pallidus bilaterally and discreet cortical damage localized to sensory motor cortex consistent with pseudolaminar necrosis, and functional imaging with β-CIT SPECT showed loss of nigrostriatal dopaminergic neurons.

As contrasted with acute, high-dose survivors, thousands of people survive with lesser overdoses from excessive consumption of cyanogenic foods on a chronic basis, particularly in the setting of overall nutritional inadequacy. Such chronic overexposure to cyanide and its metabolite thiocyanate is thought to account for prevalent peripheral nervous system disorders and perhaps also for excess goiters found within subpopulations of sub-Saharan Africa and Asia.[125,174]

In summary, most severely poisoned cyanide casualties die in the absence of early intervention. Based on limited case reports, long-term survivors may develop significant neurological morbidity arising from apoptotic demise of neurons of the basal ganglia and sensory-motor cortex. Case series from occupational settings where potentially lethal intoxications are typically identified and definitive treatment begun within minutes of exposure report early return to full duty.[175] In addition, it is likely that developing knowledge in the fields of neuroprotection and resuscitation will afford even gravely ill cyanide casualties better opportunity for excellent recovery.

Cyanide is associated with neuropathies worldwide (but not endemic to Westernized nations) that appear to result from excessive daily dietary cyanide, perhaps in combination with insufficiently varied diets with low-quality protein content. Bitter cassava root in particular is noted for this association. Cassava is a dietary staple, but it requires extensive processing to remove cyanogens prior to consumption. During food shortages or civil unrest, preparation is shortened while dependence on the staple crop increases. The upper motor neuron disorder konzo notoriously occurs in individuals—especially children—at these times.[176–178] Konzo is a persistent but nonprogressive spastic paraparesis (muscle weakness) that has been studied extensively by Rosling and colleagues.[179,180] Konzo sufferers display lower-limb dysfunction, limited mobility, and impaired fine motor function.[181] Populations recently affected by konzo have been found to have elevated urinary thiocyanate outputs and decreased inorganic sulfate excretion, consistent with high cyanide intake and low sulfur-containing amino acids intake.

Pediatric Considerations

Pediatric considerations for any toxicant must be discussed with awareness of normal development and how that toxicant interacts with specific stages of development.[182] Very little knowledge of cyanide impact on fetal development exists. Because fetal well-being is most dependent on maternal well-being, the primary therapeutic consideration for severe acute cyanide toxicity in a pregnant woman must be urgent restoration of maternal circulatory, respiratory, and neurologic status. Chronic excess of thiocyanate is thought to be thyrotoxic to both the mother and the fetus[125]; this situation is endemic in certain parts of the world where maternal-fetal wellness is already threatened by serious nutritional and socioeconomic problems. Treatment of cyanide intoxication with methemoglobin formers does induce fetal methemoglobinemia. The amount of fetal methemoglobin formed, however, is not likely to be clinically important as weighed against the necessity to treat the mother.[126]

Relatively few case reports and no epidemiological reports of survival of acute cyanide intoxication in young children are available. The few published cases resulted from consumption of cassava or apricot kernals. Children do seem to be more vulnerable to intoxication through food sources, presumably because of lower body weight.[126] In one report, two young Thai children (ages 4 and 1.5 years) became comatose

9 hours after ingesting boiled cassava. They were intubated and put on ventilatory support, but antidotes (nitrite and thiosulfate) were given several hours later upon the children's arrival at a regional intensive care unit. Both received appropriate general support for circulation and ventilation, including fluid loading and dobutamine for hypotension. The older child received nitrite and thiosulfate at 19 hours after ingestion plus gastric decontamination and recovered fully. The other child received only general supportive care because he was not sufficiently stable for transport to the regional hospital until 23 hours after ingestion; by that time he was alert and without cyanosis or serious acidosis.[183] In a second report, eight Venezuelan boys between 8 and 11 years of age consumed cyanogenic bitter cassava. Pigs that ate the remaining cassava died. On arrival at the emergency room, all were critically ill with respiratory failure, bradycardia, and hypotension. Two also displayed generalized seizures. All the children received 100% oxygen and general supportive care. The four least ill children received in addition intramuscular hydroxocobolamin (500 mg). The four sicker children received nitrite and thiosulfate on a milligram per kilogram basis. Their blood was noted to be bright cherry red with identical arteriovenous Po_2 values. All the children improved within a few minutes and were discharged in good condition in 1 day.[184] A third case suggests that methemoglobin formers should be used with particular care in children. Children have higher oxygen demands than adults, and infants in particular are unable to reduce methemoglobin efficiently because of immature methemoglobin reductase systems.[185] This case reports that a 17-month-old child died after receiving a double dose of sodium nitrite for sublethal cyanide ingestion. Antidotes were given in the absence of serious illness and were repeated without first assessing levels of methemoglobin. Furthermore, antidote dosing was not adjusted for body weight and hemoglobin. Toxicological estimates place the child's induced methemoglobin at 92%.[186]

These three case reports and principles of toxicology and pediatrics demonstrate that young children who are critically ill with cyanide overdose can be successfully resuscitated with expectation of full recovery. As with adults, resuscitation of the poisoned child involves life support and stabilization measures, followed by identification of the toxin and detoxification as appropriate. General measures include 100% oxygen and general life support, including gut decontamination with lavage and adsorbents. Antidotes should be administered in accordance with local availability and dose adjusted for weight. General dosing guidelines per package insert should be followed. In general, sodium nitrite should be dosed in the range of 4 mg/kg to 6.6 mg/kg. The former is equivalent to the standard adult dose, and the latter is recommended in the manufacturer's package insert. These doses are considerably less than the often published 10 mg/kg dose. Figure 11-5 demonstrates how the 10-mg/kg dose is unacceptably high for young children in particular. Children over approximately 40 kg body weight can receive an adult dose of sodium nitrite assuming absence of anemia. Hemoglobin levels under 12 g/100 mL dictate dose reductions.[186] It is appropriate to administer the nitrite slowly and consider partial doses so that methemoglobin levels can be carefully monitored. Methemoglobin levels must be monitored before retreatment; successful therapeutic levels appear to be well under 20%, often under 10%. If a treated child becomes cyanotic despite adequate oxygenation during nitrite therapy, methylene blue should be considered even if the methemoglobin level is less than 30%.[187] Although repeat dosing with half the original dose of antidote may be required, it should not be given until caregivers are confident that lethal exposure has occurred, that acidosis persists, that the condition remains unstable, and that adequate oxygen transport capability remains. If poor clinical state persists despite adequate methemoglobin levels, other diagnoses must be considered.

Polyintoxications

The most likely cointoxications with cyanide are alcohol and carbon monoxide. Although alcohol is frequently used before a cyanide suicide attempt and clearly complicates the clinical management of the cyanide-overdosed patient, it is not understood to directly influence outcomes of cyanide intoxication and will not be further discussed here. Of greater concern is the extent to which HCN contributes to mortality and morbidity in fire victims. The pathophysiology of smoke inhalation is complex. Thermal conditions, as well as the constituents of smoke vary not only from fire to fire, but also from one location to another within the same fire. Morbidity and mortality result from a number of interacting processes including thermal injury, carbon monoxide poisoning, trauma, reduced oxygen tension in the heated atmosphere, and other toxicants present. Cyanide is one of those toxicants that might be present in significant amounts because of incomplete combustion in hypoxic conditions.[128,188,189] Although no single factor or group of factors reliably predicts the extent to which HCN intoxication contributes to the clinical picture of any single smoke inhalation casualty, severity of carbon monoxide illness and lactic acidemia greater than 10 mmol/L are most closely associated with severe cyanide cotoxicity.[126,138,145,190–192]

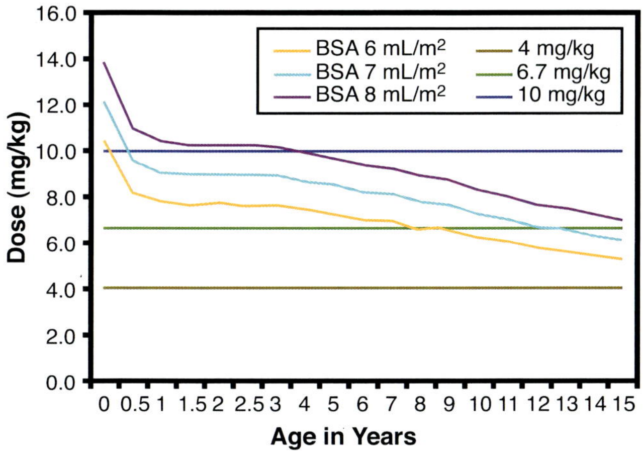

Fig. 11-5. Body surface area versus weight dosing. This figure describes the relative dose in mg/kg when charted against median weight and height for age. These data illustrate why the authors propose that dosing children with sodium nitrite at greater than the package insert recommended 6.6 mg/kg is excessive and potentially harmful. Curves were drawn after converting to dose per body surface area using 50th percentile for weights and length/stature, based on the Centers for Disease Control and Prevention 2001 weight-for-age percentiles, ages birth to 36 months and ages 2 to 20 years. For conversion purposes, 4 mg/kg is equivalent to 0.13 mL/kg of 3% solution, 6.6 mg/kg is 0.2 mg/kg of 3% solution, and 10 mg/kg is 0.33 mL/kg of 3% sodium nitrite solution. Body surface area calculated using the DuBois and DuBois formula.
BSA: body surface area
Chart: Courtesy of MAJ Thomas B Talbot, US Army Medical Research Institute of Chemical Defense, Aberdeen Proving Ground, Md.

The awareness that carbon monoxide has the dominant effect on time of survival, but that both carbon monoxide and HCN, when present, appear to synergistically affect hypoxic fatality, guides some general recommendations. Oxygen, general supportive measures, and burn and trauma management are generally indicated, with high benefit-to-risk ratios. Analysis for carboxyhemoglobin, lactic acidosis, oxygenation, and HCN levels should be accomplished at the earliest opportunity. HCN-specific treatment may be a reasonable option for severely affected smoke inhalation victims who have been properly stabilized otherwise. Thiosulfate is reasonable, effective, and safe, and appropriate for mass casualty situations. It does not diminish oxygen carrying capacity and is widely available; however, it does require a parenteral line be established. Hydroxocobalamin is also reasonable, effective, and safe. It is typically used with thiosulfate, and it does not diminish oxygen carrying capacity. It does require a parenteral line. Amyl nitrite is reasonable and effective; it does not require parenteral access and can be given to persons on supported ventilation. It does reduce oxygen carrying capacity modestly. Because treatment requires close monitoring for hypotension, amyl nitrite is not the first choice in a mass casualty situation. Similarly, sodium nitrite is effective and likely reasonably safe if a high level of oversight is available.[190] The other antidotes described in this chapter have demonstrated general effectiveness against cyanide poisoning but not necessarily against fire exposures. They also require parenteral lines and substantially more monitoring because of their side effect profiles.

In summary, clinical management of cyanide intoxications, regardless of the victim's age or source of intoxication, is based on early recognition, aggressive general support measures, and early antidotal enhancement for severely ill persons otherwise at risk for hypoxic injury. In the absence of history of cyanide exposure, clinicians have to proceed without a confirmed diagnosis, maintaining high levels of awareness for adverse effects of therapy and changes in clinical course. Successful acute intervention must be followed with sustained care directed at underlying causes of intoxication and detection of delayed sequelae.

CYANIDE-CAUSED CARDIAC TOXICITY

Histopathologic Changes

Cyanide is deposited heterogeneously in cardiac tissue, with the ventricles heavily affected. The resulting histological changes include cell swelling and hemorrhaging.[193] Cell swelling activates chloride membrane currents, as part of the ionic derangement, changing the homeostasis of the tissue. Substrate changes include formation of lactic acid and secretion of catecholamines.

One of the first manifestations of the changed electrophysiology is bradycardia, which may soon change to torsade de pointes and possibly culminate in ventricular fibrillation (Figure 11-6). Katzman and Penney and Wexler et al provide additional details.[194,195]

On the cellular level, changes in the ion concentrations become important, especially calcium overload of the cell and increase in the extracellular potassium concentration, $[K^+]_o$. The cell's energy homeostasis[196] is profoundly disturbed, and several compensatory membrane currents are activated and others diminished. Three of the most important ones are the ATP-

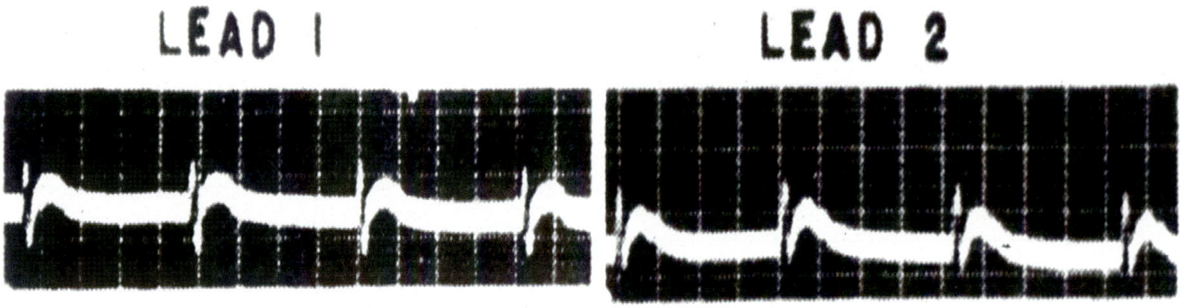

Fig. 11-6. Electrocardiogram from a cyanide-intoxicated individual. The P-wave (the atrial depolarization) is eliminated, and ST-segment deviation, usually a rise in the slope, becomes noticeable, followed by modulation of the T-wave. The changed morphology is expressed in steepening and coalescing of the QRS and the T-waves. A J-wave becomes noticeable. Reprinted with permission from: Wexler J, Whittenberger JL, Dumke PR. The effect of cyanide on the electrocardiogram of man. *Am Heart J.* 1947; 34:170.

dependent I_{KATP},[197] the osmotic swelling-activated $I_{Cl,swell}$, and the calcium-dependent $I_{Ca\text{-}L}$. The disequilibrium in the membrane currents caused by cyanide has grave implications for the cell's electrophysiology. Cyanide-caused cardiac toxicity shares some commonality with ischemia but is different in the level of acidity of the tissue and the nature of some of the activated currents. A number of ancillary effects, including enhanced catecholamine secretion where CA binds to α and β receptors that affect membrane currents, increase in free Mg^{2+}, and pH changes also occur.[54,198–200]

Computational Models

ECGs and action potential morphologies are markers of the electrophysiological state of cardiac tissue. High-performance computer simulations of the electrophysiology of the three types of cardiac cells—endocardial, midmyocardial, and epicardial—model the impact of specific changes to identified ionic currents on cardiac electrophysiology.[201–204] Usually dormant currents appear to be critical to understand-

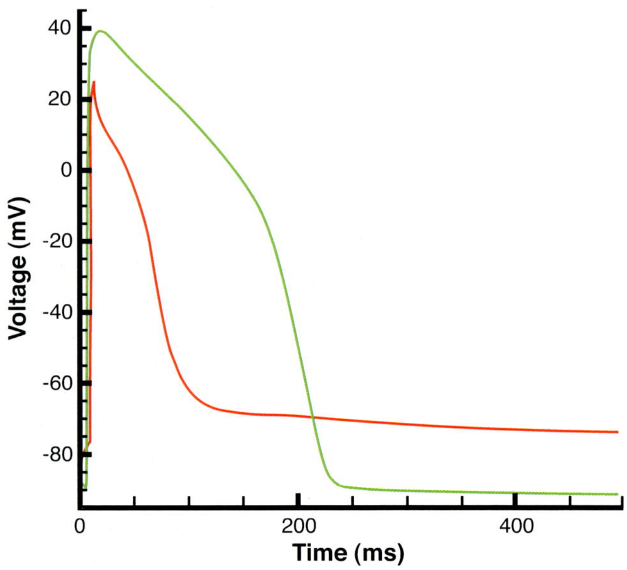

Fig. 11-7. The effect of cyanide on a ventricular cell. The red curve shows the change in the resting voltage and the drastically shortened cycle length. The green curve is the unaffected condition; the red curve shows the affected cell voltage.

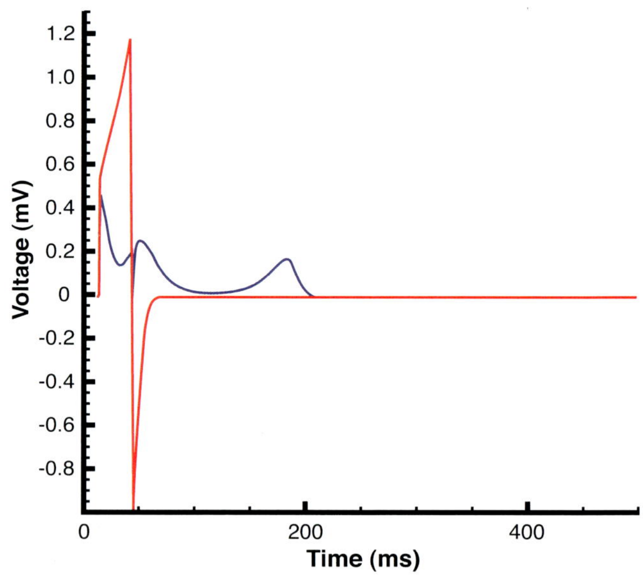

Fig. 11-8. The change in the electrocardiogram (ECG) caused by the presence of cyanide in the tissue. The red curve shows the normal ECG, with T-wave present. The blue curve shows the effect of cyanide on the ECG. The cyanide-affected tissue shows considerable morphological changes and elimination of the repolarization.

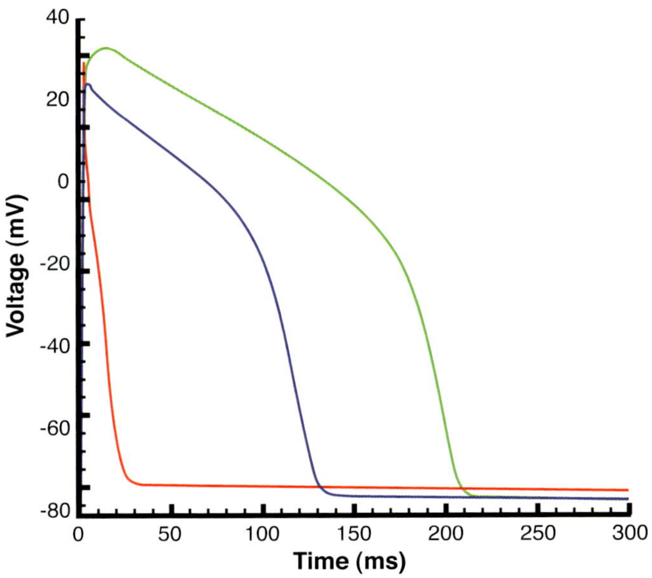

Fig. 11-9. Blocking the anionic, cell swelling-activated chloride current can restore the morphology of the cyanide affected action potential, the curve at the left (red curve), to the unaffected state. A partial block moves the curve toward the right (blue curve) and also restores the resting potential. A total block (green curve) achieves complete restoration to the normal.

ing cyanide-induced electropathophysiology. Two of the more important activated currents are the I_{KATP}, because of the decline in the ATP stores, and $I_{Cl,swell}$, when the cell volume is modulated. Change in cellular ion concentrations, also an important aspect of cyanide toxicity, includes calcium overload, which causes the activation of K^+ channels.[205] Rise in $[Na^+]_i$ and $[Ca^{2+}]_i$ enhance the I_{Ks} current, which is activated at voltage values much higher than for I_{Kr}. I_{Kr} is reduced by acidification and the presence of external divalent cations, noticeable in cyanide-affected tissue. The results were validated against the ECG of a subject under cyanide intoxication (see Figure 11-6).[195] Figures 11-7 to 11-9 demonstrate the impact of simulated changes in each current parameter. Each simulation incorporates established conductance ratios and previous modeling results.[206–210]

Disturbances of the energy homeostasis and ion concentrations in cardiac tissue from cyanide result in reversal of the normal directions and magnitude changes in cellular membrane currents. These effects in turn change the morphology of the action potential and ECG. These disturbances eventually lead to ventricular fibrillation, the usual endpoint in the effect of cyanide on the heart. The negative trending T-wave in the ECG indicates pathological behavior, the abnormal repolarization of the ventricle.

The computer simulation demonstrates that pharmacologic intervention has the potential to reverse or minimize the impact of cyanide on cardiac electrophysiology. Further research is needed to validate the conclusions of simulation. Simulation can focus research and also provide leads for successful interventions. However, no drugs have yet been assessed for their specific utility to reverse cyanide-induced perturbations in cardiac physiology. Oxygen clearly enhances antidotal efficacy, and it is possible that drugs to enhance delivery of oxygen into the mitochondria will soon improve cardiac recovery.

NEUROLOGICAL/PSYCHOLOGICAL RESPONSES TO CYANIDE AND ITS COUNTERMEASURES

Explicit understanding of the specific effects of cyanide exposure on the neuropsychology of humans or animals is limited. Impact would be expected, however, based on understood pathophysiology. Using various animal models, alterations have been observed in learning, sensory responses, and neurologic reflexes after exposure to sublethal doses of cyanide. These data have been reviewed elsewhere[176] and will not be further discussed in this clinically oriented review.

Unfortunately, EEG recordings in humans have only occasionally been reported in cases of known or suspected chronic cyanide toxicity. Sandberg described a case study of suspected chronic cyanide exposure in a goldsmith apprentice who used KCN for cleaning gold articles.[211] The patient presented with headache, general malaise, and paresis in the left arm and leg. Blood cyanide was mildly elevated at 10 to 12 μg per 100 mL of blood, and the EEG was described as exhibiting "diffuse frontal theta activity," a nonspecific finding. Treatment consisted of physical therapy and hydroxocobalamin therapy. After several months, blood cyanide levels dropped to 2 to 3 μg per 100 mL of blood, the EEG normalized, and paresis diminished, suggesting a diagnosis of chronic cyanide exposure. Diffuse frontal theta activity in the EEG is not specific to cyanide exposure, however; it has also been reported in a group of 13 people who worked with various toxic substances.[212] Zaknun et al also report EEG findings of diffuse, abnormal beta activity more pronounced in frontal and front-temporal regions but no focal epileptic activity in the case summarized previously.[163] Animal cyanide exposures provide evidence of transient EEG changes in the dog,[213] but in other studies, single or repeated IV infusions resulted in progressive deterioration in the EEGs.

The general psychological impact of terrorism and

actual or suspected chemical agent exposure on the behaviors of human populations has received much attention, particularly after September 11, 2001.[214–217] Clearly, individual psychological reactivity is a critical determinant of situational outcome. In addition, cyanide's well-earned reputation as a fear-inducing substance will likely enhance fear responses to a threatened or actual cyanide deployment. Rapid chemical detection or other means of confirming or dismissing suspicion of chemical exposure will advance application of appropriate medical and logistical procedures. Some individuals suffering from acute panic disorder have presented with symptoms similar to respiratory-distress responses, such as those seen following cyanide exposure (eg, respiratory gasp and dizziness).[65,218–220] Responders should expect some initial difficulty in distinguishing lesser cyanide intoxications from situational stress reactions.

Relatively little is known about the psychobehavioral effects of specific cyanide antidotes beyond the prevalent hypotensive response to the nitrite methemoglobin formers. In humans, the behavioral effects of p-aminopropiophenone (PAPP), a methemoglobin-forming aminophenone, have been reported. Paulet et al report no untoward effects on intellectual functioning, subjective feeling of personal comfort, or physical condition in individuals with up to 48% methemoglobin following oral administration of PAPP.[221] A small percentage of individuals were insensitive to PAPP, however, and did not develop methemoglobinemia. Bodansky and Hendley reported that up to 30% methemoglobin did not adversely affect visual detection threshold in PAPP-treated subjects, although immediately after exercise, an average of 15% methemoglobin was associated with a significant decrease in visual threshold.[222] Tepperman et al reported an interaction between exercise load and muscle oxygenation changes following PAPP administration in human volunteers.[223] Although impaired oxygenation of muscle was observed during moderate exercise in subjects with 10% to 20% with light exercise, no effect on muscle oxygenation was observed with 7% to 17% during light exercise.

SPECIFIC ANTIDOTES

The clinical use of most antidotes is based on animal experiments[224] and on extrapolations made from reported clinical cases. Antidotes are usually unnecessary, if the casualty is conscious. Comparing results from animal studies has limitations because of the differences in experimental design from one study to another, as well as marked interspecies differences in cyanide and drug metabolism. Moreover, the studies were not designed to resemble the usual emergency medical or battlefield scenario. General advantages and disadvantages of each antidote are listed in Table 11-5; however, objective comparison of antidote efficacy is hampered by the following factors[126,225]:

- the number of patients is small;
- most cyanide victims receive several treatment agents;
- readily available, adequate analysis of blood and tissue concentrations are lacking; and
- limited comparison studies are available in animal models.

Methemoglobin Formers

Sodium Nitrite and Amyl Nitrite

Sodium nitrite ($NaNO_2$) has been used successfully as a cyanide countermeasure in humans for many years,[226] usually in combination with other antidotes such as amyl nitrite, thiosulfate, and oxygen. Particular side effects include hypotension and excessive methemoglobin formation.[227–229] Kiese and Weger described serious side effects of sodium nitrite in humans. They noted that the recommended dosage for the treatment of cyanide poisoning (4.0 mg/kg) resulted in an average of 7% methemoglobin in adults. One subject who received 12.0 mg/kg developed methemoglobin levels reaching ~30% and experienced undesirable cardiovascular effects. Children must be dosed on a milligram per kilogram basis with adjustment for anemia if present. The recommended dose for children is 6.6 mg/kg (0.2 mL/kg of 3% solution) although the lesser dose of 4 mg/kg (0.13 mL/kg of 3% solution) can be used. Patients can be redosed with half the original dose, but redosing should not be done until methemoglobin levels are ascertained to be under 25%. Ideally, noninvasive monitoring for methemoglobinemia should be used if available.

Sodium nitrite for injection is made by dissolving solid sodium nitrite with water to make a final solution of 3%. Sodium nitrite is stable in light. It is incompatible with acetanilide, antipyrine, caffeine, citrate, chlorates, hypophosphites, iodides, mercury salts, morphine, oxidizing agents, permanganate, phenazone, sulfites, tannic acid, and vegetable astringent decoctions, infusions, or tinctures. The shelf life of sodium nitrite solution for injection is 5 years. The manufacturer recommends it be stored at temperatures between 15°C and 30°C; testing for stability in elevated temperatures has not been done. Sodium nitrite blood levels have not been measured during antidote therapy, and most pharmacokinetic parameters have not

TABLE 11-5

ANTIDOTES USEFUL IN ACUTE CYANIDE POISONING

Antidote	Advantages	Problems
Methemoglobin-forming agents	Potent, effective	Risk of impairment of oxygen delivery to the tissue, hypotension
Sodium thiosulfate	Efficient, safe	Delayed action
Cobalt EDTA	Very potent, effective if late	Numerous side effects
Hydroxycobalamin	Safe, no methemoglobinemia	Expensive therapy, red discoloration of urine, less potent

EDTA: ethylenediaminetetraacetate
Data sources: (1) Meredith TH, Jacobsen D, Haines JA, Berger J-C, van Heijst ANP, eds. *Anitdotes for Poisoning by Cyanide.* Vol 2. In: *International Program on Chemical Safety/Commission of the European Communities Evaluation of Antidotes Series.* Geneva, Switzerland: World Health Organization and Commission of the European Communities; 1993. Publication EUR 14280 EN. (2) Mégarbane B, Delabaye A, Goldgran-Tolédano D, Baud FJ. Antidotal treatment of cyanide poisoning. *J Chinese Med Assoc.* 2003;66:193–203.

been determined.

At least two studies suggest that sodium nitrite's efficacy is accounted for by other mechanisms in addition to methemoglobin formation. Vasodilation with improved capillary blood flow may contribute to its efficacy. Treatment of acquired methemoglobinemia from sodium nitrite poisoning in circumstances similar to those described above may involve only supplemental oxygenation and observation if the patient is asymptomatic and the methemoglobin level is 20% to 30% or less. With higher methemoglobin levels or in symptomatic patients, intravenous infusion of methylene blue at the usual dose of 0.1 to 0.2 mL/kg of a 1% solution may be necessary. Toluidine blue can also be used. Exchange transfusion may be required if severely poisoned patients are not responsive to the above measures.

Amyl nitrite is applied via inhalation and is the only simple first-aid measure for serious cyanide intoxication. Neither it nor sodium nitrite should be given to casualties who are awake and ambulant.[19] Most protocols call for 30 seconds of inhalation of an ampule per minute (30–60 seconds between ampules) by forced inhalation with attention paid to blood pressure drop or elevated heart rate. It can be delivered into the respiratory system by breaking an ampule into an Ambu Bag (Ambu, Copenhagen, Denmark) or other ventilation support system. Amyl nitrite is a less powerful producer of methemoglobin than is sodium nitrite. Its duration of action is approximately 1 hour. Amyl nitrite is usually followed by sodium nitrite infusion. Amyl nitrite is also a vasodilator, and hypotension should be treated with volume expansion. Ampules last for only 24 months. They must be protected from light and should be stored at cool (below 15°C/59 °F) conditions. Amyl nitrite capsules were shown to be stable for brief (1 day) periods of freezing.[230] Storage at high temperatures risks rupture of ampules and chemical decomposition of the drug. Amyl nitrite is highly flammable and must be stored accordingly.

Other Methemoglobin-Forming Drugs

A German-developed compound, 4-dimethylaminophenol (4-DMAP), is a methemoglobin-forming aminophenol that rapidly stimulates methemoglobin formation. It is used in the German military and by the civilian population. In humans, intravenous injection of 4-DMAP (3 mg/kg) can produce a level of 15% methemoglobin within 1 minute and 30% in 10 minutes. In dogs, a dose of 4-DMAP that produces a 30% level of methemoglobin will save animals that have received 2 to 3 LD_{50} of cyanide.[231]

The disadvantages of 4-DMAP are necrosis in the area of injection after intramuscular administration, phlebitis at intravenous infusion sites, and possible nephrotoxicity.[232] Overdoses of 4-DMAP have resulted in excessive methemoglobinemia and occasional hemolysis. Even the usual 4-DMAP dosing of 3.25 mg/kg of body weight has resulted in a methemoglobinemia of 70%. The compound must be stored in opaque containers, with a maximum storage time of 3 years.

Kiese and Weger demonstrated that 4-DMAP increased methemoglobin levels in a variety of animal species, including dog, cat, mouse, and rabbit.[228] Methemoglobinemia was also demonstrated by these authors in humans, whereby 4-DMAP (3.25 mg/kg, IV) yielded a maximum methemoglobin level of 30%, approximately 20 minutes after injection. The compound produces methemoglobinemia more rapidly than the nitrites and the aminophenones,[228] and is currently the primary specific antidote for cyanide toxicity in Germany. Although a potent and rapid methemoglobin former, 4-DMAP has been shown to produce tissue necrosis at the site of injection[57,233] and may be associated with nephrotoxicity.[234] In a recent report from Germany, 4-DMAP was administered to a subject exposed to methyl isocyanate. Excessive methemoglobinemia ensued (86.7%), followed by major organ failure.[235] The authors recommended against continued use of 4-DMAP as a treatment for cyanide toxicity.[235]

Vandenbelt et al studied a group of aliphatic phenones in dogs and identified PAPP as a potent, short-acting methemoglobin former.[236] In subsequent reports, PAPP was shown to be efficacious against cyanide toxicity in both dogs and rodents.[223,237–239] It was also demonstrated that PAPP formed methemoglobin in humans.[221,222,240] Paulet et al noted the lack of deleterious effects of PAPP on psychological and physiological parameters, although several volunteers failed to respond to PAPP and did not exhibit elevated methemoglobin levels.[221] PAPP has been described as safe and benign, with little effect on the body other than methemoglobinemia.[182] Although methemoglobin formers such as sodium nitrite are generally administered as a treatment for cyanide exposure, the toxicokinetics of the amiphenones may support preexposure prophylaxis.[241] P-aminoheptanoylphenone appears to be the safest of the amiphenones. Baskin and Fricke provide an in-depth discussion on PAPP pharmacology.[227]

Thiosulfate and Other Sulfur Donors

Thiosulfate is used for multiple conditions, including poisoning with sulfur mustard, nitrogen mustard, bromate, chlorate, bromine, iodine, and cisplatin. In combination with sodium nitrite in a fixed antidotal regimen, thiosulfate has been used for cyanide poisoning. Thiosulfate is also used in combination with hydroxocobalamin. The standard dose of sodium thiosulfate, which is supplied in the standard US cyanide antidote kit in 50-mL ampules, is 50 mL of the 250 mg/mL (12.5 g), given intravenously. A second treatment with half of the initial dose may be given. The pediatric dose is 1.65 mL per kilogram of body weight.[186] The pediatric dose equals the adult dose at about 21 kg of body weight. Thiosulfate functions as a sulfane donor to rhodanese and other sulfur transferases. However, rhodanese is located within mitochondria, and thiosulfate has poor ability to penetrate cell and mitochondrial membranes (although one rat study demonstrated that thiosulfate can utilize the dicarboxylate carrier to enter the mitochondria). Whereas rhodanese is available in excess in the body, relative deficiency of a sulfur donor capable of entering the mitochondria is the rate-limiting factor for this route of detoxification in cyanide poisoning. When a cyanide formulation is infused simultaneously with thiosulfate in dogs, a cyanide-sensitive species, the cyanide is detoxified "real time" (the actual time for the physical process of cyanide detoxification to take place in the body). The mechanism of thiosulfate protection appears to be the exceptionally rapid formation of thiocyanate in the central compartment, which limits the amount of cyanide distributed to sites of toxicity. The mechanism of action of thiosulfate, when given after cyanide exposure, is uncertain. Nevertheless, thiosulfate substantially enhances survival from cyanide. There are no specific contradictions to the use of sodium thiosulfate; its toxicity is low and adverse effects are mild. Side effects include nausea and vomiting with rapid infusion, headache, and disorientation. Rapid conversion to thiocyanate has resulted in reported hypotension. Excess thiosulfate is cleared renally. Premixed sodium thiosulfate can be stored for a maximum of 3 years. Solid thiosulfate may be stored in an airtight container for 5 years without change.

Hydroxocobalamin

Limitations associated with sodium nitrite (eg, hypotension and excessive methemoglobinemia) treatment and a desire for safer approaches to potentially cyanide-intoxicated fire casualties have increased domestic interest in identifying alternative or complementary approaches to treat cyanide poisoning.[228,242–246] Hydroxocobalamin is a major option.[145,247,248] Hydroxocobalamin is a registered antidote for cyanide poisoning in several European and Asian countries, and was approved by the Food and Drug Administration in 2006 under the animal efficacy rule. The efficacy of hydroxocobalamin versus the known effectiveness of the nitrite and thiosulfate combination in severe intoxications is still under study at the US Army Medical Research Institute of Chemical Defense. Current doctrine in France is to initially administer hydroxocobalamin (5 g in 200 mL saline, IV) over 15 to 45 minutes. Baud[249] has indicated that recovery often begins to occur before the full complement of hydroxocobalamin has been administered. Up to 15 g of hydroxocobalamin has been used in some clinical cases.[249]

The most common side effect is an orange-red discoloration of the skin, mucous membranes, and urine that lasts until the hydroxocobalamin is cleared from the body over several hours to a couple of days.[250] In rare instances, urticaria can result from hydroxocobalamin administration. Hydroxocobalamin is volumetrically inefficient, and infusion volumes are very large. The available packaging requires infusion of two full reconstituted bottles for the initial dose of 5 grams. Hydroxocobalamin must be protected from light and maintained at temperatures below 25°C. Its shelf life is 3 years. It is incompatible with reducing or basic substances such as ascorbic acid, saccharose, sorbitol, and other B vitamins. Its presence in serum can interfere with some laboratory measurements. Large volumes of hydroxocobalamin may cause significant amounts of cobalt to be released later, similar to the effect of cobalt EDTA.

Cobalt Salts

A commercial preparation of the cobalt salt of EDTA, Kelocyanor, is available in Europe but not in the United States. Cobalt salts, which are chelating agents, directly bind cyanide in the periphery but likely also cross the blood-brain barrier. Cobalt EDTA is administered intravenously.[251] In comparison studies against nitrite and hyposulfite, cobalt EDTA was thought to be superior[64]; however, in other studies the nitrite-thiosulfate combination was found to be superior.[252] No human volunteer studies or clinical trials of cobalt EDTA have been done. Following administration of cobalt EDTA, cyanide is excreted with cobalt in the urine; no follow-on treatment with thiosulfate is required.

The drawback of cobalt compounds is their severe toxicity, particularly when administered in the absence of confirmed cyanide intoxication. Massive urticaria with swelling of the face, lips and neck; convulsions; chest pains; dyspnea; and hypotension have been reported. Severe toxicity from cobalt can be seen even after initial recovery from acute cyanide poisoning. The usual dose of cobalt EDTA is one ampule followed by 50 mL of dextrose solution (500 g/L). Cobalt EDTA has a shelf life of 3 years at temperatures under 25 °C. It should be stored in the dark; if stored in the light, its color lightens, but it is otherwise unchanged.

SUMMARY

Cyanide is often associated with murders and assassinations. Because of the high amount needed to cause death and the inefficient weapons in which it was used, cyanide was not an effective chemical weapon in World War I. During World War II it was deployed effectively by the Nazi regime against internal enemies. It may have been used by Iraq against the Kurds in the Iran-Iraq War during the late 1980s, although no objective evidence supports this premise. Cyanide's widespread industrial use and ready availability provide the major opportunity for human injury today, particularly for exposure to large populations. Muslim extremists worldwide have been intercepted multiple times with cyanide and specific plans for its deployment.

Cyanide causes intracellular hypoxia by inhibiting the intracellular electron transport mechanism via binding to cytochrome-*c*-oxidase. This action stops aerobic metabolism and forces a shift to anaerobic metabolism. The nervous system and the heart are particularly intolerant of ATP deficiency. The liver is particularly tolerant of cyanide exposure, probably because of its generous supply of rhodanese. Cyanide additionally binds multiple other enzymes and nonenzymatic proteins, although the clinical consequences of these actions are less well understood. The dose toxity curve for cyanide is steep, with very large exposures, particularly respiratory, causing rapid onset of central nervous system toxicity with the potential for death within several minutes.

Rapid removal from further exposure, administration of general support measures including 100% oxygen, and administration of specific antidotes in critically impaired casualties effectively reverse the effects of exposure. Multiple antidotes are available worldwide. The most widely used are nitrites with thiosulfate. This combination has demonstrated efficacy. Hydroxocobalamin, used in France and a few other countries, has now been introduced into the US formulary. Cobalt EDTA is falling out of favor because of its high side-effect profile. The only antidote formulated for use by nonphysician emergency responders is amyl nitrite. No antidotes are currently carried by US military medics or corpsmen. Current research efforts are focused on improving the understanding of cyanide's mechanisms of toxicity and developing improved antidotes, with better safety profiles and utility in spartan environments.

Acknowledgment

The authors thank MAJ Thomas T Talbot, MC, CPT Denise Millhorn, and Dr Brain Logue of South Dakota State University for reviewing the chapter; Peter Hurst for artwork; LTC Todd Villnes and MAJ Thor Markwood for their review of cardiac electrophysiology; Paula Digenakis for library assistance; and John Portmann of Duke University for computer program aid.

REFERENCES

1. Smith S. Poisons and poisoners through the ages. *Med Leg J.* 1952;20:153–167.

2. Sykes AH. Early studies on the toxicology of cyanide. In: Vennesland B, Conn EE, Knowles CJ, Westley J, Wissing F, eds. *Cyanide in Biology*. New York, NY: Academic Press; 1981: 1–9.

3. Weider B. The assassination of Napoleon. *Georgian J Napoleonic Hist.* 2000;(Jan):138–139.

4. Maddern T. Poisoning by laurel leaves. *Philos Trans R Soc Lond Biol Sci.* 1731;37:84–99.

5. Prentiss AM. *Chemicals in War: A Treatise on Chemical War*. New York, NY: McGraw-Hill; 1937: 171–175.

6. Baskin SI. Zyklon. In: La Cleuer W, ed. *Encyclopedia of the Holocaust*. New Haven, Conn: Yale University Press; 2001.

7. Robinson JP. The problem of chemical and biological warfare. Vol 1. In: Robinson JP, ed. *The Rise of CB Weapons: A Study of the Historical, Technical, Military, Legal and Political Aspects of CBW, and Possible Disarmament Measures.* New York, NY: Humanities Press; 1971: 155–156.

8. Lang JS, Mullin D, Fenyvesi C, Rosenberg R, Barnes J. Is the "protector of lions" losing his touch? *US News & World Report.* November 1986;10:29.

9. Heylin M. US decries apparent chemical arms attack. *Chem Eng News.* 1988;23.

10. Medical expert reports use of chemical weapons in Iran-Iraq War. *UN Chronicle.* 1985;22:24–26.

11. Wolnick KA, Fricke FL, Bonnin E, Gaston CM, Satzger RD. The Tylenol tempering incident—tracing the source. *Anal Chem.* 1984;56:466A-470A, 474A.

12. Sidell FR. Chemical casualty consultant, Bel Air, Md. Personal communication, May 1996.

13. Walrath J, Li FP, Hoar SK, Mead MW, Fraumeni JF. Causes of death among female chemists. *Am J Public Health.* 1985;75:883–885.

14. Thompson RL, Manders WW, Cowan RW. Postmortem findings of the victims of the Jonestown tragedy. *J Forensic Sci.* 1987;32:433–443.

15. *Toxicological Profile for Cyanide*. Atlanta, Ga: US Department of Health and Human Services, Agency for Toxic Substances and Disease Registry; 2004.

16. Cicerone RJ, Zellner R. The atmospheric chemistry of hydrogen cyanide (HCN). *J Geophys Res.* 1983;88:689–696.

17. Li Q, Jacob DJ, Bey I, et al. Atmospheric hydrogen cyanide (HCN): Biomass burning source, ocean sink? *Geophys Res Lett.* 2000;27;357–360.

18. Vetter J. Plant cyanogenic glycosides. *Toxicon.* 2000;38:11–36.

19. Way JL. Cyanide intoxication and its mechanism of antagonism. *Annu Rev Pharmacol Toxicol.* 1984;24:451–481.

20. Towill LE, Drury JS, Whitfield BL, Lewis EB, Galyan EL. *Review of the Environmental Effects of Pollutants: V. Cyanide.* Washington DC: US Environmental Protection Agency; 1978.

21. Solomonson LP. Cyanide as a metabolic inhibitor. In: Vennesland B, Conn EE, Knowles CJ, Westley J, Wissing F, eds. *Cyanide in Biology*. New York, NY: Academic Press; 1981: 11–28.

22. Beasley V. Toxicants that inhibit the function of cytochromes. In: Beasley V, ed. *Veterinary Toxicology*. Ithaca, NY: International Veterinary Information Service; 1999.

23. Knight AP, Walter RG. Plants causing sudden death. In: Knight AP, Walter RG, eds. *A Guide to Plant Poisoning of Animals in North America*. Jackson, Wyo: Teton NewMedia; 2002.

24. Conn EE. Cyanogenic glycosides. In: Neuberger A, Jukes TH, eds. *Biochemistry of Nutrition 1*. Baltimore, Md: University Park Press; 1979: 21–43.

25. *Cyanogenic Glycosides in Cassava and Bamboo Shoots: A Human Health Risk Assessment*. Canberra, Australia: Food Standards Australia New Zealand; 2005. Technical Report Series No. 28.

26. Hall AH, Rumack BH, Schaffer MI, Linden CH. Clinical toxicology of cyanide: North American clinical experiences. In: Ballantyne B, Marrs TC, eds. *Clinical and Experimental Toxicology of Cyanides*. Bristol, England: Wright; 1987: Chap 12: 313–314.

27. Conn EE. Introduction. In: Evered D, Harnett S, eds. *Cyanide Compounds in Biology*. London, England: Wiley; 1988: 1–2. CIBA Foundation Symposium 140.

28. Hibbs CM. Cyanide and nitrate toxicoses of cattle. *Vet Hum Toxicol*. 1979;21:401–403.

29. Honig DH, Hockridge ME, Gould RM, Rackis JJ. Determination of cyanide in soybeans and soybean products. *J Agric Food Chem*. 1983;31:272–275.

30. Nartey F. Toxicological aspects of cyanogenesis in tropical foods. In: Smith RL, Bababumni ER, eds. *Toxicology in the Tropics*. London, United Kingdom: Taylor & Francis; 1980: 53–73.

31. Vennesland B, Castric PA, Conn EE, Solomonson LP, Volini M, Westley J. Cyanide metabolism. *Fed Proc*. 1982;41:2639–2648.

32. Way JL. Pharmacologic aspests of cyanide and its antagonism. In: Vennesland B, Conn EE, Knowles CJ, Westley J, Wissing F, eds. *Cyanide in Biology*. New York, NY: Academic Press; 1981: 29–49.

33. Alarie Y. Toxicity of fire smoke. *Crit Rev Toxicol*. 2002;32:259–289.

34. Chisholm IA, Bronte-Stewart J, Foulds WS. Hydroxocobalamin versus cyanocobalamin in the treatment of tobacco amblyopia. *Lancet*. 1967;2:450–451.

35. Lundquist P, Rosling H, Sorbo B, Tibbling L. Cyanide concentrations in blood after cigarette smoking, as determined by a sensitive fluorimetric method. *Clin Chem*. 1987;33:1228–1230.

36. Baker RR, Proctor CJ. The origins and properties on environmental tobacco smoke. *Environ Int*. 1990;16:231–245.

37. Guerin MR, Higgins CE, Jenkins RA. Measuring environmental emissions from tobacco combustion: Sidestream cigarette smoke literature review. *Atmos Environ*. 1987;21: 291–297.

38. Chepiga TA, Morton MJ, Murphy PA, et al. A comparison of the mainstream smoke chemistry and mutagenicity of a representative sample of the U.S. cigarette market with two Kentucky reference cigarettes (K1R4F and K1R5F). *Food Chem Toxicol*. 2000;38:949–962.

39. Bogusz M, Moroz J, Karski J, et al. Blood cyanide and thiocyanate concentrations after administration of sodium nitroprusside as hypotensive agent in neurosurgery. *Clin Chem*. 1979;25:60–63.

40. Rodkey FL, Collison HA. Determination of cyanide and nitroprusside in blood and plasma. *Clin Chem*. 1977;23:1969–1975.

41. Smith RP, Kruszyna H. Nitroprusside produces cyanide poisoning via reaction with hemoglobin. *J Pharmacol Exp Ther*. 1974;191:557–563.

42. Moertel CG, Ames MM, Kovach JS, Moyer TP, Rubin JR, Tinker JH. A pharmacologic and toxicological study of amygdalin. *JAMA*. 1981;245:591–594.

43. Ames MM, Moyer TP, Kovach JS, Moertel CG, Rubin J. Pharmacology of amygdalin (laetrile) in cancer patients. *Cancer Chemother Pharmacol.* 1981;6:51–57.

44. Keilin D. Cytochrome and respiratory enzymes. *Proc R Soc Lond B Biol Sci.* 1929;104:206–251.

45. Warburg O. Inhibition of the action of prussic acid in living cells. *Hoppe-Seyler's Z Physiol Chem.* 1911;76:331–346.

46. Alexander K, Baskin SI. The inhibition of cytochrome oxidase by diaminomalenitrile. *Biochim Biophys Acta.* 1987;912:41–47.

47. Lindahl M, Svensson LA, Liljas A. Metal poison inhibition of carbonic anhydrase. *Proteins.* 2004;15:177–182.

48. Lieske CN, Clark CR, Zoeffel LD. Temperature effects in cyanolysis using elemental sulfur. *J Appl Toxicol.* 1996;16:171–175.

49. Way JL, Gibbon SL, Sheehy M. Effect of oxygen on cyanide intoxication I. Prophylactic protection. *J Pharmacol Exp Ther.* 1966;153:381–385.

50. Jarabak R, Westley J. Steady-state kinetics of 3-mercaptopyruvate sulfurtransferase from bovine kidney. *Arch Biochem Biophys.* 1978;185:458–465.

51. Westley J. Cyanide and sulfane sulfur. In: Vennesland B, Conn EE, Knowles CJ, Westley J, Wissing F, eds. *Cyanide in Biology*. New York, NY: Academic Press; 1981: 61–76.

52. Sylvester DM, Hayton WL, Morgan RL, Way JL. Effects of thiosulfate on cyanide pharmacokinetics in dogs. *Toxicol Appl Pharmacol.* 1983;69:265–271.

53. Porter DW, Baskin SI. The effect of three alpha-keto acids on 3-mercaptopyruvate sulfurtransferase activity. *J Biochem Toxicol.* 1996;11:45–50.

54. Baskin SI, Petrikovics I, Kurche JS, et al. Insights on cyanide toxicity and methods of treatment. In: Flora SJS, Romano JA, Baskin SI, Sekhar K, eds. *Pharmacological Perspectives of Toxic Chemicals and Their Antidotes.* New Delhi, India: Narosa Publishing House; 2004: 105–146.

55. Wood JL, Cooley SL. Detoxication of cyanide by cystine. *J Biol Chem.* 1956;218:449–457.

56. Hall AH, Rumack BH. Clinical toxicology of cyanide. *Ann of Emerg Med.* 1986;15:1067–1074.

57. Way JL, Leung P, Sylvester DM, Burrows G, Tamulinas C. Methaemoglobin formation in the treatment of acute cyanide intoxication. In: Ballantyne B, Marrs TC, eds. *Clinical and Experimental Toxicology of Cyanides*. Bristol, England: Wright; 1987: 402–412.

58. Marrs TC. Antidotal treatment of acute cyanide poisoning. *Adverse Drug React Acute Poisoning Rev.* 1988;179:206.

59. Ballantyne B. Toxicology of cyanides. In: Ballantyne B, Marrs TC, eds. *Clinical and Experimental Toxicology of Cyanides*. Bristol, England: Wright; 1987: 41–126.

60. Ballantyne B, Bright J, Swanston DW, Williams P. Toxicity and distribution of free cyanide given intramuscularly. *Med Sci Law.* 1972;12:209–219.

61. Baskin SI, Wilkerson G, Alexander K, Blitstein AG. Cardiac effects of cyanide. In: Ballantyne B, Marrs TC, eds. *Clinical and Experimental Toxicology of Cyanides*. Bristol, England: Wright; 1987: 138–155.

62. Pitt BR, Radford EP, Gurtner GH, Traystman RJ. Interaction of carbon monoxide and cyanide on cerebral circulation and metabolism. *Arch Environ Health.* 1979;34:345–349.

63. Haymaker W, Ginzler AM, Ferguson RL. Residual neuropathological effects of cyanide poisoning; a study of the central nervous system of 23 dogs exposed to cyanide compounds. *Mil Surg*. 1952;111:231–246.

64. Paulet G, Chary R, Bocquet P. The comparative value of sodium nitrite and cobalt chelates in the treatment of cyanide intoxication in non-anesthetized animals. *Arch Int Pharmacodyn.* 1969;127:104–117.

65. McNamara BP. *Estimates of the Toxicity of Hydrocyanic Acid Vapors in Man.* Aberdeen Proving Ground, Md: Edgewood Arsenal; 1976. Technical Report EB-TR-78023.

66. Bark LS, Higson HG. A review of methods available for the detection and determination of small amounts of cyanide. *Analyst.* 1963:88:751.

67. Troup CM, Ballantyne B. Analysis of cyanide in biological fluids and tissues. In: Ballantyne B, Marrs TC, eds. *Clinical and Experimental Toxicology of Cyanides.* Bristol, England: Wright; 1987: 22–40.

68. Westley AM, Westley J. Voltammetric determination of cyanide and thiocyanate in small biological samples. *Anal Biochem.* 1989;181:190–194.

69. Egekeze JO, Oehme FW. Direct potentiometric method for the determination of cyanide in biological materials. *J Anal Toxicol.* 1979;3:119–124.

70. Ganjali MR, Yousefi M, Javanbakht MJ, et al. Determination of SCN^- in urine and saliva of smokers and non-smokers by SCN(-)- selective polymeric membrane containing a nickel(II)-azamacrocycle complex coated on a graphite electrode. *Anal Sci.* 2002;18:887–892.

71. Casella IG, Guascito MR, De Benedetto GE. Electrooxidation of thiocyanate on the copper-modified gold electrode and its amperometric determination by ion chromatography. *Analyst.* 1998;123:1359–1363.

72. Amini MK, Shahrokhian S, Tangestaninejad S. Thiocyanate-selective electrodes based on nickel and iron phthalocyanines. *Anal Chim Acta.* 1999;402:137–143.

73. Pasciak J, Hurek J. *Chem Anal.* 1984;29:571.

74. du Cailar J, Mathieu-Daudé JC, Deschodt J, Griffe O. Plasma level of the thiocyanate ion in sodium nitroprusside perfusion. *Ann Anesthesiol Fr.* 1976;17:519–528.

75. McAnalley BH, Lowry WT, Oliver RD, Garriott JC. *J Anal Toxicol.* 1979;3:111.

76. Cai X, Zhao Z. Determination of trace thiocyanate by linear sweep polarography. *Anal Chim Acta.* 1988;212:43–48.

77. Bjergegaard C, Moller P, Sorensen H. Determination of thiocyanate, iodide, nitrate and nitrite in biological samples by micellar electrokinetic capillary chromatography. *J Chromatogr A.* 1995;717:409.

78. Glatz Z, Novakova S, Sterbova H. Analysis of thiocyanate in biological fluids by capillary zone electrophoresis. *J Chromatogr A.* 2001;916:273–277.

79. Berlin AM. The treatment of cyanide poisoning in children. *Pediatrics.* 1971;46:793.

80. Bunn HF. Disorders of hemoglobin. In: Braunwald E, Wilson JD, Martin JB, Fauci AS. *Harrison's Principles of Internal Medicine.* 11th ed. New York, NY: McGraw-Hill; 1987: 1518–1527.

81. Groff WA, Stemler FW, Kaminskis A, Froehlich HL, Johnson RP. Plasma free cyanide and blood total cyanide: a rapid completely automated microdistillation assay. *J Toxicol Clin Toxicol.* 1985;23:133–163.

82. Lundquist P, Rosling H, Sorbo B. Determination of cyanide in whole blood, erythrocytes and plasma. *Clin Chem.* 1985;31:591–595.

83. McMillan DE, Svoboda AC. The role of erythrocytes in cyanide detoxification. *J Pharmacol Exp Ther.* 1982;221:37–42.

84. Moriya F, Hashimoto Y. Potential for error when assessing blood cyanide concentrations in fire victims. *J Forensic Sci.* 2001;46:1421–1425.

85. Ballantyne B. Blood, brain and cerebrospinal fluid cyanide concentrations in experimental acute cyanide poisoning. *J Forensic Sci Soc.* 1975;15:51–56.

86. US Department of the Army. *Assay Techniques for Detection of Exposure to Sulfur Mustard, Cholinesterase Inhibitors, Sarin, Doman, GF, and Cyanide.* Washington, DC: DA; 1996. Technical Bulletin PB-96-189295/XAB.

87. Lundquist P, Sörbo B. Rapid determination of toxic cyanide concentrations in blood. *Clin Chem.* 1989;35:617–619.

88. Sano A, Takimoto N, Takitani S. High-performance liquid chromatographic determination of cyanide in human red blood cells by pre-column fluorescence derivatization. *J Chromatogr.* 1992;582:131–135.

89. Baar S. The micro determination of cyanide: its application to the analysis of whole blood. *Analyst.* 1966;91:268–272.

90. Vesey CJ, Cole PV, Simpson PJ. Cyanide and thiocyanate concentrations following sodium nitroprusside infusion in man. *Br J Anaesth.* 1976;48:651–660.

91. Vesey CJ, Wilson J. Red cell cyanide. *J Pharm Pharmacol.* 1978;30:20–26.

92. Sunshine I, Finkle B. The necessity for tissue studies in fatal cyanide poisoning. *Arch Gewerbepath Gewerbehyg.* 1964;20:558–561.

93. Hazardous Substances Data Bank [database online]. Cyanide. Bethesda, Md: National Library of Medicine; 2004.

94. Vogel SN, Sultan TR, Ten Eyck RP. Cyanide poisoning. *Clin Toxicol.* 1981;18:367–383.

95. Rodkey FL, Robertson RF. Analytical precautions in measurement of blood cyanide. *Clin Chem.* 1978;24:2184–2185.

96. Pettigrew AR, Fell GS. Microdiffusion method for estimation of cyanide in whole blood and its application to the study of conversion of cyanide to thiocyanate. *Clin Chem.* 1973;19;466–471.

97. Ballantyne B. In vitro production of cyanide in normal human blood and the influence of thiocyanate and storage temperatures. *Clin Toxicol.* 1977;11:173–193.

98. Houeto P, Hoffman JR, Imbert M, Levillain P, Baud FJ. Relation of blood cyanide to plasma cyanocobalamin concentration after a fixed dose of hydroxocobalamin in cyanide poisoning. *Lancet.* 1995;346:605–608.

99. Lundquist P, Rosling H, Sörbo B, Tibbling L. Cyanide concentrations in blood after cigarette smoking, as determined by a sensitive fluorimetric method. *Clin Chem.* 1987;33:1228–1230.

100. Seto Y. Oxidative conversion of thiocyanate to cyanide by oxyhemoglobin by acid denaturation. *Arch Biochem Biophys.* 1995;321:245–254.

101. Seto Y. False cyanide detection. *Anal Chem.* 2002;74:134A–141A.

102. Liu X, Yun Z. High performance liquid chromatographic determination of thiocyanate anions by derivatization with pentylfluorobenzyl bromide. *J Chromatogr A.* 1993;653:348–353.

103. Baskin SI, Kurche JS, Petrikovics I, Way JL. Analysis of 2-imino-thiazolidine-4-carboxylic acid (ITCA) as a method for cyanide measurement. *Toxicologist.* 2003;72:164.

104. Pettigrew AR, Fell GS. Simplified colorimetric determination of thiocyanate in biological fluids, and its application to investigation of the toxic amblyopias. *Clin Chem.* 1972;18:996–1000.

105. Vesey CJ, McAllister H, Langford RM. A simple, rapid and sensitive semimicro method for the measurement of cyanide in blood. *Ann Clin Biochem.* 1999;36:755–758.

106. Goenechea S. Hydrogen cyanide: losses in samples of stored blood. *Z Rechtsmed.* 1982;88:97–101.

107. Ballantyne B. Changes in blood cyanide as a function of storage time and temperature. *J Forensic Sci Soc.* 1976;16:305–310.

108. Guilbault GG, Kramer DN. Specific detection and determination of cyanide using various quinone derivatives. *Anal Chem.* 1965;37:1395–1399.

109. Lundquist P, Kagedal B, Nilsson L. An improved method for determination of thiocyanate in plasma and urine. *Eur J Clin Chem Clin Biochem.* 1995;33:343–349.

110. Wu AH, McKay C; Broussard LA, et al. National Academy of Clinical Biochemistry Laboratory Medicine practice guidelines: recommendations for the use of laboratory tests to support poisoned patients who present to the emergency department. *Clin Chem.* 2003;49:357–379.

111. Dumas P, Gingras G, LeBlanc A. Isotope dilution-mass spectrometry determination of blood cyanide by headspace gas chromatography. *J Anal Toxicol.* 2005;29:71–75.

112. Calafat AM, Stanfill SB. Rapid quantitation of cyanide in whole blood by automated headspace gas chromatography. *J Chromatogr B Analyt Technol Biomed Life Sci.* 2002; 772:131–137.

113. Ishii A, Seno H, Watanabe-Suzuki K, Suzuki O, Kumazawa T. Determination of cyanide in whole blood by capillary gas chromatography with cryogenic oven trapping. *Anal Chem.* 1998;70:4873–4876.

114. Tracqui A, Raul JS, Geraut A, Berthelon L, Ludes B. Determination of blood cyanide by HPLC-MS. *J Anal Toxicol.* 2002;26:144–148.

115. Meiser H, Hagedorn HW, Schultz R. Development of a method for determination of cyanide concentrations in serum and rumen fluid of cattle. *Am J Vet Res.* 2000;61:658–664.

116. Kage S, Nagata T, Kudo K. Determination of cyanide and thiocyanate in blood by gas chromatography and gas chromatography-mass spectrometry. *J Chromatogr B Biomed Appl.* 1996;675:27–32.

117. Felscher D, Wulfmeyer M. A new specific method to detect cyanide in body fluids, especially whole blood, by fluorimetry. *J Anal Toxicol.* 1998;22:363–366.

118. Chinaka S, Takayama N, Michigami Y, Ueda K. Simultaneous determination of cyanide and thiocyanate in blood by ion chromatography with fluorescence and ultraviolet detection. *J Chromatogr B Biomed Sci Appl.* 1998;713:353–359.

119. Connolly D, Barron L, Paull B. Determination of urinary thiocyanate and nitrate using fast ion-interaction chromatography. *J Chromatogr B Analyt Technol Biomed Life Sci.* 2002;767:175–180.

120. Chen SH, Yang Z,Y, Wu HL, Kou HS, Lin SJ. Determination of thiocyanate anion by high-performance liquid chromatography with fluorimetric detection. *J Anal Toxicol.* 1996;20:38–42.

121. Hughes C, Lehner F, Dirikolu L, et al. A simple and highly sensitive spectrophotometric method for the determination of cyanide in equine blood. *Toxicol Mech Methods.* 2003;13:1–10.

122. Chattaraj S, Das AK. Indirect determination of thiocyanate in biological fluids using atomic absorption spectrometry. *Spectrochica Acta.* 1992;47:675–680.

123. Maserek WK, Rockwood GA, Platoff GE, Baskin SI, Logue BA. Feasibility of using the cyanide metabolite 2-amino-2-thiazoline-4-carboxylic acid as a retrospective marker of cyanide exposure. *Toxicol Sci.* 2006;abstract 1918:392.

124. Clark CJ, Campbell D, Reid WH. Blood carboxyhaemoglobin and cyanide levels in fire survivors. *Lancet.* 1981;1:1332–1335.

125. World Health Organization. *Hydrogen Cyanide and Cyanides: Human Health Aspects*. Geneva, Switzerland: WHO; 2004. Concise International Chemical Assessment Document 61.

126. Meredith TH, Jacobsen D, Haines JA, Berger J-C, van Heijst ANP, eds. *Anitdotes for Poisoning by Cyanide.* Vol 2. In: *International Program on Chemical Safety/Commission of the European Communities Evaluation of Antidotes Series*. Geneva, Switzerland: World Health Organization and Commission of the European Communities; 1993. Publication EUR 14280 EN.

127. Kampe S, Iffland R, Korenkov M, Diefenbach C. Survival from a lethal blood concentration of cyanide with associated alcohol intoxication. *Anesthesia.* 2000;55:1189–1191.

128. Turrina S, Neri C, De Leo D. Effect of combined exposure to carbon monoxide and cyanides in selected forensic cases.*J Clin Forensic Med*. 2004;11:264–267.

129. Chen KK, Rose CL, Clowes GHA. The modern treatment of cyanide poisoning. *J Indiana State Med Assoc.* 1944;37:344–350.

130. Graham DL, Laman D, Theodore J, Robin ED. Acute cyanide poisoning complicated by lactic acidosis and pulmonary edema. *Arch Intern Med.* 1977;137:1051–1055.

131. De Busk RE, Seidl LG. Attempted suicide by cyanide. A report of two cases. *Calif Med.* 1969;110:394–396.

132. Mascarenhas BR, Geller AC, Goodman AI. Cyanide poisoning, medical emergency. *N Y State J Med.* 1969;69:1782–1784.

133. Saincher A, Swirsky N, Tenenbein M. Cyanide overdose: survival with fatal blood concentration without antidotal therapy. *J Emerg Med.* 1994;12:555–557.

134. Henrion J, Schapira M, Luwaert R, Colin L, Delannoy A, Heller F. Hypoxic hepatitis: clinical and hemodynamic study in 142 consecutive cases. *Medicine (Baltimore).* 2003;82:392–406.

145. Isom GE, Burrows GE, Way JL. Effect of oxygen on the antagonism of cyanide intoxication— cytochrome oxidase, in vivo. *Toxicol Appl Pharmacol.* 1982;65:250–256.

136. Chen KK, Rose CL, Clowes GHA. Comparative values of several anitdotes in cyanide poisoning. *Am J Med Sci.* 1934;188:767–771.

137. Yen D, Tsai J, Wang LM, et al. The clinical experience of acute cyanide poisoning. *Am J Emerg Med.* 1995;13:524–528.

138. Barillo DJ, Goode R, Esch V. Cyanide poisoning in victims of fire: analysis of 364 cases and review of the literature. *J Burn Care Rehabil.* 1994;15:46–57.

139. Prieto I, Pujol I, Santiuste C, Poyo-Guerrero R, Diego A. Acute cyanide poisoning by subcutaneous injection. *Emerg Med J.* 2005;22:389–390.

140. Johnson WS, Hall AH, Rumack BH. Cyanide poisoning successfully treated without 'therapeutic methemoglobin levels. *Am J Emerg Med.* 1989;7:437–440.

141. Bailey B. Are there teratogenic risks associated with antidotes used in the acute management of poisoned pregnant women. *Birth Defects Res A Clin Mol Teratol.* 2003;67:133–140.

142. Forootan A. Medical notes on the chemical warfare. *Kowsar Medl L.* 1996;1:2.

143. Andrews JM, Sweeney ES, Grey TC, Wetzel T. The biohazard potential of cyanide poisoning during postmortem examination. *J Forensic Sci.* 1989;34:1280–1284.

144. Holland MA, Kozlowski LM. Clinical features and management of cyanide poisoning. *Clin Pharm.* 1986;5:737–741.

145. Mégarbane B, Delabaye A, Goldgran-Tolédano D, Baud FJ. Antidotal treatment of cyanide poisoning. *J Chinese Med Assoc.* 2003;66:193–203.

146. Baud FJ, Borron SW, Bavoux E, Astier A, Hoffman JR. Relation between plasma lactate and blood cyanide concentrations in acute cyanide poisoning. *BMJ.* 1996;312:26–27.

147. Baud FJ, Borron SW, Megarbane B. Value of lactic acidosis in the assessment of the severity of acute cyanide poisoning. *Crit Care Med.* 2002;30:2044–2050.

148. Levraut J, Bounatirou T, Ichai C. Reliability of anion gap as an indicator of blood lactate in critically ill patients. *Intensive Care Med.* 1997;23:417–422.

149. Sinex JE. Pulse oximetry: principles and limitations. *Am J Emerg Med.* 1999;17:59–67.

150. Cardozo RH, Edelman IS. The volume of distribution of sodium thiosulfate as a measure of the extracellular fluid space. *J Clin Invest* 1952;31:280–290.

151. Logue BA, Kirschten NP, Petrikovics I, Moser MA, Rockwood GA, Baskin SI. Determination of the cyanide metabolite 2-aminothiazoline-4-carboxylic acid in urine and plasma by gas chromatography-mass spectrometry. *J Chromatogr B Analyt Technol Biomed Life Sci.* 2005;819:237–244.

152. Lundquist P, Kagedal B, Nilsson L, Rosling H. Analysis of the cyanide metabolite 2-aminothiazoline-4-carboxylic acid in urine by high-performance liquid chromatography. *Anal Biochem.* 1995;228:27–34.

153. Nolan CR. *Hypertensive Crisis*. Vol 3. Philadelphia, Pa: Current Medicine Inc; 1999: 8.1–8.30.

154. Gawron O, Fernando J, Keil J, Weistman TJ. Zwitterion structure and acylative ring opening reactions of 2-aminothiazoline-4-carboxylic acid. *J Org Chem.* 1962;27:3117–3123.

155. Deim K, Lentner C, eds. *Scientific Tables*. 7th ed. Ardsely, NY: JR Geigy; 1970.

156. Ansell M, Lewis FA. A review of cyanide concentrations found in human organs. A survey of literature concerning cyanide metabolism, 'normal,' non-fatal, and fatal body cyanide levels. *J Forensic Med.* 1970;17:148–155.

157. Curry AS. *Poison Detection in Human Organs*. Springfield, Ill: Thomas; 1976: 97–98.

158. Bright JE, Inns RH, Tuckwell NJ, Marrs TC. The effect of storage upon cyanide in blood samples. *Hum Exp Toxicol.* 1990;9:125–129.

159. Chikasue F, Yashiki M, Kojima T, et al. Cyanide distribution in five fatal cyanide poisonings and the effect of storage conditions on cyanide concentration in tissue. *Forensic Sci Int.* 1988;38:173–183.

160. Vesey C J, Langford RM. Stabilization of blood cyanide. *J Anal Toxicol.* 1998; 22:176–178.

161. Wright RO, Lewander WJ, Woolf AD. Methemoglobinemia: etiology, pharmacology and clinical management. *Ann Emerg Med.* 1999:34:646–656.

162. Messing B, Storch B. Computer tomography and magnetic resonance imaging in cyanide poisoning. *Eur Arch Psychiatry Neurol Sci.* 1988;237:139–143.

163. Zaknun JJ, Stieglbauer K, Trenkler J, Aichner F. Cyanide-induced akinetic rigid syndrome: Clinical, MRI, FDG-PET, beta-CIT and HMPAO SPECT findings. *Parkinsonism Relat Disord*. 2005;11:125–129.

164. Feldman JM, Feldman MD. Sequelae of attempted suicide by cyanide ingestion: a case report. *Int J Psychiatry Med.* 1990;20:173–179.

165. Borgohain R, Singh AK, Radhakrishna H, Rao VC, Mohandas S. Delayed onset generalised dystonia after cyanide poisoning. *Clin Neurol Neurosurg*. 1995; 97:213–215.

166. Kasamo K, Okuhata Y, Satoh R, et al. Chronological changes of MRI findings on striatal damage after acute cyanide intoxication: pathogenesis of the damage and its selectivity, and prevention for neurological sequelae: a case report. *Eur Arch Psychiatry Clin Neurosci.* 1993;243:71–74.

167. Rosenberg NL, Myers JA, Martin WR. Cyanide-induced parkinsonism: clinical, MRI, and 6-fuorodopa PET studies. *Neurology.* 1989;39:142–144.

168. Fechner LD, Chen GD, Johnson DL. Potentiation of noise-induced hearing loss by low concentrations of hydrogen cyanide in rats. *Toxicol Sci.* 2002;66:131–138.

169. Tawackoli W, Chen GD, Fechner LD. Disruption of cochlear potentials by chemical asphyxiants. Cyanide and carbon monoxide. *Neurotoxicol Teratol.* 2001;23:157–163.

170. Uitti RJ, Rajput AH, Ashenhurst EM, Rozdilsky B. Cyanide-induced parkinsonism: a clinicopathologic report. *Neurology.* 1985;35:921–925.

171. Chin RG. Emergency medicine physician, Jacobi Hospital, Bronx, NY. Personal communication, September 2003.

172. Somani SM, Ramano J. Acute and chronic cyanide toxicity. In: Somani SM, Ramano J, eds. *Chemical Warfare Agents: Toxicity at Low Levels*. Boca Raton, Fla: CRC Press; 2001: Chap 10.

173. Chin RG, Calderon Y. Acute cyanide poisoning: a case report. *J Emerg Med.* 2000;18:441–445.

174. Erdoğan MF. Thiocyanate overload and thyroid disease. *Biofactors.* 2003;19:107–111.

175. Wurzburg H. Treatment of cyanide poisoning in an industrial setting. *Vet Hum Toxicol.* 1996;38:44–47.

176. Baskin SI, Rockwood GA. Neurotoxiciological and behavioral effects of cyanide and it potential therapies. *Mil Psy.* 2002;14:159–177.

177. Cardoso AP, Ernesto M, Nicala D, et al. Combination of cassava flour cyanide and urinary thiocyanate measurements of school children in Mozambique. *Intl J Food Sci Nutr.* 2004;55:183–190.

178. Cliff J, Lundqvist P, Martensson J, Rosling H, Sorbo B. Association of high cyanide and low sulphur intake in cassava-induced spastic paraparesis. *Lancet.* 1985;2:1211–1213.

179. Howlett WP, Brubaker GR, Mlingi N, Rosling H. Konzo, an epidemic upper motor neuron disease studied in Tanzania. *Brain.* 1990;113:223–235.

180. Tylleskär T, Banea M, Bikangi N, Nahimana G, Persson LÅ, Rosling H. Dietary determinants of a non-progressive spastic paraparesis (Konzo): a case-referent study in a high incidence area of Zaire. *Int J Epidemiol.* 1995;24:949–956.

181. Tshala-Katumbay D, Eeg-Olofsson KE, Tylleskar T, Kazadi-Kayembe T. Impairments, disabilities and handicap pattern in konzo – a non-progressive spastic para/tetraparesis of acute onset. *Disabil Rehabil.* 2001;23:731–736.

182. Smith RP. Toxic responses of the blood. In: Amdur MO, Doull J, Klaassen CD, eds. *Casarett and Doull's Toxicology: The Basic Science of Poisons*. 4th ed. New York, NY: Pergamon Press; 1991: 257–281.

183. Ruangkanchanasetr S, Wananukul V, Suwanjutha S. Cyanide poisoning, 2 cases report and treatment review. *J Med Assoc Thai.* 1999;82(suppl 1):162–167.

184. Espinoza OB, Perez M, Ramirez MS. Bitter cassava poisoning in eight children: a case report. *Vet Hum Toxicol.* 1992;34:65.

185. Behrman RE, Kliegman R, eds. *Nelson Essentials of Pediatrics*. 4th ed. Philadelpha, Pa: Saunders; 2002: 625.

186. Berlin CM. The treatment of cyanide poisoning in children. *Pediatrics.* 1970;46:793–796.

187. Bucaretchi F, Miglioli L, Baracat EC, Madureira PR, Capitani EM, Vieira RJ. Acute dapsone exposure and methemoglobinemia in children: treatment with multiple doses of activated charcoal with or without the administration of methylene blue. *J Pediatr (Rio J)*. 2000;76:290–294.

188. Hoffman JR, Sauter D. Methemoglobinemia resulting from smoke inhalation. *Vet Hum Toxicol.* 1989;31:168–170.

189. Bolstad-Johnson DM, Burgess JL, Crutchfield CD, Storment S, Gerkin R, Wilson JR. Characterization of firefighter exposures during fire overhaul. *AIHAJ*. 2000;61:636–641.

190. Baud FJ, Barriot P, Toffis V. Elevated blood cyanide concentrations in victims of smoke inhalation. *N Engl J Med.* 1991;325:1761–1766.

191. Yeoh MJ, Braitberg G. Carbon monoxide and cyanide poisoning in fire related deaths in Victoria, Australia. *J Toxicol Clin Toxicol.* 2004;42:855–863.

192. Shusterman D, Alexeeff G, Hargis C, et al. Predictors of carbon monoxide and hydrogen cyanide exposure in smoke inhalation patients. *J Toxicol Clin Toxicol.* 1996;34:61–71.

193. Suzuki T. Ultrastructural changes of heart muscle in cyanide poisoning. *Tohoku J Exp Med.* 1968;95:271–287.

194. Katzman GM, Penney DG. Electrocardiographic responses to carbon monoxide and cyanide in the conscious rat. *Toxicol Lett.* 1993;69:139–153.

195. Wexler J, Whittenberger JL, Dumke PR. The effect of cyanide on the electrocardiogram of man. *Am Heart J.* 1947;34:163–173.

196. Balaban RS. Cardiac energy metabolism homeostasis: role of cytosolic calcium. *J Mol Cell Cardiol.* 2002;34:1259–1271.

197. Elliott AC, Smith GL, Allen DG. Simultaneous measurement of action potential duration and intracellular ATP in isolated ferret hearts exposed to cyanide. *Circ Res.* 1989;64: 583–591.

198. Baskin SI, Brewer TG. Cyanide poisoning. In: Sidell FR, Takafuji ET, Franz DR, eds. *Medical Aspects of Chemical and Biological Warfare.* In: Zajtchuk R, Bellamy RF, eds. *Textbooks of Military Medicine.* Washington, DC: Department of the Army, Office of The Surgeon General, Borden Institute; 1997: Chap 10.

199. Leimdorfer A. About anoxia of the heart produced by intravenous sodium cyanide injections. *Arch Int Pharmacodyn.* 1950;84:181–188.

200. Van der Heyden G, Vereecke J, Carmeliet E. The effect of cyanide on the K-current in guinea-pig ventricular myocytes. *Basic Res Cardiol.* 1985;80(suppl 1):93–96.

201. Zoltani CK, Baskin SI. In silico cardiac toxicity: increasing the discovery of therapeutics through high-performance computing. In: Salem H, Katz SA, eds. *Alternative Toxicological Methods.* Boca Raton, Fla: CRC Press; 2003: Chap 42.

202. Zoltani CK, Baskin SI, Platoff GE. ECGs and metabolic networks: an in silico exploration of cyanide-caused cardiac toxicity. In: Flora SJS, Romano JA, Baskin SI, eds. *Pharmacological Perspectives of Toxic Chemicals and Their Antidotes.* New Delhi, India: Narosa Pub House; 2004: Chap 26.

203. Zoltani CK, Platoff GE, Baskin SI. Acquired Brugada-like symptoms of cyanide-caused cardiac toxicity: a computational study. *Comput Cardiol.* 2004;31:281–284.

204. Zoltani CK, Platoff GE, Baskin SI. In silico techniques aid the decryption of cellular mechanisms of cyanide-caused cardiac toxicity. In: *Proceedings of the 2004 US Army Medical Defense Bioscience Review.* Aberdeen Proving Ground, Md: US Army Medical Research Institute of Chemical Defense; 2004.

205. Inoue M, Imanaga I. Activation of Ca2+-dependent K+ channels by cyanide in guinea pig adrenal chromaffin cells. *Am J Physiol.* 1998;274:C105–C111.

206. Antzelevitch C, Zygmunt AC, Dumaine R. Electrophysiology and pharmacology of ventricular repolarization. In: Gussak I, ed. *Cardiac Repolarization: Bridging Basic and Clinical Science*. Totowa, NJ: Humana Press; 2003. Contemporary Cardiology series.

207. Carmeliet E. Cardiac ionic currents and acute ischemia: from channels to arrhythmias. *Physiol Rev*. 1999;79:917–1017.

208. Ju YK, Allen DG. Early effects of metabolic inhibition on intracellular Ca2+ in toad pacemaker cells: involvement of Ca2+ stores. *Am J Physiol Heart Circ Physiol*. 2003; 284:H1087–H1094.

209. Lukas A, Antzelevitch C. Differences in the electrophysiological response of canine ventricular epicardium and endocardium to ischemia. Role of the transient outward current. *Circulation*. 1993;88:2903–2915.

210. Mejia-Alvarez R, Marban E. Mechanism of the increase in intracellular sodium during metabolic inhibition: direct evidence against mediation by voltage-dependent sodium channels. *J Mol Cell Cardiol*. 1992;24:1307–1320.

211. Sandberg CG. A case of chronic poisoning with potassium cyanide? *Acta Med Scand*. 1967;181:233–236.

212. Roth B, Klimkova-Deutschova E. The effects of the chronic action of industrial poisons on the electroencephalogram of man. *Rev Czech Med*. 1963;90:217–227.

213. Burrows GE, Liu DH, Way JL. Effect of oxygen on cyanide intoxication. V. Physiologic effects. *J Pharmacol Exp Ther*. 1973;184:739–748.

214. Freemont WP, Pataki C, Beresin EV. The impact of terrorism on children and adolescents: terror in the skies, terror on television. *Child Adolesc Psychiatr Clin N Am*. 2005;14:429–451.

215. Garakani A, Hirschowitz J, Katz CL. General disaster psychiatry. *Psychiatr Clin North Am*. 2004;27:391–406.

216. Henderson JN, Henderson LC, Raskob GE, Boatright DT. Chemical (VX) terrorist threat: public knowledge, attitudes and responses. *Biosecur Bioterror*. 2004;2:224–228.

217. Reid WH. Psychological aspects of terrorism. *J Psychiatr Pract*. 2001;7:422–425.

218. Horwath E, Adams P, Wickramaratne P, Pine D, Weissman MM. Panic disorder with smothering symptoms: evidence for increased risk in first-degree relatives. *Depress Anxiety*. 1997;6:147–153.

219. Nicholson PJ, Vincenti GE. A case of phobic anxiety related to the inability to smell cyanide. *Occup Med (Lond)*. 1994;44:107–108.

220. Pine DS, Coplan JD, Papp LA, et al. Ventilatory physiology of children and adolescents with anxiety disorders. *Arc Gen Psychiatry*. 1998;55:123–129.

221. Paulet G, Aubertin X, Laurens L, Bourrelier J. On the methemoglobinizing effect of paraaminopropiophenone in man with an experimental supplement in the dog. *Arch Int de Pharmacodyn Ther*. 1963;142:35–51.

222. Bodansky O, Hendley CD. Effect of methemoglobinemia on the visual threshold at sea level. *J Clin Invest*. 1946;25:717–725.

223. Tepperman J, Bodansky O, Jandorf B. The effect of para-aminophenone-induced methemoglobinemia on oxygenation of working muscle in human subjects. *Am J Physiol*. 1946;146:702–709.

224. Way JL, Sylvester D, Morgan RL, et al. Recent perspectives on the toxicodynamic basis of cyanide antagonism. *Fundam Appl Toxicol*. 1984;4:(2 Pt 2)S231–S239.

225. Tadic V. Therapy of acute cyanide poisoning. *Vojnosanit Pregl*. 1981;38:117–119.

226. Chen KK, Rose CL, Clowes GHA. Cyanide poisoning and its treatment. *J Am Pharm Assoc.* 1935;24:625–630.

227. Baskin SI, Fricke. The pharmacology of p-aminopropiophenone in the detoxification of cyanide. *Cardiovasc Drug Rev.* 1992;10:358–375.

228. Kiese M, Weger N. Formation of ferrihaemoglobin with aminophenols in the human for the treatment of cyanide poisoning. *Eur J Pharmacol.* 1969;7:97–105.

229. Weiss S, Wilkins RW, Hayes FW. The nature of circulatory collapse induced by sodium nitrite. *J Clin Invest.* 1937;1673–1684.

230. Sherman CR, MD. Medical director, Hope Pharmaceuticals Inc, Scottsdale, Ariz. Personal communication with amyl nitrite drug supplier, October 2006.

231. Lorcher W, Weger N. Optimal concentration of ferrihemoglobin for the treatment of cyanide poisoning. *Naunyn Schmiedeberg's Arch Exp Pathol Pharmakol.* 1971;270:R88.

232. Szinicz L, Weger N, Schneiderhan W, Kiese M. Nephrotoxicity of aminophenols: effects of 4-dimethylaminophenol on isolated rat kidney tubules. *Arch Toxicol.* 1979;42:63–73.

233. Morocco AP. Cyanides. *Crit Care Clin.* 2005;21:691–705.

234. Szinicz L, Weger N, Schneiderhan W, Kiese M. Nephrotoxicity of aminophenols: effects of 4-dimethylaminophenol on isolated rat kidney tubules. *Arch Toxicol.* 1979;42:63–73.

235. Kerger H, Dodidou P, Passani-Kruppa D, et al. Excessive methaemoglobinemia and multi-organ failure following 4-DMAP antidote therapy. *Resuscitation.* 2005;66:231–235.

236. Vandenbelt JM, Pfeiffer C, Kaiser M, Sibert M. Methemoglobinemia after administration of p-aminoacetophenone and p-aminopropiophenone. *J Pharmacol Exp Ther.* 1944;80:31–38.

237. Bodansky O, Guttman H. Treatment of methemoglobinemia. *J Pharmacol Exp Ther.* 1947;90:46–56.

238. Jandorf BJ, Bodansky O. Therapeutic and prophylactic effect of methemoglobinemia in inhalation poisoning by hydrogen cyanide and cyanogen chloride. *J Ind Hyg Toxicol.* 1946;28:125–132.

239. Tepperman J, Bodansky O. The role of hepatic detoxification in p-aminopropiophenone induced methemoglobinemia. *J Pharmacol Exp Ther.* 1946;88:287–299.

240. Beutler E, Mikus BJ. The effect of sodium nitrite and para-aminopropiophenone administration on blood methemoglobin levels and red blood cell survival. *Blood.* 1961;18:455–467.

241. Bright JE. A prophylaxis for cyanide poisoning In: Ballantyne B, Marrs TC, eds. *Clinical and Experimental Toxicology of Cyanides.* Bristol, England: Wright; 1987: 359–382.

242. Eckstein M. Cyanide as a chemical terrorism weapon. *JEMS.* 2004;29:22–31.

243. Forsyth JC, Mueller PD, Becker CE, et al. Hydroxocobalamin as a cyanide antidote: safety, efficacy and pharmacokinetics in heavily smoking normal volunteers. *J Toxicol Clin Toxicol.* 1993;31:277–294.

244. Hall AH, Rumack BH. Hydroxyocobalamin/sodium thiosulfate as a cyanide antidote. *J Emerg Med.* 1987;5:115–121.

245. Rotenberg JS. Cyanide as a weapon of terror. *Pediatr Ann.* 2003;32:236–240.

246. Sauer SW, Keim ME. Hydroxocobalamin: improved public health readiness for cyanide disasters. *Ann Emerg Med.* 2001;37:635–641.

247. Astier A, Baud FJ. Complexation of intracellular cyanide by hydroxocobalamin using a human cellular model. *Hum Exp Toxicol.* 1996;15:19–25.

248. Borron SW, Baud FJ. Acute cyanide poisoning: clinical spectrum, diagnosis, and treatment. *Arh Hig Rada Toksikol.* 1996;47:307–322.

249. Baud FJ, Department of Medical and Toxicological Critical Care, Lariboisiere Hospital, Paris, France. Personal communication, January 2005.

250. DesLauriers CA, Burda AM, Wahl M. Hydroxocobalamin as a cyanide antidote. *Am J Ther.* 2006;13:161–165.

251. Marrs TC. Dicobalt edetate (Kelocyanor). In: Meredith TH, Jacobsen D, Haines JA, Berger J-C, van Heijst ANP, eds. *Anitdotes for Poisoning by Cyanide.* Vol 2. In: *International Program on Chemical Safety/Commission of the European Communities Evaluation of Antidotes Series*. Geneva, Switzerland: World Health Organization and Commission of the European Communities; 1993: 79–94. Publication EUR 14280 EN.

252. Rose CL, Worth RM, Kikuchi K, Chen KK. Cobalt salts in acute cyanide poisoning. *Proc Soc Exp Biol Med.* 1965;120:780–783.

Chapter 12

INCAPACITATING AGENTS

JAMES S. KETCHUM, MD,* AND HARRY SALEM, PHD†

*Colonel, MC, US Army (Retired); Clinical Assistant Professor of Psychiatry, University of California, Los Angeles, 2304 Fairbanks Drive, Santa Rosa, California 95403; formerly, Chief, Substance Abuse Program, Brentwood/UCLA VA Hospital, Los Angeles, California

†Chief Scientist for Life Sciences, US Army Edgewood Chemical Biological Center, 5183 Blackhawk Road, Aberdeen Proving Ground, Maryland 21010-5424

INTRODUCTION

In 600 BCE, soldiers of the Greek king Solon induced debilitating diarrhea in enemy troops by throwing highly poisonous hellebore roots into streams supplying their water. Today, scientists seeking new nonlethal incapacitating substances are studying neuropeptides and neuromodulators. Both then and now, the goal has been to weaken an enemy without the use of lethal force. In the last half-century, "incapacitating agent" has become the accepted military term for such unconventional weapons.

According to the US Department of Defense, an incapacitating chemical agent falls into the more general category of nonlethal weapons (NLWs) and therefore shares the following characteristics:

> [Non-lethal weapons] are explicitly designed and primarily employed so as to incapacitate personnel or materiel, while minimizing fatalities, permanent injuries to personnel, and undesired damage to property and the environment.
> Unlike conventional lethal weapons that destroy their targets principally through blast, penetration and fragmentation, non-lethal weapons only employ means other than gross physical destruction to prevent the target from functioning.
> Non-lethal weapons are intended to have one, or both, of the following characteristics:
> 1. They have relatively reversible effects on personnel or materiel.
> 2. They affect objects differently within their area of influence.[1]

Use of an incapacitating agent by conventional military forces would face political, military, medical, and budgetary constraints. Factors such as effectiveness, relative lack of toxicity or excessive persistence, logistical feasibility, predictability of behavior, manageability of casualties, availability of antidotes, limitations imposed by treaties, and cost would need to be considered. No proposed incapacitating agent has yet been acceptable.[2] Further considerations would come into play before any decision to deploy an agent. Methods and equipment must be designed to manufacture, store, and transport the agent. Troops in the field would require extensive training to operate what might be a complex delivery system. Medical personnel would need to learn how best to treat the casualties, working within the confines of the battlefield.

This chapter reviews the properties of many possible chemical incapacitating agents, as well as a few that are physical in nature, and their diagnosis, treatment, and general principles of management.

HISTORY AND MODERN DEVELOPMENT

Although few references to the historical use of drugs for military purposes appear in contemporary publications, a substantial literature describes a variety of tactical efforts to incapacitate enemy forces with mind-altering chemicals. The rarity of new publications about the incapacitating chemical agents considered most promising can be attributed in part to the exponential acceleration of pharmaceutical discovery, which has eclipsed interest in many drugs used widely in the past. In addition, computerized databases tend to include only research reports published since 1970. Consequently, the current focus is on new drugs tailored to specific nervous system targets. The "new age" neurochemicals under consideration are not new—they incorporate advances in neuropharmacology but no new modes of action; some are even less practical than those proposed in the 1960s. Even the agents attracting interest in the 1960s were not as new as they seemed.

In 1961 Ephraim Goodman, a psychologist in the Edgewood Medical Laboratories, Maryland, systematically reviewed 100 years of reports and letters appearing in four leading American and British medical journals (as well as a more limited number of several respected German medical periodicals). Goodman discovered numerous reports of deliberate administration, particularly of atropine and related drugs, to produce "behavioral toxicity" (a term introduced by Joseph Brady in 1956). Often, these substances were used by single individuals, but some can be considered examples of drugs used as "weapons of mass destruction" or "mass casualty weapons." The following excerpts from Goodman's review show that incapacitating agents are not a new approach to military conflict:

> According to Sextus Julius Frontinus, Maharbal, an officer in Hannibal's army about 200 BCE, ... sent by the Carthaginians against the rebellious Africans, knowing that the tribe was passionately fond of wine, mixed a large quantity of wine with mandragora, which in potency is something between a poison and a soporific. Then, after an insignificant skirmish, he deliberately withdrew. At dead of night, leaving in the camp some of his baggage and all the drugged wine, he feigned flight. When the barbarians captured the camp and in frenzy of delight greedily drank the

> drugged wine, Maharbal returned, and either took them prisoners or slaughtered them while they lay stretched out as if dead.[3]

His review continues, "Another example of the use of atropinic plants for military purposes occurred during the reign of Duncan, the 84th king of Scotland (1034–1040 CE), who used wine dosed with 'sleepy nightshade' against the troops of Sweno, king of Norway."[4–6] Goodman also reports:

> During his assault in 1672 on the city of Groningen, the Bishop of Muenster tried to use grenades and projectiles containing belladonna against the defenders. Unfortunately, capricious winds often blew the smoke back, creating effects opposite to those intended. As a result of this and other incidents in which chemicals were used in battle, a treaty was signed in 1675 between the French and the Germans, outlawing further use of chemical warfare.[5]

Goodman adds another incident, "In 1813 the inhabitants of an area being invaded by French troops received fortuitous help from local flora. A company of starving French soldiers was rendered helpless when they impulsively consumed wild berries containing belladonna alkaloids."[7] Finally, in reference to more recent use:

> Ironically, the first recorded 20th century use of solanaceae in a military situation occurred in Hanoi, French Indo-China (later known as North Vietnam) on 27 June 1908. On that day, two hundred French soldiers were poisoned by datura in their evening meal. One of the intoxicated soldiers saw ants on his bed, a second fled to a tree to escape from a hallucinated tiger and a third took aim at birds in the sky. The delirious troops were soon discovered and all recovered after medical attention. Two indigenous non-commissioned officers and an artilleryman were later convicted by courts-martial of plotting with ex-river pirates who had been influenced by "Chinese reformer agitators."[8,9]

The international community, particularly in the latter half of the 20th century, has repeatedly tried to find ways to make warfare more humane. Remorse and indignation were widely expressed following the use during World War I of such weapons as chlorine, mustard, and phosgene, which killed or injured hundreds of thousands of soldiers in European trenches. One consequence of these outcries was an international ban on chemical weapons adopted by the Geneva Convention in 1925.[10] The United States, although not a signatory to this document until 1975, strongly supported its purpose.

Although no chemical weapons were used during World War II, the German military had developed and stockpiled several lethal organophosphate nerve agents, which were never deployed. The Allies learned later that Hitler had a morbid fear of poisonous chemicals, having been temporarily blinded by a British gas shell in World War I; furthermore, the Nazis erroneously assumed that the Allies were in possession of the same lethal compounds and would retaliate in kind.[11]

Agents of lower lethality were used against terrorists in the 2002 Moscow theater incident (see further discussion below), reducing the potential number of deaths by more than 80%. Claims that BZ (or a related incapacitating agent) was used against defenseless civilians fleeing the Serbian genocidal purge in 1999 are difficult to confirm but considered to be true. Widespread reports of hallucinations implicate an agent related to BZ. A less credible claim by Alistair Hay,[12] although supported by the testimony of many witnesses and casualties, mentioned features uncharacteristic of BZ.

Another unsubstantiated assertion is the claim by Dr Wouter Basson, a South African political figure with a reputation for falsehoods, to having proof that BZ was used in Iraq during the Persian Gulf War.[13] His description of victims as "wide-eyed and drooling" is incongruent with the marked dryness of the mouth produced by BZ and other anticholinergic agents—proof of popular misperceptions about the pharmacological qualities of BZ and its chemical relatives.

A seemingly novel concept—using psychochemicals to produce temporary ineffectiveness—was unintentionally given credibility by Albert Hofmann's report that lysergic acid diethylamide (LSD), one of a series of ergot derivatives he had synthesized in 1938, possessed incredibly potent mind-altering effects. Hofmann realized this when he accidentally ingested an undetectable amount in 1943, while replicating the synthesis of some of his 1938 compounds. He then deliberately ingested a presumably subthreshold amount of the contents of bottle number 25 (hence, "LSD-25") and experienced a bizarre and at times terrifying "trip."[14]

LSD-25 arrived in the United States in 1949, when psychiatrist Max Rinkel brought a sample from Sandoz Pharmaceuticals in Switzerland and began work with Dr Paul Hoch at the Boston Psychopathic Hospital. Dr Harold Abramson, a New York chemist, allergist, and psychotherapist, began studying the clinical characterization of the fascinating new drug.[15] Over the next 2 decades Abramson published numerous reports describing LSD's unique effects on perception, mood, and cognitive activity. His dose/response approach quickly stimulated wider testing. Soon LSD became a multipurpose drug, used in psychiatric hospitals either to treat schizophrenics or to produce "model psychoses" in normal volunteers.[16] The Central Intelligence Agency also became involved with LSD beginning in 1951,[17] leading to serious damage to the agency's reputation when the use was uncovered during several 1977 Congressional investigations.

The head of the US Army Chemical Corps, Major General William Creasy, recognized the military potential of LSD. Creasy persuaded Congress[18] that LSD could quickly disable an enemy force, yet not destroy lives, describing a floating cloud of LSD that could disable everyone in the area for several hours without serious aftereffects. Creasy stated that the Soviet Union was spending 10 times as much as the United States on chemical weapons research and was no doubt already using LSD in covert operations. He recommended tripling the funding of Chemical Corps research and development, especially for evaluation of the military potential of LSD as an NLW. This request was endorsed by an almost unanimous vote, leading to an elaborate incapacitating agent research program.

LSD testing by both civilian contractors and at Edgewood Arsenal, Maryland (1955–1960), showed LSD's effects to be disturbingly unpredictable. However, military testing continued from 1961 to 1966 to complete LSD's characterization by various routes, evaluate treatment methods, and develop a sensitive assay technique to aid in diagnosis. Just as LSD testing was ending, the Edgewood program was reinvigorated by Hoffmann-LaRoche, Inc, who gave the Chemical Corps permission to study its patented compound, 3-quinuclidinyl benzilate.[19] (A similar "incapacitating agent" was deployed by the Soviet Union even before 1960. In 1959, the Soviets attempted to poison 1,248 employees of Radio Free Europe, covertly mixing atropine with table salt in the cafeteria. A US agent foiled the plan.[20,21]) The Edgewood program received additional support under the "blue skies" policy, first announced by President Eisenhower and later supported by President Kennedy, which brought many new personnel and funding for facilities and equipment.

POSSIBLE METHODS OF INCAPACITATION

Nonchemical Methods

After considering virtually every possible chemical technique for producing military incapacitation, and rejecting many as too toxic or unmanageable, investigators at the Edgewood Arsenal clinical laboratories examined dozens of potentially disabling but reasonably safe substances between 1953 and 1973. Although drugs that predominantly affected the central nervous system soon became of primary interest and received the most intensive study, development of nonchemical devices and techniques, protective garments, and antidotes to existing agents, as well as physician training for medical management of agent effects, were important objectives as well.

Nonpharmacological materials and techniques potentially capable of reducing an enemy's military competence were also developed in related programs that continued after volunteer testing of chemical agents was terminated in 1973. The most significant of these developments are listed below.

Auditory Methods

Several devices that produce loud or unpleasant sounds have been designed, but most have not been tested in volunteers, and none have been deployed. Some critics consider incapacitation produced by directed sound energy devices to be inhumane because none can be guaranteed not to produce injury.[22,23](Because they involve nonmedical systems, these devices will not be further discussed in this chapter.)

Microwave Devices

In the late 1960s several animal studies of microwave effects produced reversible incapacitation.[24]

Use of Light

Another proposed incapacitation modality uses high-intensity photostimulation adjusted to oscillate at certain frequencies calibrated to impair visual perception and concentration.[25] Laser light in the ultraviolet spectrum gained brief interest, but was soon judged impractical, and further light use has not been pursued.

Olfactory Devices

The notion of producing incapacitation through "olfactory assault" was briefly explored in the 1960s. Various obnoxious odors, such as those produced by derivatives of skatole (an excretory chemical) were initially thought aversive enough to impair military performance. Obnoxious odors have actually been tried as tactical weapons, but their effectiveness remains in doubt because masks that attenuate such odors would reduce their impact. Furthermore, a highly motivated soldier might not be appreciably deterred by aversive odors alone. Such considerations halted this line of investigation at Edgewood Arsenal. Research in this area was later resumed, however, and a few programs exploring the effectiveness of malodorous substances are still active.[26]

Nonlethal Mines

Incapacitating mines such as taser mines and modular land mines are examples of NLWs.[27]

Armed Robots

A group of robots capable of intelligent mobility under the control of sophisticated algorithms, armed with sublethal weapons, could act in concert as a patrolling unit. Current international humanitarian law contains very little to govern the behavior of autonomous nonhuman devices. Robots offer real promise but are not yet sufficiently advanced or dependable to be deployed.[28]

A wide range of other immobilizing devices are appearing on the market, some of which could deliver chemicals, paralyzing electric shocks, or nonlethal chemicals. However, they also carry hazards such as the risk of asphyxiation[29] (see further discussion below).

Chemical Methods

The list of possible chemical incapacitating agents has become long. Relatively unattractive for military use are those that alter a victim's physical integrity, possibly producing irreversible injury. Less objectionable are those that temporarily disturb some physiological or biochemical function. Their effects usually remit without residual disability after periods varying from minutes to months. Some agents in this latter category can be attenuated or even reversed with the help of antidotes.

Chemicals that produce injury are part of a diverse group of pharmacological agents that alter mental competence. These chemicals may affect mood or motivation, or they may interrupt the ability to process information and respond appropriately to events in the environment. "Psychochemical" is a useful term for these agents, although most of the medical community calls them "psychoactive drugs."

Psychoactivity is manifested by a variety of subgroups in the pharmacological family. The "psychoactive" umbrella covers many familiar therapeutic drugs such as stimulants, sedatives, analgesics, psychedelics, tranquilizers, and centrally active anticholinergic medications. In small doses, these drugs are useful in the treatment of either physical maladies or mental disorders. In doses greatly above therapeutic values, however, they produce incapacitation.

The safety margin or therapeutic index of psychochemicals varies greatly, as does the quantity of each required to impair the ability to function. All psychochemicals cross the blood–brain barrier with ease; some take up residence in the brain for only a few minutes or hours, whereas others are more persistent, clinging to brain receptors for days or even weeks with or without treatment. Although none of their effects is permanent at sublethal doses, at very high multiples of the incapacitating dose they can be lethal (as can any drug). Although basic concepts of drug action are familiar to physicians and pharmacologists, from a military standpoint, variations in potency, duration, safety, and mode of action require defined criteria to assess their suitability as incapacitating weapons. The following sections examine 14 categories of chemical agents, both peripheral-acting and psychochemical. The text will summarize data developed through clinical testing whenever such information is available.

A drug's mode of action is a key factor that greatly influences the decision whether or not to explore it further. Drugs that affect behavior indirectly by some aversive somatic effect, even if relatively safe, tend to be least reliable. Drugs that affect brain function directly tend to be more useful, as long as they do not compromise life-sustaining systems. Sometimes referred to as basic vegetative functions, life-sustaining systems are mostly under the control of mechanisms located in the lower brain stem or in the midbrain, which have developed phylogenetically as the most essential brain areas. These areas regulate respiration, blood pressure, body temperature, and many instinctual or well-learned reflexes.

The drugs of greatest military interest are those that tend to affect predominantly "higher integrative" or "cognitive" functions, which process sensory data or conscious decision-making, including attention, orientation, perception, memory, and motivation. Working together, these capabilities regulate conceptual thinking, planning, and judgment. These functions depend on complicated neural networks and are thus more vulnerable and easily disrupted than are basic vegetative functions. These drugs are rarely devoid of some effect on basic autonomic mechanisms, but ideally such effects are tangential to the drug's main action—impairment of the higher integrative systems. Effects on systems essential to life are side effects compared to effects on thoughts, feelings, and the anticipatory "programming" of behavior (planning).

Nerve Agents

Although lethal chemicals such as sarin or VX are not usually considered incapacitating drugs, cholinesterase inhibition can produce severe incapacitation through neuropsychological effects alone, independent of such easily recognized bodily effects as miosis, respiratory distress, muscular weakness, autonomic disturbances, and general malaise. Sarin and VX are relatively reversible; some of the other cholinesterase inhibitors are much longer acting.

A chemical worker at Edgewood Arsenal, accidentally exposed to GD (soman), provided an example of the effects of a persistent anticholinesterase agent. After receiving emergency treatment, he spent several weeks under close observation with the usual supportive measures and repeated doses of atropine and other therapeutic agents.[30] In addition to the usual life-threatening effects on respiration, cardiovascular activity, and muscle strength, all of which were reversed with atropine and 2-pralidoxime chloride, his performance of standards continued to be impaired even after his physical signs and symptoms had largely subsided.

This case of accidental poisoning presented a unique opportunity to follow the time course of GD's central nervous system effects. Through daily psychological testing the medical staff could measure the quantitative aspects of cognitive impairment produced by cholinergic excess in the brain. Of considerable interest was the greater reversal of the patient's cognitive deficits by small doses of scopolamine than by doses of atropine equivalent in peripheral potency. Scopolamine was also more effective in reducing the frequency and severity of nightmares, a common central effect of nerve agents. Recovery was gradual and took several weeks, as GD-inactivated cholinesterase was slowly replaced by newly generated, functionally normal enzyme.[30]

In a study of Australian gardeners, mental defects developed in the absence of significant peripheral physiological changes. These workers had been exposed daily to seemingly unremarkable concentrations of organophosphate pesticides. Although acute effects did not occur, the frequent, sometimes prolonged exposure to the chemicals produced cumulative effects on mental function. Hallucinations occurred and changes in cognitive efficiency became increasingly apparent, even though the men appeared otherwise normal.[31]

Irritants, Nausea-Producing Agents, and Toxins

Irritants and nauseants, including lacrimators such as CN (the original tear gas), CS (successor of CN), and DM (a nauseant) are incapacitating and generally safe when properly used.[32] These agents have the following two qualities: (1) Their duration of action is short, because adaptation to the irritant effects usually occurs after 30 minutes or less of continuous exposure, with rapid recovery when the atmosphere clears; and (2) highly motivated individuals can sometimes "fight through" their effects.

Vesicants

The vesicating agents, which include such substances as mustard, produce severe incapacitation by burning the skin and respiratory tract.[33] Vesicants have been internationally condemned, and although some nations have used them in past decades, the probability of their use solely as an incapacitant in today's conflicts is low because they have no impact on mental function.

Indole-Based Psychedelics

"Psychedelic," a term coined by Humphry Osmond in collaboration with Aldous Huxley in 1957, means "mind-manifesting" and refers to the alleged expansion of awareness that early users thought to be a unique feature of LSD and related compounds.[34] Its ability to bring forth repressed memories, fears, and fantasies supposedly made LSD a useful adjunct to traditional psychoanalysis, although few practicing psychiatrists felt comfortable using it in their practice, for the effects could be explosive and difficult to control in a doctor's office. The unmanageable flood of ideas, images, and emotions that LSD unleashes accounts for many of its disorganizing effects. A person under the influence of incapacitating doses of LSD would find it impossible to carry out complex tasks because of the sensory overload of frightening or perplexing thoughts, accompanied by a kaleidoscope of rapidly changing perceptions and emotions.[35,36]

Although many psychedelic drugs have been extracted from plants, or synthesized in the laboratory, LSD was undoubtedly the best known of these indole-based psychedelic drugs. It gained attention from diverse subcultures and scientists starting in the mid-1940s (long before it was tested systematically at the Edgewood Arsenal for possible military usefulness).[37] Chemical Corps testing of LSD as a possible incapacitating agent began in the mid 1950s.[38] When administered to volunteers, LSD produced virtually complete incapacitation. For unexplained reasons, the drug was less effective when given by the oral route than when inhaled.[39] As previously reported by civilian investigators, LSD produces bizarre and unpredictable but often well-coordinated behaviors. Individuals given larger doses usually cannot carry out a series of instructions or concentrate on a complex task. Most of the volunteers expressed the belief, moreover, that they might tend to perform unpredictable, impulsive actions.[40]

Phenothiazines and benzodiazepines have frequently been used to ameliorate LSD intoxication. One of the nation's leading psychopharmacologists, George Aghajanian, however, suggested that barbiturates would be his choice as an LSD countermeasure, based on his studies showing the effectiveness of LSD in reversing the action of barbiturates.[41] Nevertheless, an injectable benzodiazepine such as lorazepam (Ativan, Baxter Healthcare Corp, Deerfield, Ill) combined with "talking down" is now the most commonly accepted therapeutic approach.

Aghajanian has spent 5 decades studying the mode of action of LSD. Based on his findings, it seems probable that the lack of a specific antagonist to LSD's effects is attributable to its complex action.[42] LSD has affinity for several subtypes of serotonin receptor, with additional effects on locus coeruleus (alerting) neurons in the brainstem and specific glutamate (stimulating) receptors in the neocortex. Recently Aghajanian collected evidence indicating that some glutamate-producing cells in the forebrain are overstimulated by LSD, leading to a functional state of "hyperfrontality."[43] Excess glutamate "spills over" into spaces between cells and apparently impinges on adjacent neurons that subserve normally separated modalities. This may explain the synaesthesia described by some LSD-intoxicated persons, whereby specific musical notes produce specific color sensations, or numbers become associated with particular tastes or odors (less common).[42]

Before 1963 no reliable quantitative assay of LSD blood levels was available. Blood levels were assumed by many pharmacologists, relying on LSD's known half-life of 20 minutes in rats. Two possible explanations were offered for the much longer clinical effects in human subjects: either (1) the drug triggered some unusual brain activity that continued after the drug had left the body, or (2) some of it became "sequestered" in the brain, where it continued to disrupt normal neuronal activity. Aghajanian and Oscar Bing, while assigned to the Clinical Research Department at Edgewood, laid these speculations to rest in 1964 by developing a sensitive spectrophotofluorometric assay for blood levels of LSD (then one of the most fluorescent drugs known). They found the that blood elimination time of LSD was approximately 175 minutes, resolving the discrepancy between the 8- to 12-hour duration of its effect and the earlier estimates of approximately 20 minutes. Cognitive performance, using the 3-minute number facility (NF) test, revealed a striking parallelism between scores and blood levels[44] (ruling out the idea that LSD was somehow retained in the brain even after disappearing completely from the blood). A second retrospective study on the respiratory route of administration of LSD estimated that the approximate time for blood elimination was about 160 minutes. Military scientists did test administration of LSD by the oral route, but they were more interested in the effectiveness of the respiratory route.[45]

LSD analogs are numerous and vary in duration of action, but none exceeds it in potency. Many are naturally occurring psychedelics structurally related to LSD and well known to ethnopharmacologists (specialists in indigenous drug-containing plants). LSD is remarkably safe from a toxicity standpoint. Studies in several species of animals have shown that the lethal dose is at least 1,000-fold greater than the incapacitating dose.[45] An exception was the sudden death of an elephant in the Oklahoma City, Oklahoma, Lincoln Park Zoo during behavioral experiments following a dose of LSD.[46] This accidental overdose was later attributed to the rapid absorption of the injected dose (delivered by dart), creating a bolus effect that resulted in significant laryngeal spasm with subsequent asphyxiation; it probably also overwhelmed the elephant's heart.

Physiological effects of LSD are unremarkable, consisting mainly of peripheral adrenergic symptoms such as tachycardia, mildly elevated blood pressure, slight hyperthermia, and an average increase of about 2 mm in pupil diameter. Doses above certain amounts have occasionally produced grand mal seizures,[47,48] although some European recreational users claim to have ingested larger amounts without serious consequences.[49]

In the 1960s chlorpromazine (Thorazine, Smith Kline & French Laboratories, Philadelphia, Pa) was the most widely used drug to help subjects "come down" from the intense symptoms produced by LSD. However, no systematic test had determined whether chlorpromazine was a true antagonist or merely a "quieting" agent. Aghajanian and Bing explored chlorpromazine's ability to reverse performance decrements by conducting a double-blind study at clinically used dose levels to modulate LSD's effects and evaluating volunteer cognitive function using the NF test.[50] Although scores rose modestly for about 4 hours, the duration of LSD effects was not shortened. Benzodiazepines such as lorazepam, which is short-acting and injectable, have since become the preferred drugs for easing LSD effects.[51] Benzodiazepines are also nonspecific in their tranquilizing actions.

Because of the unpredictable nature of its effects, LSD was removed from consideration as a military incapacitating agent. Volunteer testing of the drug ended in 1966, after the government categorized it as a class I drug, making it illegal to use without a special research permit.

Phenethylamine-Based Psychedelics

Mescaline, derived from the peyote cactus, has long been valued for its psychedelic properties, and is legal for ceremonial use in certain Native American tribes. Unlike LSD, it is a substituted phenethylamine and thus a structural relative of norepinephrine and dopamine. Numerous synthetic relatives of mescaline with psychedelic properties exist, including 3, 4-methylene-dioxymethylamphetamine (MDMA), the drug popularly known as ecstasy. MDMA and related synthetic compounds induce dramatic alterations of consciousness similar to the effects of LSD.[52,53] Startling perceptual changes that range from frightening to enlightening can occur, depending on the user and the setting in which the drug is taken.

Some phenethylamine psychedelics are very potent, but the same limitations as with LSD apply to their use in a military situation. The potent phenethylamine derivatives were not tested in Edgewood volunteers, except for a small dose of a relatively potent amphetamine derivative given to four people.[52,53] No significant changes in performance were observed.

Cannabinoids

For a short period the Chemical Corps became interested in a potent extract of marijuana known as "red oil."[54] In 1961 oral doses were given to 12 volunteers. The dose-response regression curve had a low slope, and few of the classical cannabis effects were observed, except in one subject. Modest decrements in standardized arithmetic and word recognition tests occurred. For political as well pharmacological reasons, however, the effort was dropped, particularly after members of the press ridiculed the idea of the Army using an illegal recreational drug as a weapon of war.[55] It appears unlikely that a cannabinoid will be used as an incapacitating agent in the foreseeable future.

Stimulants

Included in this category are cocaine, caffeine, nicotine, and the unsubstituted amphetamines, as well as epileptogenic substances such as strychnine and metrazole.[56] All of these stimulants, except for the last two, increase alertness and may actually enhance performance in some tasks. At high doses D-amphetamine produces psychotic symptoms such as paranoia, and illusions develop in 50% of normal subjects. The hyperactivity produced by stimulants would probably be an undesirable effect in most situations. This group has little to offer as incapacitating agents.[57]

Sedative Hypnotics

A large variety of compounds fall under this heading, but none hold much promise as a practical agent. Barbiturates, for example, generally require doses of several hundred milligrams to produce heavy sedation. In a trial limited to four volunteers who received secobarbital (Seconal, Eli Lilly, Indianapolis, Ind), the drug caused only a 20% decline in the performance of a sensitive time-reproduction task.[58] Many civilian studies have yielded comparable results. The low safety margin of barbiturates is well known (they are frequently used for suicide attempts). As incapacitants, they probably have no useful military role.

Opioids

Originally derived from the poppy, these venerable drugs, of which morphine is the prototype, have only recently regained interest as potential incapacitating agents. Candace Pert and Solomon Snyder first isolated and characterized the morphine (μ) receptor in 1972.[58] Subsequently, δ (delta), κ (kappa), and σ (sigma) receptors were identified. The σ-receptor is no longer considered a pure opioid receptor, but is also a target of the dissociative anesthetic best known as PCP (phencyclidine).[59] The μ-receptor subserves analgesia, but also inhibits respiration.

The treatment of opioid overdose is well established. Naloxone (Narcan, Endo Pharmaceuticals, Chadds Ford, Pa) in doses of 0.4 to 1.0 mg has been the standard treatment in most emergency rooms for many years.[60,61] The antidote can be given by the intramuscular route, but if the subject appears to be deeply comatose with severely depressed respirations, it should be given by the intravenous route. Repeated injections at intervals as short as 30 to 60 minutes are usually required in the case of a large overdose to prevent relapse into coma and a possibly fatal outcome.

The morphine antagonist nalorphine (naloxone) has affinity for the κ-receptor. It also produces analgesic effects in its own right. Pentazocine (Talwin, Sanofi-Aventis, Bridgewater, NJ) is active at the κ-receptor, producing analgesia, but is dysphoric in opioid-naive subjects. However, some users have become addicted to pentazocine and are tolerant to its unpleasant effects. The role of the δ-receptor, originally isolated from the rat vas deferens, has antinociceptive, seizuregenic, and convulsive properties. It may have a role in depression. The three major opioid receptors interact in a complex manner, the details of which are beyond the scope of this chapter.

During the Cold War (1945–1991), a great deal of research was directed to chemicals that were not necessarily lethal but would incapacitate enemy personnel. The United States and the former Soviet Union, in particular, investigated a wide number of pharmacological agents for their potential as incapacitants, such as depressants, hallucinogens, belladonna drugs, and opiate derivatives.[62] The relatively recent development of several highly potent opioids is potentially significant for military use. Fentanyl, the first of these new opioids, is many times more potent than morphine. Super-potent derivatives of fentanyl have since appeared and might be used to produce incapacitation.

Since 1996 a number of different analogs of fentanyl have been introduced for use in anesthesia; the best known are carfentanil, sufentanil, and remifentanil. Their pharmacological activity is similar to that of other opiates; consequently, they produce all of the effects of heroin, including analgesia, euphoria, miosis, and respiratory depression. Because of their high lipid solubility, regardless of the route of administration, the fentanyls reach the brain very quickly, thus providing a very fast onset of action. This quality led to their popularity as illicit drugs; they were initially unregulated as controlled substances, but this loophole has since been closed by the US Drug Enforcement Agency.[63]

Among the multiple opioid receptors,[64] μ-receptors mediate analgesia, euphoria, physical dependence, and depression of ventilation, whereas κ-receptors mediate sedation and diuresis. Drugs may act at more than one opiate receptor, with varying effects. Traditionally, narcotic antagonists such as naloxone and naltrexone have been used to reverse opioid agonists' effects.[65] Also, when used clinically, longer acting opioids such as fentanyl may produce renarcotization because of differences in the pharmacokinetics of agonists and antagonists.

Because fentanyl is not listed in any of the schedules of the 1993 Chemical Weapons Convention (CWC), and is traditionally characterized by the rapid onset and short duration of 15 to 30 minutes of analgesia, some people are arguing for it to be legally considered a riot control agent according to the definition set forth in the CWC.[62] On October 23, 2002, at least 129 of the almost 800 hostages held by Chechen terrorists in the Moscow Dubrovka Theatre Center died when Russian authorities pumped what many believe was fentanyl into the building.[66–68] Although the Russian authorities insisted that emergency personnel were prepared with 1,000 doses of antidote in anticipation of the raid, controversy continues over whether local hospitals and physicians were adequately informed about the gas prior to its use in the rescue operation.[69] According to some reports, a few Russian officials suggested that a mixture of fentanyl and halothane, as well as massive doses of carfentanil, were used to produce a fully incapacitating concentration inside the theater.[70]

Carfentanil, an even more potent opioid, is often used to rapidly immobilize large wild animals, as well as horses and goats.[71] This drug produces rapid catatonic immobilization, characterized by limb and neck hyperextension. Adverse effects include muscle rigidity, bradypnea, and oxygen desaturation.

Recycling and renarcotization have been reported as possible causes of death when low doses of antagonist are used. This occurs when the antagonist has a shorter duration than the opioid it reverses. To avoid this, the treating physician must ensure close observation and may need to administer additional doses of antagonist. Recent research suggests that selective stimulation of the 5-HT_{4a} serotonin receptor might be a way to reverse or prevent μ-receptor–induced respiratory depression.[72,73] This is because the 5-HT_{4a} receptor affects the intracellular concentration of cyclic adenosine monophosphate in respiration-regulating brainstem neurons in a manner opposite to the μ-receptor.[72] Numerous investigators are currently pursuing this promising line of research, hoping to separate the anesthetic from the respiratory effects of μ-agonists.

Following antagonist treatment, residual opioid may still be present at lethal levels, even when it has partially cleared the body. Although there were naloxone syringes found in the Dubrovka theater, it is also possible that the doses given were insufficient to reverse the respiratory depression.

Dissociative Anesthetics

PCP (Sernyl, Parke Davis and Co, Detroit, Mich), introduced as an anesthetic in the 1950s, has a unique combination of pharmacological properties never seen previously.[74] Without causing loss of consciousness or respiratory depression, it prevents awareness of surgical pain. For a time it was touted as an anesthetic breakthrough, but as subsequent reports of unnatural agitation and disruptive behavior began to accumulate, its use in adults was halted. Because it prevented respiratory problems, it continued to be used in children for short procedures, but it also produces delirium and frequently caused management problems.

PCP was subsequently designated for use only in veterinary surgery, where its subjective effects are evidently less of a problem. In its place, ketamine (Ketalar, Parke Davis and Co, Detroit, Mich), a short-acting chemical relative of PCP, proved more manageable clinically and became an acceptable anesthetic for certain surgical procedures in both humans and animals.[75] Like PCP, its mode of action is complex. Also like LSD, both ketamine and PCP are attracted to 5-HT_{2A} serotonin receptors, but they also possess affinity for a number of other receptors. PCP acts as an inverse agonist at the glutamate receptor, which has been called "the PCP receptor."[76] PCP's multiplicity of receptor affinities produces a complex clinical picture, with psychedelic, delirium-producing, energizing, and analgesic elements.

Treatment for PCP, unlike for LSD, is difficult. Benzodiazepines are generally used. Physostigmine might improve cognitive functions, and antipsychotics are often given to minimize irrational behavior, but these alone do not reverse all effects. Keeping the patient in dark, quiet surroundings tends to minimize agitation and assaults. Temporary hospitalization may be necessary.[77,78]

Tranquilizers

Diazepam (Valium, Hoffmann-La Roche Inc, Nutley, NJ), successor to the popular drug meprobamate (Equanil, Wyeth-Ayerst Laboratories, Madison, NJ) was initially hailed as a wonder drug when it was introduced in 1959. Psychiatrists considered it to be a "minor tranquilizer," in contrast to "major" tranquilizers such as chlorpromazine or haloperidol (Haldol, Ortho-McNeil Pharmaceutical, Raritan, NJ). Over the next two decades, a bevy of benzodiazepines structurally related to diazepam appeared on the market.[79] The major tranquilizers were meanwhile renamed "antipsychotics," and the minor tranquilizers became "anxiolytics." In addition to their antianxiety and tranquilizing effects, benzodiazepines have muscle relaxant, anticonvulsant, amnestic, and sedative-hypnotic effects. All of these contribute to performance impairment.

Flumazenil, a benzodiazepine antagonist, is an inverse agonist at the γ-aminobutyric acid receptor with the side effect of severe anxiety[80] (which would obviously affect performance adversely, making it incapacitating in its own right). Many benzodiazepines now exist, ranging in duration of action from extremely short to very long. Some of the more recently introduced members of the family are also highly potent. Alprazolam (Xanax, Pfizer US Pharmaceuticals, New York, NY) and triazolam (Halcion, Pfizer US Pharmaceuticals, New York, NY) require small oral doses to produce sedation or tranquilization.[81]

Antipsychotic Drugs

The more potent antipsychotic drugs were previously called major tranquilizers or "neuroleptics." These drugs are valued not only for their sedative effects, but also for their ability to reduce psychotic hyperactivity. They tend to produce extrapyramidal symptoms similar to parkinsonism, which is caused by the loss of dopamine-producing neurons in the midbrain's substantia nigra. Because they block dopamine receptors, most antipsychotic drugs cause the same problems: rigidity, tremor, and reduced activity, which results in considerable impairment of movement. The potency of some antipsychotic drugs, although impressive, generally would not satisfy logistical constraints.[82] Performance decrements on the usual cognitive measures were only slightly dose related, with a shallow dose-response slope, meaning that the effects would be difficult to predict, and considerably higher doses would be required to ensure complete incapacitation.

The lethal dose of an antipsychotic drug is many times the therapeutic dose, but precise values are unavailable. Very high doses of haloperidol, for example, can be tolerated; paradoxically, such high doses may actually produce fewer parkinsonian side effects. Some clinicians, perhaps frustrated with the lack of response to ordinary doses of haloperidol, tried giving larger doses to psychotic patients. No greater therapeutic response occurred, but because haloperidol has significant anticholinergic effects at high doses, it prevented the parkinsonian side effects that are common after lower doses (working like the drug benztropine [Cogentin, Merck & Co Inc, Whitehouse Station, NJ]).[83] Malignant hyperthermia, a potentially lethal complication, occasionally occurs after repeated ingestion of much lower doses.

Parkinsonian symptoms, particularly in the form of painful spasms of neck muscles, occurred in many of the volunteers. These did not usually appear until 8 to 12 hours after ingestion, and invariably responded promptly to an injection of benztropine or diphenhydramine (Benadryl, Pfizer Consumer Healthcare, New York, NY). Delayed spasms could therefore be prevented in the field if prompt medical custody of the affected individuals were assured.

Neuropeptides and Neuromodulators

The newest potential incapacitating agents are those that operate on the central nervous system, either as surrogate neurotransmitters with unwanted effects, or as natural neuropeptide transmitters applied in ways that were unintended by nature. Military consideration of such substances was spurred by a review submitted in 2000 by the University of Pennsylvania under a government contract.[84] In 2003, three analysts from the US Defense Intelligence Agency authored a paper called

"Biotechnology: Impact on Biological Warfare and Biodefense."[85] They warned that weapons designers of the future will be able to engineer agents that produce a range of effects "...including death, incapacitation, neurological impairment." The former Soviet biological weapons effort, ostensibly halted as early as 1992, included programs to develop "bioregulators" as weapons to replace classical chemical weapons. Some chemical warfare watchers are very concerned about the growing interest in such substances. The following excerpts are illustrative:

> There is concern over the potential use of bioregulators as weapons in warfare or by terrorists. A paper in late 2001 stated that these organic compounds "... are capable of regulating a wide range of physiologic activities..." and if used as weapons "... could potentially cause profound systemic effects on multiple organ systems."[85(p3)]
>
> . . .
>
> Bioregulators of concern discussed in the paper included cytokines, eicosanoids, neurotransmitters, hormones, and plasma proteases. Neurotransmitters mediate chemical transmission in the nervous system through their interactions with specific receptors. In the central nervous system these neurotransmitter-receptor interactions have a major role in regulating consciousness, mood, anxiety, perception, and cognition.[86]

Bioregulators have sometimes been referred to as "calmatives," and some writings list as calmatives compounds that do not produce this outcome. The term has also been used by the Russians in referring to the drug (or drugs) used in the Moscow theater rescue in 2002. Most therapeutic drugs that relieve anxiety or produce some kind of sedation, including anxiolytics such as diazepam, antipsychotic neuroleptics such as chlorpromazine, muscle relaxants, and sedative-hypnotic drugs have been placed in this artificial category.

Also included in the category are serotonin 5-HT_{1a} receptor agonists and selective serotonin reuptake inhibitors, of which fluoxetine (Prozac, Eli Lilly, Indianapolis, Ind) is perhaps the most familiar. A profusion of these "biochemical" antidepressants have emerged on the psychiatric market since Prozac was released in 1987. From a pharmacological standpoint, it seems inappropriate to call them calmatives. As antidepressants they tend to produce increased energy, even though initial use may sedate some patients, especially those suffering from insomnia. Their therapeutic effects may be delayed by days to weeks. They all possess high safety margins, but their potential effectiveness as incapacitating agents is questionable.

Some researchers suggest that α-2 adrenergic agonists should also be classified as calmatives. Clonidine, the most familiar drug of this type, is effective in very low dosage and used to lower blood pressure or to help in the stabilization of hyperactivity in children. Although potent and able to produce sedation, clonidine would be a highly dangerous drug to use in the field because life-threatening hypotension can develop after even small multiples of the therapeutic dose.

The opioids can also be found in the calmative category, as can exotic drugs such as D_3 dopamine agonists and cholecystokinin-B antagonists. Pramipaxole, a D_3 dopamine agonist, is useful in treating the symptoms of Parkinson's disease, and as little as 0.125 mg supposedly helps to control restless legs syndrome. It has also been used to treat compulsive gambling. Antagonists of cholecystokinin-B (the brain counterpart of the stomach hormone gastrin) can potentiate the analgesic effects of other drugs and lower body temperature under certain conditions. Corticotropin-releasing factor antagonist is a hypothalamic hormone. It stimulates the release of adrenocorticotropic hormone from the pituitary gland. How an antagonist to this hormone would serve any useful purpose as a calmative is unclear.

The calmatives group has come to include not only the neuropeptides and neuromodulators but many preexisting drug families long recognized by pharmacologists to be distinctly different in their effects. Often belladonnoid drugs (such as BZ) or scopolamine, formerly marketed as Sleep-Eze (Whitehall Laboratories, New York, NY), an over-the-counter bedtime sedative, are barely mentioned. Sleep-Eze was a popular drug among people with insomnia until it was taken off the market because of concerns about potential abuse. Sominex (JB Williams Company, Cranford, NJ), Sleep-Eze, and Unisom (Pfizer Consumer Healthcare, New York, NY) are now over-the-counter drugs containing diphenhydramine (an antihistamine) instead of scopolamine as their active ingredient. Both antihistamines and cannabinoids have also been ignored by the calmative classifiers.

From a purely practical standpoint, administering some of the candidates with larger molecules by aerosol, or even via ingested food or water, is difficult to imagine. Not only are many neuropeptides quite large, consisting of long chains of amino acids, but they would also be extremely difficult to disseminate in the field. Even if they reach the lungs or digestive tract, they would ultimately be obliged to cross the blood–brain barrier, a difficult task for many complex molecules.

Pharmaceutical companies are currently developing methods to ferry or "piggyback" hormones, antibodies and other proteins, and large polypeptide molecules through the blood–brain barrier, but current technology can not surmount all the associated limitations of using such chemicals in a battlefield environment.[87] Nevertheless, according to Chapter V of the *Army Science and Technology Master Plan*, "...under investigation are protein carriers for transport of immunogenic peptides; vectored vaccines with multiple immunogenic properties; approaches to block the actions of threat agents on target receptor sites; and rapid evaluation of genetically altered microbes."[88] Such techniques may also be applicable to neuropeptide and neuromodulator incapacitating agents, but their relevance to field dissemination of calmatives is obscure.

Anticholinergic Deliriants

Anticholinergic deliriants, or "belladonnoids," have been and continue to be the category most likely to be considered for incapacitating agents. "Anticholinergics" is the term commonly used to refer to these drugs because their main action is to block both the central and peripheral muscarinic effects of acetylcholine. Belladonnoids are a subgroup of the anticholinergics that resemble atropine. This useful term, like opioids in the case of morphine-like compounds, refers not only to naturally occurring substances such as atropine and scopolamine, but also to synthetic glycolates that are actively antimuscarinic in the brain. Delirium is the syndrome resulting from doses of these drugs significantly above appropriate clinical doses.[89]

Many psychoactive drugs can produce delirium when given in high multiples of the therapeutic dose. In their classic 1935 monograph, Wolff and Curran enumerated more than 100 drugs and disease-altered metabolic states they had observed to produce delirium.[90] "Deliriants" as a drug category is a seemingly artificial but useful subdivision of chemical agents. It arises from the Latin "delire," meaning "to rave." By the very origin of the term, delirium is equivalent to incapacitation, because it combines confusion, hallucinosis, disorganized speech and behavior, and a variety of autonomic features.

Atropine and scopolamine are esters of tropic acid, which gives them the ability to cross the blood–brain barrier and block central cholinergic receptors of the muscarinic type by competitive inhibition of acetylcholine, the natural neurotransmitter at these sites.[91] Physician investigators at Edgewood found that scopolamine was about 7-fold stronger than atropine in terms of relative central potency. An injection of a very small amount of scopolamine hydrobromide, for example, is sufficient to produce 4 to 6 hours of incapacitating delirium in the average person. A larger dose of atropine sulfate produces a similar effect, but recovery requires 8 to 12 hours.[89,92]

In the peripheral cholinergic nervous system, both drugs cause parasympathetic blockade, resulting in tachycardia, elevation of blood pressure, hyperthermia (through blockade of sweat production), decrease in salivation, and reduction of gastrointestinal and excretory bladder functions. Impairment of near vision, attributable to a mixture of central and peripheral actions, also occurs due to loss of accommodation (from ciliary muscle paralysis) and reduced depth of field (from pupillary enlargement).

The interaction between peripheral and central effects of anticholinergic drugs at different times following administration sometimes causes biphasic changes in such variables as heart rate and peripheral spinal reflexes. For example, heart rate may be slowed initially because of brainstem influences, after which vagal blockade tends to predominate, causing tachycardia. Similarly, knee and ankle reflexes may be exaggerated at first, but are later reduced, a phenomenon mediated by Renshaw interneurons in the spinal cord. The pharmacokinetic principles that govern speed of distribution to the various drug compartments probably explain these biphasic phenomena. Although these variations in effects may seem to be academic distinctions, medical officers need to be aware of them when attempting the differential diagnosis of incapacitation (discussed later in this chapter).

BZ. The most likely incapacitating belladonnoid, and the first studied synthetic example, is 3-quinuclidinyl benzilate, referred to as QNB by neuropharmacologists, but known as "BZ" to the Chemical Corps. This designation probably derives from its benzilate structure, although some people suggest that it comes from the "buzz" it supposedly produces. BZ is a stable glycolate, an environmentally persistent crystalline solid.

Clinical Pharmacology of BZ. BZ's clinical profile closely resembles that of atropine and scopolamine, differing significantly only in duration of action and potency.[93] BZ by the oral route of administration is about 80% as effective as by either the intravenous or intramuscular routes. When applied to the skin in propylene glycol or other appropriate solvent, however, apparent absorption is only 5% to 10%. Pilot studies of percutaneously administered BZ in dimethyl sulfoxide (a solvent vehicle that facilitates the passage of some drugs through the skin) showed a delay in peak effects by approximately 24 hours; contrary to historical treatises suggesting that belladonna drugs are readily absorbed from poultices.

Inhalation studies with BZ, both under laboratory

conditions and when administered in the open air under simulated field conditions, showed it to be approximately 60% as effective as when given orally or parenterally. When breathing is regulated at 1 L per breath, 15 breaths per minute (the typical volume of respiration for a moderately active soldier), approximately 80% of 1-µm aerosol particles (the optimal diameter) is retained by the lungs. Of this quantity about 75% is actually absorbed; the remainder is inactivated within the lung or bronchial lining.[93,94]

Most absorbed BZ is excreted via the urine after hepatic metabolic processing. Edgewood chemist Albert Kondritzer studied the brain distribution of BZ and found it to be eliminated in three stages, roughly in parallel with the clinical phases of BZ symptoms.[95] It appears to be most persistent in the hippocampus and other regions that control memory and cognitive functions.

BZ produces anticholinergic drug effects similar to those produced by atropine and scopolamine, as do many related synthetic belladonnoids. To make quantitative comparisons of the growing number of related compounds subjected to testing, it became necessary to establish operational definitions of such parameters as the minimal effective dose and the incapacitating dose, as well as onset time, duration, and other important attributes. After much discussion, the following definitions were adopted:

- Minimal effective dose: dose required to produce mild cognitive impairment in 50% of the exposed population. The threshold for a minimal effect is two successive scores below 75% of baseline performance on the NF test.[39]
- Incapacitating dose (ID_{50}): dose required to produce two successive scores below 10% of baseline (at which point incapacitation is clinically obvious).[93]
- Onset time: time of first NF score below 25% of baseline, which for BZ is approximately 4 hours.
- Partial recovery time: time at which two successive scores return to 25% or higher in subjects exposed to the ID_{50}.[94]
- Duration: number of hours between onset time and partial recovery time in subjects exposed to the ID_{50}.
- Peripheral potency: dose required to elevate heart rate to a maximum of at least 100 beats per minute. This heart rate was found to be the most reliable indicator of a significant peripheral anticholinergic effect, regardless of baseline heart rate.[94]
- Relative central potency: ratio of peripheral potency to ID_{50}. This ratio was found to be useful in estimating the median lethal dose (LD_{50}) of the belladonnoids, because peripheral potency (manifested by heart rate increase) at the incapacitating dose is a predictor of belladonnoid lethality.[96]

Other operational definitions include full recovery time (the percentage of patients returning to above 75% of baseline for cognitive testing using the NF test), prolongation time (increase in duration at double the ID_{50}), and dose-onset factor (degree to which onset time is shortened as a function of dose).

Features of BZ-Induced Delirium. Delirium is a nonspecific syndrome.[90] Before the systematic study of anticholinergic delirium, however, the clinical features of delirium had not been correlated with performance of cognitive and other tasks under controlled conditions. In the following discussion, aspects of delirium produced by anticholinergic agents will be described in relation to associated impairment in cognitive performance as measured by the facility test already described.

Following the administration of BZ at the minimum effective dose, delirium appears in its mildest form, represented by a drowsy state, with occasional lapses of attention and slight difficulty following complex instructions. Recovery is usually complete by 24 hours.

Moderate delirium generally is manifested by somnolence or mild stupor, indistinct speech, poor coordination, and a generalized slowing of thought processes, along with some confusion and perplexity. Although sluggish, the subject remains in contact with the environment most of the time, with occasional illusions but rarely true hallucinations. NF test scores decline by about 50%. Recovery occurs within 48 hours, and amnesia is minimal.

Individuals receiving the ID_{50} or higher usually develop the full syndrome of delirium. There is very little variation from person to person in their response to BZ (or other belladonnoids), perhaps because these drugs operate more directly on the "hardware" of the brain—neuronal systems where all-or-none activity is more characteristic. Drugs such as LSD, in contrast, act directly at specific serotonin and glutamate receptors and indirectly on others, including dopamine, norepinephrine, and opioid μ-receptors, with effects that vary in relation to the prevailing mood, arousal, and motivational state of the subject.

During the first few hours, subjects show increasing confusion but remain oriented. When delirium is present in its full-blown state, however, the individual seems to be in a "waking dream," staring and muttering, sometimes shouting, as simple items in the environment are variably perceived as structures, animals, or people. These hallucinations may arise from some trivial aspect of the surroundings: a strip of floor molding has been called a strip of bacon; a bulky object led one subject to yell for help for an injured woman; and another described a Lilliputian baseball game on the rubber padding, evidently stimulated by uneven patches or shadows. A total lack of insight generally surrounds these misperceptions.

A striking characteristic of delirium is its fluctuation from moment to moment, with occasional lucid intervals during which appropriate answers are unexpectedly given to questions. Sometimes the correct answer gets temporarily shunted aside. An example of this unusual phenomenon was a subject who spouted gibberish when asked "who wrote Hamlet?" When asked where he lived a short time later, he answered, "Shakespeare." Phantom behaviors, such as plucking or picking at the air or at garments, are also characteristic. This behavior was termed "carphologia" in the 19th century. Sometimes two delirious individuals play off each other's imaginings. In one study one subject was observed to mumble, "Gotta cigarette?" and when his companion held out a nonexistent pack, he followed with, "S'okay, don't wanna take your last one."

Recovery from drug-induced delirium is gradual, the duration presumably paralleling the pharmacokinetic persistence of the causative agent. The more spectacular and florid hallucinations are gradually replaced by more modest distortions in perception. For example, illusions of large animals are replaced by those of smaller animals. As awareness of the time and place and recognition of people gradually returns, the subject enters a transitional phase during which he recognizes that his mental faculties are not what they should be, but suspects that something else is wrong. This may produce temporary paranoid delusions and withdrawal (or occasionally an attempt to escape from the room). A psychiatrist might be reminded of similar states observed in some schizophrenic patients.

During the period from onset of maximum effects until partial recovery at between 24 and 48 hours, the volunteers are completely unable to perform any task requiring comprehension and problem-solving. During this time and even during their gradual recovery, they are generally docile. Aggressive or assaultive behavior does not occur, except in the form of moments of irritability, sometimes punctuated by an attempted punch or other expression of annoyance. "Berserk" behavior or attack with an object is absent, contrary to some descriptions by those unfamiliar with the BZ delirious syndrome. Confusion may give way to panic in a few subjects as they near recovery, but this is always motivated by fear of imagined harm, and never by a desire to inflict severe bodily injury. Not once in several hundred drug-induced delirious states during the BZ studies was significant injury inflicted on the attending staff.

A period of restorative sleep generally precedes the return to normal cognitive function, accompanied by cheerful emotions. Many of the BZ subjects described a feeling of well-being following recovery. Initially, as reflected in their posttest write-ups, those who had been delirious can recall some events, but, as with dreams, their recollection soon fades. Thereafter, these fleeting memories are forgotten, in keeping with the clinical adage that delirium of all types is followed by amnesia.

Other glycolates. At least a dozen synthetic glycolates were provided to Edgewood Arsenal for testing in volunteer subjects. John Biel, at Lakeside Laboratories, Milwaukee, Wisconsin, prepared many of these compounds, making it possible to compare belladonnoid structures that differed only quantitatively in such parameters as potency, duration, speed of onset, and relative central potency.[96] His colleague, Leo Abood, was an early pioneer in the study of many of these compounds and formulated useful structure/activity relationships showing that duration and potency, for example, could be predicted from the position of particular features of the structure, such as the location of a hydroxyl moiety. Testing in volunteers validated many of these observations about structure. Abood's chapter in a National Academy of Sciences publication on chemical agents also contains a useful compilation of the number of volunteers tested at Edgewood Arsenal with each belladonnoid and a summary of the observed effects.[97]

Abood adds his personal knowledge of three graduate students who surreptitiously ingested up to 10 mg of BZ and were hospitalized. All three students had been in academic difficulty and had considered dropping out of school; however, after their recovery, their academic performance improved dramatically, and all went on to obtain PhDs and continue in gainful employment. In addition, several independent observers thought the students seemed happier and better adjusted. These unexpected changes tend to corroborate previous claims of psychiatric benefits from belladonna-induced coma therapy.[98–100]

Many synthetic belladonnoids were tested in the volunteers. Some of these were found to be more potent with fewer side effects, such as no significant increase in heart rate.[101–105] Testing continued to find synthetic belladonnoids with much shorter duration and with full recovery occurring within 1 to 2 days, making a convenient agent against which to test antidotes.[106–111]

Several other glycolates that were lower in potency but shorter in duration than BZ received limited testing.[112–115] BZ has often been incorrectly described as far stronger than LSD, and the reported "hundreds of compounds more potent than BZ" do not exist.[116] After the BZ program ended, enhanced glycolate formulations for use as incapacitating agents were deemed dangerous to develop and, because of their perceived slow onset time during evaluations, unsuitable for military use.

TREATMENT STUDIES

The ability to reverse the incapacitating effects of belladonnoids (or drugs such as LSD and opioids) is of paramount importance, not only for the sake of the affected individual, but also in any operation that needs to preserve fighting strength. Given in doses above their ID_{50}, belladonnoids, although eminently treatable, can be swift in action; a large number of troops in a delirious state would pose a serious problem for commanders. Fortunately in the case of BZ, during the onset and peak periods of drug action, somnolence (or even coma) would keep individuals virtually immobile for up to 24 hours—probably much longer with high doses. This somnolent period would provide time to place victims in a safe environment and treat them with an anticholinesterase to prevent the emergence of irrational behavior.

For at least 24 hours, subjects incapacitated by BZ show little inclination, and are unable, to act aggressively. This placidity is a pharmacological phenomenon. Aggression in mouse-killing rats, for example, is inhibited completely by BZ-like drugs. These rats otherwise attack and kill mice placed in their cage without delay. BZ and other belladonnoid agents could legitimately be called "calmatives." Lack of in-depth understanding of the 2- to 3-day delay between onset of delirium and partial recovery, which is the only time when behavior may become active and impulsive (though rarely aggressive), may have led to the conclusion that BZ use would provoke mayhem.

Before the mid 1960s, standard pharmacological textbooks taught that no antidotes, including cholinesterase inhibitors, were able to reverse belladonnoid delirium.[117] However, in 1963, the antidotal effectiveness of physostigmine was rediscovered at Edgewood Arsenal[118] when Goodman located and translated an 1864 report by an Austrian ophthalmologist on the successful use of Calabar bean extract (the natural source of physostigmine).[117] The report recounted the story of two prisoners who drank a quantity of tincture of belladonna, thinking it was alcohol. The physician called to attend them learned they had consumed belladonna, noted their saucer-like pupils, and suspected drug-induced delirium.[119] The doctor next reasoned that, because a few drops of Calabar extract reversed enlarged pupils and the loss of near vision caused by the belladonna drops he used for eye examinations, Calabar might have similar antidotal effects in the brain. To the most affected prisoner he gave a small amount of the extract in a spoonful of sugar and gave only plain sugar water to the other. Soon, the first man returned to a lucid state, able to describe the theft of the belladonna solution, while the second man remained unchanged.

Toward the end of the 1940s, perhaps seeking an alternative to insulin coma, a small group of psychiatrists began to use atropine to produce coma in psychiatric patients.[99–101] The physicians who introduced this unusual form of pharmacotherapy, unlike the authors of human pharmacology chapters at the time, were evidently aware that physostigmine could bring atropinized patients back to conscious awareness. They reported routinely administering 4 mg of physostigmine by injection soon after inducing a short period of atropine coma.

This useful finding received little attention from mainstream clinicians. The growing preference for neostigmine as treatment for such disorders as surgical ileus and myasthenia gravis had made physostigmine increasingly obsolescent. Neostigmine was valued for its lack of central effects, but physostigmine easily enters the brain and in fact may have been avoided because of its potential central toxicity. Anticholinesterase compounds other than physostigmine were also studied at the Edgewood clinical facility to determine their effectiveness as a BZ antidote. Even lethal nerve agents were evaluated as antidotes for BZ,[120,121] but their clinical application is highly impractical and inappropriate. Physostigmine was determined to be the safest and most appropriate antidote for BZ intoxication.

Repeated injections of physostigmine in BZ-exposed individuals, usually 2 to 4 mg at hourly intervals, maintained coherent speech and the ability to carry out tasks; without the physostigmine the individuals would have been continuously delirious for the next 2 to 3 days. In both cases, NF test scores rose dramatically when physostigmine was administered, reverted to an incapacitated level when physostigmine was temporarily withheld, and responded again when treatment was reinstituted.

In 1967 Edgewood physicians had published the first double-blind controlled study demonstrating the effectiveness of physostigmine in reversing scopolamine delirium.[118] Later they reconfirmed this finding in studies of atropine and of Ditran (Lakeside Laboratories, Milwaukee, Wis), a 2 to 1 mixture of two similar belladonnoid glycolates.[89] In the late 1950s and early 1960s, Ditran coma (like atropine coma, a decade earlier) enjoyed brief popularity as a treatment for depression.[122–124] In Edgewood studies between 1962 and 1967, physostigmine proved equally effective as an antidote to the follow-on glycolates described above. Similar findings were soon reported in civilian studies.[125–128]

Deliria produced by overdose with other drugs possessing anticholinergic side effects, such as diazepam, tricyclic antidepressants, and antihistamines, were also found to be treatable with physostigmine.[128–130] When given by the intravenous route, a dose of 30 μg/kg of physostigmine was sufficient to partially reverse the anticholinergic delirium produced by a variety of belladonnoids, although at least 45 μg/kg was the initial dose required to obtain good results.

Physostigmine has also been used and reported to be effective for morphine-induced respiratory depression; alcohol withdrawal; and the effects of heroin, ketamine, and fentanyl.[131] Its mode of action in these instances may be partially due to a direct arousal effect, rather than simple inhibition of cholinesterase. Case reports confirming its efficacy have come from the director of the Rocky Mountain Poison and Drug Center, near Denver, Colorado.[125] The use of physostigmine as an antidote was also favorably reviewed by the director of the Poison Control Center in Munich, Germany.[132] Although in undrugged patients doses of as little as 2 to 3 mg of physostigmine alone may cause nausea and other signs of cholinergic excess (eg, salivation, intestinal cramping, and diarrhea), an intramuscular dose of 4 mg is generally well tolerated without any side effects when given as an antagonist to belladonnoid intoxication. In more than 100 subjects treated by one of the authors, the only unusual side effects were transient fasciculations of the platysma (a thin superficial neck muscle) in one subject, and transient periods of nausea and vomiting in a few others.[96]

If excessive physostigmine is given in the absence of belladonnoid intoxication, adverse effects can easily be reversed by injecting 1 to 2 mg of atropine. Physostigmine, if administered intravenously, should be given gradually because a bolus effect may cause cardiac arrhythmias or even cardiac arrest. Most of these untoward outcomes, however, have occurred in patients who were in poor general health or suffering from heart disease. Back titration with atropine can usually avert or reverse disturbing anomalies of response.

When the diagnosis is in doubt, an intramuscular test dose of 1 to 2 mg of physostigmine, repeated after 20 minutes if necessary, is recommended. Once the diagnosis of delirium has been established by a definite clearing of the sensorium, improvement can be sustained by repeating the treatment at intervals of 1 to 4 hours. Changes in heart rate and intellectual performance can provide a guide to dosage. For example, if heart rate rises and confusion increases (quickly assessable by asking for serial subtraction of 7s from 100), supplemental doses can safely be given. Polish investigators studying the effects of high-dose atropine treatment of psychiatric patients reported giving as much as 15 mg of physostigmine in a single injection to terminate atropine coma.[133] They did not describe any adverse effects.

Maintenance treatment of delirium produced by BZ or other long-acting agents is best handled by the use of oral physostigmine, mixing it with fruit juice to mask its bitter taste. Dosage by the oral route is only two thirds as effective as by the parenteral route and should be adjusted accordingly. In a combat zone, the oral route may, in fact, be the only practical way to treat large numbers of casualties. Medical technicians can do the job under the supervision of a physician.

For reasons that are not fully understood, physostigmine is relatively ineffective if given during the onset phase of belladonnoid intoxication. The treatment team should therefore not be discouraged if early administration of physostigmine fails to bring about immediate, dramatic improvement. Unfortunately, use of the antagonist does not shorten the duration of the underlying intoxication. Also, if initial treatment is not maintained, final recovery may be slightly delayed.[96] Although physostigmine is probably not as highly regarded as it was during the 1970s and 1980s, it has predictable effects, and there are specific indications for its use. Test doses of 1 mg may safely be given, and minor improvement in mental status, or a decrease in tachycardia, can justify the safe use of larger titrated doses.

Whether or not physostigmine is available, supportive measures are important. It may be proper to evacuate and hospitalize patients with severe cases. Oral tetrahydroaminacridine in doses of 200 mg was also tested as an antagonist against BZ and proved to be moderately effective.[93] Its use as an anticholinesterase treatment of Alzheimer patients has since been approved by the US Food and Drug Administration. In an Edgewood pilot study, tetrahydroaminacridine caused temporary mild changes in hepatic function tests, and further testing was discontinued. Similar changes were noted in civilian patients but did not prevent its approved use.

SAFETY OF THE GLYCOLATES

As with most drugs, the per kilogram lethality of BZ (for example) is progressively less in larger species. This relationship provides an extrapolated LD_{50} of 3 to 5 mg/kg, which would suggest a very high therapeutic ratio (more than 200). Such a safety margin is probably too optimistic, however, and a ratio of 40 has been accepted as a conservative, but more likely, estimate. The latter figure was calculated by noting that preferential affinity for peripheral (such as cardiac) rather than central muscarinic receptors seems to predict the lethality of the various belladonnoids. Before the Edgewood studies, central toxicity was usually considered the cause of death from atropine-like drugs, but it is more likely that cardiotoxicity rather than central respiratory failure is the usual cause of death.

Goodman collected data from hundreds of reports of lethality and survival following high doses of atropine (most of them published in the 19th century) to estimate its LD_{50}.[134] Abood reports survival of at least one individual who ingested more than 1,000 mg of atropine.[98] Recovery took 7 days. This case alone suggests that the LD_{50} is much higher than the values given in textbooks. The LD_{50} values for the various other belladonnoids were calculated by extrapolating from Goodman's estimate from atropine, taking into account the other drugs' relative central potency.[96] The therapeutic ratio for BZ obtained by this method is approximately 40. For scopolamine and other belladonnoids with high relative central potency, the therapeutic index is probably at least 100.

In actual use, inhalation doses would be highly variable, depending to a degree on weather conditions and methods of dissemination. The Operations Research Branch at Edgewood Arsenal computed dose distribution from a point source, ignoring wind and other factors. Although difficult to apply with confidence to a real-life situation, their results showed that airborne concentration would taper rapidly from any single source, causing a gradient of dosage.

A 1964 feasibility study (Project Dork) involved 10 volunteers and a team of medical personnel at Dugway Proving Ground, Utah.[94] The subjects, standing on a flatbed trailer that moved to track the cloud, inhaled small particles of BZ disseminated from a point source. Breath samples from their modified masks were fed to spectrophotometric devices, monitored by technicians and the physician, who watched the men and gave them telephonic directions from an airtight booth mounted just behind them. Cumulative dose measurements in real time allowed the physician to terminate the exposure when the putative median incapacitating exposure was reached. At 1,000 yards, 50 pounds of BZ, floated downwind under ideal atmospheric conditions, was required to reach the desired dose.

The volunteers actually had to jog in place for most of 40 minutes to inhale the required dose. Considering that the arc subtended by the cloud of BZ was probably no more than a few degrees, it would presumably take thousands of kilograms of BZ to produce incapacitating concentrations throughout 360° at a distance of 1,000 yards. Under less than ideal weather conditions it would take much more. This study provides some idea of the limitations of point source dissemination of agents possessing potency similar to that of BZ. It also underlines the importance of accurate logistical calculations.

The operations analysis group at Edgewood developed idealized models for the dissemination of aerosolized BZ. Realistic projections, however, would require giving appropriate weights to all the geographic, terrain, and atmospheric conditions in a given tactical situation. Evasive action and protective measures taken by the target population would add further variance. Aiming at a lower target dose would be one way to minimize lethality while attaining the desired goal of disrupting a group's ability to function. Taking care of those who were completely nonfunctional would divert those who were unaffected. It would then be necessary to rely on partly incapacitated personnel whose dependability would be uncertain. A military commander, even if personally protected from the agent, would undoubtedly find it difficult to contend with such a complicated situation, even if the median dose absorbed by his troops were only a fraction of the ID_{50}.

Another theoretical possibility is the use of combinations. For example, a rapidly acting but short-lasting belladonnoid could be mixed with a longer-acting agent that would take effect later and last from 1 to 3 days (depending on the choice). A more problematic but possibly effective mixture would be a fast-acting, potent opioid combined with a slower-acting belladonnoid. Opium was used to manage the agitation of belladonna delirium for centuries before physostigmine replaced it. Whether such a mixture would increase the danger of lethal overdose more than either agent used singly could only be learned from dose-response animal studies using various combinations of candidate opioids and belladonnoids.

DIAGNOSIS OF INCAPACITATING AGENT SYNDROMES

There seems little likelihood that agents other than anticholinergics, still the only drugs known to be effective and reasonably safe, would be useful on the battlefield. Several reports suggest that BZ-like agents have already been used, in Croatia and possibly elsewhere. It is improbable, however, that such agents would be used by nations (or groups such as Al Qaeda) whose predominant goal is the destruction of life. Nevertheless, elusive maladies are invariably reported after any major conflict. The probable overestimation of the number of injuries from Agent Orange exposure in the Vietnam War and the so-called "Gulf War syndrome" are 20th century examples of this phenomenon.[135] Medical officers must therefore be able to distinguish chemical intoxication from illnesses of nonchemical origin.

Impaired performance on the battlefield is much more likely to result from stress, illicit drug use, lack of motivation, or psychiatric illness than from a chemical agent. Intoxication produced by belladonnoid agents, by contrast, should be easy to recognize if the physician maintains the proper index of suspicion. Medical students were long taught the medical adage "dry as a bone, red as a beet, hot as a hare, and mad as a hatter" as a means of remembering the features of belladonna poisoning.

As discussed, glycolate anticholinergics can vary tremendously in their potency and duration of action. Signs and symptoms may last as few as 2 hours or as long as several weeks. Differential diagnosis may be more difficult with glycolates that produce few or no peripheral antimuscarinic features, especially at the low end of the incapacitating dose range. Even the pupils may not be greatly enlarged. Familiarity with the behaviors typical of delirium, such as phantom drinking or smoking, picking or groping behavior, nonsensical speech, random disrobing, and the inability to follow simple instructions should greatly assist in making the diagnosis in such cases.

Limited or covert use of other agents (those not suitable for large-scale dissemination) makes it important to recognize the effects of LSD and other psychedelics. Because LSD is a stimulant and usually prevents sleep, medical officers should not expect to see drowsiness or sedation. Staring, enigmatic smiling, and unusual preoccupation with ordinary objects are not uncommon. Responses to commands may be superficially normal. Laughter may supervene, but so may insubordinate and oppositional behavior. There are no practical diagnostic tests for psychedelic drugs (although a sensitive fluorometric method for quantitative detection of LSD is known, and refrigerated blood samples could be useful in making a definitive diagnosis at a later time).[44]

Marijuana intoxication is common in areas where the drug is indigenous, and the presence of reddened conjunctivae, along with the lack of concern and relaxed joviality that marijuana produces, should make the diagnosis obvious. There is little likelihood that purified tetrahydrocannabinols (the active component of cannabis) would be used in a general military setting. Blood and urine can be tested if definitive proof of cannabis use is needed, but such tests are not always feasible or available.

An important, sometimes overlooked cause of bizarre symptoms and behavior is anxiety, which can manifest as dizziness, tachycardia, sweating, headache, and even loss of sensation or ability to move parts of the body. Observation and reassurance may diminish these symptoms, providing a clue to the diagnosis. Comparable syndromes such as "soldier's heart," "Da Costa's syndrome," "shell shock," "combat neurosis," "combat fatigue," and "traumatic neurosis" are terms that arose during past wars to refer to incapacitation of psychiatric origin.[135]

Another important differential diagnosis is heat exhaustion, and more importantly, heat stroke. These conditions can also impair performance and may mimic glycolate intoxication. Individuals with heat stroke will not be sweating and may have warm, flushed, skin. They have very high temperatures (106°F or higher) and may be delirious, unconscious, or have seizures. Heat stroke is a medical emergency. These patients must have their body temperature reduced quickly and be monitored closely to prevent failure of critical organ systems.

Whether covertly or overtly delivered, the differential diagnosis of incapacitation is basically the same as used in typical emergency room overdose cases. Standard textbooks and manuals provide adequate guidelines, as in Table 12-1. The possibility that secret research might produce a highly potent, unfamiliar variant of a known psychoactive drug cannot, however, be ruled out. Blood or urine analysis would probably be needed to demonstrate the drug's presence and identify its chemical structure. Medical officers in the field would probably not have access to the instruments required for precise analysis, but their probability of facing completely unfamiliar chemical substances is low. Exhibit 12-1 is a summary of signs, symptoms, field detection, decontamination methods, and medical management of BZ and fentanyl derivatives.

TABLE 12-1

DIFFERENTIAL DIAGNOSIS FOR INCAPACITATING AGENTS

Sign or Symptom	Possible Etiology
Restlessness, dizziness, giddiness, failure to obey orders, confusion, erratic behavior, stumbling or staggering, vomiting	Anticholinergics, indoles, cannabinoids, anxiety reaction, other intoxications (such as alcohol, bromides, lead, barbiturates)
Dryness of mouth, tachycardia at rest, elevated temperature, flushed face, blurred vision, pupillary dilation, slurred or nonsensical speech, hallucinatory behavior, disrobing, mumbling, picking behavior, stupor, coma	Anticholinergics
Inappropriate smiling or laughing; irrational fear; distractibility; difficulty expressing self; perceptual distortions; labile increases in pupil size, heart rate, and blood pressure; stomach cramps and vomiting	Indoles (may mimic schizophrenic psychosis in some respects)
Euphoria, relaxation, day-dreaming, unconcerned attitude, easy laughter, hypotension, and dizziness on sudden standing	Cannabinoids
Tremor, clinging or pleading, crying, clear answers, decrease in disturbance with reassurance, history of nervousness or immaturity, phobias, bodily disturbances such as blindness and paralysis	Anxiety reaction
Sleepiness, ataxia, rapid unconsciousness, miosis, reduced quality of respirations decrease with resulting respiratory depression	Fentanyl (carfentanyl)

Data sources: (1) Departments of the Army, Navy, and Air Force, and Commandant, Marine Corps. *Treatment of Chemical Agent Casualties and Conventional Military Chemical Injuries*. Washington, DC: HQ: DA, DN, DAF, Commandant, MC1995: 3–1. Field Manual 8-285, NAVMED P-5041, AFJMan 44-149, FMFM 11-11. (2) US Army Medical Research Institute of Chemical Defense. *Medical Management of Chemical Casualties Handbook.* 4th ed. Aberdeen Proving Ground, Md: USAMRICD; 2007.

EXHIBIT 12-1

SUMMARY OF BZ AND FENTANYL DERIVATIVES

- **Signs and symptoms**
  - BZ and other glycolates: mydriasis; dry mouth; dry skin; increased deep tendon reflexes; decreased level of consciousness; confusion; disorientation; disturbances in perception and interpretation (illusions and/or hallucinations); denial of illness; short attention span; impaired memory.
  - Fentanyl derivatives (carfentanil): dizziness, sleepiness, ataxia, miosis (if there is no hypoxia; with hypoxia there is pupil dilation), rapid unconsciousness, vomiting, decreased respirations, central apnea, coma.
- **Field detection:** No field detector is available for either BZ or fentanyl derivatives.
- **Decontamination**
  - BZ: gentle but thorough flushing of skin and hair with water or soap and water is all that is required. Remove clothing.
  - Fentanyl derivatives (carfentanil): No decontamination required.
- **Management**
  - BZ
    - Antidote: physostigmine.
    - Supportive: monitoring of vital signs, especially core temperature.
  - Fentanyl derivatives (carfentanil)
    - Antidote: opioid antagonist naloxone/naltrexone.
    - Supportive: monitoring of vital signs. Proper positioning of patient to maintain airway is critical until effects of central respiratory depression diminish.

Adapted from: US Army Medical Research Institute of Chemical Defense. *Medical Management of Chemical Casualties Handbook.* 4th ed. Aberdeen Proving Ground, Md: USAMRICD; 2007.

EXHIBIT 12-2

ANCILLARY SUPPORTIVE MEASURES FOR THE TREATMENT OF DELIRIUM

- Control and containment are of primary concern because delirium can easily lead to accidents and inadvertent injury to others. Comatose or stuporous casualties may emerge from immobility into a stage of persistent crawling or attempted climbing (primitive behaviors sometimes called "progresso ostinato" [obstinate progression] in 19th-century descriptions of delirium). Tethering or otherwise loosely restraining individuals who are disoriented is preferable to letting them move about freely without close supervision.
- The danger of hyperthermia must be considered if the environment is warmer than 75°F. Death from relatively low doses of anticholinergics has occurred due to impairment of sweating. Wet cloth is effective to reduce body temperature, and the casualty should be placed in the shade, if available.
- Dryness of the mouth and parching of the lips should be managed with moist swabs and small amounts of vaseline or unguents. Fluids should be given sparingly and food withheld until the individual is obviously capable of normal chewing and swallowing. If it is determined that the patient is cognizant enough to manage foods and has oral motor skills, hard candy may be given to induce sufficient salivation to keep the tongue moist.
- Significant skin abrasions can be caused by persistent repetitive movements, especially against rough surfaces. The use of wrappings or gloves may be useful. A tendency to remove clothing is common, and reflects a general regression to simple habitual behaviors. If the environment is harsh, the casualty's clothing may have to be secured so it cannot be removed.
- Evacuation from the field to more adequate medical facilities is desirable in most cases. If evacuation is not possible, separation of the affected individuals into small groups (eg, in tents) is preferable to large aggregations, in which a few confused and hyperactive individuals can lead to an escalating problem of crowd control.

Adapted from: Ketchum JS, Sidell, FR. Incapacitating agents. In: Sidell FR, Takafuji ET, Franz DR, eds. *Medical Aspects of Biological Warfare.* In: Zajtchuk R, Bellamy RF, eds. *Textbook of Military Medicine.* Washington, DC: Department of the Army, Office of The Surgeon General, Borden Institute; 1997: 301.

MEDICAL MANAGEMENT

The standard measures for management of casualties apply to victims of incapacitating agents. Following provisional diagnosis, removal of the patient from the offending environment and decontamination are required. If aggressive agitation or delirium is present, segregation and even restraint measures may be needed, which should not be regarded as punitive (a volunteer who was grossly incompetent during an indoor simulation of a military outpost later commented that in battle he should be tied to a tree, since he would at least be protected from dangerous acts and would not remember it later anyway).

During the Korean conflict, Colonel Albert Glass and colleagues concluded that treatment close to the front lines produced a better psychiatric outcome than evacuation to medical facilities further to the rear. Heavy sedation was effective in dimming the memory of traumatic aspects of injury in patients whose primary problem was emotional. More often than not, a 3-day period of treatment with sedatives and supportive measures was sufficient to restore the fighting capacity of the affected soldier. This approach to treatment applies to incapacitating agents equally well when used with the appropriate antidotal regimen. Finally, as in any emergency, good training and common sense are the most important ingredients of good care. Exhibit 12-2 lists ancillary supportive measures for the treatment of casualties with delirium.

NONLETHAL WEAPONS: A POLICY PERSPECTIVE

This section discussed the policy context and history of the proposals to use or not to use the various potential "nonlethal," "low lethality," "reduced lethality," and "incapacitating agents."[2] The end of the Cold War modified the missions faced by the US military; direct involvement in asymmetrical conflicts became more important. Peacekeeping missions (in the Balkans); intervention in regional/civil conflicts (in the Balkans, the Caribbean, and Africa); and occupation in the face of an armed insurgency (in Afghanistan and Iraq) became common and drew US military forces into conflicts in which substantial civilian populations, often hostile, were involved. At the same time, intense satellite news coverage, often by foreign news media, meant that US military interactions with civilian crowds were under immediate and intense video scrutiny.

The taking of civilian hostages by terrorist groups has highlighted the need for interventions that would not cause casualties among hostages. This resulted in an increased military interest in NLWs to minimize unnecessary civilian casualties and property damage. Following the 1995 evacuation of United Nations forces from Somalia, where Marines were issued riot control agents (RCAs), the Marine Corps was given primary responsibility in July 1996 to develop new NLWs under the Joint Non-lethal Weapons Directorate.[25] This authority included evaluation of the legality and the usefulness of proposed new NLWs.

A number of chemical and biological weapons intended to be "incapacitating agents" of low lethality had been developed during the Cold War, but all have been banned by international treaties to which the United States is a party. The CWC bans development, production, and possession of any chemical weapon intended to cause death or "temporary incapacitation." The 1975 Biological Weapons Convention similarly bans biological or toxin agents with similar effects. The United States has renounced use of such weapons under any circumstances. These treaties prohibit not only the use but also the development or possession of these chemical and biological weapons.

RCAs, nonlethal chemical agents with effects that disappear spontaneously and quickly (within minutes) after exposure ceases, remain legal. The use of these agents, typically "irritant" chemicals (such as CN, CS, and OC) commonly referred to as tear gases, is constrained by the CWC. The CWC recognizes the legitimate use of RCAs by civilian police forces, or by military forces performing police-like duties, but prohibits use of RCAs "in warfare."

This prohibition had long been established by state parties to the 1925 Geneva Protocol, and the extensive use of RCAs in the Vietnam War by the United States to augment the effects of lethal weapons resulted in their specific inclusion in the CWC.[62] The United States does not consider RCAs to be chemical weapons, and US policy reserves the right to use RCAs under some limited military circumstances. However, US policy also recognizes that other nations (including some close allies) do not recognize these reservations as valid.[136] The United States has thus far opted not to employ RCAs in engagements in which organized armed combatants are active, such as the Iraqi insurgency.

Novel chemical or biochemical NLWs face substantial legal barriers to acceptance as legal weapons. Malodorants, if effective, presumably would qualify as RCAs, but as such their use in combat would be constrained. Useful chemical/pharmacological "calmatives" face substantially greater legal barriers. To be effective in military or paramilitary operations, their effects would likely need to be severe enough or persist long enough after exposure to qualify as causing "temporary incapacitation," so their development, stockpiling, and use would be banned by the CWC.

Even if such chemical agents were found to be acceptable under US interpretations of international law, de facto acceptability would depend on acceptance by the civilian political process and, as with the use of RCAs, would be influenced significantly by world opinion. Novel NLWs using new modalities such as acoustic, microwave, and laser effects are not currently constrained by treaty law; however, the immediate and long-term safety of such devices would doubtless be debated, possibly resulting in constraints (by unilateral US policy or by international treaty agreements) being applied after their introduction. The appearance of military lasers designed to permanently blind personnel in the 1990s resulted in the addition of a protocol to the 1980 United Nations Convention on Certain Conventional Weapons banning such devices. Although the United States has not yet ratified this protocol, it has agreed to abide by its terms.[137]

Considerable controversy over the desirability of developing and employing new NLWs exists.[22] Some US military opinion fears that employment of NLWs by military forces would be interpreted by adversaries as a lack of resolve to use lethal force.[138] Many in the international arms control community fear that development of biochemical NLWs would weaken or destroy existing treaty prohibitions against chemical and biological weapons, and result in a renewed biochemical arms race involving both lethal and nonlethal agents that would not only increase the danger of chemical and biological warfare between national military organizations, but also allow proliferation of biochemical weapons technology to nonstate terrorist organizations.[139] Similarly, arms control advocates fear that development and employment of novel acoustic, microwave, and laser weapons would stimulate an arms race using these modalities, all of which lend themselves to easy modification into lethal or permanently disabling weapons.[86]

Other military and civilian opinion sees the development of modern NLWs as a method of reducing undesired and unintended collateral casualties when civilians are placed in danger during military or paramilitary operations. These advocates of new NLWs point out that restrictions or prohibitions on the use of new NLWs may result in the use of lethal weapons by default.[140] Perhaps the greatest uncertainty in NLW policy is how safe and effective new NLWs will be, and how the existing and future restrictions should be applied to their use against threats encountered in the changing circumstances of the 21st century.[140]

SUMMARY

The search for incapacitating agents capable of temporarily preventing military personnel from performing their duties (without permanent injury) has a long and colorful history. Candidate compounds offer promise, but, for a variety of reasons, they have not generally been used in overt warfare in the 20th century. Preference for conventional lethal weapons by most aggressors and the many uncertainties applying to NLW use by friendly nations has led to their elimination from the US arsenal. In the attempt to find an incapacitating agent that would meet the numerous constraints imposed by practical and political concerns, many studies were conducted, including the program at Edgewood Arsenal. Although an ideal incapacitating agent was never found, much was learned from the search.

A major medical benefit arising from the study of belladonnoids in volunteers was the demonstration that physostigmine (and other anticholinesterase agents) could be both effective and safe when properly used in healthy individuals. The usefulness of physostigmine has been recognized in mainstream medical practice; it has proven useful as an antidote for delirium brought on by belladonnoid overdose and other drugs with significant anticholinergic effects.

Reversible incapacitation by nonchemical methods or by psychedelic drugs such as LSD and other indole derivatives, as well as centrally active phenethylamines, tranquilizers, or antipsychotic drugs, are either insufficiently effective or carry risks that make their use unlikely. The recent use of potent opioids to release hostages from terrorists in Moscow resulted in high lethality, although Russia has considered the drugs safe enough for potential field use. More futuristic concepts, such as the use of agonists or antagonists at neuroregulator or neuromodulator receptor sites, do not appear to be feasible at the present time.

REFERENCES

1. US Department of Defense. *Policy for Non-Lethal Weapons*. Washington, DC: DoD; 1996. DoD Directive 3000.3. Available at: http://www.dtic.mil/whs/directives/corres/pdf/300003p.pdf. Accessed July 25, 2007.

2. Ketchum JS, Sidell, FR. Incapacitating agents. In: Sidell FR, Takafuji ET, Franz DR, eds. *Medical Aspects of Chemical and Biological Warfare.* In: Zajtchuk R, Bellamy RF, eds. *Textbook of Military Medicine.* Washington, DC: Department of the Army, Office of The Surgeon General, Borden Institute; 1997: Chap 11.

3. Frontinus SJ, Bennet CH, trans. *The Strategems*. London, England: William Heinemann; 1925. Cited by: Goodman E. *The Descriptive Toxicology of Atropine.* Edgewood Arsenal, Md; 1961.

4. Buchanan G; Watkins J, trans. *The History of Scotland.* London, England: Henry Fisher & Son and Peter Jackson; 1831. Cited by: Goodman E. *The Descriptive Toxicology of Atropine* Edgewood Arsenal, Md; 1961.

5. Lewin L. *Die Gifte in der Weltgeschichte.* Berlin, Germany: Julius Springer; 1920: 537–538. Cited by: Goodman E. *The Descriptive Toxicology of Atropine.* Edgewood Arsenal, Md; 1961.

6. Mitchel TD. *Materia Medica and Therapeutics.* 2nd ed. Philadelphia, Pa: JB Lippincott; 1857: 233. Cited by: Goodman E. T*The Descriptive Toxicology of Atropine.* Edgewood Arsenal, Md; 1961.

7. Gaultier M, trans. Narrative of the poisoning of one hundred and eighty persons by the berries of belladonna. *Med Phys J* (London). 1814;32:390–393. Cited by: Goodman E. *The Descriptive Toxicology of Atropine.* Edgewood Arsenal, Md; 1961.

8. Lewin L. *Gifte und Vergiftungen.* Berlin, Germany: Georg Stilke; 1929: 809. Cited by: Goodman E. *The Descriptive Toxicology of Atropine.* Edgewood Arsenal, Md; 1961.

9. *The Times.* July 3, 1908:8; July 9, 1908:7. Cited by: Goodman E. *The Descriptive Toxicology of Atropine.* Edgewood Arsenal, Md; 1961.

10. The 1925 Geneva Protocol for the Prohibition of the Use of Asphyxiating, Poisonous, or Other Gases and of Bacteriological Methods of Warfare, 17 June 1925. In: *United States Treaties and Other International Agreements (UST).* Vol. 26. Washington, DC: US Government Printing Office; 1976: 571 (26 UST 571). TIAS 8061.

11. Gilbert, M. *The First World War.* New York, NY: Henry Holt and Co; 2004: 478.

12. Hay A. Surviving the impossible: the long march from Srebrenica. An investigation of the possible use of chemical warfare agents. *Med ConflSurviv.* 1998;14:120–155.

13. Basson says he has proof US used hallucinogens in Gulf War. *SAPA (South African Press Association).* July 27, 2001.

14. Hofmann A. *LSD: My Problem Child.* New York, NY: McGraw-Hill; 1980.

15. Abramson HA, Jarvik ME, Kaufman MR, Kornetsky C, Levine A, Wagner M. Lysergic acid diethylamide (LSD-25): I. Physiological and perceptual responses. *J Psychol.* 1995;39:3-60.

16. Huxley A. *Doors of Perception.* New York, NY: Horizon Press; 1965.

17. Lee M, Shlain B. *Acid Dreams: The CIA, LSD and the Sixties Rebellion.* New York, NY: Grove Press; 1998.

18. Kimura KK. *Current Information From Hoffman-Laroche, Inc, on RO2-3308 as of February, 1960.* Army Chemical Center, Md: US Army Chemical Warfare Laboratories; 1960. CWL Special Publication 2-29.

19. *US News and World Report.* December 28, 1959: 10. Cited by: Goodman E. *The Descriptive Toxicology of Atropine.* Edgewood Arsenal, Md, 1961.

20. *Newsweek.* December 28, 1959: 27. Cited by: Goodman E. The descriptive toxicology of atropine. Edgewood Arsenal, Md; 1961.

21. Cook JW, Fiely DP, McGowan MT. Nonlethal weapons: technologies, legalities and potential policies. *Airpower J* [serial online]. 1995. Available at: http://www.airpower.maxwell.af.mil/airchronicles/apj/apj95/spe-ed95_files/mcgowan.htm. Accessed July 26, 2007.

22. Nonlethal weapons give peacekeepers flexibility. *Aviat Week Space Technol.* 1992;137:50.

23. Benford J, Swegle J. *High Power Microwaves.* Norwood, Mass: Artec House; 1991

24. Anderber B, Wolbarsht ML. *Laser Weapons: The Dawn of a New Military Age.* New York, NY: Plenum Press; 1992: 207.

25. Commandant of the Marine Corps. *Joint Concept for Non-Lethal Weapons.* Washington, DC: HQ, Commandant, MC. January 5, 1998.

26. Bunker RJ, ed. *Non-Lethal Weapons: Terms and References.* US Air Force Academy, Colorado: USAF Institute for National Security Studies; 1997. INSS Occasional Paper 15. Available at: http://www.angelfire.com/or/mctrl/non-lethal.html. Accessed December 29, 2005.

27. Everett HR. Representative world modeling. *Robotics Pract.* 1996;spring:31–38.

28. International Committee of the Red Cross. Ottawa Treaty. Convention on the Prohibition of the Use, Stockpiling, Production and Transfer of Anti-Personnel Mines and on Their Destruction, 18 September 1997. Available at: http://www.icrc.org/IHL.nsf/FULL/580?OpenDocument. Accessed April 13, 2006.

29. Sidell FR. Long term health effects of nerve agents and mustard. In: Sidell FR, Takafuji ET, Franz DR, eds. *Medical Aspects of Chemical and Biological Warfare.* In: Zajtchuk R, Bellamy RF, eds. *Textbook of Military Medicine.* Washington, DC: Department of the Army, Office of The Surgeon General, Borden Institute; 1997: Chap 8.

30. Gershon S, Shaw FH. Psychiatric sequelae of chronic exposure to organophosphate insecticides. *Lancet.* 1961;1:1371-1374.

31. Sidell FR. Riot control agents. In: Sidell FR, Takafuji ET, Franz DR, eds. *Medical Aspects of Chemical and Biological Warfare.* In: Zajtchuk R, Bellamy RF, eds. *Textbook of Military Medicine.* Washington, DC: Department of the Army, Office of The Surgeon General, Borden Institute; 1997: Chap 12.

32. Sidell FR, Urbanetti JS, Smith WJ, Hurst CG. Vesicants. In: Sidell FR, Takafuji ET, Franz DR, eds. *Medical Aspects of Chemical and Biological Warfare.* In: Zajtchuk R, Bellamy RF, eds. *Textbook of Military Medicine.* Washington, DC: Department of the Army, Office of The Surgeon General, Borden Institute; 1997: Chap 7.

33. Osmond H. A review of the clinical effects of psychotomimetic agents. In: Solomon D, ed. *LSD – The Consciousness Expanding Drug.* New York, NY: Putnam & Co Ltd; 1964.

34. Grinspoon L, Bakalar J. *Psychedelic Drugs Reconsidered.* New York, NY: The Lindesmith Center; 1997.

35. Ketchum JS. Clinical aspects of incapacitating agents. In: Ballinger CM, Brechner VL, eds. *Endocrines and Enzymes in Anesthesiology.* Springfield, Il: Charles C. Thomas; 1973: 158–166.

36. Shulgin A, Shulgin A. *PIHKAL: A Chemical Love Story.* Berkeley, Calif: Transform Press; 1991.

37. Sim VM. *Clinical Investigation of EA 1729.* Edgewood Arsenal, Md: Chemical Research and Development Laboratory; 1961. CRDL Technical Report 3074.

38. Ketchum JS, Aghajanian GK, Bing O. *The Human Assessment of EA 1729 and EA 3528 by the Inhalation Route.* Edgewood Arsenal, Md: Chemical Research and Development Laboratory; 1964. CRDL Technical Report 3226.

39. Ketchum JS. Incapacitating compounds. In: *Proceedings of the 1st Meeting of the Quadripartite Standing Working Group on Chemical Warfare.* Edgewood Arsenal, Md: Chemical Research and Development Laboratory; 1965.

40. Freedman DX. Chairman and Professor of Psychiatry and Pharmacology, University of Chicago Medical School, Chicago, Il. Personal communication, 1973.

41. Aghajanian GK. Serotonin and the action of LSD in the brain. *Psychiatr Annals.* 1994;24:137-141.

42. Aghajanian GK, Professor of Psychiatry and Pharmacology, Yale University. Personal communication, September 2005.

43. Aghajanian GK, Bing OH. Persistence of lysergic acid diethylamide in the plasma of human subjects. *Clin Pharmacol Ther.* 1964;5:611–614.

44. Ketchum JS. Chemical warfare: secrets almost forgotten. University of California, Los Angeles, California; 2005.

45. McNamara B. Lethality (LD_{50}) of LSD in representative animal species. Unpublished data, Edgewood Arsenal, Md; 1964.

46. West LJ, Pierce CM, Thomas WD. Lysergic acid diethylamide: its effects on a male Asiatic elephant. *Science.*1962;138:1100–1103.

47. Buckman J. Senior Medical Officer, Marlborough Day Hospital, St John's Wood, London, England. Personal communication, July 1965.

48. Leib G. Captain, Medical Corps, US Army Clinical Research Department, Medical Research Laboratory, Edgewood Arsenal, Md. Personal communication, 1968.

49. Aghajanian GK, Bing O. Unpublished report, 1963. Cited by: Ketchum JS. Incapacitating compounds. In: *Proceedings of 1st Meeting of the Quadripartite Standing Working Group on Chemical Warfare.* Edgewood Arsenal, Md; 1965.

50. Leonard BE. *Fundamentals of Psychopharmacology.* 2nd ed. Chichester, United Kingdom: John Wiley; 1997.

51. Shulgin A, Shulgin A. *TIHKAL, the Continuation.* Berkeley, Calif: Transform Press; 1997.

52. Hardman HF, Domino EF, Seevers MH. *The Chemistry and Pharmacology of EA 1476.* Army Chemical Center, Md: US Army Chemical Warfare Laboratories; 1959. Terminal Report on Contract No. DA 18-108-CML-5663.

53. Hardman HF, Domino EF, Seevers MH. *The Chemistry and Pharmacology of Certain Compounds Affecting the Central Nervous System of Animals and Man.* Army Chemical Center, Md: US Army Chemical Warfare Laboratories; 1955.

54. Ketchum JS. The marijuana story and EA 2233. Medical Research Laboratory, Edgewood Arsenal, Md; 1963.

55. Lipka LJ, Lathera CM. Psychoactive agents, seizure production, and sudden death in epilepsy. *J Clin Pharmacol.* 1987;27:169–183.

56. Griffith JD, Cavanaugh J, Held J, Oates JA. Dextroamphetamine. Evaluation of psychomimetic properties in man. *Arch Gen Psychiatry.* 1972;26:97-100.

57. Ketchum JS. Effects of secobarbital on time estimation performance. Medical Research Laboratory, Edgewood Arsenal, Md; 1962.

58. Pert CB, Snyder SH. Opiate receptor: demonstration in nervous tissue. *Science.*1973; 179:1011-4.

59. Sircar R, Zukin SR. Characterization of specific sigma opiate/phencyclidine (PCP)-binding sites in the human brain. *Life Sci.* 1983;33(suppl 1):259-262.

60. Drummond GB, Davis IT, Scott DB. Naloxone: dose dependent antagonism of repiratory depression by Fentanyl in anesthetized patients. *Br J Anaesth.* 1977;49:151-154.

61. Bradberry JC, Raebel MA. Continuous infusion of naloxone in the treatment of narcotic overdose. *Drug Intell Clin Pharm.* 1981;15:945-950.

62. Organisation for the Prohibition of Chemical Weapons. Convention on the Prohibition of the Development, Production, Stockpiling and use of Chemical Weapons and on Their Destruction. Available at: http://www.opcw.org/. Accessed April 13, 1996.

63. Mioduszewski RJ, Reutter SA, Crowley RA, Pullen R, et al. *Dissociation of Opiate-induced Sedation and Respiratory Depression by Opiate Antagonist Coadministration.* Edgewood Arsenal, Md: Chemical Research and Development Center; 1992. TR 339.

64. Mesina JE, Sylvina TJ, Hotaling LC, Pequet-Goad ME, Fox JG. A simple technique for chronic jugular catheterization in ferrets. *Lab Anim Sci.* 1988;38:89-90.

65. Leith DE. Mass transport in mammalian lungs: comparative physiology. In: Miller FJ, Menzel DB, eds. *Fundamental of Extrapolation of Inhaled Toxicants.* Washington, DC: Hemisphere Publishing Co; 1984.

66. Brown D, Baker P. Moscow gas likely a potent narcotic drug normally used to subdue big game. *Washington Post* [online edition]. November 9, 2002: A12.

67. Couzin J. Medicine. A sigh of relief for painkillers. *Science*. 2003;301:150.

68. Chemical and Biological Weapons Nonproliferation Program. The Moscow theater hostage crisis: incapacitants and chemical warfare. Center for Nonproliferation Studies Web site. Available at: http://cns.miis.edu/pubs/week/02110b.htm. Accessed April 21, 2006.

69. Miller J, Lichtblau E. U.S. investigates Moscow theatre siege, seeking Qaeda link. *New York Times*. November 18, 2003. Available at: http://query.nytimes.com/gst/abstract.html?res=F10810FB3D5F0C7A8DDDA80994DB404482&fta=y. Accessed April 13, 2006.

70. Mercadente S, Ferrera P, Villari P, et al. Hyperalgesia: an emerging iatrogenic syndrome. *J Pain Manage*. 2003;26(2):769–775. Available at: http://cns.miis.edu/iiop/cnsdataMercadente. Accessed September 10, 2005.

71. Miller MW, Wild MA, Lance WR. Efficacy and safety of naltrexone hydrochloride for antagonizing carfentanil citrate immobilization in captive Rocky Mountain elk (cervus elaphus nelsoni). *J Wildl Dis*. 1996;32:234–239.

72. Manzke T, Guenther U, Ponimaskin EG, et al. 5-HT4s receptors avert opioid-induced breathing depression without loss of analgesia. *Science*. 2003;301:226–229.

73. Eilers H, Schumacher MA. Opioid-induced respiratory depression: are 5-HT4a receptor agonists the cure? *Molecular Interventions*. 2004;4:197–199.

74. Johnstone M, Evans V, Baigel S. Sernyl (CI-395) in clinical anesthesia. *Br J Anaesth*. 1959;31:433–439.

75. Lanning CF, Harmel MH. Ketamine anesthesia. *Ann Rev Med*. 1975;26:137–141.

76. Bunney BG, Bunney WE, Carlsson A. Schizophrenia and glutamate: an update. In: Davis KL, Charney D, Coyle JT, Nemeroff C, eds. *Neuropsychopharmacology: The Fifth Generation of Progress*. Nashville, Tenn: American College of Neuropsychopharmacology; 2002.

77. Drug Enforcement Agency Intelligence Division, Office of Strategic Intelligence, Domestic Strategic Intelligence Unit and the Dangerous Drugs Strategic Intelligence Unit. PCP: the threat remains. DEA Web site. Available at: http://www.dea.gov/programs/forensicsci/microgram/mg0803/mg0803.html. Accessed on April 13, 2006.

78. Jansen K. *Ketamine: Dreams and Realities*. Sarasota, Fla: Multidisciplinary Association for Psychedelic Studies; 2004.

79. Shader RI, Greenblatt DJ. Use of benzodiazepines in anxiety disorders. *N Engl J Med*. 1993;328:1398–1405.

80. Dunton AW, Schwam E, Pitman V, McGrath J, Hendler J, Siegel J. Flumazenil: US clinical pharmacology studies. *Eur J Anaesthesiol Suppl*. 1988;2:81–95.

81. Klapper J, MD. Researcher, Bio-Medical Laboratory, Edgewood Arsenal, Md. Personal communication, 1969.

82. Tharp B, Ketchum JS. Performance effects of fluphenazine, haloperidol. Edgewood Arsenal, Md: Clinical Research Division, Medical Research Laboratories; 1965.

83. Gosselin RE, Smith RF, Hodge HC. *Clinical Toxicology of Commercial Products*. 5th ed. Baltimore, Md: Williams & Wilkins; 1984: 109.

84. Lakoski J, Bosseau MW, Kenny J. *The Advantages and Limitations of Calmatives for Use as a Non-Lethal Technique*. State College, Pa: Pennsylvania State University; 2000.

85. Davison N. Biochemical weapons: lethality, technology, development, and policy. In: Davison N, Lewer N, eds. *Bradford Non-Lethal Weapons Research Project (BNLWRP): Research Report No. 5*. Bradford, England: University of Bradford; 2004. Available at: http://www.bradford.ac.uk/acad/sbtwc/other/non_lethal.pdf. Accessed April 13, 2006.

86. Dando M. *A New Form of Warfare: The Rise of Non-Lethal Weapons*. Washington DC: Brassey's; 1966.

87. Chen Y, Dalwadi G, Benson HA. Drug delivery across the blood-brain barrier. *Curr Drug Deliv.* 2004;1:361–376.

88. US Department of the Army. *Army Science and Technology Master Plan, March 1997.* Fort Sam Houston, Tex: US Army Medical Center and School; 1998: Chap 5.

89. Ketchum JS, Sidell FR, Crowell EB, Aghajanian GK, Hayes AH. Atropine, scopolamine, and ditran: comparative pharmacology and antagonists in man. *Psychopharmacology (Berlin)* 1973;28:121–145.

90. Wolff HG, Curran D. Nature of delirium and allied states: dysergastic reaction. *Arch Neurol Psychiatr.* 1935;33:1175–1215.

91. Waelbroeck M, Taskenoy M, Camus J, Christophe J. Binding kinetics of quinuclidinyl benzilate and methyl- quinuclidinyl benzilate evantiomers at neuronal (M1), cardiac (M2), and pancreatic (M3) muscarinic receptors. *Mol Pharmacol.* 1991;40:413–420.

92. Hayes AH, Copelan H, Ketchum JS. The effect of high intramuscular doses of atropine sulfate on the human electrocardiogram. *Clin Pharmacol Ther.* 1971;12:482–486.

93. Ketchum JS. *The Human Assessment of BZ.* Edgewood Arsenal, Md: Chemical Research and Development Laboratory; 1963. Technical Memorandum 20-29.

94. Zvirblis P, Kondritzer A. *Adsorption of H3BZ and C14-Atropine to the Mitochondrial Fraction of the Rat Brain.* Edgewood Arsenal, Md: Chemical Research and Development Laboratory; 1966. Edgewood Arsenal Technical Report 4042.

95. Moran LJ, Mefferd RB. Repetitive psychometric measures. *Psychol Rep.* 1959;3:209–275.

96. Biel JH, Nuhfer PA, Hoya WK, Leiser HA, Abood LG. Cholinergic blockade as an approach to the development of new psychotropic agents. *Ann NY Acad Sci.* 1962;96:251–262.

97. Abood, LG. Structure-activity relations of the centrally active anticholinergic agents. In: National Academies of Science, Commission on Life Sciences. *Possible Long-Term Health Effects of Short-Term Exposure to Chemical Agents.* Vol 1. Washington, DC: National Academy Press;. 1982: 275–284.

98. Forrer GR. Atropine toxicity in the treatment of schizophrenia. *J Michigan State Med Soc.* 1950;49:184–185.

99. Miller JJ, Schwarz H, Forrer GR. Atropine coma therapy. Paper presented at: Michigan State Medical Society meeting, 1957.

100. Wada T, Horigome S, Sakurada T. Clinical experience of the so-called "atropine toxicity therapy [Forrer]." *Tohoku J Exp Med.* 1960;72:398–404.

101. Kitzes DL, Ketchum JS. *Estimate of Minimal Effective Dose of EA 3443 in Man.* Edgewood Arsenal, Md: Chemical Research and Development Laboratory; 1965. CRDL Technical Memorandum 2-29.

102. Crowell EB, Jr. *EA 3580A: Estimate of Incapacitating Dose in Man.* Edgewood Arsenal, Md: Chemical Research and Development Laboratory; 1965. CRDL Technical Memorandum 2-20.

103. Aghajanian GK, Kitzes DL, Harper DG, Bottiglieri NG. *EA 3580A: Estimate of Minimal Effective Dose In Man.* Edgewood Arsenal, Md: Chemical Research and Development Laboratory; 1965. CRDL Technical Memorandum 2-12.

104. Kitzes DL, Ketchum JS, Weimer JT, Farrand RL. *The Human Assessment of EA 3580 by the Aerosol Route.* Edgewood Arsenal, Md: Chemical Research and Development Laboratory; 1967. Edgewood Arsenal Technical Report 4041.

105. Sidell FR, Ketchum JS, Markis JE, Kysor KP. *Compound 302,196: Intramuscular Administration to Man.* Edgewood Arsenal, Md: Chemical Research and Development Laboratory; 1972. Edgewood Arsenal Technical Report No. 4634.

106. Tharp BR, Mershon M, Bottiglieri N. *Estimate of Intravenous MED50 of CS 27349 (219,758).* Edgewood Arsenal, Md: Chemical Research and Development Laboratory; 1964. Edgewood Arsenal Task Plan 7010.

107. Copeland HW. *MED50 of Agent 3834. Final Report, Contract No. DAAA15-68-C 0627*. Edgewood Arsenal, Md: Chemical Research and Development Laboratory; 1968.

108. Sidell FR, Braun BG. EA 3834A: *Effects in Man After a Single Oral Dose*. Edgewood Arsenal, Md: Chemical Research and Development Laboratory; 1972. Edgewood Arsenal Technical Report 4597.

109. McCarroll E, Markis J, Ketchum JS, Houff W, Sim VM. *Effects on Performance of the Administration of EA 3834 to Members of a Small Infantry Element Under Simulated Combat Conditions*. Edgewood Arsenal, Md: Chemical Research and Development Laboratory; 1971. Edgewood Arsenal Technical Report 4633.

110. Ketchum JS, Kitzes D, Copelan H. *EA 3167: Effects In Man*. Edgewood Arsenal, Md: Chemical Research and Development Laboratory; 1973. Edgewood Arsenal Technical Report 4713.

111. Hayes AH, Copelan H. *Intramuscular MED50 of 302668*. Edgewood Arsenal, Md: Chemical Research and Development Laboratory; 1967. Edgewood Arsenal Contract DA-18-035-AMC-126.

112. Copelan HW. *MED50 of Agent 302282*. Edgewood Arsenal, Md: Chemical Research and Development Laboratory;1967. Contract No. DA-18-035-AMC-126 (A) Report No. IV.

113. Arthur D Little Inc, Sterling Winthrop Research Institute. *Preclinical Pharmacology and Toxicology of Candidate Agent 226086*. Edgewood Arsenal, Md: Chemical Research and Development Laboratory; 1966. Contract No. EA 18-108-AMC-103(A) Quarterly Report 1.

114. Hayes AH, Copelan H. *Intramuscular MED50 of 302668 (Addendum)*. Edgewood Arsenal, Md: Chemical Research and Development Laboratory; 1967. Contract No. DA-18-035-AMC-126 (A).

115. Sidell FR, Ketchum JS, Markis JE, Kysor KP. *Compound 302,196: Intramuscular Administration to Man*. Edgewood Arsenal, Md: Chemical Research and Development Laboratory;1972. Edgewood Arsenal Technical Report No. 4634.

116. Federation of American Scientists. Using toxic properties of chemical substances. Adapted from Militarily Critical Technologies List Part II: Weapons of Mass Destruction Technologies. FAS Web site. Available at: http://www.fas.org/nuke/intro/cw/intro.htmsing. Accessed November 17, 2005.

117. Goodman LS, Gilman A, eds. *The Pharmacological Basis of Therapeutics*. 3rd ed. New York, NY: Macmillan; 1965: 521–545.

118. Crowell EB, Ketchum JS. The treatment of scopolamine-induced delirium with physostigmine. *Clin Pharmacol Ther*. 1967;8:409–414.

119. Kleinwachter I. Observations concerning the effectiveness of extract of Calabar against atropine poisoning. *Berl Klin Wschr*. 1864;1:369–377.

120. Sidell FR, Aghajanian GK, Groff WA, Cucinell SA. The reversal of anticholinergic intoxication in man with the cholinesterase inhibitor VX. *Proc Soc Exp Biol Med*. 1973;144:725–730.

121. Sidell FR, Groff WA. The reactivatibility of cholinesterase inhibited by VX and sarin in man. *Toxicol Appl Pharmacol*. 1974:27:241–252.

122. Gershon S. Blocking effect of tetrahydroaminacrin on a new psychotomimetic agent. *Nature*. 1960;186:1072–1073.

123. Bell C, Gershon S, Carroll B, Holan G. Behavioural antagonism to a new psychotomimetic: JB-329. *Arch Intern Pharmacodyn Ther*. 1964;147:9–25.

124. Ostfeld AM, Visotsky H, Lebonits B. A comparison of the psychotomimetic effects of scopolamine, LSD and n-ethyl-3-piperidyl benzilate (JB 318). *Clin Res*. 1958;6:416.

125. Duvoisin RC, Katz R. Reversal of central anticholinergic syndrome in man by physostigmine. *JAMA*. 1968;206:1963–1965.

126. Sidell FR. *Use of Physostigmine by the Intravenous, Intramuscular, and Oral Routes in the Therapy of Anticholinergic Drug Intoxication*. Biomedical Laboratory, EB-TR-76-12. Edgewood Arsenal, Md. 1976.

127. Daunderer M. Physostigmine salicylate as an antidote. *Int J Clin Pharmacol Ther Toxicol.* 1980;18:523–535.

128. Heiser JF, Gillin JC. The reversal of anticholinergic drug-induced delirium and coma with physostigmine. *Am J Psychiatry.* 1971;127:1050–1054.

129. Ghoneim MM. Antagonism of diazepam by physostigmine. *Anesthesiology.* 1980;52:372–373.

130. Ketchum JS. Unpublished observation. Fort Benning, GA, 1975.

131. Oguchi K, Arakawa K, Nelson SR, Samson F. The influence of droperidol, diazepam, and physostigmine on ketamine-induced behavior and brain regional glucose utilization in rat. *Anesthesiology*. 1982;57:353–358.

132. Directorate of Medical Research. *Guide to the Management of BZ Casualties*. Edgewood Arsenal, Md: Chemical Research and Development Laboratory; 1965.

133. Dolmierski R, Smoczynski S. Studies on the therapeutic value of atropine coma. *Pol Med Sci Hist Bull.* 1963;6:64–67.

134. Bliss CI. *The Statistics of Bioassay.* New York, NY: Academic Press; 1952.

135. Da Costa M. On irritable heart; a clinical study of a form of functional cardiac disorder and its consequences. *Am J Med Sci*. 1971;61:17–52.

136. US Department of the Army. *Flame, Riot control Agents, and Herbicide Operations*. Washington, DC: DA, 1996: 1–4. FM 3-11.

137. Office of Under Secretary of Defense for Acquisition, Technology, and Logistics. Treaty compliance: CCW: article by article analysis of the protocol on blinding laser weapons. ACQWeb Web site. Available at: http://www.defenselink.mil/acq/acic/treaties/ccwapl/artbyart_pro4.htm. Accessed January 3, 2006.

138. Stanton MN. What price sticky foam? *Parameters.* 1996;Autumn:63–68.

139. The Sunshine Project. Non-lethal weapons research in the US: calmatives and malodorants. Sunshine Project Web site. Available at: http://www.sunshine-project.org/publications/bk/bk8en.html. Accessed January 5, 2006.

140. Alexander J. *Future War: Non-lethal Weapons in Modern Warfare.* New York, NY: St Martin's Press; 1999.

Chapter 13

RIOT CONTROL AGENTS

HARRY SALEM, PhD*; BRADFORD W. GUTTING, PhD†; TIMOTHY A. KLUCHINSKY, Jr, PhD, MSPH‡; CHARLES H. BOARDMAN§; SHIRLEY D. TUORINSKY, MSN¥; and JOSEPH J. HOUT¶

*Chief Scientist for Life Sciences; US Army Edgewood Chemical and Biological Center, 5183 Blackhawk Road, Aberdeen Proving Ground, Maryland 21010

†Toxicologist; Naval Surface Warfare Center; Dahlgren Division (NSWCDD); Chemical, Biological, Radiological Defense Division (Code B54); Dahlgren, Virginia 22448

‡Manager, Health Hazard Assessment Program, Directorate of Occupational Health Sciences, US Army Center for Health Promotion and Preventive Medicine, 5158 Blackhawk Road, Aberdeen Proving Ground, Maryland 21010-5403

§Lieutenanat Colonel, Biomedical Sciences Corps, US Air Force; Instructor / Air Force Liaison and Occupational Therapist, US Army Medical Research Institute of Chemical Defense, 3100 Ricketts Point Road, Aberdeen Proving Ground, Maryland 21010-5400

¥Lieutenant Colonel, AN, US Army; Executive Officer, Comabat Casualty Care Division, US Army Medical Research Institute of Chemical Defense, 3100 Ricketts Point Road, Aberdeen Proving Ground, Maryland 21010-5400

¶Researcher, Uniformed Services University of the Health Sciences, 4301 Jones Bridge Road, Bethesda, Maryland 20814

INTRODUCTION

The 1993 Chemical Weapons Convention treaty defines riot control agents (RCAs) as agents that can rapidly produce sensory irritation or disabling physical effects in humans that disappear within a short time following termination of exposure.[1] More specifically, these are chemical agents that are designed to cause temporary incapacitation of the individual through intense irritation of tissues and the creation of a strong sensation of discomfort, including difficulty breathing and pain, without causing long-term disability or death. These disabling physiological effects occur when RCAs come into contact with the sensory nerve receptors at the site of contamination, resulting in local pain and discomfort with associated reflexes.

RCAs include chemicals from the following pharmacological classes: irritants, lachrymators, sternutators, emetics, sedatives, hypnotics, serotonin antagonists, hypotensives, thermoregulatory disruptors, nauseants, vision disruptors, neuromuscular blockers, and malodorous substances.[2] They are considered harassing agents, nonlethal or less than lethal agents, and although not gases, they are usually referred to as tear gas.[3] RCAs are relatively safe to use, especially when used in the open air, but have been known to cause death on occasion, particularly when used in close confines with inadequate ventilation or when the exposed individual was predisposed to cardiorespiratory compromise through disease or heavy intoxication with drugs or alcohol. Like other chemical agents, RCAs are designated with North Atlantic Treaty Organization (NATO) letter codes to label and help distinguish them. The agents covered in this chapter are those that have been used, or allegedly used, since World War II; their chemical names and respective NATO codes are *o*-chlorobenzylidene malononitrile (CS); oleoresin capsicum (OC); chloropicrin (PS); 1-chloroacetophenone (CN), diphenylaminearsine (DM), and dibenz(*b,f*)(1,4)oxazepine (CR).

Characteristics common to all of the agents discussed in this chapter are

- a rapid time of onset of effects (seconds to a few minutes);
- a relatively brief duration of effects (15–30 minutes) in most cases, once the exposed individual exits the contaminated area and is decontaminated (ie, the material is removed from the victim's clothing and skin); and
- a high safety ratio, that is, a relatively low dose of these agents is needed to cause tissue irritation or pain (effective dose or effective concentration), but a significantly larger dose is required to cause death (lethal dose or lethal concentration, LCt_{50}).[2–4]

This chapter will cover only RCAs that have been purposefully or allegedly used in recent history. Because of their prevalent use, CS and OC will be covered in greater detail than other agents.

Although the effects differ slightly among the various agents, all RCAs cause some form of eye irritation involving lacrimation and blepharospasm, which causes the eyes to close temporarily, rendering victims unable to see and dramatically reducing their ability to resist. PS, CN, CS, CR, DM, and OC also cause irritation to airways resulting in coughing, shortness of breath, and retching or vomiting.[3] DM in effective doses causes significant vomiting with resulting mental depression and malaise. These agents cause some degree of pain sensation either through irritation of peripheral nerve endings in tissue, such as the mucous membranes and skin (PS, CN, CS, CR), or by causing the sudden release of neurotransmitters, such as bradykinin or substance P, which signal the sensation of intense pain (OC).[2]

The reflex most associated with death from the inhalation exposure of irritants is the Kratschmer reflex, first reported in 1870 as the immediate response of apnea or cessation of respiration in rabbits following exposure to chemical irritants such as chloroform and carbon dioxide.[5] The response is a protective reflex or defense mechanism to prevent or reduce the amount of noxious chemical reaching the lower respiratory tract and maintain homeostasis. Accompanied by bradycardia and a biphasic fall and rise in aortic blood pressure, the reflex is mediated by the olfactory (I), trigeminal (V), and glossopharyngeal (IX) cranial nerves. It has also occurred in rodent and canine experiments following exposure to volatile solvents and was demonstrated to occur in humans.[6] The cardiopulmonary receptors involved in the reflex prevent the absorption and distribution of the inhaled irritant to the vital organs, as well as facilitating the expulsion of the irritant, and the extracardiopulmonary mechanisms promote metabolism and excretion of the absorbed chemical. These effects have been described by Aviado and Salem and by Aviado and Aviado.[7–9] During apnea or cessation of respiration, blood levels of carbon dioxide increase and drive the respiratory center to restart breathing. Individuals with compromised immune systems, nervous system depression as a result of alcohol or illicit drug consumption, or a combination of these, may not be able to restart respiration and die from asphyxia. The Kratschmer reflex may be responsible in part for some in-custody deaths attributed by law enforcement agencies to positional asphyxia following the initial use of pepper sprays in the United States in the early 1990s.[2]

Police departments throughout the world commonly use RCAs, either individually or in solutions combining several agents (OC, pelargonyl vanillylamide [PAVA or nonivamide], CS, CN, CR, and malodorous substances), as an alternative to deadly force for individual protection, subduing unruly felons, crowd control during civil disturbances, or rescuing hostages. RCAs are also regularly used by the military for mask confidence training (CS) and by military police for individual protection (OC). Because of their frequent use during peacetime operations, RCAs are repeatedly scrutinized for safety and appropriateness.

RCAs are usually solids with low vapor pressure. They can be dispersed as fine powders or in solvents as jets or streams from spray cans, tanks or larger weapons, hand grenades, or mortar artillery munitions, and also as aerosols or smoke by pyrotechnic generators.[10]

HISTORY

Irritant compounds have been used throughout history. In the 2nd century BCE, Plutarch, the Roman historian, described a Roman general using an irritant cloud to drive an enemy from caves in Spain.[3] The Byzantines also used irritants to harass opposing forces. Chinese warriors and Japanese ninjas reportedly threw or blew ground cayenne pepper powder mixtures in the faces of their opponents to temporarily disable them. Japanese police once used a lacquer or brass box, known as the *metsubichi*, to blow pepper dust in the eyes of criminals trying to flee arrest.[11,12]

Use of RCAs by Europeans in the 20th century probably began before World War I when French police used ethylbromoacetate against criminals and gangs.[13] France used the agent on the battlefield in the early part of the war, with limited success, before Germany's first use of lethal chlorine, in Ypres, Belgium, on April 22, 1915.[3] Other tear gases used in World War I included acrolein (Papite); bromoacetone (BA, B-stoff); bromobenzyl cyanide (BBC, CA); chloroacetone (A-stoff); and xylylbromide (T-stoff). Ethylbromoacetone was the most widely used potent lacrimatory agent during the war.[14]

First synthesized around 1850, PS was known as "green cross" during World War I, when it was used as a harassing agent and lethal chemical along with the other lethal agents such as chlorine, phosgene, and trichloroethyl-chlorformate. PS is no longer used as an RCA because of its toxicity, but it is used in agriculture as a soil fumigant injected below the soil surface as an effective fungicide, insecticide, and nematicide.[15,16] In 2004 an accidental release of PS in a crowded central police office in Sofia, Bulgaria, sent 49 persons to the hospital with tearing and serious respiratory complaints.[17,18] DM, an arsenic-based compound, was developed for use in the latter part of World War I. It is a vomiting and sneezing (sternutator) agent and was used as an RCA after the war; however, it is currently considered obsolete.[4] Around the year 2000 Palestinian sources accused Israel of using a chemical agent compound, possibly DM, as an RCA, although this claim has never been substantiated.[19,20] CN was invented by a German chemist, Carl Graebe, in 1869 (although some sources indicate that it was originally synthesized in 1871 or 1881). CN was used as the RCA of choice from the latter part of the First World War through the 1950s, until it was replaced by the less toxic CS as the standard RCA in the United States.[3,21] Some countries still use CN as an RCA, and it is still found in some personal defense sprays. CS, synthesized in 1928,[3] in addition to its use as an RCA, is used for individual protection, sometimes in combination with CN, OC, or PAVA.[10] CR is believed to have been deployed initially in the 1970s by the British against prison rioters. It is not in use in the United States, but some countries use the agent for riot control and security.[22] OC was originally developed as an animal repellent and used by the US Postal Service in the 1960s. In the late 1980s it was endorsed by the Federal Bureau of Investigation as a chemical agent that would be effective in subduing people.[22,23] In the 1990s OC gained wide acceptance among US law enforcement personnel, including military police, as an alternative to Mace (Smith and Wesson, Springfield, Mass) for individual protection. It now comes in a variety of forms, from liquid to dry powder.[10,12]

The United States does not consider RCAs to be chemical warfare agents as defined by the Geneva Convention in 1925. The United States ratified the Geneva Gas Protocol in January 1975, interpreting it as prohibiting the first use of lethal chemicals, but not nonlethal agents or herbicides[3] (US forces were then using CS and Agent Orange in Vietnam). On April 18, 1975, President Gerald Ford signed Executive Order 11850 renouncing first use of RCAs in war, except in defensive military modes to save lives. The executive order did allow the use of these agents against rioting prisoners and civil disturbances, during rescue operations, for nuclear weapons security operations, and to protect convoys from terrorist attacks or in similar situations.[3,10] Under current policy, the secretary of defense must ensure that RCAs are not used in warfare unless there is advance presidential approval.[10]

CS (*O*-CHLOROBENZYLIDENE MALONONITRILE)

CS (also known as 2-chlorophenyl-methylenepropanedinitrile, β,β-dicyano-*o*-chlorostyrene, and 2-chlorobenzalmalononitrile) is the US military's most widely used RCA compound in operations and training. CS was first synthesized by British scientists Corson and Stoughton (hence its name) in 1928 by condensing aromatic aldehydes with malononitrile.[24] Corson and Stoughton showed CS to have an intense nasal (sneezing) and skin irritant effect and noted that exposure to it caused the "face to smart." This outcome can be minimized by wearing a protective mask, but may be temporarily intensified if the exposed area is rinsed with water.[24] These characteristics made CS a notable candidate for widespread adoption as a military incapacitant. However, CS wasn't readily accepted for this use until well after World War II, when it was learned that the effect of CS was less toxic but more potent than that of CN. As a result, the US Army Chemical Corps declared CS its standard military RCA on June 30, 1959.[25] See Table 13-1 for a summary of CS characteristics.

Other symptoms of CS exposure, which may be associated with bradykinin release, consist of irritation and a burning sensation of the eyes, nose, skin, and throat, resulting in the need for exposed individuals to close their eyes and hold their breath, quickly rendering them incapacitated.[26,27] Recent scientific investigations into the identification of CS-derived compounds and other thermal degradation products formed during the heat dispersion of CS have raised questions about the potential health risks associated with the use of high-temperature heat dispersion devices, particularly if used in enclosed spaces.[28–31] It is critical that CS be deployed in accordance with existing training guidance to minimize its potential health hazards.

Physical Characteristics and Deployment

Physical Characteristics

CS is a gray, crystalline solid with a pepper-like odor. Additional characteristics are a molecular mass of 188.6 d; molecular formula of $C_{10}H_5ClN_2$ (Figure 13-1); melting point of 95°C to 96°C; boiling point of 310°C to 315°C; low vapor pressure of 3.4×10^{-5} mm Hg at 20°C; slight solubility in water; solubility at 25°C in the organic solvents methylene chloride, acetone, ethyl acetate, benzene, and dioxane; and half-life of 14 minutes at pH 7.4 and 25°C. Dissolved CS is rapidly hydrolyzed to form *o*-chlorobenzaldehyde and malononitrile.[32]

Deployment

CS rapidly loses its effectiveness under normal environmental conditions, making it an ideal temporary incapacitant. The US Department of Defense created at least three variations of CS—CS1, CS2, and CSX—all of which are used today. CS1 is a micronized powder consisting of 95% CS and 5% silica aerogel designed to reduce agglomeration. CS2 is a siliconized microencapsulated form of CS1 comprised of 94% CS, 5% colloidal silica, and 1% hexamethyldisilizane, whose characteristics increase shelf life, resistance to degradation, and the ability to float on water, thus providing a means of restricting key terrain during military operations.[33] CSX is comprised of 1 g CS1 dissolved in 99 g trioctylphosphite, enabling dissemination as a liquid. CS powder is usually delivered as a component of an aerosol, solution, explosive device, or smoke.[34]

The mechanism of deployment typically involves the use of storage cylinders, mortars, artillery projectiles, grenades (Figures 13-2 and 13-3), cartridges, aircraft or vehicle-mounted dispensers, portable dispensers, or personal protection dispensers.[34] Regardless of the delivery mechanism, CS exposure causes almost immediate inflammation of the conjunctivae, tearing (lacrimation), pain, and involuntary closure of the eyes and lids (blepharospasm). Respiratory effects include sneezing, nasal discharge, and throat irritation, often accompanied by violent coughing. Continued CS exposure results in tightness of chest and general breathing difficulty. These effects resolve within minutes of removal from the exposure, and only moderate tearing and redness of the eyes remain 10 minutes after exposure.[35,36]

In addition to its use by the United States in Vietnam, during demonstrations and prison riots, and for military and law enforcement training,[36] CS was used by British police to quell riots in Londonderry in August 1969.[37,38] CS has an extensive mammalian toxicology database.[2]

Thermal Degradation Products

CS is commonly used as an RCA and chemical warfare agent simulant for training, in which law enforcement and military employees are routinely exposed to heated CS. Heat assists in the dispersion process by vaporizing the CS, which then condenses to form an aerosol. Heat dispersion of CS has the potential to form CS-derived compounds that have been the focus of many recent studies. Thermal dispersion of CS from a canister in an enclosed space was shown to

TABLE 13-1

CHARACTERISTICS OF CS AND OC

Properties	CS	OC
Molecular formula	$C_{10}H_5ClN_2$	$C_{18}H_{27}NO_3$
Former/current use	RCA/RCA	Food additive/Food additive, RCA
Physical state*	White crystalline solid.	Colorless solid
Odor	Pungent pepper-like	Pungent, irritating
Freezing or melting point	Melting point: 95°C–96°C	Freezing point: 65°C
Vapor pressure	0.00034 mm Hg at 20°C	1.5×10^{-7} mm Hg at 65°C (extrapolated)
Density:		
Vapor (relative to air)	6.5 times heavier (calculated)	10.5 times heavier (calculated)
Solid	Bulk: 0.24-0.26 g/cm^3 Crystal: 1.04 g/cm^3	Data not available
Solubility:		
In water	Insoluble in water	Solubility in water is 0.090 g at 37°C
In other solvents	Moderate in alcohol; good in organic solvents such as acetone, chloroform, methylene dichloride, ethyl acetate, and benzene	Soluble in alcohol, ether, oil, chloroform, aromatic solvents, hydrocarbons, ketones, and aqueous alkali
Hydrolysis products	Data not available	Alkaline hydrolysis yields vanillylamine and isomeric decenoic acid
Decontamination:		
Clothing	Stand in front of a fan or flap arms to remove dry powder, protect airway. Wash clothing after removal	Sticks to clothing if in liquid solution. If in powder form, remove dry powder. Wash clothing after removal
Skin	Copious soap and water; do not use oil-based lotions or bleach	Copious soap and water. Can also use alcohol, baby shampoo, or flush skin with vegetable oil followed by soap and water (not for OC/CS-CN mixtures); flush eyes with copious water or baby shampoo; use milk or ice packs to reduce pain
Equipment	Wash with soap and water	Wash with soap and water or place in sun to degrade
Persistency:		
In soil	Varies	Degrades with sun and moisture
On material	Varies	Degrades with sun and moisture
Skin and eye effects	Skin irritant; itching, stinging and erythema; may cause blistering and allergic contact dermatitis. Burning and irritation to eyes with lacrimation and accompanying blepharospasm	Causes sensation of intense pain and burning through the activation of the TRPV1 sensory neuron, causing release of substance P. May cause allergic dermatitis with excessive skin exposure. Lacrimation, redness, burning sensation in the eyes and blepharospasm
Respiratory effects	Salivation, coughing, choking, and a feeling of chest tightness. May cause reactive airway disease syndrome requiring medical intervention	Tingling sensation followed by coughing and decreased inhalation rates. Pain, vasodilation, and secretion can occur in the airways depending on the dose inhaled

*At standard temperature and pressure.

RCA: riot control agent

TPRV1: transient receptor potential, vallinoid subtype 1

Data sources: (1) Sidell F. Riot control agents. In: Sidell F, Takafuji E, Franz D, eds. *Medical Aspects of Chemical and Biological Warfare.* In: Zajtchuk R, Bellamy RF, eds. *Textbook of Military Medicine.* Washington, DC: Department of the Army, Office of The Surgeon General, Borden Institute; 1997: Chap 12. (2) US Department of the Army. *Potential Military Chemical/Biological Agents and Compounds, Multiservice Tactics, Techniques, and Procedures*. Washington, DC: DA; January 10, 2005. FM 3-11.9. (3) Somani SM, Romano JA Jr, eds. *Chemical Warfare Agents: Toxicity at Low Levels*. Boca Raton, Fla: CRC Press; 2001.

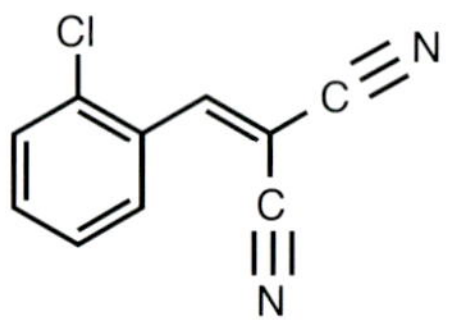

Fig. 13-1. Chemical structure of CS.

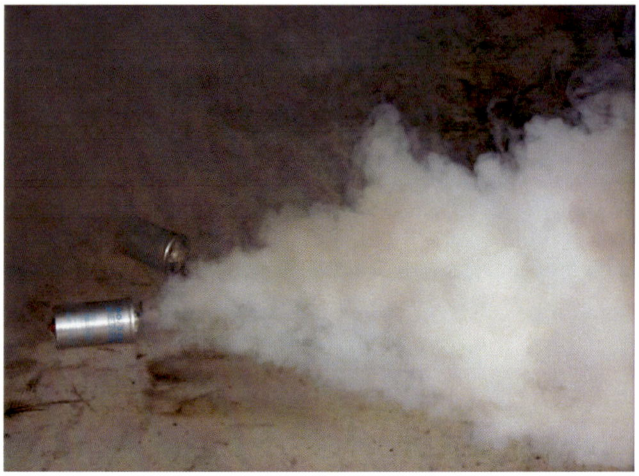

Fig. 13-2. Heat dispersion of CS canisters at Fort Meade, Maryland.
Photograph: Courtesy of TA Kluchinsky.

produce many semivolatile organic air contaminants[29]; therefore, such canisters must not be used in enclosed spaces for training. It is important for medical personnel to encourage commanders and trainers to deploy CS and other RCAs according to the most current training guidance.

The practice of heating CS capsules (national stock number 1365-00-690-8556) on an improvised aerosol generator (Figure 13-4) is currently the preferred method of CS dispersal inside a mask confidence chamber. The Uniformed Services University of the Health Sciences, Department of Preventive Medicine and Biometrics, Division of Environmental and Occupational Health is investigating this method of CS dispersal to determine the thermal degradation products produced.[39]

The metabolic effects and health issues associated with acute CS exposure and its hydrolysis products appear to have been thoroughly studied[26,40–48]; however, recent investigations into potentially harmful CS-derived compounds produced during thermal dispersion have raised new concerns. Many of these compounds have not been evaluated for their potential to produce acute or chronic effects,[28–31] and the current methods for analysis of CS and CS-derived compounds recommended by the National Institute for Occupational Safety and Health (NIOSH) are less than adequate given the current arsenal of instrumental and analytical techniques now available.

In 1961 Porter and associates[49] identified and quantified several compounds produced as a result of the thermal degradation of CS. They identified CS, CO, CO_2, Cl^-, NH_4, N_2O, C_2H_2, and water at temperatures ranging from 490°C to 625°C.[49] In 1969 McNamara et

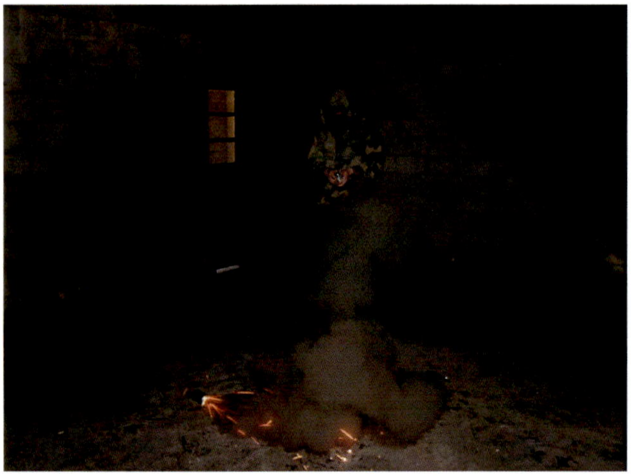

Fig. 13-3. CS canisters being dispersed inside a room at Fort Meade, Maryland. This method is neither recommended nor permitted for mask confidence training; it is being performed here for research purposes only.
Photograph: Courtesy of TA Kluchinsky.

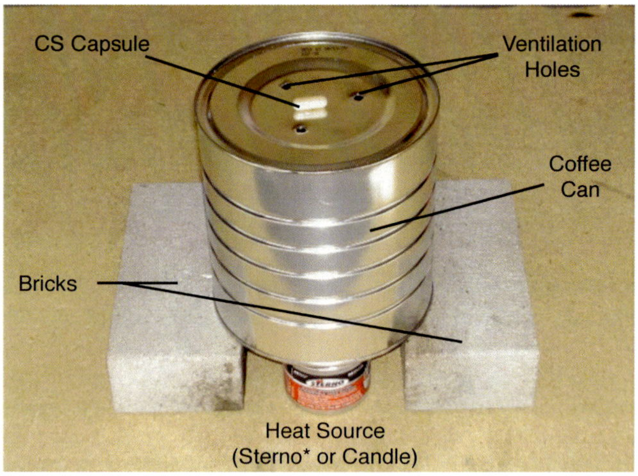

Fig. 13-4. Preferred method of heating CS capsules (national stock number 1365-00-690-8556) on an improvised aerosol generator.
Photograph: Courtesy of TA Kluchinsky and J Hout.
*Candle Corporation of America, Des Plaines, Il.

al[27] reported the pyrolytic decomposition products of CS as CS, CO, CO_2, H_2O, HCl, HCN, NH_3, N_2O_2 and C_2H_2. Further research by Kluchinsky et al[28–30] during 2000 and 2001 using heat-dispersed CS canisters (Figures 13-2 and 13-3) identified many additional thermal degradation products by trapping the contaminants on a polytetrafluoroethylene filter and analyzing them by open tubular gas chromatography coupled to mass spectrometry. Compounds observed in addition to CS and its isomer 4-chlorobenzylidenemalononitrile included 2-chlorobenzaldehyde, 2-chlorobenzonitrile, quinoline, 2-chlorobenzylcyanide, 1,2-dicyanobenzene, 3-(2-chlorophenyl)propynenitrile, *cis*- and *trans*-isomers of 2-chlorocinnamonitrile, 2,2-dicyano-3-(2-chlorophenyl)oxirane, 2-chlorodihydrocinnamonitrile, benzylidenemalononitrile, *cis*- and *trans*- isomers of 2-cyanocinnamonitrile, 2-chlorobenzylmalononitrile, 3-quinoline carbonitrile, and 3-isoquinoline carbonitrile.[28–30]

The CS-derived compounds observed were likely produced through rearrangements and by loss of cyano and chlorine substituents present on the parent CS compound. Especially noteworthy is the formation of 3-(2-chlorophenyl)propynenitrile, which is indicative of a loss of cyanide from the CS molecule. Although the metabolic effects of cyanide have been addressed in the open literature, the metabolic effects of *trans*- and *cis*-2-cyanocinnamonitrile, 3-quinoline carbonitrile, and 3-isoquinoline carbonitrile, which appear to be produced through free radical mechanisms, lack sufficient investigation.

Detailed sampling under similar conditions and analysis for inorganic salts (using the NIOSH methods 7904 and 6010 [modified] for HCN and 7903 for HCl) showed that HCN and HCl were present in air samples collected during high-temperature dispersion of CS.[28] The concentration of HCN identified during the dispersion of two CS canisters inside a 240 m^3 RCA training chamber (Figure 13-2 and 13-3) was found to be above the exposure level guidelines recommended by the American Conference of Governmental Industrial Hygienists (ACGIH) and NIOSH.

The study group hypothesized that the formation of potentially harmful CS-derived compounds produced through free radical intermediates (*cis*- and *trans*- isomers of 2-cyanocinnamonitrile, 3-quinoline carbonitrile, and 3-isoquinoline carbonitrile), and the release of HCN, evidenced by the presence of 3-(2-chlorophenyl)propynenitrile, was temperature dependent. This hypothesis led to another study in which CS was heated in an inert atmosphere using a tube furnace.[30] Pure CS was used so that the effect of temperature on CS could be analyzed independently of the other compounds present in canisters, such as potassium chlorate, sugar, magnesium carbonate, and nitrocellulose. It was assumed that the tube furnace's effect on the production of CS-derived compounds could be generalized to that formed by high-temperature dispersion of CS canisters. By assuming that neat CS behaved in a similar manner as that found in canisters dispersing at an average temperature of 798°C (Figure 13-5), standardizing residence time in the tube furnace, and using an inert nitrogen carrier gas at a constant flow, it was shown that many of the organic degradation products observed earlier in a field environment were produced through heating. Additionally, the study identified tube-furnace–induced temperature ranges associated with the formation of the CS-derived compounds.

However, generalizing conclusions drawn from laboratory-based CS data to exposures from thermal dispersion of CS in a field environment must be done with caution. CS must be deployed appropriately during operations and training to ensure optimal safety. Use of CS capsules (Figure 13-4) is the only accepted method of CS dispersal for mask confidence training performed in an enclosed space (eg, tent, chamber, or building).

Clinical Effects

Acute Effects

CS is a peripheral sensory irritant that acts primarily upon the eyes, respiratory tract, and skin; acute exposure to CS presents itself very much the same as exposures to other RCAs.[50] Exposure almost instantly results in irritation, burning, and swelling of the conjunctivae of the eye, accompanied by excessive

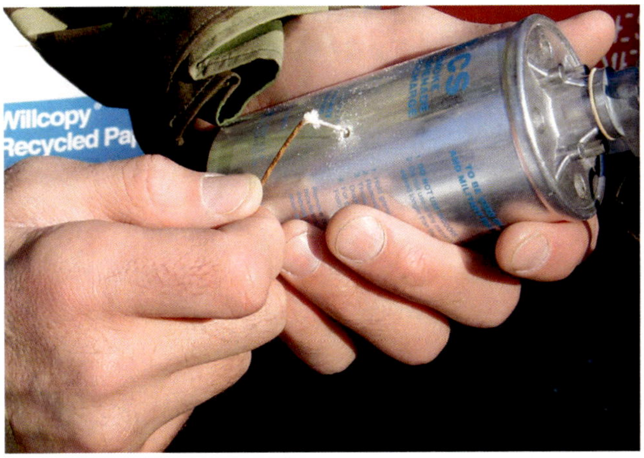

Fig. 13-5. Insertion of a thermocouple into a hole drilled in a CS canister at Fort Meade, Maryland, to determine dispersal temperature.
Photograph: Courtesy of TA Kluchinsky.

tearing and uncontrollable closure of the eyelid. In some cases, the subject experiences an aversion to light. As the agent enters the respiratory tract, it causes irritation and burning in the nose and mouth as well as excessive nasal discharge and salivation. It causes pain and discomfort in the throat and chest, resulting in sometimes violent coughing spasms and difficulty breathing.[35] The respiratory effects are the most pronounced and most capable of causing individuals to flee from the exposure.[51] Irritation and reddening of exposed skin is quite common and is more pronounced with increased temperature, humidity, and concentration of the agent.[52]

Animal Studies

Acute oral toxicology studies. Acute oral studies involving CS in alcohol or water administered by esophageal catheter to rabbits and rats yielded median lethal doses (LD_{50}s) of 401 mg/kg and 822 mg/kg, respectively.[53] When CS was administered in polyethylene glycol to various animal species, the LD_{50}s were determined to be 231 mg/kg in male rabbits, 143 mg/kg in female rabbits, 1,366 mg/kg in male rats, 1,284 mg/kg in female rats, and 262 mg/kg in female guinea pigs.[40]

Acute eye toxicology studies. Solutions of up to 10 mg CS in methylene dichloride placed into the eyes of rabbits did not produce permanent ocular damage.[54,55] Immediate effects observed following administration were conjunctivitis that lasted for 30 to 60 minutes and erythema of the eyelid. CS administered into the eyes of rabbits via solutions of 0.5% to 10% CS caused conjunctivitis, chemosis, keratitis, and corneal vascularization, as well as denudation of the corneal epithelium and neutrophilic infiltration. When administered via thermal dispersion, the solid caused tearing at all doses, uncontrolled closure of the eyelids that increased with dose, and mild chemosis at the high doses that persisted for up to 3 days. The smoke also caused excessive tearing and swelling of the conjunctiva lasting 24 hours. All tissues were normal within 7 days.[54]

Acute skin toxicology studies. When 12.5 mg of CS in corn oil or acetone was applied to the dorsal skin of rabbits, guinea pigs, and mice, the effects were erythema and edema. These effects resolved within 7 days.[40]

Mutagenic potential studies. The mutagenic potential of CS and CS2 was investigated in microbial and mammalian bioassays.[56–59] The results were equivocal, but the Committee on Toxicology of the National Research Council reported in 1984 that, taken in their totality, the test of CS for gene mutation and chromosomal damage provides no clear evidence of mutagenicity.[60] Most of the evidence is consistent with nonmutagenicity, and in the committee's judgment, it is unlikely that CS poses a mutagenic hazard to humans.

Acute inhalation toxicology studies. Acute inhalation studies of CS were conducted in several animal species with CS generated as a smoke.[40,61] The acute inhalation (vapor exposure) median lethal doses (LCt_{50}s) are presented in Table 13-2. Studies by Weimar and associates[62] indicated that toxicity of CS varies depending upon the method of dispersion, arriving at the following order of toxicity: molten dispersion > dispersion in methylene dichloride > dispersion via thermal grenade.

Repeat exposures. Repeat exposures to thermally dispersed CS were conducted in rats and dogs for 25 days. The cumulative doses received were 91,000 mg•min/m^3 and 17,000 mg•min/m^3, respectively. No lethality occurred in the dogs, while 5 of the 30 rats exposed died, 2 at the cumulative dose of 25,000 mg•min/m^3, and 3 at 68,000 mg•min/m^3. No gross pathology was observed in the rats that died, nor in the six other rats sacrificed following the 25 days of exposure. During the exposure, the rats became hyperactive and aggressive, although no changes were found in the blood chemistry. The exposed rats lost almost 1% of their body weight, whereas the unexposed rats gained 20% during the 5-week period, although there was no difference in organ to body weight ratios. It was concluded from these studies that repeated exposures did not make the animals more sensitive to the lethal effects of CS. The animals that died during the exposures showed increased numbers of goblet cells in the respiratory and gastrointestinal tracts and conjunctiva, necrosis in the respiratory and gastrointestinal tracts, pulmonary edema, and occasional hemorrhage in the adrenals. The deaths appeared to be caused by poor transfer of

TABLE 13-2

ACUTE INHALATION TOXICITY OF CS IN ANIMALS

	LCt_{50} (mg•min/m^3)	
Species	**CS Smoke**	**CS Aerosol**
Guinea pig	35,800	67,000
Rabbit	63,600	54,090
Rat	69,800	88,480
Mouse	70,000	50,110

LCt_{50}: the vapor or aerosol exposure that is lethal to 50% of the exposed population oxygen from the lungs to the blood stream, probably because of edema and hemorrhage in the lungs and obstruction of the airways.[55] In other repeat exposures to neat CS aerosols in mice, rats, and guinea pigs for 120 days, it was concluded that concentrations below 30 mg/m^3 were without deleterious effects.[63]

Subchronic toxicology studies. Punte and associates[55] exposed 30 rats and 5 dogs to molten CS aerosol dispersed via an oil bath in a 200-L exposure chamber. Both species were exposed for 5 days per week; however, the time per day was varied. Dogs were exposed for 1 minute (680 mg•min/m^3) daily, resulting in a cumulative dose of 17,000 mg•min/m^3. Rats were exposed for 5 minutes (3,600 mg•min/m^3) daily, resulting in a cumulative dose of 91,000 mg•min/m^3. The only clinical presentation of CS exposure in the dogs was salivation, which resolved itself 1 minute postexposure. Six of the thirty rats died during the 5-week period; however, no gross pathological changes were found in these rats or the others sacrificed at the end of the study. Neither species exhibited significant differences from controls in body weight ratios of the heart, kidney, lungs, liver, or spleen.[55]

Chronic toxicology and carcinogenicity studies. CS has been referred to throughout the literature as an alkylating agent, and some alkylating agents are carcinogens. McNamara and associates[64] exposed groups of mice and rats to CS daily for 20 days. Representative groups were sacrificed at 6, 12, 18, and 24 months and examined for tumors. Examinations showed no significant increase in lung tumors between the exposed animals and controls. The data suggested that CS is not a potent carcinogen.[64]

A study by Marrs and associates[63] exposed mice to 55 60-minute exposures to aerosolized CS. At 1 year postexposure, the exposed mice did not experience a statistically significant number of deaths in comparison with the control group, and pathological examinations revealed no increase in tumors. Other than an increase in chronic laryngitis and tracheitis in the exposed group, there were no pathological differences between the two groups.[63]

CS2 was evaluated for carcinogenicity in the National Toxicology Program 2-year rodent bioassay. Compound-related nonneoplastic lesions of the respiratory tract were observed. The pathological changes observed in the rats included squamous metaplasia of the olfactory epithelium and hyperplasia and metaplasia of the respiratory epithelium. In mice, hyperplasia and squamous metaplasia of the respiratory epithelium was observed. Neoplastic effects were not observed in either rats or mice, and it was concluded that the findings suggest that CS2 is not carcinogenic to rats and mice.[65]

Human Studies

Respiratory effects. CS can enter the respiratory tract as a vapor, aerosol, or solid and take action on the nasopharyngeal, tracheobronchial, and pulmonary levels of the respiratory tract. In low concentrations, it irritates the pulmonary tract; at high concentrations, it can affect the respiratory system.[50] Gongwer and associates[66] exposed volunteers to various concentrations of CS through a facemask and by total body exposure to establish the concentration that would be intolerable. Following exposure, subjects were questioned and reexamined. The concentrations varied from 2 to 360 mg/m^3 and the time from 30 to 120 seconds. Upon exposure, subjects experienced irritation of the nose, throat, and chest. They also experienced coughing and had difficulty breathing; however, airway resistance was not significantly changed. These effects were resolved within minutes in fresh air. At levels of 10 to 20 mg/m^3, 50% of the study population found the concentration intolerable.[66]

In another study, Gutentag and associates[51] exposed trained and untrained volunteers to various concentrations of CS to determine the intolerable concentration. Subjects in a wind tunnel were exposed to concentrations varying from 5 to 442 mg/m^3 of CS generated by CS-acetone spray (3 µm), CS-methylene dichloride spray (1 µm), and an M18 grenade (0.5 µm). The respiratory system effects were the most pronounced and most capable of producing incapacitation. Exposure resulted in immediate burning of the nose, throat, and lungs that soon became painful. Tightening of the chest and difficulty breathing followed shortly. Airway resistance, however, remained unchanged. A portable breathing measuring device verified that subjects involuntarily gasped and held their breath upon exposure. All symptoms resolved after removal from the environment. Of the untrained study population, 50% found a concentration of 7 mg/m^3 intolerable.[51]

Other investigators exposed human volunteers to various concentrations, particle sizes, and durations of CS. Volunteers were able to tolerate the large particle size (60 µm) for 60 seconds, but those exposed to the small particle size (0.9 µm) could not.[67] When CS was dispersed in methylene dichloride (1.0 µm) and thermally (0.9 µm), the volunteers could tolerate 1.5 mg/m^3 exposures for 40 minutes. When the concentration was increased to 11 mg/m^3, the volunteers fled the chamber within 2 minutes.[52] Respiratory effects were similar to those noted by Gutentag in 1960 for all exposures.[51] Response times (defined as tolerance) did not vary depending upon the method of dispersion; however, the duration of tolerance was reduced with increased humidity, temperature, and exercise.[52]

McNamara and associates[27] summarized six experiments to determine the incapacitating concentration of CS. The experiments varied in concentrations (5–422 mg/m^3), method of dispersal, and exposure time (30–300 seconds). The incapacitating effects were the same at that noted by Gutentag and associates. The incapacitating concentration for 50% of the population was determined to be somewhere between 0.1 and 10 mg/m^3, depending upon the motivation of the exposed population. There was no difference in tolerance times among dispersal methods or for men over age 50. This study also concluded that incapacitation time was reduced with increased temperature and humidity.[27]

Beswick and associates[35] exposed 35 men to 1-µm particles of CS dispersed in a 100-m^3 chamber by the ignition of 1-g CS pellets. The concentration varied from 0.43 to 2.3 mg/m^3 over a period of 60 minutes. Symptoms of exposure included nasal pain and discharge, rhinorrhea, throat irritation, tightness and burning of the chest, and difficulty breathing. Subjects developed tolerance to the compound and were able to remain in the chamber for 60 minutes, despite the 4-fold increase in concentration. Postexposure measurements revealed no differences in peak flow, tidal volume, or vital capacities from those made before the exposure.[35]

Cole and associates[68] exposed several male volunteers to concentrations of 0.16 to 4.4 mg/m^3 in an exposure chamber. Ventilation minute volume was observed to decrease an average of 6% in the exposed population.[68]

Based upon the data presented, a variety of health-related values have been calculated. The NIOSH recommended exposure limit ceiling value is 0.4 mg/m^3. This ceiling value should not be exceeded at any time. The OSHA permissible exposure limit is 0.4 mg/m^3. This is the concentration of CS, averaged over an 8-hour workday, to which most workers can be exposed without adverse effect. The value considered immediately dangerous to life and health (IDLH) is 2 mg/m^3.[69]

In a final report to the deputy attorney general, Heinrich[70] stated that CS can be detected by the human nose at an odor threshold value of 0.004 mg/m^3. Blain[71] stated that concentrations of 0.004 mg/m^3 are detectable by the human eye and that concentrations of 0.023 mg/m^3 are detectable in the airways. He also stated that the ICt_{50}, or the concentration that is intolerable to 50% of the exposed population for 1 minute, is 3.6 mg/m^3. This value is consistent with the work of Punte, Gutentag, and McNamara.[72,73] A summary report produced by the Directorate of Medical Research at Edgewood Arsenal, Maryland, cites the LCt_{50} for molten CS as 52,000 mg•min/m^3 and 61,000 mg•min/m^3 by thermal grenade. The same report cites the ICt_{50} as ranging from 0.1 to 10 mg•min/m^3.[53]

Dermatological effects. CS exposure can result in a multitude of cutaneous reactions, such as allergic contact dermatitis, rashes, blisters, and burns. Exposure manifests itself as a delayed (several minutes) stinging sensation that is less remarkable than the reaction of the eyes and nose. The severity of the reaction depends upon several variables including (but not limited to) the method of dispersal, CS concentration, temperature, and humidity.[72]

Gutentag and associates[51] conducted a series of patch tests on several volunteers, using CS protected from the air, CS in a porous gauze covering, a 10% CS solution in methylene dichloride, and a 20% CS solution in methylene dichloride. The porous gauze covering produced the greatest skin effect, causing four of four volunteers to develop vesicles surrounded by erythema. The 10% CS solution caused no skin reaction in three of three volunteers. The researchers also exposed subjects to wind-dispersed CS via CS-acetone spray (3 µm), CS-methylene dichloride spray (1 µm), and an M18 grenade (0.5 µm). Subjects reported burning on exposed areas of the skin that increased with the presence of moisture. The burning sensation lasted for several hours and recurred when the affected area was moistened. Heavy exposures produced vesiculation and reddening that resembled a second-degree burn.[51]

Hellreich and associates[74] exposed the arms of volunteers to an average concentration of 300 mg/m^3 for 15 to 60 minutes via thermal grenade. Within 5 minutes of exposure, subjects experienced a burning sensation of the skin; concentration multiplied by time (Ct) exposures of 4,440 and 9,480 mg•min/m^3 produced immediate reddening of the skin. Upon removal from the exposure area, subjects washed their arms and found the burning sensation to increase. Within 30 minutes of removal from the environment, all symptoms of exposure resolved.[74] In a follow-on study, Hellreich and associates[75] used patches to test the dermal effects of CS on the arms of volunteers at four temperature conditions. The patches were taken off at specified exposure times to give exposures at 37°C with 98% relative humidity (RH), 14°C with 41% RH, 20°C with 95% RH, and 22°C with 72% RH. Higher temperatures and humidity resulted in a lower Ct required to produce skin effects.[75]

Rengstorff[76] documented CS exposures in firefighters in Washington, DC, during the 1968 riots, when law enforcement agents used CS to disperse rioters from buildings. Some structures were set ablaze during the rioting; as firemen entered the building, the heat, movement, and force of the water from their hoses caused the CS to reaerosolize. This caused swelling and reddening of the exposed skin in many firemen.[76]

Weigand and associates[72] documented a case in which soldiers experienced first- and second-degree burns from exposure to CS1 during a training exercise. Upon exposure, all soldiers experience a stinging sensation on their exposed skin. At 2 hours postexposure, some soldiers cleaned their body of the agent and changed their contaminated clothing; however, many did not. Those who did not bathe or change clothes developed severe erythema and blistering of the skin 14 to 16 hours postexposure.[72]

Weimar and associates[77] conducted patch testing on four volunteers with a 1% CS trioctylphosphate solution and solutions of 0.01% to 1.0% on the forearms of five volunteers. One subject experienced a stinging sensation for the first 30 minutes of the patch test. When the CS volume was increased from 0.01 to 0.025 mL on both bare skin and patch test skin, no reactions were noted. The researchers also applied patches of CS trioctylphosphate solutions ranging from 0.1% to 1% CS to the foreheads of five volunteers, which created stinging at all concentrations. Increasing the temperature from 75°C to 105°C and duplicating the tests produced similar results.[77]

Ballantyne and associates[78] exposed the skin of 52 volunteers to concentrations of CS ranging from 0.001% to 0.005% in glyceryl triacetate by saturating their clothes and bare skin with the solutions. The skin effects presented as sunburn-like irritation that started around the eyes and spread across the body, with hands and feet being affected last. The scalp and ears were not usually affected. The symptoms diminished after 10 minutes, even with the presence of soaked clothing. Erythema was observed hours later; however, no vesication, edema, or desquamation occurred. Minor cuts and abrasions were not affected differently than healthy skin.[78]

Ophthalmologic effects. CS causes instant irritation, burning, and swelling of the conjunctivae of the eye. It is most often accompanied by lacrimation and blepharospasm and in some cases, photophobia.[54] Several studies, animal and human, have been conducted to evaluate the ophthalmologic effects of this agent.[51,52,76,78–80] An early study exposed military and civilian volunteers in a wind tunnel to CS dispersed via CS-acetone spray (3 µm), CS-methylene dichloride spray (1 µm), and an M18 grenade (0.5 µm). Eyes of the subjects were instantly affected by burning that lasted 2 to 5 minutes, followed by conjunctivitis that remained up to 30 minutes. Tearing was produced almost immediately and persisted up to 15 minutes, whereas reddening of the eyelids persisted for an hour. Uncontrollable blinking sometimes accompanied the exposure. Some subjects complained of eye fatigue lasting 24 hours postexposure. For nearly 1 hour postexposure, 5% to 10% of the subjects experienced photophobia.[51]

Punte et al[52] evaluated the effect of CS particle size on the human eye by exposing six volunteers in a wind tunnel to CS particles of small size (0.9 µm mass median diameter) disseminated from a 2% CS solution in methylene dichloride and large-size (60 µm mass median diameter) particles from a powder hopper. Only the eyes were exposed. Two of five men exposed to small particles were able to tolerate exposure for 60 seconds, while all six men exposed to large particles were able to tolerate the exposure. Postexposure, all subjects had difficulty seeing. Recovery was 90 seconds for the smaller particles and 280 seconds for the larger particles. The study concluded that small particles produce eye irritation much faster than large particles; however, larger particles prolong the eye effect.[52]

Rengstorff[76] tested the ocular effects of CS on human volunteers by exposing them to concentrations of 0.1 to 6.7 mg•min/m^3 of CS (thermally dispersed) or CS2 (powder dispersed) for 20 seconds to 10 minutes. Subjects who kept their eyes open could read a vision chart and showed no significant change in visual acuity caused by the exposure.[76] In a follow-on study, the researchers administered 0.1% or 0.25% CS solutions in water and 1% solution in trioctylphosphate directly into the eyes of several volunteers. In addition to those symptoms experienced by Gutentag's study group, the subjects were unable to open their eyes for 10 to 135 seconds postexposure. Examination revealed no corneal damage.[79,80]

Ballantyne and associates[78] evaluated the ocular effects of CS by drenching clothed military volunteers with solutions containing 0.001% CS (3 men, 2 women), 0.002% CS (3 men, 2 women), 0.003% CS (2 men, 2 women), and 0.005% CS (22 men, 11 women) in glyceryl triacetate. Subjects were either drenched individually or as a group. For individual drenching, subjects were saturated at the head, trunk, and leg level at a rate of 15 L over a 15-second period. Subjects were observed and questioned at 20 minutes postexposure. For group drenching, the spray was directed at the group for a period of 1 minute. The group exercised before and after the drenching. Individuals were questioned during the exercises and as a group after showering. CS was found to affect the eye within seconds, causing stinging, uncontrollable blinking, and tearing. The irritant did not blur vision; rather, blurred vision was caused by tears. Symptoms resolved in 3 to 5 minutes.[78]

Gray and Murray[81] and Yih[82] reported an increase in eye injury caused by the use of CS sprays in

Great Britain during the 1990s. Ocular injuries were caused by the discharge of the agent at close range, which infiltrated the conjunctiva, cornea, and sclera with CS powder. This exposure sometimes resulted in complications such as symblepharon, pseudopterygium, infective keratitis, trophic keratopathy, posterior synechia, secondary glaucoma, cataracts, hyphema, vitreous hemorrhage, and traumatic optic neuropathy.[81–83]

Gastrointestinal effects. A review of the literature revealed no human studies assessing oral toxicity of CS; however, incidents of intentional and accidental ingestion of this compound have been documented. Most cases involved children who accidentally ingested CS they found while playing in impact areas of military installations. An intentional ingestion occurred during an attempted suicide by a healthy young man. For treatment, he was given large amounts of saline cathartics, and, after abdominal cramps and diarrhea, he fully recovered. An accidental ingestion occurred when a male swallowed a 820-mg CS pellet thinking it was a vitamin. He was treated with liquid antacid and viscous lidocaine and administered droperidol intravenously. After vomiting twice and having six watery bowel movements, he recovered fully.[3]

Solomon et al[84] documented an incident in which seven people accidentally consumed CS-contaminated juice in central Israel. Five of the seven presented to a primary care clinic within minutes with complaints of eye irritation, tearing, headache, facial irritation, and burning of the mouth and throat. The other two people presented the next day with complaints of nausea, abdominal pain, and diarrhea. When inspecting the juice container, investigators found several small CS pellets partially dissolved at the bottom. Upon questioning, patients revealed that the burning sensation did not occur immediately upon consumption; rather, it presented minutes later.[84] This presentation of symptoms is consistent with research by Kemp and Willder, who found that subjects who consumed sugar contaminated with CS did not feel symptoms for 30 seconds after consumption. This delayed onset of symptoms was attributed to the masking of the CS by the sweetness of the sugar.[85] The two patients who presented with symptoms the following day did not experience any bad flavor. All patients were observed for 24 hours and released. The amount of ingestion was estimated to be less than 25 mg; the lethal amount for a 70-kg man is about 14 g. The author concluded that it might be impossible for a person to accidentally consume a lethal amount because of the low taste threshold and local irritation caused by the compound.[84]

Long-term effects and severe medical complications. Although studies show that the effects of CS are short-lived and typically resolve within minutes of exiting the contaminated area, three cases of prolonged airway dysfunction following exposure to the agent have been reported. Studies show that exposure to high levels of respiratory irritants is associated with the development of reactive airways disease syndrome (RADS) in some individuals.[86] Hu et al[87] was the first to make the association between CS and RADS in his assessment of the use of CS in South Korea, after noting that the community displayed the typical symptoms of RADS (prolonged cough and shortness of breath) after heavy exposure to CS.[87] Roth and Franzblau[88] later reported a previously healthy 53-year-old man who, after exposure to a CS/OC mixture, experienced a decreased exercise tolerance, chronic cough, fatigue, and irregular pulmonary function tests that persisted for months postexposure.[88] Hill et al[89] reported a 31-year-old prison worker who was occupationally exposed to CS during a "shake-down." In the months following exposure, the subject continued to suffer from symptoms consistent with RADS.[89] The Himsworth report on British law enforcement use of CS concluded that exposure to the agent could result in death by inflicting pulmonary damage leading to pulmonary edema; however, the authors noted that the concentration required to cause this complication is several hundred times greater than the exposure dosage that produces intolerable symptoms.[37,38] No deaths attributed to CS exposure have been documented.[72]

CS is also a powerful skin sensitizer that can cause allergic contact dermatitis with rashes or hypersensitivity upon repeated exposure to the agent.[50] A 1960 report[90] of CS exposures in plant workers by Bowers and associates revealed three general reactions to exposure: a single local reaction with no recurrence upon repeated exposure, local responses with progressively shorter latent periods, and generalized-type eruptions with progressively shorter latent periods. The author suggests that anyone who experiences one of these reactions should not return to CS-contaminated atmospheres.[90]

OC (OLEORESIN CAPSICUM)

OC is a naturally occurring mixture of compounds extracted from more than 20 different species of the capsicum plant, which include chili peppers, red peppers, jalapeno, and paprika (eg, *Capsicum frutescens, Capsicum annuum*). More than 100 different compounds have been identified in various OC extracts. The composition of the extract, and hence its precise physiological and toxicological properties, can vary depending on numerous factors, including the type and age of plant used for isolation and the method of extraction. Many of the physiological responses induced by OC are due to a family of compounds known as capsaicinoids. OC is 0.1% to 1.0% capsaicinoids by dry mass. The main capsaicinoid of interest as an irritant and RCA is capsaicin (*trans*-8-methyl-*N*-vanillyl-6-noneamide). The capsaicinoids content of OC is approximately 70% capsaicin, 20% dihydrocapsaicin, 7% norhydrocapsaicin, 1% homocapsaicin, and 1% homodihydrocapsaicin.

Historically, capsicum was used as a weapon by the ancient Chinese and Japanese police. In 1492 native Mexicans burned pepper in oil to create an irritating and suffocating smoke.[91] OC in small doses is used medicinally as a topical analgesic or counter-irritant. Capsaicin spray is also used in the pharmaceutical industry to induce cough for testing antitussive candidates.[92] Recently PAVA (nonivamide), a structural analog of capsaicin, was synthesized. PAVA, which can be used instead of naturally derived OC sprays, is believed to have similar but safer effects and more consistent ingredients than the natural form of OC.[4,93]

Physical Characteristics and Deployment

Capsaicin (Chemical Abstracts Service [CAS] registry number 404-86-4) has a molecular weight of 305.41 and a molecular formula of $C_{18}H_{27}NO_3$ (See Figure 13-6; Table 13-1). An odorless crystalline to waxy compound, capsaicin has limited solubility in water. OC is a derivative of hot cayenne peppers. PAVA (CAS 2444-46-4) has a molecular formula of $C_{17}H_{27}NO_3$ (Figure 13-7) and a molecular weight of 293.4.[93,94]

Because of its highly effective irritant properties, OC has found widespread use in various military, government, and civilian agencies for riot control and individual protection. OC is also available to the general public for personal protection. US forces deployed to Somalia carried nonlethal packages that included OC. Military police from several US Army divisions as well as several Marine Corps units, who have used OC in the past, are currently investigating its capabilities and supporting its use.[10,95] Numerous formulations of OC have been developed and marketed (commonly referred to as pepper spray, pepper mace, and pepper gas), but there appears to be no standardization.

Major factors separating one OC spray from another are the delivery device, carrier, and propellant system.[95] Currently, the most popular carrier is isopropyl alcohol. Additional carriers have included Freon, Dymel-22 (both made by DuPont, Wilmington, Del), and methylene chloride. However, with the exception of isopropyl alcohol, most OC carriers and propellants are currently banned or have use restricted by the 1987 Montreal Protocol, which attempts to regulate the use of chemicals with the potential to adversely affect the ozone layer.

The use of isopropyl alcohol as a carrier complicates the toxic effect of OC in two ways. First, isopropyl alcohol and other volatile carriers readily evaporate in the environment, and evaporation rates from OC fog and OC mist are greater than from OC streams, making it challenging to calculate the actual concentration of OC (ie, dose) on the target tissue. Second, isopropyl alcohol has physiological effects (as do the other over 100 constituents of oleoresin), causing a mild transitory injury (grade 4 on a scale of 10) when applied to rabbit eyes.[96] Additionally, the interaction of the other capsaicinoids in the oleoresin with capsaicin have not been well defined.

A variety of dissemination devices for OC exist, including many commercial preparations, and the method of choice depends largely on the number of expected subjects. These devices range from small items such as fake pens and pressurized cans, used to incapacitate subjects at close range, to grenades and cartridges for shotgun-mounted launchers, used to control groups of individuals from a distance. Some dissemination devices release OC as a fine mist or fog; others spray a stream of OC towards the subject. More recently OC has been dispensed in a "pepper ball"—a gel ball (similar to a recreational paint gun ball), fired from a high pressure air gun, that hits the individual and breaks on contact, releasing aerosolized dry OC.[97]

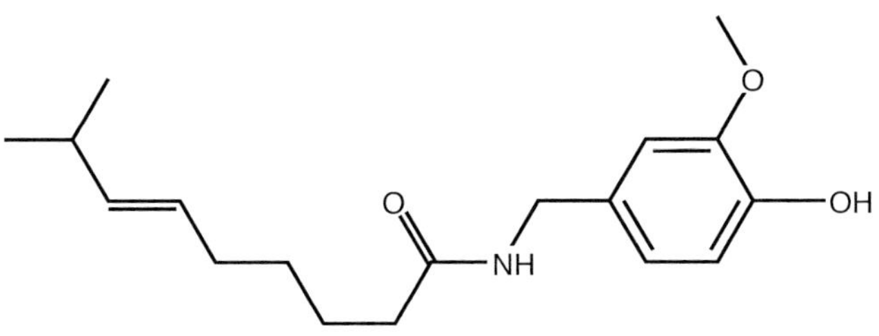

Fig. 13-6. Chemical structure of capsaicin.

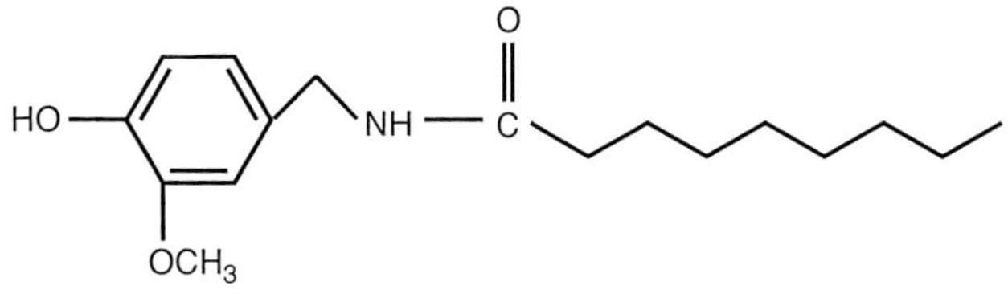

Fig. 13-7. Chemical structure of pelargonyl vanillylamide.

Physiological Effects

Capsaicin is a member of the vanilloid family of chemical compounds and binds to the vallinoid receptor subtype 1 (VR1) on sensory neurons; the VR1 receptor was discovered in 1997 using capsaicin as the ligand.[98] VR1, now known as TRPV1, is a member of the transient receptor potential (TRP) superfamily of receptors. TRPV1 is activated, in part, by excessive heat (>43°C) or abrasion, which explains why a major sensation following exposure to peppers is burning and heat. Mice deficient in TPRV1 receptors are defective in nociceptive, inflammatory, and hypothermic responses.[99] Thus, capsaicin does not cause a chemical burn, only the sensation of one. TRPV1 is also involved in purinergic signaling by the bladder urothelium, and its activation leads to a bladder distension sensation.[100]

Many of the acute respiratory effects induced by capsaicin in laboratory animals and humans are associated with the release of bioactive compounds such as substance P, neurokinin A, and calcitonin gene-related peptide from sensory nerves innervating these tissues.[4,73] The actions of these compounds result in clinical symptoms associated with exposure to capsaicin: bronchoconstriction, mucous secretion, edema of the tracheobronchial mucosa, enhanced vascular permeability, and neutrophil chemotaxis.

Clinical Effects

OC, CS, and CN are considered peripheral sensory irritants that interact with sensory nerve receptors in the skin or mucosae to produce local sensation (discomfort, itching, burning sensation, or pain) together with related local and some systemic (autonomic) reflexes. The effects subside after removal of the stimulus and do not result in any long-term adverse sequelae. The principle effects of these agents are on the eye, respiratory tract, and skin. On the eyes, depending on the concentration, the effects are local itching, discomfort, or pain with excessive lacrimation and blepharospasm as local reflexes.[2]

Pain stimuli can be suppressed through a variety of mechanisms (eg, medication and alcohol, ignored through discipline, or overcome by anger and aggression). The sensory irritation induced by OC can involve inflammation and swelling in respiratory tissues and the eyes. The ocular swelling forces the eye to involuntarily shut, which cannot be overcome or suppressed[95] (people who are described as "unaffected" by OC spray still display involuntary eye closure and temporary blindness[101]).

Acute Effects

As with any compound, the physiological and toxicological effects following acute exposure to OC are a function of the dose and route of exposure. In humans, these can range from mild irritant effects that quickly resolve following removal of the stimulant to lethality, which can occur within 1 hour of exposure. The most immediate affect following exposure to OC in a spray is in the eyes, with lacrimation and blepharospasm. Following inhalation, OC can also induce changes in the respiratory system, including nasal irritation, severe coughing, sneezing, and shortness of breath. A burning sensation in the skin is another common effect. Finally, neuromotor dysfunction and accompanying loss of motor control can result. High doses of capsaicin can induce serious and sometimes lethal toxicity on the respiratory, cardiovascular, and sensory nervous system.

The LD_{50}s for capsaicin are 0.56 mg/kg (intravenous), 7.6 mg/kg (intraperitoneal), 7.8 mg/kg (intramuscular), 9.0 mg/kg (subcutaneous), 190 mg/kg (oral), 512 mg/kg (dermal), and 1.6 mg/kg (intratracheal).[102] The most probable cause of death is respiratory paralysis. The estimated oral lethal dose in humans ranges from 0.5 to 5.0 g/kg.[102]

Respiratory Effects

The respiratory system is a major target following exposure to OC owing to the highly sensitive TRPV1 receptors located in the mucosa of the respiratory tract. These effects have been characterized in several reviews.[73,95] The initial symptoms of exposure are often a tingling sensation accompanied by the protective mechanisms of coughing and decreased inhalation rates. Thereafter, depending on dose, intense irritation accompanied by severe pain occurs. Profound vasodilatation and secretion occur in the nasal passages, both of which are considered protective mechanisms. In lower portions of the respiratory tract, capsaicin induces bronchoconstriction, pulmonary edema, and in severe cases of poisoning, apnea and respiratory arrest.

Dermatological Effects

Although OC is most effective on the eyes and mucous membranes, it does irritate the skin, which contributes to the overall unpleasant effects of the compound.[73] Following contact with skin, OC can induce intense burning pain, tingling, edema, erythema, and occasional blistering, depending on dose. The sensations usually last less than an hour following exposure. In humans, repeated applications of OC to facial skin produced initial symptoms of irritation, but the intensity and duration of the effect decreases to the point of no observable reaction.[103] Repeated short-term exposure, in a matter of minutes, can also lead to an exaggerated response to concomitant pathologies, such as experimental inflammation and allergic dermatitis.

Ophthalmologic Effects

OC is a potent ocular irritant. The clinical signs of exposure to pepper spray include lacrimation, inflammation of the conjunctiva, redness, burning, pain, swelling, and blepharospasm. As mentioned previously, victims will involuntarily shut their eyes to the inflammatory effects of OC. Although the individual may voluntarily hold their eyes shut for up to 30 minutes following exposure, visual acuity normally returns within 2 to 5 minutes following decontamination.[12] When directly applied to the eye, OC can cause neurogenic inflammation, unresponsiveness to chemical and mechanical stimuli, and loss of the blink reflex, which can last for days following exposure.[73]

Gastrointestinal Disturbances

The effects of OC on the gastrointestinal tract and its impact on nutrition have been investigated by several researchers and were recently summarized by Olajos and Salem.[73] Many of the studies have focused on direct toxicity of intestinal epithelial cells following administration of capsaicinoids and the association between toxicity and altered fat uptake. A study of the effect of intragastric capsaicin on gastric ulcer using a rat model found that 2 to 6 mL/kg aggravated existing gastric mucosal damage.[104]

Other Physiological Responses

In addition to the well-described effects of OC on the eyes and respiratory system, capsaicin has a direct effect on the thermoregulatory system. Capsaicin has a long history of use in the laboratory for studying the physiological processes of temperature regulation.

Long-Term Effects and Severe Medical Complications

When mice were fed ground *Capsicum annuum* (high dose = 0.5%-10% body weight) for a 4-week period, slight glycogen depletion and anisocytosis of hepatocytes were noted with the high-dose group, but it was concluded that *C annum* was relatively nontoxic to mice.[105] Likewise, rats fed capsaicin (50 mg/kg per day) or capsicum (500 mg/kg per day) for a period of 60 days had significant reductions of plasma urea nitrogen, glucose, phospholipids, triglycerides, total cholesterol, free fatty acids, glutamic pyruvic transaminase, and alkaline phosphatase, but these effects were considered mild.[106] Thus, although repeated doses of capsaicin are associated with some biochemical alterations, it appears to be well tolerated in experimental animals at high doses.

OTHER RIOT CONTROL COMPOUNDS

PS (Chloropicrin)

PS (CAS 76-06-2, also called nitrochloroform) was used as a tear gas (harassing agent) during World War I. Beginning in the early 1920s, PS was used commercially as an antitheft device and, since the 1950s, as a soil fumigant to kill root-destroying fungi, nematodes, and soil insects that damage delicate plants and vegetables, such as strawberries. It is currently a restricted-use pesticide in the United States but has wider use in other countries.[107] Although used as a harassing agent, PS acts much like a pulmonary agent and is often classified as such. As a security device, safes and vaults were frequently outfitted with chemical vials that released PS when breeched. Several companies produced these devices between 1920 and 1950. The number and location of PS-laden safes sold or still in circulation is unknown, and modern-day accidental exposures sporadically occur. As recently as 2003, in Beloit, Wisconsin, a safe owner was exposed to approximately 112 g of PS after the storage vial accidentally cracked; and in 1999 a pregnant worker in an Iowa bank was accidentally exposed to PS from a shattered vial.[108] Both victims sustained eye and skin irritation, with the latter victim also reporting irritation in the throat. The 2004 incident in Sofia was the most recent newsworthy deployment of PS. It was originally believed that a disgruntled individual threw a bomb containing PS into the crowded area, but Bulgarian authorities later reported that the incident occurred by accident when a 50-year-old man dropped a vial of PS from his pocket.[17,18]

The United States produces approximately 10 million pounds of PS per year for use as a soil fumigant, either by itself or, owing to its odor, as a warning agent for other odorless fumigants such as methyl bromide.[109–111] Human exposures resulting from environmental application of PS as a fumigant have been reported. Most recently, 165 persons reported symptoms consistent with PS exposure following application of 100% PS at a concentration of 36 kg per acre to 34 acres in Kern, California.[112,113] Although PS dissipates readily in the environment, trace amounts are found in drinking water disinfected by chlorination.[60,114,115] Despite its historical and current uses, PS-induced toxicity resulting from inhalation, ingestion, or direct skin or eye contact remains poorly documented.

Physical Characteristics and Deployment

The molecular weight of PS is 164.4, and its molecular formula is CCl_3NO_2 (Figure 13-8). PS is an oily, volatile, colorless to faint-yellow liquid with an intensely irritating odor. Weaponized PS is primarily disseminated through wind dispersion, the simplest technique of delivering an agent to its target. It consists of placing the agent directly on or adjacent to the target immediately before dissemination (eg, antitheft devices placed on safes). Analogous dispersion methods were used in the early 20th century for delivery of chlorine, phosgene, and mustard gases. It was learned from the 2003 Kern, California, incident that when PS was injected 17 to 18 inches into the soil, people residing one quarter of a mile downwind experienced irritating effects.[112] See Table 13-3 for a summary of the characteristics of DM and other agents.

Physiological Effects

The immediate physiological effect of PS is sensory irritation via stimulation of the trigeminal nerve endings located in the nasal mucosa, which leads to the clinical signs of exposure: a burning sensation of the nasal passages, inhibition of respiration, and lacrimation.[111,116] As an irritant, PS causes cellular lesions at the site of exposure (ie, lung lesions following inhalation, dermal lesions following contact with skin, and forestomach lesions following ingestion). Although these clinical and pathological effects have been characterized, the mechanisms of toxicity, particularly the biotransformation of the parent compound and the toxicity of the metabolites, are poorly understood.[117] It has been known for some time that PS can react directly with hemoglobin to form methemoglobin and that the toxicity of PS in mice is linked to the oxidative state of hemoglobin.[117,118] However, the contribution of these laboratory observations to the tissue damage observed in the clinic has yet to be resolved.

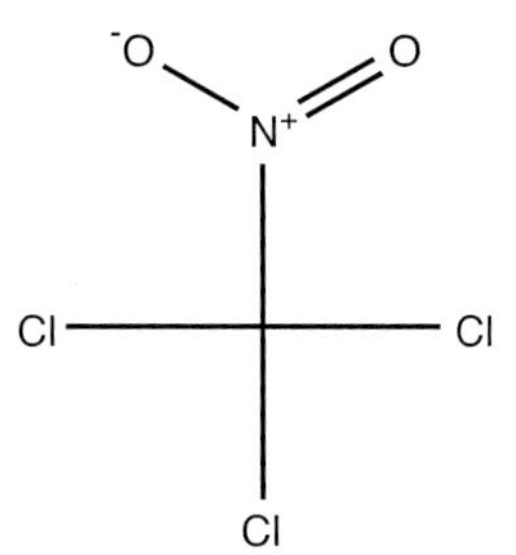

Fig. 13-8. Chemical structure of PS.

Other studies conducted in the 1940s suggested that the lacrimatory effect may be due, in part, to a selective reaction of PS with certain tissue dehydrogenases (eg, pyruvate dehydrogenase and succinate dehydrogenase).[119] Likewise, a causal relationship between these metabolic effects and toxicity has not been established. Rapid reductive dechlorination of PS to $CHCl_2NO_2$ by glutathione and other tissue thiols in vitro suggests that metabolites may be mediators of toxicity, but major differences in urinary metabolites of the compounds only partially support this hypothesis.[117] More recent evidence suggests a novel metabolic pathway for PS that involves conversion to raphanusamic acid; this study suggested that toxicity was mediated by the parent compound rather than metabolites.[117]

Clinical Effects

The major organs affected following acute exposure to PS are the eyes, skin, and respiratory tract.[69] With increasing doses or prolonged exposure times, systemic toxicity and lethality are observed. The dose of PS required to induce acute symptoms appears to be intermediate between the corresponding doses of chlorine and phosgene. Unlike with phosgene, there is no latent period between PS exposure and clinical symptoms.[60] "Chloropicrin syndrome" is characterized by unusual taste; eye tearing; nose and throat irritation; neurological symptoms (headache, nausea, and vomiting); shortness of breath; and anxiety.[111] The IDLH for PS is 2 ppm (1 ppm=6.72 mg/m^3) and the estimated LCt_{50} is 2,000 mg•min/m^3.[96] The inhalation LD_{50} in cats and pigs appears to be 800 mg/m^3 for a 20-minute exposure.[120] Acute pulmonary edema and dyspnea were observed in both species, and emphysema was reported in the pig. In mice, the LD_{50} is reported at 66 mg/m^3 for a 4-hour exposure.[120] The murine intraperitoneal LD_{50} for PS is 15 mg/kg, and the rat oral LD_{50} is 250 mg/kg.[117,121]

Respiratory effects. Inhalation of a sensory irritant causes inhibition of respiration and Kratschmer reflex. In the laboratory, inhibition of respiration is often measured by the dose required to cause a 50% decrease in respiration (RD_{50}).[122] PS exposure in mice at the RD_{50} dose (8 ppm) for 5 days, 6 hours per day, results in nasal lesions of the respiratory epithelium consisting of moderate exfoliation, erosion, ulceration, and necrosis coupled with minor squamous metaplasia and inflammation.[116] Moderate ulceration and necrosis of the olfactory epithelium, coupled with serous exudates and moderate lung pathology, were also observed. Collectively, the PS pathology was similar to that observed following an RD_{50} exposure to chlorine and displayed a distinct anterior–posterior severity gradient. The significant toxicity in the posterior nasal cavity following inhalation of PS or chlorine was likely the result of the agents' low water solubilities, which prevented significant absorption in the anterior nasal cavity.

The human toxicity of PS following inhalation is primarily restricted to the small to medium bronchi, and death may result from pulmonary edema, bronchopneumonia, or bronchiolitis obliterans.[123] As little as 1.3 ppm may cause respiratory irritation in humans.[109] The NIOSH, OSHA, and ACGIH exposure limit for PS is 0.1 ppm (time-weighted average of 0.7 mg/m^3).[69] The NIOSH IDLH level of 2.0 ppm is based partly on studies conducted in the early 1930s that determined that a few-second exposure to 4 ppm renders a man unfit for action.[69,112,124] Symptoms in humans resulting from environmental or occupational exposures to PS include pain (burning) and tightness in the chest, shortness of breath, sore throat, dyspnea, irritation, asthma exacerbation, and cough.[111,112,125] The lowest published toxic concentration in humans is 2 mg/m^3 (unknown exposure time), which produced lacrimation and conjunctiva irritation, and the lowest reported human lethal dose is 2,000 mg/m^3 for a 10-minute exposure.[69]

Dermatological effects. Direct exposure of skin to PS leads to irritation, itching, rash, and blisters.[108,111,112] The minimal dose required to cause these effects is unknown.

Ophthalmologic effects. PS causes eye irritation beginning at 0.3 to 0.4 ppm, which appears to be below the threshold of odor (approximately 1 ppm).[109,124,126] Clinical symptoms of PS-induced ocular irritation include immediate lacrimation, pain, and burning. In 1995 three dockworkers were exposed to PS that had leaked from a shipping container.[111] All three victims complained of burning and stinging in the eyes. Additionally, in the 2003 Kern, California, exposures, of the 165 persons complaining of PS-induced reactions, 99% (164) of them reported eye irritation (82% reported lacrimation, and 54% reported pain or burning of the eyes).[112]

Gastrointestinal disturbances. Following ingestion of PS, a corrosive effect on the forestomach tissue is the principal lesion.[114] Rats exposed to PS (10–80 mg/kg) for 10 days demonstrated corrosion of the forestomach with histopathological findings including inflammation, necrosis, acantholysis, hyperkeratosis, and epithelial hyperplasia. In humans, acute exposure to PS in the atmosphere from environmental sources and occupational accidents has been associated with an unusual taste, stomach and abdominal cramping, abdominal tenderness, diarrhea, vomiting, nausea, difficulty swallowing, and in rare cases, bloody stools.[111,112]

Other physiological responses. Additional clinical and toxicological observations associated with acute PS exposure in humans include neurological manifestations (headache, dizziness, and fatigue); cyanosis; general neuromuscular tenderness; peripheral numbness; painful urination; chest wall pain; elevations in creatine phosphokinase; and low-grade rhabdomyolysis.[111,112]

Long-term effects and severe medical complications. Long-term or repeated exposures to PS are associated with damage to the kidneys and heart, and may result in hypersensitivity to subsequent PS exposures. No adequate data is available to assess the mutagenic, carcinogenic, teratogenic, or reproductive toxicity of PS in humans.[60]

CN (1-Chloroacetophenone)

CN is also known as Mace from its chemical name, **m**ethyl chloro**ace**tephenone. The first chemical Mace product is widely regarded as the original tear gas.[127,128] Although it is the trademarked name for CN, the term "mace" is commonly used generically to refer to any RCA. After the United States entered the First World War, American and British chemists investigated CN and found it to be one of the most effective lacrimators known. Its lacrimatory effects and persistence were equal to or slightly greater than bromobenzyl cyanide, and its chlorine was less expensive than bromine. CN is very stable under normal conditions and does not corrode steel. It is a crystalline solid that can be dissolved in a solvent or delivered in thermal grenades.

Physical Characteristics and Deployment

CN (CAS 532-27-4, also known as *w*-chloroacetophenone, *a*-chloroacetophenone, phenacyl chloride, 2-chloro-1-phenylethanone, and phenyl chloromethyl ketone) is a gray solid with an apple blossom odor. It has a molar mass of 154.5, corresponding to a molecular formula of C_8H_7ClO (Figure 13-9). Its molar solubility at 20°C is 4.4×10^{-3} mol/L (68 mg/100 mL) in water. Hydrolysis of CN is very slow in water even when alkali is added.[71] Melting and boiling points are 54°C

TABLE 13-3

CHARACTERISTICS OF PS, CN, DM, AND CR

Properties	PS	CN	DM	CR
Molecular formula	CCl_3NO_2	C_8H_7ClO	$C_{12}H_9AsClN$	$C_{13}H_9NO$
Former/ Current use	RCA and war gas/ Preplant soil fumigant	War gas/RCA	War gas, vomiting agent/obsolete RCA	RCA/RCA
Physical state*	Colorless oily liquid	Colorless to gray crystalline solid	Light yellow to canary green crystals	Pale yellow crystalline solid
Odor	Strong, sharp, pungent and highly irritating odor	Fragrant (like apple blossoms)	Odorless or not pronounced. May be mildly irritating	Pepper-like
Freezing and/ or melting point	Melting point: -64°C Freezing point: -69°C	Melting point: 57°C	Melting point: 195°C with slight decomposition	Melting point: 72°C
Vapor pressure	20 mm Hg at 20°C	0.0041–0.005 mm Hg at 0°C	Negligible at ambient temperature. 4.5×10^{-11} mm Hg at 25°C	Data not available
Density:				
Vapor (relative to air)	5.6 times heavier	5.3 times heavier		
Liquid	1.66 g/mL	1.187 g/mL at approximately 58°C		
Solid		1.318 g /cm^3 at approximately 20°C	Bulk: < 1g/cm^3 Crystal: 1.65 g/cm^3 at 20°C	
Solubility:				
In water	Insoluble	Relatively insoluble; slow hydrolysis; 1.64 g/100 mL at 25°C	0.044 g/L at 37°C, very slow hydrolysis	Relatively insoluble and not hydrolyzed
In other solvents	Soluble in organic solvents, lipids	Soluble in carbon disulfide, ether, and benzene	Slightly soluble in benzene, xylene acetone, alcohols. Acidic solutions prevent hydrolysis	Is sometimes suspended in solutions of propylene glycol, but data on solvents not available
Hydrolysis products	Carbon dioxide, bicarbonate, chloride, nitrate, and nitrite. May also produce toxic vapors such as oxides of nitrogen, phosgene, nitrosyl chloride, and chlorine	HCl	Diphenylaminearsenious oxide and HCl	Data not available
Decontamination:				
Clothing	Move to fresh air; remove clothing, do not wear again until properly laundered or discard	Move to fresh air; remove clothing and wash before wearing again	Move to fresh air; remove clothing and wash before wearing again	Move to fresh air; remove clothing and wash before wearing again

(**Table 13-3** *continues*)

Table 13-3 *continued*

Skin	Copious soap and water	Copious soap and water	Copious soap and water	Copious soap and water or use 5% or 10% sodium bicarbonate solution, which is more effective than water
Equipment	Copious soap and water	Copious soap and water	Copious soap and water	Copious soap and water
Persistency:				
In soil	Half life from 8 hours to 4.5 days	Short	Persistent	Persistent
On material	Half-life is 20 days or less in sunlight	Short	Persistent	Persistent
Skin and eye effects	Irritation, itching, rash, and blisters on exposed skin. Eye lacrimation, pain, and burning appear below the threshold of the odor. Very potent lacrimator	Primarily skin erythema that is bradykinin-mediated and acute. Can develop blisters and burns on moist tissue due to HCl formation. Strong lacrimator with conjunctivitis, eye pain, and blepharospasm. High dose can produce chemical injury to the eyes	Significant nasal discharge. The amount needed to cause skin irritation and erythema is above that needed for irritation of respiratory and gastrointestinal tract. Repeated dose leads to sensitization. Only slight eye irritation reported when throat and chest irritation are present	Burning of skin, particularly in a hot and moist environment. Erythema and blistering are possible with lengthy exposure. Produces violent lacrimation in the eyes, with burning, conjunctivitis, and lid erythema
Respiratory effects	Immediate burning sensation in nasal passages, choking, and inhibition of respiration. Can cause lung lesions	Upper respiratory irritation, cough, dyspnea. Can also produce tissue burns of the airway and pulmonary lesions if dose is significant	Sneezing, coughing,. salivation, and congestion of the nose and upper airway to produce a feeling of suffocation	Burning sensation and pain in the upper respiratory tract with subsequent feeling of suffocation
Other effects			Produces initial nausea followed by violent retching and vomiting, which can occur 20–30 minutes after initial exposure. Can also produce perspiration, chills, mental depression, abdominal cramps, and diarrhea lasting several hours	Anxiety, fatigue

*At standard temperature and pressure.

Data sources: (1) Sidell F. Riot control agents. In: Sidell F, Takafuji E, Franz D, eds. *Medical Aspects of Chemical and Biological Warfare.* In: Zajtchuk R, Bellamy RF, eds. *Textbook of Military Medicine.* Washington, DC: Department of the Army, Office of The Surgeon General, Borden Institute; 1997: Chap 12. (2) US Department of the Army. *Potential Military Chemical/Biological Agents and Compounds, Multiservice Tactics, Techniques, and Procedures.* Washington, DC: DA; January 10, 2005. FM 3-11.9. (3) Somani SM, Romano JA Jr, eds. *Chemical Warfare Agents: Toxicity at Low Levels.* Boca Raton, Fla: CRC Press; 2001. (4) US Army Center for Health Promotion and Preventive Medicine. Detailed facts about tear Agent chloropicrin (PS). USCHPPM Web site. Available at: http://chppm-www.apgea.army.mil/dts/docs/detps.pdf. Accessed December 27, 2006. (5) Chloropicarin as a Soil Fumigant. US Department of Agriculture, Agricultural Research Service Web site. Available at: http://www.ars.usda.gov. Accessed November 2, 2005. (6) Centers for Disease Control and Prevention. Exposure to tear gas from a theft-deterrent device on a safe—Wisconsin, December 2003. *MMWR Morb Mortal Wkly Rep.* 2004;53:176–177.

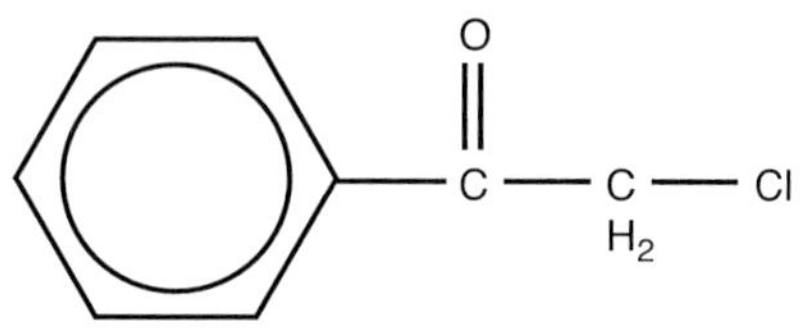

Fig. 13-9. Chemical structure of CN.

and 247°C, respectively. Density of the solid is 1.318 g/ cm^3 at 20°C, and density of the liquid is 1.187 g/ m^3 at 58°C. The vapor is 5.3 times heavier than air.[14]

Although CN was not produced in sufficient quantities to be used in World War I, Japan used the agent as early as 1930 against aboriginal Taiwanese.[128] CN was used as the tear gas of choice for the 3 decades after its introduction, but its use markedly declined after the development of CS.[96]

Physiological Effects

CN and CS are SN2 alkylating agents with activated halogen groups that react with nucleophilic sites and combine with intracellular sulfhydryl groups on enzymes such as lactic dehydrogenase to inactivate the enzymes. The effects are transient because the enzymes are rapidly reactivated. It has been suggested that tissue injury may be related to inactivation of certain of these enzyme systems. Pain can occur without tissue injury and may be mediated by bradykinin. On contact with skin and mucous membranes, CN releases chlorine atoms, which are reduced to hydrochloric acid, causing local irritation and burns.[129]

CN, which is converted to an electrophilic metabolite, reacts with sulfhydryl groups and other nucleophilic sites of biomolecules. Alkylation of sulfhydryl-containing enzymes leads to enzyme inhibition with disruption of cellular processes. Castro[130] investigated the effects of CN on human plasma cholinesterase, based on the potential to disrupt enzyme functions. He found CN to inhibit the cholinesterase via a nonsulfhydryl interaction, concluding that the toxic effects of CN may be due to alkylation of sulfhydryl-containing enzymes.[130]

Animal Studies

Toxicology. Comparative acute and repeat dose toxicity studies have been conducted in various animal species (review and summarized by McNamara et al[27]). The studies produced highly variable results, prompting subsequent studies in the mid-1960s designed to provide more quantitative data. In these studies, CN in acetone was dispersed from commercially available thermal grenades. Sublethal effects observed on exposure to CN consisted of lacrimation, conjunctivitis, copious nasal secretions, salivation, hyperactivity, dyspnea, and lethargy, which occurred in all animals. CN is considered a more toxic lacrimator than CS or CR, and at high concentrations it has caused corneal epithelial damage and chemosis. CN, as well as CS and CR, causes almost instant pain in the eyes, excessive flow of tears, and closure of the eyelids.[71]

The primary cause of death following CN inhalation appeared to be from pulmonary damage. The LCt_{50} values for various species were reported to be 8,878; 7,984; and 7,033 mg•min/ m^3 for the rat, guinea pig, and dog, respectively. The pathological observations in the animals that died from CN inhalation included pulmonary congestion, edema, emphysema, tracheitis, bronchitis, and bronchopneumonia. The pathological findings in animals following death by CN inhalation reported by Ballantyne and Swanston[40] included congestion of alveolar capillaries, alveolar hemorrhage, and excessive secretions in the bronchi and bronchioles. The researchers also reported areas of acute inflammatory cell infiltration of the trachea, bronchi, and bronchioles. McNamara et al[131] exposed guinea pigs, dogs, and monkeys to thermally generated CN on 10 consecutive days at C*t*s ranging from 2,300 to 4,000 mg•min/ m^3, for a total of 31,445 mg•min/ m^3.[131] This dosage would be expected to be lethal to about 75% of the guinea pigs and 100% of the monkeys if administered as a single dose. However, these exposures resulted in the death of only five guinea pigs and no deaths in the monkeys. When administered in divided dosages, the toxicity of CN is considerably lower. These findings were confirmed in additional studies in which dogs were exposed on 10 consecutive days to C*t*s ranging from 3,000 to 7,000 mg•min/ m^3 for a total dosage of 60,000 mg•min/ m^3. Subsequent repeated dose studies in guinea pigs, dogs, and monkeys exposed daily for 10 days to C*t*s ranging from 4,200 to 13,000 mg•min/ m^3 were lethal to the majority of the animals for all species tested. Overall, these studies demonstrated the lack of cumulative toxicity of CN when administered in divided dosages.

Kumar et al[132] subjected mice to multiple exposures of CN and CR at concentrations equivalent to 0.05 LCt_{50}—87 mg/ m^3 for CN and 1,008 mg/ m^3 for CR—for 15 minutes per day for 5 and 10 days. Biochemical endpoints measured included blood glucose, plasma urea, transaminase enzymes (serum glutamic:oxaloacetic transaminase and serum glutamic:pyruvic transaminase), liver acid phosphatase, liver glutathione levels, and hepatic lipid peroxidation (malondialdehyde formation). Clinical parameters affected by repeated exposures included decreased hepatic glutathione and increased lipid peroxidation. Hepatic acid phosphatase increased after the 5-day CN exposure, and the glutathione levels decreased after the 10-day CN exposure. CN-induced elevation in acid phosphatase levels reflected the release of lysosomal enzyme from the liver, which is indicative of tissue injury. CR exposure did not produce any significant alteration of the biochemical parameters. Additionally, hyperglycemia was observed after exposure to CN, an effect previously reported by Husain et al.[133] It was suggested that the hyperglycemia was induced by the stress-mediated release of epinephrine, which is known to elevate glucose levels. Significant decreases in body weight gain were also noted on exposure to these compounds, with CN having a more prominent effect on body weight.

The acute mammalian inhalation toxicity of CN was 3 to 10 times greater than CS toxicity in rats, rabbits, guinea pigs, and mice. Lung pathology in the CN-exposed animals was also severe, consisting of patchy acute inflammatory cell infiltration of the trachea and bronchioles, as well as of more edema and more evidence of early bronchopneumonia than with CS.[134]

Ocular effects. In a variety of studies, mice and rats exposed to CN aerosols for 13 weeks had no findings of gross clinical signs except for irritation of the eyes, including opacity. No microscopic lesions were noted compared to controls. Avoidance and the intense lacrimation and blepharospasm are indicative of defensive mechanisms caused by CN ocular irritation. High concentrations of CN may result in chemical injury to the eyes, with corneal and conjunctival edema and erosion, or ulceration, chemosis, and focal hemorrhage.[135–137] CN-induced ocular effects on the rabbit eye have been investigated by Ballantyne et al[138] and Gaskins et al.[139] The effects included lacrimation, chemosis, iritis, blepharitis, and keratitis, and the severity was dependent on the formulation.

Sublethal effects observed on exposure to CN consisted of lacrimation, conjunctivitis, copious nasal secretions, salivation, hyperactivity, dyspnea, and lethargy, which occurred in all animals. At high concentrations CN has caused corneal epithelial damage and chemosis. Like CS and CR, CN causes almost instant pain in the eyes along with excessive flow of tears and closure of the eyelids.[71] The ocular effect of conjunctivitis and dermal erythema persisted for 3 to 7 days postexposure in animal studies.[71] Lacrimation persisted for about 20 minutes postexposure; conjunctivitis and blepharospasm persisted for up to 24 hours.[27]

Cutaneous effects. Exposure to CN has been associated with primary irritation and allergic contact dermatitis.[140–142] CN is a potent skin irritant and is more likely to cause serious injury to the skin than CS. Exposure to high doses of CN results in skin injury that may consist of severe generalized itching, diffuse and intense erythema, severe edema, and vesication. CN is also considered to be a more potent skin sensitizer than CS.[140]

Carcinogenicity testing. The National Institutes of Health conducted a carcinogenicity bioassay in rats and mice with CN, finding no indication of carcinogenetic activity of CN in male rats exposed by inhalation. The evidence was equivocal in female rats based on the findings of an increase in mammary gland fibroadenomas. The 2-year inhalation study in both male and female mice did not suggest any carcinogenic activity.[143]

Human Studies and Effects

The effects caused by CN in humans are similar to those of CS, but more severe. The harassing dose and toxicity of CN are also greater than for CS. The effects of exposure to low concentrations usually disappear within 20 to 30 minutes. Based on animal toxicology of CN, the initial LCt_{50} estimated for humans was 7,000 mg•min/m^3, which was subsequently revised and established as 14,000 mg•min/m^3. Persistence of these effects (rhinorrhea, lacrimation, blurred vision, conjunctivitis, and burning of the throat) was negligible, with no clinical signs and symptoms noted approximately 10 minutes following cessation of exposure. Values for the ICt_{50} of CN range from 25 to 50 mg•min/m^3. These ICt_{50} values are comparable to those of DM. The estimated LCt_{50} for CN dispersed from solvent in grenades is 7,000 mg•min/m^3, although some researchers have reported estimates between 8,500 and 25,000 mg•min/m^3.[144]

Volunteer acute exposure studies. In human volunteer studies, the immediate effects of exposure to CN were a burning sensation or stinging in the eyes, nose, throat, and exposed skin, followed by lacrimation, salivation, rhinorrhea, and dyspnea. Common signs observed were rhinorrhea, lacrimation, and conjunctivitis, and reported symptoms included blurred vision, burning of the throat, and some less frequent but more severe symptoms of difficulty in breathing, nausea, and burning in the chest.[55] Punte et al[55] studied the effects of CN on human subjects exposed to aerosols at *Ct*s below 350 mg•min/m^3. This dosage is considered the maximum safe inhaled aerosol dosage for humans. Punte et al[55] also studied CN dispersed from solvent in grenades and found the maximum safe inhaled dose to be 500 mg•min/m^3. Other estimates range from 8,500 to 25,000 mg•min/m^3.

Respiratory effects. Exposed individuals may experience lacrimation, conjunctivitis, conjunctival edema, upper respiratory irritation, cough, dyspnea, and skin burns, as well as pulmonary lesions if exposures occur in confined spaces.[144] Hospitalizations were reported by Thorburn following the release of CN into 44 prison cells.[144] Twenty-eight inmates sought medical attention, and eight of them were hospitalized. All eight complained of malaise, lethargy, and anorexia. Five had pharyngitis, three of whom developed pseudomembranous exudates several days later. Three also developed tracheobronchitis with purulent sputum, but no infiltrates were seen on chest radiographs. Four inmates had facial burns, and three had bullae on the legs. The most severely affected had first- and second-degree burns over 25% of his body. Another inmate was admitted 5 days after the incident with a papulovesicular rash on his face, scalp, and trunk, which had appeared 2 days earlier. Ten inmates were treated as outpatients for first- and second-degree burns, and six had localized papulovesicular rashes. Ten had conjunctivitis with edema of the conjunctiva, and in some, the eyelids were closed by the swelling. None had corneal injuries or permanent eye damage. The patients with laryngotracheobronchitis were treated with bronchodilators, postural drainage, and positive-pressure exercises. Two were given short-term, high doses of steroids, but none received antibiotics. One required bronchodilator therapy 3 months later, but the others made prompt recoveries.

Stein and Kirwin[145] reported another prison incident in which inmates confined to individual cells were exposed to a "prolonged gassing" with CN estimated to last 110 minutes. The windows and doors were closed and the ventilation was off. The CN was disseminated by at least six thermal grenades of CN, fourteen 100-g projectiles of CN, and more than 500 mL of an 8% solution of CN. The calculated dosage of the exposure from just the CN projectiles was a Ct of 41,000 mg•min/m^3. Following the exposure some of the prisoners had coughing and varying degrees of illness, and at least three received medical treatment, although details were not available to the authors. One prisoner was found dead under his bunk 46 hours postexposure. Other prisoners reported that the prisoner who died had "red eyes," vomited bloody material, and had sought medical attention on several occasions. The autopsy findings included cyanosis of the face and head, edema and congestion of the lungs, alveolar hemorrhage, necrosis of the mucosal lining of the lungs, bronchopneumonia, and no evidence of physical injury. The lungs had subpleural petechiae, hyperemia, mild edema, and patchy areas of consolidation. Microscopic examination showed bronchopneumonia clustered around exudate-filled bronchioles. The larynx and tracheobronchial tree were lined with an exudative pseudomembrane, which on microscopic examination proved to be a fibrin-rich exudate containing polymorphonuclear leukocytes and their degenerating forms. There was no evidence of gastrointestinal hemorrhage, but other organs had passive hyperemia.[145]

Chapman and White[146] reported the death of an individual who had locked himself in a room in his house during an altercation with the police. A single CN grenade containing 128 g of CN was thrown into the room, which was approximately 27 m^3. The individual remained in the room for 30 minutes, for a Ct of 142,000 mg•min/m^3. This exposure is about 10 times higher than the estimated human LCt_{50}. On admission to the hospital, his respirations were 24 per minute, conjunctiva were suffused, pupils were small and unreactive, and mucoid discharge from his nose and mouth was abundant. His lungs were clear, and an occasional premature ventricular contraction was evident on the electrocardiogram. He remained in a semicomatose condition for approximately 12 hours, then suddenly developed pulmonary edema and died. The relevant findings on autopsy included cyanosis, frothy fluid in the mouth and nose, acute necrosis of the mucosa of the respiratory tract with pseudomembrane formation, desquamation of the lining of the bronchioles with edema and inflammation of the walls, and a protein-rich fluid in most of the alveolar spaces. Foci of early bronchopneumonia were also present.

Stein and Kirwan[145] also obtained information on three other cases of death following CN exposures from other medical examiners. Although details were scanty, the autopsy findings were similar in all three cases. The individuals were all confined individually in relatively small spaces, and the exposures were for 10 minutes in one case and for hours in the other two.[145]

Thus deaths from high concentrations of CN may occur and have been reported. Postmortem examinations revealed edema and congestion of the lungs, alveolar hemorrhage, necrosis of the mucosal lining of the lungs, and bronchopneumonia.[144–146]

Cutaneous effects. Although in animal studies the cutaneous effects seen consisted mainly of erythema, in humans, pain can occur without tissue injury and may be bradykinin mediated. Local tissue irritation and burns may result from the hydrochloric acid formed on moist tissues.[60]

In his 1925 textbook, Vedder stated that in field concentrations, CN does not damage human skin, although the powder might produce burning or slight rubefaction and sometimes small vesicles.[147] In 1933 Kibler[148] reported a case of primary irritant dermatitis in a soldier and three cases in civilian employees who probably had allergic dermatitis from working around

CN for years. In 1941 Queen and Stander[149] reported the case of a 43-year-old military recruit who spent 5 minutes exposed to an atmosphere of CN while masked. After removing the mask and leaving the chamber he developed a severe allergic reaction. Within 5 minutes of exiting the chamber, he complained of generalized itching, which progressively worsened until by 4 hours he had developed a diffuse and intense erythema over his entire body, except for his feet and the part of his face that was covered by the mask. His temperature was 38.9°C (102°F), which rose to 39.4°C (103°F) by the next day. By 48 hours postexposure, vesication and severe subcutaneous edema had strikingly altered his facial appearance. This was accompanied by severe generalized itching. These signs subsided over the next 4 days, and the desquamation which was profuse at day 6 gradually decreased. This recruit had been exposed to a similar CN exercise 17 years previously and developed itching, but had not been exposed in the interim.[149]

Another case of cutaneous hypersensitivity was reported by Madden in 1951,[150] in which a police officer received an initial exposure to CN, and 5 years later on repeated exposure developed recurrent attacks of what was probably allergic contact dermatitis. The source of the repeated exposures was unrecognized until the police officer realized that he was using outdated CN bombs for eradication of rodents on his property. He developed a severe dermatitis on his legs with each use over a period of 5 years. When a small area of one leg was intentionally exposed to CN, an acute contact dermatitis appeared and subsided within 8 hours.[150]

Holland and White[141] studied the skin reactions in humans following CN application. Irritation began within 10 minutes and became more severe when the agent was left in place. By 60 minutes, 0.5 mg CN had produced irritation and erythema on the skin of all the people tested. These effects disappeared when the CN was removed, but recurred transiently when the areas were washed during the subsequent 12 hours. In all cases, diffuse redness appeared in an area up to three times the original contact area. At doses of over 2 mg, localized edema occurred but subsided after 24 hours. When applied dry in doses of 0.5 to 2 mg, the redness disappeared within 72 hours. At higher doses and at all doses applied moist, the redness became raised and papular. The papules coalesced to form a ring of vesicles at about 48 hours. Two weeks later, the lesions were evident as faint areas of hyperpigmentation. These effects contrasted to those of CS also evaluated in these studies. CS at doses under 20 mg caused no irritation or erythema, and no vesiculation resulted from CS at doses of 30 mg or less. Thus CN is a more potent primary irritant on the skin than CS.

Ophthalmologic effects. The irritation caused by CN in the eye signals avoidance and, by causing lacrimation and blepharospasm, initiates a defense mechanism.[3] High levels of CN can produce chemical injury to the eyes characterized as corneal and conjunctival edema, chemosis, and loss of corneal epithelium.[136] Physical injuries may also occur following dispersion via grenade-type tear gas devices.[135,136] More lasting or permanent effects may occur when CN is released at close range (within a few meters), particularly if the dose is from a forceful blast from a cartridge, bomb, pistol, or spray.

Using records from the files of the Armed Forces Institute of Pathology in Washington, DC, Levine and Stahl[151] reviewed eye injuries caused by tear gas weapons. Although many of the histories were incomplete, in about half of the cases the injuries were self inflicted or accidental. In the other cases, the injuries were caused by a second person firing a weapon at close range with intent to injure the patient. In some instances, particles of agglomerated agent were driven into the eye tissues by the force of the blast, and a possible chemical reaction caused damage over months or years. In other instances, the injury was probably caused by the blast or other foreign particles rather than by CN. The authors carefully pointed out that features of the weapon, such as the blast force, the propellant charge, the wadding, and the age of the cartridge (in older cartridges, the powder agglomerates and forms larger particles) should be considered in evaluating eye damage from CN.[151]

Rengstorff[152] also concluded that traumatic effects of blast are a considerable factor that must be considered when determining the cause of permanent eye injury in CN exposures. Although permanent eye damage has been reported from the use of CN weapons at close range, separating the effects of the weapon from those of the compound is difficult. There is no evidence that CN at harassing or normal field concentrations causes permanent damage to the eye.[3]

Other physiological responses. The 1984 National Research Council study[60] reported histopathological changes following CN exposures including hemorrhage, perivascular edema, congestion of the alveolar capillaries, occluded bronchioles, and alveolitis. Renal histopathology demonstrated congestion and coagulative necrosis in the cortical renal tubules in CN exposed mice. Hepatic histopathology consisted of cloudy swelling and lobular and centrolobular necrosis of hepatocytes.[60]

Long-term effects and severe medical complications. Between 1958 and 1972, 99 human subjects underwent experimental exposures to CN at Edgewood Arsenal. Of these, 69 were exposed by aerosol and 30 by direct application to the skin. However, exposure data is available on only 68 subjects. The aerosol exposures ranged from 0.15 to 3.63 minutes with *Ct* dosages between 6 and 315 mg•min/m^3, and the cutaneous doses ranged from 0.01 to 0.025 mL, applied to bare or clothed arms. Effects on the aerosol-exposed subjects were transient, generally resolving within minutes of removal of the CN. Experienced subjects appeared to be tolerant, and closing their eyes often increased tolerance. Predominant effects were ocular and included lacrimation, blepharospasm, conjunctivitis, and, rarely, palpebral edema. Respiratory effects were nasopharyngeal irritation, rhinorrhea, and, rarely, dyspnea. Skin irritation was prominent on shaved areas. Other rare effects were headache and dizziness. Of the dermally exposed subjects, only one had erythema at the exposure site, which lasted 7 hours. Five had normal laboratory results, which included urinalyses, complete blood count, blood urea nitrogen, alkaline phosphatase, and serum glutamic oxalotransferases 7 days postexposure. Among the 68 subjects with exposure records, there were probably no permanent ocular or pulmonary injuries. These short, low-level exposures caused transient effects on the eyes and respiratory system, and recovery was complete within minutes. Minimal information is available on the dermal effects, but sensitization is considered likely, causing allergic contact dermatitis and possible systemic allergic reactions such as pulmonary fibrosis on reexposure, although there is no evidence that this occurred among the Edgewood subjects.[60]

DM (Diphenylaminearsine)

DM (CAS 578-94-9, also known as diphenylaminoarsine and 10-chloro-5,10-dihydrophenarsazine) is one of three arsenical war gases developed near the conclusion of World War I.[153] The other two closely related chemicals, DA (diphenylchloroarsine) and DC (diphenylcyanoarsine), proved to have much less military importance. German scientists first discovered DA in 1913 (German patent application 281049), but producing the compound proved difficult and expensive. In 1918 Major Robert Adams, working at the University of Illinois, discovered a simpler and more economical way to produce DM (which then took on the common name adamsite).[154] The United States produced DM by the end of the war but did not use it; however, very incomplete reports suggest that Italy may have used it.[155] In World War II all belligerent states produced DM, and smoke generators containing DM were developed.

After the war it was recognized that DM had applications as a possible RCA because of its harassing characteristics; it was eventually classified by the military as a vomiting agent and a sternutator. For riot control purposes, because of its minimal effects on the eye, DM was mixed with the tearing agent CN, and this preparation was used by US troops during Vietnam.[156,157] Today DM is considered obsolete as an RCA and has no other application.[73] Current US research on DM focuses on the environmental impact of the parent compound and its breakdown products near former production, storage, and disposal sites.[158,159]

Physical Characteristics and Deployment

The molecular weight of DM is 277.59, and its molecular formula is $C_{12}H_9AsClN$ (Figure 13-10). DM is a yellow-green (depending on purity), odorless (or possessing a faint bitter almond smell) crystalline substance with low volatility. It is practically insoluble in water and slightly soluble in organics such as benzene, xylene, toluene, and alcohols.[153] DM can be disseminated as a dry powder by thermal or explosive methods or by spraying the molten materials or solutions of the material.[27,153] The M6A1 (a basic Army riot control munition) and commercial grenades (such as the Spede-Heat [Defense Technology, Casper, Wyo]) are methods used to deploy DM.[153,160] Laboratory methods of dispersion include molten DM and acetone dispersions.

Physiological Effects

Only a few reports deal with the biological conversion of organoarsenical compounds. Even less data exists on the metabolism of DM. However, one recent report suggests the arsenic atom As(III) of DM is oxidized by manganese peroxide into As(V), which results in the release of chloride and the incorporation of dioxygen.[158] The relationship between this metabolism and the acute toxicity of DM in humans is unknown.

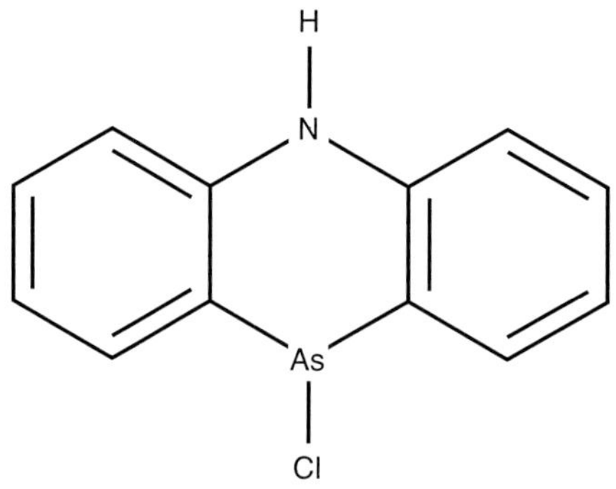

Fig. 13-10. Chemical structure of DM.

Clinical Effects

Acute effects. The acute effects in laboratory animals and human volunteers following inhalation of DM are strikingly variable.[27,161] Numerous factors can contribute to variability in laboratory studies (eg, differences in agent preparation, delivery method, dose, endpoint of interest). Clinical observations following exposure to DM have been reported as immediate or delayed; the delay in onset of pulmonary and systemic effects following DM exposure was considered advantageous because the delay meant that significant exposure could occur before the individual was warned to don a protective mask.[27,153,160]

In laboratory animals, clinical signs of toxicity immediately following exposure to high doses of DM have been studied in several species.[27] Immediately following exposure, the clinical signs of toxicity in mice (LCt_{50}: 46,245 mg•min/m^3); rats (LCt_{50}: 12,710–66,856 mg•min/m^3, depending on method of dispersion); and pigs (LCt_{50}: 6,599–29,888 mg•min/m^3, depending on the method of dispersion) included transient hyperactivity and followed within a few minutes by lacrimation and salivation. Lethargy and labored breathing were observed within 5 to 15 minutes and persisted for 1 to 2 hours.

In dogs (LCt_{50}: 13,945–28,428 mg•min/m^3, depending on the method of dispersion), immediate clinical signs of toxicity included extreme restlessness (jumping and barking) accompanied by salivation, retching, vomiting, and ataxia. Postexposure dogs also became hypoactive, with gagging and vomiting occurring periodically for 24 hours and lasting for about 1 week. Following lethal doses, most deaths in dogs occurred within the first week.

During exposure, clinical signs of toxicity in monkeys (LCt_{50}: 13,866–22,814 mg•min/m^3, depending on the method of dispersion) included salivation, vomiting, rhinorrhea, ataxia, and difficulty breathing. Postexposure monkeys exhibited wheezing, ptosis, and lethargy. Coughing and vomiting persisted for 24 to 48 hours, and depressed breathing preceded death.

During exposure to a toxic dose of DM, goats (LCt_{50}: 8,076–12,072 mg•min/m^3, depending on the method of dispersion) displayed hyperactivity, shaking of the head, rearing on hind legs, licking, chewing, frothing at the mouth, ataxia, convulsions, and bloating. Clinical signs postexposure included hypoactivity, kneeling, gagging, and vomiting. All goats were bloated upon death.

Lastly, in swine (LCt_{50}: 35,888–56,361 mg•min/m^3, depending on the method of dispersion), salivation, frothing at the mouth, ataxia, and irregular breathing were observed during exposure. During the first 2 weeks postexposure, pigs had difficulty breathing, lost weight, and appeared emaciated.

The acute lethal inhalation dose of pure DM in humans is not known but was estimated by the Chemical Research and Development Laboratories, Edgewood Arsenal, in 1959.[153] This risk assessment was based largely on lethality data collected in mice, pigs, and dogs from studies that used highly purified DM. These data were combined to produce a composite lethality dose–response curve for mammals, which was thought to capture the dose-lethality relationship in humans. From this curve, an LCt_{50} value of 14,000 mg•min/m^3 was established. Based on subsequent studies conducted between 1959 and 1965, which further characterized the lethal dose in seven species of laboratory animals and addressed different methods of dispersion, the predicted human LCt_{50} following exposure to highly purified DM was reduced to 11,000 mg•min/m^3. Given the variability in the dose–response curves in laboratory animal studies depending on the method of exposure or dissemination (as outlined above) and purity of the agent, the predicted human LCt_{50} was determined to be 44,000 mg•min/m^3 and 35,000 mg•min/m^3 for DM dispersed from the M6A1 and commercial thermal grenades, respectively.

Inhalation of DM has been linked to at least one human fatality.[153] In this incident, 22 sleeping males were exposed to the agent via a DM generator for 5 or 30 minutes at an estimated concentration of 1,130 to 2,260 mg/m^3. In the single fatality, postmortem examination revealed emphysema of the subcuataneous tissues of the neck, mediastinum, plura, and pericardium. Emphysematous bullae were scattered over the lungs, which were springy and had a bluish discoloration. Histological examination revealed pathology in the entire respiratory tract, edema and congestion of the epiglottis, superficial ulceration and acute diffuse inflammation of the trachea and bronchi, pseudomembrane formation in the trachea and bronchi, lung congestion, edema, hemorrhage, and bronchopneumonia.

The immediate incapacitating effects (irritation effects, local effects) and the delayed incapacitating effects (systemic effects) of DM in humans have been examined using volunteers. The incapacitating dose of DM following a 1-minute exposure ranged from 22 to 220 mg/m^3 (22–220 mg•min/m^3).[153] The concentration range spans an order of magnitude because intolerability is defined as the desire to leave a contaminated area, which is due, in part, to the population's degree of motivation to resist. Other researchers suggest that the effective immediate incapacitating dose of DM is as low as 0.14 mg/m^3 for a 1-minute exposure.[162] The clinical signs of immediate irritation included a burning sensation and pain in the eyes, nose, throat, and respiratory tract; uncontrollable cough; violent and persistent sneezing; lacrimation; and copious flow of saliva. In addition to irritant effects on tissues at the site of exposure, DM also has systemic incapacitating effects (ie, nausea and vomiting), which persist following termination of exposure. Based on studies using human volunteers, the inhalational ICt_{50} for systemic effects was determined to be 370 mg•min/m^3.

Postmortem observations in laboratory animals that received a lethal dose of DM have been reported in five species, and the primary cause of death for all species was lung damage.[153] In monkeys, pneumonitis; ulcerative bronchiolitis; and tracheitis, edema, and congestion of the lungs were reported. Bronchiolitis and tracheitis was also observed in guinea pigs. Dogs demonstrated hyperemia of the larynx and trachea, with signs of edema, congestion of the lung, and bronchopneumonia. In mice and rats, atelectasis, emphysema, reticular cell proliferation, respiratory epithelial proliferation, and interstitial leucocytic infiltration of the bile duct were observed. DM has also been shown to alter blood chemistry in laboratory animals.[153] Changes include alterations in leukocytes, serum enzymes, hematocrit, and prothrombin time.

Respiratory effects. In the respiratory passages and lungs, DM causes sneezing, coughing, salivation, congestion of the nose and walls of the pharynx, and a feeling of suffocation.[27,55] Viscous nasal discharge, characterized as a yellowish-orange material in monkeys, has been reported in laboratory animals and human volunteers.[156,160] A World Health Organization report characterized the clinical symptoms in the respiratory tract following DM exposure as initial tickling sensations in the nose, followed by sneezing and mucous discharge. The irritation spreads into the throat, followed by coughing and choking, with eventual affects observed in the lower air passages and lungs.[162]

Dermatological effects. Direct application of high doses of DM, 10 to 100 mg suspended in corn oil, onto rabbit skin resulted in necrosis and erythema, but neither effect was reported at a 1-mg dose.[27] Although these results identify DM as a potential skin hazard, several controlled exposures to DM aerosols in human volunteers and laboratory animals suggest that the dose required to cause acute skin irritation is well above that known to induce irritation and toxicity in other tissues.[55,153] One study in monkeys did report facial erythema following a moderate dose of aerosolized DM, but the pathology was likely the result of the animals rubbing their faces because of significant nasal discharge.[160] Repeated exposure to DM may lead to sensitization in susceptible persons.[153] Elevated environmental temperature, high relative humidity, and friction of the agent with the skin may be contributory factors to skin damage.

Ophthalmologic effects. Depending on the dose and method of administration, irritation of the eye is observed following exposure to DM, but ocular irritation is often not considered the main immediate effect at low doses.[163] For example, human volunteers exposed to airborne concentrations of DM up to 100 mg•min/m^3 (a dose causing nose, throat, and chest irritation) reported no initial eye irritation.[55] Other reports using human volunteers reported slight irritation of the eyes and lacrimation at doses causing nose and throat irritation and initial weak immediate ocular irritation.[157,162] In rabbits, a suspension of DM in corn oil was administered intraocularly to six groups of animals (0.1–5.0 mg/eye) and observed for 8 to 14 days.[27] The low dose (0.1 mg/eye) was determined to be the "no observable adverse effect" level; whereas transient conjunctivitis was observed following administration of 0.2 mg per eye; transient conjunctivitis and blepharitis were observed with the 0.5 mg per eye dose; and the high doses, 1.0 and 5.0 mg per eye, caused corneal opacity that persisted for the entire 14-day observation period. DM's weak ocular irritation at doses known to induce irritation in other sensory tissue is likely a factor contributing to the incorporation of the tearing agent CN in DM riot control preparations.

Gastrointestinal disturbances. DM is classified by the military as a vomiting agent, and several researchers have characterized that response in both humans and laboratory animals.[73,156,157] Although the human studies did not establish the minimal dose of DM required to induce these systemic incapacitating effects, the work did lead to an estimated incapacitating dose of 370 mg•min/m^3. The World Health Organization detailed the progression of symptoms resulting from DM exposure as initial nausea that soon causes violent retching and vomiting.[163] These effects can have an onset after 20 to 30 minutes of exposure.

Other physiological responses. Other systemic effects included headache, mental depression, perspiration, chills, abdominal cramps, and diarrhea.[55,147,161,163–166]

Long-term effects and severe medical complications. Prolonged exposure to DM and/or high-dose acute exposures can cause death by damage to the respiratory tract and lungs, but in general the margin of safety between irritant dose and lethal dose is great.[27] Repeated dose toxicity studies have been conducted in monkeys, dogs, and guinea pigs. Studies of aerosol DM exposures for 10 consecutive days generated by commercial thermal grenades to LCt_{20}, LCt_{25}, and LCt_{50} doses gave little indication of cumulative toxicity. The effect of repeated exposure in humans is not known.

CR (Dibenz(*b,f*)(1,4)oxazepine)

Physical Characteristics and Deployment

CR (CAS: 257-07-8, also called dibenzoxazepine) was first synthesized by Higginbottom and Suschitzkey in 1962. CR is a pale yellow crystalline solid with a pepper-like odor and a molar mass of 195.3, corresponding to a molecular formula of $C_{13}H_9NO$ (Figure 13-11). The molar solubility in water at 20°C is 3.5 × 10^{-4} mol/L (= ~7 mg/100 mL). The melting and boiling points are 73°C and 355°C, respectively. CR vapor is 6.7 times heavier than air, and the vapor pressure of the solid is 0.00059 mm Hg at 20°C. CR is a stable chemical that may persist for prolonged periods in the environment. It is hydrolyzed very slowly in water. As with CN, washing with soap and water will not inactivate CR, but will remove it from the surface. Compared to CS and CN, CR is the most potent lacrimator with the least systemic toxicity. It is the parent compound of the antipsychotic drug loxapine.[71]

CR is the newest of the C series of RCAs (CN and CR), and no in-use data has been published for this agent. However, an article in *The Observer*, on January 23, 2005, revealed that the British government secretly authorized the use of a chemical RCA in prisons at the height of the Northern Ireland troubles.[167] Documents from 1976, released under freedom of information legislation, show that beginning in 1973 the use of CR was authorized to be used on inmates in the event of an attempted mass breakout. The agent was authorized to be used in the form of an aerosol spray for the personal protection of prison officers, to be fired from water cannons, and also shot in a polyethylene capsule that would spread onto rioters after hitting the security fence. CR was alleged to have been used on October 16, 1974, to quell rioting at Long Kesh prison. The article reported CR's effects to be similar to those of CS, except that it also induces intense pain on exposed skin, and the affected areas remain sensitive for days and become painful again after contact with water.[167]

Physiological Effects

Upshall[168] reported that CR aerosols are very quickly absorbed from the respiratory tract. Following inhalation, the plasma half-life is about 5 minutes, which is about the same following intravenous administration. French et al[169] studied CR metabolism in vitro and in vivo, supporting the previous conclusions that the major metabolic fate of CR in the rat is the oxidation to the lactam, subsequent ring hydroxylation, sulfate conjugation, and urinary excretion.

Clinical Effects

Ballantyne[170] has summarized the mammalian toxicology of CR in various species. The acute toxicity by all routes of exposure (LD_{50} and LCt_{50}) indicates that CR is less toxic than CS and CR.[170] Animals exposed to CR exhibited ataxia or incoordination, spasms, convulsions, and tachypnea. In the exposed surviving animals, these effects gradually subsided over a period of 15 to 60 minutes. Death was preceded by increasing respiratory distress.

Acute effects. Studies at Edgewood Arsenal and other research centers have been conducted to assess the effects of CR on humans following aerosol exposures, drenches, and local application.[134,171–174] The 1984 National Research Council study[60] summarized the human aerosol and cutaneous studies conducted at Edgewood Arsenal from 1963 to 1972. Respiratory effects following aerosol exposures included respiratory irritation with choking and difficulty in breathing or dyspnea; ocular effects consisted of lacrimation, irritation, and conjunctivitis.

Respiratory effects. Ashton et al[171] exposed human subjects to a mean CR aerosol concentration of 0.25 mg/m^3 (particle size: 1–2 µm) for 1 hour. Expiratory flow rate was decreased approximately 20 minutes after the onset of exposure. The investigators theorized that CR stimulated the pulmonary irritant receptors to produce bronchoconstriction and increasing pulmonary blood volume by augmenting sympathetic tone.

The potential of CR aerosols to produce physiological and ultrastructural changes in the lungs was evaluated by Pattle et al.[175] Electron microscopy of rats exposed to CR aerosol of 115,000 mg•min/m^3 did not reveal any effects on organelles such as lamellated osmiophilic bodies. Studies by Colgrave et al[176] evaluated the lungs of animals exposed to CR aerosols at dosages of 78,200; 140,900; and 161,300 mg•min/m^3, and found them to appear normal on gross examination. On microscopic examination, however, the lungs revealed mild congestion, hemorrhage, and emphysema. Electron microscopy showed isolated swelling and thickening of the epithelium, as well as early

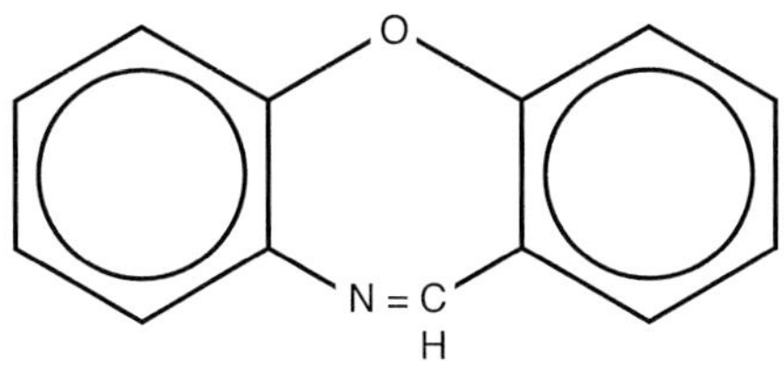

Fig. 13-11. Chemical structure of CR.

capillary damage, as evidenced by ballooning of the endothelium. The authors concluded that these very high dosages of CR aerosols produced only minimal pulmonary damage.

Dermatological effects. CR was reported by Ballantyne and Swanston[134] and by Holland[173] to produce transient erythema, but it did not induce vesication or sensitization and did not delay the healing of skin injuries. The burning sensation on exposure to CR persisted for 15 to 30 minutes, and the erythema lasted 1 to 2 hours.[134,173] Repeated dermal administration of CR was conducted in mice by Marrs et al[177] and in rabbits and monkeys by Owens et al.[178] In the latter study, CR was applied to the skin 5 days per week for 12 weeks. Both teams of investigators concluded that repeated dermal applications of CR had little effect on the skin. They further postulated that in view of the absence of any specific organ effects, absorption of even substantial amounts of CR would have little effect.

Ophthalmologic effects. Higgenbottom and Suschitzky[179] were first to note the intense lacrimation and skin irritation caused by CR. Mild and transitory eye effects such as mild redness and mild chemosis were observed in rabbits and monkeys after a single dose of 1% CR solution. Multiple doses over a 5-day period of the same solution to the eye produced only minimal effects.[179] Biskup et al[180] reported no signs of eye irritation in animals following single or multiple dose applications of 1% CR solutions. Moderate conjunctivitis following the application of 5% CR solution to the eyes of rabbits was reported by Rengstorff et al,[181] although histological examination revealed normal corneal and eyelid tissues. Ballantyne and Swanston[134] also studied the ocular irritancy of CR and arrived at a threshold concentration for blepharospasm in several species. Ballantyne et al[138] studied the effects of CR as a solid, an aerosol, and a solution in polyethylene glycol. Aerosol exposures of 10,800 and 17,130 mg•min/m^3 resulted in mild lacrimation and conjunctival injection, which cleared in 1 hour. When applied in solution, it produced reversible dose-related increases in corneal thickness. The authors concluded that CR produced considerably less damage to the eye than CN and is much safer.

Gastrointestinal disturbances. Although human data is not readily available in this area, animal studies by Ballantyne and Swanston[134] showed the repeated dose effects of orally administered CR on various animal species. The animals that died following intravenous and oral administration demonstrated congestion of the liver sinusoids and alveolar capillaries. At necropsy, the surviving animals did not show any gross or histological abnormalities. The toxic signs following intraperitoneal administration included muscle weakness and heightened sensitivity to handling. These effects persisted throughout the first day following exposure. Some animals also exhibited central nervous system effects. On necropsy, the surviving animals did not show any gross or histological abnormalities.

Other physiological responses. Ballantyne et al[172] reported the effects of dilute CR solution on humans following splash contamination of the face, or facial drench. These exposures resulted in an immediate increase in blood pressure concomitant with decreased heart rate. In subsequent studies by Ballantyne et al,[78] humans were exposed to whole body drenches that resulted in the same effects of immediate increase of blood pressure and bradycardia. The authors concluded that the cardiovascular effects in both studies were caused by the CR, theorizing that the amount of CR uptake was insufficient to produce the systemic effects on the heart. However, they did not provide an explanation for the cardiovascular changes. Lundy and McKay[182] suggested that these cardiovascular changes resulted from the CR effects on the heart via the sympathetic nervous system.

Several animal species were exposed to acute inhalation of CR aerosols and smokes for various time periods. Rats exposed to aerosol concentrations from 13,050 to 428,400 mg•min/m^3 manifested nasal secretions and blepharospasm or uncontrollable closure of the eyelids, which subsided within an hour after termination of the exposure. No deaths occurred during or following these exposures. There were also no deaths in rabbits, guinea pigs, or mice exposed to CR aerosols of up to 68,000 mg•min/m^3. Animals exposed to CR smoke generated pyrotechnically had alveolar capillary congestion and intraalveolar hemorrhage, as well as kidney and liver congestion.

Long-term effects and severe medical complications. Repeated inhalation exposures were conducted by Marrs et al,[183] who exposed mice and hamsters to concentrations of 204, 236, and 267 mg/m^3 CR for 5 days per week for 18 weeks. The high concentrations produced death in both species, but no single cause of death could be ascertained, although pneumonitis was present in many cases. Chronic inflammation of the larynx was observed in mice. Although alveologenic carcinoma was found in a single low-dose and a single high-dose group of mice, the findings and conclusions were questioned because the spontaneous occurrence of alveologenic carcinoma is high in many mouse strains.[184,185] Furthermore, this tumor type differs in many respects from human lung tumors. No lung tumors and no lesions were found in hamsters exposed to CR aerosols. Histopathology revealed hepatic lesions in mice, but these were of infectious origin and not related to the CR. The authors concluded that CR exposures at high concentrations reduced survivability and that CR produced minimal organ-specific toxicity at many times the human ICt_{50}, which has been reported as both 0.7 mg/m^3 within 1 minute[170] and 0.15 mg/m^3 within 1 minute.[183,186]

Upshall[168] studied the reproductive and developmental effects of CR on rabbits and rats. The animals were exposed to inhalation of aerosolized CR at concentrations of 2, 20, and 200 mg/m^3 for 5 and 7 minutes. Groups of animals were also dosed intragastrically on days 6, 8, 10, 12, 14, 16, and 18 of pregnancy. No dose-related effects of CN were observed in any of the parameters measured or in the number and types of malformations observed. No externally visible malformations were seen in any group, and no dose-related effects of CR were noted in any of the fetuses in any group. Based on the overall observations, the author concluded that CR was neither teratogenic nor embryotoxic to rabbits or rats.

Only one study has reported on the genotoxicity of CR. Colgrave et al[176] studied the mutagenic potential of technical grade CR and its precursor (2-aminodiphenyl ether) in the various strains of *Salmonella typhimurium*, as well as in mammalian assay systems. CR and its precursor were negative in all the assays, suggesting that CR is not mutagenic. Further testing is required to exclude the genetic threat to humans, as well as to determine the carcinogenic potential and its ability to cause other chronic health effects. Husain et al[133] studied the effects in rats of CR and CN aerosols on plasma glutamic oxaloacetic transaminase, plasma glutamic pyruvic transaminase, acid phosphatase, and alkaline phosphatase. The rats exposed to CR exhibited no change in any of these parameters, whereas significant increases in all of these parameters occurred in rats exposed to CN, suggesting that CN can cause tissue damage.

MEDICAL CARE

The effects from RCAs are typically self-limiting, and discomfort is reduced within 30 minutes upon exiting a contaminated area. Usually no medical treatment is necessary, particularly if the agent is used in an open area and the dose is minimized. Medical complications are always possible, however, so emergency services should be prepared to treat a limited number of casualties when RCAs are used for civil disturbance, civilian peacekeeping operations, and training. Injury may range from skin and eye irritation to, in rare cases, injuries sustained from exploding dispensing munitions, delayed transient pulmonary syndromes, or delayed pulmonary edema requiring hospital admission.[4]

Personal Protection

Short-term protection can be provided by dry clothing that covers the arms and legs, because sweat allows dry agents to adhere to the skin. The standard protective mask will adequately protect against the inhalation of RCA particles and vapors. When working with bulk quantities of these agents, or in mask confidence chambers with CS1, CS2, or CR, protective clothing, mask, and gloves that cover all exposed skin areas should be worn.[10] Medical providers do not require protection once an exposed patient has been decontaminated.

Decontamination

Decontamination is important to reduce injury and continued exposure from agent on the skin, hair, and clothing. This is particularly important for those in contact with RCAs in enclosed areas for long periods of time, such as individuals running mask confidence training who are in the chamber repeatedly throughout a single day. CS chamber operators have developed erythema, minor skin burns, and blistering on the neck, arms, and other areas that were not continuously protected by a mask or clothing (Figure 13-12). These problems can be avoided if operators wear adequate dermal protection during exposure and shower immediately with soap and water at the end of the training day.

When dry agents (CS, CR, CN, and DM) are dispensed in the open air in limited quantities, all that is needed to remove the agent, particularly when protective clothing is worn, is brisk movement: flapping the arms and rubbing the hair in a breeze or standing in front of a large fan. This will disperse most of the particles from the clothing and hair. The mask should be worn during this process to insure that particles blown from other people performing the same procedure upwind are not inhaled. However, agent particles adhere to sweaty skin, so completely effective decontamination requires clothing removal followed by thorough washing of exposed skin and hair.

To decontaminate an exposed patient, the contaminated clothing should be removed before admittance to a medical treatment facility. The clothing must be stored in a sealed polythene bag and, if laundered, cold water should be used to reduce vaporization of the agent.[81] Soap and water are an effective decontaminant for RCAs; they will not neutralize the agent but will wash it away. Water should be used in copious amounts. Soap helps loosen the dry particles and

a b

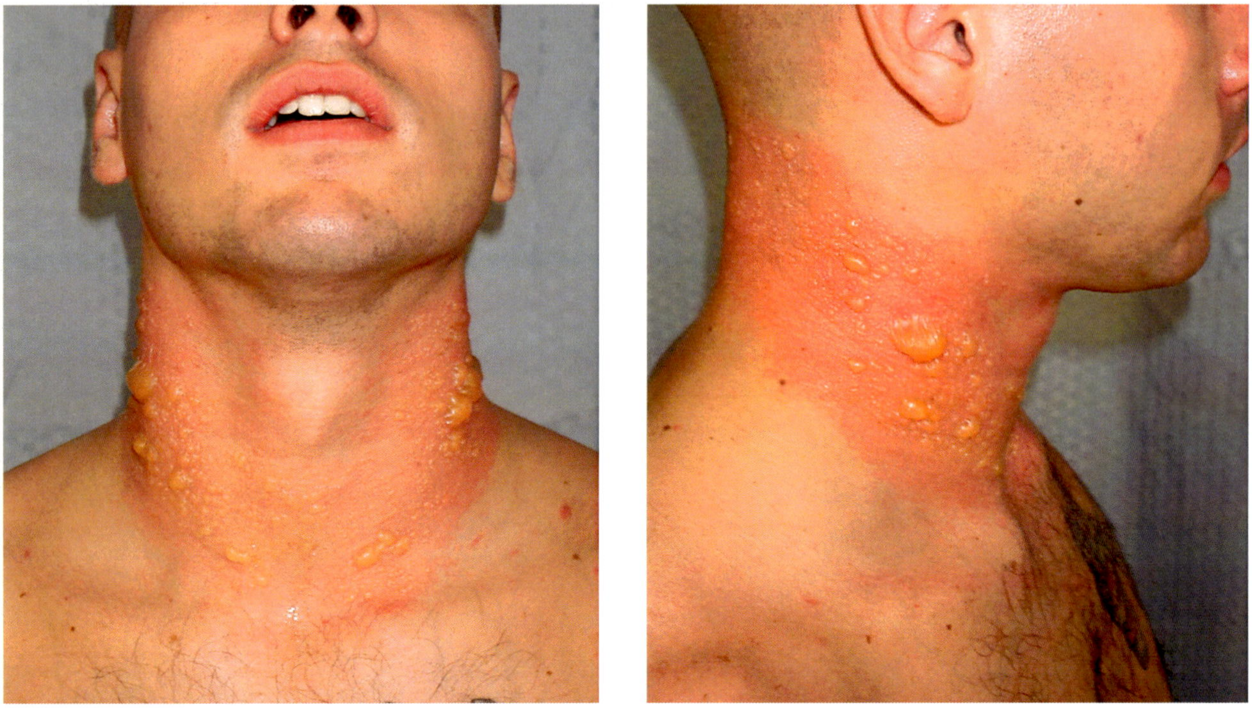

Fig. 13-12. Mask confidence chamber operator after several hours of exposure to concentrated CS. Erythema and blisters are present in areas where the skin was exposed. This service member stated that this is the first time he neglected to shower after training.
Photograph: Courtesy of CG Hurst, US Army Medical Research Institute of Chemical Defense.

remove them adequately from the skin surface. CR, CN and DM hydrolyze very slowly in water, even when alkali is present.[24] Because these agents do not decompose in water, washing with soap and water will only remove them from surfaces. Run-off may produce irritation if it gets into the eyes, so the eyes should be closed and head lowered during decontamination (if the agent is not already in the eyes). Environmental contamination from these agents may be persistent and difficult to remove. CS is insoluble in water but will hydrolyze in water at a pH of 7, with a half-life of approximately 15 minutes at room temperature, and extremely rapidly in alkaline solution with a pH of 9, with a half-life of about 1 minute.[71]

Decontamination solutions used on human skin should not be caustic to the skin. A solution containing 6% sodium bicarbonate, 3% sodium carbonate, and 1% benzalkonium chloride was found to bring prompt relief of symptoms and to hydrolyze CS.[187] No form of hypochlorite should ever be used to decontaminate CS or other RCAs because it can react with CS to produce more toxic chemical byproducts and will further irritate tissues.[51] Applying water or soap and water to skin exposed to CS or OC but decontaminated may result in a transient worsening of the burning sensation, which should dissipate with continued water flushing.[3,10] PS liquid can also be decontaminated with soap and water, and clothing, which can trap vapor, should be removed.[188]

Water in limited quantities increases the pain symptoms from OC, which has a water solubility of 0.090 g/L at 37° C.[24,189] Without decontamination, OC symptoms should dissipate over time as the body's substance P is diminished. OC resin can also be decontaminated with copious amounts of water, liquid soap and water, baby shampoo, alcohol, or cold milk.[22] OC in the eyes can be decontaminated with copious water flushing, but symptoms may not dissipate for 10 minutes. A compress of cold milk, ice water, or snow can help reduce the burning sensation once the individual has been decontaminated.[22] Substances with high fat content, such as whipped cream or ice cream, also aid in decontamination and help reduce pain.[22] Although OC is soluble in vegetable oil and other hydrocarbons, and such solutions can more easily be washed off the skin, hydrocarbons must not be used with solutions of OC and other RCAs such as CN.[24,190] Commercially available products, such as Sudecon Decontamination Wipes (Fox Labs International, Clinton Township, Mich); Bio Shield towelettes (Bio Shield, Inc, Raleigh,

NC); or Cool It! wipes and spray (Defense Technology, Casper, Wyo); claim to help decontaminate and reduce pain in people exposed to pepper sprays and other RCAs.[191–193]

Treatment

Skin

Skin erythema that appears early (up to 1 hour after exposure) is transient and usually does not require treatment. Delayed-onset erythema (irritant dermatitis) can be treated with a bland lotion such as calamine lotion or topical corticosteroid preparations (eg, 0.10% triamcinolone acetonide, 0.025% fluocinolone acetonide, 0.05% flurandrenolone, or betamethasone-17-valerate). Cosmetics, including foundation and false eyelashes, can trap agent and should be removed to insure complete decontamination.[22] When the patient has been exposed to OC, the use of creams or ointments should be delayed for 6 hours after exposure.[194] Patients with blisters should be managed as having a second-degree burn.[195] Acute contact dermatitis that is oozing should be treated with wet dressings (moistened with fluids such as 1:40 Burow solution or colloidal solution) for 30 minutes, three times daily.[3,187] Topical steroids should be applied immediately following the wet dressing. Appropriate antibiotics should be given for secondary infection, and oral antihistamines for itching. [3,187] Vesicating lesions have been successfully treated with compresses of a cold silver nitrate solution (1:1,000) for 1 hour, applied six times daily.[75] One person with severe lesions and marked discomfort was given a short course of an oral steroid. An antibiotic ointment was applied locally, but systemic antibiotics were not used.[75] With severe blistering resulting in second-degree burns, skin pigmentation changes can occur.[4]

Eye

The effects of RCAs on the eyes are self-limiting and do not normally require treatment; however, if large particles of solid agent are in the eye, the patient should be treated as if for exposure to corrosive materials.[195] The individual should be kept from rubbing the eyes, which can rub particles or agent into the eye and cause damage.[24] Contact lenses should be removed.[194]

Yih recommends that before irrigating eyes contaminated with CS, they should be blown dry, directly, with an electric fan, which helps dissolved particles evaporate and rapidly reduces pain (irrigating the eyes before drying causes additional, unnecessary, pain.[82] However, other researchers note that if Yih's recommendations are used, the care provider must be certain that the agent is CS, for such a delay in decontaminating more toxic agents such as ammonia would result in severe eye injury. With all agents, the affected eyes should be thoroughly flushed with copious amounts of normal saline or water for several minutes (some sources suggest 10 minutes) to remove the agent.[194]

Eye injury assessment should include a slit lamp examination with fluorescein staining to evaluate for corneal abrasions that could be caused by rubbing particles of the agent into the eye.[4,196] Patients should be closely observed for development of corneal opacity and iritis, particularly those who have been exposed to CN or CA. A local anesthetic can be used for severe pain, but continued anesthetic use should be restricted. If the lesion is severe, the patient should be sent for definitive ophthalmologic treatment.

Viala et al[197] reported a study of five French gendarmes who had CS exposure and were decontaminated with Diphoterine (Prevor, Valmondois, France), which dramatically resolved the effects in four of them. The researchers also recommended using it as a prophylaxis to reduce or prevent lacrimation, eye irritation, and blepharospasm.[197]

Respiratory Tract

Typically, RCA-induced cough, chest discomfort, and mild dyspnea are resolved within 30 minutes after exposure to clean air. However, both the animal data (detailed in the section on CS) and clinical experience with an infant exposed to CS[198] suggest that severe respiratory effects may not become manifest until 12 to 24 hours after exposure. If persistent bronchospasm lasting several hours develops, systemic or inhaled bronchodilators (eg, albuterol 0.5%) can be effective in reducing the condition.[4,196]

Individuals with prolonged dyspnea or objective signs such as coughing, sneezing, breath holding, and excessive salivation should be hospitalized under careful observation. Treatment in these cases may include the introduction of systemic aminophylline and systemic glucocorticosteroids.[4,55] A chest radiograph can assist in diagnosis and treatment for patients with significant respiratory complaints.[196] If respiratory failure occurs, the use of extracorporeal membrane oxygenation can be effective without causing long-term damage to the lungs.[4,199] High-pressure ventilation, which can cause lung scarring, should not be used. Although people with chronic bronchitis have been exposed to RCAs without effects, any underlying lung disease (eg, asthma, which affects one person in six) might be exacerbated by exposure to CS.[3,200] In most cases the respiratory system quickly recovers from acute exposure to RCAs, but prolonged exposure can predispose the casualty to secondary infections. Further care should be as described in Chapter 10, Toxic Inhalational Injury and Toxic Industrial Chemicals.

Cardiovascular System

Transient hypertension and tachycardia have been noted after exposure to RCAs, primarily because of the anxiety or pain of exposure rather than a pharmacological effect of the compound.[201] Whatever the cause, adverse effects may be seen in individuals with hypertension, cardiovascular disease, or an aneurysm.

Laboratory Findings

No specific laboratory study abnormalities are helpful in diagnosing RCA exposure. Appropriate tests can be ordered to guide treatment if respiratory tract or skin infection is suspected. Arterial blood gasses can be ordered if there is a concern about adequate ventilation.[196]

NEW DEVELOPMENTS AND FUTURE USE

As documented throughout this chapter, the military's interest in and occasional use of RCAs has not only kept pace with their development, but in many cases the military has spearheaded the effort. Although most of this historical activity predated the current regulations guiding research, development, and use of RCAs (ie, prior to the Chemical Weapons Convention), it is probable that this trend will continue into the future.

Recent years have witnessed a fundamental methodological shift in biomedical science research. The traditional method of identifying biologically active compounds before determining their application to disease has been replaced, in part, by identifying biological targets (ie, protein receptors) first, followed by identifying the chemical compounds capable of binding to the targets and altering their function. The advancement of microarray, proteomics, toxicogenomics, database mining techniques, and computational modeling techniques has greatly accelerated the ability to identify novel biological targets with desired physiological effects. Likewise, high-throughput technologies capable of identifying biologically active compounds such as in-vitro tissue culture systems integrated with automated robotics test stations, combinatorial chemistry, and quantitative structure activity relationship methods have accelerated new drug discovery. New RCAs are likely to be a product of this research.

Neuropharmacology is an area of biomedical research likely to yield future RCAs. The increased incidence and awareness of neurological disorders in the general population, such as Alzheimer disease in the elderly and attention deficit disorders in children, ensure a healthy research base aimed at discovering bioactive compounds capable of altering cognitive functions, perception, mood, emotions, bodily control, and alertness.

Although OC and CS, today's RCAs of choice, are very safe if deployed appropriately, more research is needed to illuminate the full health consequences of their use. The limited financial resources of the military's chemical defense programs dictate that funds be spent on measures to defend against more lethal chemical agents and toxins that could be used by America's enemies. Law enforcement agencies and manufacturers also have limited resources to thoroughly investigate the safety of these compounds. Currently, federal resources are more wisely used to prevent disease and address healthcare issues that affect the population at large.

The control of the administration of RCAs might be difficult to regulate, particularly in the areas and under the circumstances in which the use of RCAs has apparently been misused (eg, the West Bank and Gaza Strip, and Seoul, South Korea). Despite the concern about the occasional loss of life of those exposed to RCAs or the occasional injury among innocent bystanders, there is serious doubt that a prohibition of the use of RCAs would be effective. Although in some instances dialogue and negotiation should precede the use of RCAs, these agents have proved effective in curbing damage to property and persons in threatening situations. Although RCAs sometimes cause permanent injury or death, especially when used in enclosed spaces or against those with existing cardiopulmonary compromise, in most situations the amount of injury is small compared to what might have happened if more extreme measures (physical or lethal force) had been used.

SUMMARY

RCAs are intended to harass or to cause temporary incapacitation. The intended target might be rioters in a civil disturbance, or if approved by the president of the United States, the military in an armed conflict. Although developed to have a high margin of safety, RCAs can cause injury or death when used in spaces without adequate ventilation for prolonged periods, deployed incorrectly, or used against those with preexisting medical conditions. Although injuries such as burns or fragment penetration can also result from the exploding delivery device rather than from the actual agent, these injuries should not be confused. Data show that RCAs such as OC and CS are safe when used for their intended purpose.

REFERENCES

1. Article II, Definitions and Criteria. US Chemical Weapons Convention Web site. Available at: http://www.cwc.gov/treaty/treatytext_html. Accessed November 1, 2005.

2. Salem H, Ballantyne B, Katz SA. Inhalation toxicology of riot control agents. In: Salem H, Katz SA, eds. *Inhalation Toxicology*. 2nd ed. New York, NY: CRC Press; 2005.

3. Sidell F. Riot control agents. In: Sidell F, Takafuji E, Franz D, eds. *Medical Aspects of Chemical and Biological Warfare.* In: Zajtchuk R, Bellamy RF, eds. *Textbook of Military Medicine.* Washington, DC: Department of the Army, Office of The Surgeon General, Borden Institute; 1997: Chap 12.

4. Olajos EJ, Stopford W, eds. *Riot Control Agents: Issues in Toxicology, Safety, and Health*. Boca Raton, Fla: CRC Press; 2004.

5. Kratschmer F. Uber Reflexe von der Nasenschleimhaut auf athmung und Kreislaub, Sitzungsber [Minutes of the proceedings of the nasal reflexes during respirations and circulation]. *Akad Wiss*. 1870;62:147–170.

6. Allen WF. Effect on respiration, blood pressure, and carotid pulse of various inhaled and insufflated vapors when stimulating one cranial nerve and various combinations of cranial nerves. *Am J Physiol*. 1928–29; 87:319–325.

7. Aviado DM, Salem H. Respiratory and bronchomotor reflexes in toxicity studies. In: Salem H, ed. *Inhalation Toxicology: Research Methods, Applications and Evaluation*. New York, NY: Marcel Dekker; 1987.

8. Aviado DM, Guevara Aviado D. The Bezold-Jarisch reflex. A historical perspective of cardiopulmonary reflexes. *Ann N Y Acad Sci*. 2001;940:48–58.

9. Aviado DM. Kratschmer reflex induced by inhalation of aerosol propellants. In: *Proceedings of the 2nd Annual Conference on Environmental Toxicology: Toxic Hazards of Halocarbon Propellants*. Washington, DC: US Food and Drug Administration; 1971: 63–77.

10. US Department of the Army. *Flame, Riot Control Agent, and Herbicide Operations*. Fort Leonard Wood, Mo: DA; August 19, 1996. FM 3-11.11, MCRP 3–3.7.2.

11. Habanero D. A short and sordid history of pepper spray. In: *Fire in the Eyes, a Chemical Weapons Primer, Earth First Journal*. Dec/Jan 2000. Available at: http://www.nonpepperspray.org/sordid.htm. Accessed November 1, 2005.

12. Steffee CH, Lantz PE, Flannagan LM, Thompson RL, Jason DR. Oleoresin capsicum (pepper) spray and "in-custody" deaths. *Am J Forensic Med Pathol*. 1995;16:185–192.

13. Swearengen TF. *Tear Gas Munitions—An Analysis of Commercial Riot Gas Guns, Tear Gas Projectiles, Grenades, Small Arms Ammunition, and Related Tear Gas Devices*. Springfield, Ill: Charles C Thomas; 1966.

14. Salem H, Olajos EJ, Katz SA. Riot control agents. In: Somani SM, Romano JA Jr, eds. *Chemical Warfare Agents: Toxicity at Low Levels*. Boca Raton, Fla: CRC Press; 2001.

15. Chloropicrin. EXTOXNET, Extension Toxicology Network, pesticide information profiles. Web site. Available at: http://extoxnet.orst.edu/pips/chloropi.htm. Accessed April 13, 2007.

16. Wilhelm SN. Chloropicarin as a soil fumigant. US Department of Agriculture, Agricultural Research Service Web site. Available at: http://www.ars.usda.gov/is/np/mba/july96/wilhel1.htm. Accessed November 1, 2005.

17. Sofia gas poisoning was accident, police say. April 9, 2004. Bulgarian News Network Web site. Available at: http://www.bgnewsnet.com/story.php?sid=4519. Accessed November 1, 2005.

18. Forty hurt in Sofia gas accident. April 9, 2004. BBC Web site. Available at: http://news.bbc.co.uk/1/hi/world/europe/3613979.stm. Accessed November 1, 2005.

19. Brooks J. Chemical warfare on the West Bank? July 5, 2004. *Palestine.monitor* [serial online]. Available at: http://www.palestinemonitor.org/new_web/chemical_warfare_westbank.htm. Accessed November 1, 2005.

20. Brooks J. The Israeli poison gas attacks: a preliminary investigation. June 27, 2004. Vermonters for a Just Peace in Palestine Web site. Available at: http://www.vtjp.org/report/The_Israeli_Poison_Gas_Attacks_Project.htm. Accessed November 1, 2005.

21. Royer J, Gainet F. Ocular effects of ethyl bromoacetate tear gas. *Bull Soc Ophtalmol Fr*. 1973;73:1165-1171.

22. Atkinson JM. Advanced Chemical Weapons. Available at: http://www.tscm.com/mace.html. Accessed November 1, 2005.

23. The history of pepper spray. Safety Gear HQ Web site. Available at: http://www.safetygearhq.com/pepper-spray-facts.htm#1. Accessed November 1, 2005.

24. Corson BB, Stoughton RW. Reactions of alpha, beta-unsaturated dinitriles. *J Am Chem Soc*. 1928;50:2825–2837.

24. Davis SL. Riot control weapons for the Vietnam War. Historical monograph. Edgewood Arsenal, Md: US Army Munitions Command; 1970.

26. Cucinell SA, Swentzel KC, Biskup R, et al. Biochemical interactions and metabolic fate of riot control agents. *Fed Proc*. 1971;30:86–91.

27. McNamara BP, Owens EJ, Weimer JT, Ballard TA, Vocci FJ. *Toxicology of Riot Control Chemicals—CS, CN, and DM*. Edgewood Arsenal, Md: US Army Biomedical Laboratory; 1969. Technical Report EATR 4309.

28. Kluchinsky TA Jr, Savage PB, Fitz R, Smith PA. Liberation of hydrogen cyanide and hydrogen chloride during high-temperature dispersion of CS riot control agent. *AIHA J* (Fairfax, Va). 2002;63:493–496.

29. Kluchinsky TA Jr, Savage PB, Sheely MV, Thomas RJ, Smith PA. Identification of CS-derived compounds formed during heat-dispersion of CS riot control agent. *J Microcolumn*. Sep. 2001;13(5):186–190.

30. Kluchinsky TA, Sheely MV, Savage PB, Smith PA. Formation of 2-chlorobenzylidenemalonolnitrile (CS riot control agent) thermal degradation products at elevated temperatures. *J Chromatogr*. 2002;952:205–213.

31. Smith PA, Kluchinsky TA Jr., Savage PB, et al. Traditional sampling with laboratory analysis and solid phase microextraction sampling with field gas chromatograph/mass spectrometry by military industrial hygienists. *AIHA J* (Fairfax, Va). 2002;63(3):284–292.

32. Katz SA, Salem H. Synthesis and chemical analysis of riot control agents. In: Olajos EJ, Stopford W, eds. *Riot Control Agents: Issues in Toxicology, Safety, and Health*. Boca Raton, Fla: CRC Press; 2004: Chap 3.

33. Abdo K. *NTP Technical Report on the Toxicology and Carcinogenesis Studies of CS2 (94% o-chlorobenzalmalononitrile, CAS No. 2698-41-1) in F344/N Rats and B6C3F1 Mice*. Research Triangle Park, NC: US Department of Health and Human Services, Public Health Service, National Institutes of Health; 1990. NTP TR 377, NIH Publication No. 90-2832.

34. Ditter JM, Heal CS. Application and use of riot control agents. In: Olajos EJ, Stopford W, eds. *Riot Control Agents: Issues in Toxicology, Safety, and Health*. Boca Raton, Fla: CRC Press; 2004: Chap 2.

35. Beswick FW, Holland P, Kemp KH. Acute effects of exposure to orthochlorobenzylidene malononitrile (CS) and the development of tolerance. *Br J Ind Med*. 1972;29:298–306.

36. Thomas RJ, Smith PA, Rascona DA, Louthan JD, Gumpert B. Acute pulmonary effects from o-chlorobenzylidenemalonitrile "tear gas": a unique exposure outcome unmasked by strenuous exercise after a military training event. *Mil Med*. 2002;167(2):136–139.

37. Himsworth H, Black DAK, Crawford T. *Report of the Enquiry into the Medical and Toxicological Aspects of CS (orthochlorobenzylidene malononitrile). Part II. Enquiry into Toxicological Aspects of CS and Its Use for Civil Purposes*. London, UK: Her Majesty's Stationery Office; 1971. Cmnd. 4775, Home Office.

38. Himsworth H, Dornhorst AC, Thompson RHS. *Report of the Enquiry into the Medical and Toxicological Aspects of CS (orthochlorobenzylidene malononitrile). Part I. Enquiry into the Medical Situation Following the Use of CS in Londonderry on the 13th and 14th August, 1969*. London, UK: Her Majesty's Stationery Office; 1969. Cmnd. 4173, Home Office (The Himsworth Committee).

39. Hout J. Evaluation of the low temperature thermal degradation products of *o*-chlorobenzylidene malononitrile. Uniformed Services University of the Health Sciences, Department of Preventive Medicine and Biometrics, Division of Environmental and Occupational Health; 2005. Research application T087YZ-01.

40. Ballantyne B, Swanston DW. The comparative acute mammalian toxicity of 1-chloroacetophenone (CN) and 2-chlorobenzylidene malononitrile (CS). *Arch Toxicol*.1978;40:75–95.

41. Ballantyne B. The cyanogenic potential of 2-chlorobenzylidene malononitrile. *Toxicologist*. 1983;3:64.

42. Frankenberg L, Sorbo B. Formation of cyanide from o-chlorobenzylidene malononitrile and its toxicological significance. *Arch Toxicol*. 1973;31:99–108.

43. Jones GR, Israel MS. Mechanism of toxicity of injected CS gas. *Nature*. 1970;228:1315–1317.

44. Leadbeater L, Sainsbury GL, Utley D. Ortho-chlorobenzylmalononitrile: a metabolite formed from ortho-chlorobenzylidenemalononitrile (CS). *Toxicol Appl Pharmacol*. 1973;25:111–116.

45. Nash JB, Doucet BM, Ewing PL, Emerson GA. Effects of cyanide antidotes and inanition on acute lethal toxicity of malononitrile in mice. *Arch Int Pharmacodyn Ther*. 1950;84:385–392.

46. Patai S, Rappoport Z. Nucleophilic attacks on carbon-carbon double bonds. Part II. Cleavage of arylmethylenemalononitriles by water in 95% ethanol. *J Chem Soc (London)*. 1962;71:383–391.

47. Sanford JP. Medical aspects of riot control (harassing) agents. *Annu Rev Med*. 1976;27:421–429.

48. Stern J, Weil-Malherbe H, Green RH. The effects and the fate of malononitrile and related compounds in animals tissues. *Biochem J*. 1952;52:114–125.

49. Porter E, Sinkinson DV, Tees RFS. *The Pyrolysis of o-Chlorobenzylidene in a Gas Flow System*. Porton Down, Salisbury, Great Britain: Chemical Defence Establishment; 1961. Technical Paper PTP 788.

50. Olajos EJ, Stopford W. Riot control agents and acute sensory irritation. In: Olajos EJ, Stopford W, eds. *Riot Control Agents Issues in Toxicology, Safety, and Health*. Boca Raton, Fla: CRC Press; 2004: Chap 5.

51. Gutentag PJ, Hart J, Owens EJ, Punte CL. *The Evaluation of CS Aerosol as a Riot Control Agent for Man*. Edgewood Arsenal, Md: Edgewood Arsenal Medical Research Laboratory; 1960. Technical Report CWLR 2365.

52. Punte CL, Owens EJ, Gutentag PJ. Exposures to orthochlorobenzylidene malononitrile. Controlled human exposures. *Arch Environ Health*. 1963;6:366–374.

53. US Department of the Army. *The Toxicology of CN, CS, and DM*. Edgewood Arsenal, Md: Edgewood Arsenal Medical Research Laboratory; 1965. Special Summary Report by Directorate of Medical Research.

54. Ballantyne B, Gazzard, MF, Swanston DW, Williams P. The ophthalmic toxicology of o-chlorobenzylidene malononitrile (CS). *Arch Toxicol*. 1974;32:149–168.

55. Punte CL, Weimer JT, Ballard TA, Wilding JL. Toxicologic studies on o-chlorobenzylidene malononitrile. *Toxicol Appl Pharmacol*. 1962;4:656–662.

56. Rietveld EC, Delbressine LP, Waegemaekers TH, Seutter-Berlage F. 2-Chlorobenzylmercapturic acid, a metabolite of the riot control agent 2-chlorobenzylidene malononitrile (CS) in the rat. *Arch Toxicol*. 1983;54:139–144.

57. von Daniken A, Friederich U, Lutz W, Schlatter C. Tests for mutagenicity in Salmonella and covalent binding to DNA and protein in the rat of the riot control agent o-chlorobenzylidene malononitrile (CS). *Arch Toxicol*. 1981;49:15–27.

58. Wild D, Eckhardt K, Harnasch D, King MT. Genotoxicity study of CS (Ortho-chlorobenzylidenemalononitrile) in Salmonella, Drosophila, and mice. Failure to detect mutagenic effects. *Arch Toxicol*. 1983;54:167–170.

59. Zeiger E, Anderson B, Haworth S, Lawlor T, Mortelmans K, Speck W. Salmonella mutagenicity tests III. Results from the testing of 225 chemicals. *Environ Mutagen*. 1987;9:1–109.

60. National Research Council, Committee on Toxicology. *Cholinesterase Reactivators, Psychochemicals, and Irritants and Vesicants*. Vol 2. In: *Possible Long-Term Health Effects of Short-Term Exposure to Chemical Agents*. Washington, DC: National Academy Press; 1984: 221–119.

61. Ballantyne B, Callaway S. Inhalation toxicology and pathology of animals exposed to o-chlorobenzylidene malononitrile (CS). *Med Sci Law*. 1972;12:43–65.

62. Weimer JT, Wilding JL, Ballard TA, Lawson L, Punte CL. *A Study of the Acute and Sub-Acute Toxicity of Aerosols of CS in Small Laboratory Animals (U)*. Edgewood Arsenal, Md: US Army Chemical Warfare Laboratories, 1960. Technical Report CWLR 2360.

63. Marrs TC, Colgrave HF, Cross NL, Gazzard MF, Brown RF. A repeated dose study of the toxicity of inhaled 2-chlorobenzylidene malononitrile (CS) aerosol in three species of laboratory animal. *Arch Toxicol*. 1983;52:183–198.

64. McNamara BP, Renne RA, Rozmiarek H, Ford DF, Owens EJ. *CS: A Study of Carcinogenicity*. Aberdeen Proving Ground, Md: US Army Biomedical Laboratory; 1973. Edgewood Arsenal Technical Report, EATR 4760.

65. Abdo K. *Toxicology and Carcinogenesis Studies of CS2 (94% o-Chlorobenzalmalononitrile) CAS No. 2698-41-1) in F344/N Rats and B6C3F1 Mice (Inhalation Studies)*. Research Triangle Park, NC: National Toxicology Program; 1990. NTIS-PB90256280, Technical Report Series No. 377.

66. Gongwer LE, Ballard TA, Gutentag PJ, et al. *The Comparative Effectiveness of Four Riot Control Agents*. Edgewood Arsenal, Md: US Army Chemical Warfare Laboratories; 1958. Technical Memorandum CWL-TM- 24-18.

67. Owens EJ, Punte CL. Human respiratory and ocular irritation studies utilizing o-chlorobenzylidene malononitrile. *Am Ind Hyg Assoc J*. 1963;May-Jun;4:262–264.

68. Cole TJ, Cotes JE, Johnson GR, Martin HD, Reed JW, Saunders JE. Ventilation, cardiac frequency and pattern of breathing during exercise in men exposed to o-chlorobenzylidene malononitrile (CS) and ammonia gas in low concentrations. *Q J Exp Physiol Cogn Med Sci*. 1977;62:341–351.

69. *National Institute for Occupational Safety and Health (NIOSH) Pocket Guide to Chemical Hazards*. Washington, DC: US Government Printing Office; 2005. Department of Health and Human Services, Centers for Disease Control and Prevention Web site. Available at: www.cdc.gov/niosh/idlh/idhlview.html. Accessed November 2, 2005.

70. Heinrich U. Possible lethal effects of CS tear gas on Branch Davidians during the FBI raid on the Mount Carmel compound Near Waco, Texas April 19, 1993. Available at: http://www.veritagiustizia.it/docs/gas_cs/CS_Effects_Waco.pdf. Accessed August 21, 2007.

71. Blain PG. Tear gases and irritant incapacitants. 1-chloroacetophenone, 2-chlorobenzylidene malononitrile and dibenz[b,f]-1,4-oxazepine. *Toxicol Review*. 2003;22(2):103–110.

72. Weigand DA. Cutaneous reaction to the riot control agent CS. *Mil Med*. 1969;134: 437–440.

73. Olajos EJ, Salem H. Riot control agents: pharmacology, toxicology, biochemistry and chemistry. *J Appl Toxicol.* 2001;21:355–391.

74. Hellreich A, Goldman RH, Bottiglieri NG, Weimer JT. *The Effects of Thermally-Generated CS Aerosols on Human Skin.* Edgewood Arsenal, Md: Edgewood Arsenal Medical Research Laboratory; 1967. Technical Report EATR 4075.

75. Hellreich A, Mershon MM, Weimer JT, Kysor KP, Bottiglieri NG. *An Evaluation of the Irritant Potential of CS Aerosols on Human Skin Under Tropical Climatic Conditions.* Edgewood Arsenal, Md: Edgewood Arsenal Medical Research Laboratory; 1969. Technical Report EATR 4252.

76. Rengstorff RH. *The Effects of the Riot Control Agent CS on Visual Acuity.* Edgewood Arsenal, Md: Edgewood Arsenal Medical Research Laboratories; 1968. Technical Report EATR 4246.

77. Weimer JT, Owens EJ, McNamara BP, Merkey RP, Olson JS. *Toxicological Assessment of Riot Control Spray Devices and Fillings.* Edgewood Arsenal, Md: Edgewood Arsenal Biomedical Laboratory; 1975. Technical Report EB-TR-75047.

78. Ballantyne B, Gall D, Robson D. Effects on man of drenching with dilute solutions of o-chlorobenzylidene malononitrile (CS) and dibenz[b.f]1:4-oxazepine (CR). *Med Sci Law.* 1976;16:159–170.

79. Rengstorff RH, Merson MM. *CS in Trioctyl Phosphate: Effects on Human Eyes.* Edgewood Arsenal, Md: Edgewood Arsenal Medical Research Laboratories; 1969. Technical Report, EATR 4376.

80. Rengstorff RH, Merson MM. *CS in Water: Effects on Human Eyes.* Edgewood Arsenal, Md: Edgewood Arsenal Medical Research Laboratories; 1969. Technical Report EATR 4377.

81. Gray PJ, Murray V. Treating CS gas injuries to the eye. Exposure at close range is particularly dangerous. *BMJ.* 1995; 311:871.

82. Yih JP. CS gas injury to the eye. *BMJ.* 1995;311:276.

83. Hoffmann DH. Eye burns caused by tear gas. *Br J Ophthalmol.* 1967;51:265–8.

84. Solomon I, Kochba I, Eizenkraft E, Maharshak N. Report of accidental CS ingestion among seven patients in central Israel and review of the current literature. *Arch Toxicol.* 2003;77:601–604.

85. Kemp KH, Willder WB. The palatability of food exposed to o-chlorobenzylidene malononitrile (CS). *Med Sci Law.* 1972; 12:113–120.

86. Brooks SM, Weiss MA, Bernstein IL. Reactive airways dysfunction syndrome (RADS). Persistent asthma syndrome after high level irritant exposures. *Chest.* 1985;88:376–384.

87. Hu H, Fine J, Epstein P, Kelsey K, Reynolds P, Walker B. Tear gas—harassing agent or toxic chemical weapon? *JAMA.* 1989; 262(5):660-663.

88. Roth VS, Franzblau A. RADS after exposure to a riot-control agent: a case report. *J Occup Environ Med.* 1996;38(9):863–865.

89. Hill AR, Silverberg NB, Mayorga D, Baldwin HE. Medical hazards of the tear gas CS: a case of persistent, multisystem, hypersensitivity reaction and review of the literature. *Medicine (Baltimore).* 2000; 79(4):234–40.

90. Bowers MB, Owens EJ, Punte CL. *Interim Report of CS Exposures in Plant Workers.* Edgewood Arsenal, Md: US Army Chemical Warfare Laboratories; June 1960. Technical Report CWL 24-50.

91. Williams SR, Clark RF, Dunford JV. Contact dermatitis associated with capsaicin: Hunan hand syndrome. *Ann Emerg Med.* 1995;25:713–7151.

92. Dicpinigaitis PV, Alva RV. Safety of capsaicin cough challenge testing. *Chest.* 2005;128:196–202.

93. Nonivamide. Food Navigator.com Europe [serial online]. Available at: http://www.foodnavigator.com/news-by-product/productpresentation.asp?id=50&k=nonivamide. Accessed November 2, 2005.

94. Constant HL, Cordell GA, West DP. Nonivamide, a constituent of Capsicum oleoresin. *J Nat Prod* [serial online]. 1996;59(4):425–426. Available at: http://www.geocities.com/NapaValley/3378/capsaicinarticle15.htm. Accessed November 2, 2005.

95. Daroff PM, Metz D, Roberts A, Adams JA, Jenkins W. *Oleoresin Capsicum: An Effective Less-Than-Lethal Riot Control Agent.* US Army Dugway Proving Ground, Utah: Chemical Biological Defense; January,1997. Technical Report DPG/JCP-097-002. Unclassified Report (ADB225032).

96. US Army Center for Health Promotion and Preventive Medicine. *Detailed and General Facts About Chemical Agents.* Aberdeen Proving Ground, Md: USACHPPM; 1996. Technical Guide 218.

97. PepperBall Technologies, Inc, Web site. Available at: http://www.pepperball.com/. Accessed November 2, 2005.

98. Clapham DE. TRP channels as cellular sensors. *Nature*. 2003;426:517–524.

99. Caterina MJ, Schumacher MA, Tominaga M, Rosen TA, Levine JD, Julius D. The capsaicin receptor: a heat-activated ion channel in the pain pathway. *Nature*. 1997;389:816–824.

100. Birder LA, Nakamura, Kiss S, et al. Altered urinary bladder function in mice lacking the vanilloid receptor TRPV1. *Nat Neurosci*. 2002;5:856–860.

101. International Association of Chiefs of Police. Pepper Spray Evaluation Project. *Results of the Introduction of Oleoresin Capsicum (OC) Into the Baltimore County, MD, Police Department*. Alexandria, Va: IAPP; 1995. Available at: http://www.theiacp.org/documents/pdfs/Publications/peppersprayeval%2Epdf.

102. Gosselin RE, Hodge HC, Smith RP, Gleason MN. *Clinical Toxicology of Commercial Products.* 4th ed. Baltimore, Md: Lippincott Williams & Wilkins; 1976.

103. Govindarajan VS, Sathyanarayana MN. Capsicum—production, technology, chemistry, and quality. Part V: Impact on physiology, pharmacology, nutrition and metabolism; structure, pungency, pain, and desensitization sequences. *Crit Rev Food Sci Nutr*. 1991;29(6):435–474.

104. Abdel Salam OM, Mozsik G, Szolcsanyi J. Studies on the effect of intragastric capsaicin on gastric ulcer and on the prostacyclin-induced cytoprotection in rats. *Pharmacol Res.* 1995;32(4): 209–215.

105. Jang JJ, Devor DE, Logsdon DL, Ward JM. A 4-week feeding study of ground red chilli (Capsicum annuum) in male B6C3F1 mice. *Food Chem Toxicol*. 1992;30:783–787.

106. Monsereenusorn Y. Subchronic toxicity studies of capsaicin and capsicum in rats. *Res Commun Chem Pathol Pharmacol.* 1983;41:95–110.

107. Chloropicarin as a soil fumigant. US Department of Agriculture, Agricultural Research Service Web site. Available at: http://www.ars.usda.gov. Accessed November 2, 2005.

108. Centers for Disease Control and Prevention. Exposure to tear gas from a theft-deterrent device on a safe—Wisconsin, December 2003. *MMWR Morb Mortal Wkly Rep*. 2004;53:176–177.

109. Lenhart SW, Gagnon YT. Health hazard evaluation of methyl bromide soil fumigations. *Appl Occup Environ Hyg*. 1999;14:407–412.

110. Park DS, Peterson C, Zhao S, Coats JR. Fumigation toxicity of volatile natural and synthetic cyanohydrins to stored-product pests and activity as soil fumigants. *Pest Manag Sci*. 2004;60:833–838.

111. Prudhomme JC, Bhatia R, Nutik JM, Shusterman D. Chest wall pain and possible rhabdomyolysis after chloropicrin exposure: a case series. *J Occup Environ Med*. 1999;41:17–22.

112. Centers for Disease Control. Brief report: illness associated with drift of chloropicrin soil fumigant into a residential area—Kern County, California, 2003. *MMWR Morb Mortal Wkly Rep*. 2004;53:740-742. Available at: http://www.cdc.gov/mmwr/preview/mmwrhtml/mm5332a4.htm. Accessed November 2, 2005.

113. Lee S, McLaughlin R, Harnly M, Gunier R, Kreutzer R. Community exposures to airborne agricultural pesticides in California: ranking of inhalation risks. *Environ Health Perspect*. 2002;110:1175–1184.

114. Condie LW, Daniel FB, Olson GR, Robinson M. Ten and ninety-day toxicity studies of chloropicrin in Sprague-Dawley rats. *Drug Chem Toxicol*. 1994;17:125–137.

115. Tamagawa S, Irimajiri T, Oyamada M. Persistence of chloropicrin in soil and environmental effect on it. *J Pest Sci (Japan)*. 1985;10:205–210.

116. Buckley LA, Jiang XA, James RA, Morgan KT, Barrow CS. Respiratory tract lesions induced by sensory irritants at the RD50 concentration. *Toxicol Appl Pharmacol*. 1984;74:417–429.

117. Sparks SE, Quistad GB, Casida JE. Chloropicrin: reactions with biological thiols and metabolism in mice. *Chem Res Toxicol*. 1997;10:1001–1007.

118. Jackson KE. Chloropicrin. *Chem Rev*. 1934;14:251–286.

119. Mackworth JF. The inhibition of thiol enzymes by lachrymators. *Biochem J*. 1948;(42) 82–90.

120. National Institute for Occupational Safety and Health. Registry of Toxic Effects of Chemical Substances [database online]. Methane, trichloronitro-. Updated 2004. Available at: http://www.setonresourcecenter.com/MSDS_Hazcom/rtecs/pb602160.html. Accessed August 20, 2007.

121. DeBaun JR, Miaullis JB, Knarr J, Mihailovski A, Menn JJ. The fate of N-trichloro(14C)methylthio-4-cyclohexene-1,2-dicarboximide((14C)captan) in the rat. *Xenobiotica*. 1974;4:101–119.

122. Alarie Y. Sensory irritation by airborne chemicals. *CRC Crit Rev Toxicol*. 1973;2:299–363.

123. Clayton GD, Clayton FE. *Patty's Industrial Hygiene and Toxicology*. New York, NY: John Wiley & Sons; 1981; 2242-2247.

124. Amoore JE, Hautala E. Odor as an aid to chemical safety: odor thresholds compared with threshold limit values and volatilities for 214 industrial chemicals in air and water dilution. *J Appl Toxicol*. 1983;3(6):272–290.

125. Okada E, Takahashi K, Nakamura H. A study of chloropicrin intoxication. *Nippon Naika Gakkai Zasshi*. 1970;59:1214–1221.

126. American Conference of Governmental Industrial Hygienists. *Documentation of the Threshold Limit Values and Biological Exposure Indices*. 6th ed. Cincinnati, Ohio: American Conference of Governmental Industrial Hygienists; 1991.

127. Graeb C. *Berichte des Deutschem Chemisch Gesellschaft LV. Commissionsverlog von R [Report of the German chemical industry]*. Berlin, Germany: Friedlander and Son; 1881. Available at: http://awr.nti.org/e_researchprofiles/NK/Chemical/1095.html; http://www.nadir.org/nadir/initiativ/sanis/archiv/allergic/kap_01.htm. Accessed on November 2, 2005.

128. *History of Research and Development of the Chemical Warfare Service Through 1945*. Edgewood Arsenal, Md: Edgewood Arsenal Medical Research Laboratory; 1966. EASP 400–427.

129. Anderson PJ, Lau GS, Taylor WR, Critchley JA. Acute effects of the potent lacrimator o-chlorobenzylidene malononitrile (CS) tear gas. *Hum Exp Toxicol*. 1996;15:461–465.

130. Castro JA. Effects of alkylating agents on human plasma cholinesterase. *Biochem Pharmacol*. 1968;17:195-303.

131. McNamara, BP, Vocci, FJ, Owens, EJ. *The Toxicology of CN*. Edgewood Arsenal, Md: Edgewood Arsenal Medical Laboratories; 1968. Technical Report 4207.

132. Kumar P, Flora SJ, Pant SC, Sachan AS, Saxena SP, Gupta S. Toxicological evaluation of 1-chloroacetophenone and dibenz (b,f)-1,4-oxazepine after repeated inhalation exposure in mice. *J Appl Toxicol*. 1994;14:411-416.

133. Husain K, Kumar P, Malhotra RC. A comparative study of biochemical changes induced by inhalation of aerosols of o-chloroacetophenone and dibenz (b,f)-1,4-oxazepine in rats. *Indian J Med Res*. 1991;94:76-79.

134. Ballantyne B, Swanston DW. The irritant effects of dilute solutions of dibenzoxazepine (CR) on the eye and tongue. *Acta Pharmacol Toxicol (Copenh)*. 1974;35:412–423.

135. Hoffman DH. Eye burns caused by tear gas. *Br J Ophthalmol*. 1967;51:265-268.

136. Leopold IH, Lieberman TW. Chemical injuries of the cornea. *Fed Proc*. 1971; 30:92-95.

137. Macrae WG, Willinsky MD, Basu PK. Corneal injury caused by aerosol irritant projectors. *Can J Ophthalmol*. 1970;5:3–11.

138. Ballantyne B, Gazzard MF, Swanston DW, Williams P. The comparative ophthalmic toxicology of 1-chloroacetophenone (CN) and dibenz (b,f)-1:4-oxazepine(CR). *Arch Toxicol*. 1975;34:183–201.

139. Gaskins JR, Hehir RM, McCaulley DF, Ligon EW Jr. Lacrimating agents (CS and CN) in rats and rabbits. Acute effects on mouth, eyes and skin. *Arch Environ Health*. 1972;24:449–454.

140. Chung CW, Giles AL Jr. Sensitization of guinea pigs to alpha-chloroacetophenone (CN) and ortho-chlorobenzylidene malononitrile (CS) tear gas chemicals. *J Immunol*. 1972;109:284–293.

141. Holland P, White RG. The cutaneous reactions produced by o-chlorobenzyl-idenemalononitrile and -chloroacetophenone when applied directly to the skin of human subjects. *Br J Dermatol*. 1972;86:150–154.

142. Penneys NS, Israel RM, Indgin SM. Contact dermatitis due to 1-chloracetophenone and chemical mace. *N Engl J Med*. 1969;281:413–415.

143. National Toxicology Program. TR-379. Toxicology and carcinogenesis studies of 2-chloroacetophenone (CAS No. 532-27-4) in F344/N rats and B6C3F$_1$ mice (inhalation studies). *NTP Study Reports* [serial online]. 1990;379:1-191. Available at: http://ntp.niehs.nih.gov/index.cfm?objectid=0709027D-F784-3957-7B0E3F3C05F528AA. Accessed August 21, 2007.

144. Thorburn KM. Injuries after use of the lachrimatory agent chloroacetophenone in a confined space. *Arch Environ Health*. 1982;37:182–186.

145. Stein AA, Kirwan WE. Chloracetophenone (tear gas) poisoning: a clinico-pathologic report. *J Forensic Sci*. 1964;9:374–382.

146. Chapman AJ, White C. Death resulting from lachrimatory agents. *J Forensic Sci*. 1978;23:527–530.

147. Vedder EB, Walton DC. *The Medical Aspects of Chemical Warfare*. Baltimore, Md: Williams & Wilkins; 1925: 175.

148. Kibler AL. *The After-Effects of Chloroacetophenone*. Edgewood Arsenal, Md: US Department of the Army, Medical Research Laboratories; 1933. Technical Report 133.

149. Queen FB, Stander T. Allergic dermatitis following exposure to tear gas (chloroacetophenone). *JAMA*. 1941;117:1879.

150. Madden JF. Cutaneous hypersensitivity to tear gas (chloroacetophenone); a case report. *AMA Arch Derm Syphilol*. 1951;63:133–134.

151. Levine RA, Stahl CJ. Eye injury caused by tear-gas weapons. *Am J Ophthalmol*. 1968;65:497–508.

152. Rengstorff RH. Tear gas and riot control agents: a review of eye effects. *Optom Week*. 1969;60:25–28.

153. Owens EJ, McNamara BP, Weimer JT, et al. *The Toxicology of DM*. Edgewood Arsenal, Md: Edgewood Arsenal Medical Research Laboratories; 1967. Technical Report EATR 4108.

154. Prentiss AM, Fisher GJB. *Chemicals in War: A Treatise on Chemical Warfare*. New York, NY: McGraw-Hill Book Company Inc; 1937.

155. Frank S. *Chemistry of Chemical Warfare Agents*. Vol 1. In: *Manual of Military Chemistry*. US Department of Commerce, National Bureau of Standards, Institute for Applied Technology, trans. Deutscher Militirverlag: East Berlin, Germany; 1967:62–76. NTIS no. AD-849866.

156. Hersh SM. *Chemical and Biological Warfare: America's Hidden Arsenal*. Indianapolis, Ind: Bobbs-Merrill; 1968: 60–62, 185–185.

157. Prentiss AM. Respiratory irritant agents. In: Prentiss AM, Fisher GJB, eds. *Chemicals in War: A Treatise on Chemical Warfare*. New York, NY: McGraw-Hill Book Company Inc; 1937: Chap 10.

158. Haas R, Tsivunchyk O, Steinbach K, von Low E, Scheibner K, Hofrichter M. Conversion of adamsite (phenarsarzin chloride) by fungal manganese peroxidase. *Appl Microbiol Biotechnol*. 2004;63:564–566.

159. Henriksson J, Johannisson A, Bergqvist PA, Norrgren L. The toxicity of organoarsenic-based warfare agents: in vitro and in vivo studies. *Arch Environ Contam Toxicol*. 1996;30:213–219.

160. Striker GE, Streett CS, Ford DF, Herman LH, Helland DR. *A Clinicophathologic Study of the Effects of Riot Control Agents on Monkeys. III. Diphenylaminochloroarsine (DM)*. Edgewood Arsenal, Md: Edgewood Arsenal Medical Research Laboratory; 1967. Technical Report EATR 4070.

161. British Ministry of Defence, Chemical Defence Research Department. *Classified List of Compounds Examined Physiologically Since 1919*. Porton Down, Salisbury, England: Chemical Defence Experimental Station; 1941. Porton Memorandum No. 15. UK National Archives document WO 189/227 – 233 (1941 "Red Book").

162. Lawson WE, Temple JW. *Report on the Relation Between Concentration and Limit of Tolerance for Diphenylamine-chloroarsine and the Development of a Continuous Flow Apparatus for Testing*. Aberdeen Proving Ground, Md: Edgewood Arsenal; 1922. Technical Report ADB959603; EACD 92.

163. World Health Organization. *Health Aspects of Chemical and Biological Weapons*. 1st ed. Geneva, Switzerland: WHO; 1970: 24, 55.

164. Craighill MD, Folkoff AA. *A Digest of Reports Concerning the Toxic Effects of Diphenylamine Chloroarsine on Man and the Laboratory Animals*. Aberdeen Proving Ground, Md: Edgewood Arsenal; 1922. Technical Report ADB959699, EACD 145.

165. Gongwer LE, Ballard TA, Gutentag PJ, et al. *The Comparative Effectiveness of Four Riot Control Agents*. Edgewood Arsenal, Md: US Army Chemical Warfare Laboratories; 1958: 1–7. CWL-TM-24-18.

166. Kuhn HA, Henley FA. *DM, Its Penetration of the Smoke Filter and Its Effects on Man*. Aberdeen Proving Ground, Md: Edgewood Arsenal; 1921. Technical Report CB-177203, EACD 80.

167. Morrison C, Bright M. Secret gas was issued for IRA prison riot. *The Observer* [serial online]. January 23, 2005. Guardian Unlimited Web site. Available at: http://politics.guardian.co.uk/politicspast/story/0,9061,1396714,00.html. Accessed November 22, 2005.

168. Upshall DG. Effects of dibenz [b,f] [1,4] oxazepine (CR) upon rat and rabbit embryonic development. *Toxicol Appl Pharmacol*. 1974;29:301–311.

169. French MC, Harrison JM, Inch TD, et al. The fate of dibenz [b,f]-1,4-oxazepine (CR) in the rat, rhesus monkey and guinea pig. Part I. Metabolism in vivo. *Xenobiotica*. 1983;13:345-359.

170. Ballantyne B. Riot control agents. In: Scott RB, Frazer J, eds. *Medical Annual*. Bristol, United Kingdom: Wright and Sons; 1977: 7–41.

171. Ashton I, Cotes JE, Holland P, et al. Acute effect of dibenz b,f.-1:4 oxazepine aerosol upon the lung function of healthy young men [proceedings]. *J Physiol*. 1978;275:85P.

172. Ballantyne B, Beswick FW, Thomas D. The presentation and management of individuals contaminated with solutions of dibenzoxazepine (CR). *Med Sci Law*. 1973;13:265–268.

173. Holland P. The cutaneous reactions produced by dibenzoxazepine (CR). *Br J Dermatol*. 1974;90:657–659.

174. Weigand DA, Mershon MM. *The Cutaneous Irritant Reaction to Agent O-chlorobenzylidene Malononitrile (CS). I. Quantitation and Racial Influence in Human Subjects*. Edgewood Arsenal, Md: Edgewood Arsenal Medical Research Laboratory; 1970. Technical Report EATR 4332.

175. Pattle RE, Schock C, Dirnhuber P, Creasey JM. Lung surfactant and organelles after an exposure to dibenzoxazepine (CR). *Br J Exp Pathol*. 1974; 55:213–220.

176. Colgrave HF, Brown RF, Cox RA. Ultrastructure of rat lungs following exposure to aerosols of dibenzoxazepine (CR). *Br J Exp Pathol*. 1979;60:130–141.

177. Marrs TC, Gray MI, Colgrave HF, Gall D. A repeated dose study of the toxicity of CR applied to the skin of mice. *Toxicol Lett*. 1982;13:259–265.

178. Owens EJ, Weimer JT, Ballard TA, et al. *Ocular, Cutaneous, Respiratory, Intratracheal Toxicity of Solutions of CS and EA 3547 in Glycol and Glycol Ether in Animals*. Edgewood Arsenal, Md: Edgewood Arsenal Medical Research Laboratory; 1970. Technical Report EATR 4446.

179. Higginbottom R, Suschitzky H. Synthesis of heterocyclic compounds II. Cyclization of o-nitrophenyl oxygen. *J Chem Soc*. 1962;456:2367–2370.

180. Biskup RC, Swentzel KC, Lochner MA, Fairchild DG. *Toxicity of 1% CR in Propylene Glycol/Water (80/20)*. Edgewood Arsenal, Md: Edgewood Arsenal Medical Research Laboratory; May 1975. Technical Report EB-TR-75009.

181. Rengstorff RH, Petrali JP, Mershon MM, Sim VM. The effect of the riot control agent dibenz (b,f)-1,4-oxazepine (CR) in the rabbit eye. *Toxicol Appl Pharmacol*. 1975;34:45–48.

182. Lundy PM, McKay DH. *Mechanism of the Cardiovascular Activity of Dibenz (B,F) (1:4) Oxazepine (CR) in Cats*. Ralston, Canada: Defence Research Establishment; 1975. Suffield Technical Paper 438.

183. Marrs TC, Colgrave HF, Cross NL. A repeated dose study of the toxicity of technical grade dibenz-(b.f.)-1,4 oxazepine in mice and hamsters. *Toxicol Lett*. 1983;17:13–21.

184. Grady HG, Stewart HL. Histogenesis of induced pulmonary tumors in strain A mice. *Am J Pathol*. 1940;16:417–432.

185. Stewart HL, Dunn TB, Snell KC, Deringer MK. Tumors of the respiratory tract. In: Turusov SU, ed. *The Mouse*. Vol 1. In: *WHO Monographs on the Pathology of Laboratory*. Lyons, France: International Association for Research on Cancer (IARC); 1979: 251.

186. McNamara BP, Vocci FJ, Owens EJ, Ward DM, Anson NM. *The Search for an Effective Riot-Control Agent—Solvent System for Large Volume Dispersers*. Edgewood Arsenal, Md: Edgewood Arsenal Biomedical Laboratory; 1972. Technical Report EATR 4675.

187. Weigand DA. Cutaneous reaction to the riot control agent CS. *Mil Med*. 1969;134:437–440.

188. Sifton DW, Kelly GL. *PDR Guide to Biological and Chemical Warfare Response*. Montvale, NJ: Thompson/Physicians' Desk Reference; 2002.

189. Carter, RH, Knight HC. *Fundamental Study of Toxicity. Solublity of Certain Toxics in Water and in Olive Oil.* Edgewood, Md: Chemical Warfare Service; 1928. EACD 445, (ADB955216).

190. Smith T. Bear pepper spray: research and information. Alaska Science Center Biological Science Office Web site. Available at: http://www.absc.usgs.gov/research/brownbears/pepperspray/pepperspray.htm. Accessed December 22, 2005.

191. Bio Shield Towelette. Chief Supply Web site. Available at: http://www.chiefsupply.com/resources/msds/bioshield-towelettes-msds.pdf. Accessed April 9, 2007.

192. Sudecon towelettes. Fox Labs International Web site. Available at: http://www.foxlabs.net/PMarticle.htm. Accessed January 21, 2006.

193. MK-3 Cool It material safety data sheet. Chief Supply Web site. Available at: http://www.chiefsupply.com/resources/msds/DE-msds-pepper10-3050.pdf. Accessed on April 9, 2007.

194. 2% 5.3MM SHU OC protection spray with UV dye material safety data sheet. Fox Labs International Web site. Available at: http://www.chiefsupply.com/msds/FAFox2053StreamIt.pdf. Accessed January 21, 2006.

195. US Department of the Army. *Treatment of Chemical Casualties and Conventional Military Chemical Injuries*. Washington, DC: DA; 1995. FM 8-285.

196. Rega PP, Mowatt-Larssen E. CBRNE - Irritants: Cs, Cn, Cnc, Ca, Cr, Cnb, PS. *emedicine from WebMD* [serial online]. April 6, 2005. Available at: http://www.emedicine.com/emerg/topic914. Accessed December 27, 2005.

197. Viala B, Blomet J, Mathieu L, Hall AH. Prevention of CS "tear gas" eye and skin effects and active decontamination with diphoterine: preliminary studies in 5 French gendarmes. *J Emerg Med.* 2005 Jul;29(1):5–8.

198. Park S, Giammona ST. Toxic effects of tear gas on an infant following prolonged exposure. *AJAC.* 1972;123:245–246.

199. Winograd HL. Acute croup in an older child. An unusual toxic origin. *Clin Pediatr (Phila).* 1977;16(10):884–887.

200. Great Britain Home Office. *Report of the Enquiry into the Medical and Toxilogical Aspects of CS (orthochlorobenzylidene malononitrile).* London, United Kingdom: Her Majesty's Stationery Office; 1971. Cmnd 4775.

201. Beswick FW. Chemical agents used in riot control and warfare. *Hum Toxicol.* 1983;2(2):247–256.

Chapter 14

FIELD MANAGEMENT OF CHEMICAL CASUALTIES

CHARLES H. BOARDMAN, MS, ORR/L*; SHIRLEY D. TUORINSKY, MSN†; DUANE C. CANEVA, MD‡; JOHN D. MALONE, MD, MSPH§; AND WILLIAM L. JACKSON, MD, PhD¥

Lieutenant Colonel, Biomedical Sciences Corps, US Air Force; Air Force Liaison, Instructor, and Occupational Therapist, Chemical Casualty Care Division, US Army Medical Research Institute of Chemical Defense, 3100 Ricketts Point Road, Aberdeen Proving Ground, Maryland 21010-5400

†*Lieutenant Colonel, AN, US Army; Executive Officer, Combat Casualty Care Division, US Army Medical Research Institute of Chemical Defense, 3100 Ricketts Point Road, Aberdeen Proving Ground, Maryland 21010-5400*

‡*Commander, US Navy; Head, Medical Plans and Policy, Navy Medicine Office of Homeland Security, 2300 E Street, NW, Washington, DC 20372*

§*Captain, US Navy; Professor of Medicine, Uniformed Services University of the Health Sciences, Bethesda, Maryland 20814; formerly, Commanding Officer, Medical Treatment Facility, USNS Mercy*

¥*Commander, US Public Health Service; Centers for Disease Control and Prevention Quarantine Station, Honolulu International Airport, 300 Rodgers Blvd, Terminal Box 67, Honolulu, Hawaii 96819-1897; formerly, Assistant Chief Medical Officer, US Coast Guard Personnel Command, Arlington, Virginia*

INTRODUCTION

The management of casualties exposed to chemical, biological, radiological, and nuclear (CBRN) agents has long been part of military doctrine. Since the events of September 11, 2001, interest in the management of these types of casualties has extended to the civilian response network. The military mission has likewise expanded beyond the battlefield to include operations in support of homeland defense and humanitarian disaster relief. This expansion of military roles has not significantly changed the procedures for chemical casualty care. Although specific medical and decontamination equipment has changed with time, the core principles for managing contaminated casualties remain basically unchanged since World War I, when the treatment of chemical casualties was conducted on a large scale. These core principles include the early removal of hazardous agent from patients to reduce injury and contamination spread, and the provision of early and effective life-saving treatment.

To save the lives of those contaminated by hazardous agents, medical care providers, whether civilian or military, must be capable of a rapid and effective response. This involves first responders providing initial medical intervention in the contaminated area, or on the periphery, while wearing protective equipment. First responders, as well as first receivers (those who receive contaminated patients at the hospital), must have the training to carry out patient triage and life saving treatment for contaminated patients before, during, and after decontamination. This method of casualty management will reduce injury and should significantly reduce the health impact of a mass casualty event caused by the release of hazardous substances.

This chapter compares the current field management operations of the various military services (land-based and sea-based forces) and the civilian medical community. Although patient treatment strategies still vary, there are now many similarities in the decontamination procedures used by these various organizations, with key differences related to the platforms on which field management takes place (eg, on land vs. on sea-going vessels) and the specific equipment used for medical care, transport, and decontamination. The emphasis in this text is on the management of chemical casualties; however, these same processes are equally applicable to treating patients affected by biological and radiological contaminants. Doctrine and techniques continue to be upgraded, but it is expected that any future developments should continue to follow the basic principles discussed here.

HEALTH SERVICE SUPPORT AND MILITARY FORCE HEALTH PROTECTION ON THE BATTLEFIELD

Health service support (HSS) includes all services performed, provided, or arranged by the military services to promote, improve, conserve, or restore the mental or physical well-being of personnel.[1] Military doctrine and terminology are rapidly changing to better support joint operations both on the battlefield and in civil support missions at home and abroad. This brief overview of current and developing doctrine focuses on its application to the management of chemical casualties across the military.

Force health protection (FHP) consists of measures taken by all military members, from commander to the individual service member, to promote, improve, conserve, or restore mental and physical well-being of personnel.[1] FHP, the medical component of force protection, is a comprehensive approach to care that includes proactive medical services, striving to prevent casualties instead of focusing only on postcasualty intervention.[1] The basic objectives of military HSS and FHP are to promote and sustain a fit and healthy force, prevent injury and illness, protect the force from health threats, and sustain medical and rehabilitative care. The newer, more comprehensive, focus on FHP consists of three pillars of health protection (Figure 14-1), providing a continuum of military health care before, during, and after military operations.[1]

On the battlefield, medical care focuses on

- minimizing the effects of wounds, injuries, disease, environment, occupational hazards, and psychological stressors on unit effectiveness, readiness, and morale; and
- returning to duty as many service members as possible at each level of care.[2]

These objectives also apply when the military assists in homeland defense operations in support of local and state assets during a national emergency. Military and civilian HSS planning includes the medical response to CBRN agent threats.

In any setting, far-forward medical treatment is critical to reduce injury and save lives. Military medicine focuses on this far-forward care, provided initially by the military member or a fellow unit member (a "buddy"), and efficient casualty evacuation to medical facilities offering the appropriate care.[2] Table 14-1 gives an overview of the new taxonomy of care capabilities, comparing them to the current concept of levels (echelons) of care particular to the management of chemical casualties.[1,2]

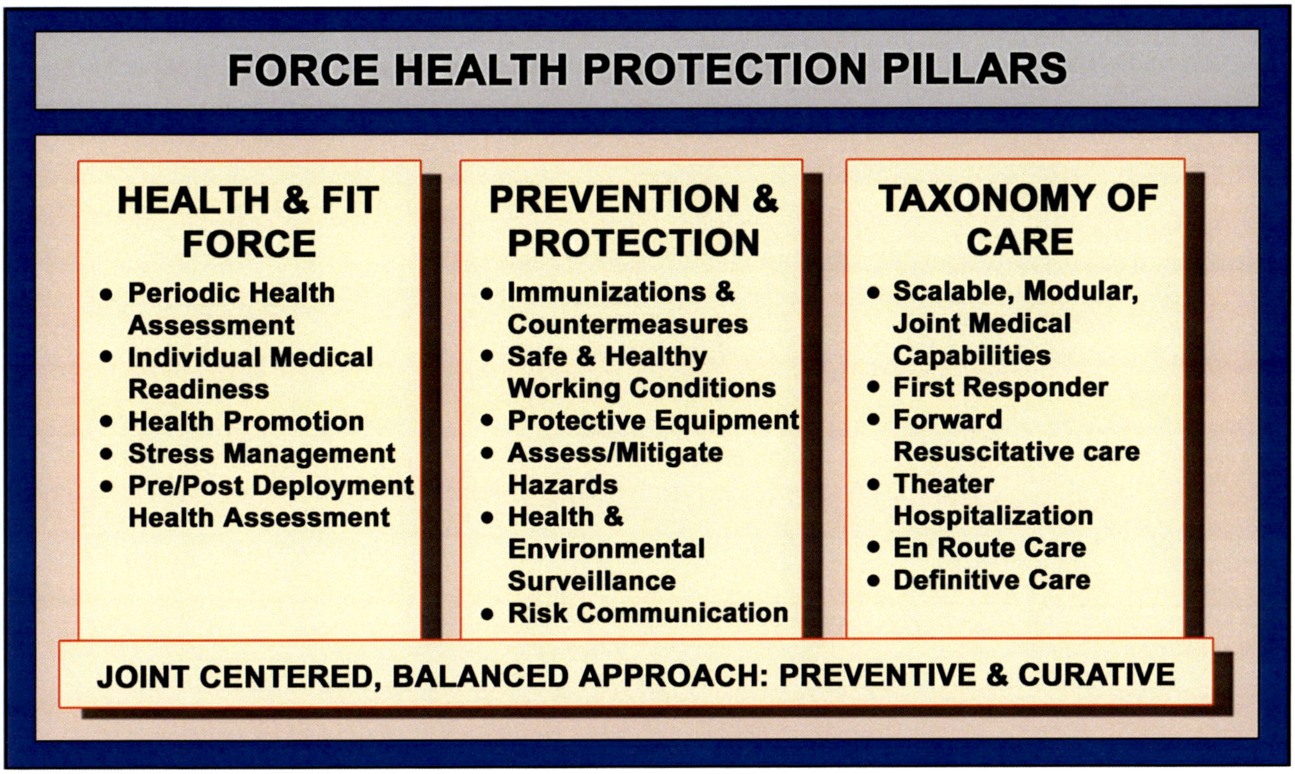

Fig. 14-1. The pillars of force health protection.
Reproduced from: US Department of Defense. *Health Service Support in Joint Operations*. Revision, Final Coordination. Washington, DC: DoD; 2005. Joint Publication 4-02: I-9.

SERVICE-SPECIFIC OPERATIONS FOR FIELD MANAGEMENT OF CHEMICAL CASUALTIES

Land-Based Forces

Land-based forces are comprised primarily of US Army and Marine Corps (USMC) personnel, land-based Navy personnel in support of land forces, and Air Force personnel in support of air operations and land forces. Land-based forces include all levels of HSS. HSS units from all services plan and train for chemical agent incidents in advance. In joint operations, all of the services move battlefield casualties through the taxonomy of care (Figure 14-2), with various service components having responsibility for particular treatment facilities as dictated by the Joint Task Force (JTF) commander.

The first responder capability (level I) for Army land-based forces at the point of injury incorporates self and buddy aid care. Units also have combat medics or treatment squads that provide first aid. Unique to the Army at this level is the combat life saver, a soldier with first-aid training. These individuals are capable of assisting the medic in field care of injured soldiers. The battalion aid station (BAS) is also part of this capability. Stabilization and emergency treatment for a limited number of contaminated casualties can be achieved at the BAS depending on its available resources to decontaminate the patients before admission to the BAS. Casualties with injuries that require further treatment, or who cannot be managed at the BAS, are evacuated to the area support medical battalion or to units capable of forward resuscitation care (FRC), which include forward surgical teams. Forward surgical teams cannot operate in a chemical environment unless supported by a unit such as the division clearing station, which provides the capability to decontaminate patients.[3] The operational tempo may not allow for the thorough decontamination of patients by first responders (level I) or units with an FRC capability (level II); therefore, medical facilities serving in a theater hospital capability (level III and IV) must be prepared for the triage and decontamination of contaminated casualties who are transported dirty (without thorough decontamination) to their facilities. The combat support hospital is the Army theater hospital asset that provides surgical care, laboratory services, and stabilization of chemical casualties. Army field medical facilities can be chemically hardened with chemically resistant inner tent

TABLE 14-1

COMPARISON OF TAXONOMY OF CARE CAPABILITIES WITH LEVELS (ECHELONS) OF CARE PARTICULAR TO CHEMICAL CASUALTY MANAGEMENT*

***Care Capability* / Level of Care**	**Care Rendered**	**Care Particular to Chemical Casualties**
First Responder Capability Compares to level I care at the unit level. Prepares patient for return to duty or transport to the next level of care.	*Initial essential stabilizing medical care rendered at the point of injury.* Self aid, buddy aid, examination, emergency lifesaving (eg, maintain airway, control bleeding, prevent shock). Use of IV fluids, antibiotics, applying splints and bandages.	Same as care rendered plus: • Decontamination of the skin and equipment. • Providing antidotes (atropine/2 PAM/diazepam) to chemical agents.
Forward Resuscitative Care Capability This compares to level II physician-directed emergency care at a small medical facility in the theater of operations. Treat patient for RTD or stabilize for movement to a larger medical treatment facility capable of providing care.	*Forward advanced emergency medical treatment performed as close to the point on injury as possible, based on current operational requirements.* Resuscitation and stabilization, can include advanced trauma management, emergency medical procedures, and forward resuscitative surgery. May have capability (depending on military service) for basic laboratory, limited radiograph, pharmacy, type O blood transfusion, and temporary holding facilities.	Same as responder capability (level I) plus: • Emergency contaminated shrapnel removal. • Intubation. • Ventilatory support (though limited). • Wound debridement. • Informal stress counseling.
En Route Care Capability	*Involves the medical treatment of injuries and illnesses during patient movement between capabilities in the continuum of essential care.*	New term not used in former doctrine. Includes support of airway, controlling bleeding, and administration of antidotes and seizure medications, if needed and available during transport.
Theater Hospitalization Capability Compares to level III and IV capabilities. Facility in theater that is larger than FRC (level II). Care requiring expanded clinical capabilities such as restorative surgery. Treat patient for RTD or begin restorative surgery and prepare for	movement to a higher level of care. *Includes theater hospitals with modular configurations to provide in-theater support and includes the HSS assets needed to support the theater.* Resuscitation, initial wound surgery, and postoperative treatment. This is the first level that offers restorative surgery and care rather than just emergency care to stabilize the patient. Has larger	variety of blood products than level II. Same as for FRC (level II) plus: • Exploratory surgery. • Initial burn care . • Bronchoscopy. • Intubation. • Ventilatory support (more assets than level II). • More extensive wound debridement. • Eye care. • Respiratory therapy.
• Formal stress counseling. Level IV Largest facility found in mature theaters. Rehabilitates those who can RTD in theater and prepares more serious	casualties for movement to level V. Provides restorative surgery, like level III, and also rehabilitative and recov-	ery therapy. Same as for level III plus: • Physical and occupational therapy rehabilitation for those with limited vesicant burns. • Full respiratory therapy . • Ventilatory support (more assets than level III). • More extensive eye care.

(**Table 14-1** *continues*)

Table 14-1 *continued*

- Psychological counseling.

Definitive Care Capability

Compares to a stateside level V.

Definitive care, which is normally provided in the continental United States, Department of Veterans Affairs hospitals, or civilian hospitals with committed beds for casualty treatment as part of the National Defense Medical System. May also be provided by overseas allied or host nation MTFs

Care rendered to conclusively manage a patient's condition, includes the full range of acute, convalescent, restorative, and rehabilitative care sites outside the theater of operations.

Includes the full range of acute convalescent, restorative, and rehabilitative care.

Same as for level IV plus:

- Longer term respiratory therapy.
- Full rehabilitative services for mental health, cognitive/memory retraining, retraining in activities of daily living/life skills, prevocational services, and post traumatic stress counseling. This incorporates a team of rehabilitation professions such as physical, occupational, speech, and mental health services as needed based on the severity of exposure and resulting disability, if any.

*Taxonomy of care terms are in italics.
FRC: forward resuscitative care
HSS: health service support
IV: intravenous
2-PAM: 2-pyridine aldoxime methyl chloride
RTD: return to duty
Data sources: (1) US Department of Defense. *Health Service Support in Joint Operations*. Revision, Final Coordination. Washington, DC: DoD; 2005. Joint Publication 4-02. (2) US Department of Defense. *Doctrine for Health Service Support in Joint Operations*. Washington, DC: DoD;

liners and fitted with air filtering units.

Land-based Naval units are divided into broad warfare areas including expeditionary warfare, forces that move to a theater of operations, and naval installations.[4] Expeditionary units include construction forces, logistic support personnel, special warfare units, and fleet hospitals. Expeditionary forces on land are typically deployed in support of USMC units. These usually include land-based FRC (level II) capability, which may initially contain as few as 10 beds but can be expanded to 500 beds with a theater hospitalization capability (ie, a combat zone fleet hospital).[1] Casualties from these facilities can then be evacuated to land-based facilities of other services or to hospital ships. Expeditionary medical units deploy as part of a landing force, with CBRN defense capabilities for individual protection, self-decontamination, and limited equipment decontamination.

Naval installations such as fleet hospitals, on the other hand, are more permanent, fixed facilities that offer FRC capabilities at level III or greater. Installation planning at these facilities involves disaster preparedness, including coordination with local authorities. Plans for operations in a contaminated environment include using shelter-in-place procedures, individual protective gear, and various types of detection equipment. The installation disaster officer directs emergency-response teams, coordinates decontamination operations, and assists in the command and control operations center.[4] In addition to triage and treating casualties from an incident, the medical department also organizes medical supplies; provides food and water inspection; conducts disease monitoring; distributes antidotes and medications as needed for CBRN incidents; and provides training on CBRN hazards, self aid, and first aid as part of FHP.[4]

The approximately 175,000-member USMC is an intrinsic part of the Department of the Navy; medical support to the Marine Corps is provided by the Navy Medical Department. USMC personnel may augment Navy medical patient decontamination operations. First responder capability (level I) is provided through self aid and buddy aid as well as by Navy corpsmen assigned to USMC units. The Marines, at this level, also utilize their intrinsic BASs, or USMC wing support squadron aid stations, staffed by Navy medical personnel. Unique to the USMC is the Chemical/Biological Incident Response Force (CBIRF) with first responder medical capabilities. CBIRF deploys domestically, particularly in the National Capital Region of Washington, DC, or overseas to pre-position or respond to a CBRN incident. Composed of USMC and Navy personnel, CBIRF has the capability to monitor, detect, identify, and analyze toxic industrial chemicals (TICs), toxic

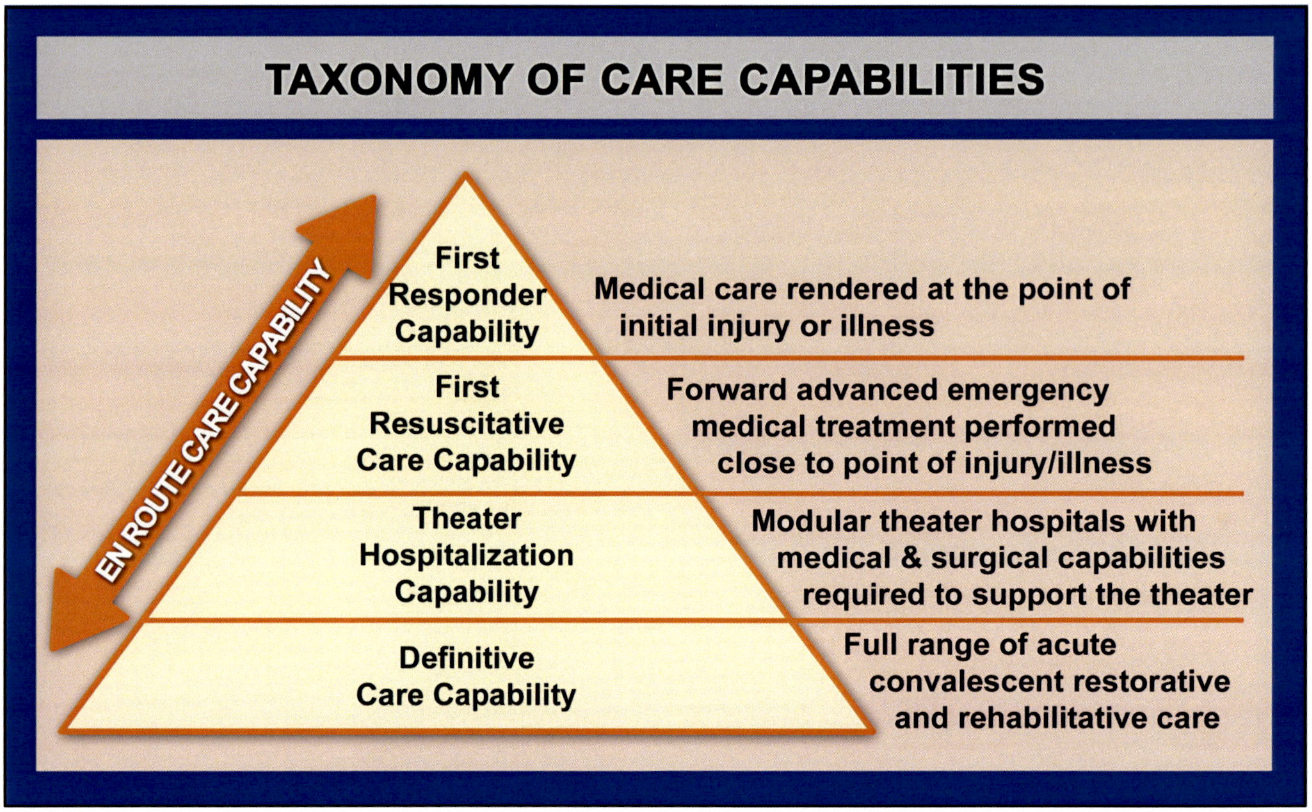

Fig. 14-2. Taxonomy of care capabilities.
Reproduced from: US Department of Defense. *Health Service Support in Joint Operations*. Revision, Final Coordination. Washington, DC: DoD; 2005. Joint Publication 4-02: I-4.

industrial materials, and other CBRN hazards. The force has casualty extraction teams, technical search and rescue teams, and patient/responder decontamination assets to support a mass casualty incident. CBIRF medical personnel are trained to conduct triage and provide emergency medical care to stabilize large numbers of contaminated casualties extracted from the incident site; then decontaminate them for transfer to local medical facilities.[4]

Air Force first responder capability (level I) consists of self aid and buddy care.[5] First responders then retrieve the patient and form a casualty collection point for transport to the base medical facility. The Air Force incorporates the split mission-oriented protective posture (MOPP) concept, dividing an air base into sectors or control zones, each operating under a different MOPP level depending on its contamination threat. Under this plan, one area of the base may be contaminated without affecting the operations of the entire base.[6] Casualties are retrieved from the contaminated zones by medical first responders in protective ensemble and transported to the base medical facility or base casualty holding area. Depending on the maturity of the base, the medical support can consist of a small portable expeditionary aeromedical rapid response package, a basic Expeditionary Medical Support (EMEDS) package, or a larger EMEDS plus 10- or 25-bed package, which evolves into an Air Force theater hospital. Casualty care includes patient decontamination, triage, clinical care, movement or quarantine on the air base, and aeromedical evacuation.[7] EMEDS can be configured to have an FRC capability (level II) or a theater hospital capability (level III or IV) based on the number of air-transportable medical equipment and personnel packages deployed to meet operational requirements. EMEDS equipment packages consist of tentage and medical equipment that can be added to an EMEDS basic package to increase service and bed capacity. The EMEDS basic package can be deployed as a "collectively protected" Air Force medical facility to provide shelter in a chemically or biologically contaminated environment.[7] In these collective protection configurations the EMEDS facilities are fitted with chemical protective liners and air handling units that filter hazardous agents. An EMEDS facility is designed to remain in operation for days after a chemical attack on the base. When collectively protected, a small-shelter patient decontamination system package is added to provide the capability to decontaminate large numbers of patients before they enter the collectively protected EMEDS.[8,9]

For all services, evacuation of land casualties is performed by the facility at the next higher level of care, which sends evacuation assets forward to retrieve the patient. Patient movement is typically carried out by rotor-winged aircraft or ground vehicles. In theater this is normally the responsibility of either the service component command that operates the particular facility or Army rotor-wing medical evacuation (MEDEVAC) units.[1,5] These units may have to designate certain assets to transport contaminated casualties from a chemical battlefield to an FRC or theater hospital. Fixed-wing Air Force aeromedical assets used for intertheater evacuation are usually reserved for patients who have been decontaminated.[1,5]

Sea-Based Forces

Sea-based forces are comprised primarily of Navy and Coast Guard assets. Medical evacuation to Naval vessels operating offshore must certainly be considered for chemical casualties with airway compromise or significant trauma. Army air ambulance, Navy, or USMC casualty evacuation helicopters provide the rotor-wing assets for these vessels (Figure 14-3).[1] In the Navy, the major designated casualty receiving and treatment ships are the dozen multipurpose large-deck amphibious landing helicopter dock assault ships of the USS *Wasp* class, such as the USS *Bon Homme Richard* or USS *Kearsage*.[10] These large, 40,000-ton vessels, 823 feet long, are designed to operate offshore in support of amphibious operations and can serve as FRC (level II) facilities.[5] They support intense helicopter activities and are designed around large, self-contained "well decks" for small boat transfers within the protected hull of the ship. Extensive command, control, communication, and computer capabilities allow for MEDEVAC coordination and patient regulating. The newly commissioned landing platform dock 17, San Antonio-class amphibious ships have similar capabilities but a smaller size.[10] These Naval platforms, connected locally with helicopter assets, can be combined with the extended 1,500-mile range of the V-22 Osprey vertical takeoff and landing aircraft to bring multiple capabilities for medical response to the severely injured, whether they have chemical or physical trauma. The medical facilities on Navy aircraft carriers provide FRC (level II) capability, although their space is limited compared with that of the casualty receiving and treatment ships.[5] The casualty receiving and treatment amphibious assault vessels are large floating facilities, with FRC (level II) capability available to land-based forces or civilian casualties during presidentially authorized military support to civil authorities.

Although they lack an enclosed "well deck" for efficient small boat transfers, the two 70,000-ton hospital ships USNS *Comfort* and USNS *Mercy* (Figure 14-4) have large helicopter landing pads and offer complete tertiary care capabilities, including 12 operating rooms, 80 intensive care beds, and 50 ventilators, providing the services of a theater hospital (level III). Naval facilities

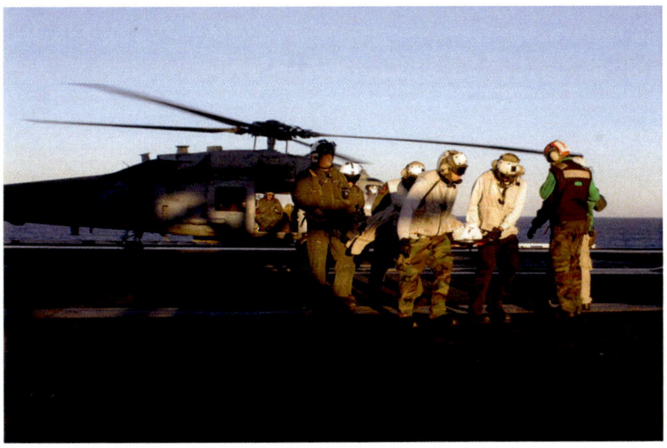

Fig. 14-3. Unloading a patient from Army MEDEVAC to a Navy ship for treatment.
Reproduced from: US Department of Defense. *Health Service Support in Joint Operations*. Revision, Final Coordination. Washington, DC: DoD; 2005. Joint Publication 4-02.

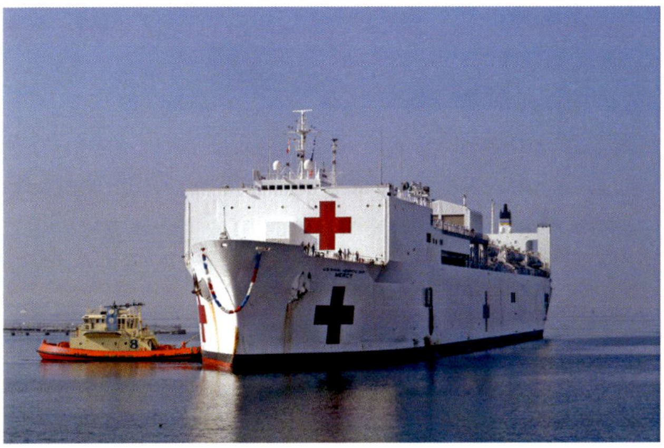

Fig. 14-4. Hospital ship USNS *Mercy*.
Reproduced from: US Department of Defense. *Health Service Support in Joint Operations*. Revision, Final Coordination. Washington, DC: DoD; 2005. Joint Publication 4-02: III-12.

capable of providing a definitive care capability (level IV and V) are located outside the theater of operations in large land-based installations.[1,11,12]

In contrast, the Coast Guard has limited capabilities to receive casualties. Coast Guard personnel can provide first aid for victims rescued from ships or the water. The primary Coast Guard role is to offer force protection and safety regulation for vessels and ports, to minimize the possibility of a chemical attack or major toxic industrial chemical incident. Their much smaller 300-foot Coast Guard cutters are staffed by independent duty corpsmen and physician's assistants capable of providing first aid for chemical casualties, including administration of atropine autoinjectors and basic decontamination with water, soap, and hypochlorite solutions. These medical assets can also participate as part of requested federal resources in response to a mass casualty event. The Coast Guard deep-draft vessels scheduled to enter operation in 2007 will have capabilities to operate in a chemical hazard environment for up to 72 hours.[13]

Medical response planning and evacuation of casualties to ships is the responsibility of the JTF surgeon, a physician of any specialty, usually embarked on the lead ship and a staff member of the JTF Commander. The JTF Commander, usually at least a one-star admiral, is responsible for coordination of Naval assets in support of land-based objectives of the operational theater commander. During shore-to-ship operations, the Army is usually responsible for medical rotary-wing support for patient transport; otherwise the Navy and USMC perform this service. The Air Force is the principal fixed-wing air asset for the transportation of patients from the theater of operations to the continental United States (ie, to level V) during joint operations.[5]

By doctrine, patients must be decontaminated before transport to Naval vessels; however, a thorough decontamination of patients may not be possible with a high operational tempo. Navy documents provide detailed instruction for the decontamination and processing of patients brought on board ship by rotor-winged aircraft and landing craft before they are brought below decks.[14] Large Navy vessels at sea have extensive water supplies for decontamination purposes. Their evaporators daily produce thousands of gallons of fresh water. Additionally, appropriately protected personnel can quickly use fire hoses to wash down external areas with salt water.

MANAGEMENT OF CHEMICAL CASUALTIES FROM A CIVILIAN PERSPECTIVE

The accidental release of toxic substances occurs regularly in the United States from fixed storage and industrial facilities and from containers during transportation. Most common among these substances are ammonia, pesticides, volatile organic compounds, acids, and petroleum products.[15] US hazardous materials (HAZMAT) response teams have gained experience in managing these accidental releases. Events such as the 1984 release of the carbaryl pesticide precursor methylisocyanate, in Bhopal, India, which killed and injured thousands, and the more limited yet lethal attacks by the Aum Shinrikyo cult in Matsumoto (1994) and later Tokyo (1995), Japan, killing less than a dozen but injuring scores more, demonstrate that intentional acts of sabotage and terrorism can create large numbers of casualties in unprotected civilian populations.[16–18]

Until recently, no effort had been made to standardize guidelines for the management of mass casualties from such events. In February 2003, Homeland Security Presidential Directive-5 was signed into law by President George W Bush, initiating the development of the National Incident Management System.[19] This system serves as the template for the management of mass casualty events in the United States, whether they are caused by a terrorist attack, accident, or natural event (such as a hurricane). It provides a framework to coordinate the response of the government, private-sector, and nongovernmental organizations. Structure is added to this framework through the National Response Plan (NRP), which provides the actual coordination mechanisms for various agencies, including fire, rescue, and emergency medical services, for effective communication and teamwork.[20] These documents, along with others developed by the Department of Homeland Security, Department of Health and Human Services, Occupational Safety and Health Administration (OSHA), Joint Commission on Accreditation of Hospital Organizations, and other agencies, have sought to foster more standardization in the disaster and medical response to mass casualty events from all hazards. This entire response plan was first fully implemented in response to Hurricane Katrina, which devastated the US Gulf Coast in August 2005, and is undergoing further modification based on the many lessons learned from the disaster.

Local responses to chemical releases vary. Typically, when a casualty-causing chemical event occurs, those who can flee the scene on foot or by private or commercial vehicle are the victims first seen at the nearest medical facility. As demonstrated in Tokyo, their arrival may be the first indicator for a medical facility, and a community, that an event has occurred.[21,22] When the event is reported to authorities, local fire departments and HAZMAT teams, if available, respond. Response time can range from 5 to 30 minutes from initial release.[23,24] Once these teams respond, the area is cordoned off. Decontamination units are established by the fire department at the periphery of the contaminated area (the hot zone). The initial processing of patients through decontamination can be 30 minutes or more after the initial toxicant release.[23] In some communities, particularly in rural areas, medical personnel do not have level II emergency medical service (EMS) or hazardous materials operations training, so they cannot accompany HAZMAT crews into contaminated areas. Frequently, local EMS personnel are not proficient in treating contaminated patients while wearing personal protective equipment (PPE), which relegates them to treating patients after decontamination.[25] Wearing appropriate self-protection ensemble while stabilizing patients before decontamination procedures is a difficult challenge for first responders. Victims are often decontaminated and only then seen by unprotected EMS personnel, who place them on ambulances for transport to hospitals. Because HAZMAT teams must take time to secure the area and muster equipment before they can begin decontamination, victims who do not flee the scene before the arrival of HAZMAT and fire department teams may not receive medical care for 30 minutes or more after their exposure.[23] A sequence of events similar to this occurred after passive release of dilute sarin nerve agent in the 1995 Tokyo attack.[17] Authors such as Okumura who studied this event closely believe that a more forward medical presence, as incorporated by the military, may save more lives in the event of a chemical release creating mass casualties, particularly if a potent warfare agent is used in the attack.[17]

Currently, many larger metropolitan fire departments are training their emergency medical technicians (EMTs) to provide life saving medical care in the contaminated area or at its periphery. This training still does not occur in many smaller rural departments, or in most private emergency services, which provide care only after patient decontamination. Without adequate first responder training in the provision of medical care while wearing PPE, first responder EMTs are relegated to the contamination-free area; in this situation medical intervention will be too late for many victims.[26] The Department of Health and Human Services is considering policy and recommendations to encourage appropriately trained and equipped first responders from all agencies to provide medical care in contaminated areas. The National Fire Protection Association has published standards for the professional competence of EMS responders in hazardous materials incidents.[25] Hospitals that receive contaminated patients now have guidance through the *OSHA Best Practices for Hospital-Based First Receivers of Victims from Mass Casualty Incidents Involving the Release of Hazardous Substances*, released in January 2005. This document establishes the baseline for medical facility response to the arrival of contaminated casualties. Its purpose is to insure that the triage, stabilization, decontamination, and treatment of contaminated casualties is successfully conducted while first receiver safety is maintained.[27]

INTEGRATION OF MILITARY SUPPORT INTO CIVILIAN HOMELAND RESPONSE

The role of the US military in national strategies for defense and homeland security is undergoing rapid development. Specific capabilities within the Department of Defense (DoD) are driven by doctrine and policy promulgated from the Office of the Secretary of Defense and operational orders from regional combatant commanders. These directives shape the forces that are organized, trained, and equipped by the services to support national strategic policies.

The primary role of military medicine, to preserve the fighting force, provides a robust, capable, HSS infrastructure that is mobile, responsive, and trained and equipped for operations in austere environments. This force, which during peacetime provides routine health care for its DoD beneficiaries, must also incorporate the needs and requirements for the post–September 11 homeland defense, the global war on terrorism strategies, and response to requests through the NRP emergency support functions. As the policy and doctrine drives development of specific capabilities, a balance is required between the goal of smaller, leaner forces with increased operational tempos engaged in supporting the strategies, and a repository of medical response in the homeland for CBRN mass casualty incidents.

Currently, military installations are required to develop and implement CBRN capabilities for response and recovery from terrorist incidents involving weapons of mass destruction (DoD Instruction 2000.18).[28] Capabilities developed for these requirements include detectors; warning and reporting technologies; decontamination equipment; triage and treatment procedures; and command, control, and communication operations. Multiple programs with overlapping capability requirements, including force protection, antiterrorism, and "all hazards" emergency management determine specific capabilities. As all military hospitals subscribe to the Joint Commission for Accreditation of Healthcare Organizations, local coordination for disaster planning is routinely required.[29] Local and state public health requirements, as well as operational orders from regional combatant commanders, also drive this interactive planning process. The military health system participation in disaster planning for the homeland occurs at city and other local, county, state, federal, and national levels.

After validation of requests by local authorities, commanders may immediately respond to local disasters to save human lives, reduce human suffering, and/or prevent significant property loss.[30–32] Although commanders must notify their chain of command of such actions as soon as reasonably possible, they do not need to seek higher authority before responding.

Medical support to the NRP, emergency support function #8, occurs through defense support of civil authority. Through a bureaucratic process, requests from state governors proceed to the president, then, upon presidential approval, to the coordinating federal agency, generally the Department of Homeland Security for most federally declared emergencies. Requests for DoD assistance are filtered through the Joint Defense Office of Military Support to ensure that requests are valid and cannot be reasonably met by non-DoD capabilities. The Joint Task Force for Civil Support then serves as the command and control element to match requirements to specific capabilities within the DoD. These assets or units are then "chopped" or change operational command from the service component to the respective regional combatant commander, usually under a specific response task force under the Joint Task Force for Civil Support. These federal assets, such as decontamination teams or medical assistance teams, then operate in support of the local incident commander under the unified command system.[30–32]

Northern Command in Colorado Springs, Colorado, and Pacific Command in Honolulu, Hawaii, represent the regional combatant commanders whose area of responsibility covers the United States and its territories. Operational orders from these commanders, through the service components, determine and influence readiness and response postures for installations under their direction.

THE MEDICAL MANAGEMENT PROCESS IN A CHEMICAL EVENT

Whether on the chemical battlefield, or in support of homeland defense in response to a terrorist mass casualty event, key measures must be taken to prepare for, manage, and recover from a chemical incident. Although not inclusive, the list below is adapted from guidelines found in several military publications.[3,4,33]

Preattack, Attack, and Postattack Measures

Preattack, or preparatory, measures include

- understanding potential local chemical threats and specific TICs, their location, specific compounds, and effects;
- preparing plans and equipment to address a chemical agent release, both warfare agents and TICs;
- developing policies to enhance patient field management in the event of a CBRN release;
- training first responders and medical providers in triage and emergency medical care while wearing protective equipment;
- training medical providers in the medical treatment of chemical casualties;
- rehearsing teams in patient decontamination methods and practicing work–rest cycles;
- acquiring appropriate decontamination equipment and PPE;
- designating shelters and practicing collective protection measures, or sheltering in place, including the use of shelters, recognition of alert states, procedures to disperse assets, and the use of appropriate levels of PPE for medical workers;
- developing and practicing communication with supporting and supported agencies;
- developing and rehearsing logistics to support the management of mass casualty events; and
- developing and rehearsing recovery plans including the management of hazardous waste from patient decontamination operations.

Attack measures, or measures to take during the event, include

- instituting plans for the evacuation and processing of casualties;
- securing medical treatment facility (MTF) entrances to maintain a contamination-free hospital environment;
- practicing individual protection and collective protection for medical and other MTF personnel in potentially contaminated areas;
- performing patient treatment and decontamination;
- instituting work–rest cycles for staff wearing protective equipment;

- providing mental health assets specific to chemical casualties and PPE utilization;
- instituting waste recovery plans for decontamination operations; and
- coordinating with supported and supporting agencies.

Postattack, or recovery, measures consist of

- practicing medical team recovery and staff technical decontamination;
- monitoring for chemical contamination;
- continuing patient evacuation if needed;
- properly disposing of hazardous waste from patient decontamination operations;
- inventorying supplies and equipment and arranging for replacements; and
- coordinating with supported and supporting agencies.

The key for effective field management of chemical casualties is to develop a workable plan and train for the event using real equipment and realistic scenarios appropriate for the location. In reality, MTFs must assume an influx of mass casualties and develop plans to effectively stabilize patients at smaller facilities and then promptly evacuate them to larger facilities with greater resources. Proper preparation for mass casualty events will ensure a smaller number of serious casualties through successful management.

Casualties may sustain additional conventional injuries; for example, blast injuries may occur when an explosive device is used to disseminate the chemical agent. The following key objectives, which also relate to military HHS and FHP, should be the focus of any field management process:

- Minimize chemical agent injuries.
- Prevent aggravation of conventional injuries during care and decontamination.
- Control the spread of chemical contamination through decontamination.
- Continue with the primary mission of caring for patients not involved with the release.

Personnel Requirements

The process of field management can be personnel intensive, requiring between 12 and 50 workers to operate triage areas, emergency treatment areas, and decontamination lines. Personnel requirements depend on a variety of the following factors: ambient temperature in which field management operations are taking place, number of casualties, type of chemical agent, level of fitness of medical and decontamination personnel wearing PPE, and decontamination equipment used.

Temperature

A critical factor in the ability to sustain decontamination operations is temperature, ambient temperature, and, most importantly, wet-bulb globe temperature (WBGT). The WBGT is a composite temperature used to estimate the effect of temperature, humidity, and solar radiation on humans. It is used by industrial hygienists, athletes, and the military to determine appropriate exposure levels to high temperatures. The WBGT index combines air temperature, humidity, air flow, and radiant heat data to provide a measure for the risk of heat stress. Typically WBGT readings are below simple thermometer readings. For example, a 78.9° F (26.1° C) WBGT could roughly be equivalent to an outdoor temperature of 95° F (35° C) in the sun or 98° F (36.7° C) in the shade.[34] WBGT measures both radiant and evaporative temperatures. A variety of WBGT devices can be purchased. Most units are lightweight, easily transportable, and have digital displays. An example of a WBGT is shown in Figure 14-5.

Wearing protective ensemble increases the WBGT index by 10° F (5.6° C).[3,4,33] Body armor (a possible requirement for the military, but not normally for civilian medical personnel) increases the index by another 5° F (2.8° C).[3,4,33] Protective clothing increases the heat load on an individual because sweat from the skin is unable to contact air and dissipate heat through evaporation. The risk of dehydration, heat cramps, heat stroke, and other heat-induced injuries is greatly increased by the hot encapsulating protective gear, and water consumption wearing a protective mask is cumbersome, if not impossible. Many civilian protective masks lack an oral rehydration tube.

A safety monitor should be appointed to prevent injury, especially heat-related injury, for teams wearing PPEs.[27] Handheld heat stress calculators are commercially available to assist in calculating the time that individuals should remain in PPE.[35,36] Both OSHA and the military joint manual covering patient decontamination emphasize the importance of preventing heat injury. OSHA recommends periodically taking the blood pressure of workers wearing protective gear or measuring core body temperature; both are difficult to accomplish while the worker remains adequately encapsulated in protective ensemble in a contaminated, or potentially contaminated, area.[27] The military incorporates a program of work–rest cycles based on the WBGT index reading (Table 14-2). During the rest cycle, team members wearing PPE rest in a shaded area

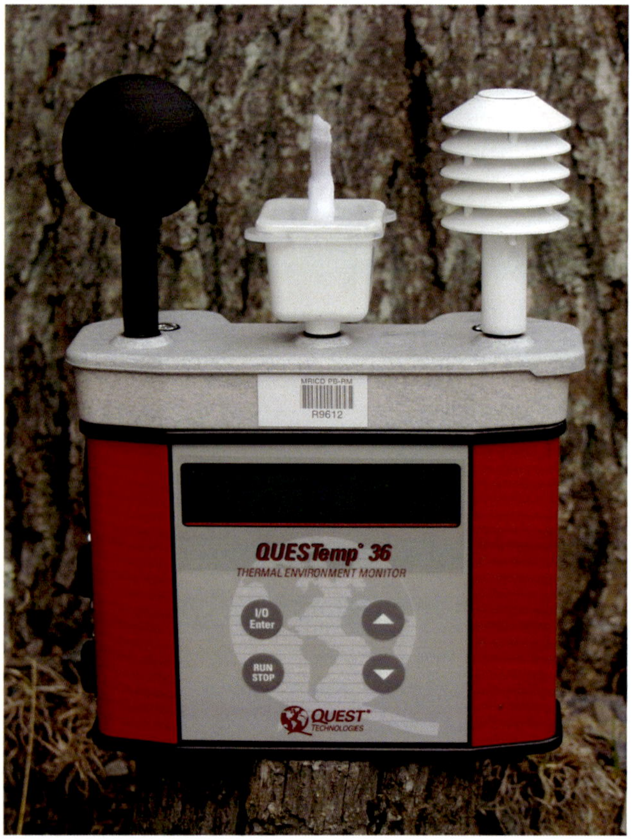

Fig. 14-5. An example of a wet-bulb globe thermometer (WBGT).
Photograph: Courtesy of US Army Medical Research Institute for Chemical Defense, Chemical Casualty Care Division, Aberdeen Proving Ground, Md.

and drink water. Masks that allow team members to drink without mask removal should be used. Hydration units, such as Camelbaks (Camelbak, Petaluma, Calif), can be worn under hooded masks and suits.

Casualty Number and Agent Characteristics

Current technology to thoroughly decontaminate patients is linear in design, and critical narrowing point "bottlenecks" are inevitable as patients are processed through a decontamination line. To reduce congestion, more decontamination lanes are added, which requires more personnel. Larger numbers of casualties also require more medical personnel to provide adequate care. Other novel ideas to hasten decontamination, particularly in a civilian setting, are to distribute personal decontamination solutions to casualties, allowing them to decontaminate themselves and others, as is done by military service members conducting immediate decontamination on the battlefield. The aim is to readily reduce the amount of contaminant on those exposed until a more through decontamination can be performed.

The type of agent encountered dictates the immediate hazard to life and limb as well as the level of decontamination necessary before a patient can enter an MTF. Many people believe that all patients exposed, or potentially exposed, to a chemical agent must be thoroughly washed. Ideally, if it does not delay life saving medical care, a comprehensive shower with warm water and soap (liquid castile soap or baby shampoo) should be performed if time and circumstances permit. Situations where clothing removal alone might suffice include (*a*) exposure to vapor only, when agent is trapped in clothing and hair but is not on the skin; (*b*) cold weather situations when individuals are wearing thick clothing and the ambient temperature is 35°F (1.6°C) or below, creating a significant risk of freezing, or even below 65°F (18.3°C), when hypothermia is a greater possibility in injured people, especially if warm water is not available. In these cases the individual should be moved promptly to a warm area for a more thorough wash after clothing removal, or decontamination should be provided for exposed skin areas only.[37,38] An appreciation of these facts and knowledge of agent characteristics listed in Table 14-3 are critical for medical and decontamination personnel.

Fitness Level

Workers who are not physically fit will fatigue faster and require more periods of rest. They may also be more prone to musculoskeletal injury. The medical management of chemical casualties can be very labor-intensive when patient lifts and litter carries are performed, especially while patient handlers are wearing PPEs or when no special ergonomic equipment (eg, roller systems, wheeled litter carriers) is available. Those who do not have adequate muscle strength will quickly fatigue after the movement of only a few litter patients. Moderate and heavy work, as is done by medical and decontamination workers, dramatically increases the strain on the cardiovascular system, and individuals who are not physically fit are at a greater risk for cardiovascular events. Those who are more physically fit will be able to wear their protective ensembles longer while incurring less cardiopulmonary risk. Personnel who are fit have enhanced pulmonary function compared to those who are less fit, allowing better oxygen exchange during exertion in protective masks. Personnel who have suffered heat stroke in the past are likely to be more susceptible to recurrence. OSHA mandates that all individuals designated to wear personal protective gear receive

TABLE 14-2

WORK–REST CYCLES AND WATER CONSUMPTION (WITHOUT PROTECTIVE ENSEMBLE)*

		Easy Work		Moderate Work		Hard Work	
Heat Category	WBGT Index (°F)	Work–Rest (Min)	Water Intake (Qt/h)	Work–Rest (Min)	Water Intake (Qt/h)	Work–Rest (Min)	Water Intake (Qt/h)
1 (White)	78–81.9	NL	½	NL	¾	40–20	¾
2 (Green)	82–84.9	NL	½	50–10	¾	30–30	1
3 (Yellow)	85–87.9	NL	¾	40–20	¾	30–30	1
4 (Red)	88–89.9	NL	¾	30–30	¾	20–40	1
5 (Black)	> 90	50–10	1	20–40	1	10–50	1

*Notes:
Wearing protective overgarments adds 10° F (5.6° C) to the WBGT index, and wearing body armor increases this by another 5° F (2.8° C).
The work–rest times and fluid replacement volumes will sustain performance and hydration for at least 4 hours of work in the specified heat category.
Hourly fluid intake should not exceed 1 quart and daily fluid intake should not exceed 12 quarts.
Rest means minimal physical activity while sitting or standing, accomplished in the shade if possible.
NL: No limit to work time per hour
Qt: quart
WBGT: wet-bulb globe temperature
Data sources: (1) US Departments of the Army, Marine Corps, Navy, and Air Force. *Health Service Support in a Nuclear, Biological, and Chemical Environment*. Draft. Washington, DC: DoD; 2004. FM 4-02.7, MCRP 4-11.1F, NTTP 4-02.7, AFTTP (I) 3-2.47. (2) US Department of the Army. *Health Service Support in a Nuclear, Biological, and Chemical Environment. Tactics, Techniques, and Procedures*. Washigton, DC: Headquarters, DA; 2002. FM 4-02.7.

an occupational health assessment, which usually includes basic pulmonary function testing for respirator utilization and determination of their physical ability to complete assigned duties while wearing protective ensemble.[27]

Decontamination Equipment

The equipment used for patient decontamination ranges from simple hoses, buckets, and sponges, to quickly erected "pop-up" decontamination tents (Figure 14-6) with intrinsic showers, to permanent decontamination systems built into hospitals. Typically, simply equipped decontamination stations are more labor intensive because water buckets and patient litters require frequent lifting. Pop-up decontamination tents and permanent hospital decontamination facilities that incorporate roller systems and integrated plumbing for litter patient decontamination help conserve energy, speed the process, and potentially reduce musculoskeletal injury in personnel. North Atlantic Treaty Organization litter carriers (Figure 14- 7), or wheeled gurneys that can be decontaminated, reduce the frequency of patient lifting; sharp, long-handled seat belt cutters (Figure 14-8) reduce the repetitive opening and closing of scissors for cutting patient garments. These and other ergonomic adaptations help reduce worker strain and subsequent risk of musculoskeletal injury. Some enclosed systems, such as pop-up tents, are frequently heated, but rarely air-conditioned. These environments in warm climates, if not air-conditioned, can become heat intense for personnel, which will necessitate more frequent work–rest cycles.

Necessary Medical Equipment and Supplies

Critical to the emergency care of chemical casualties are adequate supplies of life saving medications for individuals exposed to rapidly lethal chemicals such as nerve agents and cyanide. Initial antidotes for nerve agents are carried by all military members, in the form of three Mark I kits (Meridian Medical Technologies Inc, Bristol, Tenn; kits contain atropine and 2-pyridine aldoxime methyl chloride) and diazepam, when there is a threat of an enemy using chemical agents.[4] Military medics, corpsmen, and EMTs typically carry more of these items. Most civilians, of course, do not carry these items with them, but civilian emergency responders should have adequate supplies immediately available. Emergency airway supplies are also critical for the management of chemical casualties because most chemical agent deaths are caused by respiratory compromise. Chemical monitors can be used at decontamination stations to check for the presence of

TABLE 14-3

MINIMAL DECONTAMINATION PROCEDURES BASED ON AGENT CHARACTERISTICS

Agent Characteristics	Suggested Minimal Decontamination Procedure Before Admission To MTF
Vapors	Remove all clothing and equipment to reduce vapor trapped in cloth fibers. Wash or briskly brush hair, if exposed. Wash skin areas that were exposed to the vapor if time allows.
Liquid	Remove all clothing and equipment to reduce liquid and vapor hazard to medical staff. Decontaminate areas where liquid agent is on the skin and the protective mask.
Solid	Carefully cut off (with sharp cutting tool) and roll back overgarments to contain the solid dust particles. Patient's underclothing may need to be removed in a different area, upwind, if it is covered with solid agent. If available a HEPA-filtered vacuum can be used to vacuum garments. (Some resources suggest that an insect sprayer or mister can be used to lightly mist garments with water before removal to reduce particle aerosolization prior to protective ensemble removal. To date, this concept has not been thoroughly evaluated. Caution must be used in this process because fine agent particles could be reaerosolized with a direct flow of air or water when misting the dry material, or dry chemicals could become activated with the addition of small amounts of water). Outer clothing should always be carefully removed, followed, if possible, by a thorough washing of the skin using copious amounts of water.

HEPA: high-efficiency particulate air
MTF: medical treatment facility

contamination on casualties when they arrive, or after the cleaning process to check for completeness of decontamination. This equipment includes the improved chemical agent monitor, its nonmilitary equivalents, and M8 paper. The improved chemical agent monitor tests for vapor coming from liquid contaminants on patients and their clothing, and M8 paper is for direct testing of nonvolatile liquid chemical warfare agent contaminants. In decontamination systems with large quantities of soap and water available, use of these detection devices is often not warranted because of the thoroughness of the washing process. These detectors are also limited to the types of agents and the concentration levels they are designed to detect, and may not be appropriate for all TICs and toxic industrial materials.

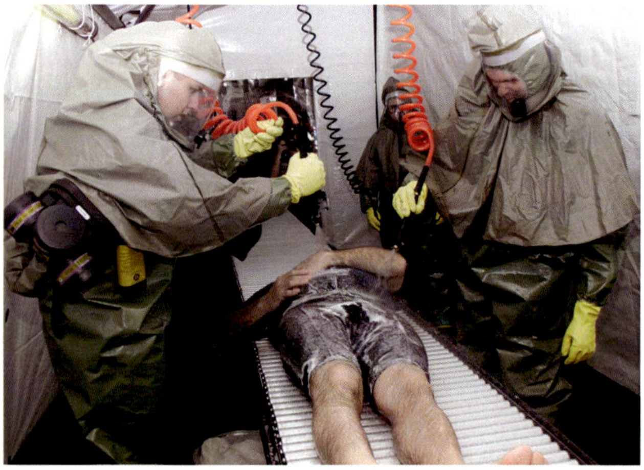

Fig.14-6. Decontamination inside a plumbed tent. The roller system supports the litter or backboard. There are many types of systems available.
Photograph: Courtesy of US Air Force.

Zones of Contamination

In interagency operations, a contaminated area is divided into zones of contamination (Figure 14-9).[25,39] To more effectively manage the contaminated area, a variety of control lines and points are designated depending upon the level of contamination. These same areas hold true on the battlefield.

Hot Zone

The hot zone is the area of chemical release. Examples include a chemical munitions impact area or an area of contamination created by an accidental or intentional TIC release from a factory storage tank. The area is determined to be contaminated with chemical agents (dry solid, liquid, or vapor). This determination is usually performed through the use of chemical monitoring devices. Individuals entering this area

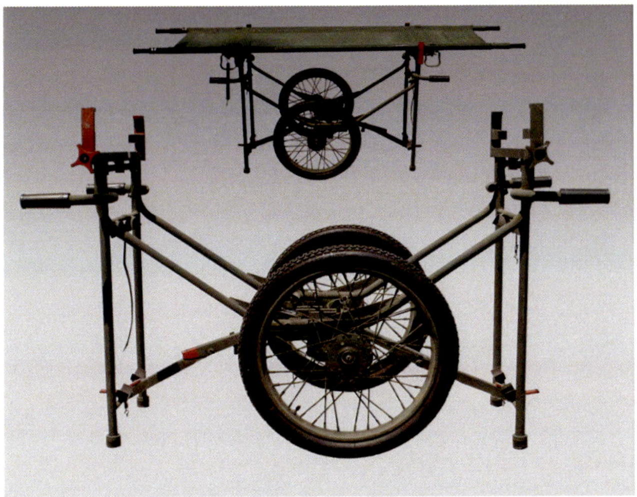

Fig. 14-7. North Atlantic Treaty Organization wheeled litter carrier. This device allows a litter to be easily handled by one or two individuals, which reduces staffing requirements and worker fatigue.
Photograph: Courtesy of US Army Medical Research Institute for Chemical Defense, Chemical Casualty Care Division, Aberdeen Proving Ground, Md.

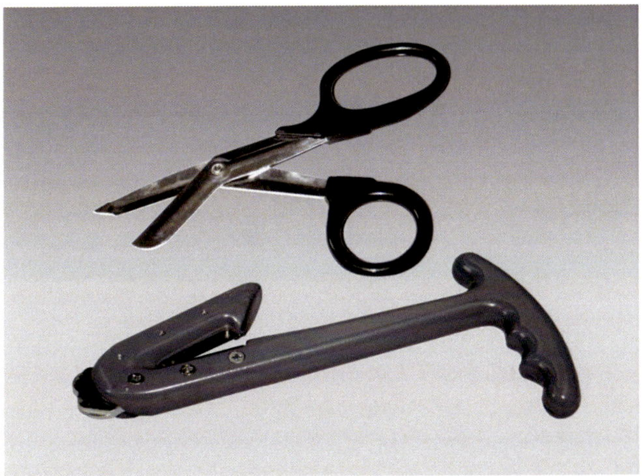

Fig. 14-8. A variety of cutting tools are available for the rapid removal of clothing. These include (from bottom to top) the two-bladed seat belt cutter and bandage scissors.
Photograph: Courtesy of US Army Medical Research Institute for Chemical Defense, Chemical Casualty Care Division, Aberdeen Proving Ground, Md.

must be in a high level of protection, OSHA level A or B (see Chapter 17, Chemical Defense Equipment, for a description of these protective levels), at least until the agent is known, after which lower levels may be appropriate. MTFs located in this area typically cease operations, shelter in place, and do not receive patients. The exception is the military collectively protected MTF which, although initially set up in a clean area, can continue to operate for a limited amount of time if the area it is in becomes contaminated. These structures have protective, chemically resistant liners and environmental control units that filter contaminated air.

Warm Zone

The warm zone is outside the hot zone. The level of contamination here is significantly lower than that found in the hot zone. Contamination in the warm zone is only that which is on the unprotected skin, clothing, and equipment of those entering from the hot zone. If the event was a release of chemical vapors (a gas plume or other passive release of vapors as in the Tokyo subway attack), the primary hazard is from the off-gassing of vapors trapped in patient clothing and hair. If the event is from a dry solid or liquid chemical release, then the contamination hazard would be from solids and liquids on clothing, equipment, and skin, as well as vapors coming from any liquid residue. As noted previously, an event involving a solid or liquid hazard would require a more intense decontamination effort.

Once an MTF begins to receive patients, the area where contaminated patients are received would be designated as part of the warm area. In the warm area medical and decontamination team members

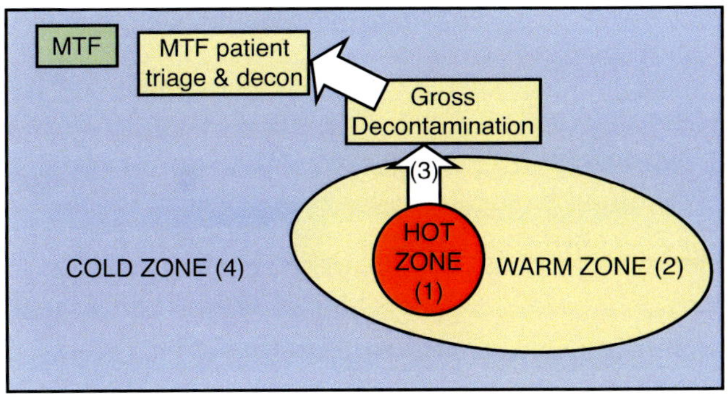

Fig. 14-9. Zones of contamination after a chemical release. (1) Hot zone: contaminated area of chemical release; (2) warm zone: contaminated individuals enter from the hot zone; (3): evacuation corridor: contains patient decontamination stations; (4) cold zone: area free of solid, liquid, and vapor contamination.
MTF: medical treatment facility
Diagram: Courtesy of US Army Medical Research Institute for Chemical Defense, Chemical Casualty Care Division, Aberdeen Proving Ground, Md.

working with the contaminated patients wear an OSHA level C protective ensemble to protect them against the limited, but still dangerous, amounts of toxic materials on the patients. This area is referred to as the contamination reduction zone, decontamination zone, or protective action zone in some references.[25,27,39]

Evacuation Corridor

The evacuation corridor, which is within the warm zone, incorporates land evacuation routes from the hot zone for casualties who may still be contaminated. Patient decontamination stations, whether located immediately outside the hot zone or near the door of a receiving MTF, are within this corridor. In some instances, particularly in a military battlefield situation, seriously injured contaminated patients who are still wearing their protective gear and have undergone only operational decontamination (see Levels of Decontamination, below) may be evacuated by rotor-wing aircraft to an MTF well outside the warm zone. In these cases a separate warm zone would be created to include the aircraft landing area and the MTF patient decontamination area.

Cold Zone

Areas free of solid, liquid, and vapor contamination are in the cold zone. All military MTFs are initially established in contamination-free areas. Before being allowed into the cold zone, individuals must go through decontamination and be determined contamination-free; this requirement applies not only to patients but also to medical workers and decontamination team members in protective ensemble. Individuals in the cold zone do not need to wear any type of protective equipment, except in the event of a nosocomially transmitted biological agent such as plague (*Yersinia pestis*) or smallpox. In these cases, respiratory and contact precautions must be followed by those in contact with the patient. The cold zone may also be referred to as the postdecontamination zone, support zone, or clean zone.[25,27,39]

Levels of Decontamination

Various stages of patient decontamination are described in the processing of a CBRN casualty.[3,14,33] The military uses the following three levels of decontamination (the official names for these levels may change, but the order of performance will remain the important focus).

Immediate

Immediate decontamination is performed by the individual who is exposed to the hazardous agent, or provided by a buddy partner immediately after the exposure event. Military members are trained to decontaminate themselves using the M291 skin decontamination kit and M295 equipment decontamination kit or reactive skin decontamination lotion, if available, as soon as possible after exposure to a chemical agent. This is the most effective time to perform decontamination to lessen the dose on the skin and significantly reduce future medical complications.

Patient Operational Decontamination

Patient operational decontamination is performed before loading a contaminated patient onto a "dirty evacuation" asset. The patient remains in a protective mask and overgarment, and any gross contamination is removed. Plastic sheeting may also be used inside the vehicle to help minimize contaminant spread during transport. This procedure would more likely be followed under operational tempos that do not allow for the removal of the patient's protective clothing until arrival at an MTF with appropriate resources to care for the individual. For example, the situation of a continued chemical threat with no replacement clothing is quite possible on the battlefield.

Patient Thorough Decontamination

Patient thorough decontamination is performed at the MTF or a consolidated troop and patient decontamination area in close proximity to the incident site, if possible. Personnel remove the patients' clothing and thoroughly clean them using either soap and water or another decontaminant. The patients are then determined to be free of contamination before being brought into the MTF.

Military Management Concepts in the Civilian Setting

The civilian setting is quite different from the military battlefield scenario. The civilian scenario described below would probably apply to the military in a situation in which service members were exposed to chemical agents while wearing their duty uniform, which offers no protection, such as in an unexpected terrorist attack on a military installation or the sudden release of toxic fumes from a nearby industrial accident. See Table 14-4 for a comparison of casualty care and decontamination

TABLE 14-4

COMPARISON OF MILITARY BATTLEFIELD AND CIVILIAN CASUALTY CARE AND DECONTAMINATION

Process	Military on Chemical Battlefield	Civilian or Unprepared Military
Immediate decontamination	Immediate decontamination takes place upon contamination using M291, RSDL, or other kit.	Casualties may wash contaminated areas if knowledgeable, otherwise they must wait for HAZMAT crews and first responders
Operational patient decontamination	Contaminated patients, wearing protective gear, can be transported on designated vehicles to decontamination facilities.	Local vehicles may have to be used if available. Ambulance services may be hesitant to transport contaminated patients.
Emergency medical care	Care can begin on the battlefield. Initiated by the individual or a buddy. Unit medics can also provide lifesaving care while they are wearing protective equipment.	Medical care is delayed in all instances by minutes. Care may not be initiated until the patient is moved from the incident site and then decontaminated. Care may be initiated earlier if medical personnel are trained to provide assistance while wearing protective equipment.
Thorough patient decontamination	Performed before patient enters the MTF, whether a small or large facility. May have gross contaminants removed at a centralized facility outside the hot zone with continued decontamination at the hospital decontamination area if indicated.	Performed before patient enters the MTF, whether a small or large facility. May have gross contaminants removed at a centralized facility outside the hot zone with continued decontamination at the hospital decontamination area if indicated.

HAZMAT: hazardous materials
MTF: medical treatment facility
RSDL: reactive skin decontamination lotion

in the military and civilian setting.

The majority of civilians are not aware of the characteristics of chemical agents or the steps to take for immediate decontamination. Many, appropriately, would probably attempt immediate decontamination of a visible or symptomatic agent by washing or wiping. They might effectively perform immediate decontamination by washing with copious amounts of water from a sink or hose, or by using bottled water. Wiping could be performed using frequently carried moistened disposable baby wipes. Liquid agent could be wiped from the skin using any nontoxic absorbent material such as clean dry sand, bread, flour, or baby powder, followed by wet wipes.[40] If the individual does not perform any of these procedures, then decontamination may not take place until the arrival of first responders, who may be delayed. Also, civilian casualties, unlike military personnel, would not have immediate access to nerve agent antidotes (or would not know how to use them). The casualties would need to wait until treated by appropriately supplied first responders.

In the civilian sector, HAZMAT crews and fire departments can take 15 minutes or longer to assess the hot zone and establish patient decontamination lanes in the warm zone[23]; during this time civilian casualties would remain contaminated and untreated. If the toxin is an organophosphate nerve agent, then antidotes would be provided, if available, by the civilian first responder. Under the best of situations in a civilian setting, casualty treatment is often administered only after the patient is evacuated by HAZMAT crews to the warm zone triage area. Local civilian EMTs could be trained to provide stabilizing patient care while wearing PPE in the warm zone's patient collection area before decontamination. In an optimal situation, first responder EMTs in PPE could accompany HAZMAT crews into a contaminated area and begin triage and treatment of victims as they are being evacuated.[26] In the military battlefield scenario, of course, initial care and decontamination is provided at the incident site, in the hot zone, before and during patient evacuation.

Patient operational decontamination would probably not be done in the civilian sector because most contract ambulance services will not take contaminated patients on their vehicles. Some semblance of operational decontamination might occur for those civilian casualties who are evacuated to hospitals in privately owned vehicles before first responders reach the area and establish boundaries. The vast majority of casualties in the Tokyo subway incident were evacuated by taxi or other private vehicles.[17] One author estimates that individuals who flee the incident area would take at least 10 minutes to locate transportation and get to an MTF, unless the facility was adjacent to the release site.[41] It is expected, however, that those who flee would try to go to the nearest medical facility they know of.

Thorough decontamination in the civilian sector would be initiated by decontamination teams immediately outside the hot zone, typically the fire department, which performs gross decontamination by hosing down the victims. Thorough decontamination would also be provided at hospital decontamination areas established outside the doors of receiving hospitals. Hospitals require these decontamination capabilities because, historically, many patients self-report to the hospital before emergency personnel arrive on the incident scene and bypass the fire department gross decontamination.[21,22] Fire department gross decontamination efforts may also not be completely effective.

Processing Patients

Whether military or civilian, all field management operations dealing with chemical casualties have the same key components, arranged approximately in linear fashion (Figure 14-10). Patients are provided with initial treatment in or on the periphery of the hot zone. In the military, individual patient decontamination can be carried out by the exposed individual or a buddy. In a civilian situation, although initial treatment would probably be delayed, it may be carried out by emergency first responders in or at the periphery of the hot zone, or by the victims themselves under instruction,

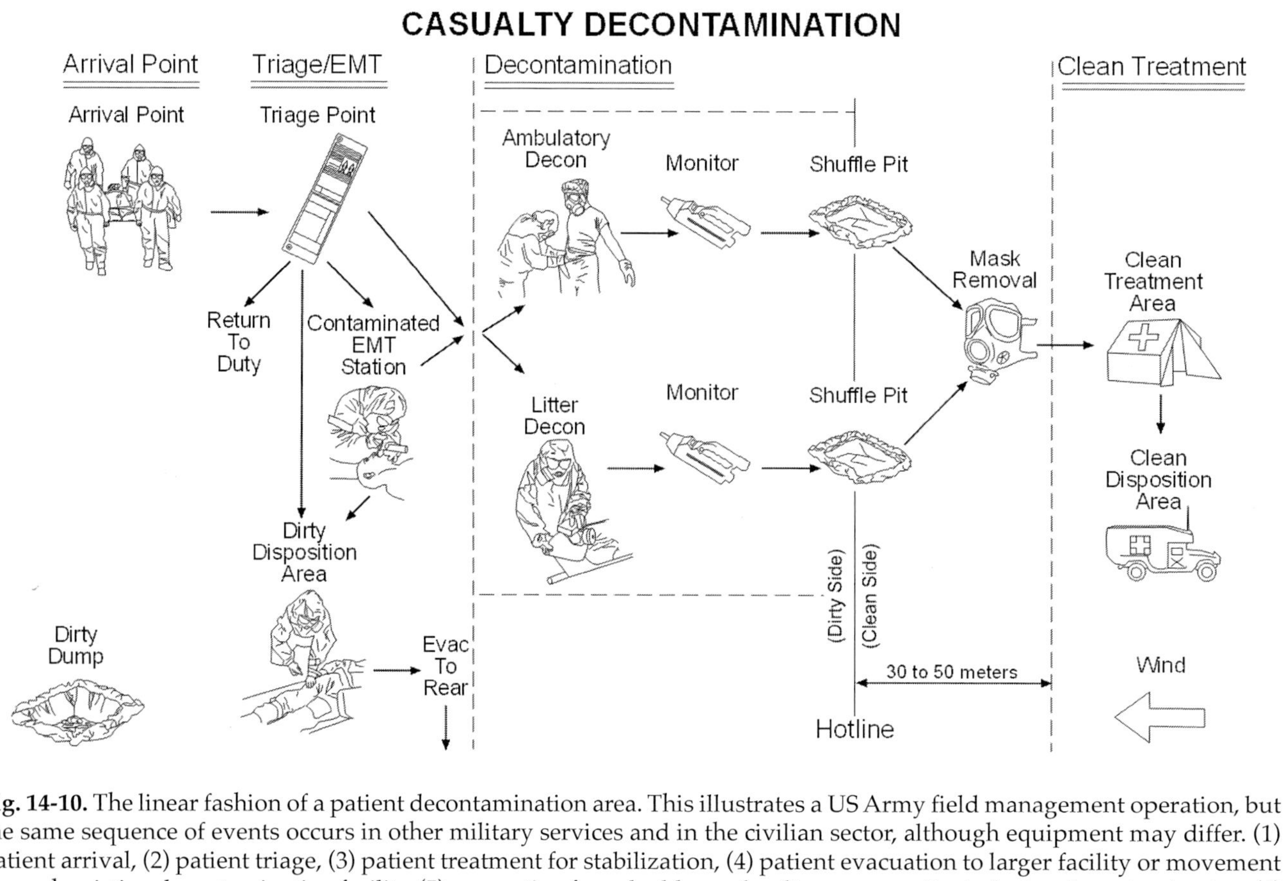

Fig. 14-10. The linear fashion of a patient decontamination area. This illustrates a US Army field management operation, but the same sequence of events occurs in other military services and in the civilian sector, although equipment may differ. (1) Patient arrival, (2) patient triage, (3) patient treatment for stabilization, (4) patient evacuation to larger facility or movement through existing decontamination facility, (5) accounting for valuables and ordinance on patients during decontamination, (6) crossing the hot line, (7) crossing the vapor control line, (8) patient mask removal, (9) treatment in the clean (contamination-free) area and evacuation.
EMT: emergency medical treatment
Diagram: Courtesy of the US Army Medical Research Institute for Chemical Defense, Chemical Casualty Care Division, Aberdeen Proving Ground, Md.

using any available materials such as bottled water, baby wipes, or reactive skin decontamination lotion.

For more thorough decontamination, civilian casualties are provided with gross decontamination in the warm zone by the fire department, using fire engine water spray or water from plumbed decontamination tents (Figure 14-11), and more complete decontamination at the MTF prior to entry into the facility. For the military casualty, thorough decontamination occurs at the patient decontamination station, which is located outside the military MTF. In both the civilian and military decontamination station, a patient moves through a sequence of substations to account for valuables, remove clothing, and wash. These same stations are established whether decontamination takes place in an area with limited resources, such as an Army BAS or civilian fire department decontamination line, or a facility with more robust capabilities, such as a moderate sized or larger military or civilian hospital (Figure 14-12). OSHA documents refer to the area outside an MTF, where contaminated patients arrive and are triaged and decontaminated, as the hospital decontamination zone.[27]

Once the patients are decontaminated, they move across the hot line into the hospital postdecontamination zone. Name designations for each area may differ depending on the setting, but the sequence of steps in the process is similar. The areas described below are adopted from several sources.[3,7,8,14,27,33,42,43]

Entry Control Point and Arrival Area

The entry control point is the doorway to the decontamination area. This entrance is typically barricaded in some way to regulate traffic flow and is usually staffed by security personnel wearing protective ensemble. Ambulances, other vehicles, and ambulatory casualties go through this control point on their way

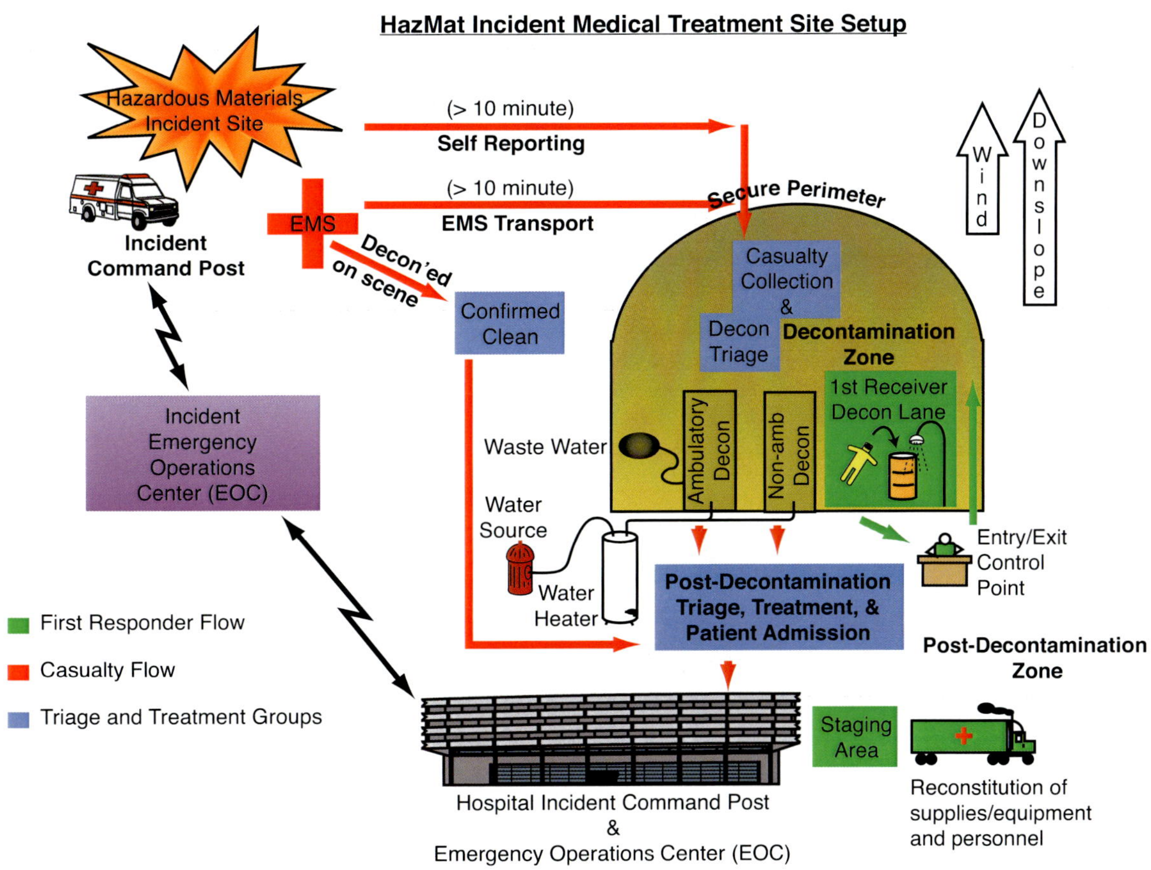

Fig. 14-11. This is one example of the layout of a civilian hazardous materials incident patient decontamination area at the periphery of the hot zone or at the entrance to the medical facility. This model takes into consideration a 10-minute lag time between incident occurrence and the self-reporting of patients. It follows the same sequence of steps noted in Fig. 14-13.
EMS: emergency medical service
Diagram: Courtesy of Commander Duane Caneva, US Navy.

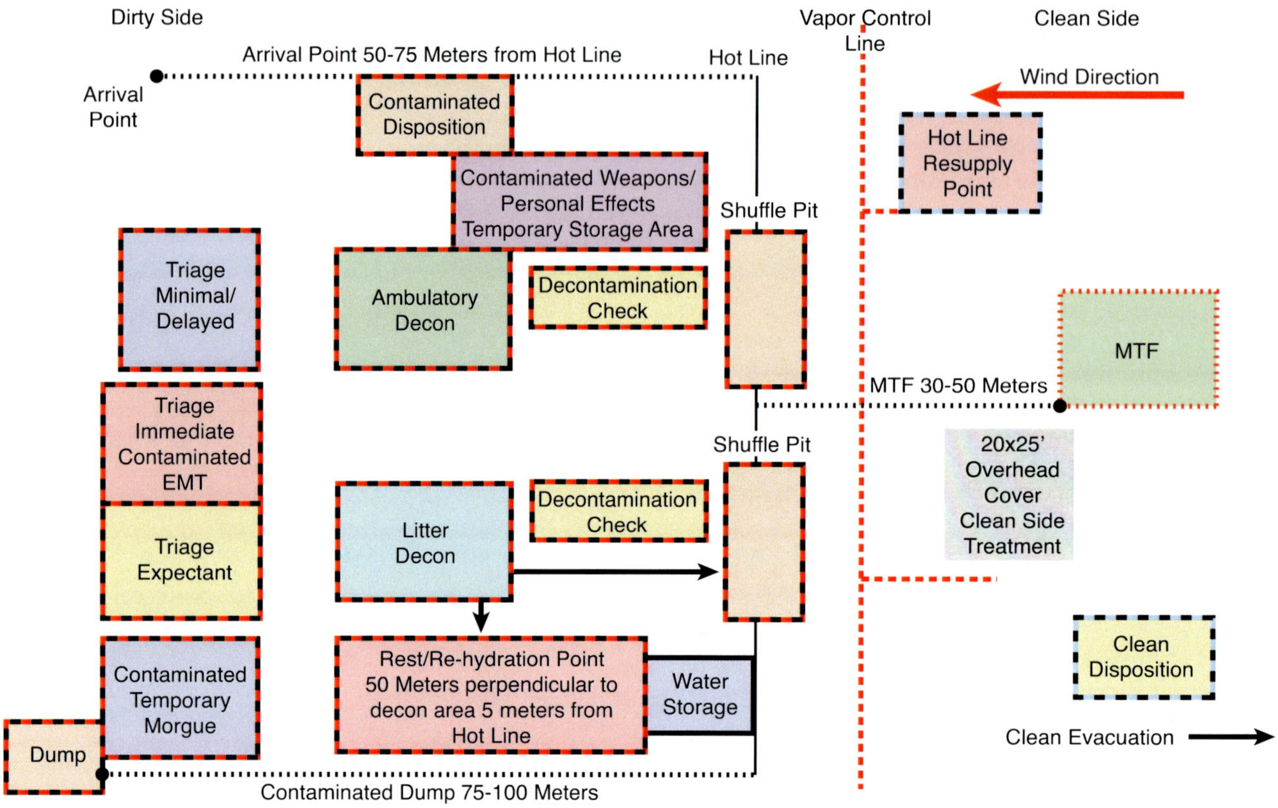

Fig. 14-12. Another, more detailed, example of the layout of a patient decontamination site at a medical treatment facility (military or civilian). Note the relative positioning of specific triage areas, the waste dump, rest/rehydration points, areas for storage of personal effects, hot line, and vapor control line.
EMT: emergency medical treatment
MTF: medical treatment facility
Diagram: Courtesy of the US Army Medical Research Institute for Chemical Defense, Chemical Casualty Care Division, Aberdeen Proving Ground, Md.

to the arrival area. On land the entry control point would be located well in front of the decontamination area, and at sea it would be at the transport aircraft or watercraft casualty loading area located on land. At the arrival area vehicles are unloaded and patients are brought to the adjacent triage area. Maintaining traffic discipline in this area is critical to ensure unimpeded flow of patients and vehicles. The arrival point on land must be large enough to accommodate ever expanding numbers of casualties; at sea the arrival point would be the aircraft or watercraft landing area. At this point monitoring devices may be used to check for contamination on patients. All personnel in these areas wear a MOPP level 4 or level C equivalent protective ensemble.

Triage Area (Warm Side)

Patients are moved to the triage area from the arrival point, where a triage officer (trained physician, nurse, EMT, physician's assistant, dentist, or veterinarian) quickly triages the patient, who is then moved to a respective immediate treatment area (also known as the warm side emergency medical treatment station). Patients are triaged according to their priority for medical treatment (immediate, delayed, minimal, or expectant); level of decontamination (high or low); and further medical evacuation required (urgent, priority, or routine). See Chapter 15, Triage of Chemical Casualties, for more detailed information. Medical workers in this area wear a level C equivalent protective ensemble.

The immediate treatment area should be located near the entrance to the litter decontamination lanes to allow direct access for patients who will be litterborne. Expectant patients are located adjacent to the dirty side emergency treatment station, but farther away from the litter decontamination lanes, so that these patients can be retriaged and stabilized for decontamination when the dirty side no longer has patients. The delayed treatment area is located near the entrances of both the litter and ambulatory patient decontamination lanes; delayed patients can be processed through either lane when available. Finally, the minimal patient triage treatment area should be positioned nearer to the ambulatory decontamination lane because these patients can walk through the lane with minimal assistance. In the military, minimal patients are typically sent back to their units after receiving medical care without needing to be decontaminated or crossing to the clean side, where the MTF is located. In the civilian sector, the movement of these patients should not interfere with the processing of more serious casualties through the decontamination line.

The warm side emergency treatment station (or immediate patient treatment area) is where life saving care is provided to stabilize the patient for decontamination or transport. Care given at this station includes the administration of antidotes, quick decontamination of contaminated skin areas, intubation, and intravenous administration of fluids. Medical staff in this area are trained in these procedures and capable of performing them while wearing OSHA level C protective ensemble.

Decontamination Area

Lanes are established in the decontamination area for litter and ambulatory patients. The number of staff required for a decontamination team is dictated, as discussed earlier, by ambient and WBGT temperature in the field management operations area, number of casualties, type of chemical agent, level of fitness of personnel wearing protective ensemble, and decontamination equipment used. Minimum staffing levels are two decontamination workers per litter patient, who must have their clothing cut off, and one per ambulatory patient, who can undress and decontaminate themselves under supervision. If only one or two patients need decontamination, it can be done with a garden hose, buckets and sponges, or built-in shower. Larger numbers of casualties require more efficient decontamination procedures. More specific suggestions for personnel are found in Chapter 16, Decontamination of Chemical Casualties.

In the Army and Navy (in support of USMC units), decontamination is carried out by nonmedical personnel from the supported military units who are supervised by medical personnel. In Air Force and some Navy shipboard decontamination teams, all the team members come from the medical unit. These personnel wear OSHA level C PPE or the military equivalent. If their garments are not completely water resistant, they also wear water repellent toxicological agent protective aprons to keep the protective overgarments dry and allow for apron decontamination before performing patient lifts.

The decontamination process usually takes up to 10 to 20 minutes for a litter patient and 5 to 10 minutes for an ambulatory patient, depending on the type of decontamination equipment and the team training level. Plumbed equipment that dispenses soap and water and roller systems for litter patients are more efficient than the more labor-intensive processes using minimal equipment such as buckets and sponges.

A final check for thoroughness of contamination is often incorporated at the end of the decontamination process. This check is more critical when water-conservative methods, such as washing with buckets and sponges, are used. In these situations, some areas of the skin might remain incompletely washed. Decontamination equipment that incorporates a large volume but a low-pressure flow of water provides a more thorough wash and can reduce the necessity for a final check. Warm water, and warm decontamination areas, are more likely to ensure thorough patient compliance and minimize the development of patient hypothermia.

Hot Line

The hot line is located at the end of the decontamination line, before the clean area. At this point, all liquid contamination has been removed from patients and decontamination team (it is sometimes referred to as the liquid control line). Patients are typically nude at this point, and decontamination station workers have removed their protective overgarments. In the civilian sector, patients undergoing gross decontamination by a fire department might still have on their undergarments. If clean covering garments are available, victims should be strongly encouraged to doff their wet undergarments, which could hold agent, particularly if exposed to liquid or potent aerosol. Patients entering an MTF should be nude but covered by a hospital gown, to insure that contamination does not enter the facility and allow for patient privacy.

Vapor Control Line

The vapor control line delineates the location where no vapor hazard remains from clothing that has been removed in the decontamination area. Although not required for biological and radiological contamination, this line is critical for chemical contamination. The vapor contol line is approximately 10 feet beyond the hot line as the patient proceeds toward the clean side. In the military, the air in this area may be monitored by a stationary vapor monitor such as the automatic chemical agent detector alarm.

Triage and Treatment Area (Clean Side)

The triage and treatment area (clean side) is part of the cold zone, located near the vapor control line (OSHA refers to this area as the hospital post-decontamination zone). The recently decontaminated patients are retriaged in this area, and wait for processing into an ambulance, if this occurs at a decontamination station separate from an MTF, or to await movement into an MTF from an adjacent decontamination station.

Additional Areas

Other areas that may be necessary, but not in all situations, include the following:

- contaminated waste dump to store contaminated waste until proper removal;
- fresh and waste water bladders if decontamination tent systems are used;
- warm side disposition areas used by the military, where casualties in protective gear have been provided operational decontamination and await dirty evacuation;
- a warm side temporary morgue for storage of the contaminated remains of those who die during field management;
- a warm side weapons and contaminated personal affects storage area for storage and eventual disposition of patient items;
- litter decontamination area for military decontamination operations with minimal equipment;
- a warm side rest area for decontamination crews and medical team members;
- a clean side supply point where medical and decontamination supplies can be apportioned as necessary; and
- a clean side disposition area for staging decontaminated patients for transport to another location.

SUMMARY

Field management of chemical casualties involves ongoing triage, treatment, and patient movement through the medical system to obtain the most appropriate care available given the situation and resources. Conducting field management in a chemically contaminated environment requires that medical and decontamination personnel wear the equivalent of OSHA level C protective ensemble for protection from contaminants on patients and hazardous vapors emitted by the contaminants.

The military's immediate medical response to a chemical event on the battlefield is identical across the services, using self and buddy aid. This response differs from the civilian response, because of lack of training in self-decontamination and treatment and lack of readily available resources. Unprotected military personnel (without PPE and individual decontaminants or antidotes) exposed to a chemical release would encounter some of the same challenges as the civilian population.

Civilian casualties unable to flee the scene of a chemical release must wait until HAZMAT teams and fire departments arrive on the scene. This initial response typically takes 10 minutes or longer, and victims may not encounter a medical care provider for 30 minutes or more after their initial exposure. Typically medical treatment is not provided until after the victim has undergone decontamination. This process is changing for civilian medical responders, particularly in larger metropolitan communities; many fire department medical responders wearing PPE are now prepared to provide early life saving medical triage and care to contaminated casualties before decontamination. This alignment of civilian and military medical response should improve response capabilities and patient outcomes in the event of a mass casualty incident.

Although the positioning of up-front medical care in the warm zone may differ, the process of patient decontamination is similar for civilian and military. It includes the following: accounting for patient valuables, clothing removal, washing, and movement across the hot line; evidence recognition and proper chain of custody procedures; recognition of secondary explosive devices; clean side triage and treatment; and patient disposition from the decontamination site. The procedures may vary slightly depending on the decontamination platform (land vs sea) and type of equipment used (eg, buckets and sponges vs robust plumbed systems or designated permanent decontamination facilities). Decontamination typically takes from 5 to 20 minutes, depending on the medical condition of the casualty, the type of decontamination equipment, and the level of training of the decontamination team.

REFERENCES

1. US Department of Defense. *Health Service Support in Joint Operations*. Revision, Final Coordination. Washington, DC: DoD; 2005. Joint Publication 4-02.

2. US Department of Defense. *Doctrine for Health Service Support in Joint Operations*. Washington, DC: DoD; 2001. Joint Publication 4-02.

3. US Departments of the Army, Marine Corps, Navy, and Air Force. *Health Service Support in a Nuclear, Biological, and Chemical Environment*. Draft. Washington, DC: DoD; 2004. FM 4-02.7, MCRP 4-11.1F, NTTP 4-02.7, AFTTP (l) 3-2.47.

4. US Departments of the Army, Marine Corps, Navy, and Air Force. *Multiservice Tactics, Techniques, and Procedures for Nuclear, Biological, and Chemical Defense Operations*. Washington, DC: DoD; 2003. FM 3-11, MCWP 3-37.1, NWP 3-11, AFTTP (I) 3-2.42.

5. US Department of Defense. *Joint Tactics, Techniques and Procedures for Patient Movement in Joint Operations*. Washington, DC: DoD; 1996. Joint Publication 4-02.2.

6. US Department of the Air Force. *Airman's Manual*. Washington, DC: USAF; 2004. Air Force Manual 10-100.

7. US Department of the Air Force. *Health Services*. Washington, DC: USAF; 2002. Air Force Doctrine Document 2-4.2.

8. US Department of the Air Force. *Expeditionary Medical Decontamination Team*. Washington, DC: USAF; 2005. AFTTP 3-42.33.

9. US Department of the Air Force. *Patient Decontamination Shelter System for Expeditionary Medical Support, Military Utility Assessment Final Report*. Washington, DC: USAF; 2003.

10. GlobalSecurity.org. LHD-1 Wasp class. Available at http://www.globalsecurity.org/military/systems/ship/lhd-1.htm. Accessed November 22, 2005.

11. USNS *Comfort*. US Navy Web site. Available at: http://www.comfort.navy.mil. Accessed November 22, 2005.

12. USNS *Mercy*. US Navy Web site. Available at: http://www.mercy.navy.mil. Accessed November 22, 2005.

13. Myers T. Commander, US Coast Guard, Division Chief for Float Safety. Telephone conversation, July 2005.

14. US Department of the Navy. *Surface Ship Survivability*. Washington, DC: DN; 2004. NTTP 3-20.31.555; NSTM Chap 555.

15. Hall I H, Haugh GS, Price-Green P, Dhara VR, Kaye WE. Risk factors for hazardous substances releases that result in injuries and evacuations: data from 9 states. *Am J Public Health*. 1996;86:855–857.

16. Dhara VR, Dhara R. The Union Carbide disaster in Bhopol: a review of health effects. *Arch Environ Health*. 2002;57:391–404.

17. Okumura T, Suzuki K, Fukuda A, et al. The Tokyo subway sarin attack: disaster management, Part 1: Community emergency response. *Acad Emerg Med*. 1998;5:613–617.

18. Okudera H, Morita H, Iwashita T, et al. Unexpected nerve gas exposure in the city of Matsumoto: report of rescue activity in the first sarin gas terrorism. *Am J Emerg Med*. 1997;15:527–528.

19. FEMA Independent Study Program: IS-700 National Incident Management System (NIMS), An Introduction. Available at: http://training.fema.gov/emiweb/is/is700.asp. Accessed November 22, 2005.

20. Federal Emergency Management Agency. What is the NRP? FEMA web site. Available at: http://faq.fema.gov/cgi-bin/fema.cfg/php/enduser/std_adp.php?p_faqid=290&p_created=1110828264&p_sid=TpOCcfNh&p_lva=335p_sp-=cF9zcmNoPTEmcF9zb3J0X2J5PSZwX2dyaWRzb3J0PSZwX3Jvd19jbnQ9NiZwX3Byb2RzPTMwJnBfY2F0cz0mcF9wdj0xLjMwOzIudTAmcF9jdj0mcF9wYWdlPTEmcF9zZWFyY2hfdGV4dD1OUlA*&p_li=&p_topview=1. Accessed November 22, 2005.

21. Okumura T, Suzuki K, Fukuda A, et al. The Tokyo subway sarin attack: disaster management, Part 2: Hospital response. *Acad Emerg Med*. 1998;5:618–624.

22. Macintyre AG, Christopher GW, Eitzen E Jr, et al. Weapons of mass destruction events with contaminated casualties: effective planning for health care facilities. *JAMA*. 2000;283:242–349.

23. Broughton, R. CBRNE incident response. Lecture presented at: Uniformed Services University of the Health Sciences Chemical Warfare and Emergency Management Course; March 1, 2005; Bethesda, Md.

24. Cathey T. Medical Director, Oklahoma State Department of Health, Protective Health Services, Emergency Medical Services, Oklahoma City, Okla. Telephone conversation, September 2005.

25. US Department of Health and Human Services, Agency for Toxic Substance and Disease Registry. *Emergency Medical Services, A Planning Guide for the Management of Contaminated Patients*. Vol 1. In: *Managing Hazardous Materials Incidents*. Atlanta, Ga: DHHS; 2001: Chap 9.

26. Baker D. Civilian exposure to toxic agents: emergency medical response. *Prehospital Disaster Med*. 2004;19:174–178.

27. Occupational Safety and Health Administration. *The OSHA Best Practices for Hospital-Based First Receivers of Victims from Mass Casualty Incidents Involving the Release of Hazardous Substances*. Washington, DC: OSHA; 2005.

28. US Department of Defense. *Department of Defense Installation Chemical, Biological, Radiological, Nuclear, and High-Yield Explosive Emergency Response Guidelines*. Washington, DC: DoD; 2002. DoD Instruction 2000.18.

29. JCAHO standards. Management of the environment of care. Walter Reed Army Medical Center Web site. Available at: http://www.wramc.army.mil/JCAHO/Division.cfm?D_Id=6. Accessed January 6, 2006.

30. US Department of Defense. *Military Support to Civil Authorities (MSCA)*. Washington, DC: DoD: 1993. DoD Directive 3025.1.

31. US Department of Defense. *Military Assistance for Civil Disturbances (MACDIS)*. Washington, DC: DoD: 1994. DoD Directive 3025.12.

32. US Department of Defense. *Military Assistance to Civil Authorities*. Washington, DC: DoD: 1997. DoD Directive 3025.15.

33. US Department of the Army. *Health Service Support in a Nuclear, Biological, and Chemical Environment. Tactics, Techniques, and Procedures*. Washigton, DC: Headquarters, DA; 2002. FM 4-02.7

34. Saskatchewan Department of Labor, Canada. Working under hot conditions. Available at: http://www.labour.gov.sk.ca/safety/thermal/hot/INDEX.HTM. Accessed August 30, 2007.

35. Geomet Technologies, LLC. PPE heat stress calculator. Available at: http://www.geomet.com/heatstresspda.com/. Accessed on January 19, 2006.

36. Technical support working group. TSWG Web site. Available at: http://www.tswg.gov/tswg/cbrnc/cbrnc_currpr.htm. Accessed January 19, 2006.

37. US Department of Health and Human Services, Technical Support Working Group. *Best Practices and Guidelines for CBR Mass Personnel Decontamination*. 2nd ed. Washington, DC: DHHS; 2004.

38. U S Army Soldier and Biological Chemical Command. *Guidelines for Cold Weather Mass Decontamination During a Terrorist Chemical Agent Incident*. Revision 1. Aberdeen Proving Ground, Md: SBCCOM; 2003.

39. US Department of Transportation, Office of Hazardous Materials Safety. *The 2004 Emergency Response Codebook: A Guidebook for First Responders During the Initial Phase of a Dangerous Goods/Hazardous Materials Incident*. Washington, DC: DOT; 2004.

40. van Hooidonk C. CW agents and the skin: penetration and decontamination. In: *Proceedings of the International Symposium on Protection Against Chemical Warfare Agents, Stockholm, Sweden, June 6-9, 1983.* Stockholm, Sweden: National Defense Research Institute; 1983.

41. Georgopoulos PG, Fedele P, Shade P, et al. Hospital response to chemical terrorism: personal protective equipment, training, and operations. *Am J Ind Med*. 2004;46:432–445.

42. Stutz DR, Ulin S, eds. *Hazardous Materials Injuries: A Handbook for Pre-Hospital Care, Basic and Advanced Life Support.* 4th ed. Bowie, Md: Bradcomm Inc; 1997.

43. Secretary of the Air Force. *In-Place Patient Decontamination Capability (IPPDC).* Washington, DC: DAF; 2004.

Chapter 15

TRIAGE OF CHEMICAL CASUALTIES

SHIRLEY D. TUORINSKY, MSN*; DUANE C. CANEVA, MD†; AND FREDERICK R. SIDELL, MD‡

*Lieutenant Colonel, AN, US Army; Executive Officer, Combat Casualty Care Division, US Army Medical Research Institute of Chemical Defense, 3100 Ricketts Point Road, Aberdeen Proving Ground, Maryland 21010-5400

†Head, Medical Plans and Policy, Navy Medicine Office of Homeland Security, 2300 E Street, NW, Washington, DC 20372

‡Formerly, Chief, Chemical Casualty Care Division, and Director, Medical Management of Chemical Casualties Course, US Army Medical Research Institute of Chemical Defense, Aberdeen Proving Ground, Maryland

INTRODUCTION

The term "triage" has come to have different meanings depending on the situation in which it is used. Derived from the French word *trier,* meaning to sort, categorize, or select, its initial use is thought to have been in reference to the sorting of crops according to quality. Triage soon became used on the battlefield as the sorting of casualties into three groups: (1) those needing immediate care, (2) those who could wait for treatment, and (3) those not expected to survive. Military triage has certain definitions codified in doctrine and policy. The term also refers to the initial screening and prioritization process in emergency departments.

Triage is one of the most important tools in the handling of mass chemical casualties. Triage criteria must be relevant to the available medical units' capabilities, and triage process should be planned in advance and practiced. In general, triage is performed at naturally occurring bottlenecks, where delays in medical care may occur, and when medical requirements exceed capabilities or resources, which may cause a breech in the standard of care. The ultimate goal of triage is to optimize the use of available medical resources to provide the best medical care possible by identifying the correct priority of patients.[1] This chapter will focus on the process of triage in chemical agent mass casualties. Specific chemical warfare agent classes, current triage systems, and classifications of triage will be reviewed, with discussion of issues specific to the battlefield and installation setting.

TRIAGE PRINCIPLES AND PROCESSES

In a mass casualty situation, whether in peacetime or on a battlefield, triage is carried out to provide immediate and appropriate care for casualties with treatable injuries, to delay care for those with less immediate needs, and to set aside those for whom care would be too timely or asset-consuming. Triage ensures the greatest care for the greatest number and the maximal utilization of medical assets: personnel, supplies, and facilities. To effectively triage a given population, a triage officer should know the following essential information:

- The current environment and potential threat, course, and harm. Situational awareness must include current tactical goals and conditions, the potential evolution of hazardous materials or conditions, and the impact these might have on the patients and providers.
- The ongoing medical requirements, including the number and type of current casualties and potential population at risk.
- The medical resources on hand.
- The natural course of a given injury.
- The current and likely casualty flow.
- The medical evacuation capabilities.
- The decontamination requirements in a chemical incident.

According to FM 8-10, *Health Service Support in a Theater of* Operations,[2] the triage officer should be a highly experienced medical provider who can make sound clinical judgments quickly. Ideally, a surgeon experienced with combat trauma would be used in this capacity; however, once casualty flow progresses, surgeons must spend time in the operating suite, and their available time to perform triage will be limited beyond the initial efforts and between operations. Additionally, the expertise of surgical triage applies to traumatic injuries, and may not be as applicable to chemical incidents. Commonly, the most experienced combat medic performs triage; however, other physicians, dentists, or nurses with appropriate training and experience can also accomplish this arduous task.

Part of the triage process is the evaluation of the benefit that immediate assistance will provide. This evaluation is based, in part, on the natural course of the injury or disease. For example, dedicating medical assets to a casualty with an injury that will either heal or prove fatal no matter what immediate care is given would be of little benefit. Another part of the process is considering the overall tactical mission requirements, which may change rapidly in the battlefield setting. The ultimate goal of combat medicine is to return the greatest possible number of soldiers to combat and the preservation of life, limb, and eyesight in those who must be evacuated.[3]

Setting aside casualties who are in need is unpopular among medical care providers, and poses an ethical dilemma on how to provide the ultimate care for each patient. The Hippocratic Oath is not helpful in this sorting process, because the modern interpretation of the Oath states that the duty of physicians and nurses is to protect and promote the welfare of their patients. Furthermore, according to the Oath, caregivers must focus their full attention on that patient until the patient's needs are met, before turning their attention to another patient. Additionally, in peacetime, every patient who enters the hospital emergency room receives the full attention of all personnel needed to provide optimal care. For these reasons, the thought of setting aside a critically sick or injured patient may well be repugnant to someone who has not been in a mass casualty situation or who has given little thought to such situations.[4]

In addition to knowing the natural course of the disease or injury, the triage officer should also be aware of current medical assets, the current casualty population, the anticipated number and types of incoming casualties, the current status of the evacuation process, and the assets and casualty population at the evacuation site. Committing assets to the stabilization of a seriously injured casualty in anticipation of early evacuation and more definitive care would be pointless if evacuation could not be accomplished within the time needed for the casualty's effective care, or if the assets at the evacuation site were already committed. The officer might also triage differently if, for example, he or she knew that the 10 casualties present would need care in the next 24 hours, or, on the other hand, that those 10 casualties were to be followed by 50 more within an hour.[5] In an unfavorable tactical situation, another consideration may arise: casualties with minor wounds, who otherwise may be classified minimal, might have highest priority for care to enable them to return to duty. The fighting strength thus preserved could save medical personnel and casualties from attack.

Levels of Care

Triage is a dynamic rather than a static process, in which casualties are periodically reevaluated for changes in condition and retriaged at various levels of medical care, ranging from the battlefield to the battalion aid station to the combat support hospital. The first triage is done by the corpsman, medic, or unit combat lifesaver in the field. The medic first evaluates the severity of injury and decides whether anything can be done to save life or limb. If the answer is no, the medic moves on, perhaps after administering an analgesic. More commonly, the medic decides that care is indicated. Can the medic provide that care on the spot to return the service member to duty quickly? Can the care wait until the battle is less intense or an ambulance arrives? Or must the care be given immediately if the casualty is to survive? In the latter case, the medic ensures that the casualty is transferred to the medical facility if possible.

A casualty is triaged once more upon entry into a medical care facility, followed by repeated triage within the facility as circumstances (eg, the casualty's condition and the assets available) change. For example, a casualty set aside as expectant (see Triage Categories for Chemical Casualties, below, for definitions of classification groups) because personnel are occupied with more salvageable casualties might be reclassified as immediate when those personnel become free. On the other hand, a casualty with a serious but not life-threatening wound, initially classified as delayed, could suddenly develop unanticipated bleeding and, if treatment assets were available, might be retriaged as immediate.

Even in the most sophisticated medical setting, a form of triage is usually performed (perhaps not always consciously): separation of those casualties who will benefit from medical intervention from those who will not be helped even by maximal care. However, in most circumstances in a large medical facility, care is administered anyway; for instance, an individual with a devastating head injury might receive life-support measures. The realization that in some settings assets cannot be spent in this manner is an integral part of triage.[6]

Decontamination

At the first level of medical care, the chemical casualty is contaminated, and both the casualty and the triage officer are in protective clothing (mission oriented protective posture [MOPP] level 4 or Occupational Safety and Health Administration level C). Furthermore, the first medical care given to the casualty is in a contaminated area, on the "hot" or dirty side of the "hotline" at the emergency treatment station (see Chapter 14, Field Management of Chemical Casualties). This situation is in contrast to any level of care in which casualties were previously decontaminated, and to a conventional situation with no contamination involved. Examination of the casualty is not as efficient or effective as it might be in a clean (not contaminated) environment, and very little care can be given to a casualty in the emergency treatment section in the contaminated area. In a chemically contaminated environment, in contrast to other triage situations, the most experienced medical staff work in the clean treatment area, where they can provide maximum care.

It is extremely unlikely that immediate decontamination at the first level of medical care will change the fate of the chemical casualty or the outcome of the injury. Various estimates indicate that the casualty usually will not reach the first level of care for 15 to 60 minutes after the injury or onset of effects, except when the medical treatment facility (MTF) is close to the battle line or is under attack and the injury occurs just outside. The casualty is unlikely to seek care until the injury becomes apparent, which is usually long after exposure. For example, mustard, a vesicant, may be on the skin for many hours before a lesion becomes noticeable. Thus, it is likely that the agent has been completely absorbed or has evaporated from the skin by the time the casualty reaches the MTF, and the small amount unabsorbed, or absorbed during a wait for decontamination, is very unlikely to be significant.

The process of patient decontamination must be factored into the triage decision. (It must be remembered that triage refers to priority for medical or surgical care, not priority for decontamination. All chemical casualties require decontamination. Although a casualty exposed to vapor from a volatile agent such as cyanide, phosgene, or a nerve agent may not appear to need decontamination, verifying that no liquid is present on the casualty is difficult.) In a contaminated environment, emergency care is given by personnel in MOPP 4, the highest level of protective gear, which limits their capabilities. After receiving emergency care, a casualty must go through the decontamination station before receiving more definitive care in a clean environment. Decontamination takes 10 to 20 minutes. As a rule no medical care is provided during this time or during the time spent waiting to begin the decontamination process. Therefore, before leaving the emergency care area, patients must be stabilized to an extent that their condition will not deteriorate during this time. If stabilization cannot be achieved, the triage officer must consider this factor when making the triage judgment. If the casualty has torn clothing or a wound suspected to be the source of contamination, a different type of decontamination—immediate decontamination—must be performed at the triage or emergency treatment station in the dirty or chemically contaminated area.

Casualties exposed to certain chemical agents such as nerve agents may be apneic or nearly apneic; one of the first interventions required is assisted ventilation. Special, air-filtering assisted ventilation equipment, a chemical mask-valve-bag device (called resuscitation device, individual chemical), is available for use in a chemical environment. However, personnel available to provide ventilator assistance in the contaminated environment are likely to be limited. Also, if a brisk wind is present and the medical facility is far upwind from the source of contamination, very little agent vapor will remain in the air. If no air-filtering ventilation equipment is available, medical personnel must decide whether to ventilate with air that is possibly minimally contaminated or let the casualty remain apneic. Once assisted ventilation is begun, the care provider is committed to the process and cannot care for other casualties, so the number of medical personnel available in the contaminated area influences the ventilation decision. However, a walking wounded casualty (in the minimal category) can quickly be taught how to ventilate other casualties.[7]

Treatment, Decontamination, and Transport Linkage

Triage is always linked to treatment; in a mass casualty event, triage and treatment are also linked to transport. In a chemical weapons mass casualty event, decontamination is also linked, and transport is from the contaminated environment. This linked process occurs at the incident site, and is somewhat duplicated at the MTF; however, different statutory codes, policies, and requirements are relevant in each place. As the preparedness and response efforts for homeland security mature, the tactics, techniques, and procedures used in military settings or homeland settings are converging. Likewise, the regulatory statutes, including best practices, certification processes for equipment, training, and competencies, are showing a pattern of convergence. Further alignment should be driven by such initiatives as development of national resource typing systems (discussed in Other Triage Systems, below) in support of national preparedness goals.

During response preparations, the triage and treatment teams are best placed at naturally occurring bottlenecks as patients are processed through the decontamination corridor (Figure 15-1). At least three triage locations should be placed at the incident site. Triage and treatment teams must integrate their work with patient transport teams (litter bearers and ambulance staff). They must also integrate with decontamination teams, which may be comprised of personnel with very limited medical training. Medical oversight of the patients must be clearly defined and understood by all personnel, including recognition of and proper alerts for changes in patient condition, continuation of any supportive measures, and strict adherence to protocol and procedure.

The initial casualty collection point is located near the border of the hot and warm (contamination reduction) zones. This location allows for initial collection of nonambulatory victims from the incident site in the hot zone and provides shorter distances and cycle times for teams retrieving the casualties from the incident site. It also provides a working environment for medical personnel who are initially uncontaminated. Antidote administration and airway management are the mainstays of treatment at this point. The next bottleneck generally occurs on both sides of the decontamination shelter. Current methods for mass casualty decontamination allow for very limited throughput, even by the most experienced of teams with the best technology, leading to a backup of patient flow at the entrance. These "decon triage" teams provide retriage and basic treatment including airway management, additional administration of antidote, and perhaps more invasive medical intervention.

On the clean side of the decontamination shelter is another typical bottleneck as patients await transport from the incident scene to more definitive treatment facilities. Here, medical personnel are not encumbered with personal protective equipment and are able to evaluate patients in an uncontaminated environment. More invasive medical intervention is possible without concern for further contaminating the patient. A balance among condition, transport times, medical resources, and interventional requirements must be sought in the prioritization and triage of the patients. In incidents conducted in a noncombat situation, such as might occur on an installation during peacetime, first responders adhere to federal statutes for training qualifications.[8]

A somewhat similar scenario occurs at the MTF (see Figure 14–12**)**. At the MTF, training requirements are governed by different regulations than those for the incident site. For example, current Occupational Safety and Health Administration guidelines require 8 hours of hazardous waste operations and emergency response (HAZWOPER) first responder operations level training for first receivers who are expected to decontaminate victims or handle victims before they are thoroughly decontaminated at the MTF. The guidelines include additional criteria for the personal protective equipment levels recommended (level C), no more than a 10-minute time period from patient exposure at the incident site to presentation to the MTF, and a thorough hazard vulnerability assessment to identify specific threats or hazards that might drive additional requirements. Additionally, the hazardous zones are recognized as different from those at the decontamination incident site, referred to as the "warm (contamination reduction) zone" and "cold (postdecontamination) zone" (see Figure 14-12). At

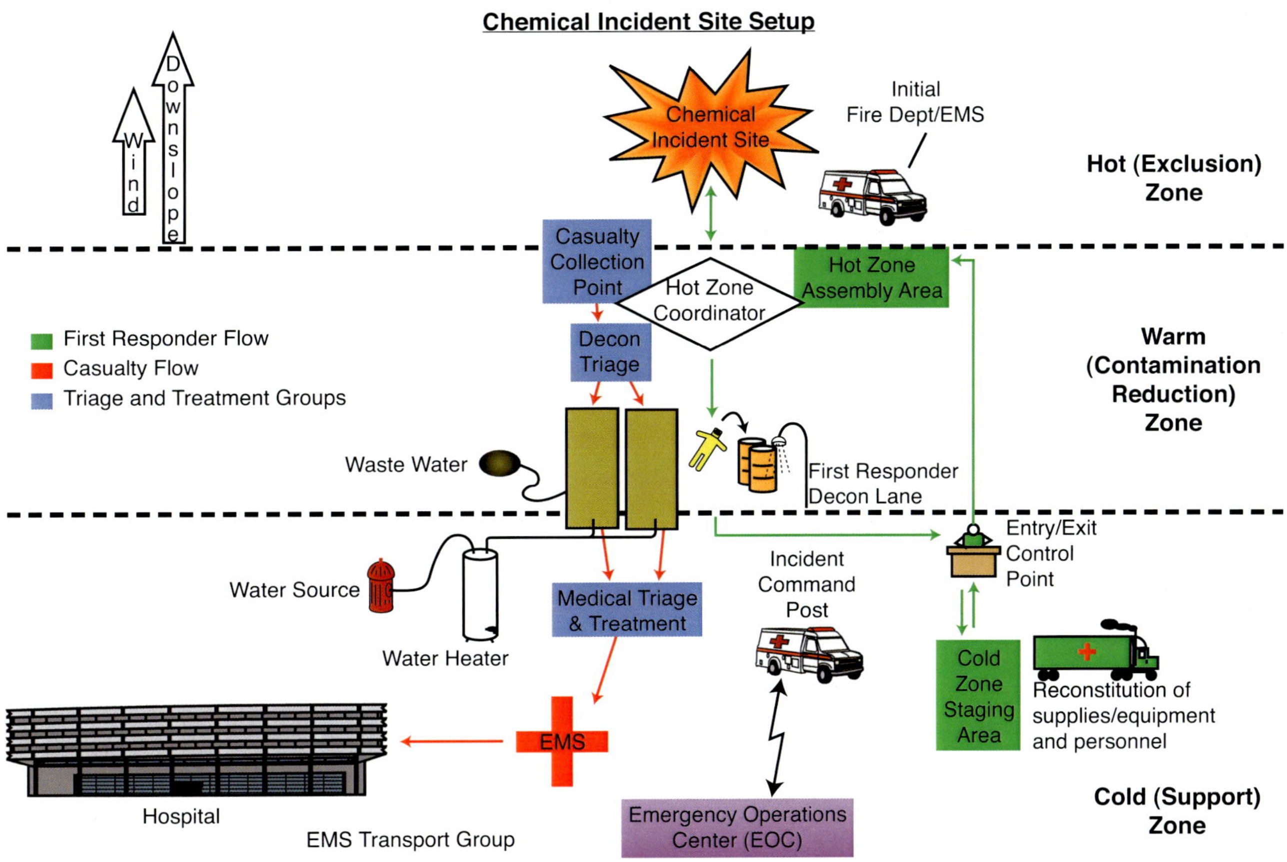

Fig. 15-1. National site setup and control zones for a hazardous materials site. All distances are notional.
EMS: emergency medical service
Diagram: Courtesy of Commander Duane Caneva, US Navy.

the MTF, the casualty receiving and decontamination triage areas are likely to be co-located or simply combined. Additionally, a separate evaluation area may be needed where those who received thorough decontamination at the warm or contamination reduction zone are confirmed clean.[9]

TRIAGE CATEGORIES FOR CHEMICAL CASUALTIES

Chemical casualty triage poses unique challenges beyond the normal triaging of patients with traumatic injuries. Current triage systems are designed for traumatic injuries and, to the degree that they are evidence-based, are based on trauma data. Criteria used, such as respiratory rate and effort, pulse, mental status, and motor function, are specifically affected by many chemical weapons agents; however, correlation with degree of abnormality, course of injury, and survivability is not as well understood as in cases of traumatic injury. Complicating the situation may be the occurrence of combined injury, both poisoning and trauma, if the chemical agent was dispersed through explosive ordnance (see Casualties with Combined Injuries, below). Such a situation requires decisions to be made balancing emergency medical treatments with chemical decontamination: airway management or control of hemorrhage may be equally urgent or more urgent than the treatment for chemical agent poisoning. Emergency medical treatment triage measures may need to be performed simultaneously or in rapid sequence with decontamination procedures.

The simplest form of triage is placing the casualties into treatment priority categories. In a conventional situation (uncontaminated environment), casualties who require immediate intervention to save their lives usually have injuries affecting the airway, breathing, or circulation—the "ABCs"—that can be treated effectively with the assets available within the time available. The second conventional category consists of casualties with injuries that pose no immediate danger of loss of life or limb. Casualties in this group might include someone with a minor injury who merely needs suturing and a bandage before being returned to duty, or someone who has an extensive injury necessitating long-term hospitalization, but who at present is stable. The third conventional category consists of those for whom medical care cannot be provided because of lacking medical assets or time or because the triage officer knows from experience that the casualty will die no matter what care is given. Again, a casualty's classification might change as assets become available or when later reevaluation shows that the casualty's condition was not as serious as first anticipated.

US Military Triage Categories

The triage system commonly used by US military medical departments and by many civilian medical systems, based on the North Atlantic Treaty Organization mass casualty triage standard, contains four categories:

1. Immediate treatment (T1): Casualties who require emergency life-saving treatment. This treatment should not be time consuming or require numerous or highly trained personnel, and the casualty should have a high chance of surviving with the medical treatment.
2. Delayed treatment (T2): Casualties whose condition permits some delay in medical treatment. However some continuing care and pain relief may be required before definitive care is given.
3. Minimal treatment (T3): Casualties with relatively minor signs and symptoms who can care for themselves or who can be helped by untrained personnel.
4. Expectant treatment (T4): Casualties with a low chance for survival whose life-threatening condition requires treatment beyond the capabilities of the medical unit. Placing casualties into this category does not necessarily mean that no treatment will be given; rather, the category determines the priority in which treatment will be given.

These are the categories that will be used in this chapter. This chapter will not cover triage of the conventionally wounded casualty except in the context of combined injury.

Alternative triage categories are emergent (historically subdivided into immediate and urgent), nonemergent (historically subdivided into delayed and minimal), and expectant. Sometimes the term "chemical intermediate" is used for a casualty who requires an immediate life-saving antidote (as in nerve agent or cyanide poisoning).

Triage categories are based on the need for medical care, and they should not be confused with categories for evacuation to a higher-level MTF for definitive care. However, the need for evacuation and, more importantly, the availability of evacuation assets influences the medical triage decision. For example, if a casualty at a battalion aid station is urgently in need of short-term surgery to control bleeding, and evacuation is not possible for several hours, the triage category might be expectant instead of immediate. The evacuation categories are urgent (life immediately threatened), "urgent-surg" (must receive surgical intervention to save life and stabilize for further evacuation), priority (life or limb in serious jeopardy), routine, and convenience (evacuation is matter of medical convenience).[10] The distinction between the urgent and immediate groups has often been ignored, as has the separation of the chemical immediate and immediate groups.

Other Triage Systems

In an attempt to eliminate subjectivity from the triage process, various systems have been created to identify specific criteria for categorization and to correlate these criteria to data from trauma registries; however, very few systems address the impact of chemical toxidromes. Cone and Koenig provide a comprehensive summary of various systems and propose algorithms for chemical, biological, radiological, and nuclear incident types.[11] The commonly used simple triage and rapid treatment (START) system, based on the respiratory rate, pulse, and motor function (collectively referred to as the "RPMs"), provides an algorithm that allows for a patient to be evaluated, classified by color, and receive minimal lifesaving measures within about 30 to 60 seconds. The START process begins with an initial safety survey, followed by the identification of ambulatory patients considered "green," or having minimal injury, to be moved to a safe gathering place, and the evaluation of the remaining nonambulatory victims. These victims are then triaged as immediate (red), delayed (yellow), minimal (green), or expectant (black).[12] Largely objective, the START algorithm is correlated with a trauma registry that identifies which field-measurable physiological parameters correlate with survival and severity of injury. The RPMs are used to determine the revised trauma score for a predictable outcome.[13]

The Sacco triage method (STM) builds on this concept through a more complex algorithm. Using the criteria developed for START, the RPMs are used to provide a revised trauma score ranging from 0 to 12. STM then considers the available resources (eg, receiving hospital beds), transport times, and scoring distribution of all known patients, and optimizes the order of patients by their revised trauma score. For example, if an incident occurs with long transport times, the model predicts that patients with lower scores will not survive. Higher scored patients are thus prioritized for transport first so as to not use limited resources on patients who are statistically unlikely to survive.

Although STM is more complex than other systems, it has several advantages.[14] Like START, its basic evaluation is fairly objective, using criteria correlated to actual trauma data registry. Unlike other systems, STM accounts for other critical factors such as transport times and receiving hospital resources. It also provides a better stratification of critical patients, with a more practical, realistic spectrum of severity of condition. Furthermore, STM recognizes that patients with more severe injury tend to decompensate faster and sooner and considers differing transport times to separate hospitals, as well as the availability of hospitals to receive patients. Through use of an incident management system, STM links on-scene triage and treatment, transport, and patient reception at the hospital, providing the data for a unified command system to secure transport routes. The system can therefore be customized for specific municipalities or operational scenarios, as well as providing strategies to maximize survivability during preparedness and response phases.

Current military doctrine provides limited insight into specific criteria for mass casualty triage in a chemical environment. Although the triage criteria for casualties exposed to a chemical agent may be similar or even the same as those for traumatic injury, substantial differences in the triage process exist. Additional steps in the process of care for casualties exposed to a chemical agent include, for example, the administration of antidote, if efficacious; extraction from the area of chemical exposure; proper management and removal of any personal protective equipment worn by the patient; and medical management through a decontamination corridor. Medical personnel must carry out these procedures while wearing personal protective equipment.

Furthermore, changes in vital signs of chemical casualties are generally predictable given the severity of exposure, but their correlation with injury is not nearly as well understood as that for traumatic injury and vital signs. No easily measurable, dose-response parameters have been predictably correlated to survivability with a known time course for decompensation. No criteria are available, therefore, to prioritize, for example, the evacuation of an unconscious, nearly apneic casualty versus one who is alert and dyspneic. Applying these criteria to an algorithm is further complicated by differing toxicity levels across the general population.[15]

MEDICAL MANAGEMENT OF CHEMICAL CASUALTIES

The initial management and treatment of contaminated chemical agent casualties varies according to the agent as well as the tactical situation. For this reason, each MTF must have a plan that can be modified as needed for specific situations. Unless the chemical agent is dispensed downwind or at the site of the incident, casualties will probably take at least 15 minutes after the exposure to reach a medical treatment area. Furthermore, some casualties will not seek medical attention until effects from the agents are apparent, and an appreciable amount of time may elapse before the casualty is seen.

Nerve Agents

In a unit-level MTF, nerve agent casualties might be classified as immediate, minimal, delayed, or expectant. In a full-care MTF, a nerve agent casualty is unlikely to be classified as expectant because treatment should be available. A nerve agent casualty who is walking and talking can generally be treated and returned to duty within a short period (see Chapter 5, Nerve Agents for a more complete discussion of nerve agent effects and treatment). In most cases, rather than reporting to the triage point, military personnel exposed to nerve agents should self-administer the Mark I or antidote treatment nerve agent autoinjector (ATNAA), either of which should reverse the respiratory effects of vapor exposure. Casualties who appear at the triage station should be classified as minimal because they are able to self-administer the antidote (or it can be administered by a medic), evacuation is not anticipated, and they can return to duty shortly.

Casualties who have received the contents of all three Mark I or ATNAA kits and continue to have dyspnea, have increasing dyspnea, or begin to have other systemic symptoms (such as nausea and vomiting, muscular twitching, or weakness) should be classified as immediate. A source of continuing contamination with liquid agent, such as a break in protective clothing or a wound, should be given immediate decontamination and irrigated with water or saline solution (this procedure is not included in the general advice about decontamination in Warrior Task Training[16]; however, the newest version of FM 8-285[5] directs caregivers to provide treatment as described here). If the casualty is conscious, has not convulsed, and is still breathing, prevention of further illness will ensure a quick return to duty. The casualty will survive unless he or she continues to absorb agent. Also, administration of more atropine should help considerably. With these measures, the progression of nerve agent illness can be stopped or reversed with a minimal expenditure of time and effort in the emergency treatment area.

At the other end of the spectrum, casualties who are seriously poisoned will usually not survive long enough to reach an MTF. However, there are exceptions. If the attack is near an MTF, casualties who are unconscious, apneic, and convulsing or postictal might be seen within minutes of exposure. Or, if the casualties have taken soman nerve agent pyridostigmine bromide pretreatment, they might remain unconscious, convulsing, and with some impairment (but not cessation) of respiration for many minutes to hours. These patients, as well as those in a similar condition who have not used the pretreatment, require immediate care. If they receive that care before circulation fails and convulsions have become prolonged (see Chapter 5, Nerve Agents), they will eventually recover and be able to return to duty.

Supporting this view is a report from the Tokyo subway terrorist incident of 1995. One hospital received two casualties who were apneic with no heartbeat. With vigorous cardiopulmonary resuscitation, cardiac activity was established in both. One resumed spontaneous respiration and walked out of the hospital several days later; the other was placed on a ventilator but did not start breathing spontaneously and died days later. These anecdotes suggest that when circumstances permit, resuscitation should be attempted, for recovery by such patients after nerve agent exposure is clearly possible. In a contaminated area where resources, including personnel, are limited, the use of ventilatory support and closed chest cardiac compression must be balanced against other factors (discussed above), but the immediate administration of diazepam and additional atropine requires little effort and can be very helpful in the casualty who still has recoverable cardiopulmonary function.

Cyanide

Symptoms of cyanide poisoning depend upon the agent concentration and the duration of exposure. High concentrations of cyanide gas can cause death within minutes; however, low concentrations may produce symptoms gradually, causing challenges for the triage officer. Generally, a person exposed to a lethal amount of cyanide will die within 5 to 10 minutes and will not reach an MTF. Conversely, a person who does reach the MTF may not require therapy and could possibly be in the minimal group, able to return to duty soon. If the exposure occurs near the treatment area, a severely exposed casualty might appear for treatment. The casualty will be unconscious, convulsing or postictal, and apneic. If circulation is still intact, antidotes will restore the person to a reasonably functional status within a short period of time. The triage officer, however, must keep in mind that it takes 5 to 10 minutes to inject the two antidotes needed. In a unit-level MTF, a cyanide casualty might be immediate, minimal, or expectant; the last classification would apply if the antidote could not be administered or if circulation had failed before the casualty reached medical care.

In a full-care facility, the casualty might be classified as immediate or minimal.

Vesicants

Most casualties from mustard exposure require evacuation to a facility where they can receive care for several days to months. The exceptions are those with small areas of erythema or with only a few small, discrete blisters. However, even these guidelines are not absolute. If the casualty is seen early after exposure, erythema may be the only manifestation, but it may be the precursor of blister formation. Small, discrete blisters may appear innocuous, but on certain areas of the body they can be incapacitating, rendering a soldier unfit for duty (see Chapter 8, Vesicants, for a more complete discussion).

Mustard casualties, especially those with eye involvement, are often classified as immediate for purposes of decontamination. However, immediate decontamination within 2 minutes can decrease the damage of mustard to the tissues. This classification is not helpful unless the casualty presents to the MTF within 2 minutes of exposure, which is very unlikely because of mustard's latent effects. By the time the mustard lesion forms, the agent has been in contact with the skin, eye, or mucous membrane for a number of hours, and irreversible effects have already begun.

Casualties who have liquid mustard burns over 50% or more of body surface area or burns of a lesser extent but with more than minimal pulmonary involvement pose a challenge for the triage officer. The medial lethal dose (LD_{50}) of liquid mustard, estimated at 100 mg/kg, covers 20% to 25% of body surface area. It is unlikely that a casualty will survive twice the LD_{50}, which would cover about 50% of body surface area, because of the tissue damage from the radiomimetic effects of mustard. Casualties with a burn this size or greater from liquid mustard should be considered expectant. They require intensive care (which may include care in an aseptic environment because of leukopenia) for weeks to months, which can be provided only at the far-rear level of care or in the continental United States. Chances of survival are very low in the best of circumstances and are decreased by delays in evacuation. Furthermore, even in a major hospital during wartime, long-term care will require assets that might be needed for casualties more likely to survive.

Under battlefield or other mass casualty conditions, casualties with conventional thermal burns covering greater than 70% of body surface area are usually put in the expectant group when medical facilities are limited. This percentage is subject to downward modification (in increments of 10%) by other factors, including further restriction of healthcare availability, coexisting inhalational injury, and associated traumatic injury. However, differences exist between conventional burns and mustard burns: conventional burns are likely to have a larger component of third-degree burns, whereas mustard burns are mostly second-degree. On the other hand, exposure to mustard causes problems not seen with conventional burns, such as hemopoietic suppression and the ensuing susceptibility to systemic infection, which is greater than that seen with conventional burns.

Mustard casualties are generally classified as delayed for both medical attention and decontamination. Exceptions are casualties with a very small lesion (< 1% of body surface area) in noncritical areas, who are usually classified as minimal and returned to duty, and those with large burn areas from liquid mustard (> 50% of body surface area) and moderate to severe pulmonary involvement, who are usually classified as expectant. In a more favorable medical environment, every effort should be made to provide care for these casualties; at least those in the latter group should be classified as immediate.

In a unit-level MTF, a mustard casualty might be categorized as minimal, delayed, or expectant, but probably not immediate, because required care would not be available. Even if immediate evacuation is possible, the eventual cost in medical care for a casualty needing evacuation must be compared to the probable cost and outcome of care for a casualty of another type. In a large medical facility where optimum care is available and the cost is negligible, a mustard casualty might be classified as minimal, delayed, or immediate.

Lung-Damaging Agents

Casualties exposed to lung-damaging agents (toxic industrial chemicals) may also present a dilemma to the triage officer. A casualty who is in marked distress, severely dyspneic, and productive of frothy sputum might recover in a fully equipped and staffed hospital; however, such a casualty would not survive without ventilatory assistance within minutes to an hour. This assistance is not possible in the forward levels of medical care, nor is it possible to transport the casualty to a hospital within the critical period. Casualties with mild or moderate respiratory distress and physical findings of pulmonary edema must also be evacuated immediately; if evacuation to a full-care MTF is not forthcoming in a reasonably short period, the prognosis becomes bleak. (These casualties would not be triaged as immediate because the required immediate care is probably unavailable at the forward levels of medical care.) Thus, with lung-damaging agent casualties, availability of both evacuation and further medical care is important in the triage decision.

Peripherally acting lung-damaging agents induce pulmonary edema that varies in severity; a casualty might recover with the limited care given at the unit-level MTF. However, a casualty who complains of dyspnea but has no physical signs presents a triage dilemma: to evacuate this casualty might encourage others to come to the MTF with the same complaints, anticipating evacuation from the battle area, but refusing to evacuate might preclude timely care and potentially cause an unnecessary fatality, and observing the individual until signs of illness appear might also delay medical intervention until the damage is irreversible. Knowledge about the following physical manifestations of peripherally acting lung-damaging agent intoxication may be helpful to the triage officer if a reliable history of the time of exposure is available:

- The first physical signs, crackles (rales) or rhonchi, occur at about half the time it takes for the injury to become fully evident. Thus, if crackles are first heard 3 hours after exposure, the lesion will increase in severity for the next 3 hours.
- If no signs of intoxication occur within the first 4 hours, the chance for survival is good, although severe disease may ultimately develop. In contrast, if the first sign occurs within 4 hours of exposure, the prognosis is not good, even with care in a medical center. The sooner after exposure that symptoms develop, the more ominous the outlook.

Casualties with crackles or rhonchi 3 hours after exposure must reach a medical facility that can provide care as soon as possible. Even with optimal care, the chances of survival are not good. It should be emphasized that these guidelines apply only to objective signs, not the casualty's symptoms (such as dyspnea). In a contaminated area, where both medical personnel and casualties are wearing MOPP 4 gear, it will not be easy and may not be possible to elicit these signs.

In a unit-level MTF, casualties from peripherally acting lung-damaging agents might be triaged as minimal or expectant, with a separate evacuation group for those who require immediate care, if timely evacuation to a higher-level facility is possible. In a large, higher-level MTF, these casualties might be classified as minimal or immediate because full care can be provided on-site.

Incapacitating Agents

An incapacitating agent is a chemical warfare agent that produces temporary disabling conditions that can last hours or even days after exposure. Casualties showing the effects of exposure to an incapacitating agent may be confused, incoherent, disoriented, and disruptive. They cannot be held at the unit-level MTF, but they should not be evacuated ahead of casualties who need lifesaving care unless they are completely unmanageable and threatening harm to themselves or others. Casualties who are only mildly confused from exposure to a small amount of agent, or whose history indicates they are improving or near recovery, may be held and reevaluated in 24 hours. In a unit-level MTF, a casualty from exposure to an incapacitating agent might be minimal or delayed, with little need for high priority in evacuation. In a higher-level MTF, these casualties would be cared for on a nonurgent basis.[7]

Riot Control Agents

Riot control agents, which include irritant agents (eg, CN [chloroacetophenone]) and vomiting agents (eg, DA [diphenylchlorarsine]), have been available for many years and are used in uncontrolled disturbances to render people temporarily incapacitated without injury, although use of the agents includes risks of persistent skin effects, eye effects, and allergic reaction after exposure. Decontamination can relieve irritation of symptoms and decrease risk of injury or delay effects of contact dermatitis. Casualties exposed to riot control agents will most likely not be seen at an MTF, but if they do present with complications, triage according to the nature of the injuries.[17]

TRIAGE BY CATEGORY AND AGENT

Immediate

Nerve Agents

A nerve agent casualty in severe distress would be classified as immediate. The casualty may or may not be conscious; may be in severe respiratory distress or may have become apneic minutes before reaching the facility; may not have convulsed or may be convulsing or immediately postictal. Often the contents of three Mark I or ATNAA kits (or more) plus diazepam and, possibly, short-term ventilatory assistance will be all that is required to prevent further deterioration and death. In addition, a casualty with involvement of two or more systems (eg, neuromuscular, gastrointestinal, and respiratory, but excluding effects on the eyes and nose) should be classified as immediate and administered the contents of three Mark I or ATNAA kits plus diazepam.

Phosgene and Vesicants

Casualties of phosgene (or any peripherally acting lung-damaging agent) or vesicants who have moderate or severe respiratory distress should be placed in the immediate group when intense ventilatory and other required support is immediately available. In a battalion aid station or other unit-level MTF, these support systems may not be available immediately, and would probably not be available during transport to a large medical facility. In general, limited assets would best be used for casualties more likely to benefit from them.

Cyanide

A cyanide casualty who is convulsing or who has become apneic minutes before reaching the medical station and has adequate circulation should be in the immediate group. If circulation remains adequate, the administration of antidote may be all that is required for complete recovery. However, since death may occur within 4 to 5 minutes of exposure to a lethal dose of cyanide unless treatment is immediate, this type of casualty is unlikely to be seen in an MTF.

Incapacitating Agents

Casualties with cardiovascular collapse or severe hyperthermia following the exposure to incapacitating agents such as BZ (3-quinuclidinyl benzilate) should be placed in the immediate category.

Delayed

Nerve Agents

Casualties who require hospitalization but have no immediate threat to life should be placed in the delayed group. This is generally limited to a casualty who has survived a severe nerve agent exposure, is regaining consciousness, and has resumed spontaneous respiration. These casualties will require further medical care but cannot be held in the unit-level MTF for the time necessary for recovery.

Vesicants

Casualties with a vesicant burn between 5% and 50% of body surface area (if by liquid) or with eye involvement require hospitalization but not immediate lifesaving care. These casualties must be observed for pulmonary symptoms and hemopoietic complications. Pulmonary complications generally occur about the same time that dermal injury becomes apparent.

Peripherally Acting Lung-Damaging Agents

Casualties who have been exposed to peripherally acting pulmonary agents such as phosgene with delayed onset of respiratory distress (> 4 hours after exposure) can be placed in the delayed category. For casualties with significant exposure, evacuation should not be delayed because pulmonary edema can rapidly become life threatening. Medical intervention must be initiated quickly for the casualty to survive (as noted above; however, this care may not be available).

Cyanide

Casualties exposed to cyanide vapor who have survived for 15 minutes can be categorized as minimal or delayed.

Incapacitating Agents

Casualties showing signs of exposure to an incapacitating agent (such as BZ; see Chapter 12, Incapacitating Agents) usually does not have a life-threatening injury, but must be evacuated because of long recovery times. A casualty who has had a very large exposure, however, and is convulsing or has cardiac arrhythmias requires immediate attention if it can be made available.

Minimal

Nerve Agents

A nerve agent casualty who is walking and talking and has only mild effects from the agent vapor (such as miosis, rhinorrhea, or mild-to-moderate respiratory distress) should be categorized as minimal. If any treatment is indicated, the contents of one or more Mark I or ATNAA kits will suffice. A casualty who has administered self-aid for these effects may need no further therapy and can often be returned to duty in 24 hours or sooner, if the degree of miosis does not interfere with performance of duty.

Vesicants

A vesicant casualty with a small area of burn—generally less than 5% of body surface area in a noncritical site (but the critical size depends on the site [see Chapter 8, Vesicants])—or minor eye irritation can be placed in the minimal category and possibly returned to duty after treatment. Lesions covering larger areas or evidence suggesting more than minimal pulmonary involvement would place this casualty in another triage group.

Peripherally Acting Lung-Damaging Agents

A casualty exposed to phosgene or other peripherally acting lung-damaging agents rarely belongs in the minimal group. If development of pulmonary edema is suspected, the casualty is placed in a different triage group. On the other hand, if a casualty gives a reliable history of exposure several days before, reports mild dyspnea in the intervening time, and is now improving, the triage officer should consider holding the casualty for 24 hours for reevaluation and determination of return-to-duty status.

Cyanide

A casualty who has been exposed to cyanide but has not required therapy will recover quickly.

Incapacitating Agents

Casualties exposed to an incapacitating agent should be evaluated in a similar manner as those exposed to peripherally acting lung-damaging agents. If the casualty's condition is worsening, evacuation is necessary. On the other hand, if there is a reliable history of exposure with an intervening period of mild symptoms and evidence of recovery, the casualty may be observed for 24 hours on-site and returned to duty.

Expectant

Nerve Agents

Any nerve agent casualty who is pulseless or apneic (duration unknown) should be categorized as expectant. (However, as noted above, some of these casualties may survive if prolonged, aggressive care is possible.)

Vesicants

A vesicant casualty who has burns covering more than 50% of body surface area from liquid exposure, or who has signs of more than minimal pulmonary involvement, can survive only with extensive medical care. This care may be available at rear levels of medical care, but advanced treatment should be initiated for those with the greatest chance of survival.[7]

Peripherally Acting Lung-Damaging Agents

A casualty with moderate or severe dyspnea and signs of advanced pulmonary edema from exposure to phosgene or other peripherally acting lung-damaging agents requires a major expenditure of rear-area medical assets.[7]

Cyanide

A cyanide casualty who is pulseless belongs in the expectant group.

CASUALTIES WITH COMBINED INJURIES

Combined injury casualties have wounds caused by conventional weapons and have been exposed to a chemical agent. The conventional wounds may or may not be contaminated with chemical agent. Limited experimental data on this topic exists, and little has been written about the treatment for combined injury chemical casualties in World War I or the Iran–Iraq War. Uncontaminated wounds should be dressed and treated in the usual way. The wound should be covered with agent-proof (nonporous) material (for additional information, see Chapter 16, Decontamination of Chemical Casualties), and if a pressure bandage is needed, it should be applied after the protective covering. These safety measures may prevent the patient from becoming a combined chemical and conventional casualty. This section will consider the effects of chemical agent poisoning on conventional wounds, the results of treatment for such poisoning, and possible drug interactions of the treatments.

Nonpersistent Nerve Agents

Nerve agents interact with anesthetic drugs, causing increased respiratory depression and reduced cholinesterase activity, which affects metabolism. Blood loss complicates respiratory failure, so casualties may require supplemental oxygen or resuscitation with positive pressure ventilation. Need for replacement of blood lost through conventional injury is increased in the presence of respiratory depression. The action of anticholinesterase (including pyridostigmine pretreatment, to a lesser extent) may potentiate or prolong the action of depolarizing relaxants (eg, succinylcholine).

With nondepolarizing relaxants (eg, vecuronium), the actions are opposed, leading to a higher effective dose. Opiates and similar drugs reduce respiratory drive and should be used with caution in cases of nerve agent poisoning.

Persistent Nerve Agents

When a conventional injury is contaminated by a persistent nerve agent, the danger of absorbing a lethal dose is great and the prognosis is poor. The skin surface surrounding the wound must be decontaminated, followed by application of a surface dressing with a protective cover to prevent further contamination. In a superficial wound the entire skin surface would be decontaminated. Surgery on contaminated wounds poses minimal danger to medical staff when butyl rubber gloves are worn. If these gloves are not available, two pair of latex rubber gloves, washed at short intervals in hypochlorite solution and changed frequently, should suffice. These casualties require careful observation during evacuation to the surgical unit. If signs of poisoning persist or worsen, Mark I or ATNAA treatment should be continued (for further information see Chapter 5, Nerve Agents).

If the wound is not directly contaminated by liquid agent on the skin but the surrounding skin is affected, the casualty should be decontaminated and given the appropriate agent therapy. If the injury is not directly contaminated but skin absorption is thought to have occurred, the skin must be decontaminated. Because liquid nerve agent can penetrate the skin within 2 minutes but the effects from agent absorption into the bloodstream may be delayed up to 18 hours after exposure, the casualty should be kept under close observation during this period and given an autoinjector when indicated.

Vesicants

Vesicant agents weaken those exposed, and the agent's systemic effects could lead to serious delay in the healing of any wound because of depression of the immune system (see Chapter 8, Vesicants, for more information) even if the wound is not directly contaminated. Casualties with a Lewisite-contaminated wound will feel immediate pain disproportionate to the severity of the wound. Early treatment with dimercaprol (BAL) is required. The first responder (medic or buddy) should decontaminate the area around the wound and dress it with a protective material to prevent further contamination.

Thickened vesicant agent may be carried into conventional wounds on fragments and debris. These wounds need to be carefully explored using the no-touch technique. Wounds should be irrigated using a solution containing 3,000 to 5,000 ppm free chlorine for approximately 2 minutes, followed by irrigation with saline (this can be done by squeezing the fluid from intravenous bags into the wound). This technique should not be used in the abdominal or thoracic cavities, or in casualties with intracranial head injuries.

Lung-Damaging Agents

A conventional wound in a casualty exposed to a lung-damaging agent is compounded by development of pulmonary edema. The latent period between exposure and the onset of pulmonary edema may be short. The resultant pulmonary edema may be servere. Casualties exposed to lung-damaging agents should be kept at rest. When indicated, steroid treatment should be started early. The use of opiates and other systemic analgesics to treat pain or shock from the conventional injury is not contraindicated. Oxygen therapy is required; however, fluid replacement should be used with caution to avoid precipitating or increasing pulmonary edema.

Cyanide

Contamination of conventional injuries with cyanide can result in respiratory depression and reduction of oxygen-carrying capacity of the blood. Urgent use of cyanide poisoning antidote is required (see Chapter 11, Cyanide Poisoning). Oxygen therapy combined with positive pressure resuscitation may be required sooner in the presence of marked hemorrhage from the conventional injury. Opiates and other drugs that reduce respiratory drive must be used with extreme caution.

Incapacitating Agents

A casualty presenting with a major wound and intoxication by an incapacitating compound might be delirious and unmanageable. If the compound is a cholinergic-blocking agent such as BZ, the administration of physostigmine may temporarily calm the patient (the effects diminish in 45–60 min) so that care can be given. However, physostigmine may have a limited effect on muscle relaxants used during anesthesia. At various stages the incapacitating compounds cause tachycardia, suggesting that heart rate may not be a reliable indication of cardiovascular status. Otherwise, review of these compounds indicates that they do not interfere with wound healing or further care.[7]

SUMMARY

Triage of chemical agent casualties is a dynamic process based on the same principles as the triage of conventional casualties, with the same goal of maximizing survival. The triage officer must provide immediate care to those who need it to survive; however, the officer is also faced with the task of deferring treatment for some casualties or delaying the treatment of those with minor injuries or who do not need immediate medical intervention. The triage officer should judiciously use valuable resources on casualties who are certain to die or those who will survive without medical care. At the first level of medical care on a battlefield, medical capabilities are very limited. When chemical agents are present or suspected, medical capabilities are further diminished because early care is given by the medical care provider and to the casualty in protective clothing. Decontamination, a time-consuming process, must be carried out before the casualty receives more definitive care, even at this initial level. At the rear level of care, or at a hospital in peacetime, medical capabilities are much greater, and decontamination is anticipated to have been accomplished prior to casualty arrival.

Triage should be based on knowledge of medical assets, the casualty load, and, at least at unit-level MTFs, the evacuation process. Most importantly, the triage officer must have full knowledge of the natural course of an injury and its potential complications.

REFERENCES

1. Rund DA. *Triage*. St. Louis, Mo: Mosby Company; 1981: 310.

2. US Department of the Army. *Health Service Support in a Theater of Operations*. Washington, DC: DA; 1991. FM 8-10.

3. US Department of the Army. *Force Health Protection in a Global Environment*. Washington, DC: DA; 2003. FM 4-02.

4. Veatch RM. Disaster preparedness and triage: justice and the common good. *Mt Sinai J Med*. 2005; 72(4):236-241.

5. Medical management and treatment in chemical operations. In: US Departments of the Army, Navy, Air Force, and Marine Corps. *Treatment of Chemical Agent Casualties and Conventional Military Chemical Injuries*. Washington, DC: DoD; 1995: Appendix C. FM 8-285, NAVMED P-5041, AFJMAN 44-149, FMFM 11-11.

6. Triage. In: Burris DG, FitzHarris JB, Holcomb JB, et al, eds. *Emergency War Surgery*. 3rd rev ed. Washington, DC: Department of the Army, Office of The Surgeon General, Borden Institute; 2004: Chap 3.

7. US Departments of the Army, Navy, and Air Force. *NATO Handbook on the Medical Aspects of NBC Defensive Operations*. Washington, DC: DoD; 1996: Chap 11. AMedP-6(B), FM 8-9, NAVMED P-5059, AFJMAN 44-151. Available at: http://www.fas.org/nuke/guide/usa/doctrine/dod/fm8-9/toc.htm. Accessed on October 18, 2007.

8. 29 CFR, Part 1910.120.

9. Occupational Safety and Health Agency. *OSHA Best Practices for Hospital-Based First Receivers of Victims from Mass Casualty Incidents Involving the Release of Hazardous Substances*. Washington, DC: OSHA; 2005. Available at: http://www.osha.gov/dts/osta/bestpractices/html/hospital_firstreceivers.html. Accessed September 10, 2007.

10. US Department of the Army. *Medical Evacuation in a Theater of Operations: Tactics, Techniques, and Procedures*. Washington, DC: DA; 2000. FM 8-10-6.

11. Cone DC, Koenig KL. Mass casualty triage in the chemical, biological, radiological, or nuclear environment. *Eur J Emerg Med*. 2005;12:287-302.

12. START triage plan for disaster scenarios. *ED Manag*. 1996;8:103-104.

13. Champion HR, Sacco WJ, Copes WS, Gann DS, Gennarelli TA, Flanagan ME. A revision of the trauma score. *J Trauma*. 1989;29:623-629.

14. Sacco WJ, Navin DM, Fiedler KE, Waddell RK 2nd, Long WB, Buckman RF Jr. Precise formulation and eEvidence-based application of resource-constrained triage. *Acad Emerg Med*. 2005;12:759-770.

15. Sommerville DR, Reutter SA, Crosier RB, Shockley EE, Bray JJ. *Chemical Warfare Agent Toxicity Estimates for the General Population*. Aberdeen Proving Ground, Md: US Army Edgewood Chemical Biological Center; 2005. AD B311889.

16. US Department of the Army. *Soldier's Manual of Common Tasks, Warrior Skills, Level 1*. Washington, DC: DA; 2006. STP 21-1-SMCT.

17. Liudvika J, Erdman, DP. CBRNE—evaluation of a chemical warfare victim. *Emedicine* [serial online]. Available at: www.emedicine.com/emerg/topic892.htm. Accessed September 15, 2004.

Chapter 16

DECONTAMINATION OF CHEMICAL CASUALTIES

ERNEST H. BRAUE, JR, PhD*; CHARLES H. BOARDMAN, MS, ORR/L†; AND CHARLES G. HURST, MD‡

*Scientist, US Army Medical Research Institute of Chemical Defense, 3100 Ricketts Point Road, Aberdeen Proving Ground, Maryland 21010-5425

†Lieutenant Colonel, US Air Force; Instructor, Air Force Liaison, and Occupational Therapist, US Army Medical Research Institute of Chemical Defense, 3100 Ricketts Point Road, Aberdeen Proving Ground, Maryland 21010-5425

‡Colonel (Retired), Medical Corps, US Army; Director, Chemical Casualty Care Division, US Army Medical Research Institute of Chemical Defense, 3100 Ricketts Point Road, Aberdeen Proving Ground, Maryland 21010-5425

INTRODUCTION

Decontamination is the process of removing or neutralizing hazardous substances from people, equipment, structures, and the environment.[1,2] This chapter focuses on the safe decontamination of medical casualties exposed to chemical agents; however, the patient decontamination process discussed here also is appropriate for those exposed to biological and radiological hazards (although procedures, operator protective ensemble, and detectors may vary slightly).

Decontamination performed within the first few minutes after exposure is the most effective for protecting the patient, although later skin decontamination, which can benefit the patient by reducing the agent dose, should not be ignored. Early skin decontamination can often mean the difference between patient survival (or minimal injury) and death (or severe injury). Patient decontamination serves two primary purposes: (1) protecting the casualty by removing harmful agents from the skin, thus reducing the dose and severity of the agent's hazardous effects, and (2) protecting emergency responders, transport personnel, medical personnel, and other patients from secondary exposure. Cross contamination from dry or liquid agent on the patient's clothing or skin can sicken others or make equipment temporarily unusable. Cloth fibers can hold agent liquid and vapors. The off-gassing of liquid contaminants, or vapor trapped in clothing and hair, can cause those who work near the casualty to become symptomatic if they are not wearing respiratory protection. Often removing clothing and brushing the hair greatly reduces the level of contaminant carried on the patient; in some instances, these actions are the only necessary decontamination.

Contaminated persons who present for decontamination may additionally have conventional wounds, psychological stress reactions, physiological reactions to heat or cold, or any combination of these. Persons wearing individual protective ensemble (IPE) are particularly prone to heat injuries caused by extended time in this gear.

MILITARY AND CIVILIAN DECONTAMINATION PROCEDURES

The decontamination of chemical casualties is a challenging task that may require large numbers of personnel, water and equipment resources, and time. Casualty decontamination takes place at all levels of patient care, from the exposure site to the door of the medical treatment facility (MTF). In the military, there are three levels of patient decontamination (these same processes may differ in the civilian sector)[3]:

1. *Immediate decontamination* is conducted by the individual exposed to the agent, or another individual (a buddy), who comes to assist the victim, as soon as possible after exposure. Ideally it is performed within minutes after exposure. The individual decontaminates exposed skin and garments using a military decontamination kit. If a kit is not available, any material, dry or wet, that can be applied or used to physically remove agent from the skin is beneficial. This process is very effective in reducing the hazard posed by agent on the skin, particularly if IPE is already being worn.
2. *Patient operational decontamination* is carried out by members of the individual's unit to prepare the individual for transport. At this level the casualty is kept in IPE, from which any large concentration of agent is removed. The casualty is placed on a litter covered with plastic and loaded into a transport vehicle dedicated to evacuating contaminated patients. Evacuation vehicles are kept well ventilated, and crew members wear protective ensemble. Operational decontamination helps to reduce the level of contamination on the patient, thereby reducing the level of cross contamination to the transport vehicle. This level of decontamination allows for large numbers of contaminated casualties to be quickly evacuated to patient decontamination facilities that are prepared to handle them.
3. *Patient thorough decontamination* is performed outside the MTF that receives the contaminated patients. At the decontamination station the patients' clothing is removed and their skin and hair are thoroughly decontaminated. It is critical that patients are prevented from entering a medical facility until patient thorough decontamination has been conducted.

In civilian industry, workers are usually trained in self-decontamination methods pertinent to the hazards for that setting. In a civilian or homeland defense scenario, however, immediate decontamination by the victims themselves may not be possible because they may not have access to decontaminants or know what to do. Immediate decontamination in a civilian setting is often referred to as emergency decontamination, self decontamination, or buddy rescue. The first decontamination in the civilian setting may not occur until a fire department decontamination unit arrives. Patient operational decontamination might not readily apply in the civilian setting because private ambulance services may refuse to accept contaminated patients and civilian patients do not have IPE.

Individuals who escape the scene of the release before the arrival of the first responders may manage to access transportation while still in contaminated clothing. This was the case during the Tokyo subway sarin attack, in which many victims either walked or took taxis to hospitals.[4] Otherwise, contaminated individuals must be moved to a decontamination station established by the fire department or set up at a hospital for patient thorough decontamination. Decontamination stations near the incident site are often referred to as mass casualty decontamination stations or gross decontamination areas.[2,5] Victims might also be moved to a water source, such as a hose or shower, for buddy decontamination. Because fleeing casualties might bypass decontamination, or responding fire departments may fail to perform adequate decontamination, it is important that every hospital has the capability of establishing its own patient thorough decontamination area outside its entrance.

Since the events of September 11, 2001, military and civilian agencies have sought to improve their patient decontamination capabilities.[6] Industry has responded with a wide array of decontamination equipment and materials for simplifying this process. Civilian and military sectors are now much better prepared for the challenges of patient decontamination.

ACTION OF CHEMICAL AGENTS ON THE SKIN

Crone described the function of the skin as a barrier and the possible effect of chemical agents on tissues:[7,8]

> The skin consists of a number of layers of living cells of varied function bounded on the outside by a thin layer of dead cells, the stratum corneum. This layer is the main diffusion barrier to the entry of foreign substances. The blood supply to the skin does not reach directly to the epidermis. Therefore, a liquid contacting the skin surface first has to penetrate the stratum corneum, and then diffuse through the largely aqueous medium of the cell layers to the nearest blood capillaries, from whence it is carried round the body. There is opportunity for a chemical to be bound to the outer skin layers, so that further delay and storage can occur.[7]

Chemicals that act directly on the skin, such as sulfur mustard, need little penetration for their effects to begin; they act directly on the integrity of the skin cells. This same process occurs with other highly reactive chemicals such as acids and alkalis. More systemically acting chemicals, such as nerve agents, may need to cross the skin barrier before they can affect body systems. Generalizations about the permeability of skin are often inadequate.[8] The skin is not a simple system, and its permeability depends on many factors including temperature and the skin's thickness, integrity, and hydration.

The stratum corneum retains moisture and provides a barrier to outside hazards. This barrier is very effective against water-soluble chemicals. However, it is more permeable to fat-soluble (lipophilic) chemicals because of the layers of lipids in the epidermis that underlie and surround the keratinized dead skin cells making up the stratum corneum.[8] When tracing agent progress from the surface of the skin to the bloodstream, three skin "compartments" must be considered: (1) the outer application layer, where the agent lies on the skin; (2) the boundary layer, where the agent is moving through the skin; and (3) the area where a dermal reservoir of agent that has diffused into the lipid area of the stratum corneum may form.[9] Rapid decontamination seeks to prevent large doses of agent from penetrating to the lipid area of the stratum corneum and subsequently into the circulation. Later decontamination seeks to remove any agent that remains on the surface of the skin.

A liquid chemical warfare agent (CWA) is often thought to be accessible on the surface of the skin for up to 3 minutes, taking approximately 30 minutes for the agent to cross the skin barrier and enter the capillaries. Some of the hazardous agent is likely to be temporarily sequestered in the skin during this transit. According to Buckley et al,[10] inappropriate skin treatments could theoretically aid in the dermal transit of agent, and the resulting store of hazardous agent could potentially make the situation worse for the victim.[10]

Most CWAs (particularly VX and mustard) are moderately fat-soluble, enabling them to be absorbed through the stratum corneum over time. Lipid-soluble chemical agents move quickly throughthe lipids surrounding the cells in the stratum corneum and then more slowly into the hydrophilic (water-soluble) bloodstream.

Contact time, concentration, solubility, temperature, hydration state, and physical condition of the skin are all factors that affect the absorption of agent through the skin's epithelial layer. Vascularity of tissue plays an important part in the rate at which agents access the bloodstream and act systemically on the body. Studies by Lundy et al[11] administering VX dermally to juvenile male Yorkshire-Landrace cross pigs and earlier experiments on dermal VX exposure on human subjects by Sim[12] showed that skin that was highly vascularized led to more rapid systemic agent effects as indicated by reduced levels of acetylcholinesterase. Sim's study also noted that VX spread thinly over areas of the skin had much less of an effect on acetylcholinesterase, a reduced systemic effect, than the agent concentrated in one area, which increased the penetration rate (see Exhibit 16-1).

BARRIER SKIN CREAMS

History

Improving the skin as a barrier to chemical agents has been a concern since at least World War I, when sulfur mustard (HD) was first used in warfare. Applying a topical protectant to vulnerable skin surfaces before entry into a chemical combat arena was proposed as a protective measure against percutaneous CWA toxicity soon after Germany used HD at Ypres, Belgium, in 1917.[13] The US Army began examining various soaps and ointments for protective capabilities in the summer of that year. Although several simple formulations were found to be effective in reducing "skin redness" produced by agents such as hydrogen sulfide, no product was available before the end of the war.[13] Research continued but did not produce a fielded product before World War II began. During World War II, a concentrated effort to develop ointments for protection against HD took place at the Chemical Warfare Service, Edgewood Arsenal, Maryland. The Army produced the M-5 protective ointment, which was manufactured in 1943 and 1944. However, because of limited effectiveness, odor, and other cosmetic characteristics, the M-5 ointment was no longer issued to soldiers by the mid 1950s.[14]

EXHIBIT 16-1

VX STUDIES

Lundy et al[1] conducted a study in which 31 Yorkshire-Landrace cross pigs were exposed to pure liquid VX, and VX in isopropyl alcohol. Both of these exposures were at the calculated median lethal dose. In some animals the nerve agent was placed on the ventral surface of the ear (thin tissue with generous blood flow), and on others the agent was placed on the belly just above the naval (thicker tissue with a less pervasive blood flow). Liquid agent absorption was measured by blood cholinesterase inhibition. Those swine with VX applied to the ear showed more than 90% cholinesterase inhibition within 45 minutes, resulting in apnea (within 2 hours) requiring ventilatory assistance thereafter and death within 45 minutes after ventilatory support was initiated. Those animals with belly VX exposure showed only 75% cholinesterase inhibition within the 6-hour timeframe of the experiment, but developed the same progression of symptoms requiring ventilatory support. In neither case were the animals provided with antidotes within the time period that would have slowed or ameliorated the effects. This study demonstrates, in part, that death from liquid VX can be delayed by up to several hours depending on a variety of factors, one being the specific body area exposed. Earlier human studies by Sim[2] also show the variable and delayed effects of exposure to liquid VX.

Data sources: (1) Lundy PM, Hamilton MG, Hill I, Conley J, Sawyer TW, Caneva DC. Clinical aspects of percutaneous poisoning by the chemical warfare agent VX: effects of application site and decontamination. *Mil Med*. 2004;169:856-862. (2) Sim VM. *VX Percutaneous Studies in Man*. Aberdeen Proving Ground, Md: US Army Chemical Research and Development Laboratories; 1960. Technical Report 301.

Skin Exposure Reduction Paste Against Chemical Warfare Agents

Between 1950 and the early 1980s, research focus shifted to medical countermeasures rather than protective creams. Then, a limited research effort at the successor to the Chemical Warfare Service, the US Army Medical Research Institute of Chemical Defense (USAMRICD), produced two non-active barrier skin cream formulations based on a blend of perfluorinated polymers. The two formulations were transferred to advanced development in October 1990.[15] The best formulation was selected and progressed through development as an investigational new drug filed with the US Food and Drug Administration in 1994 and approval of a new drug application in 2000. This new product was called skin exposure reduction paste against chemical warfare agents (SERPACWA). SERPACWA consisted of fine particles of polytetrafluoroethylene solid (Teflon; DuPont, Wilmington, Del) dispersed in a fluorinated polyether oil. The excellent barrier properties of this polymer blend were related to the low solubility of most materials in it. Only highly fluorinated solvents like Freon (DuPont, Wilmington,

Del) were observed to show appreciable solubility. SERPACWA is now a standard issue item to US forces facing a threat of CWA use.

Function

SERPACWA is an antipenetrant barrier cream for use by service members to protect against the toxic effects of CWAs (eg, blister [vesicant] and nerve agents) and percutaneously active biological agents. When used in conjunction with IPE, or mission-oriented protective posture (MOPP) gear, SERPACWA will prevent or significantly reduce the toxicity following percutaneous exposure to such agents. It is used as an adjunct to IPE, not as a substitute. The effective barrier of SERPACWA also has been found to protect against poison ivy and poison oak.

Effectiveness

SERPACWA was developed to extend the protection afforded by the current protective garments and allows a longer window for decontamination. It provides for excellent protection against liquid challenges of GD (soman), VX, and HD, but its protection against HD and GD vapor is less than optimal. It does not neutralize CWAs into less toxic products.

Application

SERPACWA is used at the direction of the commander. Each service member is issued six packets of SERPACWA, sufficient material for six applications or for 2 days of use. Its effectiveness depends on the thickness and integrity of the layer applied and the length of time between application and agent exposure (wear time). The cream should be applied first to skin areas adjacent to IPE closures (such as at the neck, wrists, and lower legs around the top of the boots). If the situation permits, SERPACWA should also be applied to the armpits, groin area, creases and crack of the buttocks, and around the waist. It is not applied to open wounds. It should never be applied to the entire body, because its occlusiveness can interfere with the ability to dissipate heat. Under normal conditions, SERPACWA is effective when spread over the skin as a thin layer (0.1 mm thick, or 0.01 mL / cm^2). One packet of SERPACWA contains 1.35 fluid ounces (about 2.7 weight ounces or 84 g) for one application. This amount of SERPACWA is sufficient to cover the indicated skin areas with a smooth coating that has a barely visible cream color and is slightly detectable by touch.

SERPACWA is not water soluble, so it cannot be washed off by water or removed by sweat without brushing and scrubbing, but it may physically wear off with time. Abrasion of SERPACWA by clothing or other contacts, such as sand or dirt, will reduce the wear time. SERPACWA must be reapplied if the coating becomes embedded with particulate matter (dirt or sand), if the sites are decontaminated, or after 8 hours on the skin. Normally, SERPACWA is effective for 4 hours in preventing CWAs from contacting and penetrating the skin. Insect repellents such as DEET (N,N-diethyl-meta-toluamide) decrease its effectiveness. If DEET is wiped off before application using a dry towel, gauze, or piece of cloth, SERPACWA can still provide significant protection.

Effects on Decontamination

The use of SERAPCWA makes decontamination easier in areas protected by the barrier. It is easier to physically remove CWA from a SERPACWA layer than from the skin. Service members should still perform skin decontamination immediately after chemical contamination, because SERPACWA's effectiveness decreases with time. SERPACWA can be removed by brushing and scrubbing the skin areas with soap and water. SERPACWA has no vapors, so it does not register a false alarm with automatic vapor detectors such as the improved chemical agent monitor (ICAM), nor does it register with systems that detect chemical liquid such as M8 paper. M8 paper, however, detects agent on the surface of the SERPACWA layer (however, it has been noted that if moist SERPACWA paste coats the surface of M8 paper, it can prevent CWA from contacting the paper).

Active Barrier Creams

In 1994, to overcome the limitations of SERPACWA, USAMRICD began development of an improved substance that would act as both a protective barrier and an active destructive matrix to detoxify CWAs. The types of molecules that could potentially neutralize or detoxify CWAs have been known for a long time. These compounds fall into three general classes: oxidizers, reducers, and nucleophiles. The USAMRICD researchers were required to find a final formulation that does not irritate the skin, however, which eliminated many of the most reactive species. The aprotic nonpolar environment of SERPACWA provides a unique but challenging medium for active moieties to neutralize CWA. Reaction mechanisms that do not involve charged transition states are favored in this medium. The improved SERPACWA containing a reactive matrix became known as active topical skin protectant (aTSP). Four criteria were established for aTSP: (1) the protectant must neutralize CWAs including HD, GD, and VX; (2) the barrier properties of SERPACWA must be maintained or increased; (3) protection against HD and GD vapor must be increased; and (4) the cosmetic characteristics (eg, odor, texture) of SERPACWA must be maintained.[16] Additionally, aTSP could not degrade a soldier's performance.

Using the two components of SERPACWA, perfluorinated polyether oil and polytetrafluoroethylene solid, as a base cream, USAMRICD scientists evaluated over 150 different active components. Classes of compounds tested included organic polymers, enzymes, hybrid organic-inorganic materials, polyoxometalates, inorganic composites, inorganic oxides, metal alloys, and small organic molecules. These compounds were incorporated into the base cream to produce over 500 candidate formulations (see Table 16-1).[17]

Two candidate formulations were selected for transition to advanced development. The lead aTSP formulation, a mixture of organic polymers, surfactants, and the base cream of perfluorinated-polyether oil and polytetrafluoroethylene solid, was ready for advanced development in 2004. Although it is not currently funded for further research, this new product is expected to dramatically improve protection from CWAs when it is fielded, and it may reduce the need for a full protective ensemble.

METHODS OF DECONTAMINATION

The first and most effective method of decontamination is timely physical removal of the chemical agent. To remove the substance by the best means available is the primary objective of effective decontamination. Chemical destruction (detoxification) of the offending agent is a desirable secondary objective (but is not always possible). Physical removal is imperative because none of the chemical means of destroying these agents work instantaneously.

The US military has actively explored personnel and

TABLE 16-1

PATENTS COVERING WORK ON ACTIVE TOPICAL SKIN PROTECTANT AT THE US ARMY MEDICAL RESEARCH INSTITUTE OF CHEMICAL DEFENSE

Name	Authors	US Patent No.	Date
Active Topical Skin Protectants Containing OPAA Enzymes and CLECs	Braue EH Jr et al (Hobson, Govardhan, and Khalaf)	6,410,603	6/25/2002
Active Topical Skin Protectants Containing S-330	Braue EH Jr et al (Mershon, Braue CR, and Way)	6,472,438	10/29/2002
Active Topical Skin Protectants Using Polyoxometalates	Braue EH Jr et al (Hobson, White, and Bley)	6,420,434	7/16/2002
Active Topical Skin Protectants Using Polyoxometalates and/or Coinage Metal Complexes	Braue EH Jr et al (Hobson, Hill, Boring, and Rhule)	6,414,039	7/2/2002
Active Topical Skin Protectants	Braue EH Jr, Hobson ST, Lehnert EK	6,472,437	10/27/2002
Active Topical Skin Protectants Using Polymer Coated Metal Alloys	Hobson ST, Braue EH. Jr, Back D	6,437,005	8/20/2002
Active Topical Skin Protectants Using Reactive Nanoparticles	Hobson ST et al (Braue, Lehnert, Klabunde, Koper, and Decker)	6,403,653	6/11/2002
Active Topical Skin Protectants Using Organic Inorganic Polysilsesquioxane Materials	Hobson ST, Braue EH Jr, Shea K	6,417,236	7/9/2002
Active Topical Skin Protectants Using Combinations of Reactive Nanoparticles and Polyoxometalates or Metal Salts	Hobson ST et al (Braue, Lehnert, Klabunde, Decker, Hill, Rhule, Boring, and Koper)	6,410,603	6/25/2002
Polyoxometalate Materials, Metal-Containing Materials, and Methods of Use Thereof	Hill CL et al (Xu, Rhule, Boring, Hobson, and Braue)	6,723,349	4/20/2004

a b

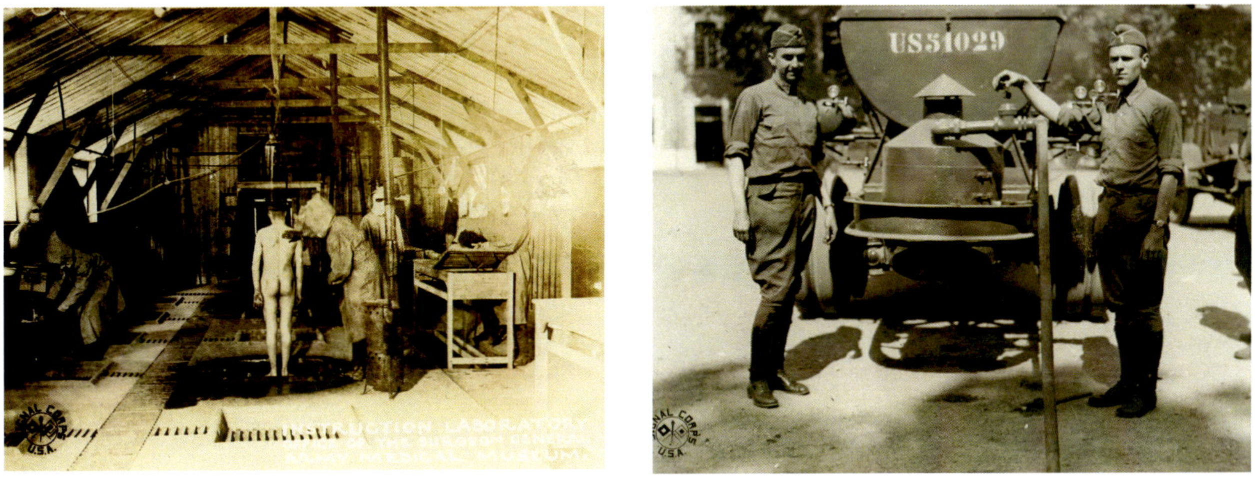

Fig. 16-1. (a) Treatment barracks for gas cases. Evacuation Hospital #2 [ca World War I]. **(b)** Mobile degassing unit #1. Tours, France. November 21, 1918.
Photographs: Courtesy of the National Museum of Health & Medicine, Armed Forces Institute of Pathology (a: Reeve 1179; b: Reeve 12196).

patient decontamination methods since World War I, the beginning of modern chemical warfare (Figure 16-1). Many substances have been evaluated for their usefulness in skin decontamination. The most common problems with potential decontaminants are irritation of the skin, toxicity, ineffectiveness, or high cost. An ideal decontaminant would rapidly and completely remove or detoxify all known chemical (as well as biological and radiological) warfare agents from both skin and equipment (Exhibit 16-2). Decontaminants used for equipment have often been considered for human skin but are found unsuitable because they cause chemical burns.[18]

Recent research has explored the use of water, soap and water, polyethylene glycol and polyvinylpyrrolidone[19]; polyethylene glycol (PEG 300, PEG 400) and glycerol or industrial methylated spirit mixtures[20]; hydrogen peroxide foam mixtures (Sandia foam, Modec Decon Formula)[21]; immobilized enzymes (Gordon sponge)[22–25]; cyclodextrines[26]; ozones (L-Gel)[27]; organophosphorus acid anhydrolases[28]; phosphotriesterases[29]; chloroperoxidases[30]; a mixture of bovine hemoglobin, gelatin, and poi[31]; blends of catitonic and anionic tensides[32]; hydroperoxides and hydroperoxycarbonate anions, dichloroisocyanurate, and oxidants such as sodium hypochlorite and calcium hypochlorite[33]; polyglycol and corn oil[34]; and technology such as the use of atmospheric pressure plasma jets[35] and postexposure cooling.[36]

Currently recommended decontamination materials for US service members that are safe for human skin include soap and water (hydrolysis is probably the most economical choice if water is readily available in ample quantities); dry decontaminants (eg, fuller's earth, M291 skin decontamination kit [SDK]); packaged liquid decontaminants (eg, the Canadian-manufactured Reactive Skin Decontamination Lotion [RSDL; E-Z-EM Canada Inc, Anjou, Quebec, Canada]); and chemical decontaminants that create an oxidative reaction with the agent (eg, dilute 0.5% hypochlorite solution [dilute bleach]). Table 16-2 gives the suggested applications for the various decontamination materials.

HD and the persistent nerve agent VX contain sulfur atoms that are readily subject to oxidation and/or dehydrochlorination reactions. VX and the other nerve agents (GD, GA [tabun], GB [sarin], and GF [cyclosarin]) contain phosphorus groups that undergo alkaline hydrolysis. HD can also be neutralized by hydrolysis or other nucleophilic substitution, but the rate is generally slow. Therefore, most chemical decontaminants are designed to neutralize CWAs by either oxidative chlorination or hydrolysis.[1]

Soap and Water: Hydrolysis

Many classes of CWA, including HD, V agents, and G agents, can be detoxified by reaction with nucleophiles (water is the nucleophile). Chemical hydrolysis reactions are either acid or alkaline. Acid hydrolysis is of negligible importance for agent decontamination because the hydrolysis rate of most chemical agents is slow, and adequate acid catalysis is rarely observed.[8] Alkaline hydrolysis is initiated by the nucleophilic attack of the hydroxide ion on the phosphorus atoms

EXHIBIT 16-2

DESIRABLE TRAITS OF A SKIN DECONTAMINANT

- Effective against chemical, biological, radiological, and nuclear agents, toxic industrial material, toxic industrial chemicals, and new threat agents.
- Neutralizes all chemical and biological agents.
- Safe (nontoxic and noncorrosive) for skin, eyes, and wounds.
- Removes agent from below the skin surface.
- Applied easily by hand.
- Readily available.
- Acts rapidly over a wide temperature range.
- Produces no toxic end products.
- Stable in long-term storage.
- Stable in the short term (after issue to unit / individual).
- Affordable.
- Does not enhance percutaneous agent absorption.
- Nonirritating.
- Hypoallergenic.
- Disposed of easily.

Data sources: (1) Chang M. *A Survey and Evaluation of Chemical Warfare Agent Contaminants and Decontamination*. Dugway Proving Ground, Utah: Defense Technical Information Center; 1984. AD-202525. (2) Baker JA. Paper presented at: COR Decontamination / Contamination Control Master Plan Users' Meeting; 11–13 September 1985. (3) Joint Requirements Office for Chemical, Biological, Radiological and Nuclear Defense. *Joint Service Personnel / Skin Decontamination System (JSPDS)*. Washington, DC: Joint Requirements Office, 2004.

found in VX and the G agents. The hydrolysis rate is dependent on the chemical structure and reaction conditions such as pH, temperature, the kind of solvent used, and the presence of catalytic reagents. The rate increases sharply at pH values higher than 8, and increases by a factor of 4 for every 10°C rise in temperature.[37] Many nucleophilic agents are effective in detoxifying chemical warfare agents; unfortunately, many of these (eg, sodium hydroxide) are unacceptably damaging to the skin. Alkaline pH hypochlorite hydrolyzes VX and the G agents quite well.[1,38,39]

The rate of detoxification of HD in water, however, is slow and depends more on the limited solubility of HD in water (approximately 0.8 g/L at room temperature) than on the reaction rate of hydrolysis (half-life at 20°C is 14.7 min). HD is highly soluble in oils and fats.[40] The hydrolysis rate is not affected by pH and decreases with increasing salt concentration in aqueous solutions (seawater and saline intravenous bag). Using stronger nucleophiles such as sulfides and amines does not increase the reaction rate, because the rate-determining step is the initial formation of the cyclic ethylene sulfonium ion, which forms directly from the HD molecule. Thus, while nucleophilic detoxification of HD is possible, oxidative chlorination is much more effective, although still slow.[8]

Liquids are best for decontaminating large or irregular surface areas. Soapy water solutions are well suited for MTFs with adequate water supplies. Soap and water are low-cost materials that remove agents by hydrolysis and by simply washing them away if used in copious amounts. These solutions do not kill biological agents or neutralize radiological or chemical agents; therefore, water run-off must be collected. Liquid soap acts as a surfactant. The surfactant molecule reduces the water surface tension, making it "wetter" so that it spreads out. Also, one end of the surfactant molecule is soluble in oily substances, and the other end is soluble in water.[41,42] This enables water to better loosen and suspend agent particles in the water so they can be washed away. Fat-based soaps and emulsifiers/surfactants (eg, Dawn dishwashing liquid [Procter & Gamble, Cincinnati, Ohio],[43] baby shampoo, castile liquid soap, or soft soap) are much more effective than detergents that dry the skin (the latter should not be used).[44] Soap and water is best used during patient thorough decontamination, but also can be used for immediate and operational patient decontamination if available and practical. Copious amounts of soap and water should not be used on the joint service lightweight integrated suit technology or similar MOPP garments, because dampening the fabric reduces its protective abilities.

Dry Decontaminants

Any material that can absorb a liquid and then be brushed or scraped off without abrading the skin can be used as an effective skin or equipment decontaminant to remove liquid agents. Clean sand, baking powder, fuller's earth, diatomaceous earth, and baby wipes (dry or wet) can be applied to the agent, allowed to absorb it, and then carefully wiped away. Initially, large quantities of thickened liquid agent can be removed from clothing and skin by scraping it off with an uncontaminated stick or similar device.

Van Hooidonk[45] conducted animal studies to determine the effectiveness of common household compounds for decontamination of liquid agents on

TABLE 16-2

APPROPRIATE USES FOR MILITARY DECONTAMINANTS

Decontaminant	Types of Patient Decontamination Station (PDS)	When and Where Used
M291 Skin Decontamination Kit	All types of PDS with limited water or freezing temperature conditions	For dry decontamination of liquid chemical agents only; very useful if water is not available or ambient temperature is freezing; used on skin and equipment
M295 Decontamination Kit	All types of PDS with limited water or freezing temperature conditions	For the dry decontamination of liquid chemical agents only, used on equipment
Soap and water	Used at all PDSs; the primary decontaminant used at PDSs with plumbed tentage and on water vessels. It is very cost effective.	Used for • skin (copious amounts) • equipment (copious amounts) • washing down decontamination team's TAP aprons and rinsing their gloves after washing with 5% bleach • best for washing away radiological, biological, and most chemical agents, but does not neutralize or kill them
0.5% hypochlorite (bleach) solution	PDSs with minimal equipment.	Used on skin, also can be used to wipe down TAP aprons.
5% hypochlorite (bleach) solution	PDSs with minimal equipment: to wash patient mask hood; decontamination team member gloves. All PDSs: to soak cutting tools (chemical and biological agents only; for radiation use soap and water).	Used only on equipment, NOT skin. Not used with radiological agents. Used for chemical and biological agents to • wipe down rubber mask hoods • wash gloves of patients and decontamination team members (then rinse with fresh water) • fill pail for cutting tools • wash decontaminated litters (then rinse with fresh water) • wipe down equipment (30 min contact time, then rinse)
Locally available absorbent material: • clean sand • baking powder • fuller's earth • baby wipes • flour • bread • other dry, non-toxic, absorbent items	Any PDS	Used for the dry decontamination of liquid chemical agents only on skin and equipment; used if water and M291 or M295 are not available or ambient temperature is freezing.
Reactive skin decontamination lotion (RSDL)	Any PDS	Expected to replace or supplement the M291 kit. Used on skin and equipment for all types of agents. It wipes away contaminants and oximes and neutralizes some chemical agents and biological toxins.

PDS: patient decontamination station
TAP: toxicological agent protective

the skin. They found that wiping the skin with a dry absorbent object (such as paper, aseptic gauze, toilet paper, or a towel) or covering the liquid with absorbent powders, such as flour, talcum powder, diatomaceous earth, fuller's earth, or Dutch powder (the Dutch variation of fuller's earth), and then wiping the residue off with wet tissue paper were reasonably effective for removing both nerve agent and mustards. Either procedure had to be performed within 4 minutes, before the agent permeated the epidermis, to be maximally effective. The study also found that washing with small amounts of water or soap and water was effective for removing nerve agents, but not effective for mustard agents.[45] Fuller's earth and Dutch powder are decontamination agents currently fielded by some European countries to absorb liquid agents.[1]

Developed to absorb and slowly neutralize liquid chemical agent, the M291 SDK (Figure 16-2) was first issued to US forces in 1989 and is the current method of battlefield decontamination used by individual service members. The M291 kit was extensively tested in a rabbit model and proved effective for immediate decontamination of skin.[46,47] Recent studies in the clipped-haired guinea pig model, however, demonstrated that the M291 SDK is only marginally effective against GD, GF, VX, and VR.[48]

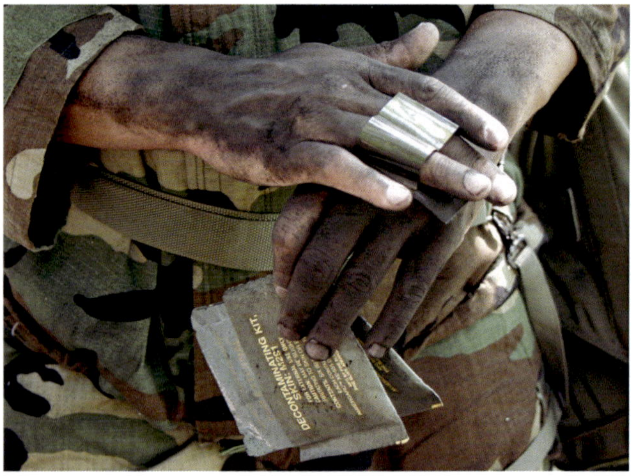

Fig. 16-2. The six individual decontamination pads of the M291 kit are impregnated with the decontamination compound Ambergard XE-555 resin (Rohm and Haas Co, Philadelphia, Penn), a black, free-flowing, resin-based powder. Each pad has a loop that fits over the hand. Holding the pad in one hand, the user scrubs the pad over contaminated skin. The chemicals are rapidly transferred into and trapped in the interior of the resin particles. The presence of acidic and basic groups in the resin promotes the destruction of trapped chemical agents by acid and base hydrolysis. Because the resin is black, the area that has been decontaminated is easy to see.

The M291 SDK consists of a wallet-like carrying pouch containing six individual decontamination packets. Each packet contains a nonwoven, fiberfill, laminated pad impregnated with the decontamination compounds: a carbonaceous adsorbent, a polystyrene polymeric, and ion-exchange resins. The resultant black powder is both reactive and adsorbent. Each pad provides the individual with a single-step, nontoxic, nonirritating decontamination application, which can be used on intact skin, including the face and around wounds, but should not be used in wounds or on abraded skin.[1] Instructions for its use are marked on the case and packets. Small, dry, and easily carried, the M291 SDK is well suited for field use and is particularly useful in areas where water is scarce. It is not effective for removing dry chemical, biological, or radiological agents or for neutralizing them. Early intervention with the use of this kit will reduce liquid chemical agent injury and save lives in most cases.

Packaged Wet Decontaminants

In 2004 the joint services established an operational requirements document to procure an effective skin decontaminant, referred to as the joint service personnel decontamination system, that could be used effectively on the skin and eyes, around wounds, and on equipment against all CBRN agents as well as other toxic industrial materials.[49] In March 2007, RSDL was selected as the joint service personnel decontamination system and is scheduled to replace the M291 SDK.

RSDL is a bright yellow viscous liquid dispensed on a sponge that washes away chemical agent contamination (Figure 16-3). The lotion is a solution of potassium 2,3-butanedione monoximate and free oxime in a mixture of water and polyethyleneglycol monoethylether.[11,50] RSDL can be used to decontaminate intact skin around wounds, but it is not approved for the decontamination of wounds or eyes. Testing at USAMRICD demonstrated that RSDL is superior to the M291 SDK, 0.5% hypochlorite solution, and 1% soapy water against a broad spectrum of chemical agents.[48] It was even effective against a 5–medial-lethal-dose challenge of VX when applied up to 25 minutes after exposure.[51] In addition to VX, RSDL neutralizes the effects of G agents, HD, and T-2 micotoxin.[52] After breaking down the chemical agent or toxin, it becomes a nontoxic liquid that can be washed from the skin with water.[53] RSDL is approved by the Food and Drug Administration as a medical device.[54]

a b

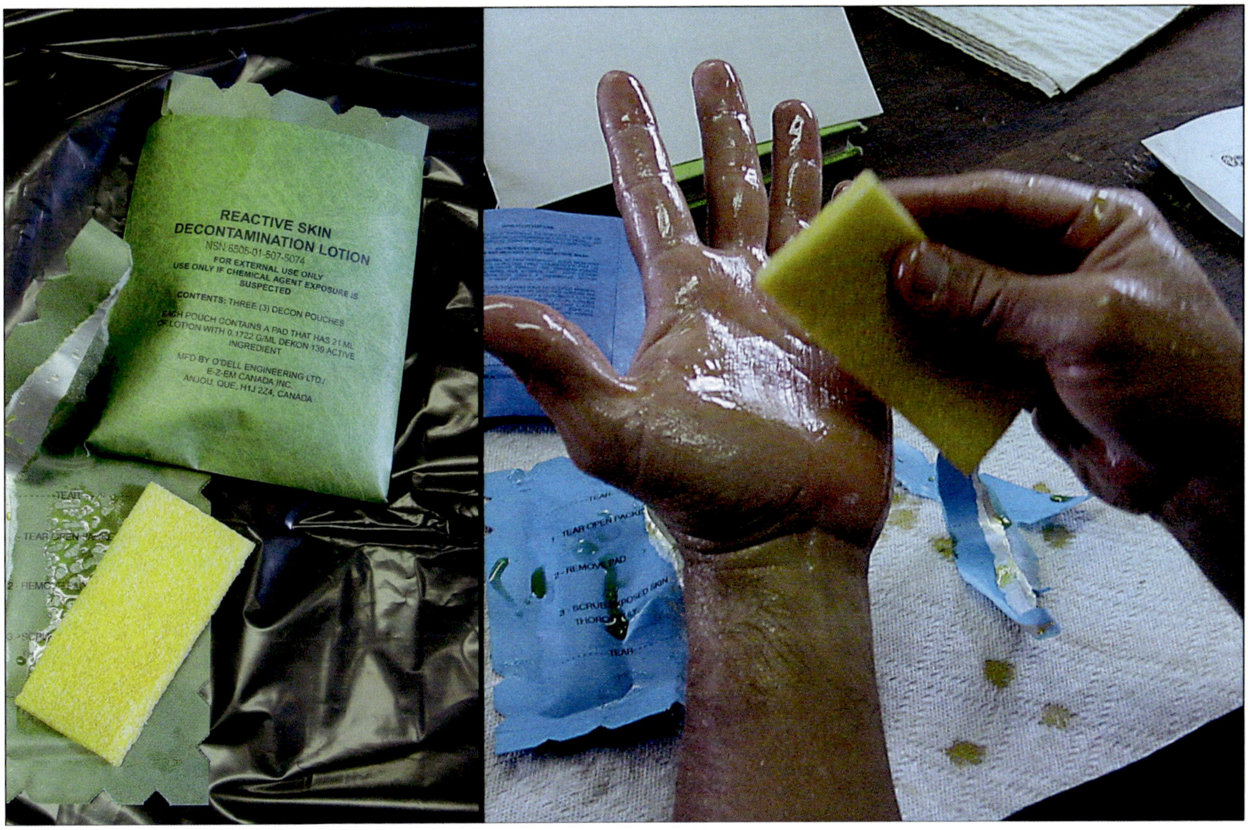

Fig. 16-3. (a) Reactive Skin Decontamination Lotion (E-Z-EM Canada Inc, Anjou, Quebec, Canada) packets and **(b)** blue training packets.
Photographs: Courtesy Lt Col Charles Boardman, US Air Force, US Army Medical Research Institute of Chemical Defense.

The manufacturer (E-Z-EM Inc, Lake Success, NY) also produces a training stimulant (Figure 16-3[b]) without oxime, packaged in a blue pouch, that allows for realistic training and the incorporation of human decontamination into civil defense scenarios.

Chemical Decontaminants: Oxidation

Electrophilic reactions are the oxidative processes associated with CWA detoxification. The most important category of chemical decontamination reactions is oxidative chlorination. This term covers active chlorine chemicals (such as hypochlorite), which under the proper conditions generate the positively charged chloride ion, a very reactive electrophile. The pH of a solution is important in determining the amount of active chlorine concentration; an alkaline solution is advantageous. Hypochlorite solutions act universally against the organophosphorus and mustard agents.[1,8]

Both VX and HD contain sulfur atoms that are readily subject to oxidation. Current US doctrine specifies the use of 0.5% sodium or calcium hypochlorite solution for decontamination of skin and a 5% solution for equipment.[1] Decontamination preparations such as fresh hypochlorite solution (either sodium or calcium hypochlorite) react rapidly with some chemical agents (eg, the half-time for destruction of VX by hypochlorite at pH 10 is 1.5 min), but the half-times of destruction of other agents such as mustard are much longer. If a large amount of agent is initially present, more time is needed to completely neutralize the agent.

Dilute hypochlorite (0.5%) is an effective skin decontaminant for patient use. The solution should be made fresh daily with a pH in the alkaline range (pH 10–11). Plastic bottles containing 6 ounces of calcium hypochlorite crystals are currently fielded for this purpose.[1] Dilute hypochlorite solution is contraindicated for the eye; it may cause corneal injuries. It also is not recommended for brain and spinal cord injuries. Irrigation of the abdomen with hypochlorite solution, which can cause adhesions, is also contraindicated. The use of hypochlorite in the thoracic cavity may be less of a problem, but the hazard remains unknown.[1]

WOUND DECONTAMINATION

All casualties entering a medical unit after experiencing a chemical attack must be considered contaminated unless they have been certified as noncontaminated. The initial management of a casualty contaminated by chemical agents requires removal of IPE and decontamination before treatment within the field MTF.

Initial Wound Decontamination

During thorough patient decontamination at a patient decontamination station, all bandages suspected of contamination are removed and the wounds are flushed with isotonic saline solution or water. Bandages are replaced only if bleeding begins after decontamination. Tourniquets suspected of being contaminated are replaced with clean tourniquets, and the sites of the original tourniquets decontaminated. Both bandage replacement and tourniquet replacement are performed by medical personnel. Splints are thoroughly decontaminated but removed only by a physician or under physician supervision. Once the patient has been thoroughly decontaminated and enters the medical facility, the new dressings are removed and submerged in 5% hypochlorite or sealed in a plastic bag.[55]

General Considerations

Three classes of chemical agent (vesicants, nerve agents, and cyanide) might present a hazard from wound contamination. Hydrogen cyanide is a blue-white liquid with a boiling point of 26°C (79°F). It can be absorbed slowly through unbroken skin but much more rapidly through an open wound. Cyanide may be delivered as pure hydrogen cyanide (liquid or gas depending on temperature), pure solid salt (sodium cyanide), or an aqueous solution of the metal salt. Cyanide is very toxic but less so than vesicants and nerve agents, and therefore less of a concern in open wounds.

Mustard converts to a reactive cyclic intermediate compound within a few minutes of absorption into a biological milieu, and the cyclic intermediate reacts rapidly (within a few minutes) with blood and tissue components.[13] In a wound, the compound reacts with blood, the necrotic tissue, and the remaining viable tissue. If the amount of bleeding and tissue damage is small, mustard will rapidly enter the surrounding viable tissue, where it will quickly biotransform and attach to tissue components, and its biological behavior will be similar to an intramuscular absorption of the agent.

Although nerve agents cause their toxic effects by very rapid attachment to the enzyme acetylcholinesterase, they also quickly react with other enzymes and tissue components. As with mustard, the blood and necrotic tissue of the wound "buffers" the nerve agents. Nerve agent that reaches viable tissue will be rapidly absorbed, and because of the high toxicity of nerve agents (a small fraction of a drop is lethal), casualties with wounds contaminated by liquid nerve agent are unlikely to reach medical care alive.[56] The potential risk from contaminated wounds arises from chemical agent on foreign bodies in the wound and from thickened agents.[57]

Thickened Agents

Thickened agents are chemical agents mixed with another substance (commonly an acrylate) to increase their persistency. They do not dissolve as quickly in biological fluids, nor are they absorbed by tissue as rapidly as other agents. (VX, although not a thickened agent, is absorbed less quickly and may persist in a wound longer than other nerve agents.) Thickened agents are not known to be stockpiled by any country. In a chemical attack, the intelligence and chemical staff should be able to identify thickened agents and alert medical personnel of their use.

Casualties with thickened agents in wounds (eg, from pieces of a contaminated battle-dress uniform or protective garment being carried into the wound tract) require more precautions and are unlikely to survive to reach surgery. Thickened mustard has delayed systemic toxicity and can persist in wounds even when large fragments of cloth have been removed. Although the vapor hazard to surgical personnel is low, contact hazard from thickened agents remains and should always be assumed.[56]

Foreign Material and Off-Gassing

The contamination of wounds with mustard, nerve agents, or cyanide is mostly confined to the pieces of contaminated fabric in the wound tract. The removal of this cloth from the wound effectively eliminates the hazard. Little chemical risk is associated with individual fibers left in the wound. No further decontamination of the wound for un-thickened chemical agent is necessary.[56] Cooper et al[56] reported that the risk from vapor off-gassing of chemically contaminated fragments and cloth in wounds is low or nonexistent, and that off-gassing from a wound during surgical exploration is negligible. Eye injury is not expected from off-gassing from any of the chemical agents, and chemical-protective masks are not required for surgical personnel. However, recent studies[58] indicate that swine exposed to 400 μL of neat HD continue to off-gas up to 48 hours postexposure.

Wound Exploration and Debridement

No single glove material protects against every substance. Butyl rubber gloves generally provide better protection against chemical warfare agents and most toxic industrial chemicals (but not all) than nitrile gloves, which are generally better than latex surgical gloves. Surgeons and assistants are advised to wear two pairs of gloves[44]: a nitrile (latex if nitrile is not available) inner pair covered by a butyl rubber outer pair. Thicker gloves provide better protection but less dexterity. Latex and nitrile gloves are generally 4 to 5 mils thick (1 mil = 1/1,000 of an inch). The recommended butyl rubber glove is 14 mils thick; if greater dexterity is needed a 7-mil butyl glove may be worn. A study at the US Army Soldier and Biological Chemical Command[59] showed breakthrough times for HD and GB depended on glove material and thickness. N-Dex (Best Manufacturing, Menlo, Ga) nitrile gloves (4 mil) had a breakthrough time of 53 minutes for HD and 51 minutes for GB. North (North Safety Products, Cranston, RI) butyl gloves (30 mil) had a breakthrough time of over 1,440 minutes for both HD and GB. The safety standard operating procedure at USAMRICD[60] for working with neat agents requires a maximum wear time of 74 minutes for HD and 360 minutes for G agents and VX when wearing 7-mil butyl rubber gloves over 4-mil N-Dex nitrile gloves. Wearing this glove combination is recommended until users ascertain that no foreign bodies or thickened agents are in the wound. Double latex surgical gloves have no breakthrough for 29 minutes in an aqueous medium; they should be changed every 20 minutes[61] (changing gloves is especially important when bone spicules or metal fragments can cause punctures).[56]

The wound should be debrided and excised as usual, maintaining a no-touch technique (explore the wound with surgical instruments rather than with the fingers). Pieces of cloth and associated debris must not be examined closely but quickly disposed of in a container of 5% hypochlorite. Recent studies at USAMRICD by Graham[58] demonstrated significant off-gassing during laser debridement of HD-exposed skin in swine. Removed fragments of tissue should be dropped into a container of 5% to 10% hypochlorite. Bulky tissue such as an amputated limb should be sealed in a chemical-proof plastic or rubber bag.[56] Penetrating abdominal wounds caused by large fragments or containing large pieces of chemically contaminated cloth will be uncommon. Surgical practices should be effective in the majority of wounds for identifying and removing the focus of remaining agent within the peritoneum.

Cooper et al[56] suggest checking a wound with an ICAM, which may direct the surgeon to further retained material. However, this process is slow (a stable reading takes about 30 seconds; a rapid pass over the wound will not detect remaining contamination) and is not effective unless vapors are emanating from wound debris. A single bar reading on an ICAM with the inlet held a few millimeters from the wound surface indicates that a vapor hazard does not exist; more than one bar is needed to indicate a vapor has been detected.[56]

Dilute hypochlorite solution (0.5%) should not be used to flush wounds. Isotonic saline or water may be instilled into deep, noncavity wounds following the removal of contaminated cloth. Subsequent irrigation with saline or other surgical solutions should be performed.[1] Saline, hydrogen peroxide, or other irrigating solutions do not necessarily decontaminate agents but may dislodge material for recovery by aspiration with a large-bore suction tip. The irrigation solution should not be swabbed out manually with surgical sponges; rather, it should be removed by suction to a disposal container and handled like other agent-contaminated waste within a short time (5 min). Although the risk to patients and medical attendants is low, safe practice suggests that any irrigation solution should be considered potentially contaminated. Following aspiration by suction, the suction apparatus and the solution should be decontaminated in a solution of 5% hypochlorite. Superficial wounds should be subjected to thorough wiping with normal saline or sterile water.[1]

Instruments that have come into contact with possible contamination should be placed in 5% hypochlorite for 10 minutes before normal cleansing and sterilization. Reusable linen should be checked with the ICAM, M8 paper, or M9 tape for contamination. If found to be contaminated, the linen should be soaked in a 5% to 10% hypochlorite solution or discarded.[1]

PATIENT THOROUGH DECONTAMINATION

Need

The focus of patient decontamination is identical throughout the services and in the civilian sector: it is the removal of hazardous substances from the contaminated individual to protect that person and subsequently reduce the incidence of cross contamination to others. Early removal of the hazardous substance is key to significantly reducing the dose of agent an individual is exposed to. When early removal (within the first 15 minutes—ideally within the first 2 minutes) is not possible, later removal can reduce the effects from a chemical agent but to a lesser degree. Removal at any time reduces the threat that others may be cross-contaminated. Patient thorough decontamination, performed before allowing a contaminated patient inside the confines of a hospital, provides two benefits. First, it can potentially reduce the dose the patient receives, and, second, it protects hospital staff from exposure to the hazardous agent and its vapors.

In the United States, healthcare workers are the 11th most common group injured in hazardous materials incidents, but injury to emergency department workers is even more infrequent, only 0.2% of some 2,562 events from 1995 to 2001 documented in the Agency for Toxic Substances and Disease Registry Hazardous Substance Emergency Events Surveillance System.[44] In these instances, the injured workers were not wearing respiratory protection and suffered eye and respiratory tract irritation.[62]

Several studies and reports illustrate the need for the thorough decontamination of patients before hospital admission. Okumura et al[63] published a survey of the staff of Saint Luke's International Hospital in Tokyo. This facility was closest to the Tokyo subway sarin release and received 640 patients, the largest number of victims from the event. The study indicated that 110 staff members, 23% of the 472 medical personnel in the hospital at the time, reported acute poisoning symptoms including headache, blurred vision, dyspnea, nausea, and dizziness. None of the staff at this facility wore respiratory protection, and none of the patients were decontaminated in any way. Particularly affected were staff working in the hospital temporary triage area, which was located in the poorly ventilated hospital chapel, and those in the intensive care unit.[63]

Nozaki et al[64] conducted a retrospective study of care providers at another facility, the University Hospital of Metropolitan Japan, who also attended to subway victims. Of the 15 physicians who worked in the emergency room, none wore any protective equipment; 13 became aware of symptoms of exposure while resuscitating two of the casualties. Eleven of these doctors complained of dim vision lasting several days, and eight showed significant miosis (pupils < 2 mm). Eight had rhinorrhea (runny nose), four had dyspnea (shortness of breath or tightness of the chest), and two had a cough. Six of the symptomatic care providers were given atropine sulfate, and one, who had more predominant dim vision than the others, was also given pralidoxime methiodide. Subsequent removal of the patients' contaminated clothing and ventilation of the emergency room helped reduce exposure.[64] Table 16-3 summarizes the signs and symptoms displayed by medical personnel at St Luke's and University hospitals.

Similarly, reports by Foroutan[65] indicate that unprotected medical staff caring for contaminated Iranian victims of an Iraqi poison chemical gas bombardment also became ill. In one instance, a doctor and a nurse providing patient resuscitation in a busy treatment area became dizzy, were short of breath, and had severe headaches and cough. Within 5 minutes the remainder of the medical staff in the emergency room developed the same symptoms, could no longer stand up, and had to sit on the floor. The staff was evacuated to another hospital and the emergency room closed and ventilated for 3 hours. In this case both cyanide antidotes and later atropine were administered, which reduced the providers' symptoms.[65]

Another documented relevant example took place in 2001 in the emergency room of a hospital in an agricultural area of Great Britain. Pesticides are among the top choices for those committing suicide and homicide, particularly in agricultural regions of the world.[66] A man who attempted suicide by ingesting an organophosphate pesticide was brought into the emergency room, where he vomited, causing a chemical spill. The incident caused 25 hospital workers to seek medical attention, and 10 complained of symptoms indicative of toxic exposure.[67] These events illustrate the importance of thorough decontamination for contaminated patients, prompt clean-up of pesticide-tainted vomit, and adequate protection, particularly respiratory protection, for hospital workers when vapor hazard from contamination exists.

Personnel

Patient thorough decontamination operations are personnel intensive. Typically from 7 to 20 personnel are needed to staff decontamination teams, not including medical treatment personnel. In the military, with the exception of the US Air Force and some ship-based units that deploy trained patient decontamination teams composed of medical personnel, the military patient decontamination process is carried out by nonmedical augmentees supervised by trained medical personnel.[3] In the civilian sector gross decontamination is often performed by fire departments or hazardous materials (HAZMAT) teams, and thorough decontamination at medical facilities is carried out by hospital personnel assigned to perform the job as an additional duty.[2,68]

TABLE 16-3

SIGNS AND SYMPTOMS REPORTED BY TOKYO HOSPITAL WORKERS TREATING VICTIMS OF SARIN SUBWAY ATTACKS*

Symptom	Number/percentage of the 15 physicians who treated patients at UH		Number/percentage of 472 care providers reporting symptoms at SLI	
Dim vision	11	73%	66	14%
Rhinorrhea	8	53%	No information	
Dyspnea (chest tightness)	4	27%	25	5.3%
Cough	2	13%	No information	
Headache	No information		52	11%
Throat pain	No information		39	8.3%
Nausea	No information		14	3.0%
Dizziness	No information		12	2.5%
Nose pain	No information		6	1.9%

*Data reflect reported survey of self-reported symptomatology of physicians at the University Hospital of Metropolitan Japan emergency department and all hospital workers at Saint Luke's International Hospital exposed to sarin vapors from victims of the Tokyo subway attack.
SLI: Saint Luke's International Hospital
UH: University Hospital
Data sources: (1) Nozaki H, Hori S, Shinozawa Y, et al. Secondary exposure of medical staff to sarin vapor in the emergency room. *Intensive Care Med.* 1995;21:1032-1035. (2) Okumura T, Suzuki K, Fukuda A, et al. The Tokyo subway sarin attack: disaster management, Part 1: community emergency response. *Acad Emerg Med.* 1998;5:613-617. (3) Okumura T, Suzuki K, Fukuda A, et al. The Tokyo subway sarin attack: disaster management, Part 2: Hospital response. *Acad Emerg Med.* 1998;5:618-624.

Close medical monitoring and treatment of casualties before, during, and after thorough decontamination must be an integral part of all patient decontamination operations. Medical conditions can change as individuals undergo the stressful process of decontamination. If the exposure is to a liquid agent, it may take time for the agent to transit the skin layers. A patient exposed to a liquid chemical agent may appear stable or well during decontamination but can become worse during or after the decontamination process.

Decontamination Operator Protection

Heat and musculoskeletal injury are primary concerns for decontamination team members. Individuals must perform heavy work (patient treatment, triage, and litter movement) while wearing IPE. Working in a hot environment lowers individual mental alertness and physical performance. Increased body temperature and physical discomfort can cause workers to overlook safety procedures or divert their attention from hazardous tasks. These critical issues must be addressed before and throughout decontamination operations.

Musculoskeletal injury can occur from lifting patients, carrying litters, or falling while wearing protective ensemble. Injury reduction strategies such as removing tripping hazards, policing the decontamination area for debris, working at a safe pace, rehearsing ergonomically correct patient lifts, enforcing frequent rest breaks, using special equipment to reduce lifting (such as wheeled litter carriers), and insuring adequate staffing are all useful strategies to prevent worker injury.

The chemical protective ensemble prevents an individual's sweat from readily making contact with the air, which inhibits heat transfer from the body, making it difficult for the body to cool itself, which can lead to heat injury. The National Institute for Occupational Safety and Health publication *Working in Hot Environments* describes a variety of heat conditions including heat stroke (the most life threatening), heat exhaustion, heat cramps, fainting, heat rash, and transient heat fatigue.[69] All decontamination personnel must be trained in preventative measures for these conditions, be able to identify their signs and symptoms, and know what to do when they occur. It typically takes humans 5 to 7 days to adjust to working in hot temperatures. Heat stress can be reduced by reducing prolonged exposure to heat. Effective measures include enforcing work–rest cycles; providing shaded work and rest areas; reducing the amount of protective ensemble worn (eg, wearing level C during decontamination operations or only respiratory protection if the principal chemical hazard is vapor); and maintaining adequate supplies of potable water and encouraging its consumption by decontamination team members.

A safety officer must be appointed whose primary duty during decontamination operations is to monitor the health status of decontamination team members in IPE. This individual enforces safe patient lifting techniques, insures the decontamination area is free from debris that can cause a tripping hazard, manages team member work–rest cycles, stays abreast of temperature conditions, and insures that adequate fluids are available and used by decontamination team members.

Occupational Safety and Health Administration (OSHA) first receiver guidance suggests that medical monitoring of decontamination personnel should be conducted before protective ensemble is donned or soon after, during rest breaks in the warm area, and after decontamination operations. These measures are particularly important when temperatures in the work area exceed 70°F (21°C). Monitoring may not be practical on the battlefield or in the fast-paced mass casualty environment; however, it is a useful measure to prevent heat injury during training and should be integrated into exercises when feasible. The American Heart Association–recommended safe limits are noted in Table 16-4. Automated wrist cuffs are now available that make ongoing blood pressure monitoring of workers in IPE much easier. Readings taken through IPE, however, may not be accurate. Individuals with elevated readings who are not under work or anxiety duress should receive particular attention.[44]

In the field, a more practical way to reduce both heat and musculoskeletal injury is to distribute the

TABLE 16-4

AMERICAN HEART ASSOCIATION RECOMMENDED VALUES FOR SAFE CARDIOVASCULAR FUNCTION

Function	Value
Blood pressure (max)	140 bpm systolic / 100 bpm diastolic
Pulse rate (max)	100 bpm
Temperature	min: 98.0°F (36.6°C) max: 99.2°F (37.3°C) or +/- 0.6°F (1.08°C) from normal

bpm: beats per minute

EXHIBIT 16-3

OCCUPATIONAL SAFETY AND HEALTH ADMINISTRATION LEVELS OF PERSONAL PROTECTIVE EQUIPMENT

Level A Provides the greatest level of skin and respiratory protection. Level A consists of a totally encapsulating suit with gloves and boots attached. A self-contained breathing apparatus (SCBA) is worn inside the suit, or a supplied-air system (with escape SCBA) is used for respiratory protection.

Level B Used when the highest level of respiratory protection is necessary, but a lesser level of skin and eye protection is needed. This level consists of nonencapsulating, chemical-resistant suits, often called splash suits or rain suits. The SCBA or a supplied-air system is worn either inside or outside the suit, depending on the configuration.

Level C Worn when the concentration and type of airborne substance is known and the criteria for using air purifying respirators are met. The level C ensemble consists of a full facepiece, an air-purifying respirator, and a chemical agent-resistant suit. Military MOPP 4 is similar to level C. Level C is the preferred IPE for decontamination operators (first receivers).

Level D A work uniform affording minimal protection. The military battle dress uniform, Army combat uniform, or coveralls meet the requirements for level D protection.

IPE: individual protective ensemble
MOPP: mission-oriented protective posture
SCBA: self-contained breathing apparatus
Adapted from: US Departments of the Army, Marine Corps, Navy, and Air Force, and Marine Corps. *Multiservice Tactics and Procedures for Nuclear, Biological, and Chemical (NBC) Protection*. Washington, DC: DoD; 2003. FM 3-11.4, MCWP 3-37.2, NTTP 3-11.27, AFTTP (I) 3-2.46.

workload among team members. Failure to enforce appropriate work–rest cycles increases the risk of injury and ultimately depletes personnel pools on subsequent days. Work–rest cycles insure adequate hydration, give the body an opportunity to disperse excessive heat, and slow down the production of internal body heat created during physical work. Chapter 14, Field Management of Chemical Casualties, provides further discussion on work–rest cycles and a table for calculating them.

EQUIPMENT FOR PATIENT THOROUGH DECONTAMINATION

Individual Protective Equipment

All decontamination team members must wear IPE for their protection.[3,44] OSHA and the Federal Chemical Stockpile Emergency Preparedness Program recommend OSHA level C as the most appropriate wear for first receivers, which include decontamination team members.[44,70,71] In the military, MOPP level 4 is roughly equivalent to OSHA level C. OSHA levels A and B (Exhibit 16-3) are normally worn at an incident site (hot zone; Exhibit 16-4) when the contamination is unknown. This high level of protection, which creates an additional heat burden on the worker and restricts mobility, is not necessary for decontamination operations in the warm zone, where the chemical risk is greatly reduced. For more information on OSHA levels see Chapter 17, Chemical Defense Equipment.

Decontamination team members using dry decontaminants, water, soap and water, or other liquid decontaminants must wear IPE that allows for easy operator wipe down. The IPE must also prevent undergarments from being saturated with water if water is used during decontamination. Torngren et al[72] showed that aerosolized agent simulants and their vapors penetrate protective equipment that becomes saturated with water during patient decontamination operations.[72] In this study, the wet underwear of the decontamination operators became contaminated. Preventing this saturation is best accomplished by

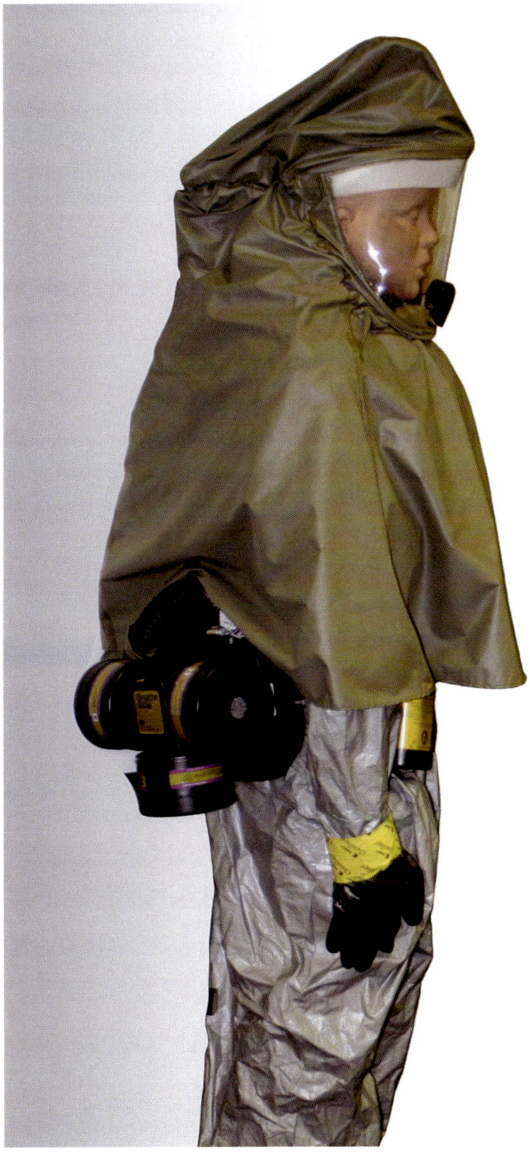

Fig. 16-4. An example of a hooded, powered air pressure respirator with a Tyvek F [(DuPont, Wilmington, Del) overgarment. Note the filter power unit worn at the waist. Photograph by Peter Hurst, US Army Medical Research Institute for Chemical Defense.

EXHIBIT 16-4

ZONES OF CONTAMINATION

Hot zone: Area of agent release that is directly contaminated.

Warm zone (or decontamination zone): Area outside the hot zone where contamination consists only of that brought into the area by contaminated patients and workers from the hot zone.

Cold zone (postdecontamination zone): Area beyond the warm zone that is free of solid, liquid, and vapor contamination. Patients are decontaminated before entering this area.

wearing a butyl rubber toxicological agent protective apron over IPE or wearing IPE that is impermeable to water (eg, Tyvek F [DuPont, Wilmington, Del]). These impermeable garments, however, increase the heat load on the worker. Protective aprons serve several purposes: they allow team members to easily decontaminate themselves between patients, keep undergarments free from contaminated moisture, and allow workers the option to remove this layer and more easily cool themselves in a rest area.

Military decontamination team members may wear the standard military M40 series, MCU2P, or new joint service general-purpose mask (see Chapter 17, Chemical Defense Equipment, for more information). An alternative is to wear a powered-air purifying respirator, which has a blower motor that pulls air through filters and into the mask hood (Figure 16-4). The circulated air blown into the mask hood helps keep the wearer cool, eliminates the effort to inhale air through filters, and reduces carbon dioxide buildup in the mask during heavy work. Produced by several companies, these masks must be rated at a protective factor of 1,000, per OSHA first receiver guidance, and should be approved by the National Institute of Occupational Safety and Health.[44] OSHA also dictates that all individuals must be medically cleared to wear full-face protective masks and equipment.[73] A variety of voice amplifiers that fit to the mask, throat or voice-activated microphones that work with head-mounted radios, and other types of communications systems that improve communication with mask use are available on the market.

Transport Equipment

Only litters or backboards made of plastic material that can be readily and thoroughly decontaminated should be used to hold contaminated patients. Cloth litters will hold agent, cannot be decontaminated effectively, and rapidly deteriorate when decontaminated with bleach solution.

Detection Devices

Detectors and monitors can be used at the arrival point, to assess which patients require decontamination, or after the decontamination process, to check for thoroughness of decontamination. In some instances the thoroughness of the decontamination process may make detectors less necessary (for example, when plumbed tent systems are used and ample supplies of soapy water and rinse water are available). The use of detectors is dictated by unit operating plans and specific service concepts of operation and tactics, techniques, and procedures.

Currently fielded chemical warfare agent detection and monitoring equipment does not identify all possible CWAs or toxic industrial chemicals (see Chapter 17, Chemical Defense Equipment for more detail). Existing military chemical detectors that can be useful during patient decontamination operations include M8 chemical detector paper, M9 chemical detector paper, the ICAM, the M22 automatic chemical agent detector alarm, and the HAPSITE Smart Chemical Identification System (INFICON, East Syracuse, NY).[55]

Decontamination Shelters

Decontamination equipment varies from the simple use of buckets and sponges, or the use of fire trucks to spray down victims, to the more complex deployment of pop-up shelters or patient decontamination systems built on existing medical facilities. The variety of decontamination equipment has dramatically expanded since the terrorist events of September 11, 2001. Most decontamination systems use soap and water as the primary decontaminant. Some examples are shown in Figures 16-5 through 16-7. Shelters differ in construction, method of erection, plumbing, and system for moving litters. All of these factors can impact on overall system weight, durability, ease of set-up and tear down, and shelter footprint.

Decontamination shelters are useful for a variety of reasons. They protect decontamination workers and patients from wind and poor weather conditions, as well as providing privacy for patients during the decontamination process. Shelters provide a framework to support built-in plumbing, which makes set-up and processing of patients faster and easier than using buckets and sponges. Some degree of water pressure is necessary to operate the systems. Each system requirement is different, but the ideal system incorporates a high volume of water at low pressure.[2] Air and water heaters should be added to improve patient comfort. Roller systems can be incorporated to more rapidly process litter patients while reducing the incidence of musculoskeletal injuries among decontamination workers. Roller systems also reduce the number of workers necessary to perform decontamination procedures. A crew of 12 is recommended by the Air Force for decontamination shelter operations, but the process can be performed with a staff (not including medical personnel) of four individuals for the litter line, one for the ambulatory line, and two for the clean (cold) side of the hot line (or liquid control line).[74,75] More individuals, encompassing several shifts, are needed to insure adequate rest cycles to reduce injury to decontamination operators. A variety of roller systems that differ in weight, ease of portability, and ease of

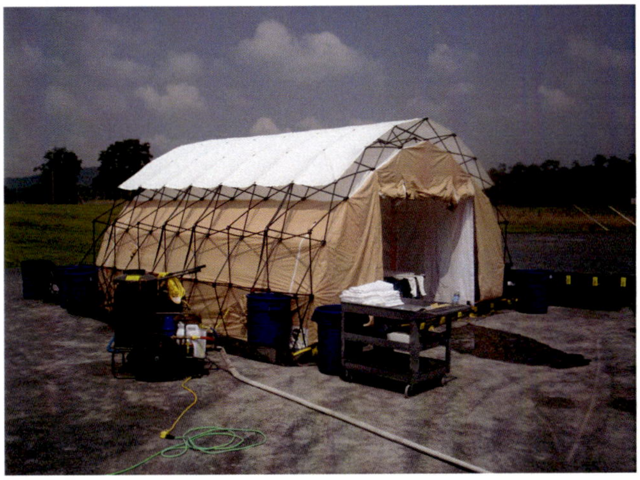

Fig. 16-5. TVI (TVI Corporation Inc, Glenn Dale, Md) decontamination pop-up shelter consisting of a light-weight scissor frame tent, integrated plumbing, heater, water bladder, and quickly expandable light-weight roller system with backboard. It can easily be erected within a few minutes by two individuals. Shown is a small size tent. Can be configured for both ambulatory and litter patients.
Photograph: Courtesy TVI Corporation.

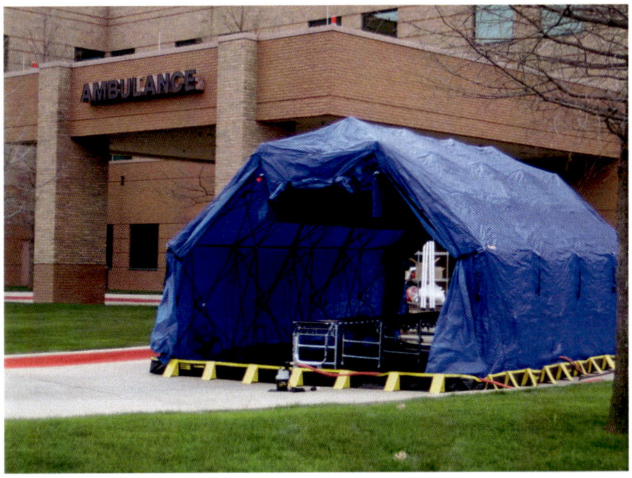

Fig. 16-6. A medium sized Reeves DRASH (deployable rapid assembly shelter). The scissors construction allows for tent expansion similar to the TVI tent but with the framework on the inside of the shelter. It also has integrated plumbing and a litter roller system. Can be configured for both ambulatory and litter patients.
Photograph: Courtesy of Lt Col Charles Boardman, US Air Force, US Army Medical Research Institute of Chemical Defense. Reproduced with permission from Reeves EMS LLC, Orangeburg, NY.

assembly are on the market.

OSHA's recommended best practice for fixed facilities such as hospitals is to build decontamination facilities outside the building or near the emergency entrance.[44] Fixed decontamination facilities allow for immediate decontamination of casualties because no set-up time is required. A well trained crew can typically set up a pop-up decontamination shelter in 10 to 20 minutes, depending on the type of equipment used.[76] For units expected to assist in decontamina-

a

b

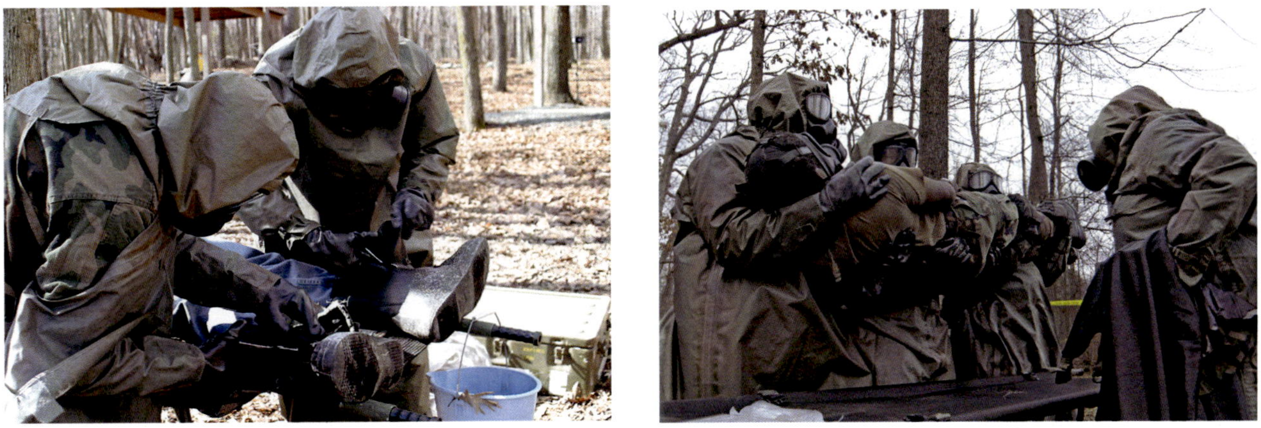

Fig. 16-7. The US Army's method of using litter stands, buckets, and sponges. This process requires more frequent lifting of patients and water buckets than shelters with roller systems. The advantage, on the battlefield, is that this decontamination equipment is easy to carry. Ample quantities of water are still needed unless dry decontamination is used. This method is currently preferred by Army field units that cannot carry large quantities of equipment.
Photographs: Courtesy of Lt Col Charles Boardman, US Air Force, US Army Medical Research Institute of Chemical Defense, and Peter Hurst, US Army Medical Research Institute of Chemical Defense.

tion operations near an incident site, pop-up shelters or covered configurations of fire trucks that allow for privacy and some protection from the elements are preferred.

ESTABLISHING A PATIENT THOROUGH DECONTAMINATION AREA

Patient thorough decontamination areas are established in locations considered to be free from contamination. Once contaminated patients arrive, these areas become designated as warm areas because low levels of dry, liquid, and vapor contamination may be brought in on the clothing, equipment, hair, and skin of patients admitted to the area. The direct hazard to workers is much reduced compared to the hot zone, but decontamination team members must wear protective ensemble because vapors and particles, even in small amounts, pose a hazard to those working directly with the contaminated patients. For more information on zones of contamination and the relationship of the decontamination area to triage and treatment areas see Chapter 14, Field Management of Chemical Casualties.

Water Concerns

Decontamination operations may use dry decontaminants, such as the M291 kit or diatomaceous earth; prepackaged wet decontaminants such as RSDL; soap and water; or chemical decontaminants such as 0.5% hypochlorite solutions. Critical to operations using soap and water is the availability of an adequate supply of water and a way to collect waste water run-off. Water trucks or water buffalos are needed for locations where water is scarce and fire hydrants are not available. In an urban setting, such as the civil response to a homeland incident, ample water is usually available through access to fire hydrants. Water is typically, however, not easily available in a battlefield situation.

If casualties are wearing full MOPP ensemble, as in a battlefield environment, the need for a comprehensive washing of the whole body is reduced, because much of the body is protected by the IPE. Casualties without protective clothing will have greater dermal exposure, because liquid chemical agents penetrate regular clothing, and subsequently will usually require washing of the whole body.

The disposition of waste water is an issue both on the battlefield and during homeland operations. Failure to contain contaminated waste water will pollute an area and prevent its later use. Federal regulations that apply to homeland operations in emergency situations allow for water run-off, as long as the action is not performed intentionally as a way of ignoring waste disposal regulations. Environmental Protection Agency regulation 550-F-00-009,[77] which addresses first responder liability to mass decontamination run-off, considers the release of chemical or biological warfare agents from a terrorist event to be the same as a HAZMAT event and therefore covered under the Comprehensive Environmental Response, Compensation, and Liability Act of 1980, section 107.[77] This act notes that under the good Samaritan provision, which would apply to emergency response HAZMAT operations, "No person shall be liable under this sub chapter for costs or damages as a result of actions taken or omitted in the course of rendering care, assistance, or advice in accordance with the National Contingency Plan or at the direction of an on-scene coordination with respect to an incident creating a danger to public health or welfare or the environment as a result of any release of a hazardous substance or the threat thereof."[77]

The decontamination of patients with large amounts of water is expected to result in waste water run-off containing a minimal concentration of chemical agent.[78] Currently most response agencies have received funding to purchase adequate decontamination equipment, which would include the use of waste water containment systems. In the United States in particular, failure to use these systems could be seen as negligence, if a response agency washed contamination down a sewer as an alternative to avoiding the extra costly and sometimes problematic effort of appropriate waste water collection and disposal using containment berms and bladders. The provisions cited above do not protect an agency against failing to develop a plan for collection and disposal of contaminated water during an incident. Plans may be overcome by events, but if no plans exist, a unit could be liable for damages. Even when protected by the Comprehensive Environmental Response, Compensation, and Liability Act, agencies can still be sued by state agencies, private agencies, and private individuals or groups. Tort reform is different in each state, so it is important for response agencies to participate in their local area planning committee early to work out these issues in writing.[77] It is critical that military units responding to homeland events follow these guidelines.

Training exercises should be used to determine the number of waste water bladders needed for expected mass casualty decontamination operations. If bladders are filling during exercises, additional ones should be purchased. Decontaminating one individual is estimated to take 10 gallons of water, so a 200-gallon water bladder will become full sometime during the decontamination of the 20th patient. Bladders in a variety of sizes are made by several manufacturers; some models are now available with handles that can be lifted onto a truck. Site plans should include the staging of additional bladders so that an empty bladder is always available when needed. Training water decontamination crews to turn off water sprayers when they are not needed will keep bladders from filling as quickly. Procedures for cleaning bladders and disposing of waste material should be practiced. Written contracts should be made with hazardous waste disposal agencies before an incident occurs.

Handling Patients

Writings by Foroutan[65] and others[63,79] note the importance of triage and treatment to stabilize patients before they undergo more thorough decontamination. Medical facilities must also be prepared for walk-in contaminated casualties who have bypassed emergency response teams. These patient triage and treatment areas should be established at the front of patient thorough decontamination operations. Decontamination can take time, typically from 10 to 20 minutes for litter patients and at least 5 minutes for ambulatory patients. In mass casualty situations medical personnel will be needed to manage patients awaiting decontamination. Because patients can also become medically unstable during decontamination, medical personnel are also needed to follow patients through the decontamination line.

Whether shelters, fixed facilities, or buckets and sponges are used, the thorough decontamination process is similar: patient arrival, triage, medical stabilization, securing of personal effects, clothing removal, washing, checking for any remaining contamination (where dictated), crossing the hot line, drying and re-clothing or covering the patient, and finally disposition of the patient to the medical treatment area on the clean side of the hot line. See Chapter 14, Field Management of Chemical Casualties, for more information.

Removal of contaminated IPE from patients should be done by carefully cutting and rolling the ensemble away from the patient's underclothing and skin. This process helps to contain any agent on the garment and prevents cross contamination of the patient's undergarments and now unprotected skin. If the patient is not wearing protective clothing, the containment of contamination is not as critical, and the clothing should be cut off as quickly as possible. During a suspected terrorist incident, clothing should be individually bagged and labeled for forensic investigation by law enforcement agencies.

Sharp, long-handled seat belt cutters (not listed in medical equipment sets) and bandage scissors are ideal for quickly cutting off clothing and IPE; however, they typically become dull after cutting three to five garments, so operators should have a dozen or more of each cutter available (placed in a bucket of 5% bleach). To reduce the possibility of cross contamination, the cutting tools should be dipped into the bleach or exchanged after every long cut.

Additionally, litters used on the warm side should not cross the hot line. Rather, the patient is transferred to a clean litter at the hot line, and the warm-side litter is cleaned and reused. This process further reduces any cross-contamination hazard. Medical information should be transferred from contaminated patient triage cards to clean ones as the patient is moved across the hot line. A variety of patient card systems are available. In the battlefield, the military currently uses the field medical card (DD Form 1380).

Night Operations

Night operations make patient triage, treatment, and decontamination more challenging. Floodlights are not appropriate in a battlefield situation where blackout conditions are imposed, but in a noncombat environment their use should be encouraged to enhance visibility. Also, fluorescent light sets are available for use inside decontamination shelters to improve visibility.

To reduce the incidence of accidents under light-restricted conditions, decontamination lanes should be set up during daylight hours, if possible. The lanes should be clearly marked with reflective tape or waist-high, hanging chemical lights that glow in the dark. Lanes must be kept free from debris and should be familiar to litter bearers. Effective traffic control and off-load procedures are critical at the arrival point to prevent vehicles from hitting patients or operators.

To help identify personnel, operators should have their names and job clearly marked on the front and back of their protective ensemble. If available, reflective vests are ideal and serve to both enhance visibility and identify personnel. Voice amplifiers or other communication devices fitted to protective masks will help communications. Adequate flashlights, with red lens filters, are essential for operators during tactical scenarios.

Night operations require careful planning and additional resources; even in optimal weather conditions such operations pose great challenges. To minimize the challenges and risks associated with night operations, leaders should develop night plans to meet their organizational mission objective and train their personnel accordingly. These plans should then be incorporated into the organization's tactical standing operating procedures.

DECONTAMINATION IN COLD WEATHER

Although cold temperatures can decrease the effectiveness of deploying some chemical agents, various chemical formulations have been developed for cold-weather use, such as Lewisite, which can remain a liquid at freezing temperatures. A more realistic threat today is the purposeful or accidental release of hazardous industrial chemicals during cold weather. Accidents of this type regularly occur in the United States through ground and rail transportation mishaps, such as the January 2005 train derailment in Graniteville, South Carolina, which released chlorine gas.[80] On a cold day, chemical agents can also be dispersed in warm areas such as buildings. In the event of a building evacuation, casualties might be required to report to an outside assembly area or decontamination station. Additionally, nighttime temperature drops and rainy conditions produce reduced temperature situations even in warm climates.

Cold Shock and Hypothermia

Cool temperatures greatly increase the risk of cold shock and hypothermia.[81] Cold shock occurs when an individual is suddenly exposed to cold temperatures, such as cold water in a decontamination shower.[82] Cold shock can cause death by triggering peripheral vasoconstriction, a gasp reflex, hyperventilation, and rapid heart rate leading to heart failure.[83] Casualties who are medically compromised, elderly, or have heart disease are particularly at risk. Hypothermia, though less of a threat than cold shock, occurs when the body core temperature drops below its normal 98.6°F (37°C) range.[82]

Giesbrecht, who studied hypothermia extensively, identified its symptoms and stages (Table 16-5).[83] Mild hypothermia begins when victims are no longer able to shiver and their motor responses begin to become impaired. A narrow window of only 7°C (13°F) below normal core body temperature exists before severe hypothermia can develop. A rapid drop in core body temperature will occur in patients who are already medically compromised (eg, have symptoms of chemical agent exposure or coexisting traumatic injuries). Trauma itself causes hypothermia.[84] Those with hypothermia who are already medically compromised are at much higher risk of death than those who are normothermic.[85,86] The use of benzodiazepines (eg, diazepam), the anticonvulsant for exposure to nerve

TABLE 16-5

STAGES AND SYMPTOMS OF HYPOTHERMIA

Stage	Core Temp °C	Core Temp °F	Status	Symptoms
Normal	35.0–37.0	95.0–98.6	Muscle and mental control and responses to stimuli fully active.	Cold sensation; shivering.
Mild	32.0–35.0	89.6–95.0		Physical (fine and gross motor) and mental (simple and complex) impairment.
Moderate	28.0–32.0	82.4–89.6	Muscle and mental control and responses to stimuli reduced or cease to function.	At 86°F (30°C) shivering stops, loss of consciousness occurs.
Severe	< 28.0	< 82.4	Responses absent.	Rigidity; vital signs reduced or absent; risk of ventricular fibrillation/cardiac arrest (especially with rough handling).
	< 25.0	< 77.0	Spontaneous ventricular fibrillation; cardiac arrest.	

Data sources: (1) Giesbrecht GG. Pre-hospital treatment of hypothermia. *Wilderness Environ Med.* 2001;12:24-31. (2) US Army Soldier and Biological Chemical Command. *Guidelines for Cold Weather Mass Decontamination During a Terrorist Chemical Agent Incident.* Revision 1. Aberdeen Proving Ground, Md: SBCCOM; 2003.

agents, can cause an acute and transient hypothermia.[87] Individuals in wet clothing, or those who are stationary, will lose body heat more rapidly. Heat is conducted out through cool, damp clothing,[88] and wind convection against wet skin also facilitates rapid body cooling and, in cooler temperatures, hypothermia.[89]

Those who are not medically compromised can tolerate ambient temperatures down to 65°F (18.3°C) for several minutes. Colder ambient temperatures, however, are uncomfortable and may cause shivering. Shivering, although it heats the body and is a sign of healthy thermoregulation, is very uncomfortable and depletes a patient's available energy stores.

Protection for Decontamination Team Members

Cold climates reduce the risk of heat injury for decontamination team members, but heat injury can occur if individuals wear excessive thermal undergarments under their protective ensemble and fail to anticipate the heat their bodies generate once they begin working. Cold injuries also can result if personnel sweat heavily and then rest in the cold. Larimer[90] suggests wearing a complete uniform under protective overgarments in extremely cold climates to increase insulation. Thin long underwear made of polypropylene or other materials can wick sweat away from the body,[90] which is particularly helpful when temperatures fall below 30°F (–1°C). Keeping active warms the body, and layered clothing, although difficult to remove while in IPE, can be worn under a rubber protective apron. In cool conditions cotton or wool liners worn under rubber gloves help insulate workers' hands against the cold. Teams should train at various temperatures to gain a better understanding of the amount of layered underclothing appropriate for their work level, so that they do not become overheated while working.

A warming tent is important for decontamination staff to use when needed.[82] If a heated warming tent is not available, blankets must be made available for staff in the rest area. Ideally, heated triage and treatment tents as well as heated decontamination shelters should be used in operations where cold temperatures are frequent. Available buildings can be used if the situation permits. Heated tents and buildings will reduce both staff and patient exposure to the cold. If contaminated clothing is not removed from patients before they are brought into heated areas, these areas must be well ventilated so hazardous chemical vapors do not build up inside the enclosed space. Ideally, patient clothing should be removed just inside or outside the entrance to these facilities. Shelter air heaters and water heaters are available from most pop-up tent manufacturers.

Other cold weather risks are dehydration and ice. In a cold environment individuals may not feel as thirsty as they would in warm weather, fail to drink the necessary amount of water, and become dehydrated.[90] Rehydration is critical for decontamination team members, and warm liquids should always be available. At freezing temperatures slips and falls on ice can pose a real hazard to patients and decontamination team members, especially around decontamination shelters where soap and water are used. In freezing conditions rock salt or a similar deicing material should be applied to ice patches around shelters and along routes of travel.

Protection for Patients

The Department of the Army suggests four decontamination methods based on the ambient temperature (Table 16-6).[82] The closer the ambient temperature is to freezing, the more patient operations are conducted inside a heated enclosure. Regardless of the ambient temperature, individuals who have been exposed to a known life-threatening level of chemical contamination should disrobe, undergo decontamination, and be sheltered as soon as possible. Water heaters and decontamination shelter air heaters make decontamination operations in cold temperatures possible, although 6 to 20 minutes are needed to set up this equipment.

IPE worn by patients should not be removed until the patient appears medically stable enough to undergo decontamination. Asymptomatic patients may be left in IPE, still masked, and moved to a warm and well-ventilated holding area, or they may have IPE removed, be promptly decontaminated with warm water, and be moved directly to a warm holding area free of contamination. If clothing is removed, replacement clothing or blankets must be provided. If the patient may have been exposed to a liquid agent, clothing can be removed and areas not covered by clothing can be decontaminated. Thicker, layered winter clothing worn during exposure provides more protection against chemical agents than thin summer clothing, and thicker clothing should provide adequate protection against dry particles. Once clothing removal begins, decontamination should be accomplished as quickly as possible so that the patient can be covered again with a blanket and moved to a warm area.

If temperatures are near freezing, a dry decontaminant such as sand, paper towels, an M291 or M295 kit, or other absorbent material should be used for immediate decontamination before the patient is moved into a warm tent or room for clothing removal. Heavily contaminated outer protective clothing should be removed in a ventilated area immediately outside or near the entrance to the heated room. Ample sup-

TABLE 16-6

DECONTAMINATION METHODS BASED ON AMBIENT TEMPERATURE

Temperature	Method*	Warm Side Triage and Treatment	Clothes Removed	Location/Technique	After decontamination, patient moved to...
65°F (18°C) and above	1	Outside	Outside	Decontaminate outside	Outside clean side triage area OR Heated clean side triage area*
64°F to 36°F (17°F to 2°C)	2	Outside	Inside	Heated decontamination enclosure	Heated clean side triage area
35°F (1.6°C) and below	3	Inside	Inside	Dry decontamination such as flour, sand, paper towel; M291 or M295 kit for immediate decontamination	Transport to indoor heated decontamination area, preferably in a building

*Grey areas indicate activities performed inside a heated enclosure.
Adapted from: US Army Soldier and Biological Chemical Command. *Guidelines for Cold Weather Mass Decontamination During a Terrorist Chemical Agent Incident*. Revision 1. Aberdeen Proving Ground, Md: SBCCOM; 2003.

plies of blankets are critical during cold weather decontamination to cover patients as soon as they are decontaminated and while they are in assembly areas (this important detail is sometimes neglected in response operations).[91]

An air heater can keep the temperature comfortable for operators and patients. Air heaters should be placed at the clean side of the tent and blow toward the showering and disrobing area; this will move the air away from clean areas and also encourage patients to move toward the heat.[91] A local gym or indoor swimming pool near the site of the incident can serve as a warmed treatment and decontamination area,[82] but clean-up operations in commandeered buildings may be difficult.

If decontamination operations are typically conducted in ambient temperatures below 65°F (18°C), a decontamination system that heats the water is essential. Water may have to be heated to 100°F (38°C) or greater so that it is comfortably warm, but not hot, by the time it reaches the patient.[92] Heaters are also needed for water and waste water bladders in below freezing temperatures. Water transport lines should be covered and insulated to prevent freezing and rupture.[93] Power generators should remain on or be kept warm so that they do not freeze. Once operations have ceased, all pumps, lines, water heaters, and tent plumbing must be thoroughly drained before they freeze and rupture. These items should then be moved to a warm area to prevent freezing.

Additionally, chemical vapor detectors such as the automatic chemical agent detector alarm and ICAMs do not work effectively in the cold because agents give off few vapors in low temperatures. Also, battery life is significantly reduced, especially at temperatures below freezing. Chemical vapor detectors can be placed in warm shelters or tents to measure any vapors in these areas.[90]

SPECIAL POPULATIONS

In the past, military decontamination doctrine has not addressed the medical management and decontamination of special populations such as infants, children, the disabled, or elderly. Recent operations in southwest Asia, relief efforts throughout the world, and the military's involvement with homeland defense have made it imperative that military decontamination teams are familiar with managing these special populations.

Pediatric Patients

Children and infants will inevitably be among those exposed to chemical agents during an industrial accident or purposeful attack, and they are at greater risk of injury for several reasons. Their small size and position close to the ground make them more susceptible to agent clouds that hang low to the ground, a classic characteristic of most chemical agents. Their respiratory rate is faster than adults (increased minute ventilation), so they will inhale a greater quantity of toxins.[94] Children have a reduced fluid reserve, so diarrhea and vomiting can rapidly lead to shock.[95] They will also absorb a greater dose of agent than adults because of their thinner skin, reduced weight, and larger body surface area related to volume of agent.[94]

Children have limited vocabulary and may be nonverbal or crying, which makes assessing their needs difficult and complicates the decontamination process.[95] Young children will also be anxious about the unfamiliar and inhuman appearance of decontamination operators dressed in IPE. An additional challenge is identifying children; a patient numbering system incorporating photographic identification in combination with an identification bracelet that is difficult to remove is ideal.

If possible, parents and children should be decontaminated as a family so parents can assist in the process, although staff will need to direct them. If children are unaccompanied, provisions must be made for appropriate custodial care through the decontamination line and for several hours thereafter, and operators need to wash younger children who cannot bathe independently. Ideally, these operators should have some training and be comfortable working with children.

Soap and water is the safest decontaminant for children. Chemical decontaminants may cause skin breakdown.[94,95] Wet agents with components that can transit the skin, such as RSDL, should be used with caution with this population until their safety is proven, and any use should be followed by a soap and water wash. Children have greater difficulty maintaining body temperature, so warm showers, ample towel supplies, and other means to warm them before and after decontamination are critical.

Other Special Populations

Individuals with physical or mental disabilities may require escorts during decontamination. If these patients can walk independently, they should be processed through the ambulatory decontamination line. Ideally, relatives or acquaintances among fellow ambulatory patients can help individuals with special needs wash themselves; otherwise decontamination operators or other staff members must guide these patients. Hands-on assistance will probably be required for those with limited comprehension or movement limitations that impede their ability to shower independently.

Patients in wheelchairs, using walkers, or with limited mobility are more safely processed through the decontamination line as litter patients because floor grates, slippery floors, and water collection berms can pose hazards or barriers. Individuals with limited vision will need to be escorted through the decontamination line. Plastic chairs, which can be readily decontaminated, can be placed in disrobing, showering, and redressing areas as room allows to help those with limited mobility undress themselves. They should be washed off between patients. Canes, crutches, and other assistive devices should be thoroughly washed with soap and water, dried, and returned to the patients or caregivers after the decontamination process is complete. Eyeglasses can be worn during decontamination but must be thoroughly washed.

Wheelchairs must be decontaminated with special attention paid to cracks, crevices, movable joints, and water-resistant cushions. Contaminated cushions and other items that absorb water should be discarded. If a wheelchair cannot be decontaminated at the same time as its owner, it should be labeled for later decontamination and returned.

Communication challenges may occur with those who are deaf, blind, or nonverbal; additional staff will be required to assist these individuals through the decontamination line. Professionals with occupational therapy, physical therapy, mental health, or nursing backgrounds are ideal as members of decontamination teams to assist those with special needs. They should be trained, qualified to wear IPE, and integrated into decontamination operations.

SUMMARY

Decontamination is a process in which hazardous materials are removed from an individual, used in some form since World War I. Chemical liquids, dry powders, and vapors pose a significant risk to contaminated patients and individuals they come in contact with. Early removal prevents or reduces a patient's injury from a chemical agent. Later removal also protects the patient, but its primarily purpose is to reduce any contamination in an MTF and reduce injury to medical staff.

Current doctrine specifies the use of soap and water, the M291 kit, or 0.5% hypochlorite solution to decontaminate skin. RSDL was recently selected to replace the M291 kit. Fabric and other foreign bodies that have entered a wound can present a hazard to both the patient and medical personnel. These objects should be irrigated with fresh water or saline solution and removed carefully using a no-touch technique.

A variety of decontamination shelters have recently been developed to protect patients and workers from the weather, provide privacy, and provide a framework for plumbing. Most shelters use soap and water as the decontaminant. Various patient litter roller systems are available to reduce the risk of musculoskeletal injury for workers and speed the decontamination process. All decontamination operations, whether using buckets and sponges or plumbed shower systems, follow the same sequence of steps: patient arrival, triage, patient stabilization, securing of personal effects, clothing removal, washing, checking for any remaining contamination (where dictated), crossing the hot line, drying and reclothing or covering the patient, and finally disposition of the patient to the medical treatment area on the clean side of the hot line. Both military and civilian decontamination processes will benefit from additional streamlining and, as the military plays a greater role in homeland defense, increased integration.

REFERENCES

1. Hurst CG. Decontamination. In: Sidell FR, Takafuji ET, Franz DR, eds. *Medical Aspects of Chemical and Biological Warfare.* In: Zajtchuk R, Bellamy RF, eds. *Textbook of Military Medicine*. Washington, DC: Department of the Army, Office of The Surgeon General, Borden Institute; 1997: Chap 15.

2. US Department of Health and Human Services, Technical Support Working Group. *Best Practices and Guidelines for CBR Mass Personnel Decontamination.* 2nd ed. Washington, DC: DHHS; 2004.

3. US Departments of the Army, Marine Corps, Navy, and Air Force, and Marine Corps. *Multiservice Tactics, Techniques, and Procedures for Chemical, Biological, Radiological, and Nuclear Decontamination.* Washington, DC: DoD; 2006. FM 3-11.5, MCWP 3-37.3, NTTP 3-11.26, AFTTP (I) 3-2.60.

4. Okumura T, Suzuki K, Fukuda A, et al. The Tokyo subway sarin attack: disaster management, Part 1: community emergency response. *Acad Emerg Med.* 1998;5:613–617.

5. US Department of Health and Human Services, Agency for Toxic Substance and Disease Registry. *Emergency Medical Services, A Planning Guide for the Management of Contaminated Patients.* Vol 1. In: *Managing Hazardous Materials Incidents.* Atlanta, Ga: DHHS; 2001: Chap 9.

6. Vogt BM, Sorensen JH. *How Clean is Safe? Improving the Effectiveness of Decontamination of Structures and People Following Chemical and Biological Incidents.* Oak Ridge, Tenn: Oak Ridge National Laboratory; 2002. ORNL/TM-2002/178.

7. Crone HD. Simple methods for the removal of chemical agents from the skin. In: *Proceedings of the International Symposium on Protection Against Chemical Warfare Agents, 6-9 June 1983.* Stockholm, Sweden: National Defense Research Institute; 1983: 169–171.

8. Trapp R. *The Detoxification and Natural Degradation of Chemical Warfare Agents*. Stockholm, Sweden: Stockholm International Peace Research Institute; 1985: 44–75.

9. McHargue CA, Commander, MC, US Navy Reserve, Chemical/Biological Incident Response Force, email, February 24, 2004.

10. Buckley JT, Sapkota A, Cardello N, Dellarco MJ, Klinger TD, of Colormetric Laboratories Inc. A rational approach to skin decontamination. Unpublished document; 2004.

11. Lundy PM, Hamilton MG, Hill I, Conley J, Sawyer TW, Caneva DC. Clinical aspects of percutaneous poisoning by the chemical warfare agent VX: effects of application site and decontamination. *Mil Med*. 2004;169:856–862.

12. Sim VM. *VX Percutaneous Studies in Man*. Aberdeen Proving Ground, Md: US Army Chemical Research and Development Laboratories; 1960. Technical Report 301.

13. Papirmeister B, Feister A, Robinson S, Ford R. *Medical Defense Against Mustard Gas: Toxic Mechanisms and Pharmacological Implications.* Boca Raton, Fla: CRC Press; 1991: 2–3.

14. Romano JR, US Army Medical Research Institute of Chemical Defense, Aberdeen Proving Ground, MD, personal communication, 2001.

15. McCreery MJ. Topical Skin Protectant. US patent 5,607,979. March 4, 1997.

16. Braue EH. Development of a reactive topical skin protectant. *J Appl Toxicol*. 1999;19(suppl 1):47–53.

17. Hobson ST, Lehnert EK, Braue EH Jr. The US Army reactive topical skin protectant (rTSP): challenges and successes. *MRS Symp Ser CC: Hybrid Org Inorg Mater* [serial online]. 2000;628:CC10.8.1-CC10.8.8.

18. Chang M. *A Survey and Evaluation of Chemical Warfare Agent Contaminants and Decontamination*. Dugway Proving Ground, Utah: Defense Technical Information Center; 1984. AD-202525.

19. Monteiro-Riviere NA, Inman AO, Jackson H, Dunn B, Dimond S. Efficacy of topical phenol decontamination strategies on severity of acute phenol chemical burns and dermal absorption: in vitro and in vivo studies. *Toxicol Ind Health*. 2001;17:95–104.

20. Brown VK, Box VL, Simpson BJ. Decontamination procedures for skin exposed to phenolic substances. *Arch Environ Health*. 1975;30:1–6.

21. *Formulations for the Decontamination and Mitigation of CB Warfare Agents, Toxic Hazardous Materials, Viruses, Bacteria and Bacterial Spores*. Denver, Colo: Modec Inc, 2001. Technical Report MOD2001-1008-M. Available at: http://www.deconsolutions.com/pdf_files/TECHNICAL%20REPORT%20MOD2001-1008-M. Accessed December 20, 2007.

22. Gordon RK, Feaster SR, Russell AJ, et al. Organophosphate skin decontamination using immobilized enzymes. *Chem Biol Interact*. 1999;119–120:463–470.

23. Gordon RK et al. Preparation of enzymatically active sponges or foams for detoxification of hazardous compounds. US patent 6,642,037. November 4, 2003.

24. Gordon RK et al. Detoxification with sponges or foams containing plurality of enzymes and encapsulated indicator. US patent 6,541,230. April 1, 2003.

25. Gordon RK et al. Immobilized enzymes biosensors for chemical toxins. US patent 6,406,876. June 18, 2002.

26. Cabal J, Kuca K, Sevelova-Bartosova L, Dohnal V. Cyclodextrines as functional agents for decontamination of the skin contaminated by nerve agents. *Acta Medica (Hradec Kralove)*. 2004;47:115–118.

27. Raber E, McGuire R. Oxidative decontamination of chemical and biological warfare agents using L-Gel. *J Hazard Mater*. 2002; 93:339–352.

28. Cheng TC, DeFrank JJ, Rastogi VK. Alteromonas prolidase for organophosphorus G-agent decontamination. *Chem Biol Interact*. 1999;119–120:455–462.

29. Ghanem E, Raushel FM. Detoxification of organophosphate nerve agents by bacterial phosphotriesterase. *Toxicol Appl Pharmacol*. 2005;207(2 Suppl):459–470.

30. Amitai G, Adani R, Hershkovitz M, Bel P, Rabinovitz I, Meshulam H. Degradation of VX and sulfur mustard by enzymatic haloperoxidation. *J Appl Toxicol*. 2003;23:225–233.

31. Cerny LC, Cerny ER. The effect of biological media on the hydrolysis of mustard simulants. *Biomed Sci Instrum*. 1997;33:535–540.

32. Cabal J, Kassa J, Severa J. A comparison of the decontamination efficacy of foam-making blends based on cationic and nonionic tensides against organophosphorus compounds determined in vitro and in vivo. *Hum Exp Toxicol*. 2003;22:507–514.

33. Fitch JP, Raber, E, Imbro DR. Technology challenges in responding to biological or chemical attacks in the civilian sector. *Science*. 2003;302:1350–1354.

34. Wester RC, Xialing H, Landry TD, Maibach HI. In vivo evaluation of MDI skin decontamination procedures. Paper presented at: Polyurethane Expo Sponsored by the International Isocyanate Institute, September 1998; Des Plaines, Ill.

35. Neutralizing chemical and biological warfare agents—a new approach. *Environmental Health*. 1999;62(1):52.

36. Sawyer TW, Nelson P, Hill I, et al. Therapeutic effects of cooling swine skin exposed to sulfur mustard. *Mil Med*. 2002;167:939–943.

37. Chang AMH, Ciegler A. Chemical warfare: part 1–chemical decontamination. *Nucl Bio Chem Defense Technol Int*. 1985;1:59–65.

38. Yurow HW. *Decontamination Methods for HD, GB, and VX: A Literature Survey*. Aberdeen Proving Ground, Md: Army Armament Research and Development Command, Chemical Systems Laboratory; 1981. AD-B057349L.

39. Block F, Davis GT. *Survey of Decontamination Methods Related to Field Decontamination of Vehicles and Material.* Dugway Proving Ground, Utah: Defense Technical Information Center; 1978: 59–60. AD-B031659.

40. US Departments of the Army, Marine Corps, Navy, and Air Force, and Marine Corps. *Potential Military Chemical / Biological Agents and Compounds*. Fort Monroe, Va: US Army Training and Doctrine Command; 2005. FM 3-11.9, MCRP 3-37.1B, NTRP 3-11.32, AFTTP (I) 3-2.55.

41. Swanson MB, Davis GA, Perhac DG. *Environmentally Preferable Cleaners: All Purpose Cleaners, Glass Cleaners, and Dishwashing Liquids.* Knoxville, Tenn: Center for Clean Products and Clean Technologies, University of Tennessee; 1995.

42. Hunt B. Surfactants. Available at: http://www.spraytec.com/articles/octnov97/surfactants.asp. Accessed June 20, 2006.

43. Bryndza HE, Foster JP, McCartney JH, Lundberg B, Lober JC. Surfactant efficacy in removal of petrochemicals from feathers. Available at: http://www.ibrrc.org/pdfs/ibrrc_policy.pdf. Accessed June 18, 2006.

44. Occupational Safety and Health Administration. *The OSHA Best Practices for Hospital-Based First Receivers of Victims from Mass Casualty Incidents Involving the Release of Hazardous Substances*. Washington, DC: OSHA; 2005.

45. Van Hooidonk C. CW agents and the skin: penetration and decontamination. In: *Proceedings of the International Symposium on Protection Against Chemical Warfare Agents, 6–9 June 1983*. Stockholm, Sweden: National Defense Research Institute; 1983.

46. Hobson D, Blank J, Menton R. *Comparison of Effectiveness of 30 Experimental Decontamination Systems and Evaluation of the Effect of Three Pretreatment Materials Against Percutaneous Application of Soman, Thickened Soman, VX, and Sulfur Mustard in the Rabbit*. Edgewood Area, Aberdeen Proving Ground, Md: US Army Medical Research Institute of Chemical Defense; 1985. MREF Task 85-12: Final Report.

47. Hobson D, Blank J, Menton R. *Testing of Candidate CSM Decontamination Systems*. Edgewood Area, Aberdeen Proving Ground, Md: US Army Medical Research Institute of Chemical Defense; 1986. MREF Task 86-25: Final Report.

48. Braue E. Unpublished test results at the US Army Medical Research Institute of Chemical Defense, Edgewood, Md. 2006.

49. Joint Requirements Office for Chemical, Biological, Radiological and Nuclear Defense. *Joint Service Personnel/Skin Decontamination System (JSPDS)*. Washington, DC: Joint Requirements Office, 2004. Operational Requirements Document.

50. Bide RW, Burczyk AF, Risk DJ. *Comparison of Skin Decontaminants for HD: Canadian Reactive Skin Decontamination Lotion, Canadian Decontaminating Mitt and US Skin Decontaminant Kit.* Medicine Hat, Alberta, Canada: Defence Research Establishment; nd.

51. Hanssen KA, Doxzon BF, Lumpkin HL, Clarkson E, Braue EH Jr. Evaluation of decontamination systems challenged with nerve agents. In: *Proceedings of the 25th Army Science Conference, 27–30 November 2006* [CD-ROM]. Arlington, Va: Assistant Secretary of the Army (Acquisition, Logistics and Technology); 2006. Paper KP-16.

52. FDA clears skin lotion for military to protect against chemical burns [press release]. Washington, DC: US Food and Drug Administration; March 28, 2003.

53. Sweeney R, Director, Government Contracting, O'Dell Engineering Ltd. Personal e-mail communication with Boardman CH, 2004.

54. Letter from the Food and Drug Administration to the US Army authorizing the marketing of RSDL in the United States, March 25, 2003, archived at Joint Program Executive Office for Chemical and Biological Defense, Falls Church, Va.

55. US Departments of the Army, Marine Corps, Navy, and Air Force. *Health Service Support in a Nuclear, Biological, and Chemical Environment.* Draft. Washington, DC: DoD; 2004. FM 4-02.7, MCRP 4-11.1F, NTTP 4-02.7, AFTTP (I) 3-2.47.

56. Cooper GJ, Ryan JM, Galbraith KA. The surgical management in war of penetrating wounds contaminated with chemical warfare agents. *J R Army Med Corps.* 1994;140:113–118.

57. Hobson D, Snider T. *Evaluation of the Effects of Hypochlorite Solutions in the Decontamination of Wounds Exposed to Either the Organophosphate Chemical Surety Material VX or the Vesicant Chemical Surety Material HD*. Columbus, Ohio: Battelle Memorial Institute; 1992. Task 89-04.

58. Graham JS, Research Biologist, US Army Medical Research Institute of Chemical Defense, Aberdeen Proving Ground, Md. Unpublished research.

59. Lindsay RS. *Swatch Test Results of Phase 2 Commercial Chemical Protective Gloves to Challenge by Chemical Warfare Agents: Executive Summary*. Aberdeen Proving Ground, Md: Defense Technical Information Center; 2001. AD-A440407. Available at: http://stinet.dtic.mil/cgi-bin/GetTRDoc?AD=ADA440407&Location=U2&doc=GetTRDoc.pdf. Accessed December 20, 2007.

60. US Army Medical Research Institute of Chemical Defense. *General Provisions for Neat Research Chemical Agent (NRCA).* Aberdeen Proving Ground, Md: USAMRICD; 2006. SOP No. 96-124-RS-02.

61. Smith W, PhD. US Army Medical Research Institute of Chemical Defense, Aberdeen Proving Ground, Md. Personal communication with Charles Hurst, 1996.

62. Horton DK, Berkowitz Z, Kaye WE. Secondary contamination of ED personnel from hazardous materials events, 1995–2001. *Am J Emerg Med.* 2003;21:199–204.

63. Okumura T, Suzuki K, Fukuda A, et al. The Tokyo subway sarin attack: disaster management, Part 2: Hospital response. *Acad Emerg Med*. 1998;5:618–624.

64. Nozaki H, Hori S, Shinozawa Y, et al. Secondary exposure of medical staff to sarin vapor in the emergency room. *Intensive Care Med*. 1995;21:1032–1035.

65. Foroutan A. Medical notes on the chemical warfare: part IX. Trans. *Kowsar Med J*. Fall 1997;2(3).

66. World Health Organization. The impact of pesticides on health. Available at: http://www.who.int/mental_health/prevention/suicide/en/PesticidesHealth2.pdf. Accessed June 12, 2006.

67. Stacey R, Morfey D, Payne S. Secondary contamination in organophosphate poisoning: analysis of an incident. *Q J M*. 2004;97:75–80.

68. Cox R. Hazmat. *Emedicine* [serial online]. Available at: http://www.emedicine.com/emerg/topic228.htm. Accessed August 17, 2005.

69. National Institute for Occupational Safety and Health. *Working in Hot Environments.* Washington, DC: NIOSH; 1992. Available at: http://www.cdc.gov/niosh/hotenvt.html. Accessed June 12, 2006.

70. US Department of Health and Human Services, Centers for Disease Control and Prevention. CDC recommendations for civilian communities near chemical weapons depots: guidelines for medical preparedness. *Federal Register* 60, no. 123 (June 27, 1995): 3308.

71. Hick JL, Hanfling D, Burstein JL, Markham J, Macintyre AG, Barbera JA. Protective equipment for health care facility decontamination personnel: regulations, risks, and recommendations. *Ann Emerg Med.* 2003;42:370–380.

72. Torngren S, Persson SA, Ljungquist A, et al. Personal decontamination after exposure to simulated liquid phase contaminants: functional assessment of a new unit. *J Toxicol Clin Toxicol.* 1998;36:567–573.

73. 29 CFR, Part 1910.134. Available at: http://www.osha.gov/pls/oshaweb/owadisp.show_document?p_table=STANDARDS&p_id=12716. Accessed June 14, 2006.

74. Bocek TJA, Reed T, Walker WW. *USAF Concept of Operations, In-Place Patient Decontamination Capability (IPPDC).* Langley Air Force Base, Va: HQ Air Combat Command, SGPM; 2004.

75. Boardman CH. Notes from final demonstration of Contamination Avoidance at Seaports of Debarkation Advanced Concept Demonstration Exercise, 2005, and from observations at Field Management of Chemical and Biological Casualties Course, June 2006.

76. Boardman CH. Personal communication with vendors and personal experience during Field Management courses, 2006.

77. US Environmental Protection Agency. *First Responders' Environmental Liability Due to Mass Decontamination Runoff.* Washington, DC: EPA; 2000. 550-F-00-009.

78. National Association of Clean Water Agencies. *Planning for Decontamination Wastewater: A Guide for Utilities.* Washington, DC: NACWA; 2005.

79. Macintyre AG, Christopher GW, Eitzen E, et al. Weapons of mass destruction events with contaminated casualties: effective planning for health care facilities. *JAMA.* 2000;283:242–249.

80. US Department of Health and Human Services, Agency for Toxic Substances and Disease Registry. Train derailment and chemical release in Graniteville, South Carolina, January 2005. Available at: http://www.atsdr.cdc.gov/HS/HSEES/sctrain.html. Accessed June 6, 2006.

81. Hudson TL, Reilly K, Dulaigh J. Considerations for chemical decontamination shelters. *Disaster Manag Response.* 2003;1:110–113.

82. US Army Soldier and Biological Chemical Command. *Guidelines for Cold Weather Mass Decontamination During a Terrorist Chemical Agent Incident.* Revision 1. Aberdeen Proving Ground, Md: SBCCOM; 2003.

83. Giesbrecht GG. Pre-hospital treatment of hypothermia. *Wilderness Environ Med.* 2001;12:24–31.

84. Segers MJ, Diephuis JC, van Kesteren RG, van der Werken C. Hypothermia in trauma patients. *Unfallchirurg.* 1988;101:742–749.

85. Shafi S, Elliott AC, Gentilello L. Is hypothermia simply a marker of shock and injury severity or an independent risk factor for mortality in trauma patients? Analysis of a large national trauma registry. *J Trauma.* 2005; 59:1081–1085.

86. Wang HE, Calloway CW, Peitzman AB, Tisherman SA. Admission hypothermia and outcome after major trauma. *Crit Care Med.* 2005;33:1296–1301.

87. Echizenya M, Mishima K, Satoh K, et al. Enhanced heat loss and age-related hypersensitivity to diazepam. *J Clin Psychopharmacol.* 2004;24:639–646.

88. Rav-Acha M, Heled Y, Moran DS. Cold injuries among Israeli soldiers operating and training in a semiarid zone: a 10-year review. *Mil Med*. 2004;169:702–706.

89. Irwin BR. A case report of hypothermia in the wilderness. *Wilderness Environ Med*. 2002;13:125–128.

90. Larimer E. Extreme cold weather decontamination–the challenge–chemical warfare. *CML Army Chemical Review*. 2001;Aug. Available at: http://www.findarticles.com/p/articles/mi_m0IUN/is_2001_August/ai_79855465. Accessed September 26, 2007.

91. Bocek T. Representative for TVI Corporation and Reeves Corporation. Personal communication, 2006.

92. Boardman CH. Personal notes from Contamination at Seaports of Debarkation Advanced Concept Demonstration, 2005.

93. Fitzgerald DJ, Sztajnkrycer MD, Crocco TJ. Chemical weapon functional exercise—Cincinnati: observations and lessons learned from a "typical medium-sized" city's response to simulated terrorism utilizing Weapons of Mass destruction. *Public Health Rep*. 2003;118:205–214.

94. Rotenberg JS, Burklow TR, Selanikio JS. Weapons of mass destruction: the decontamination of children. *Pediatr Ann*. 2003;32:260–267.

95. Department of Health and Human Services, Agency for Healthcare Research and Quality. *The Decontamination of Children: Preparedness and Response for Hospital Emergency Departments* [DVD]. Rockville, Md: AHRQ; 2006.

Chapter 17

CHEMICAL DEFENSE EQUIPMENT

LAUKTON Y. RIMPEL*; DANIEL E. BOEHM†; MICHAEL R. O'HERN‡; THOMAS R. DASHIELL§; AND MARY FRANCES TRACY¥

*Sergeant First Class, US Army (Retired); Consultant, Battelle Scientific Program Office, 50101 Governors Drive, Suite 110, Chapel Hill, North Carolina 27517

†Field Medical Education Specialist, US Army Medical Research Institute of Chemical Defense, 3100 Ricketts Point Road, Aberdeen Proving Ground, Maryland 21010-5400

‡Sergeant First Class, US Army (Retired); PO Box 46, Aberdeen, Maryland 21010; formerly, Noncommissioned Officer in Charge, Chemical Casualty Care Office, US Army Medical Research Institute of Chemical Defense, Aberdeen Proving Ground, Maryland 21010-5425

§Formerly, Director, Environmental and Life Sciences, Office of the Director of Defense Research, Office of the Secretary of Defense, Department of Defense, Washington, DC; Deceased

¥Research Scientist, Chemical, Biological, Radiological & Nuclear Defense Information Analysis Center, Aberdeen Proving Ground, Maryland 21010-5425

INTRODUCTION

A number of countries around the world have the capability to use chemical weapons, and terrorist groups around the world display great interest in these weapons and the willingness to use them. Within the past 2 decades, incidents of chemical weapons use in armed conflict, most notably during the Iran-Iraq War, have been well documented. The most recent threat of such use was during the Persian Gulf War, when US forces were possibly exposed to both chemical and biological agents.[1] However, the threat is no longer restricted to the battlefield. Recent events such as the September 11, 2001, terrorist attack on the World Trade Center in New York City and the Pentagon in Washington, DC, and subsequent national threat warnings, have raised fears of a future terrorist incident involving chemical agents. An essential part of preparedness to ensure continued operations in a chemical environment, whether in armed conflict or during a terrorist attack, is adequate equipment. Such equipment must encompass detection and warning, personal protection, decontamination, and treatment. Only an integrated approach to these aspects of protection can ensure an effective response in a chemical warfare environment with a minimum degradation in human performance.[1,2]

The primary item of protection is the personal respirator, designed to protect individuals against volatile agents and aerosols. The respirator must be carefully fitted to ensure minimal leakage, and individuals must be well trained in donning masks (a maximum time of ≤ 9 sec is desirable). In addition to the respiratory hazard, many chemical agents are dermally active, requiring that a proper overgarment, usually containing an activated charcoal layer to adsorb chemical agent, be donned, along with protective gloves and footwear. The complete ensemble can seriously degrade individual performance; a 50% reduction in mission-related task performance has routinely been measured in tests. In addition to physical performance degradation, psychological problems in some individuals wearing the complete ensemble, owing to its claustrophobic effects, have been reported.[3] This subject is discussed separately in the attachment at the end of this chapter.

The rapid "detection and warning" of chemical agent use is critical to force protection.[4,5] Usually, the chemical agent will be delivered via an aerial or missile attack, or in an upwind release causing a cloud of agent to pass over a troop concentration. Because the effects of agents can sometimes occur in less than a minute, timely detection is required to permit all potentially exposed forces to adopt an adequate posture. Detection equipment is also used to confirm agent hazard reduction, which facilitates reducing the mission-oriented protective posture (MOPP) level and removal of protection equipment—the "all clear" signal.

Decontamination of equipment, facilities, and personnel is also required after an attack if effective military operations are to be maintained. Some of this decontamination burden can be mitigated by the use of effective collective protection equipment, which can allow continuing operations, such as communications and medical care, within protected facilities.

This chapter is not intended as an all-encompassing overview of chemical defense equipment; rather, it will describe the items and operations of greatest interest to the medical community. The following sections address in detail each of the protection areas described above. Current equipment items are featured, and items in development that are designed to overcome the deficiencies of current equipment are briefly described. Sufficient technical data are included to allow healthcare professionals to become familiar with the equipment's operation, components, and the limitations. Several sources that provide additional detail are available, including the written references and expert consultants to this chapter. Possibly of more value to the healthcare professional are chemical, biological, radiological, and nuclear (CBRN) officers who are an integral part of each combat element and can provide detailed advice as well as hands-on assistance.

One criterion for the selection of protective equipment items is suitability for joint service use; differences between the missions of air and ground crews must be accommodated. As new and better chemical defense equipment is developed and made available to the forces, several principles must be followed for an optimal outcome:

- Intelligence must continually identify new agents that may be used against combat forces and ensure that the defense equipment meets the new threats.
- A viable, active training program must be maintained.
- Medical input into operations while participants are wearing protective equipment is vital to maintenance of a combat operation. Planned rest periods consonant with work loads and MOPP gear will allow continuing operations even in a contaminated environment.

INDIVIDUAL PROTECTIVE EQUIPMENT

Agents of chemical warfare can exist in three physical forms: gas, liquid, and aerosol (ie, a suspension in air of liquid or solid particles). These agents can gain entry into the body through two broad anatomical routes: (1) the mucosa of the oral and respiratory tracts and (2) the skin. Protection against chemical agents includes use of the gas mask, which protects the oral and nasal passages (as well as the eyes), while the skin is protected by the overgarment. An integrated approach to total individual protection, with respiratory protection as the primary goal, combined with an overgarment, gloves, and footwear, all properly fitted and used correctly, can provide excellent protection against chemical agents of all known types.[1]

Respiratory Protection

The general principles of respiratory protection are documented in four primary source documents:

1. "Chemical Warfare Respiratory Protection: Where We Were and Where We Are Going," an unpublished report prepared in 1918 for the US Army Chemical Research, Development, and Engineering Center[6];
2. *Jane's NBC Protection Equipment* (the most recent edition available), particularly the chapter titled "Choice of Materials for Use With NBC Protection Equipment"[7];
3. *Basic Personal Equipment,* volume 5 in the *NIAG Prefeasibility Study on a Soldier Modernisation Program,* published by the North Atlantic Treaty Organization (NATO) in 1994[8]; and
4. *Worldwide NBC Mask Handbook,* published in 1992.[9]

The fundamental question of protective mask design, first addressed in World War I, is whether the mask should completely isolate the soldier from the poisonous environment or simply remove the specific threat substance from the ambient air before it can reach the respiratory mucosa. The first approach requires that a self-contained oxygen supply be provided. Because of logistical constraints (eg, weight, size, expense), this approach is not used by the typical service member except for specialty applications in which the entire body must be enclosed.

The more common practice has been to follow the second approach: to prevent the agent from reaching the respiratory mucosa by chemically destroying it, removing it in a nonspecific manner by physically adsorbing it, or both. Destruction by chemical reaction was adopted in some of the earliest protective equipment such as the "hypo helmet" of 1915 (chlorine was removed by reaction with sodium thiosulfate) and the British and German masks of 1916 (phosgene was removed by reaction with hexamethyltetramine).[6] More commonly, the removal of the agent was brought about by its physical adsorption onto activated charcoal. (Charcoal, because of its mode of formation, has an extraordinarily large surface area, approximately 300–2,000 m^2/g, with a correspondingly large number of binding sites.[10]) Impregnation of charcoal with substances such as copper oxide, which reacts chemically with certain threat agents, further increases protection.[6]

The effectiveness of modern masks is based on both physical adsorption and chemical inactivation of the threat agent. For example, in the older M17 series protective mask, the adsorbent, known as ASC Whetlerite charcoal, is charcoal impregnated with copper oxide and salts of silver and hexavalent chromium (Figure 17-1). The Centers for Disease Control and Prevention and the National Institute for Occupation Safety and Health have identified hexavalent chromium as a potential human carcinogen.[11] Subsequently, newer protective masks in the M40 series began using an ASZ impregnated charcoal, which substitutes zinc for the chromium. A filter layer to remove particles and aerosols greater than 3 μm in diameter is also a component of all currently produced protective masks.

The location of the filters and adsorbent in relation to the respiratory tract was also addressed by mask designers in World War I. In the standard British mask (the small box respirator of 1916), the filter and adsorbent were housed in a separate container worn around the soldier's trunk and connected to the mask by a hose. In contrast, the standard German mask, introduced in late 1915, was directly attached to a small canister containing the filter and adsorbent. The canister arrangement was lighter and required less effort to breathe, but these advantages were gained at the expense of smaller protective capacity and a degree of clumsiness with head movement.[1] The canister (Figure 17-2) is attached directly to the mask in the majority of modern protective masks.

Several other essential features of modern protective mask design also originated during World War I, for example, designing the inside of the mask so that inhaled air is first deflected over the lenses (which prevents exhaled air, saturated with water vapor, from fogging the lenses) and the use of separate one-way inlet and outlet valves (to minimize the work of breath-

a

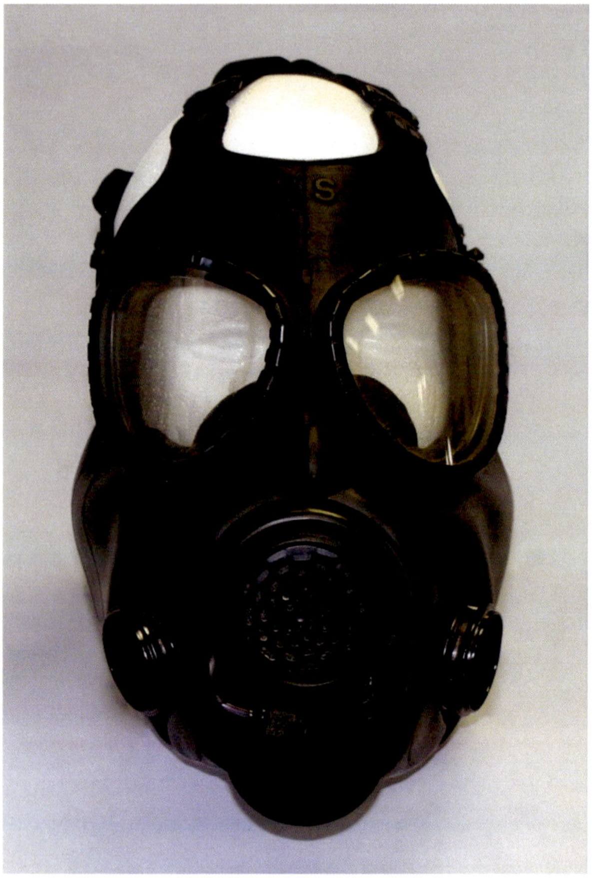

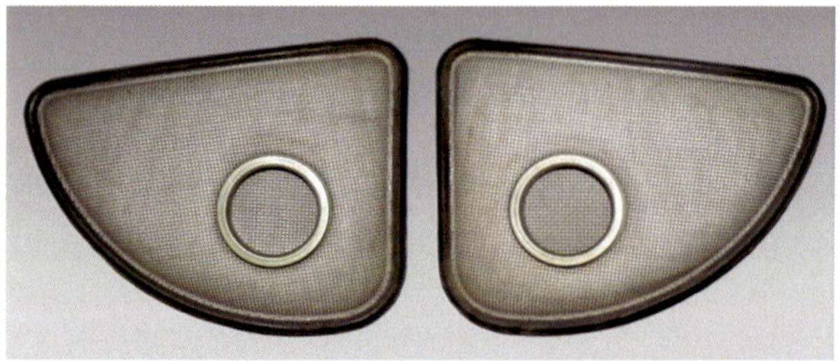

b

Fig. 17-1. (a) The M17A2 chemical-biological field mask. **(b)** M13A2 filter elements are located inside the right and left cheek in the M17 series and can only fit inside in the appropriate opening in the facepiece.
Photographs: Courtesy of the Chemical Casualty Care Division, US Army Medical Research Institute of Chemical Defense, Aberdeen Proving Ground, Md.

ing). World War I mask designers also recognized the need for masked soldiers to speak with each other but failed to solve the problem. After the war, the US Navy introduced the first useful communication solution: a moveable diaphragm held in place by perforated metal plates in the front of the mask. This device ultimately became the "voicemitter" found in today's protective masks.[6]

An important part of mask design is the composition of the elastic material used to cover the face (the "faceblank"). The first World War I masks were made of rubberized cloth or leather. Subsequent masks used natural rubber; recently, sophisticated synthetic polymers using silicone, butyl, and perfluorocarbon rubbers have been used.[6] Silicone rubber has the advantage of making a tight fit or seal between the mask and skin possible, with a correspondingly decreased leakage potential (a factor thought to be responsible for about 5% of mask failures).[12] Unfortunately, silicone rubber offers rather low resistance to the penetration of common chemical agents. Perfluorocarbon rubber is very impermeable but is expensive and tears easily. Butyl rubber, providing both good protection and good seal, has become the material of choice.[7]

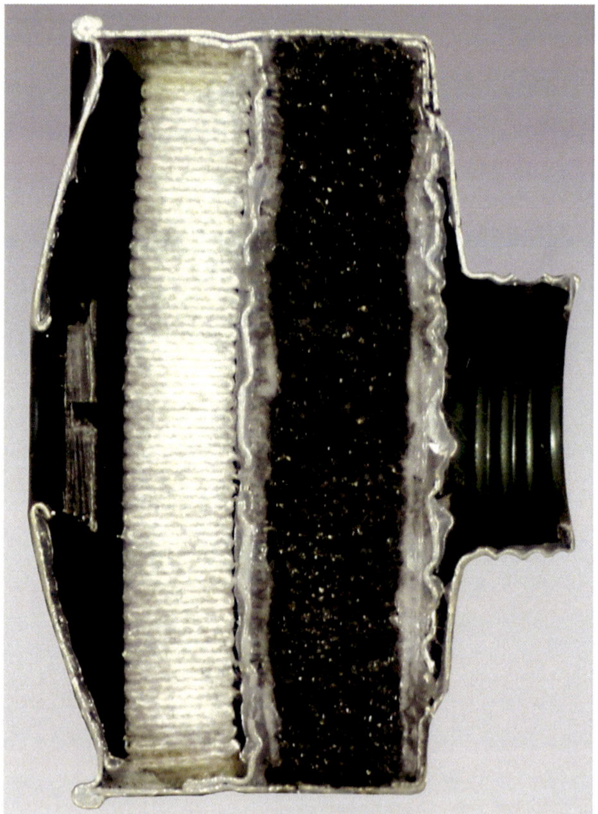

Fig. 17-2. The C2A1 canister is used with the M40 series protective mask. After entering through the orifice on the left side, ambient air passes first through the pleated white filter (where aerosols are removed), then through the layer of ASZ charcoal, then through a second filter (to remove charcoal dust), finally exiting the canister through the orifice on the right side.
Photograph: Courtesy of the Chemical Casualty Care Division, US Army Medical Research Institute of Chemical Defense, Aberdeen Proving Ground, Md.

The faceblank in current standard US military masks consists of two separate layers: an inner layer made of silicone rubber for maximum seal and an outer layer made of butyl rubber for maximum protection (Figure 17-3).[1] However, recent advancements in technology have resulted in the construction of a faceblank with elastic material composed of a mixture of butyl and silicone rubber, thus eliminating the need for an outer layer of butyl rubber. The joint service general purpose mask (JSGPM), the latest generation of protective mask to be issued to the US military, is built on a butyl/silicone rubber faceblank. This mask will be discussed later in the chapter.

The sophisticated design of modern protective masks is most evident in the recognition of the dictates of respiratory physiology: specifically, the importance of dead space. The greater the space between the back of the mask and the face of the wearer in relation to the tidal volume, the smaller the proportion of inhaled air that will reach the alveoli. To minimize dead-space ventilation, modern protective masks have a nose cup— the equivalent of a second mask—fitted separately from the mask proper and inserted between the main mask and the wearer's midface (Figure 17-4). The smaller volume encompassed by the nose cup, rather than the total volume enclosed by the entire mask, is responsible for most of the dead space added by the mask. Furthermore, the nose cup provides an extra seal against entry of threat agents.[6]

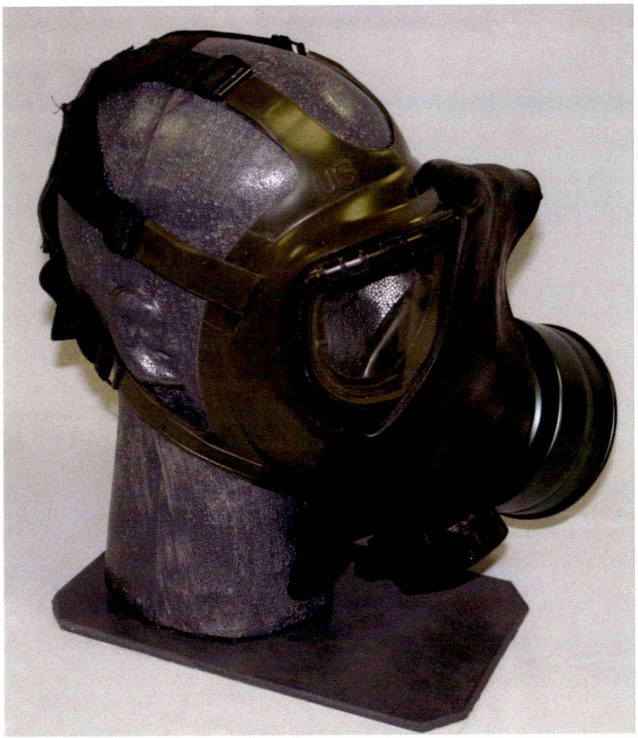

Fig. 17-3. The M40A1 protective mask facepiece has two skins. The inner skin is composed of silicone rubber, and the outer skin is composed of butyl rubber. This arrangement maximizes both mask-to-skin seal and chemical agent impermeability.
Photograph: Courtesy of the Chemical Casualty Care Division, US Army Medical Research Institute of Chemical Defense, Aberdeen Proving Ground, Md.

The work of breathing added by the mask is an important factor; it determines not only soldiers' acceptance of a given mask, but more importantly, the degree that a soldier's exercise tolerance is degraded. Because the pressure gradient required to move a given mass of air is flow-rate dependent, a specific flow rate must be specified to make a quantitative comparison between the work of respiration needed for different masks. For example, at a flow rate of 85 L/min, a pressure gradient of about 8 cm H_2O is observed in World War II–vintage masks. At the same flow rate, the gradient for the M17 series is 4.5 cm H_2O, and for the M40 series it is 5 cm H_2O.[6] By way of contrast, breathing at a rate of 85 L/min without a mask requires a pressure gradient of 1.5 cm H_2O.[13] Some mask wearers perceive the 3-fold increase in the work of breathing as "shortness of breath."[1]

The developmental objectives in personal respiratory protection equipment generally encompass factors such as personal comfort, breathing resistance, mask weight, and the ability to provide protection from new chemical warfare agents and toxic industrial material (TIM). Current equipment was designed to meet a number of these objectives, but much remains to be done to protect adequately against TIM and toxic industrial chemicals (TICs), to incorporate the use of more chemically resistant materials, to utilize advanced manufacturing methods, and to incorporate scratch-resistant lenses. All of these items must be integrated into a new, reliable, less cumbersome, and less degrading system.[1]

The equipment described below is generally suitable for use by all services, although oceanic environments may require that other construction materials be developed for the US Navy and Marine Corps. The masks protect against all known chemical and biological agents, whether in droplet, aerosol, or vapor form. However, a protective mask is only as good as its fit. In the past, the degree of fit was assessed by field-expedient qualitative indices (eg, the degree to which the mask collapsed with its inlet valve obstructed). Modern technology incorporated into the M41 protection assessment test system (PATS) and the joint service mask leakage tester allows the degree of fit to be quantified.[14,15]

a

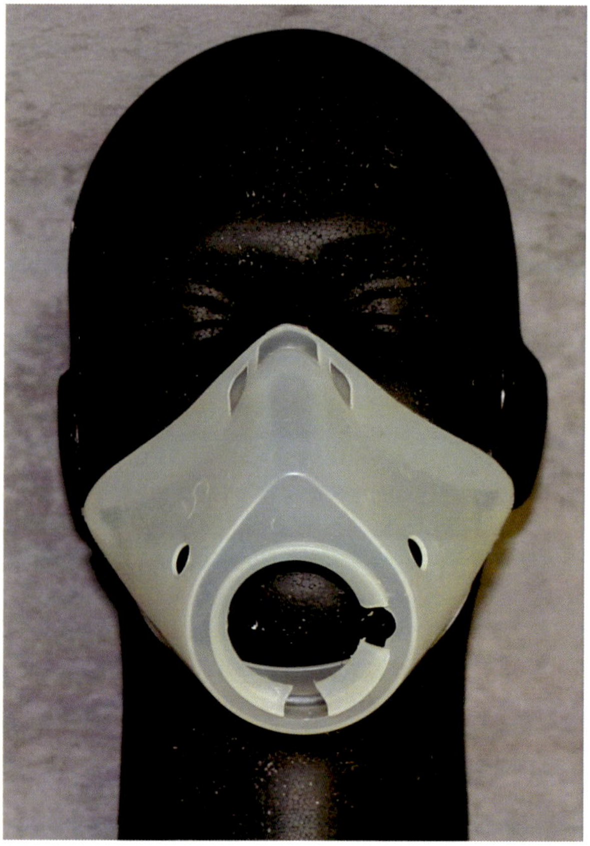

b

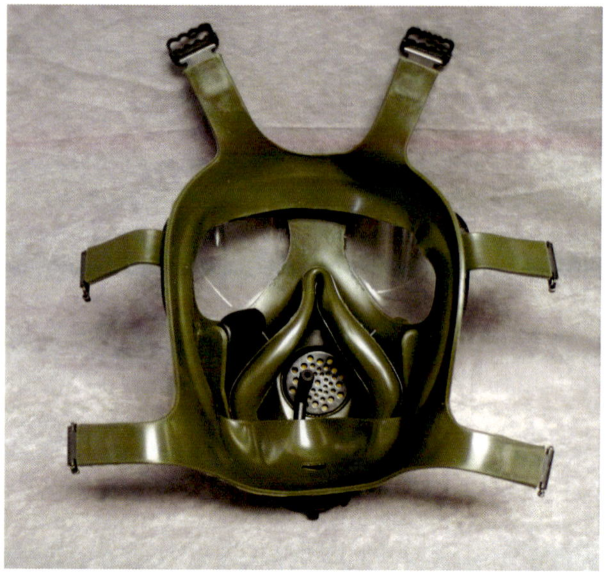

Fig. 17-4. (a) Modern protective masks have a nose cup with a single large hole in the center through which exhaled air is expelled on its way to the exit valve in the main mask. Inhaled air, which has passed through the canister, passes up and around the side of the nose cup, preventing fogging of the mask's lenses, after which it passes through the valve on its way to the user's respiratory tract. **(b)** Location of the nose cup of the M40A1 mask.
Photographs: Courtesy of the Chemical Casualty Care Division, US Army Medical Research Institute of Chemical Defense, Aberdeen Proving Ground, Md.

M41 Protection Assessment Test System

The protective masks issued to members of the US armed forces protect the individual's face, eyes, and respiratory tract from field concentrations of chemical and biological agents, toxins, and radioactive fallout particles. Several critical steps must be taken to ensure that an assigned mask will function properly in a toxic chemical environment:

- select the correct mask size,
- properly fit the selected mask,
- validate the mask protection,
- train the user in the proper wear and use of the mask, and
- perform preventive maintenance checks on the mask as required.

The M41 PATS, designed to validate the protection afforded by the M40, M45, MCU-2/P series and JSPGM masks, is a miniature, continuous flow, condensation nuclei counter. PATS samples particles from ambient air and compares them with particles in the air contained inside the wearer's mask. The resulting numerical values are then used to determine the protection factor of the mask. To pass the test, a mask must to provide a protection factor of at least 1,667 for the Army, Navy, and Air Force, and at least 2,000 for the Marine Corps.[14,15]

PATS ensures that the mask is the proper size for the individual wearer and that the mask system has no critical leaks caused by missing or defective parts or improper maintenance.[1] PATS is compatible with masks that have a NATO drink tube quick disconnect. Two PATS, located at the headquarters company, are fielded for each battalion-sized unit. One PATS is fielded for each separate company-sized unit. PATS is used by the Army, Navy, Air Force, Marine Corps, US surety sites, and foreign military sales clients.[14,15]

Joint Service Mask Leakage Tester

The joint service mask leakage tester (JSMLT) is a portable device capable of determining serviceability and proper fit, and identifying defective components of current and future chemical, biological, and radiological (CBR) negative pressure protective masks. This system combines all these features in one unit, providing a capability currently not available in the field to quantitatively test protective masks for defects and to assess the fit on any individual. The device provides the operator with an audible and visual indication if a component is defective or if the fit does not meet accepted service-specific standards.

The JSMLT currently works with M40 series and MCU-2/P masks. Future capabilities are planned to include M42, M45, and the JSGPM. Key features of the JSMLT include ability to locate leaks so repair or replacement decisions can be made; preventive maintenance checks and services serviceability testing for leakage in the mask, outlet valve, and drink tube; option to perform a fit test on human subjects with the same protocol used by the M41 PATS; and two test heads that allow testing for various mask sizes. The US Marine Corps, Air Force, and Navy are current users of the JSMLT.[14,15]

M40A1 Chemical-Biological Field Mask

The M40 series chemical-biological (CB) field mask (Figure 17-5) replaced the M17 series mask as the standard protective mask issued to the US military. The inner layer of the facepiece is composed of molded silicone rubber that fits tightly against the face, and has an in-turned peripheral seal, which increases comfort and fit. The mask's two-ridged eye lenses are approximately 35% larger than the type used in the M17 series, providing a better field of view. Filtration is provided in the M40A1 mask by one C2A1 filter canister, which can be mounted on either cheek. Two canisters may be mounted on both cheeks for special-purpose activities such as explosive ordnance disposal or technical escort. Any other standard-thread canister issued by NATO countries will fit the M40A1 mask.[14,15]

Communication is provided by two voicemitters. One is mounted in the front to allow face-to-face communication; the second is located in the cheek to permit the use of a radio telephone handset. A drinking system consists of internal and external drink tubes; the external tube has a quick-disconnect coupling that connects with the M1 canteen cap. The system allows personnel to hydrate while wearing the respirator (Figure 17-6). A six-point, adjustable harness with elastic straps located at the forehead, temples, and cheeks comes together at a rectangular head pad for ease of fitting.[14,15]

The M40A1 mask comes in three sizes: small,

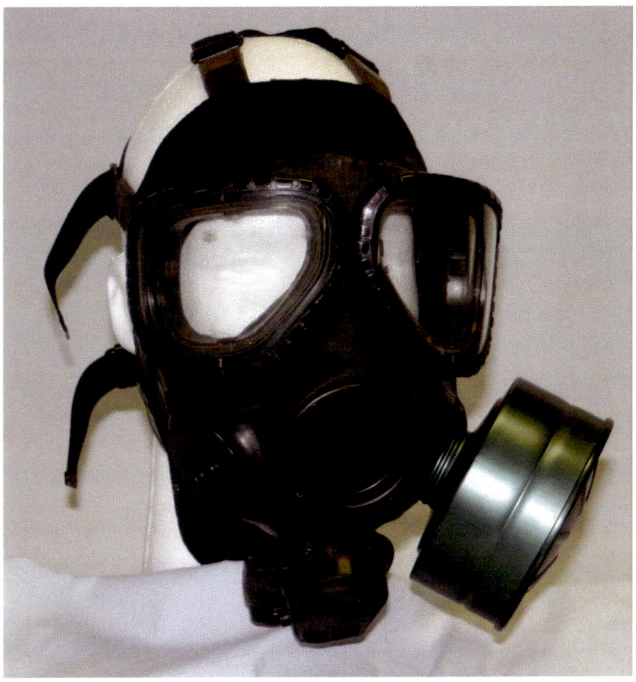

Fig. 17-5. The M40A1 chemical-biological field mask.
Photograph: Courtesy of the Chemical Casualty Care Division, US Army Medical Research Institute of Chemical Defense, Aberdeen Proving Ground, Md.

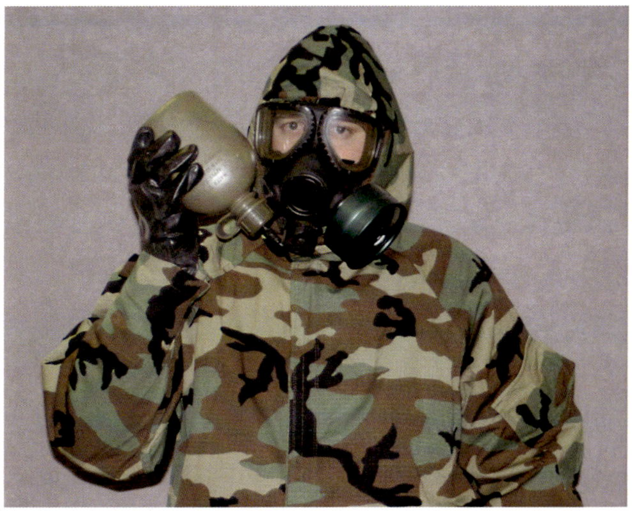

Fig. 17-6. The M40A1 chemical-biological field mask with drinking tube assembly allows the soldier to drink without unmasking. Soldiers wearing mission-oriented protective posture gear must drink water to prevent heat stress. The drinking tube, essentially a flexible straw, couples with the canteen cap. The user holds the canteen upright and inverted, then sips water through the tube. After every few sips, the user must blow exhaled air back into the canteen to equalize the atmospheric pressure without introducing contaminated air.
Photograph: Courtesy of the Chemical Casualty Care Division, US Army Medical Research Institute of Chemical Defense, Aberdeen Proving Ground, Md.

medium, and large. Optical inserts are provided for vision correction, and outserts are available to reduce fogging and sun glare and to protect against scratching. A check valve on the nose cup prevents exhaled air from fogging the lenses inside, and an air deflector directs inhaled air over the lenses, which also helps prevent fogging.[14,15] Other components include a carrier, a waterproof bag, and a quick-doff hood to protect the neck and head areas (Figure 17-7).[16] The quick-doff hood is not used when the mask is worn with parka overgarments.

M42A2 Chemical-Biological Combat Vehicle Mask

The M42A2 CB mask, in the same series as the M40A1, is used by combat vehicle crews (Figure 17-8). The materials of construction and the basic features are identical to the M40A1. Filtration is provided by a C2A1 canister attached to the mask by a corrugated hose; the canister is housed in a specially designed canister carrier. The M42A2 integrates with the combat vehicle filtration protection system. The M42A2 also has a dynamic microphone that integrates with the combat vehicle via a microphone cable.[14,15,17]

MCU-2/P Chemical-Biological Mask

The MCU-2/P CB mask is used by US Air Force ground crews and air crews when not in flight, and also by the Navy onboard ship for CBR defense. This mask has a facepiece constructed of molded silicone rubber material, and an integral, molded, polyurethane, one-piece panoramic lens bonded to the facepiece. Filtration is provided by one C2A1 canister mounted on either side of the facepiece. The primary voicemitter is located over the mouth area; a secondary voicemitter in the cheek area can be used with telephone handsets. The mask incorporates a drinking tube, which connects to the M1 canteen cap for hydration while wearing the mask. The mask has a six-point, adjustable head harness suspension made of elastic, which comes together in the center in the back of the head into a rectangular patch of woven material. The mask comes in three sizes: small, medium, and large. Accessories include a carrier bag, a butyl-coated nylon cloth hood, a large outsert to protect the lens in storage, a neutral gray outsert to protect against sun glare, and a waterproof bag.[14,15]

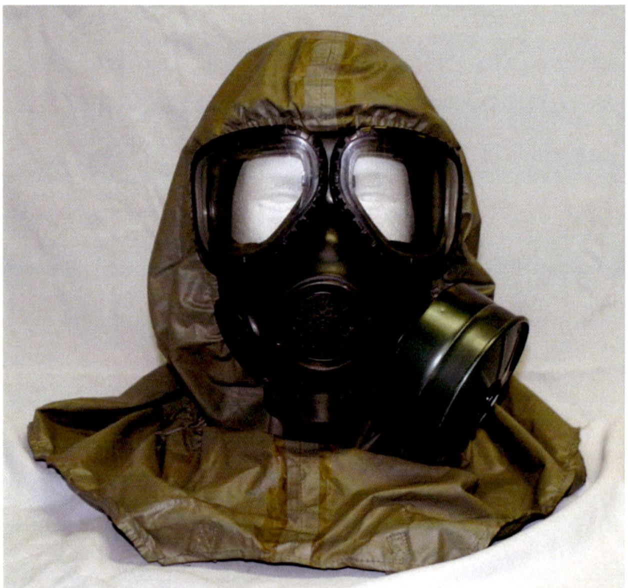

Fig. 17-7. The M40A1 chemical-biological field mask with the quick-doff hood.
Photographs: Courtesy of the Chemical Casualty Care Division, US Army Medical Research Institute of Chemical Defense, Aberdeen Proving Ground, Md.

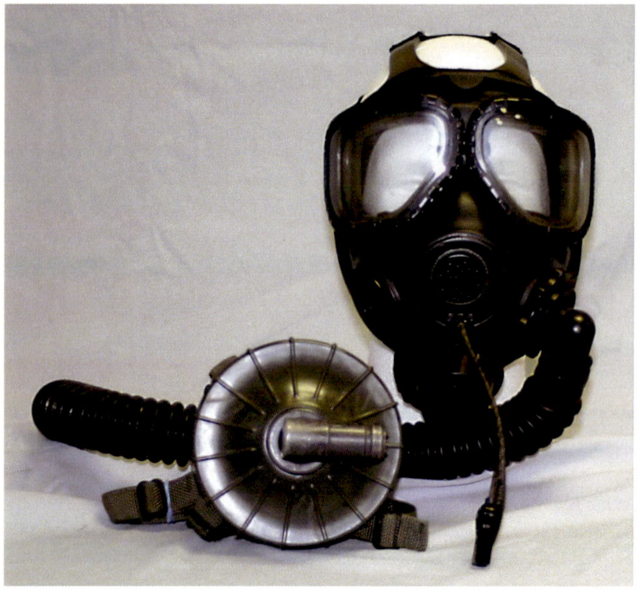

Fig. 17-8. The M42A2 chemical-biological field mask.
Photograph: Courtesy of the Chemical Casualty Care Division, US Army Medical Research Institute of Chemical Defense, Aberdeen Proving Ground, Md.

M45 Chemical-Biological Mask

The M45 mask consists of close-fitting eye lenses shaped to improve peripheral vision and compatible with most optical sighting and night-vision devices; vision-corrective inserts that can be fitted inside the facepiece; front and side voicemitters for face-to-face and telephone communication; a low profile canister

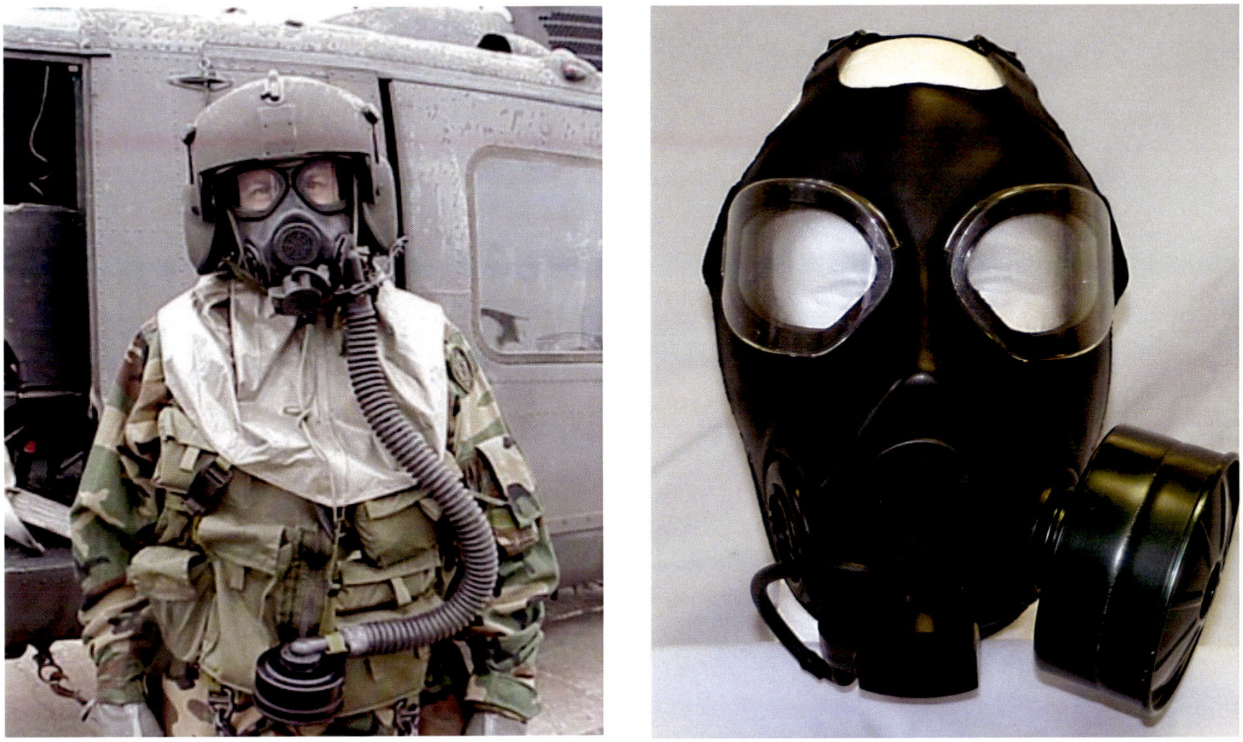

Fig. 17-9. (a) The M45 mask (aircrew configuration) with hose assembly. **(b)** The M45 Land Warrior mask.
Photographs: Courtesy of the Chemical Casualty Care Division, US Army Medical Research Institute of Chemical Defense, Aberdeen Proving Ground, Md.

interoperability hose assembly to allow both hose- and face-mounted configurations; a rubber facepiece with an in-turned peripheral seal; a second skin; and a hood (Figure 17-9). The mask provides the required CB protection without the aid of forced ventilation air. It is used by all Army air crew members, except AH-64 Apache helicopter pilots, in the conduct of aviation missions anywhere in a CB environment.[14,15]

The M45 mask supports the Land Warrior program, as well as Joint Special Operations Command requirements, and serves as the mask for personnel who cannot be fitted with the standard M40A1, M42A2, or MCU-2/P protective masks. The M45 Land Warrior mask does not include the hose assembly, hood, canister baffle, microphone, or microphone cable.[14,15,18]

Joint Service General Purpose Mask

The JSGPM (Figure 17-10) is provided in two models with individual national stock numbers to support major operational modes: the M50 for field use, the M51 for use in combat vehicles. The M50 and M51 components are configured to reduce the overall profile of the mask and to improve integration with future protective systems. Common to both models are the mask carrier, bag, individual equipment carrier, facepiece assembly, sunlight outsert, primary CBR filters, waterproof bag, and operator cards.[14,15,19]

The M50 and M51 facepiece assemblies are built on a butyl/silicone rubber faceblank with an inverted peripheral face seal and an integrated chin cup. The facepiece assembly forms a comfortable seal on the wearer's face and protects the face, eyes, and respiratory tract from chemical and biological agents, designated TICs, and radiological particulates. The facepiece assembly incorporates a flexible, single, polyurethane eye lens that provides an overall field of vision greater than 80%. A front module assembly provides a direct speech capability and integrates the exhalation disk valve, drinking system components, and communications interface. Filtration is provided by two filter mount assemblies (left and right) that integrate the air inlet disk valves and self-sealing disk valves, and a nose cup that controls the flow of air throughout the mask and prevents fogging of the eye lens while breathing.[14,15]

The M51 includes the following items: combat vehicle hose assembly (connects the mask to the vehicle collective protection system), protective hood, microphone, microphone adapter, and microphone lead (connects the microphone and microphone adapter to the individual's combat vehicle crew helmet). One

a

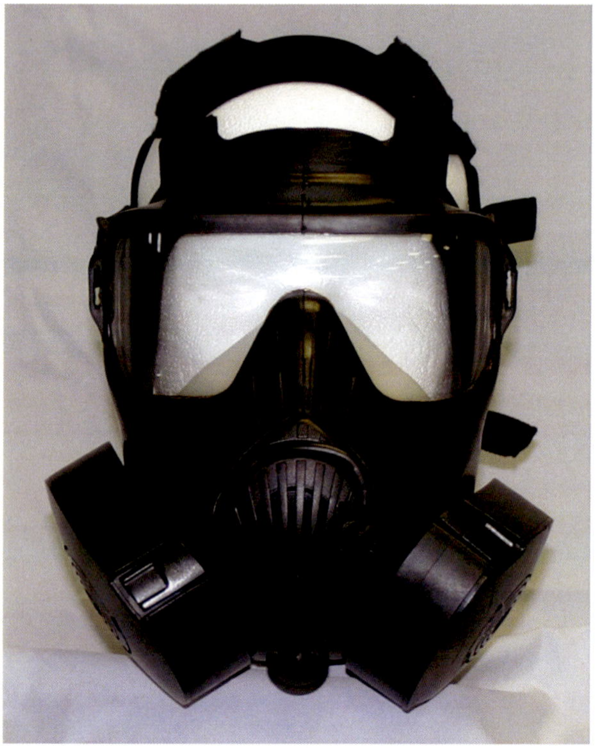

b

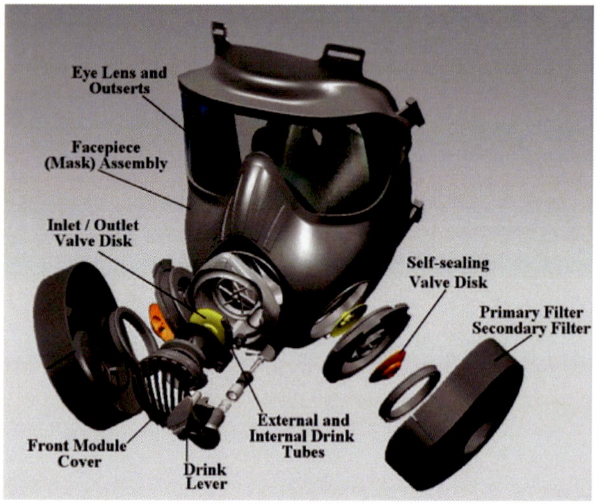

Fig. 17-10. (a) The joint service general purpose mask incorporates state-of-the-art technology to protect US forces from anticipated threats. **(b)** Illustration of the mask's technical design.
Photograph (a): Courtesy of the Chemical Casualty Care Division, US Army Medical Research Institute of Chemical Aberdeen Proving Ground, Md. Drawing (b): Courtesy of the Respirator Engineering and Acquisition Team, ECBC-RDECOM, Aberdeen Proving Ground, Md.

end of the hose assembly connects directly to the CBR or secondary TIC filter, if used. The other end has a quick-connect fitting that interfaces with the vehicle's collective protection system.

The M50 and M51 are manufactured in three sizes: small, medium, and large. The masks are equipped with a sunlight outsert for eye protection from bright sunlight. A laser outsert is available as an additional authorization list item for laser eye protection. Both masks use twin primary CBR filters, positioned on either side of the face, to provide protection against CBR threats. Supplemental twin secondary TIC filters are available as additional authorization list items. The secondary filters provide protection from designated TICs and are used in conjunction with the primary filters, as required for mission/operations.[14,15]

M53 Chemical-Biological Protective Mask

The M53 mask (Figure 17-11) is specially designed to meet US Special Operations Command requirements; it is not a standard mask issued to other service members. The M53 facepiece assembly is built on a butyl/silicone rubber faceblank with an inverted peripheral face seal and an integrated chin cup. The facepiece assembly forms a comfortable seal on the wearer's face and protects the face, eyes, and respiratory tract from CB agents, certain TICs, and radiological particulates. The facepiece assembly incorporates a single, flexible, polyurethane eye lens; a variable resistance exhalation unit that allows for operations in negative pressure, powered air purifying respirator, self-contained breathing apparatus, and closed circuit breathing apparatus modes; drinking system components; a communications interface; single filter mount assemblies with a 40-mm NATO thread that integrate the inlet disk valve and air deflector; and a nose cup that controls the flow of air throughout the mask and prevents fogging of the eye lens during operation.[14,15]

The M53 is manufactured in four sizes (extra-small, small, medium, and large) and in either a left- or right-handed version. The mask also incorporates interchangeable nose cups in five sizes: extra-small, small, medium, large, and extra-large. Each mask is equipped with a sunlight outsert for eye protection from bright sunlight and lens protection. A clear outsert is provided for lens protection when the sunlight outsert is not required. A laser outsert is also available as an additional authorization item for laser eye protection. The mask uses a single CBR filter, positioned on the side of the face, to provide protection against nuclear, biological, and chemical threats and certain TICs. A particulate filter, also available as an additional authorization list item, provides protection from biological and riot control agents.[20] A protective hood is provided for

a

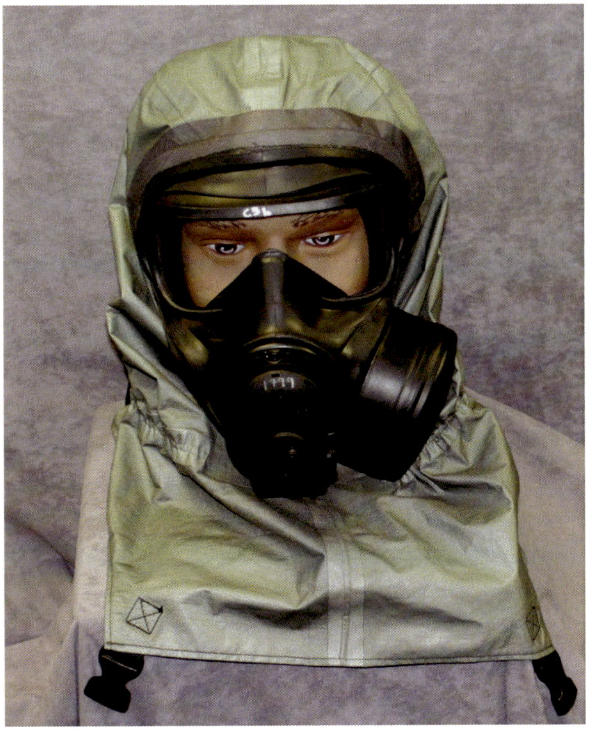

b

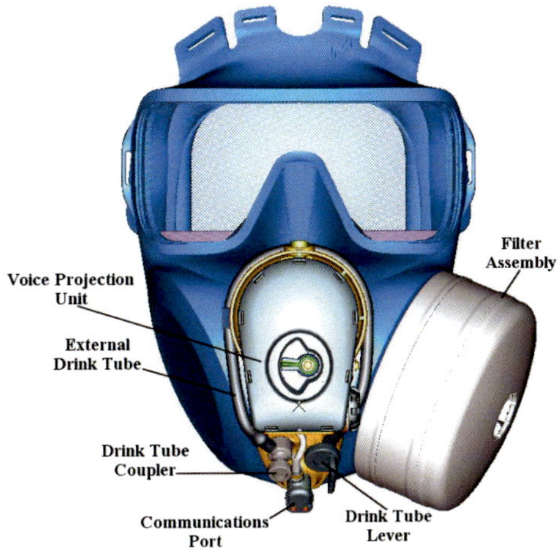

Fig. 17-11. (a) The M53 chemical-biological protective mask is positive-pressure capable and provides an internal variable resistance exhalation unit for operations with self-contained, closed-circuit and powered-air breathing systems. **(b)** Illustration of the M53 mask front facepiece assembly.
Photograph (a): Courtesy of the Chemical Casualty Care Division, US Army Medical Research Institute of Chemical Defense, Aberdeen Proving Ground, Md. Drawing (b): Courtesy of the Respirator Engineering and Acquisition Team, ECBC-RDECOM, Aberdeen Proving Ground, Md.

joint service lightweight integrated suit technology (JSLIST) type VII users to protect the head and neck from exposure to agents, because these suits lack a hood. An audio frequency amplifier and microphone assembly (microphone and microphone adapter) are provided for amplified voice communication. Each facepiece assembly has serial number bar code as well as human-readable lot and serial numbers located on the filter mount assembly.[14,15]

Protective Clothing

An overgarment can be made to protect skin from chemical agents by either physical or chemical means, depending on the type of fabric:

- the fabric may be impermeable to most molecules, even to air and water vapor, or
- the fabric may be permeable to most molecules but chemically alters or physically removes chemical agents before they reach the skin.

An overgarment made of the first type of fabric, which can be butyl rubber or an impermeable plastic, offers complete protection against threat agents but places a significant heat load on the wearer and limits movement. Because the individual's skin does not contact the outside air, sweating does not cool the body and heat is retained. Most fielded military garments utilize the second type of fabric technology, which allows some limited air exchange through the fabric but filters the air through a charcoal lining, which also absorbs agent.

The decision to place a service member into full chemical protective equipment—mask, overgarment, gloves, and boots—must take into account not only the provided protection but also the added heat stress and potential for dehydration.[1] To guard against dehydration, personnel must begin a drinking regimen before encapsulation. The physical burden of a full ensemble can add 5 to 7 lbs to a normal load; this added weight combined with heat stress, dehydration, and physical exertion can cause significant impairment to any mission. Because of these factors, the military developed MOPP levels to stratify the levels of required protection based on the anticipated threat risk (Figure 17-12). There are seven MOPP levels; Exhibit 17-1 describes each level in detail. More information on the applications of the various MOPP levels can be found in Field Manual 3-11.4, *Multiservice Tactics, and Procedures for NBC Protection*.[14] The MOPP level must be coordinated with the workload if personnel are to remain effective. Overgarments are continuously redesigned to reduce heat stress, reduce weight and bulk, and provide increased comfort as well as reduce the logistical burden.

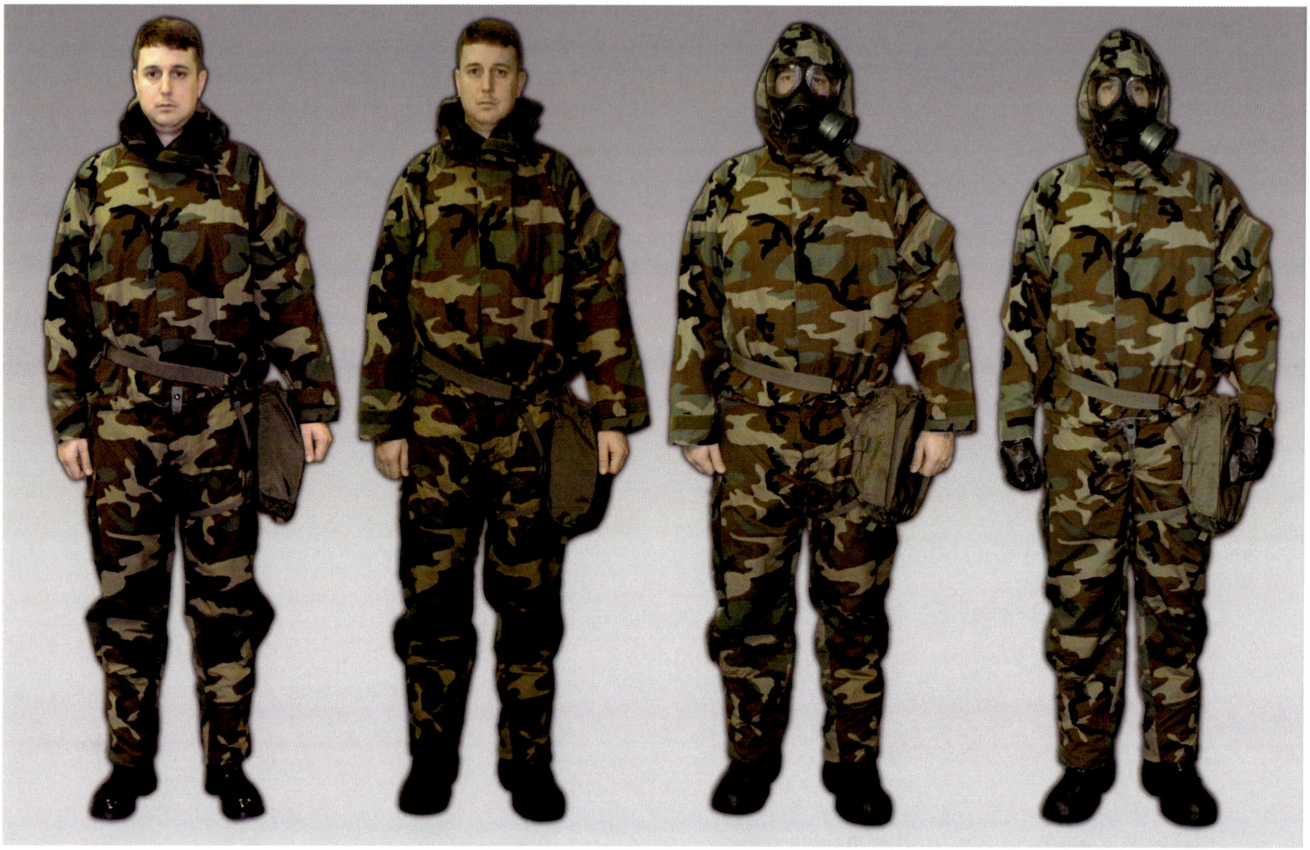

Fig. 17-12. Mission-oriented protective posture gear, from left to right: levels 1, 2, 3, and 4.
Photograph: Courtesy of the Chemical Casualty Care Division, US Army Medical Research Institute of Chemical Defense, Aberdeen Proving Ground, Md.

EXHIBIT 17-1

LEVELS OF MISSION-ORIENTED PROTECTIVE POSTURE

MOPP Ready Applies to US Army/Marine Corps only. Personnel carry their protective masks with their load-carrying equipment. Individual mission-oriented protective posture (MOPP) gear is labeled and stored no farther back than a logistics site (eg, brigade support area) and is ready to be brought forward to the individual when needed. The time necessary to bring the MOPP gear forward should not exceed 2 hours. Units at MOPP ready are highly vulnerable to persistent agent attacks and will automatically upgrade to MOPP 0 when they determine or are notified that chemical, biological, radiological, or nuclear (CBRN) weapons have been used or that the threat exists for CBRN weapons use. When a unit is at MOPP ready, personnel have field-expedient items, such as wet weather gear, identified for use in the event of an unanticipated CBRN attack. Additionally, Air Force personnel stationed in or deployed to CBRN medium- and high-threat areas are issued individual protective equipment (IPE) capable of bringing them to the MOPP 4 level of protection. Therefore, when the theater commander declares MOPP ready, Air Force personnel will automatically assume MOPP 0 as opposed to MOPP ready.

(Exhbit 17-1 *continues)*

Exhibit 17-1 *continued*

MOPP 0 IPE is issued to and inspected by the individual and prepared for use. Personnel carry their protective masks with their load-carrying equipment. The standard-issue overgarment and other IPE are carried or are readily available. To be considered readily available, equipment must be carried by each individual, stored within arm's reach, or be available within 5 minutes; for example, within the work area, vehicle, or fighting position. Units at MOPP 0 are highly vulnerable to persistent agent attacks and will automatically upgrade to MOPP 1 when they determine or are notified that persistent chemical agents have been used or that the threat exists for CBRN weapons use. The primary use for MOPP 0 is during periods of increased alert when an enemy has a chemical-biological (CB) employment capability, but there is no indication of use in the immediate future. MOPP 0 is not applicable to forces afloat.

MOPP 1 When directed to MOPP 1, personnel immediately don the overgarment. In hot weather, the overgarment jacket may be left open and the overgarment may be worn directly over underwear and other IPE making up the individual MOPP gear (eg, footwear, mask, and gloves are readily available or carried). M8 or M9 paper is attached to the overgarment; the nerve agent antidote kit and decontamination kit must be carried or kept on hand. MOPP 1 provides a great deal of protection against persistent agents. MOPP 1 is primarily used when a CB attack in theater is possible. Personnel must remove contact lenses and wear protective mask optical inserts. Leaders also monitor hydration levels. For forces afloat, MOPP 1 means IPE is available.

MOPP 2 Personnel wear and/or put on their footwear, overgarment, and protective helmet cover. As in MOPP 1, the overgarment jacket may be left open, but trousers must remain closed. The mask with mask carrier and gloves are carried. The primary use for MOPP 2 is when a CB attack in theater is possible.

MOPP 3 Personnel wear the overgarment, footwear, protective mask, and protective helmet cover. Again, flexibility is built into the system to allow for relief at MOPP 3, particularly in hot weather. Personnel may open the overgarment jacket, and those with hood attached to the mask can roll the protective mask hood for ventilation, but the trousers must remain closed. The primary use of MOPP3 is for personnel operating inside areas where a chemical-agent contact hazard does not exist. MOPP 3 is not appropriate if a contact hazard is present. At MOPP 3, forces afloat don protective suits and boots and activate intermittent countermeasure washdown.

MOPP 4 Personnel completely encapsulate themselves by closing their overgarments, adjusting all drawstrings to minimize the likelihood of any openings, and putting on their protective gloves. MOPP 4 is used when the highest degree of protection is required, or if CB agents are present but the actual hazard is not determined. As with every other MOPP level, flexibility is built into the system to provide relief to the individual. Once the hazard is identified and risk assessment measures are employed, the overgarment may be left open. During coalition operations, US forces familiarize themselves with the protection levels used by personnel from other nations.

MOPP Options A MOPP option involves the mask only. The mask is worn with the long-sleeve duty uniform (for limited skin protection). The mask-only command may be given under these situations: (*a*) When riot control agents are being employed and no CB threat exists. (*b*) In a downwind vapor hazard of a nonpersistent CB agent. Mask only is not normally an appropriate command when blister agents (vesicants) or nerve agents are involved.

Adapted from: Departments of the Army, Marine Corps, Navy, and Air Force, and Marine Corps. Multiservice Tactics, Techniques, and Procedures for Chemical, Biological, Radiological, and Nuclear (NBC) Protection. Washington, DC: DoD; 2003. FM 3-11.4, MCWP 3-37.2, NTTP 3-11.27, AFTTP (I) 3-2.46.

Protective Ensembles

Several types of chemical protective clothing are available, depending on the protection required to perform a specific mission and whether the fabric should be permeable or impermeable. Most military units use permeable protective clothing, which allows air and moisture to pass through the fabric without hindering the chemical protection capabilities of the clothing.[1]

The standard CB protective overgarment is the JSLIST, which provides protection from the effects of liquid, solid, and vapor CB agents, toxins, radioactive alpha and beta particles, and TIM (Figure 17-13). The JSLIST is a two-piece garment (coat and trousers), weighing between 5 and 7 lb, depending on size (approximately 1 lb lighter per size than previous generation protective garments). The JSLIST overgarment has an outer shell made of a 50% nylon and 50% cotton poplin ripstop material with a durable water-repellant finish. Its liner layer consists of a nonwoven front laminated to activated carbon spheres and bonded to a tricot knit back that absorbs chemical agents. This overgarment provides increased durability, reduced weight, improved fit, enhanced suit closures, and a 15% reduction in heat stress for the wearer compared to previous protective garments. The overgarment can be worn over individual underwear or a conventional duty uniform.[21]

The JSLIST is designed to permit efficient communications and to be compatible with existing and planned clothing and equipment, including load-bearing equipment, helmets, handwear, footwear, body cooling systems, and protective masks of each service and the special operations forces. The garments are launderable up to six times by field methods, can be

a

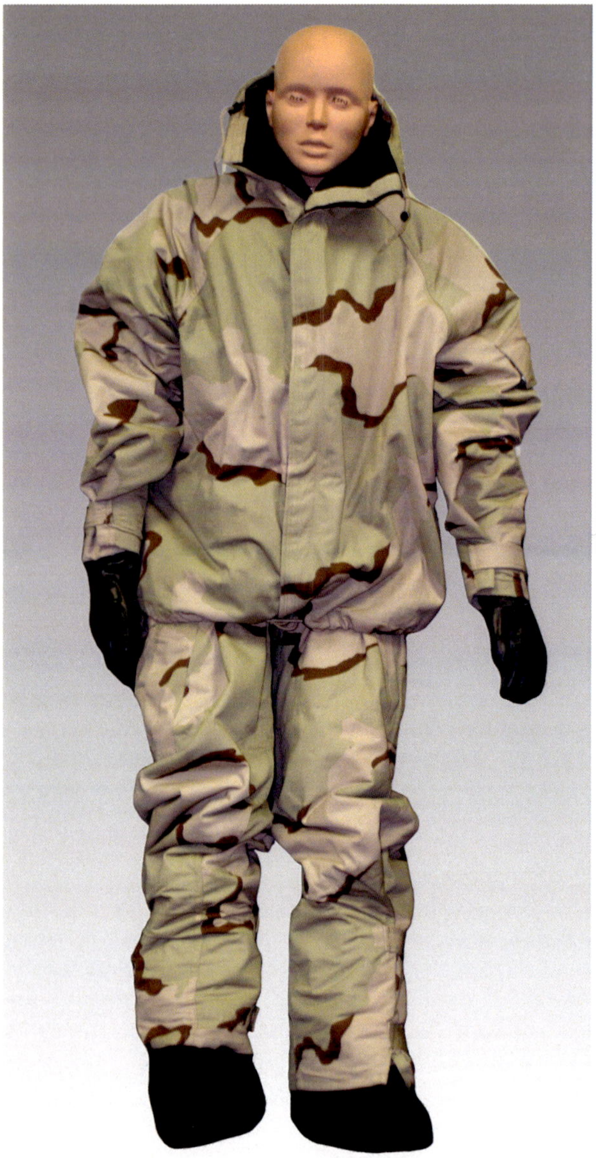

b

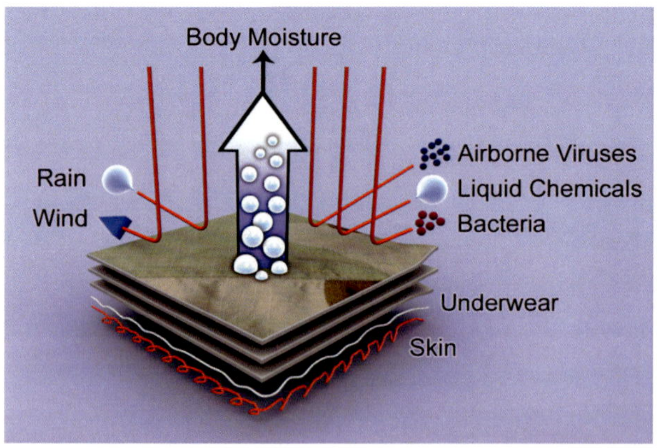

Fig. 17-13. (a) The joint service lightweight integrated suit technology overgarment type II (type II has an integrated hood). **(b)** The garments allow body moisture to evaporate while repelling rain, wind, airborne viruses, liquid chemicals, and bacteria. Personnel wearing the overgarment and an Army combat uniform are afforded five layers of protection: (1) The overgarment's outer layer, made of 50% nylon and 50% cotton poplin ripstop material, in woodland or desert camouflage pattern with a durable water-repellant finish; (2) the garment's inner layer, consisting of a nonwoven front laminated to activated carbon spheres and bonded to a tricot knit back; (3) the Army combat uniform, made of a 50% cotton and 50% nylon rip-stop fabric; (4) drawers and undershirt made of 100% cotton; and (5) human skin surface.
Photograph and drawing: Courtesy of the Chemical Casualty Care Division, US Army Medical Research Institute of Chemical Defense, Aberdeen Proving Ground, Md.

worn for a maximum of 45 days, and provide up to 24 hours of protection against CB challenges within the stated maximum wear time.[22]

Two distinct versions of the suit exist: type II and type VII. The JSLIST type II overgarment (see Figure 17-13) has an integrated hood, bellows-type pockets, high-waist trousers, adjustable suspenders, an adjustable waistband, and a waist-length jacket. This design improves system compatibility, user comfort, and system acceptance by wearer, as well as maximizing individual equipment compatibility. The JSLIST type II is used for most applications. The JSLIST overgarment type VII has a similar design but no integrated hood; this type also has eyelets with a drawstring at the leg cuff. Type VII coats and trousers must be paired to maintain their effectiveness. It is used by special operations personnel and, on an interim basis, by combat vehicle crew personnel.[21,23]

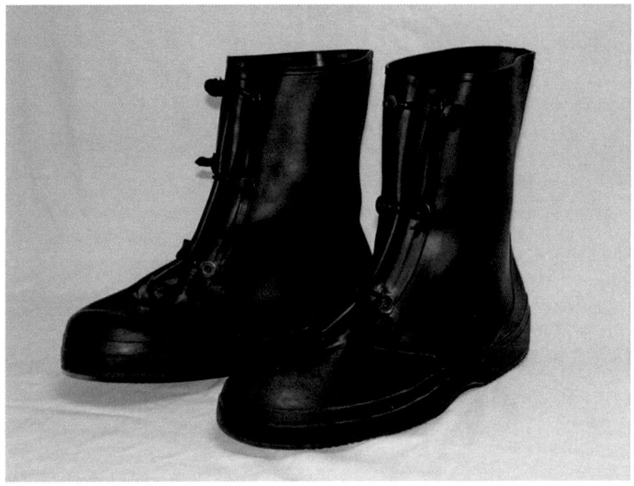

Fig. 17-14. The black vinyl overboot.
Photograph: Courtesy of the Chemical Casualty Care Division, US Army Medical Research Institute of Chemical Defense, Aberdeen Proving Ground, Md.

Protective Boots and Gloves

A service member wearing the chemical protective boots and gloves discussed here will soon realize that mobility is compromised by the boots and tactile ability is degraded by the gloves. Also, the protective overboots currently worn by service members, although providing good protection against chemical warfare agents, cause serious risk of falls because of the lack of adequate traction, and their weight contributes to the increased fatigue from complete protection ensemble wear. Furthermore, the overboots do not protect against heat or cold; in some cases they may contribute to medical problems such as trench foot, frostbite, or other cold weather injuries. The military hopes to develop a new boot that provides chemical protection while being easy to don, comfortable, able to provide steady footing, and capable of rapid and thorough decontamination for reuse. The current protective gloves, in addition to degrading tactility, also fail to protect against heat or cold. Failing to wear a work glove over the protective glove may increase the chance of cold weather injuries.[1,21]

Black vinyl overboot. The black vinyl overboot (Figure 17-14) is used to protect the individual's combat boots against all known chemical and biological agents, vectors, and radioactive (alpha and beta) particles. The overboots also provide protection from the environmental effects of snow, rain, and mud. However, vinyl overboots issued and worn for environmental protection should not be used for CBR protection; a new pair should be issued with CBR protective gear. Following contamination by liquid agent, the overboots will provide protection for a limited time. Subsequently, they should be decontaminated with a 5% household bleach or a 5% high-test hypochlorite solution. If signs of deterioration occur after decontamination, the overboots should be replaced.[21] Additional information about wear-times and protective capabilities can be found in Field Manual 3-11.4, *Multiservice Tactics, and Procedures for NBC Protection.*[14]

Alternative footwear system. The alternative footwear system (AFS) is a lightweight, low-volume overboot for use by ground and shipboard forces. AFS is worn over standard combat boots and provides a minimum of 24 hours protection from chemical agents in liquid and vapor form. The overboot has an antislip ridge tread pattern for improved traction, an antistatic surface, and fully sealed and vulcanized seams, as well as three sets of buttons with a butyl rubber securing strap for each set (Figure 17-15). The adjustable securing strap is symmetrical and can be released from either side of the overboot. Other features include mobility, agility, and reduced combat load.[15,21]

Chemical protective glove set. The chemical protective glove set consists of an outer glove for chemical protection and an inner glove for perspiration absorption. The outer glove is made of impermeable butyl rubber, and the inner glove is made of white cotton. The gloves come in three thicknesses: 7, 14, and 25 mil. Service members such as medical, teletypist, and electronic repair personnel, whose tasks require extreme tactility and sensitivity and who do not expose the gloves to harsh treatment, use the 7-mil glove set. Aviators, vehicle mechanics, weapons crews, and other personnel whose tasks require tactility and sensitivity use the 14-mil glove set. Personnel who perform close

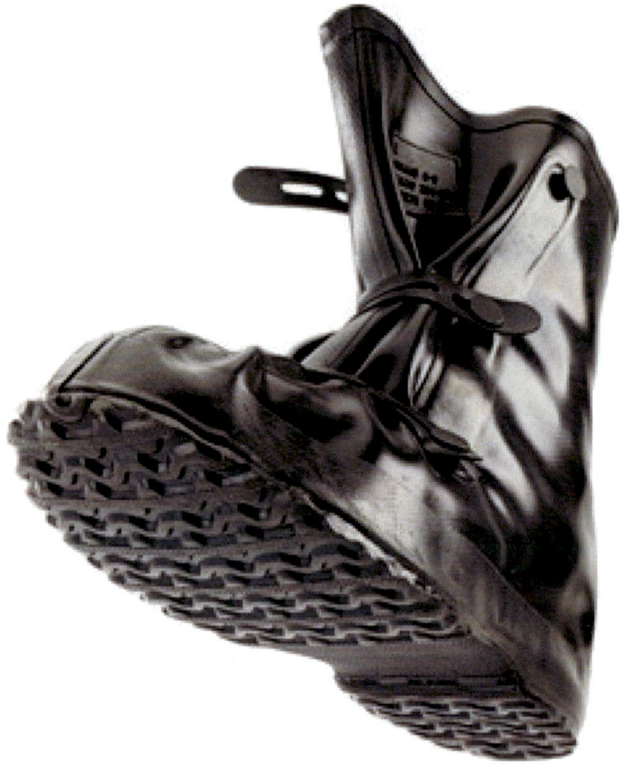

Fig. 17-15. The alternative footwear system.
Photograph: Courtesy of the Joint Program Management Office-Individual Protection (JPMO-IP), Quantico, Va.

combat tasks and other heavy labor tasks use the 25-mil glove set (Figure 17-16). All of the sets protect against liquid chemical agents and vapor hazards. However, if the 7-mil set is contaminated, it must be replaced or decontaminated within 6 hours after exposure. The 14-mil and 25-mil sets will provide protection following contamination for 24 hours. All three glove sets can be decontaminated with a 5% bleach or a 5% high-test hypochlorite solution, then inspected and reused. All gloves become sticky and soft if exposed to petroleum-based fluids and must be replaced. Gloves must be replaced after any damage or degradation.[14,21]

Joint service lightweight integrated suit technology block 2 glove upgrade. The JSLIST block 2 glove upgrade (JB2GU) provides 24 hours of CB protection from battlefield concentrations of all known agents for up to 30 days of wear. The glove provides enhanced tactility, dexterity, durability, and comfort over existing systems and can be worn in all climates. These qualities satisfy a broader spectrum of ground, shipboard, and aviation requirements. The JB2GU comes in two variants (Figure 17-17): flame-resistant (FR) and non–flame-resistant (nFR). The FR variant combines a Nomex (DuPont, Wilmington, Del)/leather outer glove with an inner chemical protective liner for aviators and combat vehicle crews. The nFR variant is a molded glove made from compounded butyl rubber and comes with a removable protective liner for sweat management. The nFR glove is primarily for ground forces.[15]

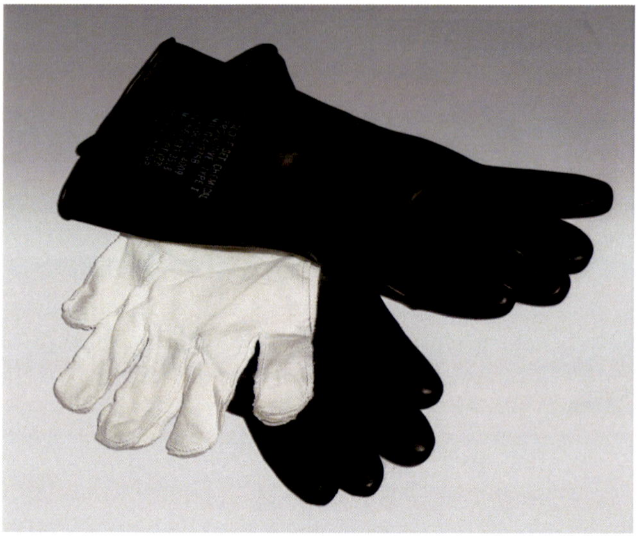

Fig. 17-16. The 25-mil chemical protective glove set with cotton liners.
Photograph: Courtesy of the Chemical Casualty Care Division, US Army Medical Research Institute of Chemical Defense, Aberdeen Proving Ground, Md.

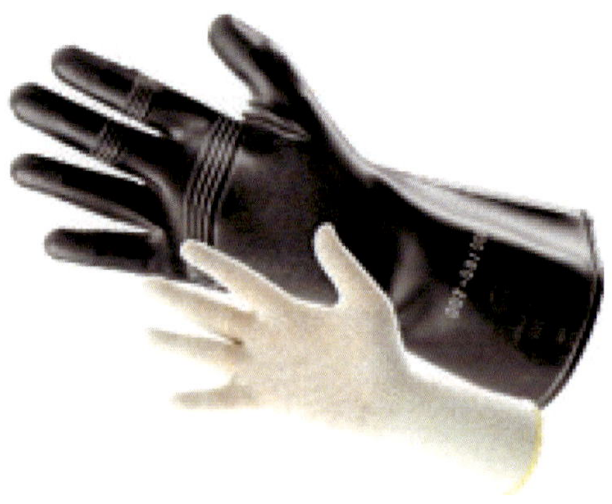

Fig. 17-17. The joint service lightweight integrated suit technology block 2 upgrade glove, non–flame-resistant variant.
Photograph: Courtesy of AirBoss Defense (Acton Vale, Québec, Canada).

Psychological Factors

The threat of CBRN warfare creates unique fears in personnel, and protective gear isolates them from the environment. Individuals encapsulated in MOPP ensembles are subject to both physiological and psychological stresses. MOPP 4 reduces the ability to see and hear clearly and makes it more difficult to recognize and communicate with others, which creates or increases feelings of isolation and confusion. Chemical filters in the protective mask make breathing more difficult, which can create feelings of claustrophobia or panic in many personnel.[14] In some cases, these personnel hyperventilate, causing the eyelenses to fog up, which further inhibits the ability to carry out tasks. As a result, many service members either break the seal and lift the protective mask off the face or remove it completely.[1] Such problems can be corrected by training personnel to relax and avoid taking deep or rapid breaths while wearing the protective mask.

Personnel wearing MOPP 4 will take about one-half times longer to perform most tasks,[14] which can cause frustration and stress. The adverse impact of psychological stress during MOPP operations can be minimized by the experience and confidence provided by realistic training in MOPP gear with the protective mask. Training in MOPP gear should allow for gradual increase of wear time and should focus on tasks personnel are expected to accomplish while encapsulated in MOPP ensemble in CBRN environments.

DETECTION AND WARNING

Detection of a chemical attack, with subsequent warning of affected forces downwind, can allow adoption of an effective protective posture and continuation of military operations with minimal degradation. This section will discuss instruments that have the greatest impact on military medical operations; special purpose items are not discussed.[1] The Army has a wide range of chemical agent detectors and alarms available to protect the force. These detectors are divided into two groups: point detectors and standoff detectors.

Point Detectors

Point detectors sample the immediate area to determine the presence of chemical agents. The sample is most often taken from the atmosphere; however, specialized detection kits can be used to sample soil or water. In addition to monitoring the atmosphere, point detectors provide monitoring after an attack, identify the contaminated area, monitor collective protection areas, monitor effectiveness of decontamination, and identify chemical contamination during reconnaissance efforts.[1,14,24]

M8 Chemical Agent Detection Paper

M8 chemical agent detection paper detects and identifies liquid chemical agents. The tan paper comes in a booklet containing 25 perforated sheets (2 × 3 in), which are heat sealed in a polyethylene envelope. Three sensitive indicator dyes are suspended in the paper matrix. The paper is blotted on a suspected liquid agent and observed for a color change, which will occur within 30 seconds: VX turns the paper dark green, the G series agents turn the paper yellow, and blister agent turns it red (Figure 17-18). M8 paper will change color with many interferents, such as sodium hydroxide and petroleum products; thus, it is not a reliable way to check the completeness of personnel decontamination, which should always be verified with another means. The M8 paper has a 10-year shelf life from the manufacture date, which is stamped on the back cover of the booklet (the integrity and the quality of the paper is compromised past the shelf life).[14,24]

M9 Chemical Agent Detection Paper

M9 chemical agent detection paper is a portable, single roll of paper that comes with a Mylar (DuPont, Wilmington, Del) adhesive-backed and -coated tape.

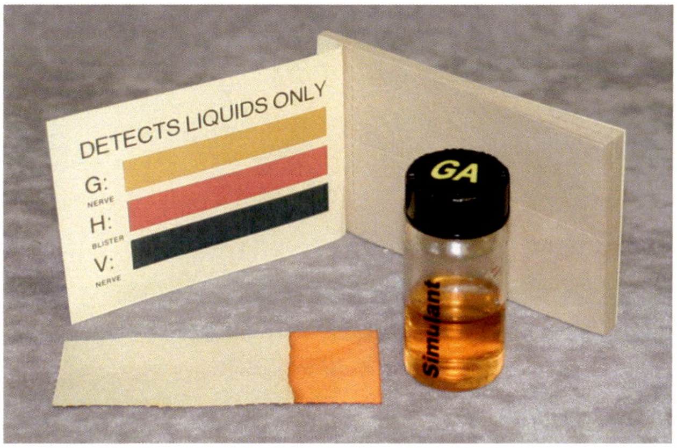

Fig. 17-18. The M8 chemical agent detection paper detects and identifies GA (G series nerve agent) simulant from the vial by changing color in less than 30 seconds.
Photograph: Courtesy of the Chemical Casualty Care Division, US Army Medical Research Institute of Chemical Defense, Aberdeen Proving Ground, Md.

It contains a suspension of an agent-sensitive dye in a green-colored paper matrix. The dye turns pink, red, reddish brown, or red-purple when exposed to agent but does not identify the specific agent. M9 paper, which is similar to masking tape, is used by attaching strips to an overgarment or equipment such as vehicle controls, then inspecting the strips routinely for color change (Figure 17-19). The paper should not be attached to surfaces above 125°F (52°C). Excessive heat will discolor the tape and lead to a false positive reaction. M9 paper is more sensitive to nerve and blister agents and reacts more rapidly than M8 paper, although it also reacts to a wide range of interferents such as petroleum products, brake fluid, aircraft cleaning compounds, insect repellent, defoliant, and antifreeze.[14,24]

Improved Chemical Agent Monitor

The improved chemical agent monitor (ICAM) is a hand-held device designed for monitoring chemical agent contamination on personnel, equipment, and surfaces (Figure 17-20). It uses ion mobility spectrometry technology to detect and discriminate between mustard and nerve agent vapor. The concentrations of agents detected by the ICAM areas are as follows: for sarin (GB), 0.03 mg/m^3; for VX, 0.1 mg/m^3; and for mustard (HD), 0.1 mg/m^3.[1,14,24]

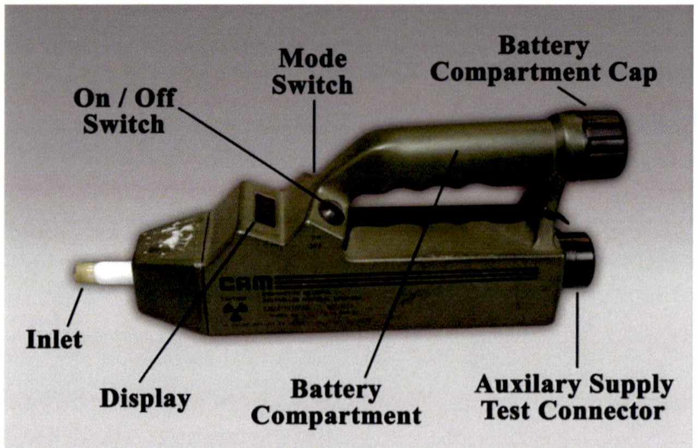

Fig. 17-20. The improved chemical agent monitor.
Photograph: Courtesy of the Chemical Casualty Care Division, US Army Medical Research Institute of Chemical Defense, Aberdeen Proving Ground, Md.

The unit is simple to operate, can be held in either hand while the user is wearing chemical protective equipment, and can be operated day or night. Relative vapor hazard and malfunction information is displayed by bars on a liquid crystal display. The ICAM is a point monitor only and cannot give an assessment of an area vapor hazard. It may give false readings when used in enclosed spaces or near strong vapor sources such as dense smoke, aromatic vapors, cleaning compounds, exhausts from some rocket motors, and fumes from some munitions. Because of the technology employed, the ICAM is subject to saturation; it must be cleared before each use to function properly.[14,24–26]

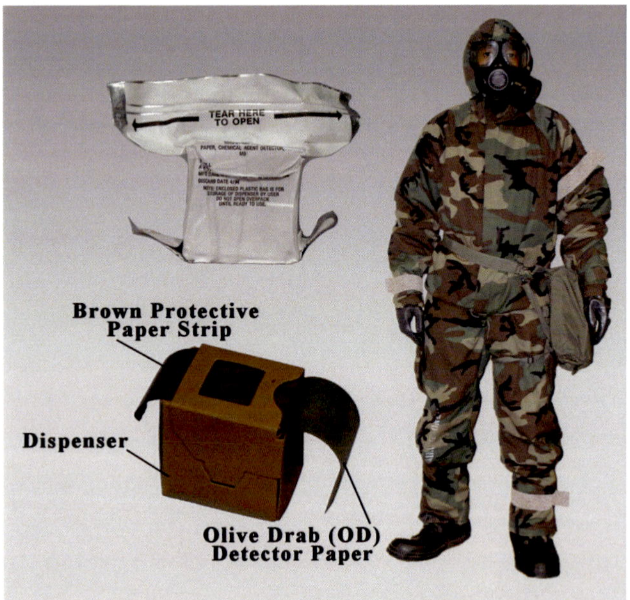

Fig. 17-19. M9 paper is attached to a protective overgarment to detect the presence of liquid chemical warfare agents. Note: The paper should not be attached to hot surfaces, which will discolor the tape and lead to a false positive reaction.
Photograph: Courtesy of the Chemical Casualty Care Division, US Army Medical Research Institute of Chemical Defense, Aberdeen Proving Ground, Md.

Chemical Agent Detector Kit

The M256A1 chemical agent detector kit is a portable, expendable item capable of detecting and identifying hazardous concentrations of nerve and blister agents and cyanide. The kit is used after a chemical attack to determine whether personnel can safely unmask or reduce the protective posture level. Each kit consists of 12 disposable plastic sampler-detectors (ticket or card), one booklet of M8 paper, and a set of instruction cards (Figure 17-21). Each ticket or card contains laboratory filter paper test spots for the various agents. The technology used is wet chemistry, enzymatic substrate-based reactions, in which the presence of agents is indicated by a specific color change. Response time is about 15 minutes. Some smokes, petroleum products, and high temperatures may produce false readings.[27] The M256A1 kit cannot be used to detect

a

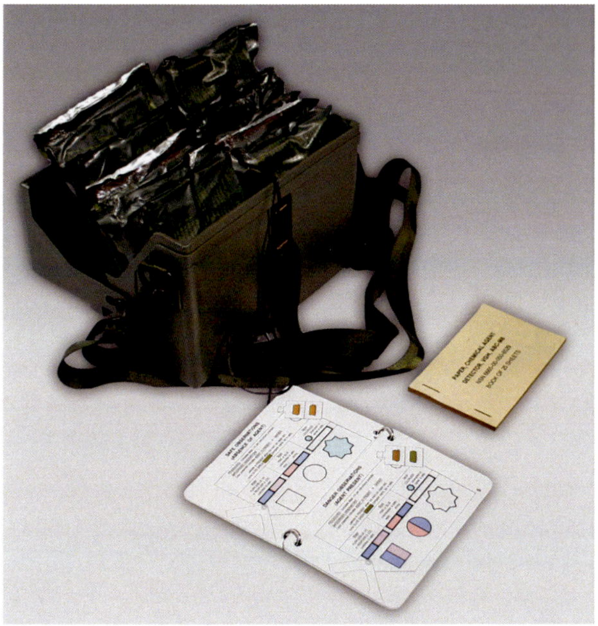

b

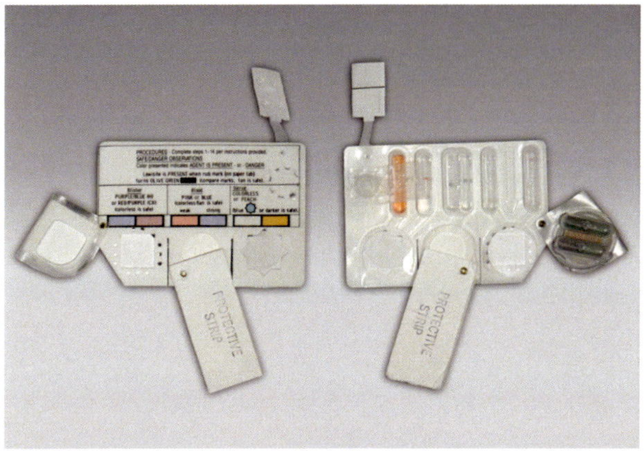

Fig. 17-21. (a) The M256A1 chemical agent detector kit. **(b)** The sampler/detector is used to test for vapor contamination.
Photographs: Courtesy of the Chemical Casualty Care Division, US Army Medical Research Institute of Chemical Defense, Aberdeen Proving Ground, Md.

agent in water. It can, however, be used to check an area before a military unit moves in or to define clean areas or routes. Some chemical ingredients in the kit are considered possible carcinogens and should be handled as such. The emissions produced by the kit are also toxic; a mask and gloves must be worn while the kit is being used.[1,14,24]

The detection limits for the M256A1 are as follows: for the G series nerve agents, 0.005 mg/m^3; for VX, 0.02 mg/m^3; for the vesicants mustard (HD) and lewisite, above threshold concentrations of 3.0 mg/m^3 and 14 mg/m^3, respectively; for hydrogen cyanide (AC), 11 mg/m^3; and for cyanogen chloride (CK), 10 mg/m^3.

Chemical Agent Water Testing Kit

The M272 chemical agent water testing kit is designed to detect and identify, via colorimetric reactions, hazardous levels of nerve agents, mustard, lewisite, and cyanide in treated or untreated water. A full kit contains enough supplies to perform 25 tests for each agent, and simulants are included for training use (Figure 17-22). About 20 minutes is required to perform all four tests. Some kit chemicals can be very harmful; all bodily contact with the chemicals should be avoided, and the kit should only be handled while wearing protective gloves and equipment. Detection limits are as follows: for the G-series nerve agents and VX, 0.02 mg/L; for the vesicants lewisite and mustard (H and HD), 2.0 mg/L; and for the cyanides (AC and CK), 20 mg/L.[14,24]

M22 Automatic Chemical Agent Detector and Alarm

The M22 automatic chemical agent detector and alarm is an off-the-shelf automatic chemical agent alarm system capable of detecting and identifying standard blister and nerve agents simultaneously. The M22 system is portable and operates independently after system start-up. The system consists of the M88 detector and up to five M42 alarms, which provide both an audible and visible warning (Figure 17-23). The M22 system is used primarily to alert stationary units when a cloud of nerve agent vapor has arrived or is about to arrive at their position, providing a communications interface for automatic battlefield warning and reporting. The M22 can be located within a hospital complex, with alarm units placed to cover all critical care, treatment, and support areas. It can also augment the ICAM as a survey instrument.[14,24]

Standoff Detectors

Early warning of chemical agents provides troops the necessary time to increase protective posture and to avoid contaminated areas. Standoff detectors provide this early warning at line-of-sight distances. Optical remote sensing technologies, employing infrared spectral analysis techniques, have been used in the development of chemical agent standoff detection technologies, including two types of remote sensing systems: passive and active (laser). The passive system discussed below employs a Fourier transform infrared spectrometer.[1,14,24]

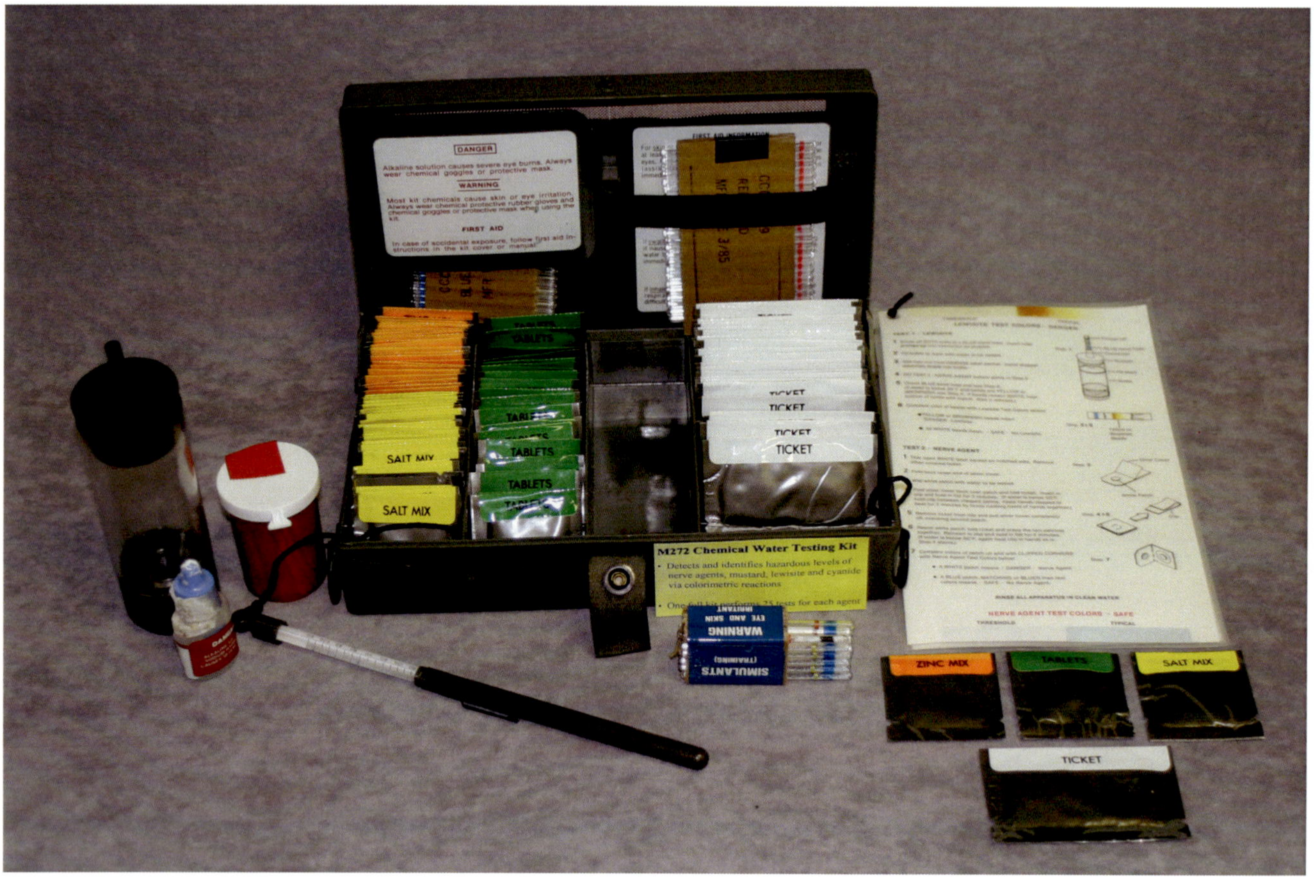

Fig. 17-22. The M272 chemical agent water testing kit and its components. New kits have a test strip instead of a thermometer.
Photograph: Courtesy of the Chemical Casualty Care Division, US Army Medical Research Institute of Chemical Defense, Aberdeen Proving Ground, Md.

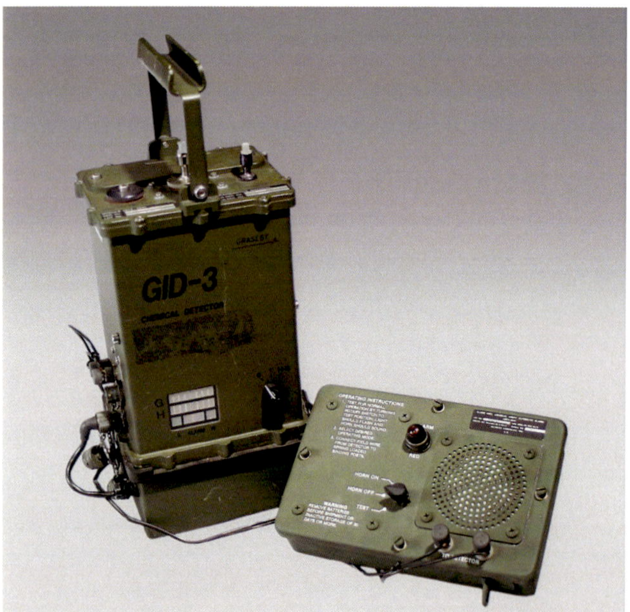

Fig. 17-23. The M22 automatic chemical agent detector and alarm consists of the M88 detector (left) and the M42 alarm (right).
Photograph: Courtesy of the Chemical Casualty Care Division, US Army Medical Research Institute of Chemical Defense, Aberdeen Proving Ground, Md.

M21 Remote Sensing Chemical Agent Alarm

The M21 remote sensing chemical agent alarm is the first standoff chemical agent detector approved for fielding to military personnel. The M21 is a passive infrared device that detects nerve and blister agent clouds based on changes in the background infrared spectra caused by the presence of the agent vapor. In a stationary position, the M21 alarm automatically scans a horizontal 60° arc and can recognize agent clouds at line-of-sight ranges up to 5 km (Figure 17-24). It reacts both audibly by horn and visually by illuminating

a

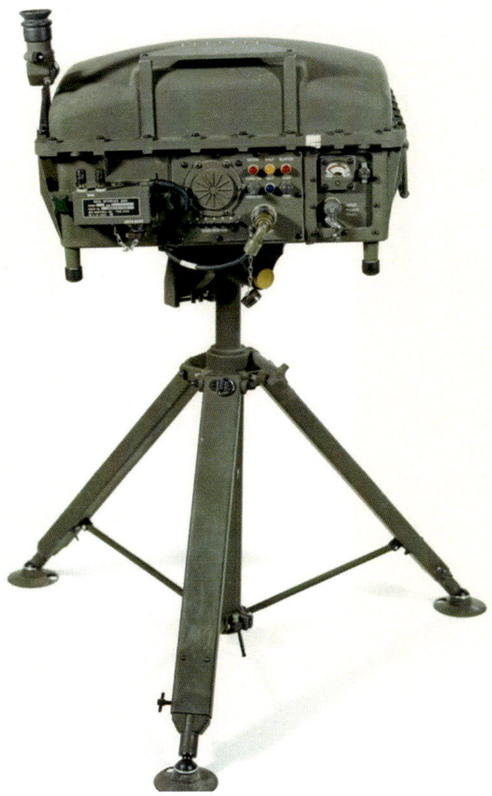

b

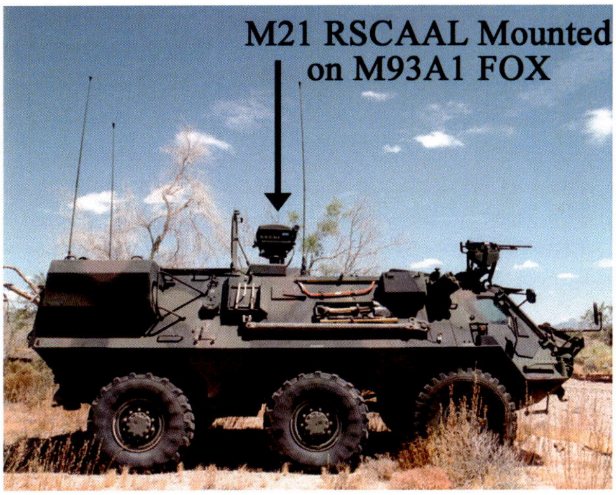

Fig. 17-24. (a) The M21 remote sensing chemical agent alarm (RSCAAL) deployed in a stationary position. **(b)** The RSCAAL mounted on a Fox nuclear, biological and chemical reconnaissance system allows commanders to identify contaminated areas and maneuver around them.
Photographs: Courtesy of Joint Product Manager, NBC Contamination Avoidance, Aberdeen Proving Ground, Md.

either a blister or nerve agent light.[14,24]

Usually, the M21 is placed facing into the wind. It measures and stores a background spectrum that is then analyzed by an onboard microcomputer, which makes agent/no agent decisions based on ambient radiance levels. Response time is 1 minute or less. The sensitivity of the M21 for detecting nerve agents (GA, GB, and GD) is 90 mg/m^3; for vesicants its sensitivity is 500 mg/m^3 for lewisite and 2,300 mg/m^3 for sulfur mustard.[14,24]

Joint Services Lightweight Standoff Chemical Agent Detector

The joint services lightweight standoff chemical agent detector is a state-of-the-art detection system designed to provide US forces with enhanced capability in detecting chemical warfare agents, significantly improving on the capabilities of the currently fielded M21 alarm. The lightweight, passive, and fully automatic system scans the surrounding atmosphere for chemical warfare agent vapors. The detector provides standoff detection and warning for nerve, blister, and blood agent vapor clouds. It furnishes on-the-move, 360° coverage from a variety of tactical and reconnaissance platforms at distances up to 5 km (Figure 17-25). This system will provide enhanced early warning to allow personnel to avoid chemically contaminated battlespace or, when avoidance is not possible, provide extra time to don MOPP gear or achieve the appropriate MOPP level.[14,24,28]

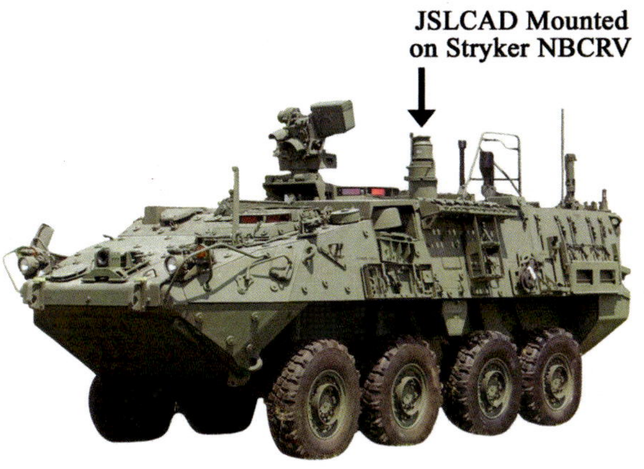

Fig. 17-25. Joint services lightweight standoff chemical agent detector (JSLSCAD) mounted on a Stryker nuclear, biological, chemical reconnaissance vehicle (NBCRV).
Photograph: Courtesy of Joint Product Manager, NBC Contamination Avoidance, Aberdeen Proving Ground, Md.

TOXIC INDUSTRIAL MATERIAL PROTECTION

TIM, especially TICs, are often available in enormous quantities, do not require extensive research, and can be mass-produced. TIM, which can be released from industrial plants or storage depots through accidental or deliberate damage, can be used as improvised weapons and have the potential for inclusion in clandestine weapons programs or contingency plans. Deliberate or inadvertent release of TIM significantly increases hazards to the indigenous population and deployed US forces. Military personal protection, detection, and medical countermeasures are not specifically designed for TIM hazards. Often there are no specific antidotes for TICs. Each TIM should be evaluated individually to establish protection and response procedures and to select associated equipment requirements.[29]

Individual Protection

Military individual protective equipment (IPE) is designed to protect personnel from CBR agents in a combat environment, but it provides only limited protection from other hazards. Personnel equipped with standard military IPE are not protected in a TIC environment and should seek a clean area as soon as possible. The military chemical protective mask does not afford sufficient protection within the immediate hazard zone, where extremely high concentrations of industrial chemicals such as ammonia may occur and where the lack of oxygen requires a self-contained breathing apparatus (Figure 17-26). The military respirator should only be used for emergency protection against the immediate effects of a toxic release and during evacuation from the immediate hazard zone.[30] When planning for operations in areas where TIM may be present, commanders must include considerations of the potential hazards and the appropriate level of protection and equipment for effective response.

The US Environmental Protection Agency has established four levels of protection, A, B, C, and D, according to 29 CFR 1910.120. The Occupational Safety and Health Administration and the National Fire Protection Agency have developed guidelines for each level. The level of skin and respiratory protection provided by the selected chemical protective ensemble determines the protection furnished to the responder (see Chapter 16, Decontamination of Chemical Casualties, Exhibit 16-3).[14]

Detection and Identification

Numerous technologies are available for the detection and identification of TIM. The applicability of this equipment to potential user groups depends on the characteristics of the detection equipment, the type of TIM, and the objective of the user.[31] Standard military chemical detectors are designed only to detect chemical agents. Detection of TICs can, in some circumstances, be made by in-service military chemical detection systems.

Several industrial detectors are available for the rapid detection of specific industrial chemicals. Detectors such as Dräger-Tubes (Draeger Safety Inc, Luebeck, Germany) can be used for detecting and determining the concentration of a large number of dan-

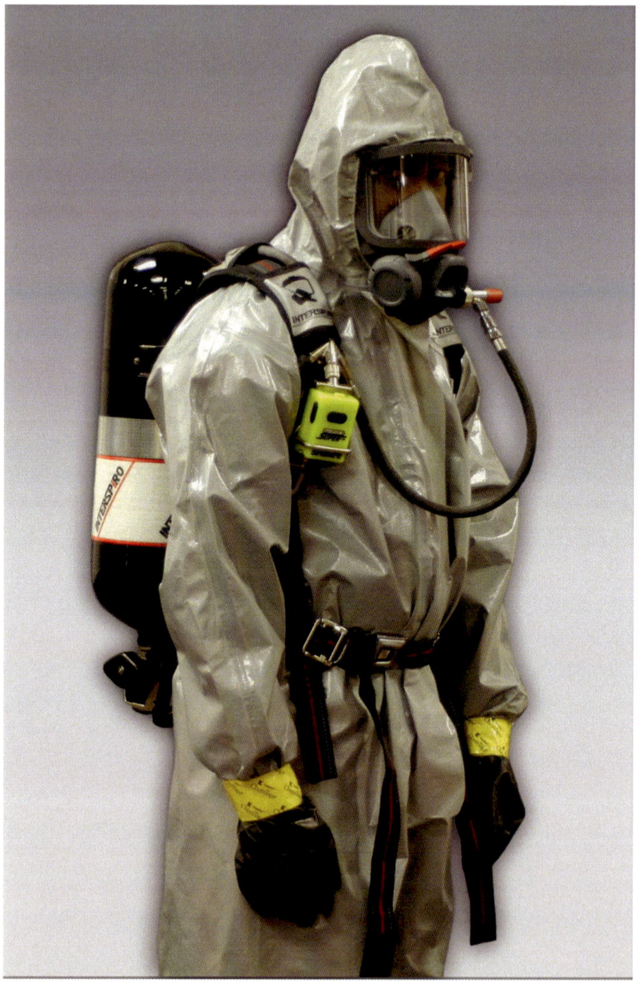

Fig. 17-26. The self-contained breathing apparatus is used when the highest level of respiratory protection is necessary.
Photograph: Courtesy of the Chemical Casualty Care Division, US Army Medical Research Institute of Chemical Defense, Aberdeen Proving Ground, Md.

gerous chemicals. This detector comes in the form of a simply operated kit using individual reagent tubes to detect a variety of specific industrial chemicals. Such detectors can be supplied to units operating in an area with a known hazard from industrial chemicals.[30]

TIC and TIM detector technology is constantly being upgraded as developers seek devices that are easier to use, provide more accurate readings, and can identify a wider array of hazards. The National Institute of Justice's *Guide for the Selection of Chemical Agent and Toxic Industrial Material Detection Equipment for Emergency First Responders*[31] is more practical than technical and provides information on a variety factors to be considered when purchasing detection equipment, including sensitivity, detection states, and portability.

DECONTAMINATION EQUIPMENT

The physical properties of chemical agents are highly variable. Chemical agents range from nerve agent vapor, which usually dissipates in a few minutes to a few hours, to vesicants such as mustard, which can remain active for weeks (or in some cases, years; buried and recovered World War I mustard projectiles are often still toxic). These various properties make timely decontamination of skin and personal equipment that has been exposed to agent, especially liquid agent, imperative. Skin decontamination should ideally take place within 2 minutes, and equipment decontamination should be completed within 1 hour. For more detailed information on decontamination and decontamination equipment used for the thorough decontamination of patients, refer to Chapter 16, Decontamination of Chemical Casualties.

Personnel Decontamination

Personnel decontamination, performed to reduce the level of contamination so it no longer presents a hazard to the individual, consists of removing contaminated clothing and decontaminating the skin. To expedite this procedure, personnel decontamination kits are used to remove gross contamination. Thorough decontamination, which is conducted by specialized decontamination units, is provided to troops to reduce the requirement for wearing complete IPE. Additionally, when both crews and equipment are contaminated, combined complete personnel and equipment decontamination operations are scheduled as the situation and mission permit, bearing in mind the lengthy time required for such an operation. During this complete decontamination commanders can give their soldiers rest and a change of IPE.[33] The personnel decontamination items described below would be used to quickly decontaminate the skin of an exposed individual. Open wounds, however, should be decontaminated with water or saline.[32–35]

M291 Skin Decontamination Kit

The M291 kit consists of a wallet-type pouch containing six individual packets. Each packet contains a non-woven fiber-fill laminated pad impregnated with the decontamination compound (Ambergard XE-555 resin [Rohm and Haas Co, Philadelphia, Penn]) that reacts with chemical agents to absorb and neutralize in a single step (Figure 17-27). Decontamination is accomplished by opening the packet and scrubbing the skin surface with the applicator pad until an even coating of the resin is achieved. As the pad is scrubbed over the exposed/contaminated skin area, the chemicals are rapidly transferred into, trapped, and retained in the interior of the resin particles. The presence of acidic and basic groups in the resin promotes the destruction of trapped chemical agents. The kit can also be used to decontaminate the outside of protective masks, butyl rubber gloves, and the hood of individual protective equipment.[36] The powder should be kept away from wounds, the eyes, and the mouth. The M291 kit has a 10-year shelf life from the manufacture date stamped on the upper right corner of each packet. Expired or unserviceable kits can not be used for training; they must be discarded according to organization standing operating procedures.[32–35]

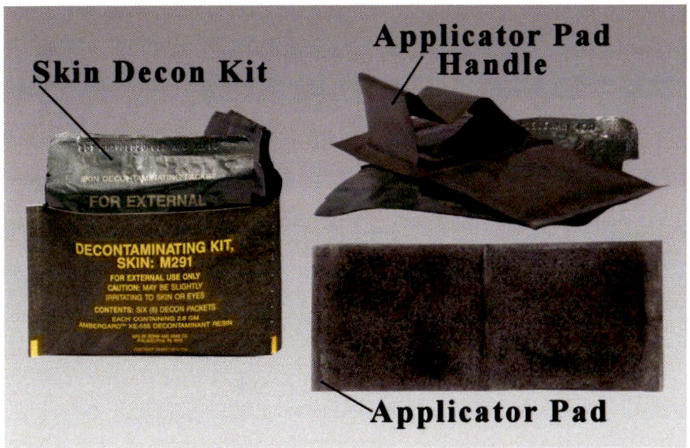

Fig. 17-27. The M291 skin decontamination kit.
Photograph: Courtesy of the Chemical Casualty Care Division, US Army Medical Research Institute of Chemical Defense, Aberdeen Proving Ground, Md.

Joint Service Personnel Skin Decontamination System

The joint service personnel skin decontamination system consists of decontaminants and applicators required to immediately reduce morbidity and mortality resulting from chemical warfare agent contamination of the skin. It is expected to receive US Food and Drug Administration approval as an individually carried skin decontamination kit. The system's applicators are preimpregnated with reactive skin decontamination lotion, a potassium solution dissolved in a special solvent and water (Figure 17-28) that facilitates the reaction of decontamination between the potassium salt and the chemical agent. The lotion decontaminates the warfare agents HD, soman (GD), and VX as well as T-2 mycotoxins on skin to a level that eliminates toxic effects better than the M291 kit. Each packet will decontaminate an area of 1,300 cm^2. The system can be used in temperatures ranging from −25°F/−32°C to 130°F/54°C. When approved, the system will be used by service members to perform immediate decontamination of skin, field protective masks, mask hoods, chemical protective gloves, chemical protective boots, and individual and crew-served weapons under .50 caliber.[37] It is expected that the military services will use this system to replace or augment the M291 kit.[32–35]

Equipment Decontamination

Equipment decontamination items are used to destroy, remove, or neutralize most of the CBRN hazards from personal gear or unit equipment. Of the many items available to decontaminate equipment, those most useful to the medical community are described below.

M295 Equipment Decontamination Kit

The M295 is a hand-held kit used to apply decontaminant to an individual's personal equipment, including mask, hood, and boots. Each kit consists of a carrying pouch containing four sealed, soft-pack packets designed to fit comfortably within a pocket of the chemical protective overgarment. Each individual wipe-down mitt in the kit is comprised of 22 g of decontaminating powder (A-200-SiC-1005S) contained within a pad material and a polyethylene film backing (Figure 17-29). In use, powder from the mitt is allowed to flow freely through the pad material. Decontamination is accomplished through sorption of contamination by both the pad and the decontaminating powder.[32–35]

M100 Sorbent Decontamination System

The M100 sorbent decontamination system replaces the M11 and M13 portable decontamination appara-

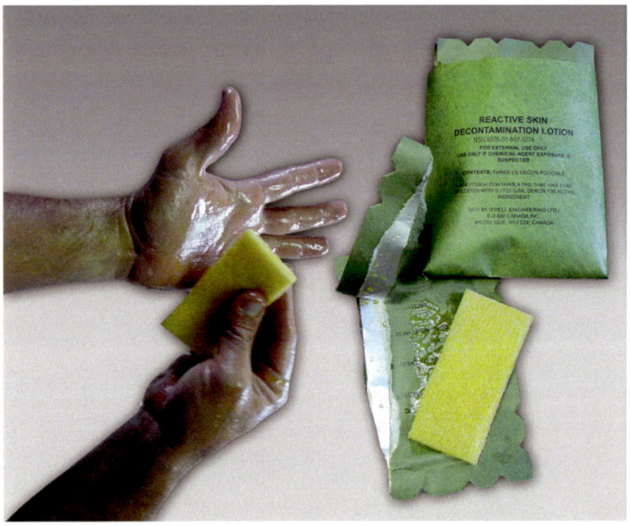

Fig. 17-28. A service member using the joint service personnel skin decontamination system with reactive skin decontamination lotion to decontaminate his hands.
Photograph: Courtesy of the Chemical Casualty Care Division, US Army Medical Research Institute of Chemical Defense, Aberdeen Proving Ground, Md.

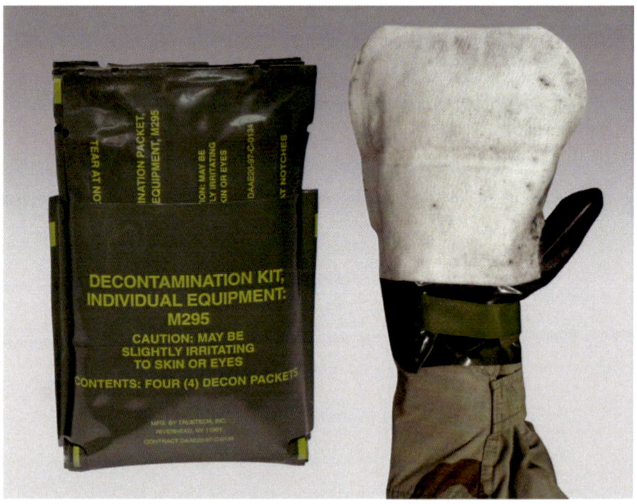

Figure 17-29. The M295 individual equipment decontamination kit. Wipe-down mitt on right.
Photograph: Courtesy of the Chemical Casualty Care Division, US Army Medical Research Institute of Chemical Defense, Aberdeen Proving Ground, Md

tuses previously employed in spray-down procedures associated with operational decontamination. Each M100 system consists of two 0.7-lb packs of reactive sorbent powder, two wash mitt-type sorbent applicators, a case, straps, and detailed instructions (Figure 17-30). The system uses the same nontoxic and noncorrosive reactive sorbent powder as in the M295 kit to remove and neutralize chemical agent from surfaces. The sorbent powder is first poured onto the palm of the mitt, then the mitt is used to rub and wipe the contaminated surfaces until target areas are visually dry. The system removes gross liquid contamination, limits the spread of chemical agent, preserves the integrity of MOPP gear, and minimizes casualties while decreasing decontamination time and eliminating the need for water.[32–35]

M17 Lightweight Decontamination System

The M17 lightweight decontamination system is a rugged, simple-to-use, powerful, multipurpose CB system for decontaminating and preserving military materiel in a contaminated environment. The system is designed to draw water from any source and deliver it to the two installed spray wands at pressures up to 100 psi and temperatures up to 120°C (Figure 17-31). The M17 can also be used as a personnel showering system and for cleaning vehicles and food handling and hospital equipment.[32–35]

The M17 is capable of dispensing Easy DECON 200 (Envirofoam Technologies Inc, Huntsville, Ala) as a liquid or as a foam (using a foam nozzle), and it can be used in an anticorrosion mode. It is designed for ease of operation, with one soldier operating each of its two outfitted wands. The M17 has a 3,000-gallon collapsible water tank that can be prepositioned and filled for hot water showers or hospital use.[38,39] A diesel version—a portable, lightweight, compact, engine-driven pump and multifuel-fired water heating system—is under development and will be capable of performing the same immediate and operational decontamination procedures as required of any of the M17 series systems.[32–35]

Decontamination Methods in Development

A need still exists for an effective and environmentally safe reactive decontaminant that does not harm equipment and personnel. Bacterial enzymes, catalytic-type compounds, and other stable decontaminants (eg, quaternary ammonium complexes) are under consideration. Sorbent compounds and nonaqueous decontaminants are also being investigated for use on electronic components and other sensitive equipment.[1] A joint platform interior decontamination system is being investigated for use in decontaminat-

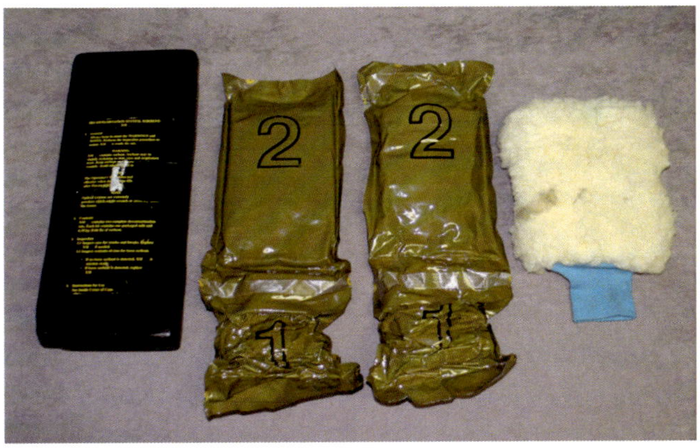

Fig. 17-30. The M100 sorbent decontamination system provides vehicle and crew-served weapon (≥ .50 caliber) operators the capability to perform operator wipe-down (previously referred to as operator spray-down) during immediate decontamination operations.
Photograph: Courtesy of the Chemical Casualty Care Division, US Army Medical Research Institute of Chemical Defense, Aberdeen Proving Ground, Md.

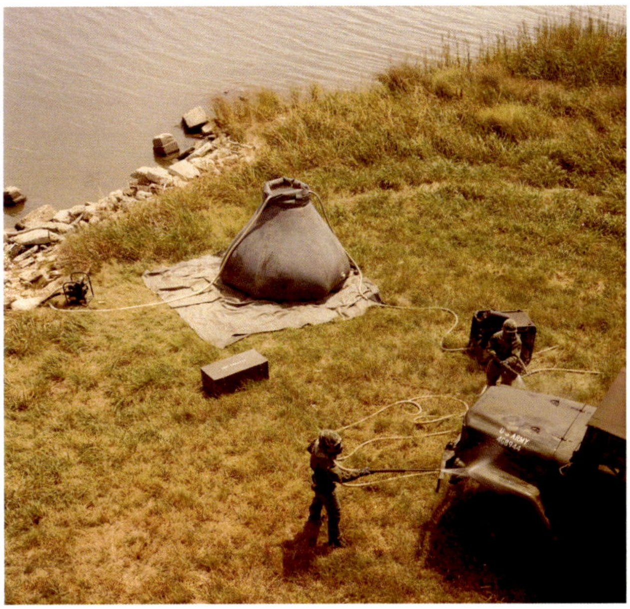

Fig.17-31. The M17 lightweight decontamination system. The system is designed to decontaminate equipment but can also be used as a personnel showering system.
Photograph: Courtesy of the Chemical Casualty Care Division, US Army Medical Research Institute of Chemical Defense, Aberdeen Proving Ground, Md.

ing chemical and biological warfare agents on the interior of aircraft, vehicles, ships, and buildings. This system will have two increments: increment I will provide capabilities to decontaminate interior areas and equipment, and increment II will focus on improving decontamination processes, speed, efficacy, TIM decontamination, and other system capabilities.[32–35]

COLLECTIVE PROTECTION

Collective protection (COLPRO) provides a protective capability to personnel who must operate in an environment where wearing IPE is not possible. COLPRO is typically incorporated into chemically protected medical treatment facilities, command centers, or rest areas. The use of COLPRO allows for sustained operations in a contaminated environment.

COLPRO systems are categorized according to their tactical application: fixed-site, transportable, and mobile. Fixed-site COLPRO consists of hardened, semihardened, or unhardened systems. Transportable COLPRO shelters can be moved as needed to achieve mission requirements. Transportable shelters are generally unhardened. Mobile COLPRO shelters include facilities that are armored or soft-skinned; this type of system may or may not have the capability to be used on the move. Mobile systems may not have integrated airlocks or contamination control areas. COLPRO shelters are constructed of rigid-wall, soft-wall, or hybrid materials and should include design features that will facilitate tactical functions without the restrictions of IPE.[14, 29] This section addresses COLPRO systems that have been specifically designed for, or systems that are ideally suited for, applications in health service support.

Chemically Protected Deployable Medical System

The chemically protected deployable medical system (DEPMEDS) was fielded in 2003 under the Mission Force 2000 configuration, which protects 236 beds of a 298-bed DEPMEDS hospital (Figure 17-32). All Mission Force 2000 chemically protected DEPMEDS will be upgraded to the medical reengineering initiative configuration, which protects a complete 248-bed DEPMEDS combat support hospital. This configuration also allows simultaneous split-base hospital operations through 84-bed and 164-bed hospital companies. The 84-bed company will use the Army Medical Department shelter system. The 164-bed company will use the tent, extendable, modular personnel system. The 248-bed DEPMEDS combat support hospital uses both types of shelter from each hospital company. Chemically protected DEPMEDS consists of the M28 collective protection equipment, designed to protect areas within the hospital from CB contamination. The M28

a

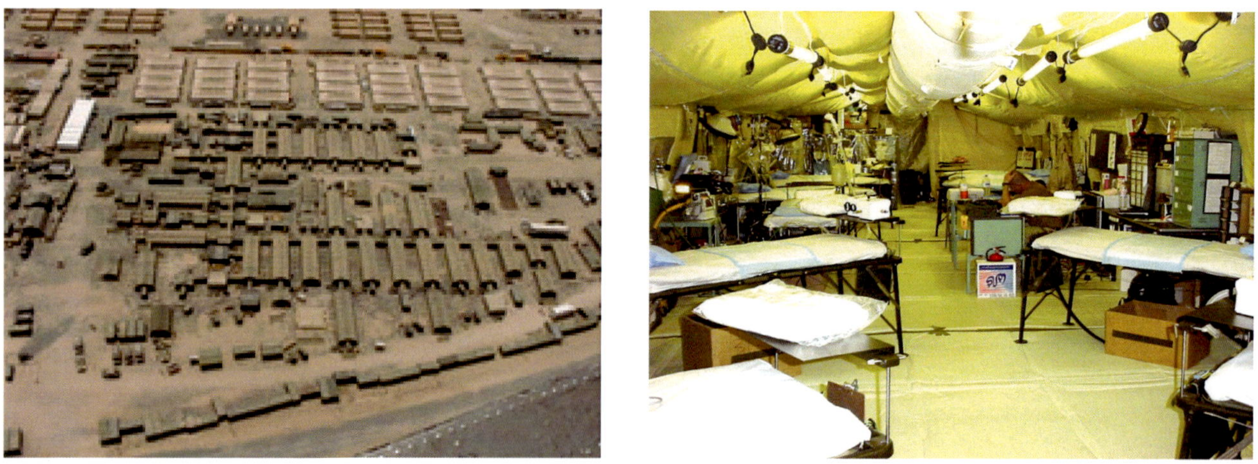

b

Fig. 17-32. (a) The chemically protected deployable medical system as shown in the 236-bed configuration is capable of sustaining continuous operations for up to 72 hours in a contaminated environment. This system provides medical personnel a contamination-free work space allowing them to operate without wearing cumbersome individual protective equipment items. The system is also equipped with two 12-person latrines and 20,000 gallons of water. **(b)** Intensive care units in the system are equipped to perform complex lifesaving medical procedures. This figure illustrates the inside of a treatment unit.
Photographs: Courtesy of the Joint Program Management Office for Nuclear Biological Chemical Collective Protection, Naval Surface Warfare Center Dahlgren, Dahlgren, Va.

collective protection equipment is used with both shelter systems. The entire composite hospital ensemble consists of expandable tentage, passageways, environmental control units, and International Organization for Standardization shelters.[40]

The M28 collective protection equipment consists of the following items: end section liners; center section liners; 32.5-ft liners; 19.5-ft liners; vestibule liners fabricated from a plastic film that is resistant to liquid and vapor agents; a protective entrance airlock (Figure 17-33) for ambulatory personnel made from a butyl-coated material and hung in a collapsible aluminum frame, creating a triangular shape; a tunnel airlock for litter-borne patients consisting of a collapsible frame with entry and exit doors at opposite ends fabricated from a CBR protective cover; a supply airlock for mission resupply while operating under collective protection; a hermetically sealed filter canister and the accessory package, which support the purge requirement during collective protective entry; and a a portable self-contained recirculation filter designed to filter any chemical agent vapors brought in through the entry or exit.[40,41]

Collectively Protected Expeditionary Medical Support

The US Air Force uses the collectively protected expeditionary medical support (CP EMEDS) system (Figure 17-34), a direct replacement for the chemically hardened air transportable hospital. CP EMEDS provides an air transportable medical facility that allows healthcare providers, support staff, and patients to interact in a protected environment without the need for individual protection equipment. Composed of an Air Force small shelter system with a CB liner to harden the shelter, CP EMEDS provides filtered air with slight positive pressure to keep out vapor. The system was designed to be adaptable and can be deployed in a variety of configurations, ranging from a single 32-ft shelter to a complex of ten 32-ft shelters with a 25-bed hospital; its capabilities can be extended to include surgical operations and additional capacity. CP EMEDS is capable of providing medical care to a population of 3,000 to 5,000 service members.[40,42]

Chemical and Biological Protected Shelter

The chemical and biological protective shelter is designed to provide a highly mobile, 300-sq-ft, contamination-free, environmentally controlled work area for forward deployed medical treatment. This shelter is employed at levels I and II medical treatment facilities and forward surgical teams. The system is comprised of a modified high-mobility multipurpose wheeled vehicle, lightweight multipurpose shelter, air beam shelter, and a high-mobility trailer with a 10-kW tacti-

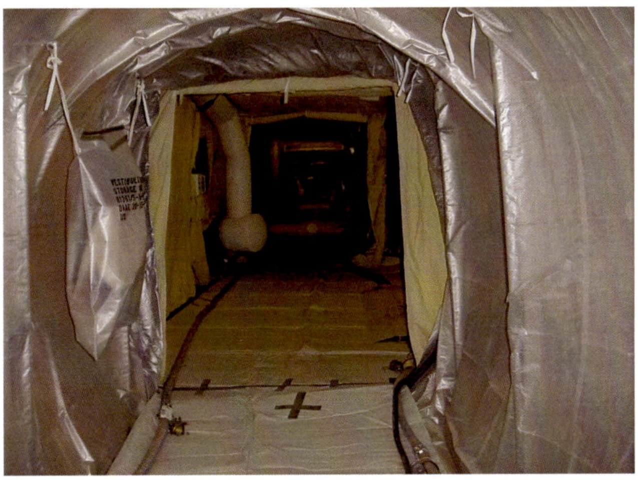

Fig. 17-33. The M28 collective protection equipment is outfitted with multiple entry points capable of receiving litter and ambulatory casualties. These entry points function as positive pressure airlocks; thoroughly decontaminated casualties are directed through the airlocks for an air purge and decontamination check prior to receiving medical treatment.
Photograph: Courtesy of the Joint Program Management Office for Nuclear Biological Chemical Collective Protection, Naval Surface Warfare Center Dahlgren, Dahlgren, Va.

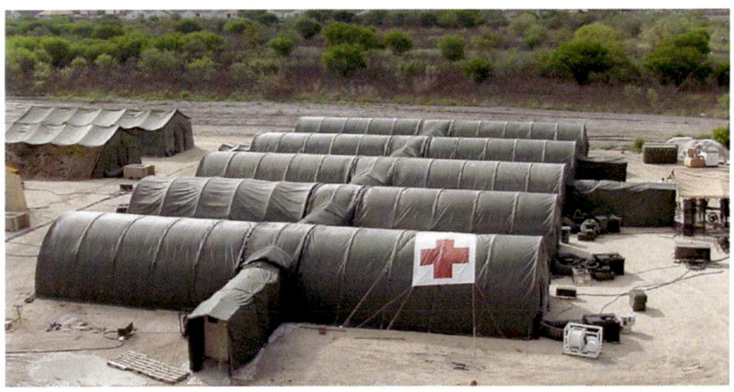

Fig. 17-34. The collectively protected expeditionary medical support system provides protection from chemical and biological warfare agents to health care providers and patients in a contaminated environment. The system provides filtered air that allows occupants to operate without the need for individual protective equipment while inside the shelter. It has been designed for maximum versatility and can be configured to meet the demands of many mission requirements.
Photograph: Courtesy of the Joint Program Management Office for Nuclear Biological Chemical Collective Protection, Naval Surface Warfare Center Dahlgren, Dahlgren, Va.

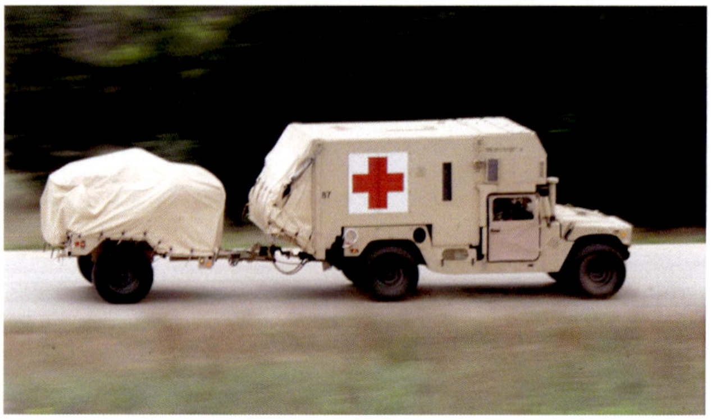

Fig. 17-35. The chemical and biological protective shelter is a highly mobile system that can be established or disestablished by a crew of four in fewer than 20 minutes. Systems are fielded to meet demands of various modified table of organization and equipment requirements. Outfitted with organic medical equipment sets unique to a specific level of care, the system is employed at levels I and II medical treatment facilities.
Photograph: Courtesy of the Joint Program Management Office for Nuclear Biological Chemical Collective Protection, Naval Surface Warfare Center Dahlgren, Dahlgren, Va.

cally quiet generator with frame (Figure 17-35).

The vehicle serves as a power platform for the system; it includes an environmental control unit and CBR filtration system. The lightweight multipurpose shelter, mounted on the rear of the vehicle, contains controls and indicators for inflating and pressurizing the air beam shelter; it also provides a platform for radio communication (Figure 17-36). The 18-sq-ft semicylindrical air-beam–supported shelter, constructed of chemical-agent–resistant fabric, is clamped to an aluminum retainer attached to the rear of the multipurpose shelter. The system is equipped with two air locks that allow passage of both ambulatory and litter bound patients, as well as removable side entrances that permit systems to be joined together as needed to meet mission requirements. The trailer carries the generator, medical supplies, and other items if needed. The generator is available to provide supplemental power to the system.[40]

M20 Simplified Collective Protection Equipment

The M20 simplified collective protective equipment provides 200 cu ft of contamination-free work space. The M20, an inflatable shelter designed for use in a fixed structure, provides protection from chemical and biological agents and radioactive particles, allowing personnel to perform duties without wearing IPE. The system consists of a recirculation filter, shelter assembly, protective entrance, air ducts, and other basic issue items. Tactical application may include command and control, rest relief, communication, and intelligence.

a b

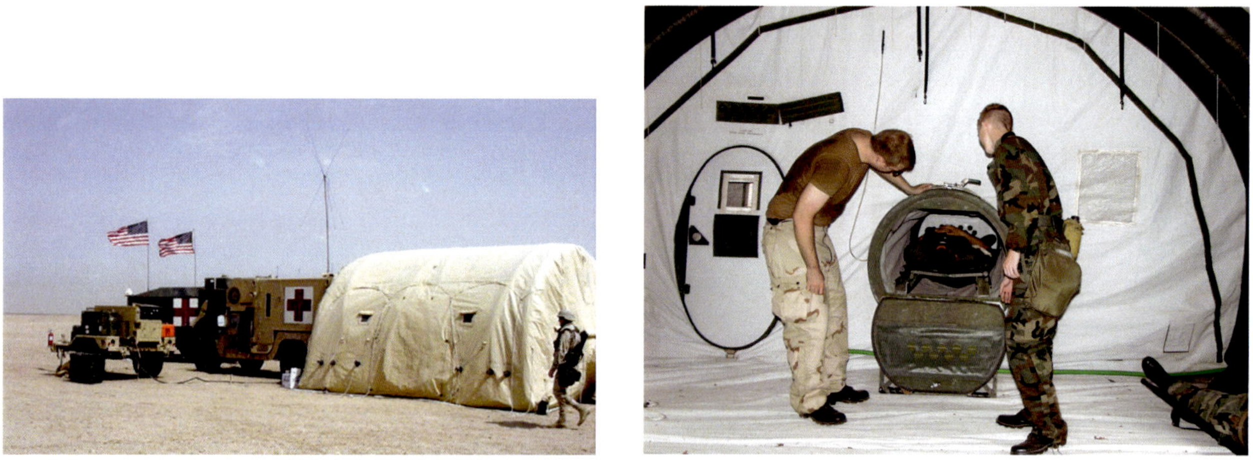

Fig. 17-36. (a) The high-mobility multipurpose wheeled vehicle serves as the main power platform for the chemical and biological protective shelter. The vehicle, which includes the environmental controls and chemical, biological radiological, and nuclear filtration systems, is attached to the tent structure and may not be separated to perform patient evacuation or other vehicular missions. When the shelter is pressurized personnel inside can work without encumbrances of individual protective equipment. This allows healthcare providers ease of movement while providing emergency lifesaving treatment. **(b)** Casualties enter the shelter for treatment through either the ambulatory or litter entrance. These entry points function as positive-pressure airlocks; thoroughly decontaminated casualties are directed through the airlocks for an air purge and decontamination check prior to receiving medical treatment.
Photographs: Courtesy of the Joint Program Management Office for Nuclear Biological Chemical Collective Protection, Naval Surface Warfare Center Dahlgren, Dahlgren, Va.

a

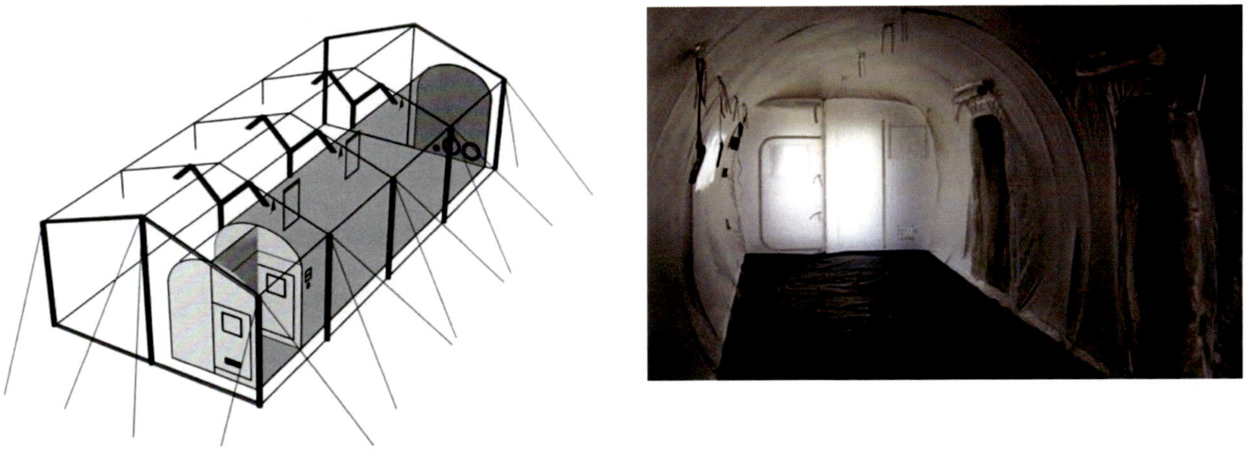

b

Fig. 17-37. **(a)** The modular general purpose tent system chemical-biological protective liner can be placed in operation in approximately 60 minutes and prepared for movement in approximately 30 minutes. **(b)** The liner is equipped with an integrated airlock that functions as an air purge, allowing decontaminated personnel or casualties requiring treatment, rest, rehydration, or command control to enter the system.
Drawing (a): Courtesy of the Chemical Casualty Care Division, US Army Medical Research Institute of Chemical Defense, Aberdeen Proving Ground, Md. Photograph (b): Courtesy of the Joint Program Management Office for Nuclear Biological Chemical Collective Protection, Naval Surface Warfare Center Dahlgren, Dahlgren, Va.

Primary users of this system are the US Army and Marine Corps.[40,43]

Modular General Purpose Tent System Chemical-Biological Protective Liner System

The modular general purpose tent system CB protective liner system (general purpose tent system, CB liner, and filtration system) provides 324 sq ft of toxic-free space, allowing occupants to conduct operations without IPE (Figure 17-37). Its positive-pressure environment provides filtered air for protection against chemical and biological warfare agents and radioactive particles. The liner system occupies half of the tent system; depending on mission requirements, the system is capable of accommodating two liners per tent to provide additional space as needed. Each liner system is equipped with pressure gauges, a high/low pressure alarm, a motor blower, a filtration unit, and an integrated air lock. Tactical applications for this equipment may include rest and relief, command and control, and medical treatment.[40,44]

ADDITIONAL PATIENT PROTECTION AND TRANSPORT EQUIPMENT

Patient Protective Wrap

Patient protective wrap is designed to protect a patient during evacuation after the chemical protective overgarment has been removed and the patient has received medical treatment. A patient can remain in the wrap for up to 3 hours. Whenever a patient is evacuated in the wrap, the M48 motor blower must be attached to provide fresh air to the patient and reduce carbon dioxide build-up (Figure 17-38). Patient protective wrap is for one patient only, weighs approximately 5.5 lb, and comes in woodland and desert camouflage patterns. It incorporates layered fabric with a charcoal lining. The top layer is made of a material similar to that used in the battle dress overgarment, and the bottom layer is made of chemically resistant plastic material. The wrap has a continuous zipper along the outer edge for ease of patient insertion; a large, transparent window in the top to view the patient (or for the patient to see out); and a pocket for medical records.[40]

Individual Chemical Patient Resuscitation Device

Developed according to US military specifications, the individual chemical resuscitation device is a ventilatory system consisting of a compressible butyl rubber bag, a NATO standard C2A1 canister filter, a nonrebreathing valve, a cricothyroid cannula adapter, and a flexible hose connected to an oropharyngeal mask (Figure 17-39). The mask is removable from the distal end of the flexible hose for connection of the hose to the cannula adapter. The butyl rubber bag resists the penetration of liquid chemical agent that may be on the

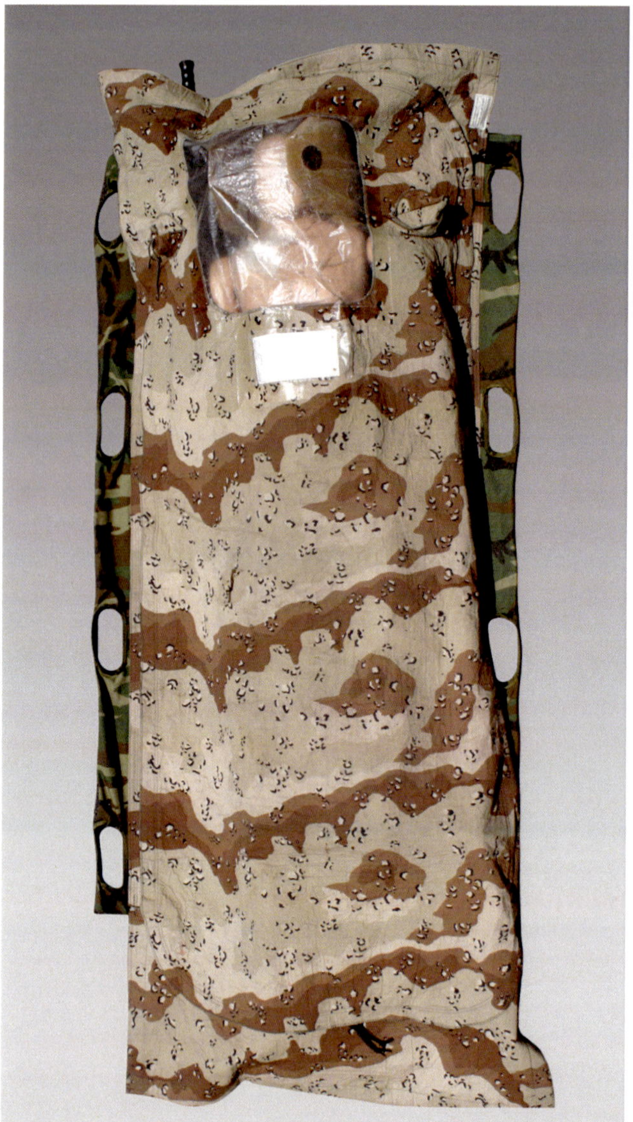

Fig. 17-38. Patient protective wrap with motor blower attached. The blower is used to provide fresh air to the patient and reduce carbon dioxide build-up
Photograph: Courtesy of the Chemical Casualty Care Division, US Army Medical Research Institute of Chemical Defense, Aberdeen Proving Ground, Md.

gloves of operator and is easily decontaminated. The elasticity of the outer cover limits airway pressure to a maximal value of 70 cm H_2O (70 mbar). The device can deliver up to 600 mL of filtered air per cycle at a rate of 30 cycles per minute, and it can be used in contaminated environments as well as all conventional ventilation emergencies.[40]

Decontaminable Litter

Contaminated casualties arriving at the medical

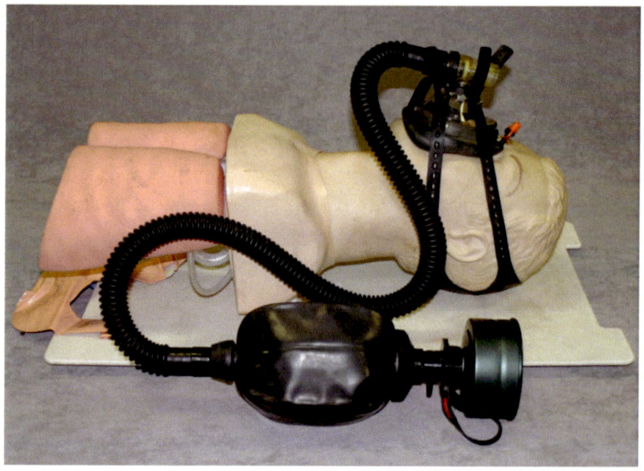

Fig. 17-39. The individual chemical resuscitation device application is demonstrated on a mannequin.
Photograph: Courtesy of the Chemical Casualty Care Division, US Army Medical Research Institute of Chemical Defense, Aberdeen Proving Ground, Md.

treatment location will, in most cases, require decontamination prior to definitive care. Traditional canvas litters exposed to liquid blister agents, when decontaminated, still desorb vapors for 72 hours after all surface contaminants are removed. Consequently, the

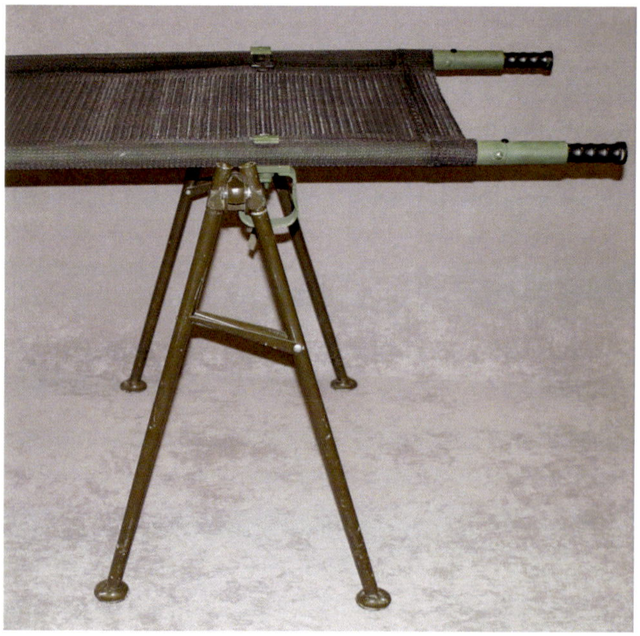

Fig. 17-40. The decontaminable litter allows liquid to pass through openings in the fabric.
Photograph: Courtesy of the Chemical Casualty Care Division, US Army Medical Research Institute of Chemical Defense, Aberdeen Proving Ground, Md.

decontaminable litter (Figure 17-40) was developed to replace the canvas litters currently in use. The decontaminable litter is made of a monofilament polypropylene with high tensile strength and low elasticity. The fabric does not absorb liquid chemical agents and is not degraded by decontaminating solutions. The fabric is flame retardant, highly rip resistant, and treated to withstand exposure to weather and sunlight. It has a honeycomb weave, which results in a rough, no-slip surface through which liquids easily pass (40% of the surface is open).[40]

The litter's carrying handles retract into the metal pole frame for a closed total length of 83.5 in (212.1 cm), to allow for loading the litter onto the UH-60 helicopter. The handle lengths are adjustable to conform to NATO standards as well as to allow for litter bearers' comfort. The aluminum poles are designed to provide direct gripping surfaces for litter stanchions as well. All metal parts have been painted with chemical agent resistant coating.[40]

SUMMARY

An integrated system of available chemical defense equipment is necessary to adequately protect military personnel. This system includes the following principal elements:

- Real-time detection and warning, preferably from remote sensors, to allow personnel more time to assume the appropriate protective posture and provide for the identification of the specific agent.
- Personal protective equipment consisting of a properly fitted mask and overgarment with gloves and boots as required. This equipment is the most critical component of chemical defense equipment, the first line of defense.
- Collective protection, which is necessary for optimal combat casualty care in a contaminated environment, whether the casualty's injuries are from exposure to CB weapons alone or are combined with injuries from conventional weapons.
- Decontamination, which is required for personnel and equipment to maintain combat operations in a contaminated environment.

Although the focus of this chapter is not on the medical treatment of chemical casualties, it is critical that medical personnel develop a good understanding of chemical defense equipment. Some medical personnel will need to provide care in the contaminated area, others will need to know how to operate equipment in the patient decontamination area, and still others will need to know the limitations of the collective protective environment. Without an adequate understanding of their protective equipment and proper training in its use, medical personnel will become casualties of the same agents that have incapacitated those they treat.

ACKNOWLEDGMENT

The authors thank the following organizations and experts for their technical assistance and generous help in illustrating and preparing this chapter: the Joint Program Management Office for Nuclear Biological Chemical Collective Protection; the Joint Program Management Office—Decontamination, Marine Corps System; the Joint Program Management Office—Individual Protection; Jeffrey S Hofmann, Deputy Program Manager, Respirator Engineering and Acquisition Team, ECBC-RDECOM; SFC Jeffrey Dawson, US Army Medical Research Institute of Chemical Defense; SFC Larry Harris, US Army (Ret); and Peter Hurst.

REFERENCES

1. O'Hern MR, Dashiell TR, Tracy MF. Chemical defense equipment. In: Sidell FR, Takafuji ET, Franz DR, eds. *Medical Aspects of Chemical and Biological Warfare.* In: Zajtchuk R, Bellamy RF, eds. *Textbook of Military Medicine.* Washington, DC: Department of the Army, Office of The Surgeon General, Borden Institute; 1997: Chap 16.

2. US Army Armament Munitions and Chemical Command. *Chemical Defensive Equipment (General Information Booklet).* Rock Island, Ill: Materiel Management Directorate, HQ, US Army Armament Munitions and Chemical Command; 1984.

3. Department of the Army. *NBC Field Handbook*. Washington, DC: DA; 1994. FM 3-7.

4. Ramirez TL, Rayle ME, Crowley PA, Derringer, CV. *The Thermal Effects of the Chemical Defense Ensemble on Human Performance.* San Antonio, Tex: US Air Force, Human Systems Division, Brooks Air Force Base; 1988. CB-010358. ADB131 710.

5. Department of the Army. *Chemical and Biological Contamination Avoidance*. Washington, DC: DA; 1992. FM 3-3.

6. Weiss RA, Weiss MP, Church JK Jr, Strawbridge JB, Decker RW II, Martin FA. Chemical warfare respiratory protection: where we were and where we are going. Aberdeen Proving Ground, Md: US Army Chemical Research, Development, and Engineering Center; 1918. Unpublished report.

7. Gander TJ, ed. *Jane's NBC Protection Equipment, 1992–93*. Alexandria, Va: Jane's Information Group Inc; 1992: 21–25.

8. North Atlantic Treaty Organization, Industrial Advisory Group, Sub-Group 48. *Basic Personal Equipmen*t. Vol 5. In: *NIAG Prefeasibility Study on a Soldier Modernisation Program*. Brussels, Belgium: NATO Industrial Advisory Group; 1994. NATO unclassified document NAIG-D(94)3.

9. Brletich NR, Tracy MF, Dashiell TR. *Worldwide NBC Mask Handbook*. Edgewood, Md: Chemical Warfare / Chemical and Biological Defense Information Center; 1992.

10. McHenry R, ed. *The New Encyclopedia Britannica*. Vol 3, Micropædia. 15th ed. Chicago, Ill: Encyclopedia Britannica, Inc; 1993: 98.

11. Bender TR, MD, MPH. Director, Division of Safety Research, Centers for Disease Control, National Institute for Occupation Safety and Health, Morgantown, WV. Letter to all respirator manufacturers; June 15, 1990.

12. Klenke WJ. Lieutenant Colonel, Medical Service, US Army. Medical NBC Defense Staff Office, Office of The Surgeon General. Personal communication, June 1996.

13. Phillips YY. Colonel, Medical Corps, US Army; Chief, Department of Medicine, Walter Reed Army Medical Center, Washington, DC. Personal communication, July 1996.

14. Departments of the Army, Marine Corps, Navy, and Air Force, and Marine Corps. *Multiservice Tactics, Techniques, and Procedures for Chemical, Biological, Radiological, and Nuclear (NBC) Protection.* Washington, DC: DoD; 2003. FM 3-11.4, MCWP 3-37.2, NTTP 3-11.27, AFTTP (I) 3-2.46.

15. Joint Program Management Office-Individual Protection (JPMO-IP), Quantico, Va. Telephone and email correspondence, July 2005.

16. Department of the Army. *Operator's Manual for Chemical-Biological Mask: Field, M40A1*. Washington, DC: DA; 1998. TM 3-4240-346-10.

17. Department of the Army. *Unit Maintenance Manual for Chemical-Biological Mask: Combat Vehicle, M42A2*. Washington, DC: DA; 1998. TM 34240-346-20&P.

18. Department of the Army. *Unit Maintenance Manual for Mask Chemical-Biological: Land Warrior, M45*. Washington, DC: DA; 2001. TM 3-4240-348-20&P.

19. Department of the Army. *Operator and Unit Maintenance Manual for Mask Chemical-Biological: Joint Service General Purpose Field and Combat Vehicle, M50 / M51*. Washington, DC: DA; 2006. TM 3-4240-542-12&P.

20. Department of the Army. *Operator and Unit Maintenance Manual for Mask Chemical-Biological: Protective, M53 Right / Left*. Washington, DC: DA; 2005. TM 3-4240-541-12&P.

21. US Army Natick Research, Development, and Engineering Center. *Items of Combat Clothing and Equipment*. Natick, Mass: US Army Natick Research, Development, and Engineering Center; 1991. Natick P-32-1.

22. Department of the Army. *Operator's Manual for Joint Service Lightweight Integrated Suit Technology (JSLIST) Chemical Protective Ensemble.* Washington, DC: DA; 1998. TM 10-8415-220-10.

23. Joint Service Project Managers, Joint Program Executive Office for Chemical and Biological Defense. *Joint Service Lightweight Integrated Suit Technology (JSLIST) Garment*. Quantico, Va: Joint Program Executive Office for Chemical/ Biological Defense; 2005. Available at: http://www.jpeocbd.osd.mil/documents/IP-JSLIST_(L).doc. Accessed April 25, 2006.

24. Brletich NR, Waters MJ, Bowen GW, Tracy MF. *Worldwide Chemical Detection Equipment Handbook.* Edgewood, Md: Chemical Warfare/Chemical and Biological Defense Information Analysis Center; 1995.

25. Department of the Army. *Chemical Agent Monitor (CAM) Users' Guide*. Ft Leonard Wood, Mo: US Army Maneuver Support Center; 1999. GTA 03-06-004.

26. Department of the Army. *Unit and Direct Support Maintenance Manual for the Improved Chemical Agent Monitor (ICAM).* Washington, DC: DA; 1998. TM 3-6665-343-23&P.

27. Department of the Army. *Operator's Manual for Chemical Agent Detector Kit, M256/M256A1*. Washington, DC: DA; 1995. TM 13-6665-307-10.

28. Joint Service Project Managers, Joint Program Executive Office for Chemical and Biological Defense. *Joint Services Lightweight Standoff Chemical Agent Detector (JSLSCAD).* Quantico, Va: Joint Program Executive Office for Chemical/ Biological Defense; 2005. Available at: http://www.jpeocbd.osd.mil/documents/CA-JSLSCAD_(L).doc. Accessed May 3, 2006.

29. US Departments of the Army, Marine Corps, Navy, and Air Force. *Health Service Support in a Nuclear, Biological, and Chemical Environment*. Washington, DC: DoD; 2004. FM 4-02.7, MCRP 4-11.1F, NTTP 4-02.7, AFTTP (I) 3-2.47.

30. US Departments of the Army, Marine Corps, Navy, and Air Force, and Marine Corps. *Multiservice Tactics, Techniques, and Procedures for Nuclear, Biological, and Chemical Aspects of Consequence Management.* Washington, DC: DoD; 2001. FM 3-11.21, MCRP 3-37.2C, NTTP 3-11.24, AFTTP (I) 3-2.37.

31. US Department of Justice, National Institute of Justice. *Guide for the Selection of Chemical Agent and Toxic Industrial Material Detection Equipment for Emergency First Responders.* Vol 1. Washington, DC: DoJ; 2000. NIJ Guide 100-00. Available at: http://www.ojp.usdoj.gov/nij/. Accessed April 25, 2006.

32. Edgewood Research Development and Engineering Center. *Decontamination of Chemical Warfare Agents.* Aberdeen Proving Ground, Md: Edgewood Research Development and Engineering Center; 1992. ERDEC-TR-004.

33. US Departments of the Army, Marine Corps, Navy, and Air Force, and Marine Corps. *Multiservice Tactics, Techniques, and Procedures for Chemical, Biological, Radiological, and Nuclear Decontamination*. Washington, DC: DoD; 2006. FM 3-11.5, MCWP 3-37.3, NTTP 3-11.26, AFTTP (I) 3-2.60.

34. Joint Program Management Office—Decontamination, Marine Corps System Command, Quantico, Va. Telephone and email correspondence, June 2005.

35. US Army Tank-Automotive and Armaments Command—Soldier Biological Chemical, Rock Island, Ill. Telephone and email correspondence, June 2005.

36. Department of the Army. *Operator's Manual for Skin Decontamination Kit, M291*. Washington, DC: DA; 1989. TM 34230-229-10.

37. Joint Service Project Managers, Joint Program Executive Office for Chemical and Biological Defense. *Joint Service Personal Decontamination System, JSPDS (RSDL)*. Quantico, Va: Joint Program Executive Office for Chemical and Biological Defense; 2005. Available at: http://www.jpeocbd.osd.mil/documents/DC-JSPDS-RSDL_(L).doc Accessed April 28, 2006.

38. Joint Service Project Managers, Joint Program Executive Office for Chemical and Biological Defense. *Lightweight Decon System (LDS): M17A3*. Quantico, Va: Joint Program Executive Office for Chemical and Biological Defense; 2005. Available at: http://www.jpeocbd.osd.mil/documents/DC-LDS-M17A3_(L).doc. Accessed April 28, 2006.

39. Joint Service Project Managers, Joint Program Executive Office for Chemical and Biological Defense Web site. Available at: https://secureweb.hqda.pentagon.mil/jpeocbd_secure/page_manager.asp?pg=0. Accessed April 25, 2006.

40. Joint Program Management Office for Nuclear Biological Chemical Collective Protection, Naval Surface Warfare Center Dahlgren, Dahlgren, Va. Telephone and email correspondence, July 2005.

41. Green TG. Collective Protection Team, US Army Tank-Automotive and Armaments Command—Soldier Biological Chemical, Rock Island, Ill. Email correspondence, August 2005.

42. Dougherty J, Poehling K, Holloran N. Collectively Protected Field Hospitals, A Continuing Evolution. *CHEM-BIO DEFENSE Quarterly*. 2005;2:8-9.

43. Department of the Army. *Operator's Manual for Simplified Collective Protection Equipment: M20A1*. Washington, DC: DA; 1995. TM 3-4240-313-10.

43. US Marine Corps. *Collective Protection System (CPS) Modular General Purpose Tent System (MGPTS) (Medium)*. Washington DC: USMC; 2004. TM-10935A-OR.

Chapter 18

OCCUPATIONAL HEALTH AND THE CHEMICAL SURETY MISSION

CLAUDIA L. HENEMYRE-HARRIS, PhD*; MELANIE L. MURROW†; THOMAS P. LOGAN, PhD‡; BRENT R. GIBSON, MD, MPH§; and ROBERT GUM, DO, MPH¥

* *Major, Medical Service Corps, US Army; US Army Medical Research Institute of Chemical Defense, Physiology and Immunology Branch, 3100 Ricketts Point Road, Aberdeen Proving Ground, Maryland 21010-5400*

† *Safety and Occupational Specialist, Safety, Surety, and Security Office, Office of the Commander, US Army Medical Research Institute of Chemical Defense, 3100 Ricketts Point Road, Building E3101, Room 104, Aberdeen Proving Ground, Maryland 21010-5400*

‡ *Chemist, Medical Diagnostics Branch, Analytical Toxicology Division, US Army Medical Research Institute of Chemical Defense, 3100 Ricketts Point Road, Building E3081, Room 293, Aberdeen Proving Ground, Maryland 21010-5400*

§ *Captain, Medical Corps, US Army; Army Medical Department Center and School, 3151 Scott Road, Suite 3507, Fort Sam Houston, Texas 78234*

¥ *Chief of Bio Surety, Barquist Army Health Clinic, 1434 Porter Street, Fort Detrick, Maryland 21702*

INTRODUCTION

Medical officers assigned to US Army arsenals, depots, or other installations that store chemical warfare agents face a number of unique challenges concerning chemical surety. The clinics supporting these installations, although frequently staffed by occupational medicine specialists, may still be managed by primary care physicians or even general medical officers with no specialty training. These providers must care for both military and civilian workers as well as master myriad additional duties unique to chemical weapons storage sites, including managing complex medical programs that support chemical surety and accident or incident response. In addition, many installations are actively demilitarizing chemical munitions. These operations run parallel with, but independent of, chemical surety operations. Chemical surety systems manage chemical agents throughout their life cycles while maintaining operational performance, which adds other challenges to chemical surety medical support program directors (CSMSPDs)—one of many titles physicians may earn as they provide medical support to employees working on tasks from storage to the final disposal of chemical agents. Providers must be on orders from their medical commanders to perform CSMSPD duties, as well as those duties outlined below, in ways that ensure accountability and responsibility for operations.

In this chapter, a chemical agent is defined as a chemical substance intended for use in military operations to kill, seriously injure, or incapacitate a person through its physiological effects. Riot control agents, chemical herbicides, smoke, and flames are not officially defined as chemical agents, but installations with chemical agents may contain varying amounts of these substances. Chemical surety (a term that encompasses both safety and security) operations employ a system of controls, procedures, and actions that contribute to the safe and secure storage, transportation, and demilitarization of chemical agents and their associated weapon systems. Chemical surety material is defined in Army Regulation (AR) 50-6, *Chemical Surety*, as "chemical agents and their associated weapon system, or storage and shipping containers that are either adopted or being considered for military use."[1(p43)]

Although the chemical agents discussed are unique to the military, the hazards to employees are common to many industries. Examples include acetylcholinesterase inhibitors (the operative mechanism of nerve agents) used in pesticides and carbonyl chloride (phosgene) used in the production of foams and plastics. Both are transported daily on the nation's highways and railways. In addition to these chemical threats, chemical storage depots carry out other operations that pose potential physical hazards similar to those found in other industries (eg, excessive noise, heat stress, and lifting). When they were being produced, military chemical munitions had different intended uses, packaging, and methods of storage than industrial chemicals (and are typically more hazardous), so they required different controls.

Military chemical agent workers can find information on chemical surety operations in a variety of resources, including ARs, which implement Army laws, and Department of the Army pamphlets (DA PAMs), which provide additional technical guidance. The most useful documents for the CSMSPD are AR 50-6, *Chemical Surety*[1]; DA PAM 50-6, *Chemical Accident or Incident Response and Assistance* [*CAIRA*] *Operations*[2]; DA PAM 40-8, *Occupational Health Guidelines for the Evaluation and Control of Occupational Exposure to Nerve Agents GA, GB, GD, and VX*[3]; and DA PAM 40-173, *Occupational Health Guidelines for the Evaluation and Control of Occupational Exposure to Mustard Agents H, HD, and HT*.[4] Safety publications AR 385-61[5] and DA PAM 385-61[6] also contain medical guidance. The installation medical authority (IMA) must be aware of any interim or implementation guidance or Department of Defense directives, instructions, or memoranda that affect operations. The IMA should maintain a close relationship with the installation and legal offices of the supporting medical treatment facility.

Military installations are often physically isolated and are located a considerable distance from the medical center or medical department activity responsible for providing support and consultation. The preventive/occupational medicine physicians at these hospitals are responsible for providing the necessary support and are a source of information and guidance. The level of chemical and occupational-specific medical expertise at the supporting treatment facility varies; however, the depot-level physician should be a subject-matter expert on the treatment of chemical surety exposures and perhaps even on occupational medicine. Assets and time are seldom available to train a general medical officer in the unique occupational setting of depot operations (Exhibit 18-1).

According to DA PAM 50-6,[2] medical officers supporting chemical surety operations are required to complete the Toxic Chemical Training Course for Medical Support Personnel (given by the US Army Chemical Materials Agency) and the Medical Management of Chemical and Biological Casualties Course (given by the US Army Medical Research

Institute of Chemical Defense [USAMRICD]). Both courses are offered at Aberdeen Proving Ground, Maryland, and provide the basic concepts needed to recognize the clinical signs and symptoms of chemical agent exposure and the appropriate therapeutic interventions for treating and managing chemical agent casualties. The Toxic Chemical Training Course also presents material on the medical challenges of supporting demilitarization operations.

Understanding patients' occupational healthcare needs is an integral part of a physician's practice. This responsibility includes identifying occupational and environmental health risks, treating disease and injury, and counseling patients on preventive behavior. Occupational health alone is time consuming; the occupational health nurse, the industrial hygienist, and other clinic staff members can help perform required tasks. Although industrial hygienists are not often assigned to health clinics, they are an essential part of the healthcare team. The industrial hygienist maintains a hazard inventory that contains conventional hazards as well as a list of chemical agents located at the installation. They routinely design primary prevention strategies and frequently oversee hearing conservation, respiratory protection, and occupational vision programs. The information provided by the hygienist is necessary to evaluate a work environment and to determine the appropriate frequency of periodic medical examinations. Close and frequent coordination with this individual is imperative for developing knowledge of the worksite and the subsequent development of a medical surveillance program.

In addition to the industrial hygiene and safety personnel, medical personnel must work in accord with the command, supervisors, personnel officers, and employees who handle chemical agents. Maintaining these relationships is frequently difficult, but by identifying and addressing concerns of both management and individual workers, medical personnel can establish a basis for formulating appropriate preventive medical measures.

EXHIBIT 18-1

ADVISING AGENCIES FOR THE TREATMENT OF CHEMICAL AGENT INJURY

Agency	Contact Information
The preventive or occupational medicine department of the supporting medical department activity or medical center	Specific to location
US Army Center for Health Promotion and Preventive Medicine	Director, Occupational and Environmental Medicine/ MCHB-TS-M 5158 Blackhawk Road Aberdeen Proving Ground, Maryland 21010-5403
US Army Chemical Materials Agency	Command Surgeon/AMSCM-RD 5183 Blackhawk Road, Bldg E-4585 Aberdeen Proving Ground, Maryland 21010-5424
Proponency Office for Preventive Medicine	Surety Medicine Consultant/DASG-PPM-NC 5111 Leesburg Pike, Suite 538 Falls Church, Virginia 22041-3258
US Army Medical Research Institute of Chemical Defense	MCMR-CDM 3100 Ricketts Point Road Aberdeen Proving Ground, Maryland 21010-5400
US Army Reserve Unit for Chemical/Biological Consequence Management	Detachment Surgeon 1309 Continental Avenue, Suite K Abingdon, Maryland 21009-2336
US Army Materiel Command	AMCSG/Deputy Command Surgeon 9301 Chapek Road Fort Belvoir, Virginia 22060

THE CHEMICAL AGENT WORKPLACE

Chemical agent operations are conducted in a variety of job settings, including storage depots, demilitarization facilities, research laboratories, and transportation units. Before a chemical agent employee can be placed in a job, a physician must consider the occupational and environmental health risks associated with the position. The physician must understand the various workplaces in which chemical agent operations are performed to effectively identify the corresponding risks.

The chemical agent worker uses different kinds of personal protective equipment (PPE) and engineering controls based on the work environment. The use of protective clothing itself can create significant hazards, such as heat stress, physical and psychological stress, and impaired vision, mobility, and communication. The physician must understand these PPEs and engineering controls in order to select the most appropriate preplacement examination and medical surveillance for the initial and continued safety of the worker. DA PAM 385-61[6] defines the protection levels (A through D) for chemical agent workers and lists the personal protective clothing and equipment required for each level. The following text and accompanying figures describe the various types of chemical agent workplaces.

The purpose of the US Army Chemical Materials Agency is to protect and safely store the nation's aging chemical weapons. The agency works toward the effective recovery, treatment, and ultimate elimination of the nation's chemical warfare materials, and it manages a national inventory control point and national maintenance point to ensure that the stockpile is maintained safely during its remaining storage life. Chemical depot workers routinely check storage containers for potential degradation and leaks. During these inspections, the workers operate in Level A protective clothing, the demilitarization protective ensemble, which consists of a totally encapsulated, positive-pressurized suit (Figure 18-1). A mask (manufactured by Mine Safety Appliances Company, Pittsburgh, Pa) and backpack, both certified by the National Institute of Occupational Safety and Health and the Occupational Safety and Health Administration, are contained within the suit to provide a continual air supply via an umbilical cord. The suit is also equipped with a self-contained emergency breathing system in case the hose air supply is compromised. The workers wear butyl rubber boots and gloves over the ensemble as an additional layer of protection and can communicate with each other and the control station by way of a radio internal to the demilitarization protective ensemble.

Another mission of the Chemical Materials Agency is to manage the safe treatment and disposal of chemical agents and weapons. To accomplish this mission, the agency uses various technological tools, many of

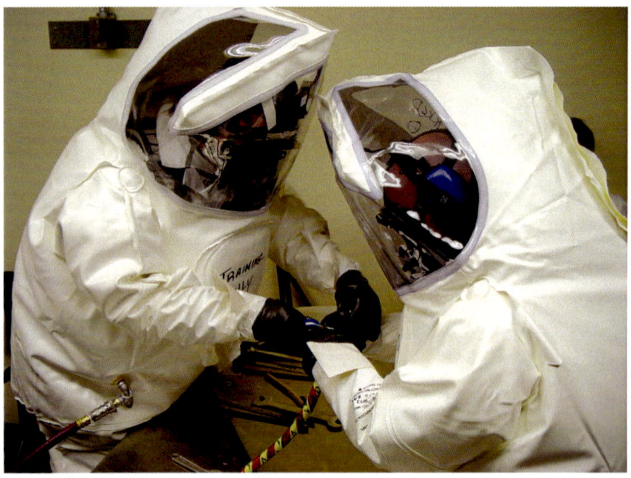

Fig. 18-1. A team of chemical workers wears Level A protective clothing, the demilitarization protective ensemble, which provides the greatest level of protection against agent exposure.
Photograph: Courtesy of US Army Chemical Materials Agency, Aberdeen Proving Ground, Md. Available at http://www.cma.army.mil/multimediagallery. Accessed December 2005.

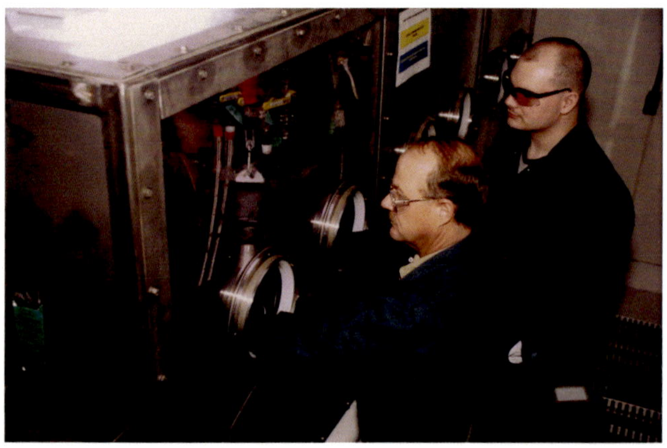

Fig. 18-2. Two chemical agent operators wear Level C protective clothing and use a glovebox as they drain mustard agent from ton containers in the neutralization process at the Aberdeen Chemical and Biological Agent Disposal Facility.
Photograph: Courtesy of US Army Chemical Materials Agency, Aberdeen Proving Ground, Md. Available at http://www.cma.army.mil/multimediagallery. Accessed December 2005.

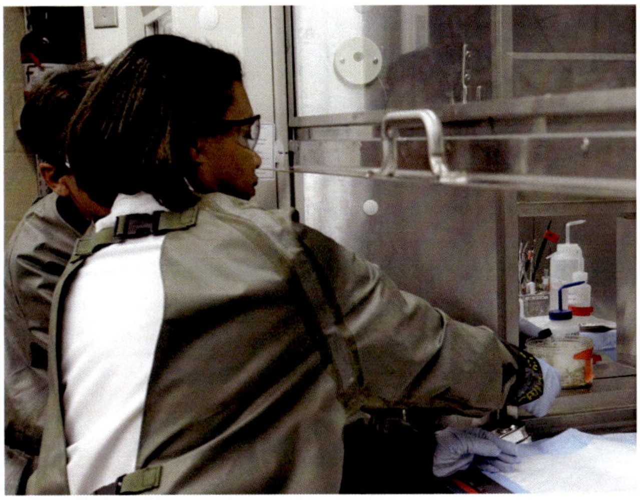

Fig. 18-3. Chemical agent operators wear Level C protective clothing in a professional laboratory research setting to discover and develop medical countermeasures and therapeutics to chemical warfare agents.
Photograph: Courtesy of US Army Medical Research Institute of Chemical Defense, Aberdeen Proving Ground, Md.

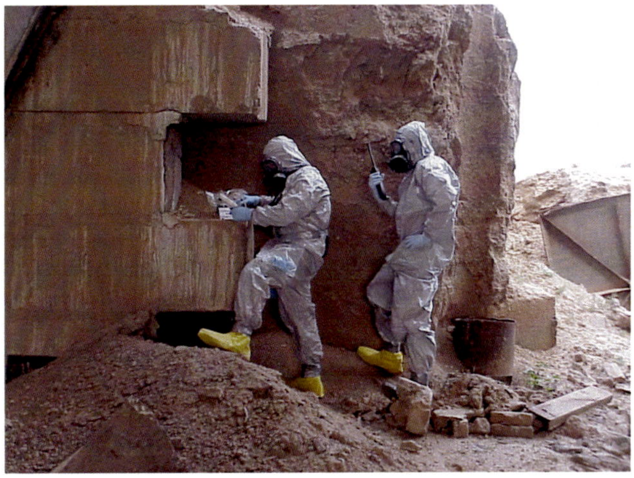

Fig. 18-4. Soldiers from the 22nd Chemical Battalion (Technical Escort) work in Level C protective clothing to conduct a sampling mission.
Photograph: Courtesy of Major Chadwick T Bauld, 22nd Chemical Battalion, Technical Escort, US Army 20th Support Command, CBRNE.

which are at least partially automated. However, the worker must handle chemical agents during other phases of the treatment and disposal process. For example, operators at the Aberdeen Biological Chemical Agent Disposal Facility drain mustard agent from ton containers using a glovebox in the neutralization process (Figure 18-2). During this procedure, workers don Level C protective clothing consisting of work coveralls, safety glasses with side shields, and M40A1 protective masks worn in the slung position.

In a research laboratory setting such as USAMRICD, chemical agent operators conduct experiments to discover and develop medical countermeasures to and therapeutics for chemical warfare agents. The experimental parameters, and therefore the working conditions, are tightly regulated to maintain a climate-controlled environment. Agent operators conduct studies in a certified chemical fume hood, and preliminary airflow measurements are taken using a worker's velometer. Operators wear several layers of PPE, as shown in Figure 18-3, and work in Level C protective clothing. The first layer of PPE is a laboratory coat and nitrile gloves. The second, outer layer of PPE consists of a 7-mm–thick butyl rubber apron and butyl rubber gloves. Many operators wear a second pair of nitrile gloves over the butyl rubber gloves to improve dexterity. Laboratory safety glasses with side shields are worn at all times and protective masks are kept readily available or are worn in a slung position.

The mission of the 22nd Chemical Battalion is to deploy task-organized teams throughout the world to conduct technical escort and chemical, biological, radiological, and nuclear hazard characterization, monitoring, disablement, and elimination support operations. The 22nd Chemical Battalion provides emergency response to incidents involving weapons of mass destruction and chemical, biological, radiological, and nuclear hazards, homeland defense, contingency support operations to combatant commanders and lead federal agencies, and site remediation and restoration support operations for the Department of Defense. The battalion works at a high operational tempo in a wide variety of settings, including hostile and austere environments. In addition to the PPE and engineering controls described above, battalion members use specialized protective measures unique to each mission (Figure 18-4). If the members are faced with an unknown agent or unsafe oxygen level, they require a higher respiratory protection level (Level B or Level A, with self-contained breathing apparatus).

MEDICAL SURVEILLANCE FOR CHEMICAL AGENT WORKERS

Medical surveillance is the systematic collection, analysis, and dissemination of disease data on groups of workers. It is designed to detect early signs of work-related illness.[7] A chemical worksite medical program should provide the following surveillance: preplacement screening, periodic medical examinations (with follow-up examinations, when appropriate), and termination examinations. Additional follow-up examinations are required if an individual has potentially or actually been exposed. An efficient medical surveillance program helps determine if a relationship exists between exposure to a hazard and development of a disease, and it can identify an occupational disease at an early stage, when medical intervention can be most

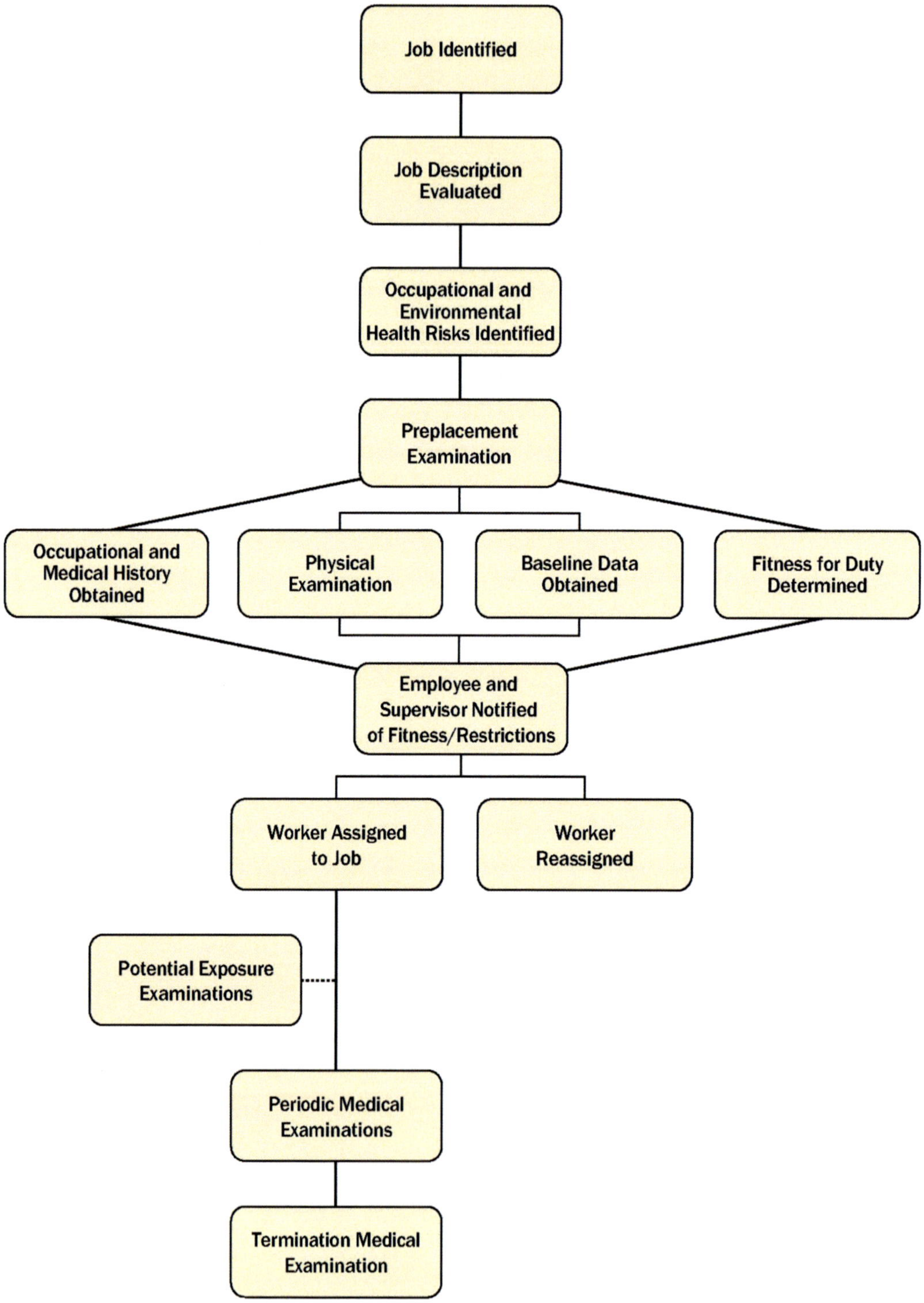

Fig. 18-5. Medical surveillance for chemical agent workers.

beneficial (Figure 18-5).

"Screening" is defined as the search for a previously unrecognized disease or pathophysiological condition at a stage when intervention can slow, halt, or reverse the progression of the disorder. Medical surveillance is considered a type of screening because it seeks to identify work-related disease at an early stage.[7] Screening for medical and physical standards, a practice distinct from yet related to medical surveillance for occupational exposure to toxic chemicals, is sometimes necessary for a worker to be placed, or remain in place, in a particular position. In addition to this duty, another related function of the CSMSPD is to provide medical support for the administrative chemical personnel reliability program (CPRP). An officially designated physician or other qualified medical staff member (physician's assistant, dentist, or dental assistant) must screen personnel for medical aspects of reliability for the CPRP. When making medical recommendations related to reliability, the CSMSPD may offer guidance to a non-medically trained certifying or reviewing official, whereas the treating provider has complete discretion and authority (as allowed by his or her current clinical privileges) in the medical evaluation and treatment of chemical injuries. Additional examinations, independent of medical surveillance, may also be required. These include evaluating a potential worker's fitness for PPE and ability to meet the functional requirements of the job.

Administrative and engineering controls, followed by individual protective measures such as PPE, are the primary disease prevention methods; medical screening is an adjunct method. The importance of this hierarchy must be continually stressed. An individual who shows signs or complains of symptoms of occupationally related illness should be identified as a possible sentinel case. Not only must the individual be treated, but the cause of the complaint must also be thoroughly investigated by the IMA, the industrial hygienist, and safety personnel. The cause may be related to improper work practices of the affected individual or to a failure of engineering devices or personal protective measures. In the latter case, further morbidity can be avoided if the problem is promptly identified.

The IMA (usually the CSMSPD) or contract physician is responsible for establishing and supervising the medical surveillance system for toxic chemicals, including nerve and mustard agents. Not all individuals working at the installation, or even in a particular work area, need to be on the same surveillance program. The type of work, work area, and required PPE are factors that determine the type and frequency of surveillance. Determining the level of medical surveillance is an important step, usually achieved with input from medical and safety personnel. In accordance with DA PAM 40-8[3] and DA PAM 40-173,[4] the ultimate determination of appropriate medical surveillance categories is the responsibility of surety or safety personnel.

The distinction between medical surveillance and personnel reliability is often overlooked. The level of medical surveillance is determined by the occupational hazards of the job, whereas the placement of a worker in the CPRP is a function of the level of responsibility and critical functions of his or her job. A worker may be in a medical surveillance program, a personnel reliability program, in both, or in neither. For example, a locksmith working at an office far from a chemical storage area may not require medical surveillance, but his or her position is critical to safe chemical operations. Therefore, the locksmith must be included in the CPRP. When making medical recommendations regarding chemical surety issues, providers are referred to as the competent medical authority.

For additional information on occupational medicine programs, the installation medical authority (IMA) should seek advice from the regional medical center or medical department activity. The Occupational and Environmental Medicine Division of the US Army Center for Health Promotion and Preventive Medicine at the Edgewood Area of Aberdeen Proving Ground, Maryland, may also be of assistance. Moreover, the Code of Federal Regulations, title 5, part 339[8] contains detailed guidance on determining physical and medical requirements and conducting medical examinations. Medical personnel should have at least a basic working knowledge of the Americans with Disabilities Act[9] to ensure that their programs do not discriminate based on a disability.

Preplacement Examination

Before evaluating a worker's history and completing a physical examination, physicians should acquire an accurate and current job description listing the specific tasks the worker will be required to do. The civilian personnel office can usually provide this information. The type of respiratory protection and protective clothing required must also be ascertained, because these will affect an individual's ability to perform the job. Position descriptions with physical requirements should be viewed carefully; supervisors are responsible for ensuring that position descriptions are current and accurate.

Not all individuals are required to wear protective clothing all the time. Frequency of use, exertion level, and environmental conditions have a dramatic influence on how well an individual performs in PPE. For example, a worker in a temperate desert climate such as the American Southwest may be very comfortable in protective clothing during winter but unable to tolerate the same level of protection in the heat of summer. Therefore, it is very important to observe work–rest cycles.

Preplacement examination has two major functions: (1) to determine an individual's fitness for duty, including his or her ability to work while wearing PPE; and (2) to provide baseline medical surveillance for comparison with future medical data.[10] Chemical agent workers must be evaluated to ensure that they are not predisposed to physical, mental, or emotional impairment that may result in an increased vulnerability to chemical warfare agent exposure. This examination is performed at no cost to the applicant. Abnormalities identified during the course of the preplacement examination, however, need to be followed up by the applicant, at his or her expense, with a private physician.

The first step in acquiring necessary information from a prospective worker is an occupational and medical history questionnaire. The medical officer is required to conduct a thorough review to identify past illnesses and diseases that may prevent satisfactory job performance. It is particularly important to inquire about skin, lung, cardiovascular, and psychiatric disease to evaluate the ability of an individual to work in protective ensemble. Questions concerning shortness of breath or labored breathing on exertion, asthma or other respiratory symptoms, chest pain, high blood pressure, and heat intolerance provide helpful information, as do questions about hypersensitivity to rubber products and cold-induced bronchospasms. The medical officer should also take a brief psychiatric history to determine the individual's ability to be encapsulated in PPE; questions about panic attacks, syncopal episodes, or hyperventilation can supply valuable information.

A potential employee's physical examination should follow the medical history questionnaire. It should be comprehensive and focus on the skin and the cardiovascular, pulmonary, and musculoskeletal systems. Obesity, lack of physical strength, and poor muscle tone are indicators of increased susceptibility to heat injury, a condition that is amplified by working in chemical protective clothing. Factors that restrict the wearing of protective clothing include (*a*) the inability to obtain a seal with the protective mask, (*b*) an allergy to protective clothing and equipment, (*c*) any medical condition that precludes correct wear of protective clothing, and (*d*) poor visual acuity that requires the use of glasses unless mask optical inserts are used. Facial hair, scarring, dentures, and arthritic hands or fingers can affect a worker's ability to wear a respirator and protective clothing. Acne scarring and pseudofolliculitis barbae are common facial skin conditions that may interfere with proper mask seal. Mask fit testing should be used to augment fitness determination in these cases.

Baseline data acquired during the preplacement screening can be used following an exposure event to determine the extent of the exposure. This data can also be used to verify the engineering controls in effect, and it may be used to determine if the worker has been adversely affected by exposure. Red blood cell cholinesterase (RBC-ChE) baseline levels are essential for workers assigned to areas in which nerve agent munitions are stored. Workers are categorized by the area they are assigned to and how frequently they are in a chemical environment, and the frequency of follow-up examinations is determined by this category. These categories are in a state of flux; the current regulatory guidance is discussed in the following section. As of the date of this writing, RBC-ChE baseline levels must be determined every 3 years by a two-draw series, with the draws taking place within 10 days of each other. This test may be performed at the installation level or at the cholinesterase reference laboratory of the US Army Center for Health Promotion and Preventive Medicine. This reference laboratory serves as a central repository of RBC-ChE baseline values and provides enhanced quality control and record management. RBC-ChE measurement is necessary throughout a worker's employment to monitor for nerve agent exposure. The surety officer, safety officer, and IMA are jointly responsible for determining who will be monitored and how often. Certifying officials and other supervisors are responsible for supplying information about the worker's duties, and an accurate job description is essential.

Periodic Medical Examinations

Periodic medical examinations should be used in conjunction with preplacement screening examinations.[10] Comparing the data obtained through periodic monitoring with the baseline data is essential for identifying early signs of occupationally induced diseases. The periodic medical examination is intended to identify any conditions for which early intervention can be beneficial.

The frequency and extent of the periodic medical examination should be determined by the toxicity of the potential or actual exposures, frequency and duration of the contact, and the information obtained in the preplacement history and physical examination. The data obtained from these periodic examinations can guide the future frequency of physical examinations or tests. Data consistently within acceptable limits for several months may indicate that the frequency of medical examinations can be safely decreased, provided the work situation remains constant.

The interval medical history and physical should focus on changes in health status, illness, and possible work-related signs and symptoms. To effectively identify occupational conditions or disease, the examining physician must be aware of the work environment and potentially hazardous exposures; if chemical surety workers show a change in health status in the periodic evaluation, it is necessary to evaluate the worksite. Depending on the identified conditions, additional workers may require examination. At a minimum, examining physicians should communicate with industrial hygiene personnel to determine whether there has been a change in the work environment that could be causally related.

Previously, DA PAM 40-8, modified November 2007, *Occupational Health Guidelines for the Evaluation and Control of Occupational Exposure to Nerve Agents GA, GB, GD, and VX*,[3] dictated that four categories of personnel are required to have RBC-ChE measured (Exhibit 18-2).[3,11] As of 2006 installations with chemical surety missions are required to adhere to the *Implementation Guidance Policy for Revised Airborne Exposure Limits for GB, GA, GD, GF, VX, H, HD, and HT*.[4] RBC-ChE baseline monitoring is one significant change in these documents; using soap and water in place of dilute bleach for personnel decontamination is another. Currently, an individual in category I must have a monthly measurement of the RBC-ChE level; an individual in category II must have an annual RBC-ChE measurement.

Termination Examinations

At the termination of employment or duty in a chemical surety position, all employees must have a medical examination. Unless otherwise specified by a local regulation, this examination may be done up to 30 days before or after termination of employment. If an employee is exposed after the termination examination, it will be necessary to thoroughly document and evaluate that specific exposure. In most cases, such exposure is unlikely; completing the termination examination within the 30 days before departure is advisable so that the employee does not have to return to the worksite. Employees have the right to refuse any examination, but the provider should encourage those terminated to undergo the final examination before separation.

Workers whose surveillance category changes as a result of a job change must receive a medical exami-

EXHIBIT 18-2

CATEGORIZATION OF WORKERS BASED ON THEIR LIKELIHOOD OF EXPOSURE TO CHEMICAL AGENTS

Category	Includes
I (formerly Category A)	Personnel with a high risk of potential exposure due to the nature of the agent operations being conducted. Examples of such operations might include (but are not limited to) storage monitoring inspections of M55 rockets, periodic inspections, toxic chemical munitions maintenance operations that involve movement of munitions from storage locations, work in known contaminated environments, and first-entry monitoring. Personnel may be routinely required to work for prolonged periods in areas with high levels of nerve agents where the use of either toxicological agent protective ensembles or protective ensembles with a self-contained or supplied-air breathing apparatus may be required.
II (formerly Category B)	Personnel with both a low risk or infrequent potential exposure to nerve agents in routine industrial, laboratory, or security operations. Examples of such operations might include (but are not limited to) daily site security checks and accident/incident response by initial response force members. Prolonged wear of protective ensembles during training and emergency responses may be required.
III (formerly Category C)	Personnel with minimal probability of exposure to nerve agents, even under accident conditions, but whose activities may place them in close proximity to agent areas.
IV (formerly Category D)	Transient visitors to agent areas where a potential for exposure exists and who are not included in the medical surveillance program for nerve agents at the visited installation.

nation appropriate for their new category. In general, employees who move up or down in category must be treated as though they are entering initial surveillance or terminating surveillance. In addition, workers may move into and out of surveillance categories without actually leaving employment. These transitions, often overlooked, are a difficult aspect of managing chemical surety. Overall, there is growing interest in simplifying medical surveillance categories. Meanwhile, the surety officer must ensure that the IMA is aware of changes in employment duties that may affect medical surveillance. Inaccurately categorizing workers can result in inadequate surveillance as well as excessive cost and effort.

Potential Exposure Evaluations

Any agent exposure, suspected exposure, agent spill or release, or other abnormal situation that may result in personnel injury must be reported to supervisory personnel immediately after emergency action is taken. Personnel with possible agent exposures must report for medical evaluation as soon as possible. The scope and frequency of examination and the retention of physical examination records should follow the guidance of DA PAM 40-8[3] and DA PAM 40-173.[4] All personnel exposed or potentially exposed to nerve agent must have a cholinesterase level drawn the day prior to release from duty. All personnel working with chemical agents should be given an off-duty telephone number to report suspected exposures. Employees who have been in areas of possible chemical agent exposure (for example, downwind of an agent release or in known areas of agent contamination) must remain at the installation for at least 30 minutes after leaving the contaminated area, during which the supervisor or designated representative will observe them for symptoms of agent exposure. If signs of agent exposure are noted, the worker will be immediately referred to the medical facility.

Respirator Clearances

Once workers have passed the medical history and physical exams, the medical officer must determine their ability to function in respiratory protective equipment. This check can be done by either pulmonary function testing or a "use" test. Both tests are easily performed in an occupational health clinic, and each provides important data. The pulmonary function test provides vital information about lung capacity and may expose underlying clinical disease, such as early chronic obstructive pulmonary disease. However, pulmonary function tests may be subject to operator error and depend on patient cooperation, and they do not predict how well employees will actually perform their duties. A use test, on the other hand, is highly subjective but provides a real-world measure of performance. Although it is impractical to simulate every possible job function and level of PPE in the clinic, an innovative provider can devise physical performance measures that simulate actual employee tasks. For example, a worker can don PPE and carry objects around the clinic while staff records signs and symptoms of cardiovascular or pulmonary stress. The physician must be available during such tests to provide advanced care if the worker does not tolerate the testing. If testing tolerance is in doubt, it should be deferred until a more controlled testing environment can be provided, or omitted altogether. For example, a worker with a questionable history (eg, with angina or a previous myocardial infarction) should not be required to complete a use test prior to pulmonary function testing. Input from industrial hygienists and supervisors concerning the employee's required tasks will produce more useful results than a generic use test. The outcome of either test must be documented in the individual's medical record.

Screening for Substance Abuse and Dependency

Substance abuse is inconsistent with the high standards of performance, discipline, and attention to detail necessary to work with chemical agents. The Army Substance Abuse Program[12] promotes healthy life choices, quality of life, and Army values through substance abuse prevention and risk-reduction education and training. All soldiers receive a minimum of 4 hours of alcohol and other drug awareness training per year, and Army civilian employees receive a minimum of 3 hours of such training per year.

All active duty soldiers are randomly drug tested at least once a year. Civilian drug abuse testing is conducted according to statutory and applicable contractual labor relations. However, Army civilian employees must refrain from alcohol abuse or using drugs illegally, whether on or off duty. Supervisors must refer any civilian employee found violating the rule to the installation employee assistance program coordinator.

Army Substance Abuse Program policies are designed to fully support the CPRP. Both military and Army civilian employees undergo drug screening prior to placement in the CPRP. Thereafter, CPRP military personnel are drug tested at least once in a 12-month period. Army civilian employees enrolled in the CPRP serve in sensitive positions called testing-designated positions. By Executive Order 12564, *The Drug-free*

Workplace,[13] these employees are also subject to random drug testing.

The physician who reviews positive urine drug tests for the Army is currently a certified medical review officer. If the IMA fills this position, it is important for the physician to review drug tests independently of his or her surety duties. The IMA is legally bound to perform an impartial review of the medical evidence for a federally mandated positive test and then release the results only through proper channels. This task may be difficult, given the responsibility of surety duties; the physician must always use sound medical judgment backed by legal advice.

Heat Stress Physiologic Monitoring

Heat stress is a constant and potentially severe health threat to employees wearing toxicological protective clothing. The combination of exposure to solar radiant energy or enclosed areas with high temperatures, metabolic heat production, and the use of impermeable clothing (which prevents evaporative cooling) places the chemical worker at high risk for heat injury.

Encapsulating uniforms increase the heat strain associated with most environments and work rates by creating a microenvironment around the worker. The suit's impermeability to vapor (the characteristic that makes it protective) creates high local humidity, restricting evaporative cooling and conductive/convective cooling. In effect, the suit creates an environment at the body surface hotter and wetter, under almost any circumstances, than the environment outside the suit. Moderating the heat strain associated with an encapsulating ensemble is accomplished in the following ways:

- microclimate cooling by direct removal of heat, water vapor, or both from the worker's microenvironment;
- heat sinks in the suit, such as ice vests;
- increasing the temperature gradient across the suit by shielding workers from radiant heat sources, cooling the work space, or, in dry environments, wetting the surface of the suit; and
- work–rest cycles to permit cooling and rehydration.

Heat-induced occupational injury or illness occurs when the total heat load from the environment and metabolism exceeds the cooling ability of the body. The resulting inability to maintain normal body temperature results in heat strain (the body's response to total heat stress).[14]

Adverse health effects can be reduced by training and acclimatization, measuring and assessing heat stress, medical supervision, heat-protective clothing and equipment, and properly applying engineering and work-practice controls.[14] Training and adequate supervision are basic requirements that need constant reinforcement. The occurrence of heat-induced illness or injury is an indication that (*a*) the worker has engaged in an act that should have been avoided by adequate training and supervision, (*b*) the individual's medical status has changed and requires further or more frequent evaluations, or (*c*) supervisory enforcement of work–rest cycles or adequate hydration is lacking. In all cases, the healthcare provider must investigate the cause. If the individual's health status has changed, further medical evaluation is needed. The worker may require temporary duties commensurate with his or her present health status or a permanent change of duties. If the injury appears to be the result of carelessness or lack of attention to changing environmental conditions, further training is needed. Eliciting the worker's support may be necessary to acquire the appropriate cooperation of intermediate supervisors.

Numerous textbooks and other sources discuss thermoregulation and physiological responses to heat, and healthcare providers may benefit from a review of these subjects. This chapter, however, will address the evaluation of heat stress and preventive measures.

The preplacement physical examination is designed for workers who have not been employed in areas exposed to heat extremes. It should be assumed that such individuals are not acclimatized to work in hot climates. Therefore, the physician should obtain the following information[14]:

- A medical history that addresses the cardiovascular, respiratory, neurological, renal, hematological, gastrointestinal, and reproductive systems and includes information on specific dermatological, endocrine, connective tissue, and metabolic conditions that might affect heat acclimatization or the ability to eliminate heat.
- A complete occupational history, including years of work in each job, the physical and chemical hazards encountered, the physical demands of these jobs, the intensity and duration of heat exposure, and any nonoccupational exposures to heat and strenuous activities. The history should identify episodes of heat-related disorders and evidence of successful adaptation to work in heat environments as part of previous jobs or in nonoccupational activities.

- A list of all prescribed and over-the-counter medications used by the worker. In particular, the physician should consider the possible impact of medications that can affect cardiac output, electrolyte balance, renal function, sweating capacity, or autonomic nervous system function. Examples of such medications include diuretics, antihypertensive drugs, sedatives, antispasmodics, anticoagulants, psychotropic medications, anticholinergics, and drugs that alter the thirst (haloperidol) or sweating mechanism (phenothiazines, antihistamines, and anticholinergics).
- Information about personal habits, including the use of alcohol and other social drugs.
- Data on height, weight, gender, and age.

The direct evaluation of the worker should include the following[14]:

- physical examination, with special attention to the skin and cardiovascular, respiratory, musculoskeletal, and nervous systems;
- clinical chemistry values needed for clinical assessment, such as fasting blood glucose, blood urea nitrogen, serum creatinine, serum electrolytes (sodium, potassium, chloride, and bicarbonate), hemoglobin, and urinary sugar and protein;
- blood pressure evaluation; and
- assessment of the ability of the worker to understand the health and safety hazards of the job, understand the required preventive measures, communicate with fellow workers, and have mobility and orientation capacities to respond properly to emergency situations.

A more detailed medical evaluation may be required. Communication between the physician performing the preplacement evaluation and the worker's private physician may be appropriate and is encouraged.

The phenomenon of heat acclimatization is well established, but for an individual worker, it can be documented only by demonstrating that after completion of an acclimatization regimen, the person can perform without excessive physiological heat strain in an environment that an unacclimatized worker could not withstand. Follow-up evaluations may be warranted during the acclimatization period for selected workers, and the IMA must be intimately involved in developing the acclimatization program for the installation.

Annual or periodic examinations should monitor individuals for changes in health that might affect heat tolerance and for evidence suggesting failure to maintain a safe work environment. Education of workers and supervisors, however, is the single most important preventive measure in avoiding heat casualties.

Personnel required to wear toxic agent protective clothing are also at high risk for dehydration, which is a contributing factor for developing heat injury. A worker may lose as much as a liter of water per hour in sweat, and the thirst mechanism is not adequate to stimulate this much water consumption. If an individual loses 1.5% to 2.0% body weight, heart rate and body temperature increase while work capacity (physical and psychological) decreases.[15] Workers should be required to consume at least 8 oz of cool water at each break period; for moderate work in greater than 80°F wet-bulb-globe temperature, the average fluid replacement recommendation is 1 quart per hour. More water may be required depending on the ambient temperature, humidity, and the physical size and exertion level of the worker. Workers should not exceed 1½ quarts per hour or 12 quarts per day.[16]

The average US diet provides adequate salt intake for an acclimatized worker, but an unacclimatized worker may excrete large amounts of salt. Individuals on medications that further deplete sodium, such as diuretics, need even closer monitoring and medical follow up. The judicious use of sodium replacement may be required during the acclimatization period.

TRAINING AND EDUCATION FOR CHEMICAL AGENT WORKERS

All personnel who work with or have some association with chemical agents and munitions, or who have a potential for exposure, must receive enough training to enable them to work safely and to understand the significance of agent exposure. Employees must know the procedures necessary to help a coworker and to summon assistance in the event of a chemical accident. Moreover, visitors who enter an area where chemical munitions are stored must be briefed on basic procedures that will enable them to visit safely, including how to properly wear a mask.

Training programs for chemical agent workers should make them aware of potential hazards and provide the knowledge and skills necessary to work with minimal risk. At the very least, chemical agent workers are required to demonstrate proficiency in the following areas before being assigned to operations:

- knowledge of operating procedures, including safety requirements;

- recognition of hazards involved in the operation;
- recognition of signs and symptoms of agent exposure;
- administration of first aid and self/buddy aid, including CPR;
- knowledge of personnel decontaminating procedures;
- execution of emergency procedures; and
- donning and doffing of protective clothing and equipment (such as self-contained breathing apparatus).

Refresher training should be conducted at least annually, and the IMA must review and approve the courses' contents and the training personnel.

Training programs may focus on chemical warfare agents, but they should also address any additional physical and chemical hazards. One example of these hazards is heat stress caused by wearing butyl protective gear, as discussed earlier in this chapter. The level of training should be commensurate with employees' job functions and responsibilities. When feasible, the training program should consist of both classroom instruction and hands-on practice. Dry runs of operational and emergency procedures are often an effective training tool.

During training, emphasis must be given to the first rule of protection—to protect oneself from injury. Workers should also know the procedure for requesting medical assistance and should be aware of any predetermined format for reporting emergencies that will expedite the report and response time. Teaching employees a logical system in which to present this information is extremely helpful. Their reports should include the nature of the accident or incident as well as what has been done for the victims (for example, the number of Mark I kits [Meridian Medical Technologies Inc, Bristol, Tenn] administered). Support personnel can request additional information as the situation progresses. The installation will greatly benefit from active involvement of the IMA and clinic staff in this training.

MEDICAL SUPPORT OF THE CHEMICAL PERSONNEL RELIABILITY PROGRAM

The CPRP is a management tool used within the Army to identify chemical surety duty positions and to manage the personnel assigned to these positions, as discussed earlier. It also provides a way to assess the reliability and acceptability of employees who are being considered for or assigned to chemical duty positions.

The program was established to ensure that personnel assigned to positions involving access to, or responsibility for, the security of chemical surety material are emotionally stable, loyal to the United States, trustworthy, and physically fit to perform assigned duties. The certifying official is the commander's representative for the CPRP and is ultimately responsible for its administration. This official, with input from the personnel officer and medical personnel, decides whether to qualify or disqualify personnel for CPRP duties. He or she must also help determine the appropriate medical surveillance category for each worker (see above) based on the worker's potential for exposure.

During each part of the screening process, evaluators look for evidence of potentially disqualifying factors that may affect personnel reliability or suitability for CPRP duties. Disqualifying factors of medical relevance include alcohol abuse, drug abuse, inability to wear protective clothing and equipment required by the assigned position, or any significant physical or mental condition that might be prejudicial to the reliable performance of CPRP duties.

The examining physician must notify the certifying official orally and in writing of any medical conditions, including the use of any prescribed medications, that may detract from an individual's ability to perform assigned chemical surety duties. In addition, the physician must provide a recommendation on the employee's suitability to continue CPRP duties. Information that may affect reliability is referred to as potential disqualifying information. These communications should be documented on Standard Form 600. As in all healthcare, documentation is extremely important and, in this case, subject to examination during a chemical surety inspection (Exhibit 18-3).

Simply supplying a diagnosis or excerpt from the medical record is not enough to enable the certifying official to make an informed decision; the competent medical authority must provide a sound medical interpretation and recommendation. The recommendation and supporting documents must be succinct and decisive, and should also note any lack of potential disqualifying information. The recommendation should state one of the following: (*a*) no restriction, (*b*) restrictions or limitations on duties, (*c*) temporary disqualification, or (*d*) permanent disqualification. Potentially disqualifying information must be provided in a sealed envelope marked "EXCLUSIVE FOR" the certifying official. Temporarily disqualified personnel remain in the CPRP, and their medical records must be treated in the same manner as the medical records of other employees in the program.

A chemical-duty position roster lists all individuals

EXHIBIT 18-3

ADMINISTRATIVE DOCUMENTATION TO SUPPORT A CHEMICAL SURETY INSPECTION

Army Regulations

AR 11-34, 15 Feb 90	*The Army Respiratory Protection Program*
AR 40-3, 18 Oct 07	*Medical, Dental and Veterinary Care*
AR 40-5, 25 May 07	*Preventive Medicine*
AR 40-13, 1 Feb 85	*Medical Support—Nuclear/Chemical Accidents and Incidents*
AR 40-63, 1 Jan 86	*Ophthalmic Services*
AR 40-66, 21 Jun 06	*Medical Record Administration and Health Care Documentation*
AR 40-68, 26 Feb 04	*Clinical Quality Management*
AR 40-400, 13 Oct 06	*Patient Administration*
AR 50-6, 26 Jun 01	*Chemical Surety*
AR 385-10, 23 Aug 07	*Army Safety Program*
AR 385-40, 1 Nov 94	*Accident Reporting and Records*
AR 385-61, 12 Oct 01	*The Army Chemical Agent Safety Program*
AR 385-64, 1 Feb 00	*US Army Explosives Safety Program*
AR 600-85, 24 Mar 06	*Army Substance Abuse Program (ASAP)*

Department of the Army Pamphlets and Technical Bulletins Medical

DA PAM 40-8, 4 Dec 90	*Occupational Health Guidelines for the Evaluation and Control of Occupational Exposure to Nerve Agents GA, GB, GD, and VX*
DA PAM 40-173, 03 Jun 03	*Occupational Health Guidelines for the Evaluation and Control of Occupational Exposures to Mustard Agents H, HD, and HT*
DA PAM 40-501, 10 Dec 98	*Hearing Conservation Program*
DA PAM 50-6, 26 Mar 03	*Chemical Accident or Incident Response and Assistance (CAIRA) Operations*
DA PAM 385-61, 27 Mar 02	*Toxic Chemical Agent Safety Standards*
TB MED 502, 15 Feb 82	*Respiratory Protection Program*
TB MED 507, 7 Mar 03	*Heat Stress Control and Heat Casualty Management*
TB MED 509, 24 Dec 86	*Spirometry in Occupational Health Surveillance*

Field Manuals

FM 3-11.5, Apr 06	*CBRN Decontamination*
FM 402.285, Sep 07	*NBC Decontamination*
FM 4-02.7, 2004	*Health Service Support in a Nuclear, Biological, and Chemical Environment*

Personnel Documents

- Table of Distribution and Allowances with mission statement for medical treatment facility or activity
- Intraservice support agreement between tenant health clinic and the host installation
- Job descriptions with performance standards (or support forms for active duty)
- Scopes of practices
- Individual or categorical credentials for health care practitioners
- Current certificates of licensure for physicians and nurses
- Advanced Trauma Life Support / Advanced Cardiac Life Support certification for physicians (nurses optional)
- Basic life support certification for all personnel with patient care responsibilities
- Certificate of completion of Medical Management of Chemical and Biological Casualties Course for physicians

Memoranda of Understanding and Mutual Aid Agreements

- With local civilian hospitals or ambulance services
- With the supporting medical center or medical department activity
- Between Army Medical Command and Army Medical Research and Materiel Command (or other major Army commands, if appropriate)

Standing Operating Procedures

- Spirometry
- Audiometry
- Vision screening

(**Exhibit 18-3** *continues*)

(**Exhibit 18-3** *continued*)

- Optical insert program for protective masks
- Medical surveillance examination (agent-specific)
- Pregnancy surveillance / reproductive hazards
- Medical screening of CPRP records
- Illness absence monitoring via CPRP records
- Incorporation of air monitoring results into the medical record
- Interface with alcohol and drug control officer
- Ambulance operation and stockage
- Preparation and review of first aid briefings
- Chemical accident and incident response
- Handling contaminated casualties at the clinic

Medical Directives

- Administration of nerve agent antidotes in the clinic
- Administration of intravenous solutions
- First aid for minor illnesses or injuries

Other Documents

- *Medical Management of Chemical Casualties Handbook*, July 2007. Available from Chemical Casualty Care Division, US Army Medical Research Institute of Chemical Defense, Aberdeen Proving Ground, Maryland 21010-5400.
- US Department of the Army. *Implementation Guidance Policy for Revised Airborne Exposure Limits for GB, GA, GD, GF, VX, H, HD, and HT.* Washington, DC: DA; 2004.

CBRN: chemical, biological, radiological, and nuclear
CPRP: chemical personnel reliability program
NBC: nuclear, biological, and chemical

assigned to chemical-duty positions in the CPRP by name, social security number, and job title. This roster also contains the name of the certifying official, the organization, and the medical surveillance exposure category of each worker. The roster must be periodically reviewed to verify that changes in duty position resulting in changes in category are incorporated into medical records and that periodic surveillance is changed to match. Medical records for personnel in the CPRP must be identified in accordance with AR 40-66, *Medical Record Administration*,[17] and segregated from records of personnel not in the CPRP.

MEDICAL ASPECTS OF A CHEMICAL ACCIDENT OR INCIDENT RESPONSE AND ASSISTANCE

Each installation with a chemical surety mission is required to develop detailed plans and procedures to be implemented by the emergency actions community in response to a chemical (surety material) accident or incident (CAI). Health services support during chemical accident or incident response and assistance (CAIRA) involves personnel with a wide range of medical expertise who will be involved in providing emergency care. When functioning as the medical leader in response to a CAI, the provider is referred to as the medical response team (MRT) leader. The MRT leader, an installation-level asset, is supported at the medical department activity or medical center level by a medical augmentation team composed of additional personnel to supplement or replace the MRT as needed. The composition of these teams and their training must be clearly documented and maintained. At the regional and national levels, there are special medical augmentation response teams composed of subject-matter experts as well as a service response force surgeon, a non-Army Medical Department asset, who supports the Chemical Materials Agency and the Army Materiel Command. There is also a chemical casualty site team deployed from USAMRICD.

The planning phase is essential to any successful medical operation; however, the plan is useless if the personnel involved are not familiar with their responsibilities or if the plan is not kept current. A routinely scheduled review and update of the clinic's standard operating procedures, in addition to maintaining current documentation, ensures that healthcare personnel review the plan and reacquaint themselves with operating procedures.

In addition to producing viable internal standard operating procedures, external coordination dictates memoranda of agreement with local agencies. The nature of the chemical agents being stored or demilitarized requires that preparations be made for receiving and treating casualties beyond the capability of the installation clinic. Although stabilization may be handled at the clinic, hospitalization will require outside facilities. Local hospitals may be reluctant to accept chemical casualties even after decontamination, and existing memoranda of agreement should facilitate the transfer and encourage the hospitals to do preaccident planning and training. Ultimately, the MRT leader is responsible for certifying that a patient as decontaminated.

Much of the coordination required for outside agreements is managed through command channels. The medical officer and medical administrator can accomplish much, however, through contact with the medical facilities and emergency medical personnel who will respond to an installation emergency. Coordination and interaction between civilian and military medical resources should be a continuous process. The IMA must take the lead to ensure that limited post resources are adequately augmented by off-post medical facilities. The staffing and treatment capabilities of off-site emergency medical facilities should be verified to ensure that appropriate resources are available. Although an IMA has limited time to coordinate with local healthcare providers and administrators, such communication is extremely valuable.

The IMA, having completed the Toxic Agent Training Course and the Medical Management of Chemical and Biological Casualties Course prior to reporting for duty, is responsible for training enlisted personnel and civilian healthcare providers. Evacuation plans, coordination with off-post civilian medical facilities, memoranda of agreement, and periodic inventories (with restocking of supplies and equipment) are also the responsibility of the IMA. In addition to individual training, collective training in the form of drills should become a routine part of the clinic schedule. Training of civilian resources is coordinated through the Chemical Stockpile Emergency Preparedness Program, centered at the Edgewood Area of Aberdeen Proving Ground, Maryland. Only the successful completion of all these types of planning and training ensure readiness for proper management of a chemically contaminated patient. Clinics at depots with a chemical surety mission should have an area designated for the decontamination of exposed patients; this area is necessary to provide early medical care that will limit the degree of the casualty's exposure. Generally, the treatment area for these patients is separate from the normal patient treatment areas. Although these facilities are rarely used for an actual chemically contaminated patient, an ongoing effort must be made to keep these rooms at 100% operational capability. To maintain this capability, the medical staff must develop comprehensive and detailed standard operating procedures.

In the event of a CAI, emergency medical care will initially be provided by nonmedical workers responsible for removing casualties from the site of injury through a personnel decontamination station and to the waiting medical team. Further evacuation may be required, either to the installation medical facility or to an off-post medical treatment facility. The fundamental pathophysiological threats to life (namely, airway compromise, breathing difficulties, and circulatory derangement) are the same for chemical casualties as they are for casualties of any other type, but all personnel treating chemical injuries require additional training. At the least, nonmedical workers require training in self/buddy-aid. The installation response force is responsible for providing the immediate safety, security, rescue, and control at the CAI site to save lives and reduce exposure to hazards. The IMA must approve the training program for both workers and the installation response force and must review their lesson plans for accuracy and completeness. The essentials of this training include recognizing signs and symptoms of agent exposure, first aid, self/buddy-aid, individual protection, personnel decontamination (including decontamination of a litter patient), and evacuation of casualties.

To develop appropriate emergency medical plans, it is necessary to know the chemical agents included, number of personnel involved in the incident, location of the work area, a summary of work procedures, and the duration of the operation. This information is available through the installation commander or the certifying official. In addition, the most probable event (MPE) and maximum credible event (MCE) must be defined to determine the anticipated casualty loads in either situation. When dealing with large amounts of dangerous agents, an MPE is the worst potential event likely to occur during routine handling, storage, maintenance, or demilitarization operations that results in the release of agent and exposure of personnel. An MCE is the worst single event that could reasonably occur at any time, with maximal release of agent from munitions, bulk container, or work process as a result of an accidental occurrence. The Office of The Surgeon General is developing guidance for installations to estimate the chemical agent casualties expected from an MPE or an MCE. For planning purposes, medical staffing requirements are based on the MPE for the installation. Because an MCE is expected to exceed the capabilities of the installation medical facility, medical contingency plans and coordination with local, state, and federal emergency medical authorities are essential.

The procedure for the decontamination of litter patients can be found in FM 4-07.7, *Health Service Support in a Nuclear, Chemical and Biological Environment*.[18] The installation response force decontaminates patients and passes them across a hotline to the MRT. At that point, the casualty should be completely clean. Civilian officials may require a casualty to be "certified clean" before moving the patient off the military installation. This requirement may be addressed through coordination and training prior to an exercise or an actual CAI. Coordination with the civilian sector through education and communication is essential to providing a rapid and adequate medical response.

CAIRA encompasses actions taken to save lives and to preserve health and safety. This support involves a continuum of medical care, ranging from self/buddy aid in the field to treatment at a tertiary care facility. Because of the nature of some chemical warfare agents, proper care and adequate decontamination must be provided early to avoid serious injury or death. CAIRA includes the following levels of medical care:

Level I: composed of installation response force nonmedical installation personnel. The local commander appoints the incident response force members and ensures they are provided initial and ongoing training as described in DA Pamphlet 50-6, *Chemical Accident or Incident Response and Assistance (CAIRA) Operations*.[2] The Office of The Surgeon General and the US Army Medical Department Center and School are developing a list of essential medical tasks for this group. Additional tasks may be added at the discretion of the IMA or the local commander.

Level II: the MRT (composed of installation medical personnel). The MRT leader is a physician and is responsible for training the team in triage, treatment, stabilization, and evacuation of casualties from the accident site to the appropriate medical treatment facility. The MRT must have adequate personnel, supplies, and equipment to provide healthcare to casualties generated by an MPE. The specific tasks for the MRT leader and members are specified in DA PAM 50-6, Tables 6-3 and 6-4.[2] One MRT member should be issued toxicological agent protective gear so he or she may cross the hotline and provide emergency medical care to casualties. The remaining members should be available on the clean side of the hotline to perform triage and to provide immediate care. Current guidance requires forward medical personnel to be trained in advanced airway skills such as intubation. For military medics, these skills should be (but are not always) taught during advanced individual training. Ambulances should be staffed with at least one paramedic, a level of training more advanced than a military medic.

Level III: the medical augmentation team, provided by the medical department activity or the medical center to an installation with a chemical surety mission. This team must have the capability to augment the MRT in the event of an MCE. The medical augmentation team leader's responsibilities are also outlined in DA PAM 50-6, Table 6-5.[2]

Level IV: the chemical casualty site team, provided by USAMRICD, which provides clinical consultation and subject-matter experts in chemical casualty care. A veterinarian may also be a designated member of this team. During the initial phases of an exercise, concern is primarily for casualties. In previous service response force exercises, however, questions have been asked about the safety of livestock, pets, and wildlife. The veterinarian has proven to be a valuable source of information and an asset to this team.

The installation commander looks initially to the IMA for medical support and advice. If the CAI exceeds the installation's capability, a service response force is provided to assume control of the situation. The service response force surgeon assumes operational control of the MRT, the medical augmentation team, and the medical chemical advisory team at the accident site.

DEMILITARIZATION OF CHEMICAL WARFARE AGENTS

The United States has produced and stored a stockpile of chemical warfare agents since World War I. These projectiles, rockets , mines, and ton containers have been maintained at eight depots in eight states: Aberdeen Proving Ground, Maryland (demilitarization completed); Anniston Army Depot, Alabama; Blue Grass Army Depot, Kentucky; Newport Chemical Depot, Indiana; Pine Bluff Arsenal, Arkansas; Pueblo Chemical Depot, Colorado; Deseret Chemical Depot, Utah; and Umatilla Chemical Depot, Oregon. In the event of a large release of agents, two neighboring states, Washington and Illinois, might also be affected.

The majority of chemical agents are stored in bulk containers that do not have explosive components, and leaking chemical agents have not presented a health threat to areas surrounding these depots. However, continuing to store the aging munitions may present a risk of chemical agent exposure. Of the chemical munitions, the M55 rocket is the most hazardous; under certain accidental circumstances, it could deliver its chemical payload into the community.

In 1985 Congress initiated a program to dispose of the entire US stockpile of lethal chemical agents. There were multiple reasons for destroying these chemical warfare agents:

- Ratification of the multilateral Chemical Weapons Convention treaty in April 1997 required the destruction of the weapons by April 2007, with an extension to April 2012, if necessary.
- The need for the stockpile no longer exists.
- The stockpile is slowly deteriorating with age.
- The stockpile is a potential target for terrorism.

In 1988 the US Army chose incineration as the method of destruction for the stockpile because it allows safe treatment of all the components of a chemical weapon, including the agent, fuses, bursters, explosives, motors, metal parts, and metal bodies. The prototype incineration destruction plant for lethal agents, the Johnston Atoll Chemical Agent Destruction System, was erected on Johnston Island in the South Pacific. The plant completed its mission in 2000 after destroying more than 2,000 tons of chemical agents and 410,000 chemical munitions. Incineration is currently in use at four of the storage depots: Deseret, Anniston, Umatilla, and Pinebluff. All destruction facilities were engineered with redundant safety features designed to prevent the release of agent. The US Public Health Service reviews plans and monitors operations of these chemical destruction plants. The appropriate state environmental authorities must issue permits before incineration can begin.

During the incineration process, the agent and all metal parts are destroyed at 2,700°F. Exhaust gases are passed through extensive, state-of-the-art pollution control systems, including a pollution abatement filtration system. Personnel dismantle the weapons in explosive containment rooms designed to withstand detonation. Explosives are separated from the liquid agent and metal parts with each waste stream and destroyed in separate furnaces. Unconfined explosives are consumed in the fire. The solid residue remaining from ash, fiberglass, and wooden dunnage is evaluated for contamination and transported to approved landfills. Brine (a by-product waste) is packaged and also sent to approved landfills. There is no water discharge resulting from the incineration process. Stack effluent must meet all requirements of the Clean Air Act,[19] especially the amendments passed in 1970,[20] 1977,[21] and 1990[22] (these last three versions were codified in the US Code in 1990[23]). Special precautions have been taken to reduce and eliminate the formation of furans and dioxans from the incineration process. Discharges from the stack are continuously monitored to ensure that the Clean Air Act requirements are met. Even though the possibility of an event leading to the contamination of an area surrounding a community is remote, extensive planning and preparation have been accomplished. The US Army and the Federal Emergency Management Agency have jointly enhanced the emergency preparedness of these communities.

Despite the extensive precautions in building the destruction plants, the Chemical Stockpile Emergency Preparedness Program and the Federal Emergency Management Agency are working with emergency responders to enhance their capabilities. Through the Chemical Stockpile Emergency Preparedness Program, first responders and emergency management officials are trained to manage chemical casualties specific to the installation. Extensive security and safety measures have been adopted to avoid accidents or incidents involving chemical agents and chemical surety. Some containers are transported in large overpack containers (a container within a heavier container) designed to withstand an explosion and stored in an igloo (a storage building topped with, for example, 3 to 4 ft of earth and concrete). These measures have been strengthened against acts of terrorism since the attacks on the United States on September 11, 2001.

The US Army has also investigated and developed alternatives to incineration. The Alternative Technologies and Approaches Project developed and implemented neutralization disposal technologies of bulk container stocks of the nerve agent VX in Newport, Indiana, and the blister agent HD (mustard gas) at the Edgewood Area of Aberdeen Proving Ground. Destruction of VX was carried out with sodium hydroxide and hot water. Destruction of HD was accomplished by neutralization followed by biotreatment involving the microbial destruction of biodegradable organic material, such as thiodiglycol found in the hydrolysate. As of fall 2006, the Army has neutralized 100% of the stockpile at the Aberdeen Proving Ground facility and as of May 2008, 90% of the stockpile at the Newport facility. The Aberdeen facility was officially closed in June 2007.[24]

The Assembled Chemical Weapons Alternatives Program is responsible for the safe destruction of chemical weapons stockpiles at Pueblo, Colorado, and Blue Grass, Kentucky. Neutralization followed by biotreatment was selected for the Pueblo stockpile; neutralization followed by supercritical water oxidation will be used to destroy the Blue Grass stockpile. Construction of full-scale pilot test disposal facilities is underway in both states.

Critics of the Army's high-temperature incineration believe that the method is undesirable. The disagreement among scientific experts and the concerns of people surrounding the eight US depots have created numerous debates over the chemical agent destruction program, presenting a risk communication challenge for the Army. This communication challenge has lead to the development of active public outreach offices staffed with knowledgeable teams to answer questions and provide informational materials. These outreach teams have fostered an environment of trust and cooperation among the Department of Defense and the citizens that it serves.

SUMMARY

The unique challenges of handling chemical warfare agents and aging munitions while protecting the health of chemical workers requires thorough knowledge of occupational medicine and of chemical agents. It also involves the interaction of multiple professional groups, such as physicians, industrial hygienists, safety officers, surety officers, and certifying officials. Lack of communication between these groups and the community can pose significant risk, especially in the chemical demilitarization process. Healthcare providers can play an important role in reducing this risk by providing information to communities and building confidence in the US Army's ability to safely destroy chemical agents.

REFERENCES

1. US Department of the Army. *Chemical Surety*. Washington, DC: DA; 2001. Army Regulation 50-6.

2. US Department of the Army. *Chemical Accident or Incident Response and Assistance (CAIRA) Operations*. Washington, DC: DA; March 2003. DA PAM 50-6.

3. US Department of the Army. *Occupational Health Guidelines for the Evaluation and Control of Occupational Exposure to Nerve Agents GA, GB, GD, and VX*. Washington, DC: DA; 1990. DA PAM 40-8.

4. US Department of the Army. *Occupational Health Guidelines for the Evaluation and Control of Occupational Exposure to Mustard Agents H, HD, and HT*. Washington, DC: DA; 2003. DA PAM 40-173.

5. US Department of the Army. *The Army Chemical Agent Safety Program*. Washington, DC: DA; 2001. Army Regulation 385-61.

6. US Department of the Army. *Toxic Chemical Agent Safety Standards*. Washington, DC: DA; 2002. DA PAM 385-61.

7. McCunney RJ. *Handbook of Occupational Medicine*. Boston, Mass: Little, Brown and Co; 1988.

8. 5 CFR, Part 339.

9. Americans with Disabilities Act, 42 USC §12101 (1990).

10. National Institute of Occupational Safety and Health. *Occupational Safety and Health Guidance Manual for Hazardous Waste Site Activities*. Cincinnati, Ohio: NIOSH; 1985.

11. US Department of the Army. *Interim Guidance for Decontamination and Medical Services in Support of Nerve and Mustard Agent Operations*. Washington, DC: DA. Memorandum, 10 June 2003.

12. US Department of the Army. *Army Substance Abuse Program (ASAP)*. Washington, DC: DA; 2006. Army Regulation 600-85.

13. Executive Order 12564, "Drug-Free Workplace," *Federal Register* 51 (1986): No. 180.

14. National Institute of Occupational Safety and Health. *Criteria for a Recommended Standard: Occupational Exposure to Hot Environments. Revised Criteria*. Cincinnati, Ohio: NIOSH; 1986.

15. Greenleaf JE, Harrison MH. Water and electrolytes. In: Layman DK, ed. *Exercise, Nutrition and Health*. Washington, DC: American Chemical Society; 1986: 107–123.

16. US Department of the Army. *Prevention of Heat and Cold Casualties.* Washington, DC: DA; 2003. TRADOC Regulation 350-29.

17. US Department of the Army. *Medical Record Administration*. Washington DC: DA; 2004. Army Regulation 40-66.

18. US Department of the Army. *Medical Platoon Leaders' Handbook: Tactics, Techniques and Procedures*. Washington, DC: August 2001. Field Manual 4-02.4.

18. Clean Air Act of 1963. Pub L No. 88-206.

20. Clean Air Act of 1970. Pub L No. 91-604.

21. Clean Air Act of 1977. Pub L No. 95-95.

22. Clean Air Act of 1990. Pub L No. 101-549.

23. Clean Air Act, 42 USC §7401–7671 (1990).

24. US Army Chemical Materials Agency Web site. Available at http://www.cma.army.mil. Accessed June 2008.

Chapter 19

TOXINS: ESTABLISHED AND EMERGENT THREATS

PATRICK WILLIAMS, MS*; SCOTT WILLENS, DVM, PhD†; JAIME ANDERSON, DVM, PhD‡; MICHAEL ADLER, PhD§; AND COREY J. HILMAS, MD, PhD¥

*Research Biologist, Department of Neurobehavioral Toxicology, US Army Medical Research Institute of Chemical Defense, 3100 Ricketts Point Road, Aberdeen Proving Ground, Maryland 21010

†Major, Veterinary Corps, US Army; Chief of Department of Neurobehavioral Toxicology, Analytical Toxicology Division, US Army Medical Research Institute of Chemical Defense, 3100 Ricketts Point Road, Aberdeen Proving Ground, Maryland 21010

‡Division Chief, Analytical Toxicology Division, Department of Neurobehavioral Toxicology, US Army Medical Research Institute of Chemical Defense, 3100 Ricketts Point Road, Aberdeen Proving Ground, Maryland 21010

§Research Pharmacologist, Neurobehavioral Toxicology, Department of Neurobehavioral Toxicology, US Army Medical Research Institute of Chemical Defense, 3100 Ricketts Point Road, Aberdeen Proving Ground, Maryland 21010

¥Research Physiologist and Pharmacologist, Analytical Toxicology Division, Department of Neurobehavioral Toxicology, US Army Medical Research Institute of Chemical Defense, 3100 Ricketts Point Road, Aberdeen Proving Ground, Maryland 21010

INTRODUCTION

In its definition of "toxin," the 1993 Chemical Weapons Convention includes "any chemical which through its chemical action on life processes can cause death, temporary incapacitation or permanent harm to humans or animals," regardless of its origin or method of production.[1] Because there is no consensus on the inclusion criterion for toxins, international law regards a wide range of biological and chemical substances as toxins.

An array of toxins exists among the species of all kingdoms (Table 19-1). Many of these toxins have well-characterized and therapeutic effects and have been employed as medical treatments and scientific tools. However, many can have nefarious applications, especially when used outside of their therapeutic indices.

The wide spectrum of toxins includes the following three categories: 1) bacterial toxins (eg, botulinum neurotoxin and staphylococcal enterotoxin), which are high-molecular–weight proteins produced in large quantity by industrial microbiological methods; 2) snake poisons, insect venoms, plant proteins, and marine algae, which are either naturally occurring or chemically synthesized (eg, curare, batrachotoxin [BTX], and ricin); and 3) small molecules, such as potassium fluoroacetate, which are synthesized by chemical processes and produced by living organisms. This chapter focuses on the second toxin group.

Nature of the Threat

An attack involving a mass-casualty–producing weapon, whether biological or chemical, can no longer be anticipated only from hostile states. Some nonstate and terrorist entities have limited moral or social reservations about attacking civilian populations with the intent of causing large numbers of casualties. Agents considered "classical" chemical or biological weapons, such as mustard gas, organophosphorous nerve agents, botulinum toxin, and anthrax, threaten the health and safety of civilian and military populations. Throughout the 20th century, numerous countries have developed and stockpiled chemical and biological agents. Changes in the geopolitical climate over the last 30 years have made it possible for these weapons to fall into terrorists' hands.

Any toxin is a putative, mass-casualty–producing weapon, and to objectively estimate the threats they might pose, toxins must be evaluated against several criteria. First, the potential weapon agent must be suitably toxic. Groups who intend to injure or kill will not waste time or limited resources on agents that are harmless irritants to humans. Marginally toxic compounds must be stockpiled in very large quantities (tons) to produce an effective weapon. Similarly, toxins that produce mild effects following intoxication, or effects for which there are readily available treatments or antitoxins, are less likely threats. Many toxins can be discounted as potential candidates for weaponization based on this criterion alone.

Second, the requirement to stockpile toxin suggests that terrorists must possess the storage capability to maintain toxin potency and prevent toxin degradation. Unstable toxins with short half-lives or toxins that require special handling or storage conditions are typically undesirable. Terrorists' surroundings must be considered when assessing the stability of a potential toxin threat. For example, terrorists operating out of caves in mountains or tent encampments in the desert will not possess the necessary equipment to handle and store some toxins, but a small cell of college students or a state-sponsored group might have access to storage containers, a variety of solvents and acids to properly buffer a toxin for long-term storage, temperature- and humidity-controlled environments, and other special handling equipment.

Third, for a toxin to create mass casualties, a source of the toxin must be readily available. It is unlikely that terrorist groups would tend large snake farms, for example, to harvest snake toxin for weaponization. In addition to other logistical challenges, such an undertaking would be conspicuous and time consuming. However, if a commercial source of a particular toxin is available, the toxin becomes more attractive to a terrorist organization, particularly if the organization has the secure infrastructure available to acquire, purify, concentrate, and properly store toxin stocks. Many toxins have been chemically synthesized and are commercially available to researchers and scientists. Commercially available toxins are typically sold in small quantities for research purposes and are not cost prohibitive; however, some terrorist organizations are able to purchase and store toxins for future weaponization, and the chemical reactions for the synthesis of many toxins have been published in scientific literature and are therefore available to these organizations. Chemical synthesis begins with readily available, simple, and nontoxic compounds, which could be easily and inexpensively obtained from many scientific supply houses. In many cases, the requisite knowledge, skills, and apparatus to perform such synthesis are not trivial; however, for the well-equipped and skilled terrorist, there are no impediments to the synthesis and storage of very large quantities of toxin.

A suitable delivery method must also be designed in advance of bioweapon deployment for toxins to cause a significant threat. While some toxins are lipid soluble

TABLE 19-1

LIST OF KNOWN TOXINS AND THEIR SOURCES

Toxin	Source
α-Aminitin	Death cap mushroom, *Amanita phalloides*
α-Latrotoxin	Black widow spider venom, *Latrodectus mactans*
Abrin, crystalline	Jequirity beans, the seeds of *Abrus precatorius*
Aconitine	Roots of monkshood, *Aconitum napellus*
Aerolysin	*Aeromonas hydrophila*
Aflatoxin	Molds *Aspergillus flavus* and *A parasiticus*
Anatoxin	Cyanobacteria, *Anabaena flosaquae*
Atelopidtoxin	*Atelopus zeteki*
Batrachotoxin	Frogs, *Phyllobates terribilis* and *P aurotaenia*
Bee venom (apamin)	Honey bees, *Apis mellifera*
Botulinum toxin type A-G	*Clostridium botulinum* bacteria
Brevetoxin	Dinoflagellate algae, *Ptychodiscus brevis* or *Gymnodinium breve*
Brown recluse spider venom	*Loxosceles reclusa*
C2 toxin, C3 toxin	*Clostridium botulinum*
C-alkaloid E	Calabash-curare arrow poison
Cholera toxin	*Vibrio cholerae*
Ciguatoxin	Dinoflagellate *Gambierdiscus toxicus*
Clostridium difficile toxin A and B	*Clostridium difficile*
Cobra neurotoxin	Indian cobra venom, *Naja naja*
Conotoxins	Pacific cone snails
Dendrotoxin	Green mamba snake, *Dendroaspis anguisticeps*
Dermonecrotic toxin, pertussis toxin	*Bordetella pertussis*
Diphtheria toxin	*Corynebacterium diphtheriae*
d-Tubocurarine	Tube-curare arrow poison
Edema factor	*Bacillus anthracis*
Enterotoxins, exfoliative toxins, toxic-shock toxin	*Staphylococcus aureus*
Epsilon toxin	*Clostridium perfringens*
Escherichia coli toxins (cytotoxic necrotizing factors, heat-labile toxin, heat-stable toxin, cytolethal distending toxin, heat-stable enterotoxin-1)	*Escherichia coli*
Exotoxin A	*Pseudomonas aeruginosa*
Fasciculin	Venom of the green mamba snake
Grayanotoxin	Rhododendron and other Ericaceae
Hemolysin	*Escherichia coli*
Histrionicotoxin	Colombian frog, *Dendrobates histrionicus*
Israeli scorpion venom (charybdotoxin)	*Leiurus quinquestriatus hebraues*
Kokór arrow poison	Colombian frog, *Phyllobates aurotaenia*
Lethal factor	*Bacillus anthracis*
Listeriolysin O	*Listeria monocytogenes*
Maitotoxin	Marine dinoflagellate, *Gambierdiscus toxicus*
Microcystin	Cyanobacteria, *Microcystis aeruginosa*
Nicotine	*Nicotiana* tobacco plants
North American scorpion venom	*Centruroides sculpturatus*
Ouabain	*Strophanthus gratus* seeds
Palytoxin	Soft coral, *Palythoa toxica*
Perfringolysin O	*Clostridium perfringens*
Picrotoxin (cocculin)	*Cocculus indicus, Anamirta cocculus*
Pneumolysin	*Streptococcus pneumoniae*
Pumiliotoxin	Formicine ants of genera *Brachymyrmex* and *Paratrechina* and frog *Dendrobates pumilio*
Pyrogenic exotoxins	*Streptococcus pyogenes*

(**Table 19-1** *continues*)

Table 19-1 *continued*

Ricin, amorphous and crystalline	Castor beans, the seeds of *Ricinis communis*
Russell's viper venom	*Vipera russelli*
Salmonella toxin, cytotoxin, enterotoxin	*Salmonella Typhimurium* and *S Enteritidis*
Saxitoxin	Dinoflagellate marine algae, *Gonyaulax catenella and G tamarensis*
Shiga toxin	*Escherichia coli/Shigella dysenteriae*
Staphylococcus aureus α-toxin	*Staphyloccocus aureus*
Streptolysin O	*Streptococcus pyogenes*
Strychnine	*Stryhnos nuxvomica* bark or seeds
Taipoxin	Australian taipan snake, *Oxyuranus scutellatus*
Tetanus toxin	*Clostridium tetani bacteria*
Tetrodotoxin	Puffer fishes and certain salamanders
Textilotoxin	Australian common brown snake, *Pseudonaja textilis*
Tityustoxin	Brazilian scorpion, *Tityus serrulatus*
Trichothecene Mycotoxin (T-2)	Fusarial species of fungus
Veratridine	Liliaceae
Western diamondback rattlesnake venom	*Crotalus atrox*

and readily absorbed through dermal layers (posing contact hazards), most are water soluble. Water-soluble toxins can be aerosolized for delivery to target populations, which allows toxin access to the more vulnerable inner surfaces of the lung. Aerosol particles between 0.5 and 5 μm in diameter are typically retained within the lung, but smaller particles are not retained in the airway and most are exhaled. Particles between 5 to 15 μm are generally sequestered in nasal mucosa or in the trachea. A large percentage of aerosol particles larger than 15 μm drop to the ground or onto flat surfaces in the environment. Water-soluble toxins are generally not volatile, and those particles falling onto the ground no longer pose a respiratory threat.[2]

Many cases of accidental exposure to toxins in humans, especially from marine toxins, occur by ingestion. Intoxication by agents such as tetrodotoxin (TTX; isolated from the Japanese puffer fish) or brevetoxin (PbTx), implicated in neurotoxic shellfish poisoning (NSP), suggest that water or food supplies could be targeted for large-scale delivery of weaponized toxins to civilian populations. Several recent publications have presented mathematical models of toxin weapons delivered into food or water supplies.[3] These data suggest that this means of toxin delivery would impose a significant financial burden to diagnose and treat the affected population, a compromise to key infrastructure, and a reallocation of resources to deliver clean supplies to the effected population.

Established Threats

Toxins of concern to the US military and the Department of Homeland Security comprise a group of structurally diverse substances that share many features with chemical warfare agents. Toxins and chemical warfare agents interfere with important biological processes (eg, synaptic transmission, DNA replication, and protein synthesis) and produce incapacitation and death following acute exposure.[4] Toxins that are generally considered to be battlefield or bioterrorist threats include anthrax, botulinum neurotoxin, staphylococcal enterotoxin B, T-2 mycotoxin, and ricin. These five biotoxins are thought to be most likely used in the event of warfare or bioterrorism, although they represent a small subset of all lethal toxins known.[5] Potency, ease of production, stability, and prior history of weaponization are all factors hostile forces must consider before deploying bioweapons.[4–6] The Centers for Disease Control and Prevention (CDC) have designated anthrax and botulinum neurotoxin as category A threat agents, and staphylococcal enterotoxin B and ricin as category B agents (Table 19-2).[7] Category A agents are defined as those that "can be easily disseminated or transmitted from person to person; result in high mortality rates and have the potential for major public health impact; might cause public panic and social disruption and require special action for public health preparedness."[7] Category B agents are defined as those that "are moderately easy to disseminate; result in moderate morbidity rates and low mortality rates; and require specific enhancements of CDC's diagnostic capacity and enhanced disease surveillance."[7] For example, T-2 mycotoxin, a category B agent, is specifically addressed by the CDC as a select agent and toxin and additionally regarded as a threat because of its documented use in Laos, Vietnam, and Cambodia during 1975–1978.[8] Category C agents, the third highest priority, "include emerging pathogens that could be engineered for mass dissemination in

TABLE 19-2

CENTER FOR DISEASE CONTROL AND PREVENTION CLASSIFICATION OF BIOTERRORISM AGENTS/DISEASES

Category A	Category B	Category C
Anthrax	Brucellosis	Emerging future toxin threats
Botulism	Epilson toxin of *Clostridium perfringens*	
Plague	Food safety threats (*Escherichia coli, Salmonella species,* O157:H7, *Shigella*)	
Smallpox	Glanders	
Tularemia	Meloidosis	
Viral Hemmoragic Fevers	Psittacosis	
	Q Fever	
	Ricin toxin from *Ricinus communis*	
	Staphylococcal enterotoxin B	
	Typhus	
	Viral encephalitis	
	Water safety threats (eg, *Vibrio cholerae, Cryptosporidium parvum*)	

Data source: Bioterrorism agents/diseases: emergency preparedness & response Web site. Available at: http://www.bt.cdc.gov/agent/agentlist-category.asp. Accessed February 10, 2007.

the future because of availability; ease of production and dissemination; and potential for high morbidity and mortality rates and major health impact."[7] These emerging toxin threats are the focus of this chapter, toxins that possess the properties of the more well-known category A and B agents but that have not been considered likely threats to date (see Table 19-2).

Emergent Threats

The group of biotoxins not considered immediate threats with the potential to cause human illness and death is potentially very large and includes the sodium channel toxins BTX,[9] PbTx,[10] saxitoxin (STX),[11] TTX,[12] and pumiliotoxin.[13] Others include palytoxin (PTX), which alters the sodium-potassium exchanger (sodium-potassium ATPase),[14] and the nicotinic receptor agonist, anatoxin-A.[15] Because these toxins are employed as pharmacological tools for studying ion channel properties, active efforts to optimize their synthesis are being developed.[16] If these efforts are successful in generating large quantities of toxin, members of this group will need to be reevaluated for their potential as threat agents.

TOXINS

Palytoxin

Synthesis

PTX is an extremely potent marine neurotoxin that acts on sodium-potassium ion pumps. First isolated from the zoanthid coral (genus *Palythoa*) by Moore and Scheuer,[17] PTX has long been categorized as a marine animal toxin. It has been identified in several species living in close contact with zoanthid anemones (eg, some dinoflagellates, *Ostreopsis* species);[18] Polychaete worms;[19] several species of xanthid crab (*Lophozozymus pictor* and *Demaina toxica*),[20] and several species of fish.[21–23] PTX is found in the red alga *Chondria aramata*.[24,25] PTX has also been associated with the blue humphead parrotfish,[26] filefish, and serranid fish.[27] The primary source is most likely a bacterium associated with soft corals that inhabit the digestive tract of filefish (Figure 19-1). PTX is a large (molecular weight 2,678.5), water-soluble, nonproteinaceous polyether, with molecular formula $C_{129}H_{223}N_3O_{54}$. PTX has an exquisitely complex structure (see Figure 19-1). It was first elucidated and synthesized in 1982[28] and is currently available from several commercial sources.

Mechanism of Action and Toxicity

PTX affects all excitable cells by inducing the activity of a small conductance (9–25 pS), nonselective, cationic channel, which triggers secondary activations of voltage-dependent calcium channels and of sodium-calcium exchange. In addition to electrically excitable

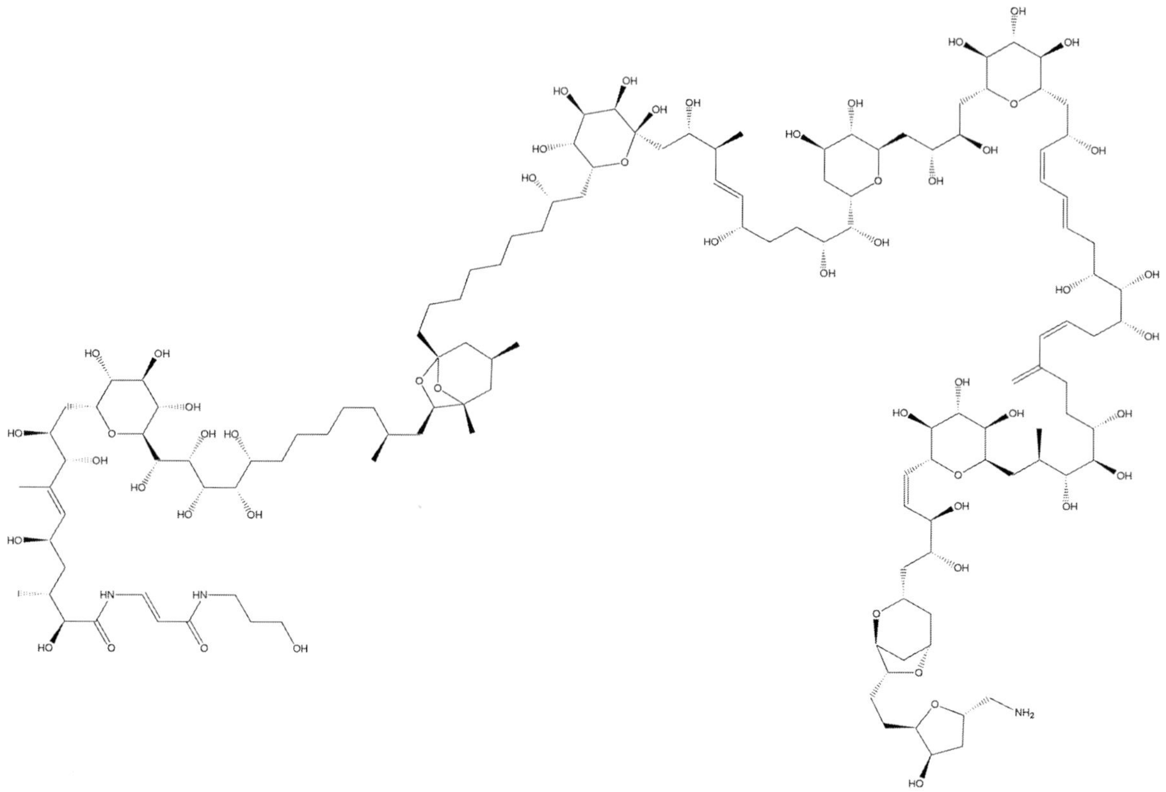

Fig. 19-1. Structure of palytoxin.
Illustration: Courtesy of Richard Sweeny.

cells (muscle, heart, neurons), PTX affects virtually all cell types that rely on the sodium-potassium ATPase exchanger to maintain electrolyte balance, membrane potential, and electrical/ionic gradients. The sodium-potassium ATPase exchanger pump has been suggested to be a major molecular target of PTX.[29] PTX leads to contractions of striated skeletal and smooth muscle cells, neurotransmitter release by nerve terminals,[30] potassium release and hemolysis of red blood cells, and blood vessel vasoconstriction. PTX leads to contraction in both smooth and skeletal muscle as a result of slow and irreversible depolarization of the plasma membrane in these cells from an induction of an inward, sodium-dependent current.[25,30] A cardiotonic effect in cardiac muscle and depolarization of muscle membranes occurs as a result of PTX intoxication.[30] PTX causes a depolarization and a decrease in the amplitude, upstroke velocity, and duration of action potential in papillary muscle of the heart secondary to an increase in sodium permeability of the cardiac cell membrane. Membrane depolarization of the plasma membrane drives sodium into the cells, promoting calcium influx through L-type calcium channels and by the sodium-calcium exchanger. Evidence suggests PTX binds to the sodium-potassium ATPase exchanger at ouabain receptor sites. This active transport ion pump is converted to an open ion channel, diminishing ion gradient across the membrane.[22,29–31]

PTX affects adrenergic neurons and red blood cells, increasing norepinephrine and potassium release, respectively.[30] PTX also effects blood vessels through its interactions on vascular smooth muscle, nerve terminals, and vascular endothelial cells, leading to vasoconstriction, an increase in systemic blood pressure, and massive pulmonary hypertension. In addition, depolarization of the plasma membrane opens L-type calcium channels, promoting calcium influx and contractions.[25] Perivascular nerve terminals undergo membrane depolarization, releasing norephinephrine that binds to alpha-1-adrenoceptors on smooth muscle cells. Activation of phospholipase C by norephinephrine binding induces mobilization of intracellular calcium stores and activates protein kinase.[25] PTX also acts on vascular endothelial cells by releasing nitric oxide and induces the release of prostaglandins from the aorta.[25]

PTX is a rapid-acting, lethal neurotoxin most commonly introduced by ingestion. The median lethal dose

(LD_{50}) in humans is estimated to be 0.15 μg/kg body weight. Intoxication by PTX affects the sodium-potassium ATPase exchanger pump by converting the active ion transport process into a relatively nonspecific cation channel.[25,29] At the cellular level, PTX action leads to membrane depolarization, the most likely cause of smooth muscle contraction in vitro and vasoconstriction in vivo.[14] Clinical signs and symptoms of PTX intoxication include vasoconstriction, hemorrhage, ataxia, muscle weakness, ventricular fibrillation, ischemia, and death.[25,30] Challenge by intravenous (IV) or subcutaneous injection has been shown to be the most effective route of exposure for inducing intoxication by PTX in test animals, although a number of fatalities involving human intoxication by ingestion have been reported.[27,32–34]

Toxin Exposure, Health Effects, and Treatment

PTX can cause a diverse array of clinical signs and symptoms, including skin irritation, generalized weakness, muscle spasms, sweating, skin irritation, abdominal cramps, nausea, vomiting, diarrhea, temperature dysesthesia, and paresthesias ("pins and needles"). More severe signs and symptoms include acute respiratory distress, vasoconstriction, hemorrhage, ataxia, generalized muscle weakness, tonic contraction of all muscle groups, elevated muscle enzymes, myoglobinuria, rhabdomyolysis, tremors, seizures, cyanosis, bradycardia, ventricular fibrillation, ischemia, renal and cardiac failure, and death. Because PTX is an extremely potent vasoconstrictor, it affects all muscle and neuronal cell types. A depolarization of membrane potential occurs in cells, with sodium entering the cells in exchange for potassium.[31]

Physical Examination. After PTX intoxication, an initial decrease in blood pressure followed by a rise in systemic blood pressure has been observed.[35] In addition, after ingesting PTX, some poison victims have reported tasting metal.[34] Bradycardia has been reported in acute poisonings. PTX can also lead to myocardial damage. Furthermore, PTX displays cardiotonic properties in cardiac muscle, leading to depolarization of excitable membrane, including cardiac muscle, as described above.[22,34] Electrocardiograms (EKGs) have shown negative T waves in leads III and aVf following human ingestion of PTX; however, echocardiography remained normal during the clinical course.[26] In one clinical case report of PTX intoxication, serum cardiac enzyme, creatine kinase MB isozyme, was reported to be 8% on the fourth hospital day.[26] On respiratory examination, patients may experience acute dyspnea, tachypnea, and shallow breathing.[22,34] While coronary vasoconstriction is usually a primary factor leading to death, respiratory failure can result in death when the essential muscles of respiration stop working.[36] Neurological examination may show seizures, tremors,[22,36] muscle spasms, and generalized weakness[23,34] secondary to depolarization of muscle or nerve membranes.[22] In addition, a cold-to-hot temperature reversal dysesthesia has been noted in ciguatera fish poisoning.[34,37] Circumoral and limb paresthesias have also been reported in patients,[22,34,37] in addition to restlessness and dizziness.[34]

Gastrointestinal symptoms are the earliest symptoms to manifest in PTX intoxication. Nausea, vomiting, abdominal cramps, and diarrhea are common complaints.[22,34] Patients may complain of dark brown to black urine, secondary to myoglobinuria,[36] anuria, and renal failure.[34] PTX can also cause eye and skin irritation,[38] cold sweats,[34] and excessive perspiration.[22] While contractile responses are seen in both smooth and skeletal muscle,[22] increased skeletal muscle tone, cramps, and severe myalgya[23,36] are hallmarks of PTX intoxication. A prominent rhabdomyolysis may also occur, leading to myoglobinuria.[26] Additionally, PTX has caused a dose-dependent contraction of the human umbilical artery,[39] but there is no data concerning teratogenicity. PTX is also a known tumor promoter, even at low levels.[40]

Laboratory Findings and Monitoring. Laboratory examination can reveal elevated liver enzymes in serum creatine phosphokinase (CPK), aspartate aminotransferase, and lactate dehydrogenase.[22,26,36] These should be monitored as indicators of muscle damage. One case report showed that serum aspartate aminotransferase was elevated to 3,370 IU/L on the third day after ingestion of PTX-containing fish, and serum lactate dehydrogenase was elevated to 7,100 IU/L on the fourth day.[26] Serum levels should be monitored for hyperkalemia and hyponatremia due to PTX effects on the sodium-potassium exchanger. In addition, hemolysis has been shown to develop within hours after potassium release from human erythrocytes.[31] Urinalysis is typically positive for blood but with few or no red blood cells, an early indicator of hemolysis. A dark urine color and myoglobinuria may also be present. Serum aldolase, serum myoglobin, and urinary myoglobin should all be monitored.

PTX may be isolated using successive column chromatography or thin layer chromatography.[34,36,40] In addition, a nuclear magnetic resonance spectrometry method can be used, in combination with gradient enhancement and 3D Fourier transform, to elucidate hydrogen and carbon nuclear magnetic resonance signals of PTX.[41] A rapid and sensitive neutralization assay has been developed to detect PTX.[42] This assay uses the hemolytic properties of the toxin to specifically induce neutralizing monoclonal antibody.

PTX toxicity has been studied in several animal species, each showing similar sensitivities[43,44] and clinical effects to humans. In general, most experimental animals show clinical signs of drowsiness, weakness, vomiting, respiratory distress, diarrhea, convulsions, shock, hypothermia, and death within 30 to 60 minutes of IV injection. Early signs of PTX poisoning in dogs include defecation and vomiting.[30] Rats and nonhuman primates have demonstrated similar sensitivity to IV PTX challenge with 24-hour LD_{50} of 89 ng/kg and 78 ng/kg, respectively.[43] Following IV administration of PTX, nonhuman primates become drowsy, weak, and ataxic. Vomiting sometimes occurs (incidence not reported),[43] followed by collapse and death.

PTX causes a moderate skin reaction in rabbits[45] as well as an increase in histidine decarboxylase activity in mice after topical PTX application to the skin.[46] Based on histamine release data in rat mast cells, PTX may have immunological effects.[47] It causes a depolarization of the membranes of myelinated fibers, spinal cord, and squid axons; induced norepinephrine release from adrenergic neurons[48] and clonal rat pheochromocytoma cells[49]; and causes a temperature-dependent potassium loss from rat erythrocytes, followed by hemolysis in a matter of hours.[50]

PTX also leads to dysrhythmias and vasospasm in animals. It exerts cytotoxic effects in rat aortic smooth muscle, leading to surface granularities, vacuoles, rounding, and cell death; increased release of lactate dehydrogenase; increased ionic conductance to sodium and potassium; and profound membrane depolarization on electrophysiological recording.[14] Finally, PTX has a direct cardiotoxicity in vivo, resulting in atrioventricular block, extrasystoles, ventricular tachycardia, coronary vasoconstriction, and ventricular fibrillation. The shape and rhythm of the EKG is abnormal, showing S-T segment elevation most likely due to coronary vasoconstriction.[35] Death from PTX appears to be secondary to coronary artery vasoconstriction, reducing blood flow to cardiac tissues, resulting in necrosis. This leads to cardiac failure and progressive myocardial ischemia, ventricular fibrillation, and cardiac arrest observed by EKG in nonhuman primates following IV exposure to PTX.[43]

Food poisoning incidents by accidental PTX ingestion are not uncommon in Japan,[26,36] and clinical signs and symptoms have been reported after cases of human PTX ingestion.[26,27,34,36] The patients in a Taniyama et al case report suffered severe muscle pains, dyspnea, apnea, and discharge of black urine.[27] Symptom onset occurred 3 to 36 hours following ingestion. On laboratory findings, serum CPK levels were above the normal range and were reported to be 700–23,800 IU/L. All of the patients observed in the study recovered. Reported muscle pains abated, CPK levels returned to normal, and urine color resolved, although recovery took approximately 1 month (Exhibit 19-1).

In cases of accidental poisoning it is difficult to ascertain how much PTX the victim ingested. Toxin distribution and concentration, the precise quantity of food consumed, and the amount of toxin ingested cannot be adequately determined, as PTX toxicity by ingestion has not been thoroughly studied. An Okano case report involved a 55-year-old male who consumed the raw meat and liver of a blue humphead parrotfish contaminated with PTX. The patient developed progressive weakness and myalgia in his extremities 5 hours after ingesting the toxin. Rhabdomyolysis and myocardial damage developed with serum CPK levels elevated to 40,000 IU/L by the third day following ingestion. Serum aldolase, serum myoglobin, and urinary myoglobin were similarly elevated. Elevated myosin light chain levels and alterations in the EKG were noted.[26] After mannitol-alkaline diuresis once daily for a period of 4 days, the patient recovered. Weakness and myalgias subsided within 4 weeks.

PTX is less toxic by ingestion than by other routes of exposure.[51] Its stability and the potency differences from various routes of entry must be further studied to estimate the threat of PTX.

Treatment. Life support may be required to minimize respiratory and cardiovascular compromise after PTX intoxication. Treatment of PTX-intoxicated victims consists of rapid diagnosis, decontamination with copious amounts of water, and general supportive care. Any patient suspected of ingesting PTX should be monitored in a controlled setting until all signs and symptoms of toxicity have abated. In cases of oral exposure, syrup of ipecac is not recommended due to the rapid nature of PTX absorption. Activated charcoal should be given emergently in aqueous slurry for suspected ingestion only in patients who are awake and able to protect their airways. In patients at risk for seizures or mental status changes, activated charcoal should be administered by personnel capable of airway management to prevent aspiration in the event of spontaneous emesis. Activated charcoal is only useful if administered within approximately 30 minutes of ingestion. Cathartics are not recommended due to the vomiting, diarrhea, and electrolyte imbalance caused by PTX.

Oxygenation, hemoglobin, hematocrit, plasma free hemoglobin, urinalysis, and other indices of hemolysis should be monitored. Transfusion of blood or packed red blood cells may be necessary to treat hemolysis. Early treatment should be aimed at controlling acute metabolic disturbances (hyperkalemia, hyponatremia,

EXHIBIT 19-1

ADVERSE EFFECTS OF HUMAN PALYTOXIN INTOXICATION

- A 49-year-old Filipino male fell ill minutes after ingesting crab containing PTX. Early symptoms were dizziness, nausea, fatigue, cold sweats, and an oral metallic taste. The patient complained next of paresthesias in the extremities, restlessness, vomiting, and severe muscle cramps. The patient suffered episodes of severe bradycardia (heart rate 30 bpm), rapid and shallow breathing, cyanotic hands and mouth, anuria, and eventual renal failure at the hospital. He was treated with atropine, diphenhydrimine, meperidine, and epinephrine without success. The patient died 15 hours after ingestion.

- A 54-year-old Asian male and a 79-year-old Asian female ingested parrotfish (*Ypiscarus ovifrons*) containing PTX. Both patients presented with dyspnea, myalgia, convulsions, and myoglobinuria on the first day of admission. Labs revealed elevated serum creatine phosphokinase, lactate dehydrogenase, and serum glutamic-oxaloacetic transaminase. The male patient recovered after 1 week, and the female patient died 3 days later after complications of respiratory arrest.

- PTX-contaminated mackerel was ingested by a 35-year-old male. Within hours, he experienced excessive sweating, weakness, nausea, abdominal discomfort, diarrhea, circumoral and extremity paresthesias, temperature reversal dysesthesia, muscle spasms, and tremor. The patient was hospitalized 48 hours after ingestion when he developed tonic contractions. Endotracheal intubation was started after he developed respiratory distress. Creatine phosphokinase, lactate dehydrogenase, and serum glutamic-oxaloacetic transaminase levels were extremely elevated, and his urine was dark brown. The patient recovered 11 days after ingestion and received only symptomatic therapy throughout his hospital stay.

Data sources: (1) Alcala AC, Alcala LC, Garth JS, Yasumura D, Yasumoto T. Human fatality due to ingestion of the crab *Demania reynaudii* that contained a palytoxin-like toxin. *Toxicon*. 1988;26:105–107. (2) Noguchi T, Hwang DF, Arakawa O, et al. Palytoxin is the causative agent in the parrotfish poisoning. In: Gopalakrishnaknoe P, Tan CT, eds. *Progress in Venom and Toxin Research. Proceedings of the First Asia-Pacific Congress on Animal, Plant and Microbial Toxins* Singapore, China: National University of Singapore; 1987: 325–335. 3) Kodama AM, Hokama Y, Yasumoto T, Fukui M, Manea SJ, Sutherland N. Clinical and laboratory findings implicating palytoxin as cause of ciguatera poisoning due to *Decapterus macrosoma* (mackerel). *Toxicon*. 1989;27:1051–1053.

hyperthermia, hypovolemia). Subsequent treatment should focus on the control of seizures, agitation, and muscle contraction. Urine alkalinization with sodium bicarbonate and maintenance of adequate urine output may help prevent nephrotoxicity from red blood cell breakdown products. One case report involved gastric lavage with activated charcoal and forced mannitol-alkaline diuresis therapy.[26] In this case, the patient recovered without long-term sequelae (eg renal failure). However, urine alkalinization can cause alkalemia, hypocalcemia, and hypokalemia.

If central nervous system and respiratory depression occur, intubation, supplemental oxygenation, and assisted ventilation should be rapidly administered. Rapid administration of steroids may reduce the severity of effects. In case of seizure activity, benzodiazepines (diazepam or lorazepam) should be administered first. If seizures persist, phenobarbital should be considered. One should also monitor for hypotension, dysrhythmias, and respiratory depression and the possible need for endotracheal intubation. Healthcare providers should evaluate for hypoxia, electrolyte disturbances, and hypoglycemia, and consider starting IV dextrose. In the case of rhabdomyolysis, early aggressive fluid replacement is the definitive treatment and may prevent renal insufficiency. Diuretics (eg, mannitol or furosemide) may be needed to maintain urine output. Vigorous fluid replacement with 0.9% saline is necessary if there is no evidence of dehydration. The hypovolemia, increased insensible losses, and third spacing of fluid increase the fluid requirements associated with managing a patient with PTX intoxication. In addition, one should monitor for evidence of fluid overload, compartment syndrome, and CPK, and perform renal function tests.

Decontamination should be administered immediately in cases of PTX intoxication. For ocular exposure, the eyes should be irrigated with copious amounts of saline or water for at least 15 minutes. If symptoms of eye irritation, pain, swelling, lacrimation, or photophobia persist after irrigation, obtain an ophthalmology consult for further examination. In cases of dermal exposure, remove contaminated clothing and wash exposed areas thoroughly with soap and water.

Intoxication by PTX in laboratory animals can be managed by the administration of vasodilator agents. Intraventricular cardiac injections of papaverine or isosorbide dinitrate in animals will ameliorate the vasoconstrictive actions of PTX. IV injection of vasodilators is ineffective because of PTX's rapid lethality. Laboratory animals die within 3 to 5 minutes of receiving a lethal dose of PTX,[43] during which time the animals' circulation is compromised because PTX prevents adequate delivery of the vasodilator to effected tissues. There have been reports of some success protecting laboratory animals by pretreatment with hydrocortisone, but at most half of the test subjects showed resistance to the toxin following pretreatment.

Stability

PTX is soluble in water, pyridine, dimethylsulfoxide, and aqueous acidic solutions. The chemical stability and activity of dilute PTX, stored in glass or plastic, are unaffected by exposure to light and room temperature for short periods (up to several hours).[52] Reconstituted PTX can be stored at 4°C for 3 to 6 months, but no stability data exists for longer term storage. Lyophilized PTX from a commercial source is recommended to be stored at $< 0°C$ and protected from light.

These storage and stability recommendations indicate that PTX is not a particularly stable substance, although the storage conditions are very mild. These mild storage requirements could make PTX desirable to potential terrorists who have limited specialized equipment to reconstitute and store PTX. The storage conditions are somewhat restrictive but not necessarily prohibitive, allowing a small but sufficient window of opportunity for terrorists to disperse a PTX weapon.

Protection

PTX is extremely potent once it is introduced to the body; however, it is not lipid soluble and therefore not likely to present a contact hazard by absorption through the skin. The probable routes of human exposure to PTX in a bioterrorism incident would be inhalation of PTX vapor or ingestion of contaminated food or water. Human fatalities due to accidental PTX intoxication have been reported[22,34,36]; however, more testing must be done to fully understand how to protect against PTX intoxication.

Surveillance

Currently, there are no specific PTX surveillance programs in place, but several public health surveillance programs may be adapted to monitor specifically for potential bioterrorist events. The CDC, in conjunction with state and local health departments, is developing the Enhanced Surveillance Program, which is designed to monitor data on hospital emergency department visits during special events to establish a baseline of patient symptoms. The goal of this program is to identify deviations from the normal patient visit data and report to state and local health departments for confirmation and appropriate epidemiological follow up. Data from patient visits was collected at the 1999 World Trade Organization Ministerial in Seattle, the 2004 Republican and Democratic National Conventions held in Philadelphia and Los Angeles, respectively, and the 2001 Super Bowl in Tampa, Florida, to test the Enhanced Surveillance Program. If the Enhanced Surveillance Program proves successful, it could serve as a model for a national surveillance program to quickly identify casualties from the types of weaponized toxins presented in this chapter.

Tetrodotoxin and Saxitoxin

Synthesis

TTX, and to some extent STX, have been used as tools in physiology and pharmacology research for many years, allowing investigators to study the physiological properties of ion channels, action potential generation and propagation, cellular membranes, and various aspects of neuroscience. TTX, a selective sodium channel blocker and potent neurotoxin, has been isolated from a wide variety of marine animals. Puffer fish and toadfish, members of Tetraodontiformes, are the best known sources of TTX, although the toxin has been detected in more than 40 species of fish.[53] TTX has also been found in the Australian blue-octopus (*Hapalochlaena maculosa*), xanthid crabs (*Eriphia* species), horseshoe crabs (*Carcinoscorpius rotundicauda*), two Philippine crabs (*Zosimus aeneus* and *Atergatis floridus*), mollusks (*Nassarius* species), marine algae (*Jania* species), epiphytic bacterium (*Aleromonas* species), *Vibrio* species, and from *Pseudomonas* species.[54] Additionally, TTX has been isolated in some terrestrial organisms, including Harlequin frogs (*Atelopus* species), Costa Rican frogs (*Atelopus chiriquiensis*), three species of California newt (*Taricha* species), and members of the family Salamandridae.[33,55,56] STX is the best-understood member of a much larger group of structurally related neurotoxins, the paralytic shellfish poisoning (PSP) toxins, which are found in dinoflagellates.[57–59] PSP is similar to NSP but more severe because paralysis is not a typical feature of NSP.[60] PSP is associated with red tide blooms but also may occur without red tide (Figure 19-2).[61]

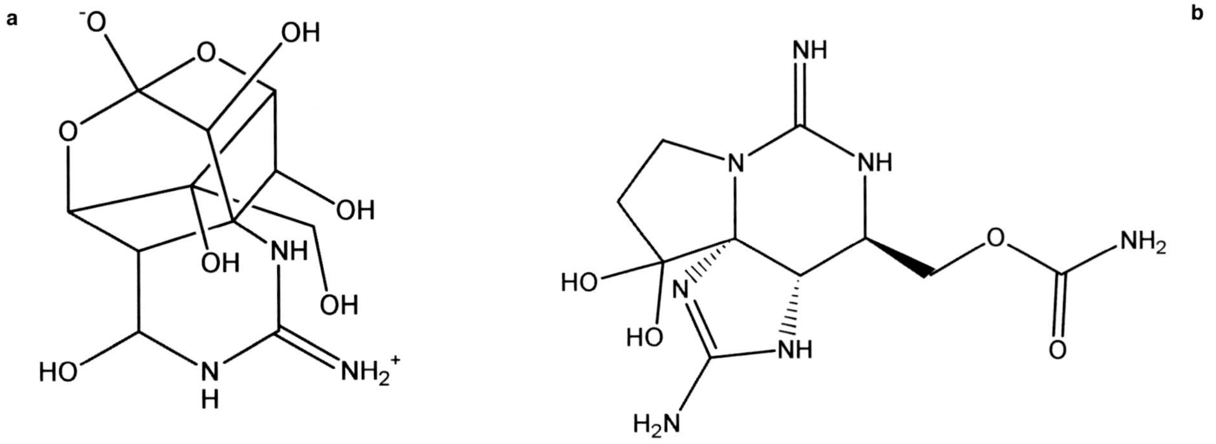

Fig. 19-2. Structures of tetrodotoxin (left) and saxitoxin (right).
Illustration: Courtesy of Richard Sweeny.

From 1956 to 1958, nearly 500 Japanese citizens died from puffer fish ingestion, prompting the immediate elucidation of the toxin.[62] The structure of TTX (see Figure 19-2, left) was determined in 1964,[63–65] and Kishi synthesized the toxin.[66] TTX remains widely used in research today and is available to scientists from many commercial sources. STX synthesis (see Figure 19-2, right) was first published in 1977.[67] Like TTX, STX is a potent, selective, sodium channel blocker. STX, only one component of PSP toxins, is the product of the dinoflagellates *Gonyaulax catenella* and *Gonyaulax tamarensis*. STX has been isolated in certain mollusks that feed on *Gonyaulax catenella*[68] and is believed to bioaccumulate to cause toxicity in humans.

Mechanism of Action and Toxicity

Both TTX and STX are water-soluble, heat-stable molecules[61,69–72] and can be absorbed through the mucous membranes and small intestine.[73,74] Both inhibit neuromuscular transmission by binding to the voltage-gated sodium channel (Figure 19-3). As selective, voltage-dependent, sodium channel blockers, both toxins exert major neurotoxic effects by preventing action potential generation and propagation (see Exhibit 19-1). Six different binding sites on the voltage-gated sodium channel have been identified, each site corresponding to a locus on the protein where groups of neurotoxins can bind (Figure 19-4). Both TTX and STX occupy binding site 1,[75] which is on the S6 transmembrane domain. This domain forms the mouth of the pore in the three-dimensional structure of the channel on the extracellular face (see Figure 19-3). TTX and STX will bind irreversibly to the sodium channel, occluding the pore. In this way, TTX and STX act as sodium channel blockers, sterically preventing sodium ion access through the channel. In the context of the brief description of action potential generation above, prevention of sodium ion movement by either toxin has catastrophic effects on normal neuronal function. The end result is blockade of nerve conduction and muscle contraction (see Figure 19-4). The toxins are reversible and do not lead to damage of the nerve or skeletal muscle.[73,74,76] Another similar feature is that these toxins inhibit cardiac and smooth muscle at higher concentrations. One difference between the two toxins is that STX lacks the emetic and hypothermic action of TTX[77]; the mechanism behind this difference is not well understood. Other cardiovascular effects for these sodium channel toxins have been noted. STX has been demonstrated to induce hypotension by direct action on vascular smooth muscle or through blocking vasomotor nerves.[78] It also decreases conduction at the AV node.[79] Both toxins have effects in the brain. STX inhibits the respiratory centers of the central nervous system[79] while TTX action produces blockade of sodium channels in the axon of the magnocellular neurons of the neurohypophysis, inhibiting release of vasopressin. Children appear to be more sensitive to STX than adults.[80,81]

As a selective sodium channel blocker, TTX binds its molecular target tightly with extremely strong kinetics (Kd = 10-9 nM). Toxicology of TTX and STX is reported in the literature based primarily on mouse data. Both toxins are extremely potent, with an approximate LD_{50} 8 to 10 μg/kg in mice.[69] Toxicity studies in mice examined intoxication by IV administration, while the route of exposure in humans is generally through ingestion. Deaths have been reported following human ingestion of both toxins,[61,70] and it is estimated that 1 to 2 mg

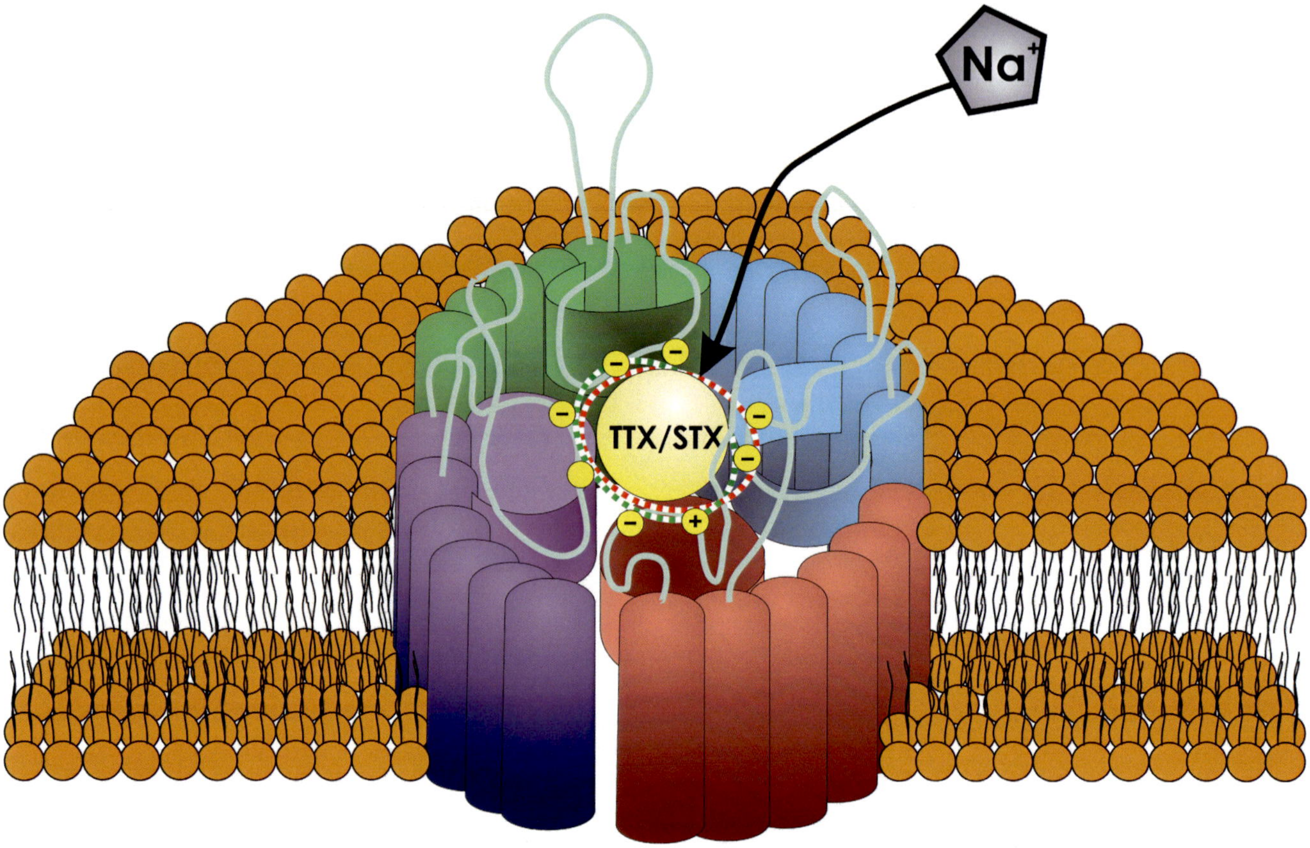

Fig. 19-3. Three-dimensional representation of a voltage-gated sodium channel sitting in a phospholipid bilayer membrane. The linear protein folds to form a pore in the cell membrane, providing a central, electrically charged aperture through which sodium ions can pass. The toxins bind to regions of the channel structure occluding the pore, preventing sodium ions from entering and traversing the channel pore.
Na^+: sodium ion
STX: saxitoxin
TTX: tetrodotoxin

of TTX is a lethal dose for an average adult human.[69] Respiratory toxicity of STX is less well understood in every model system than systemic toxicity; however, data from aerosol deposition studies in mice exposed to STX aerosol give LC_{50} (lethal concentration; the concentration of the chemical in air that kills 50% of the test animals in a given time) values < 1 μg/kg.[71] Thus, in these studies, STX is at least 10-fold more toxic to mice by aerosol exposure than by systemic administration. The mechanism of this enhanced toxicity is unknown.

Toxin Exposure, Health Effects, and Treatment

Intoxication by TTX is the most common lethal marine poisoning[82] and most often occurs by the consumption of contaminated food. Ingestion of TTX-contaminated foods occurs throughout Southeast Asia and the Pacific, most commonly in Japan, where puffer fish is a delicacy. Additionally, neurologic illnesses associated with ingestion of Florida puffer fish have been reported since 2002. Signs and symptoms of TTX intoxication usually begin within 30 to 60 minutes after ingestion of the toxin. Anxiety, nausea, vomiting, and paresthesias of the lips, fingers, and tongue are all common. In cases of severe poisoning, clinical signs and symptoms include marked paresthesias, loss of consciousness, generalized flaccid paralysis, respiratory arrest, and death. Dizziness, dyspnea, and fixed, dilated pupils have also been reported. Patients with more moderate poisoning generally retain consciousness. There are reports of unresponsive patients who were nonetheless fully cognizant of events around them.[83]

PSP typically results from the consumption of mussels, clams, oysters, mollusks, starfish, sand crabs,

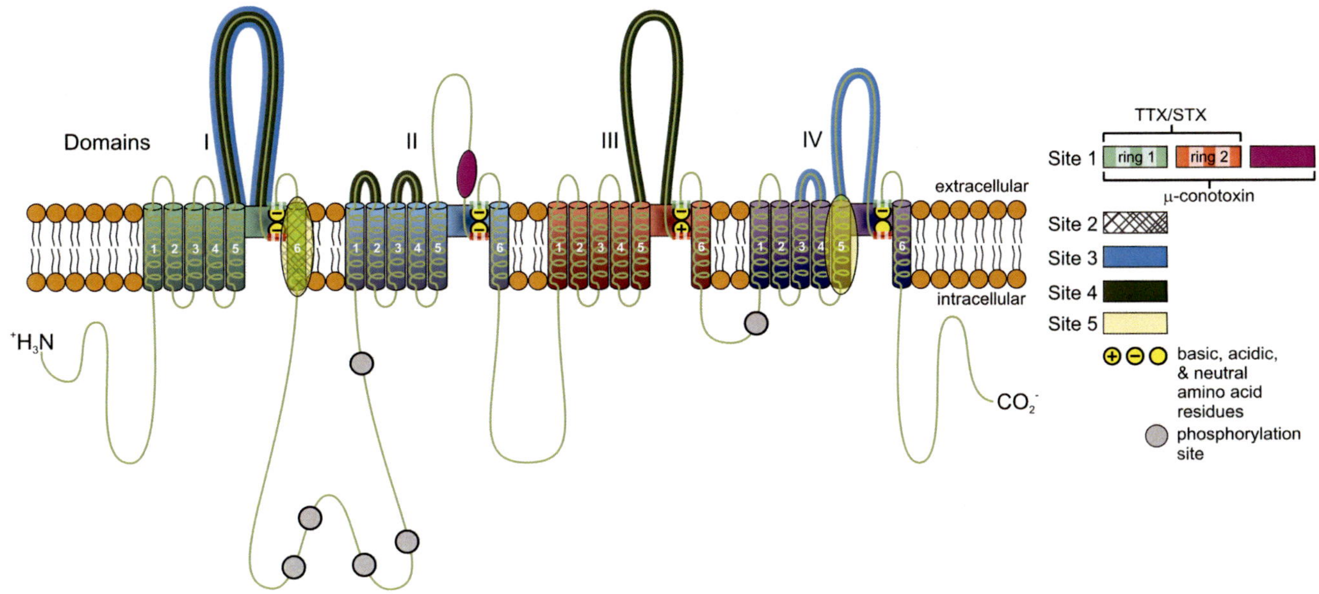

Fig. 19-4. Structure of the α-subunit of the voltage-gated sodium channel. The six transmembrane portions for each colored domain (I-IV) insert into the cell membrane and form the charged pore (shown above) through which ions can travel. The known toxin binding sites are color-coded and numbered, as are the phosphorylation sites and charged residues that form the selectivity filter of the channel. The lipid bilayer is illustrated in orange. Transmembrane segments 5 and 6 from each domain contribute to the channel pore and contributions from segment 4 form the voltage sensor. Amino acids between segments 5 and 6 from each domain form the filter (or gate) for ionic selectivity. The α-subunit illustrated here folds into four transmembrane domains (I–IV), colored green, blue, orange, and purple. The transmembrane domains are themselves comprised of six α-helical segments designated S1 through S6. Within each domain, the S4 segment has a primary structure containing positive charged amino acid residues at every third position. The S4 segment functions as the voltage sensor, detecting the depolarization of the cell membrane and initiating channel opening. When the α-subunit is properly folded in three dimensions, segments S5 and S6 form the channel pore. Amino acid residues between transmembrane segments S5 and S6 are predominately acidic (negatively charged) or neutral, which creates an electrically favorable tunnel to allow the passage of positively charged ions (eg, sodium ions) of a particular radius.

Six different binding sites on the voltage-gated sodium channel have been identified, each site corresponding to a locus on the protein where groups of neurotoxins can bind. TTX and STX bind to site 1 on the extracellular face of the sodium channel, occluding the pore and thereby preventing the movement of sodium ions through the pore. Batrachotoxin and the brevetoxins have similar physiological effects, mainly causing activation of the channel at more negative membrane potentials. Batrachotoxin binds to site 2 and brevetoxins to site 5.

STX: saxitoxin

TTX: tetrodotoxin

xanthid crabs, and various fish that have consumed the toxic marine algae dinoflagellates. Eating shellfish contaminated with STX, readily absorbed through the oral and gastrointestinal mucosa, can cause paralytic, neurotoxic, and amnestic symptoms.[80,84] STX causes symptoms very similar to several other dinoflagellate toxins (eg, PbTxs). Because STX and TTX share very similar mechanisms of action, as discussed above, it is not surprising that the symptoms of STX intoxication are almost indistinguishable from TTX intoxication. PSP can produce paralytic, neurotoxic, and amnestic symptoms in the range of mild to severe. Neurologic symptoms can include sensory, cerebellar, and motor. Mild symptoms of STX intoxication begin with paresthesia of the lips, tongue, and fingertips. These symptoms start within minutes of toxin ingestion. Nausea, headache, and the initial spread of paresthesias to the neck and extremities are common features. Moderate symptoms include limb weakness, dyspnea, hypersalivation, diaphoresis, and more neurologic involvement (eg, incoherent speech, ataxia, floating sensation, extremity paresthesias). Giddiness, rash, fever, tachycardia, hypertension, dizziness, and temporary blindness have been reported. Severe symptoms include muscle paralysis, severe dyspnea, choking sensation, and respiratory failure. As STX poisoning progresses, muscular paralysis and respiratory distress develop, and death from respiratory arrest occurs within 2 to 12 hours, depending upon the severity of STX intoxication. As with TTX poisoning, many patients appear calm and remain conscious throughout the episode.[82]

Physical Examination. Fever has been associated with PSP,[85] hypothermia and sweating occur with TTX intoxication,[83,86–88] and both neurotoxins cause lip paresthesias.[89] TTX-induced circumoral paresthesia of the tongue and mouth occur within 10 to 45 minutes of ingestion.[90,91] Oral paresthesia, typically the first presenting symptom of TTX intoxication,[92] is followed by dysphagia,[90] aphagia, and aphonia.[93] STX causes ocular symptoms like temporary blindness,[61,94] nystagmus,[94,95] ophthalmoplegia, and iridoplegia.[96] TTX produces ophthalmoparesis,[97] blurred vision,[87,98] early stage miosis,[92,99,100] late stage mydriasis,[92,101] and absence of papillary light reflex.[91] TTX was reported to cause laryngospasm and dysgeusia.[36] PSP is associated with loss of the gag reflex, jaw and facial muscle paralysis, tongue paralysis,[96,102] dysphagia, and dysphonia.[94]

PSP can also cause tachycardia, T-wave changes on EKG,[94] hypertension,[103,104] or hypotension.[84] The cardiac enzyme creatine kinase MB has been shown to be elevated after PSP intoxication,[105] and mild tachycardia has been reported.[106] Puffer fish toxin may cause bradycardia, hypotension or hypertension,[92] dysrhythmias, and conduction abnormalities.[92,97,107,108] Chest pain is a common feature of both toxins.[93,99,106] TTX can also lead to cardiopulmonary arrest.[92,109]

Death from TTX or STX intoxication is caused by respiratory depression and paralysis of effector muscles of respiration.[79,96,107,108,110,111] Both TTX and STX intoxication cause dyspneic symptoms.[91,92,111,112] Apnea has been noted to occur within the first 2 hours after TTX ingestion[92,101] and even earlier with PSP,[113] suggesting the need for endotracheal intubation and mechanical ventilation. TTX blocks neuromuscular transmission, leading to skeletal muscle paralysis. Ascending paralysis may develop within 24 hours for either toxin.[91,99,106,114] Both toxins lead to the diminution of the gag reflex.[88,89,94] TTX has also been associated with acute pulmonary edema secondary to hypertensive congestive heart failure[115] and aspiration pneumonia.[99]

In addition to respiratory effectors, all voluntary muscles rapidly weaken with either toxin due to their effect on neuromuscular transmission; typically the upper extremities become weak, followed by the lower extremities.[89,92] Ascending paralysis follows[99] and patients may drop deep tendon reflexes, including absent Babinski signs.[90,91,100,112,113,116,117] Neurologic symptoms, such as paresthesias of the lips, tongue, face, neck and extremities, are the hallmarks of early intoxication, occurring within the first 30 minutes of ingestion.[95,96,104,107,109,114,118] Paresthesias of the lips, tongue, and throat usually precede the spread to the fingertips, neck, arms, and legs.[79,81] Lack of coordination, progressing to ataxia and dysmetria, has been reported for both toxins.[79,90,95,103] Seizures have been documented for puffer fish intoxication; these typically occur later in the progression of toxicity.[92,99] STX has also been associated with generalized giddiness, dizziness, incoherent speech, aphasia,[104] headaches,[81,104,113] asthenia,[79,113] and cranial nerve disturbances (eg, dysarthria, dipopia, dysphagia, fixed dilated pupils, absent ciliary reflex,[95,113] temperature reversal dysesthesia,[60] and neuropathies). STX-induced neuropathies consist of prolongation in distal motor and sensory latencies, decreased motor and sensory amplitudes, and reduced conduction velocities.[96] EEG abnormalities showing posterior dominant alpha waves intermixed with trains of short duration and diffuse theta waves have been demonstrated in TTX intoxication.[91] TTX causes central nervous neuropathies as well, manifested as blurred vision, ophthalmoplegia, dysphagia, and dysphonia.[93,97] Coma has been reported only after severe TTX poisoning but is less common.[112,117,119] Other symptoms reported with TTX intoxication include dizziness,[99] headaches,[110] and diabetes insipidus.[86]

Similar gastrointestinal complaints are experienced by patients early in TTX and STX poisoning by ingestion. Nausea, vomiting, diarrhea, epigastric pain, and hypersalivation are common to both TTX[83,88–90,92,93,99,100,107,112,114,117] and STX[96,103,104,120,121] intoxication. Xerostomia has been reported in up to 20% of STX patients in one study.[103]

Hematologic abnormalities have been documented with puffer fish intoxication. Petechial hemorrhages and hematemesis are attributed to increased intrathoracic and intraabdominal pressure from violent episodes of emesis and wretching.[92,97] An isolated case of leukocytosis has been documented following TTX ingestion.[114] Hematologic abnormalities have not been reported for STX.

Laboratory findings and monitoring. Because TTX- and STX-intoxicated patients are diagnosed based on a high index of suspicion, clinical signs, and symptom presentation, laboratory findings and tests may be useful to determine etiology when patient history is inadequate and to monitor recovery. As a minimum, hemodynamic, acid-base, and fluid status, as well as serum electrolytes, blood urea nitrogen, creatinine, calcium, magnesium, phosphorous, urine output, CPK, EKG, and pulse oximetry should be monitored. Blood gases are helpful to monitor adequate oxygenation and ventilation. Lactic acidosis has also been reported in animals exposed to STX[105] and may be a useful parameter to monitor. Electromyography may show marked abnormalities and the cardiac enzyme creatine kinase MB can be elevated. Serum electrolytes can be monitored for abnormalities due to dehydration, vomiting, and diarrhea. In addition, serum sodium, serum osmolality, and urine osmolality are useful for diagnosing suspected secondary diabetes insipidus in TTX intoxication.[86] CPK levels, which maybe elevated in STX intoxication, should be monitored. Urinary levels of TTX have been detected from suspected intoxication.[122]

STX has a direct action on the conducting system of the frog heart, producing decreases in heart rate and contractile force with severe bradycardia, bundle branch block, or complete cardiac failure. In cats, STX produces a reversible depression in contractility of papillary muscle.[77] In rats, TTX given intraarterially produces a rapid hypotension, beginning within 1 to 2 minutes and lethal by 6 minutes.[108] In several animal models, large doses of TTX cause conduction slowing, AV dissociation, and failure of myocardial contractility.[83] Seizures have been reported in several animals intoxicated with TTX.[35,83]

Dermatologic abnormalities, including pruritis, excessive diaphoresis,[104] and rash,[85] are reported for STX, while pallor,[93] bullous eruptions, petechiae, desquamation,[92,123] and diaphoresis[92,99] occur in puffer fish poisoning. Other abnormalities shared by both toxins include low back pain, muscle weakness, and elevated CPK levels.[102] Progression of any symptom is dependent on dose, route of exposure (ingestion or dermal), and rate of elimination, and not all individuals will react the same way to intoxication. Outbreaks of contamination may involve multiple toxins, so symptoms may appear to be characteristic of one toxin but clinical evidence may suggest the involvement of other toxins, further contributing to morbidity and mortality.[124]

Treatment. While there are no antidotes for TTX and STX intoxication, treatment is predominantly supportive and symptomatic. Good cardiovascular and respiratory support is critical,[83] and prognosis is excellent if supportive care is instituted early.[83,97] Activated charcoal can be administered after ingestion of either toxin, especially within 1 hour of ingestion of either toxin.[104,125] Cathartics and syrup of ipecac are not recommended for treatment of toxin ingestion. Most patients will recover with supportive care alone, but they should be monitored for signs of respiratory depression and neurotoxicity, requiring endotracheal intubation and mechanical ventilation. Electrolytes should be replaced, and fluids should be regulated according to arterial blood pressure and urinary output.[93,126] Fluid therapy can improve renal elimination of STX[105] because it is excreted into the urine.[106]

Hypoxia, acidemia, and conduction abnormalities should be corrected with careful EKG and blood gas monitoring. Bolus sodium bicarbonate may reverse ventricular conduction, slowing and dysrhythmias. Lidocaine IV can be given for ventricular tachycardia and ventricular fibrillation.[127] Bradycardia can be managed with supplemental oxygen and atropine; however, atropine alone may increase the lethality of TTX.[88,97] Adrenergic antagonists may prolong neuromuscular blockade of TTX and are not recommended.[128] Atropine can be given for asystolic cardiac arrest. Treatment with cholinesterase inhibitors has been attempted for TTX-induced muscle weakness, but data concerning their efficacy is scant. One study shows improvement of muscle weakness after TTX ingestion using IV edrophonium (10 mg) or intramuscular neostigmine (0.5 mg).[97,116]

Hemodialysis might aid recovery, but there is little data concerning the effectiveness of this treatment for TTX and STX intoxication. Hemodialysis was attempted because both toxins are low molecular weight, water-soluble molecules that are significantly bound to protein.[119] For example, an uremic woman who received regularly scheduled hemodialysis developed severe symptoms of TTX intoxication after eating fish soup. An hour after hemodialysis (and 21 hours after symptom onset), the patient recovered.[119] Hemodialysis was tried with mixed results for STX intoxication; one patient recovered and the other did not.[79] Desmopressin IV has been shown to be effective for TTX-induced central diabetes insipidus.[86] All other symptoms (hypotension, seizures, etc) can be managed as discussed previously.

Stability

TTX is water soluble at neutral pH and soluble in a dilute citrate or acetate buffer at acidic pH. In citrate or acetate buffers, it can be stored at −20°C for extended periods without loss of efficacy. It is unstable both in strong acid and alkaline solutions, and is rapidly destroyed by boiling at pH 2. TTX is likewise unstable in dilute hydrochloric or sulfuric acid, slowly protonating into the less toxic anhydrotetrodotoxin at equilibrium. It is relatively heat stable in neutral and organic acid solutions. Lyophilized TTX, available from commercial sources, should be refrigerated to maintain stability for long periods.

STX is remarkably stable[129,130] and readily soluble. Lyophilized STX is stable under the same storage conditions as TTX. Solutions of STX in acidic, aqueous solvent, or aqueous methanol, stored at a range of −80° to 4°C, are stable for several years. STX solutions stored at higher temperatures (37°C) are much less stable.

Protection

Cases of human poisoning by TTX and STX most commonly occur by ingestion of toxin-contaminated food, and poisoning by either toxin can result in paralysis, respiratory arrest, and death. Similar to PTX ingestion, it is often difficult to estimate the amount of toxin actually consumed. Relatively little toxin is usually consumed per accidental food poisoning case, yet deaths are not uncommon because of the toxicity of these compounds. Both TTX and STX are water soluble and stable under mild storage conditions, making them exceptional options for bioterrorist attacks targeting water, milk, or food supplies, especially fresh meats or vegetables.

The credibility of an aerosol TTX or STX threat is difficult to estimate, given the lack of inhalation toxicity research. It appears, however, that STX exhibits greater toxicity by inhalation[71] than by other routes of administration by a factor of 10. Whether this is a property of STX in particular or of all such toxins in general is not known at this time, and indeed the feasibility of weaponizing these toxins has not been explored. Given the known toxicity data, the threat cannot be discounted.

No antidote to TTX or STX poisoning is currently available for clinical use. Neostigmine has been suggested in some reports as a potential treatment for TTX poisoning;[83] however, no controlled trials have been conducted to investigate its efficacy.

Upon admission to intensive care facilities, treatment for TTX or STX intoxication involves careful observation and management of symptoms to avert respiratory arrest or cardiac failure.[131] In severe poisoning cases, atropine can be used to treat bradycardia,[107] and respiratory support may be indicated for periods of up to 72 hours. For cases of relatively mild intoxication, life-threatening complications are unlikely to develop after 24 hours following intoxication.

Surveillance

TTX and STX are presented together here because of the similarity in their sources, mechanisms of action, and clinical signs and symptoms of intoxication. Both are designated by the CDC as select agent toxins, or agents that have the potential to pose a severe threat to human health. STX was rumored to have been employed as the toxin in suicide capsules and injections provided to Central Intelligence Agency officers during the Cold War, notably U2 pilot Francis Gary Powers.[132] In 1969 President Nixon ordered the destruction of STX stockpiles.[133]

The extent of surveillance programs for TTX or STX is currently limited to state public health department monitoring for TTX- or STX-related food poisoning outbreaks, and no national program exists.

Brevetoxin

Synthesis

PbTxs are a family of marine neurotoxins found in the dinoflagellate *Karenia brevis*. *K brevis* produces nine known endotoxins, designated PbTx-1 through PbTx-9. During periods of algal blooms, like red tides, populations of the toxin-producing organism multiply, resulting in such high concentrations that they have been associated with human and animal intoxication. During these tidal blooms, the toxins are particularly poisonous to fish. Approximately 100 tons of fish per day were killed in a 1971 bloom off the Florida coast.[134] Other blooms have been noted in the Gulf Coast areas of Mexico, California,[135] and North Carolina (Figure 19-5).[136]

The PbTx family is composed of lipid soluble polyethers[137] and based on two different structural backbones (see Figure 19-5), PbTx-1 (brevetoxin A) and PbTx-2 (brevetoxin B). The other members of the family are derivatives of these parent chains and their chemical differences lie in the composition of the R-side chains. Each toxin subtype is an 11-member, heterocyclic, oxygen-containing, fused ring system ending with an unsaturated lactone on one end and an unsaturated aldehyde at the other. PbTx-1 is the only known toxin that is composed of five-, six-, seven-, eight-, and nine-member rings.[138] Synthesis of PbTx-1 and PbTx-2 was first accomplished by Nicoloau and colleagues.[139,140] PbTx-2 was the first to be synthesized,[139] validating the proposed structure of the molecule first advanced by Lin et al.[141] PbTx-1 was synthesized by the same group in 1998.[140] It is likely that the seven derivatives, PbTx-3 to PbTx-9, represent metabolites or biosynthetic modifications of one of the two parent chains, although at this time no specific pathways have been suggested.

Laboratory synthesis of PbTx-1 and PbTx-2 has been documented. These syntheses require many serial reactions to complete the complex macromolecule because, while the reactions are of moderate complexity, the overall yield is not very high. This last point is significant in the context of bioweapon production because terrorists might select compounds that could be easily synthesized with high yield, minimizing the skills and expertise required to produce toxin. PbTx-1 synthesis begins using D-glucose and D-mannose to synthesize two advanced intermediates, which are combined over Horner-Wittig conditions.[140] A total of 23 chemical reactions on D-glucose produces yields that range from 64.5% to 94% per reaction. An additional six reactions on D-mannose, with approximately 90% yield per reaction, yields two advanced intermediate products, which are then bonded in four more synthesis reactions. Proper functionality and stereochemistry are established, and this synthetic PbTx-1 is identical to naturally occurring PbTx-1. The total synthesis of PbTx-2 has been reported by the molecular assembly of three subunits, requiring 108 total steps with similar step yields as PbTx-1 and an overall yield of 0.28%.[142]

Mechanism of Action and Toxicity

Similar to the mechanism of action of TTX and STX, PbTx also targets voltage-gated sodium channels. Active PbTx molecules bind on the α-subunit of the sodium channel at site 5, near the binding site of TTX and STX.[143,144] Binding of PbTx to the sodium channel alters the normal channel kinetics in two ways. First, it encourages the channel to open at more negative membrane potentials, which elicits sodium currents and causes the action potential to fire in the absence of membrane depolarization, a process that normally occurs in response to neurotransmitter binding to receptors. Second, PbTx inhibits the ability of the channel to inactivate itself.[138] Taken together, these effects can cause hyperactivity of the intoxicated neuron through increased duration of action potential firing because sodium channels open earlier (or spontaneously) and stay open longer. PbTx-induced sodium channel activation leads to acetylcholine release in the smooth muscles surrounding the airways, which leads to contraction and bronchospasm.[145,146,147]

PbTx-2 causes respiratory arrest and death in fish and mice.[148] PbTx-2 and PbTx-3 both produce symptoms of muscarinic-induced cholinergic crisis.[149] PbTx-3 is thought to be responsible for NSP and is more potent than PbTx-2 in mice, regardless of the route of exposure.[149] In contrast, PbTx-2 is more potent than PbTx-3 at neuromuscular blockade.[150] The principle mechanism of action appears to involve sodium-channel–mediated depolarization[151] rather than acetylcholine depletion.[150] PbTx produces a stimulatory effect on the nervous system and keeps sodium channels in their open states, while STX closes them.[151,152] PbTx also produces airway contraction and depolarization of airway smooth muscle.[145]

Toxin Exposure, Health Effects, and Treatment

Physical Examination. Human exposure to PbTx usually coincides with the red tide phenomenon and generally occurs through one of two routes: ingestion or inhalation. Intoxication by ingestion occurs through consumption of seafood containing high concentrations of PbTx and can result in NSP. Symptoms of NSP are generally mild, clinically resembling ciguatera, and include paresthesias of the face, throat, and extremities as well as a burning of the mucous membranes.[153–156] Abdominal pain, ataxia, seizures, and respiratory arrest may also develop. These toxins are heat stable and remain poisonous even after meals have been thoroughly cooked. PbTx is less potent than some of the neurotoxins presented here (eg, mouse LD_{50} of PbTx-1 is 95.0 μg/kg and the LD_{50} of PbTx-2 is 500 μg/kg intraperitoneal)[155]; therefore, PbTx ingestion is not lethal to humans.[156,157]

Exposure by inhalation occurs during red tide episodes, when wind can aerosolize PbTxs from the water-air interface.[158] These aerosols may contain additional contaminants, including subcellular fractions,

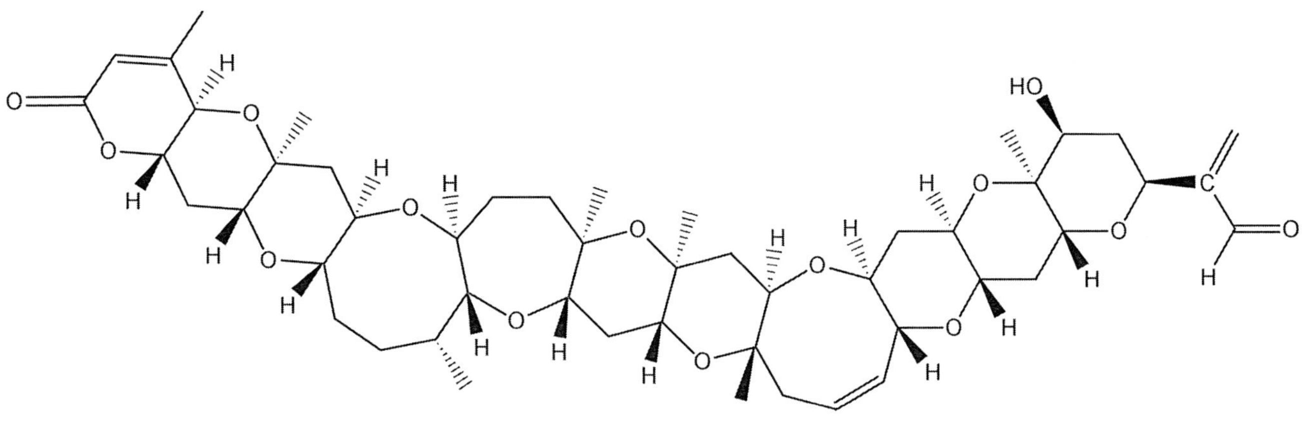

Fig. 19-5. Structure of brevetoxin A (PbTx-1).
Illustration: Courtesy of Richard Sweeny.

as well as bacteria, fungi, spores, and other materials. Symptoms of inhalation exposure include mydriasis,[159] ocular irritation,[157] lacrimation,[149] rhinorrhea,[160] coughing,[157] sneezing,[161] salivation,[149] bronchospasm, dyspnea, and burning sensations of the pharyngeal and nasal mucosa[162,163] in a concentration-dependent manner. PbTx-induced bradycardia can persist up to 12 hours in humans,[164] and the bronchospasms induced by PbTx may elicit an asthmatic attack in those with a preexisting history of exposure or hypersensitivity,[165] and respiratory irritation in the general population. The respiratory irritant zone of offshore red tide that has aerosolized has been estimated within a few kilometers of the beach.[161] In a study of 59 patients with asthma, exposure to aerosolized PbTx after walking along the beach for 1 hour during red tide was associated with significant increases in cough, wheezing, chest tightness, and eye and pharyngeal irritation, as well as abnormal pulmonary functional tests (eg, decreased forced expiratory volume 1[FEV1] and forced midexpiratory flow rate [FEF25–75]) compared to control subjects.[163]

Perioral, facial, and extremity paresthesias are common following PbTx ingestion.[136,157,166] A distorted or clouded sensorium,[159] dystaxias and generalized weakness,[136,157] temperature reversal dysesthesia (eg, warm objects feel cold), tremors,[136] seizures,[157,166] and coma have all been reported following PbTx ingestion.

The earliest symptoms of PbTx intoxication are gastrointestinal or dermatological, depending on the route of exposure. Ingesting these endotoxins can cause nausea, vomiting, abdominal discomfort, and diarrhea.[136,157,159,166] Swimming in red tides can produce pruritus.[157]

Although symptoms of PbTx exposure itself are relatively mild, the effects of inhalation exposure highlight the potential use of aerosolized neurotoxins during a bioterror attack. Toxicity in animal models by oral and parenteral routes has been shown to occur in the nanomolar to picomolar range.[137] Studies of atmospheric PbTx concentration in locations near red tide episodes have shown that concentrations less than 27 ng/m^3 are sufficient to cause symptoms in recreational beachgoers.[167]

PbTx released at a high concentration into a confined space with mechanically circulated air, such as shopping malls or subways, could have deadly effects, especially in individuals with respiratory ailments. Human deaths attributed to PbTx have never been reported,[157] so a minimum lethal dose in humans has not been determined.

Laboratory Findings and Monitoring. While no existing laboratory tests are useful for diagnosing PbTx intoxication, multiple methods are available to detect the toxin, including thin layer chromatography,[148] liquid chromatography/mass spectrometry, and immunoassay. A radioimmunoassay, synaptosomal assay using rat brain synaptosomes,[168] and an enzyme-linked immunoassay[169] have additionally been developed to detect PbTx.

A wealth of animal toxicity data exists for PbTx. This data shows that blood pressure responds biphasically depending on the dose. Low doses of IV PbTx lead to hypotension, while higher doses (160 $\mu g/kg$ IV) cause hypertension.[170] Bradycardia has been demonstrated in both cats and dogs.[159] Labored breathing and death have been reported in mice exposed to PbTx-2 or PbTx-3 by ingestion or injection.[149] Cat studies demonstrated bradypnea following PbTx intoxication,[170] and guinea pigs showed a biphasic tachypnea followed by bradypnea.[171] It is thought that PbTx-3 induces greater respiratory symptoms during red tide than PbTx-2.[149] A cholinergic syndrome (salivation, lacrimation, urination, and defecation) similar to nerve agent intoxication has been shown in mice injected with PbTx-2 or PbTx-3.[172] Both toxin subtypes produce tremors and muscle fasciculations in mice.[149] While a hemolytic agent has been associated with red tide dinoflagellates,[173] hemolysis is not a feature of PbTx in contrast to PTX intoxication.

Treatment. The route of exposure to PbTx should guide patient management. Inducing emesis is not recommended for PbTx ingestion. Activated charcoal can adsorb large molecules and is effective within 1 hour of ingestion, but it is ineffective once neurologic symptoms have occurred. Use of a cathartic with activated charcoal is not recommended because cathartics can cause gastrointestinal symptoms, electrolyte imbalances, and hypotension. Atropine has been suggested to reverse the bronchoconstriction induced by PbTx-3 as well as rhinorrhea, lacrimation, salivation, urination, and defecation.[149] No human data exists on the use of atropine in PbTx intoxication. Atropine does reverse PbTx-induced bradycardia in dogs but has no effect on blood pressure changes.[159] In the case of seizures, benzodiazepine treatment with diazepam, lorazepam, or midazolam should be administered, and the patient should be monitored for respiratory depression, hypotension, dysrhythmias, serum drug levels, and possible endotracheal intubation. If seizures continue, phenobarbital can be administered. In case of hypotension, isotonic fluids should be started while the patient is supine. Dopamine or norepinephrine can be used if hypotension persists.

In case of inhalation exposure, the patient should first be removed from the exposure, decontaminated, and monitored for respiratory distress. If cough or dyspnea develops, monitor for hypoxia, respiratory tract irritation, bronchitis, or pneumonitis. Symptomatic treatment should consist of 100% humidified supplemental oxygen. The patient should be monitored for systemic signs of toxicity as well as the need for endotracheal intubation and assisted ventilation. Bronchospasm can be reversed using beta-2 adrenergic agonists. Ipratropium and systemic corticosteroids for bronchospasm should be started with continued monitoring of peak expiratory flow rate, hypoxia, and respiratory failure, or nebulized albuterol or ipratropium added to the nebulized albuterol. Systemic corticosteroids, such as prednisone, can reduce the inflammation associated with bronchospasm and asthma. For ocular or dermal exposure, eyes and skin should be flushed with copious amounts of water.

Stability

PbTx derivatives exhibit remarkably stable properties. In aqueous or organic solvent solutions, PbTx remains potent for months; culture media that contained growing *Karenia brevis* maintained its ability to intoxicate for similar periods. PbTxs are reportedly sensitive to air,[174] so commercial source PbTx is shipped in nitrogen-blanketed or evacuated containers. Lyophilized PbTx is stable for months without special storage conditions, and certain derivatives, such as PbTx-2 and PbTx-3, have been reported to be heat stable at extreme temperatures (300°C). The relative stability of PbTx and the ease with which lyophilized PbTx can be reconstituted make PbTx an attractive toxin to be weaponized.

Protection

No cases of paralysis or death from NSP have been reported.[157] Symptoms of PbTx intoxication as detailed above generally begin within 15 minutes of exposure, but may occur as late as 18 hours post-exposure, with symptoms potentially persisting for several days. Treatment for NSP or PbTx poisoning consists of supportive care; there is no antidote or antitoxin for PbTx exposure.

For individuals sensitive to PbTx inhalation exposure, a respiratory barrier or particle filter mask and departure from the area of exposure to an air conditioned or filtered environment should provide relief from inhalation exposure symptoms. The bronchoconstricitve airway response to inhaled PbTx in a sheep asthma model can be relieved by the use of histamine H1 antagonist diphenhydrimine, atropine, and the natural polyether brevenal.[165,175] This may direct further research and provide treatment options for both asthmatics and other susceptible persons exposed to aerosolized PbTxs. PbTxs can be easily oxidized by treatment with potassium permanganate ($KMnO_4$). This reaction is irreversible, proceeds quickly, leaves a nontoxic compound,[176] and is a potential means of detoxification.

Surveillance

Significant information is available on morbidity and mortality in aquatic animal populations exposed to red tide toxins, including domoic acid, PbTxs, STXs, and ciguatoxins. Much of what is known about gross and histopathologic analyses, diagnostics, and therapeutic countermeasures for these toxins has been gleaned from environmental population exposure studies.[177] Historically, marine mammals (pinnipeds, cetaceans, and sirenians), aquatic birds, sea turtles, fish, and invertebrates are environmental sentinel species. All are susceptible to toxin exposure via ingestion and immersion; however, marine mammals and sea turtles are particularly susceptible to respiratory exposure at the air-water interface, where aerosolization and concentration occurs. In addition, marine mammals have poor tracheobronchial mucociliary clearance compared to terrestrial mammals.

Although human and environmental impacts on coastal seawater quality and temperature can result in significant algal blooms, it is unlikely that a terrorist attack would attempt to directly impact red tides. However, an intentional chemical spill or factory attack could lead to subsequent algal blooms. Communication with marine mammal and sea turtle stranding networks, as well as other environmental agencies (eg, the Environmental Protection Agency, National Oceanic and Atmospheric Administration, etc), is critical in the early identification of adverse health effects on sentinel species.

A tampered freshwater source, such as a reservoir, would also have effects on fish, aquatic birds, and mammals in that system. A real-time, automated, biomonitoring, portable ventilatory unit developed by the US Army Center for Environmental Health Research measures gill rate, depth, purge (cough rate), and total body movement determined by amplified, filtered, electrical signals generated by opercular (gill) movements in bluegill (*Lepomis macrochirus*) and recorded by carbon block electrodes.[178] Biomonitor studies have already been conducted to determine the effects of PbTx-2 and toxic *Pfiesteria piscicida* cultures on bluegill.[179] Applications for this biomonitoring system have included watershed protection, wastewater treatment plant effluent, and source water for drinking water protection.

Batrachotoxin

Synthesis

BTX (Figure 19-6) is a steroidal alkaloid and the primary poison of the so-called Colombian Poison Dart Frogs of the genus *Phyllobates*. These frogs are brightly colored golden yellow, golden orange, or pale metallic green and they release BTX, as well as four other steroid toxins, through colorless or milky secretions from the granular glands in response to predatory threats. It is believed that *Phyllobates* do not produce BTX, but accumulate the poison by eating ants or other insects in their native habitats that have obtained BTX from a plant source. The natural sources of BTX have not been reported; however, frogs raised in captivity do not contain BTX and thus may be handled without the risk of intoxication,[180,181] suggesting that the toxin is the product of another organism. Recent field work has identified BTX in tissues of other, unexpected species, including the skin and feathers of some birds from New Guinea, *Ifrita kowaldi*, and three species of the genus *Pitohui*. The link between the toxin-bearing birds and frogs was hypothesized to be Melyrid beetles of the genus *Choresine*.[9,182–185] These beetles contain high concentrations of BTX and have been discovered in the stomach contents of captured toxin-bearing bird and frog species (see Figure 19-6).

BTX is commonly used by Noanamá Chocó and Emberá Chocó Indians of western Colombia for poisoning blowgun darts used in hunting. The most toxic member of *Phyllobates*, (*P terribilis*, *P aurotaenia*, and *P bicolor*), is *P terribilis*, which can bear a toxic load up to 1900 μg of toxin.[185] *Phyllobates* generally contain approximately 50 μg of toxin. Toxin is extracted by Chocó Indians by roasting captured frogs over a fire.[186,187] BTX is harvested from blisters that form on the frog from the heat of the fire and is weaponized by touching dart or arrow tips to the toxin. The toxin can be stockpiled by collection and fermentation in a storage container, and toxin stocks prepared in this way are reported to be potent for up to 1 year.[185]

Mechanism of Action and Toxicity

BTX is a neurotoxin that affects the voltage-gated sodium channels in a manner similar to the PbTx discussed above. Pathologic effects from BTX intoxication are due to the depolarization of nerve and muscle cells, which results from an increased sodium ion permeability of the excitable membrane.[188] BTX is lipid soluble, and activity is temperature dependent and pH sensitive. The maximum activity of BTX occurs at 37°C[185] and at an alkaline pH.[189]

BTXs bind sodium channels both in muscle cells and in neurons, modifying both their ion selectivity and voltage sensitivity.[188] The effect of toxin on the sodium channel is to make it constitutively open, causing the irreversible depolarization of cells.[190] However, effects are not observed in experiments where sodium ions are absent in intracellular and extracellular compartments. In addition, BTX alters the ion selectivity of the ion channel by increasing the permeability of the channel toward larger cations.[189] In-vitro muscle preparations treated with BTX have shown massive acetylcholine release in response to depolarization, as predicted. Ultrastructural changes have been observed in nerve and muscle preparations and are due to the massive influx of sodium ions that produce osmotic alterations.[191]

Toxin Exposure, Health Effects, and Treatment

BTX-tipped darts have been used to hunt game by several Indian groups with very effective results, although few Indian groups, notably the Chocó, have adopted its use in warfare. The Chocó fiercely resisted the Spanish in the late 16th Century, and it is not unlikely that BTX weapons were employed in warfare during that period.[185]

Physical Examination. Few published reports have described the systemic effects of BTX intoxication; however, the Chocó Indians claim that a human shot with a BTX-poisoned dart could run only a few hundred meters before dying.[185] In 1825 Captain Charles Stuart Cochrane, a Scottish explorer, described his encounters with the Chocó during an expedition around the lowland tropical rain forests of Colombia.

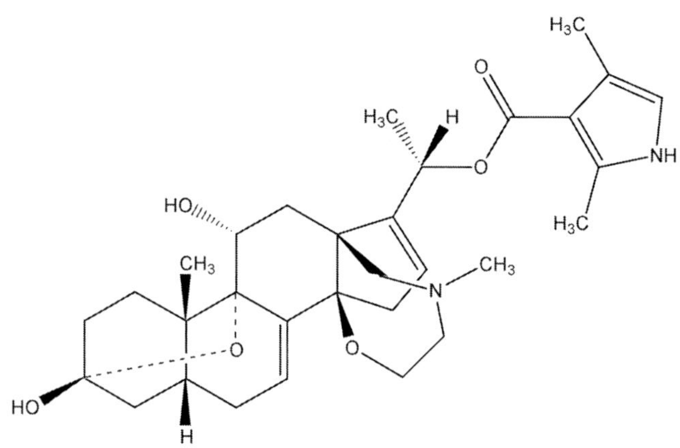

Fig. 19-6. Structure of batrachotoxin, the poison dart frog poison.
Illustration: Courtesy of Richard Sweeny.

In his work, Captain Cochrane writes that a dart envenomed with BTX will cause "certain death to man or animal wounded by it; no cure as yet having been discovered."[186]

Laboratory Findings and Monitoring. BTX is one of the most potent nonprotein poisons. It is cardiotoxic and neurotoxic to humans and animals. Cardiotoxic actions lead to irreversible depolarization of nerves and muscles, causing arrhythmias, fibrillation, and cardiac failure.[192] BTX produces a rapid succession of symptoms when given to animals, including ataxia, weakness, convulsions, paralysis, and cyanosis. Respiratory arrest from paralysis of respiratory effector muscles and cardiac arrest are the causes of death in cases of BTX poisoning.[187] At sublethal doses, symptoms in animals include strong muscle contractions, convulsions, salivations, dyspnea, and death,[193] death ensuing in mice of lethal challenge within minutes. BTX effects on cardiac muscle are similar to the cardiotoxic effects of digitalis, including interference with heart conduction causing arrhythmias, ventricular fibrillation, and other changes that can lead to cardiac arrest.[188]

Treatment. While there is no known antidote for BTX intoxication, treatment has been suggested by using an approach similar to that for treating toxins and chemicals with comparable mechanisms of action (eg, DigiBind [GlaxoSmithKline, SpA, Parma, Italy]).[194]

Stability

Collecting large quantities of the frog-based alkaloid toxins is difficult because a microgram-load of toxin is contained in a single specimen and because frogs bred and raised in captivity lose their toxic properties. Therefore, stockpiling BTX from natural sources may not be practical. BTX is notable because humans have weaponized it under primitive conditions and have successfully employed it in both hunting and warfare. However, the practicality of using such toxins as weapons of mass destruction is questionable.

Protection

BTX is a particularly deadly toxin; the LD_{50} in mice (subcutaneous) is 2 μg/kg.[195] Membrane depolarization can be blocked, or in some cases reversed, by treatment with sodium channel blockers (eg, TTX or STX), which allosterically block sodium currents through voltage-gated channels.[189] This presents an additional complication, because nerve conduction and action potential generation will be compromised.

Surveillance

As with several of the other toxins reviewed here, public health surveillance programs for BTX intoxication have not been established.

SUMMARY

The potential use of disease-producing microorganisms, toxins, and chemical agents has been of concern in both ancient and modern military conflicts, especially during the last century.[4–6] As of 2000, public reports assert that at least two dozen countries either have such chemical or biological weapons or actively seek them.[196] Covert attacks against unsuspecting civilian populations with any of the toxins reviewed here have the potential to produce large numbers of casualties. Management of these casualties will be difficult because treatment for exposure to the presented toxins generally only consists of supportive care. The key to mitigating the effects of a bioterror weapon is the realization that one has been used. Early characterization of the attack will allow appropriate steps to be taken to mediate the effects of the weapon both physically and psychologically on the civilian population. These critical measures include decontamination and evacuation of the affected area, early administration of antitoxin or treatments where available, and the allocation of clean food, water, or air supplies. Early determination of a bioterror attack by a weaponized toxin becomes more difficult when surveillance programs for these kinds of toxins are lacking.

Given a sufficient quantity of even mildly toxic material, bioterrorist attacks, in theory, could be conducted with virtually any toxin, resulting in numerous casualties and chaos in civilian populations. The potential of a toxin to be employed as an effective bioweapon, and therefore the need for a surveillance program for that toxin, should be evaluated using several criteria, including the toxicity of the compound, the ease of synthesis or commercial availability, and the ease of weaponization and delivery (ie, getting the bulk toxin into an appropriate form to introduce into the target population). The toxins reviewed here are sufficiently toxic, if employed effectively, to cause large numbers of casualties in populations unprepared for their release and without advance warning. In addition, most of these compounds are stable enough to be stockpiled with minimal specialized equipment and are also water soluble, allowing for easy dispersal of the toxins in food or water sources or via aerosol dispersion (Figure 19-7).

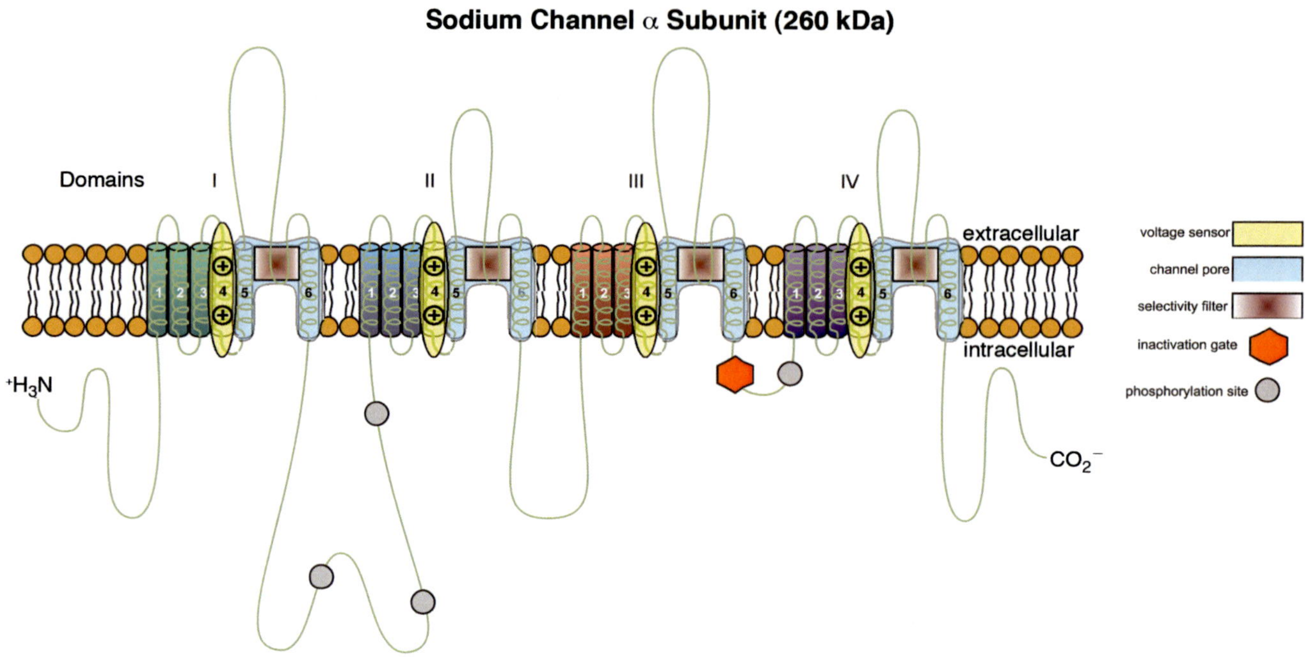

Fig. 19-7. Sodium channel proteins play an essential role in action potential generation and propagation in neurons and other excitable cell types. The resting membrane potential of a neuron remains around - 80 mV. When the neuron membrane becomes excited by the binding of neurotransmitters to their appropriate receptor molecules for example, the cell begins to depolarize and these voltage-gated sodium channels are activated. In response to membrane depolarization, these channels open, increasing cell membrane conductance and a large influx of sodium ions travels down the sodium concentration gradient. This large sodium current drives the membrane potential of the cell towards the reversal potential for sodium, approximately + 55 mV and is recognizable on electrophysiological recordings of neuron activity as the "spike" or action potential. Membrane potential is returned to resting by a combination of the termination of sodium influx due to loss of driving force on sodium, the eventual inactivation of the voltage-gated sodium channels, and the opening of potassium channels. The inactivated state is different from the closed channel state, with the inactivated-to-closed transition driven by the slight hyperpolarization of the cell membrane, which occurs in response to potassium current. Only closed channels are available to open.

Voltage-gated sodium channels are protein complexes composed of a 260 kDa α-subunit and one or more smaller, auxiliary β-subunits (β1, β2, or β3). The variable combinations of the α-subunit with multiple β-subunits allow the creation of a number of functionally distinct channels. The α-subunit illustrated here folds into four transmembrane domains (I–IV), colored green, blue, orange, and purple. The transmembrane domains are composed of six α-helical segments designated S1 through S6 (see Figure 19-4).

The use of biological agents against civilian populations is a legitimate issue of concern; attacks using biological agents have already occurred in the United States and abroad. We must anticipate terrorist groups employing toxins or other agents that are not considered classical weapon agents. Understanding the real strengths and weaknesses of toxins as weapons allows an educated and realistic assessment of the threat posed by toxins and can guide the administration of surveillance programs and contingency plans.

ACKNOWLEDGMENT

The authors thank Lieutenant Colonel Charles Millard, Walter Reed Army Institute of Research, and Dr Mark Poli, US Army Medical Research Institute of Infectious Diseases, for their insight and editorial contributions.

REFERENCES

1. Convention on the Prohibition of the Development, Production, Stockpiling and Use of Chemical Weapons and on their Destruction Web site. Article II, definitions and criteria page. Available at: http://www.opcw.org/html/db/cwc/eng/cwc_article_II.html. Accessed January 15, 2008.

2. Garland T, Bailey EM. Toxins of concern to animals and people. *Rev Sci Tech*. 2006;25:341–351.

3. Wein LM, Liu Y. Analyzing a bioterror attack on the food supply: the case of botulinum toxin in milk. *Proc Natl Acad Sci U S A*. 2005;102:9984–9989.

4. Christopher GW, Cieslak TJ, Pavlin JA, Eitzen EM. Biological warfare. A historical perspective. *JAMA*. 1997;278:412–417.

5. Aas P. The threat of mid-spectrum chemical warfare agents. *Prehospital Disaster Med*. 2003;18:306–312.

6. Franz D. Defense against toxin weapons. In: Sidell FR, Takafuji ET, Franz DR, eds. *Medical Aspects of Chemical and Biological Warfare*. In: Zajtchuk R. Bellamy RF, eds. *Textbook of Military Medicine*. Washington, DC: Department of the Army, Office of The Surgeon General, Borden Institute; 1997: Chap. 30.

7. Centers for Disease Control and Prevention. Bioterrorism agents/diseases: emergency preparedness & response Web site. Available at: http://www.bt.cdc.gov/agent/agentlist-category.asp. Accessed February 10, 2007.

8. Watson SA, Mirocha CJ, Hayes AW. Analysis for trichothecenes in samples from Southeast Asia associated with "Yellow Rain." *Fundam Appl Toxicol*. 1984;4:700–717.

9. Dumbacher JP, Wako A, Derrickson SR, Samuelson A , Spande TF, Daly JW. Melyrid beetles (Choresine): a putative source for the batrachotoxin alkaloids found in poison-dart frogs and toxic passerine birds. *Proc Natl Acad Sci U S A*. 2004;101:15857–15860.

10. Deshpande SS, Adler M, Sheridan RE. Differential actions of brevetoxin on phrenic nerve and diaphragm muscle in the rat. *Toxicon*. 1993;31:459–470.

11. Taroncher-Oldenburg G, Kulis DM, Anderson DM. Coupling of saxitoxin biosynthesis to the G1 phase of the cell cycle in the dinoflagellate Alexandrin fundyense: temperature and nutrient effects. *Nat Toxins*. 1999;7:207–219.

12. Sato K, Akai S, Sugita N, et al. Novel and stereocontrolled synthesis of (+/-)-tetrodotoxin from myo-inositol. *J Org Chem*. 2005;70:7496–7504.

13. Sheridan RE, Deshpande SS, Lebeda FJ, Adler M. The effects of pumiliotoxin-B on sodium currents in guinea pig hippocampal neurons. *Brain Res*. 1991;556:53–60.

14. Sheridan RE, Deshpande SS, Adler M. Cytotoxic actions of palytoxin on aortic smooth muscle cells in culture. *J Appl Toxicol*. 2005;25:365–373.

15. Rogers EH, Hunter ES, Moser VC, et al. Potential developmental toxicity of anatoxin-a, a cyanobacterial toxin. *J Appl Toxicol*. 2005;25:527–534.

16. Kibayashi C. Development of new synthetic methods and its application to total synthesis of nitrogen-containing bioactive natural products. *Chem Pharm Bull (Tokyo)*. 2005;53:1375–1386.

17. Moore RE, Scheuer PJ. Palytoxin: a new marine toxin from a coelenterate. *Science*. 1971;172:495–498.

18. Usami M, Satake M, Ishida S, Inoue A, Kan Y, Yasumoto T. Palytoxin analogs from the dinoflagellate Ostreopsis siamensis. *J Am Chem Soc*. 1995;117:5389–5390.

19. Gleibs S, Mebs D, Werding B. Studies on the origin and distribution of palytoxin in a Caribbean coral reef. *Toxicon*. 1995;33:1531–1537.

20. Yasumoto T, Nagai H, Yasumura D, et al. Interspecies distribution and possible origin of tetrodotoxin. *Ann N Y Acad Sci*. 1986;479:44–51.

21. Fukui M, Murata M, Inoue A, Gawel M, Yasumoto T. Occurrence of palytoxin in the trigger fish Melichtys vidua. *Toxicon*. 1987;25:1121–1124.

22. Kodama AM, Hokama Y, Yasumoto T, Fukui M, Manea SJ, Sutherland N. Clinical and laboratory findings implicating palytoxin as cause of ciguatera poisoning due to *Decapterus macrosoma* (mackerel). *Toxicon*. 1989;27:1051–1053.

23. Hashimoto Y, Fusetani N, Kimura S. Aluterin: a toxin of filefish, Alutera scripta, probably originating from a zonatharian Palythoa tuberculosa. *Bull Jpn Soc Sc Fisheries*. 1969;35:1086–1093.

24. Budavari S. *The Merck Index*. 12th ed. Rahway, NJ: Merck & Co Inc; 1996.

25. Frelin C, Van Renterghem C. Palytoxin. Recent electrophysiological and pharmacological evidence for several mechanisms of action. *Gen Pharmacol*. 1995;26:33–37.

26. Okano H, Masuoka H, Kamei S, et al. Rhabdomyolysis and myocardial damage induced by palytoxin, a toxin of blue humphead parrotfish. *Intern Med*. 1998;37:330–333.

27. Taniyama S, Mahmud Y, Terada M, Takatani T, Arakawa O, Noguchi T. Occurrence of a food poisoning incident by palytoxin from a serranid *Epinephelus sp*. in Japan. *J Nat Toxins*. 2002;11:277–282.

28. Cha JK, Christ WJ, Finan JM, et al. Stereochemistry of palytoxin. Part 4. Complete structure. *J Am Chem Soc*. 1982;104:7369–7371.

29. Artigas P, Gadsby DC. Na+/K+-pump ligands modulate gating of palytoxin-induced ion channels. *Proc Natl Acad Sci U S A*. 2003;100:501–505.

30. Hirata Y, Uemura D. Chemistry and pharmacology of palytoxin. In: Tu A, ed. *Handbook of Natural Venoms*. New York, NY: Marcel Dekker; 1988: 241–258.

31. Ozaki H, Nagase H, Urakawa N. Sugar moiety of cardiac glycosides is essential for the inhibitory action on the palytoxin-induced K^+ release from red blood cells. *FEBS Lett*. 1984;173:196–198.

32. Llewellyn LE, Dodd MJ, Robertson A, Ericson G, de Koning C, Negri AP. Post-mortem analysis of samples from a human victim of a fatal poisoning caused by the xanthid crab, *Zosimus aeneus*. *Toxicon*. 2002;40:1463–1469.

33. Mebs D. Occurrence and sequestration of toxins in food chains. *Toxicon*. 1998;36:1519–1522.

34. Alcala AC, Alcala LC, Garth JS, Yasumura D, Yasumoto T. Human fatality due to ingestion of the crab *Demania reynaudii* that contained a palytoxin-like toxin. *Toxicon*. 1988;26:105–107.

35. Walker DG. Survival after severe envenomation by the blue-ringed octopus (*Hapalochlaena maculosa*). *Med J Aust*. 1983;2:663–665.

36. Noguchi T, Hwang DF, Arakawa O, et al. Palytoxin is the causative agent in the parrotfish poisoning. In: Gopalakrishnaknoe P, Tan CT, eds. *Progress in Venom and Toxin Research. Proceedings of the First Asia-Pacific Congress on Animal, Plant and Microbial Toxins* Singapore, China: National University of Singapore; 1987: 325–335.

37. Arcila-Herrera H, Castello-Navarrete A, Mendoza-Avora J, Montero-Cervantes L, Gonzalez-Franco MF, Brito-Villanueva WO. Ten cases of Ciguatera fish poisoning in Yucatan. *Rev Invest Clin*. 1998;50:149–152.

38. Fujiki H, Suganuma M, Nakayasu M. Palytoxin is a non-12–0-tetradecanoylphorbol-13-acetate type tumor promoter in two–stage mouse skin carcinogenesis. *Carcinogenesis*. 1986;7:707–710.

39. Ishida Y, Satake N, Habon J, Kitano H, Shibata S. Inhibitory effect of ouabain on the palytoxin-induced contraction of human umbilical artery. *J Pharmacol Exp Ther*. 1985; 232:557–560.

40. Fukui M, Yasumura D, Murata M. Occurrence of palytoxin in crabs and fish. In: Gopalakrishnakone P, Tan CK, eds. *Progress in Venom and Toxin Research. Proceedings of the First Asia-Pacific Congress on Animal, Plant and Microbial Toxins*. Singapore, China: National University of Singapore; 1987: 51–57.

41. Kan Y, Uemura D, Hirata Y. Complete NMR signal assignment of palytoxin and N-acetylpalytoxin. *Tetrahedron Lett.* 2001;42:3197–3202.

42. Bignami GS. A rapid and sensitive hemolysis neutralization assay for palytoxin. *Toxicon.* 1993;31:817–820.

43. Vick JA, Wiles JS. The mechanism of action and treatment of palytoxin poisoning. *Toxicol Appl Pharmacol.* 1975;34:214–223.

44. Vick JA, Wiles JS. Pharmacological and toxicological studies of palytoxin. In: Hall S, ed. *Marine Toxins: Structure and Molecular Pharmacology*. Washington, DC: American Chemical Society; 1990: 241–254. Chapter 19.

45. Centers for Disease Control and Prevention, National Institute for Occupational Safety and Health. Registry of Toxic Effects of Chemical Substances (RTECS) Web site. Available at: http://www.cdc.gov/niosh/rtecs/default.html. Accessed March 30, 2007.

46. Kitamura Y, Taguchi T, Yokoyama M, Tamai M, Yamatodani A, Watanabe T. Increase in histidine decarboxylase activity in mouse skin after application of tumor promoters. *Princess Takamatsu Symp.* 1983;14:327–334.

47. Chhatwal GS, Ahnert-Hilger G, Beress L, Habermann E. Palytoxin both induces and inhibits the release of histamine from rat mast cells. *Int Arch Allergy Appl Immunol.* 1982;68:97–100.

48. Habermann E. Palytoxin acts through Na+,K+-ATPase. *Toxicon.* 1989;27:1171–1187.

49. Tatsumi M, Takahashi M, Ohizumi Y. Mechanism of palytoxin-induced (3H) norepinephrine release from a rat pheochromocytoma cell line. *Mol Pharmacol.* 1984;25:379–383.

50. Ahnert-Hilger G, Chatwal GS, Hessler HJ, Habermann E. Changes in erythrocyte permeability due to palytoxin as compared to amphotericin B. *Biochim Biophys Acta.* 1982;688:486–494.

51. Wiles JS, Vick JA, Christensen MK. Toxicological evaluation of palytoxin in several animal species. *Toxicon.* 1974;12:427–433.

52. Taylor TJ, Parker GW, Fajer AB, Mereish KA. Non-specific binding of palytoxin to plastic surfaces. *Toxicol Lett.* 1991;57:291–296.

53. Fuhrman FA. Tetrodotoxin. It is a powerful poison that is found in two almost totally unrelated kinds of animal: puffer fish and newts. It has been serving as a tool in nerve physiology and may provide a model for new local anesthetics. *Sci Am.* 1967;217:60–71.

54. Yotsu M, Yamazaki T, Meguro Y, et al. Production of tetrodotoxin and its derivatives by *Pseudomonas sp*. Isolated from the skin of a pufferfish. *Toxicon.* 1987;25:225–228.

55. Hwang DF, Tai KP, Chueh CH, Lin LC, Jeng SS. Tetrodotoxin and derivatives in several species of the gastropod Naticidae. *Toxicon.* 1991;29:1019–1024.

56. Yasmasuto T, Nagal H, Yasumura D, et al. Interspecies distribution and possible origin of tetrodotoxin. *Ann N Y Acad Sci.* 1986;479:44–51.

57. Durborow RM. Health and safety concerns in fisheries and aquaculture. *Occup Med.* 1999;14:373–406.

58. Chen CY. Paralytic shellfish poisoning toxins accumulation in purple clam *Hiatula rostrata* and toxic effect on milkfish Chanos chanos larval fish. *J Nat Toxins.* 2001;10:299–305.

59. Goldfrank LR, Flomenbaum NE, Lewin NA. *Goldfrank's Toxicologic Emergencies*. 7th ed. New York, NY: McGraw-Hill, Medical Publishing Division; 2002.

60. Dembert ML, Strosahl KF, Bumgarner RL. Disease from fish and shellfish ingestion. *AFP.* 1981;24:103–108.

61. Lehane L. Paralytic shellfish poisoning: a potential public health problem. *Med J Aust*. 2001;175:29–31.

62. Woodward RB. The structure of tetrodotoxin. *Pure Appl Chem.* 1964;9:49–74.

63. Tsuda K, Tachikawa R, Sakai K, et al. On the structure of tetrodotoxin. *Chem Pharm Bull (Tokyo)*.1964;12:642–645.

64. Goto T, Kishi Y, Takahashi S, Hirata Y. Tetrodotoxin. *Tetrahedron*. 1965;21:2059–2088.

65. Tsuda K, Ikuma S, Kawamura M, Tachikawa R, Sakai K. Tetrodotoxin. VII. On the structure of tetrodotoxin and its derivatives. *Chem Pharm Bull (Tokyo)*. 1964;12:1357–1374.

66. Kishi Y, Fukuyama T, Aratani M, Nakatsubo F, Goto T. Synthetic studies on tetrodotoxin and related compounds. IV. Stereospecific total syntheses of DL-tetrodotoxin. *J Am Chem Soc*. 1972;94:9219–9221.

67. Tanino H, Nakata T, Kaneko T, Kishi Y. A stereospecific total synthesis of d, l-saxitoxin. *J Am Chem Soc*. 1977;99:2818–2819.

68. Schantz EJ. Chemistry and biology of saxitoxin and related toxins. *Ann N Y Acad Sci*. 1986;479:15–23.

69. Sharma R, Taylor J. Animal toxins. In: Haley T, Berndt W, eds. *Handbook of Toxicology*. Cambridge, England: Hemisphere Publishing; 1987.

70. Isbister GK, Son J, Wang F, et al. Puffer fish poisoning: a potentially life-threatening condition. *Med J Aust*. 2002;177:650–653.

71. Creasia D, Neally M. *Acute Inhalation Toxicity of Saxitoxin to Mice*. Fort Detrick, Md: US Army Medical Research Institute of Infectious Diseases Pathophysiology Division; 1988. AD-A203 563.

72. Meier J, White J. *Handbook of Clinical Toxicology of Animal Venoms and Poisons*. Boca Raton, La: CRC Press; 1995.

73. Evans MH. Tetrodotoxin, saxitoxin, and related substances: their applications in neurobiology. *Int Rev Neurobiol.* 1972;15:83–166.

74. Henderson R, Ritchie JM, Strichartz G. The binding of labelled saxitoxin to the sodium channels of nerve membranes. *J Physiol.* 1973;235:783–804.

75. Cestele S, Catterall WA. Molecular mechanisms of neurotoxin action on voltage-gated sodium channels. *Biochimie*. 2000;82:883–892.

76. Louzao MC, Vieytes MR, Baptista de Sousa JM, Leira F, Botana LM. A fluorimetric method based on changes in membrane potential for screening paralytic shellfish toxins in mussels. *Anal Biochem.* 2001;289:246–250.

77. Casarett LJ, Klaassen CD, Curtis D, Andur MO, Doull J. *Casarett and Doull's Toxicology: the Basic Science of Poisons*. 5th ed. New York, NY: McGraw-Hill, Health Professions Division; 1996.

78. Kao CY. Pharmacology of tetrodotoxin and saxitoxin. *Fed Proc.* 1972;31:1117–1123.

79. Acres J, Gray J. Paralytic shellfish poisoning. *Can Med Assoc J*. 1978;119:1195–1197.

80. Morse EV. Paralytic shellfish poisoning: a review. *J Am Vet Med Assoc.* 1977;171:1178–1180.

81. Rodrigue DC, Etzel RA, Hall S, et al. Lethal paralytic shellfish poisoning in Guatemala. *Am J Trop Med Hyg*. 1990;42:267–271.

82. Isbister GK, Kiernan MC. Neurotoxic marine poisoning. *Lancet Neurol*. 2005;4:219–228.

83. Torda TA, Sinclair E, Ulyatt DB. Puffer fish (tetrodotoxin) poisoning: clinical record and suggested management. *Med J Aust*. 1973;1:599–602.

84. *Aquatic (Marine and Freshwater) Biotoxins*. Geneva, Switzerland: World Health Organization, 1984. Environmental Health Criteria Monograph 37.

85. National Library of Medicine. Hazardous Substances Data Bank (HSDB) Web site. Available at: http://toxnet.nlm.nih.gov/cgi-bin/sis/htmlgen?HSDB. Accessed March 30, 2007.

86. Tambyah PA, Hui KP, Gopalakrishnakone P, Chin NK, Chan TB. Central-nervous-system effects of tetrodotoxin poisoning. *Lancet*. 1994;343:538–539.

87. Oda K, Araki K, Totoki T, Shibasaki H. Nerve conduction study of human tetrodotoxication. *Neurology*. 1989;39:743–745.

88. Kao CY. Tetrodotoxin, saxitoxin and their significance in the study of excitation phenomena. *Pharmacol Rev*. 1966;18:997–1049.

89. Bradley SG, Klika LJ. A fatal poisoning from the Oregon rough-skinned newt (*Taricha granulosa*). *JAMA*. 1981;246:247.

90. Kiernan MC, Isbister GK, Lin CS, Burke D, Bostock H. Acute tetrodotoxin-induced neurotoxicity after ingestion of puffer fish. *Ann Neurol*. 2005;57:339–348.

91. Lan MY, Lai SL, Chen SS. Tetrodotoxin intoxication in a uraemic patient (letter). *Br Med J*. 1999;127.

92. Noguchi T, Ebesu JSM. Puffer poisoning: epidemiology and treatment. *J Toxicol-Toxin Rev*. 2001;20:1–10.

93. Halstead BW. *Poisonous and Venous Marine Animals of the World*. Rev ed. Princeton, NJ: Darwin Press; 1978.

94. Sakamoto Y, Lockey RF, Krzanowski JJ Jr. Shellfish and fish poisoning related to the toxic dinoflagellates. *South Med J*. 1987;80:866–872.

95. de Carvalho M, Jacinto J, Ramos N, de Oliveira V, Pinho e Melo T, de Sa J. Paralytic shellfish poisoning: clinical and electrophysiological observation. *J Neurol*. 1998;245:551–554.

96. Long RR, Sargent JC, Hammer K. Paralytic shellfish poisoning: a case report and serial electrophysiologic observations. *Neurology*. 1990;40:1310–1312.

97. Chew SK, Goh CH, Wang KW, Mah PK, Tan BY. Puffer fish (tetrodotoxin) poisoning: clinical report and role of anticholinesterase drugs in therapy. *Singapore Med J*. 1983;24:168–171.

98. Gage PW, Dulhunty AF. Effects of toxin from the blue–ringed octopus (*Hapalochlaena maculosa*). *Marine Pharmacognosy*. 1973;36:85–105.

99. Yang CC, Liao SC, Deng JF. Tetrodotoxin poisoning in Taiwan: an analysis of poison center data. *Vet Hum Toxicol*. 1996;38:282–286.

100. Field J. Puffer fish poisoning. *J Accid Emerg Med*. 1998;15:334–336.

101. Tibballs J. Severe tetrodotoxic fish poisoning. *Anaesthesia Intensive Care*. 1988;16:215–217.

102. Paralytic shellfish poisoning—Massachusetts and Alaska, 1990. *MMWR Morb Mortal Wkly Rep*. 1991;40:157–161.

103. Gessner BD, Middaugh JP. Paralytic shellfish poisoning in Alaska: a 20-year retrospective analysis. *Am J Epidemiol*. 1995;141:766–770.

104. Lehane L. Paralytic shellfish poisoning: a potential public health problem. *Med J Aust.* 2001;175;29–31.

105. Cheng HS, Chua SO, Hung JS, Yip KK. Creatine kinase MB elevation in paralytic shellfish poisoning. *Chest.* 1991;99:1032–1033.

106. Centers for Disease Control and Prevention. Neurologic illness associated with eating Florida pufferfish, 2002. *MMWR Morb Mortal Wkly Rep.* 2002;51:321–323.

107. How CK, Chern CH, Huang YC, Wang LM, Lee CH. Tetrodotoxin poisoning. *Am J Emerg Med.* 2003;21:51–54.

108. Flachsenberger WA. Respiratory failure and lethal hypotension due to blue-ringed octopus and tetrodotoxin envenomation observed and counteracted in animal models. *J Toxicol Clin Toxicol.* 1986–1987;24:485–502.

109. Laobhripatr S, Limpakarnjanarat K, Sangwonloy O, et al. Food poisoning due to consumption of the freshwater puffer *Tetraodon fangi* in Thailand. *Toxicon.* 1990;28:1372–1375.

110. Ahasan HA, Mamun AA, Karim SR, Bakar MA, Gazi EA, Bala CS. Paralytic complications of puffer fish (tetrodotoxin) poisoning. *Singapore Med J.* 2004;45:73–74.

111. Fenner P. Marine envenomation: an update—A presentation on the current status of marine envenomation first aid and medical treatments. *Emerg Med.* 2000;12:295–302.

112. Mahmud Y, Tanu MB, Noguchi T. First occurrence of a food poisoning incident due to ingestion of Takifugu oblongus, along with a toxicological report on three marine puffer species in Bangladesh. *J Food Hyg Soc Japan.* 1999;40:473–480.

113. Gessner BD, Middaugh JP, Doucette GJ. Paralytic shellfish poisoning in Kodiak, Alaska. *West J Med.* 1997;167:351–353.

114. Sun K, Wat J, So P. Puffer fish poisoning. *Anaesth Intensive Care.* 1994;22:307–308.

115. Deng JF, Tominack RL, Chung HM, Tsai WJ. Hypertension as an unusual feature in an outbreak of tetrodotoxin poisoning. *J Toxicol Clin Toxicol.* 1991;29:71–79.

116. Chew SK, Chew LS, Wang KW, Mah PK, Tan BY. Anticholinesterase drugs in the treatment of tetrodotoxin poisoning. *Lancet.* 1984;2:108.

117. Hwang DF, Hsieh YW, Shiu YC, Chen SK, Cheng CA. Identification of tetrodotoxin and fish species in a dried dressed fish fillet implicated in food poisoning. *J Food Prot.* 2002; 65:389–392.

118. Shui LM, Chen K, Wang JY, et al. Tetrodotoxin-associated snail poisoning in Zhoushan: a 25-year retrospective analysis. *J Food Prot.* 2003;66:110–114.

119. Lan MY, Lai SL, Chen SS, Hwang DF. Tetrodotoxin intoxication in a uraemic patient (letter). *J Neurol Neurosurg Psychiatry.* 1999;67:127–128.

120. Akaeda H, Takatani T, Anami A. Mass outbreak of paralytic shellfish poisoning due to ingestion of oysters at Tamano–ura, Goto Islands, Nagasaki, Japan. *J Food Hyg Soc Japan.* 1998;39:272–274.

121. Garcia C, del Carmen Bravo M, Lagos M, Lagos N. Paralytic shellfish poisoning: post-mortem analysis of tissue and body fluid samples from human victims in the Patagonia fjords. *Toxicon.* 2004;43:149–158.

122. Kawatsu K, Shibata T, Hamano Y. Application of immunoaffinity chromatography for detection of tetrodotoxin from urine samples of poisoned patients. *Toxicon.* 1999;37:325–333.

123. Leber A. Uber tetrodonvergiftung. *Arb Trop Grenzgebiete.* 1972;26:641–643.

124. Mahmud Y, Arakawa O, Noguchi T. An epidemic survey on freshwater puffer poisoning in Bangladesh. *J Nat Toxins.*

2000;9:319–326.

125. Chyka PA, Seger D. Position statement: single-dose activated charcoal. American Academy of Clinical Toxicology; European Association of Poisons Centers and Clinical Toxicologists. *J Toxicol Clin Toxicol.* 1997;35:721–741.

126. Sims JK, Ostman DC. Pufferfish poisoning: emergency diagnosis and management of mild human tetrodotoxication. *Ann Emerg Med.* 1986;15:1094–1098.

127. Guidelines 2000 for cardiopulmonary resuscitation and emergency cardiovascular care. Part 6: advanced cardiovascular life support: section 4: devices to assist circulation. The American Heart Association in collaboration with the International Liaison Committee on Resuscitation. *Circulation.* 2000;102(suppl 8):1–383.

128. Kohane DS, Lu NT, Crosa GA, Kuang Y, Berde CB. High concentrations of adrenergic antagonists prolong sciatic nerve blockade by tetrodotoxin. *Acta Anaesthesiol Scand.* 2001;45:899–905.

129. Alfonso A, Vieytes MR, Botana AM, Goenaga X, Botana LM. Preparation of mixtures of paralytic shellfish toxin (PSP) standards from mussel hepatopancreas. *Fresenius J Anal Chem.* 1993;345:212–216.

130. Alfonso A, Louzao MC, Vieytes MR, Botana LM. Comparative study of the stability of saxitoxin and neosaxitoxin in acidic solutions and lyophilized samples. *Toxicon.* 1994; 32:1593–1598.

131. Benton BJ, Keller SA, Spriggs DL, Capacio BR, Chang FC. Recovery from the lethal effects of saxitoxin: a therapeutic window for 4-aminopyridine (4–AP). *Toxicon.* 1998;36:571–588.

132. Toxin tocsin. *Time Magazine.* September 22, 1975:31.

133. Tucker JB. *War of Nerves, Chemical Warfare for World War I to Al–Qaeda.* New York, NY: Pantheon Books; 2006:216–217.

134. Sasner JJ Jr. Comparative studies or algal toxins. In: Martin DF, Padilla GM, eds. *Marine Pharmacognosy.* New York, NY: Academic Press; 1973: 127–177.

135. Cortez-Altamirano R, Hernandez-Becerril DU, Luna-Soria R. Red tides in Mexico: a review. *Rev Latinoam Microbiol.* 1995;37:343–352.

136. Morris PD, Campbell DS, Taylor TJ, Freeman JI. Clinical and epidemiological features of neurotoxic shellfish poisoning in North Carolina. *Am J Public Health.* 1991;81:471–474.

137. Baden DG. Brevetoxins: unique polyether dinoflagellate toxins. *FASEB J.* 1989;3:1807–1817.

138. Baden DG, Bourdelais AJ, Jacocks H, Michelliza S, Naar J. Natural and derivative brevetoxins: historical background, multiplicity, and effects. *Environ Health Perspect.* 2005; 113:621–625.

139. Nicoloau K, Rutjes F, Theodorakis E, Tiebes J, Sato M, Untersteller E. Total synthesis of brevetoxin B. 2. Compilation. *J Am Chem Soc.* 1995;117:1173–1174.

140. Nicoloau K, Yang Z, Shi G, Gunzner J, Agrios K, Gartner P. Total synthesis of brevetoxin A. *Nature.* 1998;392:264–269.

141. Lin Y, Risk M, Ray S, et al. Isolation and structure of brevetoxin B from "red tide" dinoflagellate *Gymnodinium breve.* *J Am Chem Soc.* 1981;103:6773–6776.

142. Kadota I, Takamura H, Nishii H, Yamamoto Y. Total synthesis of brevetoxin B. *J Am Chem Soc.* 2005;127:9246–9250.

143. Poli MA, Mende TJ, Baden DG. Brevetoxins, unique activators of voltage-sensitive sodium channels, bind to specific sites in rat brain synaptosomes. *Mol Pharmacol.* 1986; 30:129–135.

144. Catterall WA, Gainer M. Interaction of brevetoxin A with a new receptor site on the sodium channel. *Toxicon.* 1985;23:497–504.

145. Richards IS, Kulkarni AP, Brooks SM, Pierce R. Florida red-tide toxins (brevetoxins) produce depolarization of airway smooth muscle. *Toxicon.* 1990;28:1105–1111.

146. Shimoda T, Krzanowski, Lockey R, et al. Lower airway smooth muscle contraction induced by Ptychodiscus brevis (red tide) toxin. *J Allergy Clin Immunol.* 1987;79:899–908.

147. Watanabe T, Lockey RF, Krzanowski JJ Jr. Airway smooth muscle contraction induced by Ptychodiscus brevis (red tide) toxin as related to a trigger mechanisms of bronchial asthma. *Immunol Aller Practice.* 1988;10:25–32.

148. Baden DG, Mende TJ, Lichter W. Crystallization and toxicology of T34: a major toxin from Florida's red tide organism (Ptychodiscus brevis). *Toxicon.* 1981;19:455–462.

149. Baden DG, Mende TJ. Toxicity of two toxins from the Florida red tide marine dinoflagellate, *Ptychodiscus brevis*. *Toxicon.* 1982;20:457–461.

150. Baden DG, Bikhazi G, Decker SJ, Foldes FF, Leung I. Neuromuscular blocking action of two brevetoxins from the Florida red tide organism *Ptychodiscus brevis*. *Toxicon.* 1984;22:75–84.

151. Wu CH, Huang JM, Vogel SM, Luke VS, Atchison WD, Narahashi T. Actions of *Ptychodiscus brevis* toxins on nerve and muscle membranes. *Toxicon.* 1985;23:481–487.

152. Sheridan RE, Adler M. The actions of a red tide toxin from *Ptychodiscus brevis* on single sodium channels in mammalian neuroblastoma cells (letter). *FEBS Lett.* 1989;247:448–452.

153. Baden DG, Mende TJ, Bikhazi G, Leung I. Bronchoconstriction caused by Florida red tide toxins. *Toxicon.* 1982;20:929–932.

154. Gervais A, MacLean J. Management. In: Anderson D, White A, Baden D, eds. *Toxic dinoflagellates: proceedings of the Third International Conference on Toxic Dinoflagellates, St. Andrews, New Brunswick, Canada, June 8-12, 1985.* New York, NY: Elsevier; 1985: 530–533.

155. Baden DG. Marine food-borne dinoflagellate toxins. *Int Rev Cytol.* 1983;82:99–150.

156. Hemmert W. The public health implications of *Gymnodinium breve* red tides, a review of the literature and recent events. In: LoCicero V, ed. *The First International Conference on Toxic Dinoflagellate Blooms.* Wakefield, Mass: Massachusetts Science and Technology Foundation; 1975:489–498.

157. Ellis S. Introduction to symposium-brevetoxins, chemistry and pharmacology of "red tide" toxins from *Ptychodiscus brevis* (formerly *Gymnodinium breve*). *Toxicon.* 1985;23: 469–472.

158. Pierce RH, Henry MS, Blum PC, et al. Brevetoxin concentrations in marine aerosol: human exposure levels during a *Karenia brevis* harmful algal bloom. *Bull Environ Contam Toxicol.* 2003;79:161–165.

159. Johnson GL, Spikes JJ, Ellis S. Cardiovascular effects of brevetoxins in dogs. *Toxicon.* 1985;23:505–515.

160. Hughes JM, Merson MH, Gangarosa EJ. The safety of eating shellfish. *JAMA.* 1977;237: 1980–1981.

161. Pierce RH. Red tide (*Ptychodiscus brevis*) toxin aerosols: a review. *Toxicon.* 1986;24:955–965.

162. Backer LC, Kirkpatrick B, Fleming LE, et al. Occupational exposure to aerosolized brevetoxins during Florida red tide events: effects on a healthy worker population. *Environ Health Perspect.* 2005;113:644–649.

163. Fleming LE, Backer LC, Baden DG. Overview of aerosolized Florida red tide toxins: exposures and effects. *Environ Health Perspect.* 2005;113:618–620.

164. McFarren EF, Silva FJ, Tanabe H, Wilson WB, Campbell JE, Lewis KH. The occurrence of a ciguatera-like poison in oysters, clams and *Gymnodinium breve* cultures. *Toxicon.* 1965;3:111–123.

165. Abraham WM, Bourdelais AJ, Sabater JR, et al. Airway responses to aerosolized brevetoxins in an animal model of asthma. *Am J Respir Crit Care Med.* 2005;171:26–34.

166. Poli MA, Musser SM, Dickey RW, Eilers PP, Hall S. Neurotoxic shellfish poisoning and brevetoxin metabolites: a case study from Florida. *Toxicon.* 2000;38:981–993.

167. Cheng YS, Zhou Y, Irvin CM, et al. Characterization of marine aerosol for assessment of human exposure to brevetoxins. *Environ Health Perspect.* 2005;113:638–643.

168. Trainer VL, Baden DG. An enzyme immunoassay for the detection of Florida red tide brevetoxins. *Toxicon.* 1991;29:1387–1394.

169. Whitefleet-Smith J, Boyer GL, Schnoes HK. Isolation and spectral characteristics of four toxins from the dinoflagellate *Ptychodiscus brevis*. *Toxicon.* 1986;24:1075–1090.

170. Thampi S, Domer N, Haarstad VB. Pharmacological studies of norphenyl hemicholinium 3. *J Pharm Sci.* 1966;55:381.

171. Franz DR, LeClaire RD. Respiratory effects of brevetoxin and saxitoxin in awake guinea pigs. *Toxicon.* 1989;27:647–654.

172. Thampi S, Domer N, Haarstad VB, Schueler FW. Pharmacological studies of norphenyl hemicholinium 3. *J Pharm Sci.* 1966;55:381-386.

173. Kim YS, Padilla GM. Purification of the ichthyotoxic component of *Gymnodinium breve* (red tide dinoflagellate) toxin by high pressure liquid chromatography. *Toxicon.* 1976;14: 379–387.

174. Baden DG, Mende TJ, Szmant AM, Trainer VL, Edwards RA, Roszell LE. Brevetoxin binding: molecular pharmacology versus immunoassay. *Toxicon.* 1988;26:97–103.

175. Abraham WM, Bourdelais AJ, Ahmed A, Serebriakov I, Baden DG. Effects of inhaled brevetoxins in allergic airways: toxin-allergen interactions and pharmacologic intervention. *Environ Health Perspect.* 2005;113:632–637.

176. Hua Y, Cole RB. Solution reactivity of brevetoxins as monitored by electrospray ionization mass spectrometry and implications for detoxification. *Chem Res Toxicol.* 1999; 12:1268–1277.

177. Dierauf LA, Gulland FM, eds. *CRC Handbook of Marine Mammal Medicine.* 2nd ed. New York, NY: CRC Press; 2001.

178. van der Schalie WH, Shedd TR, Widder MW, Brennan LM . Response characteristics of an aquatic biomonitor used for rapid toxicity detection. *J Appl Toxicol.* 2004;24;387–394.

179. US Environmental Protection Agency. *Real-time Monitoring for Toxicity Caused by Harmful Algal Blooms and Other Water Quality Perturbations.* Washington, DC: EPA; 2001. EPA/600/R–01/103.

180. Daly JW, Myers CW, Warnick JE, Albuquerque EX. Levels of batrachotoxin and lack of sensitivity to its action in poison-dart frogs (*Phyllobates*). *Science.* 1980;208:1383–1385.

181. Daly JW, Secunda SI, Garraffo HM, Spande TF, Wisnieski A, Cover JF. An uptake system for dietary alkaloids in poison frogs (Dendrobatidae). *Toxicon.* 1994;32:657–663.

182. Weldon PJ. Avian chemical defense: toxic birds not of a feather. *Proc Natl Acad Sci U S A.* 2000;97:12948–12949.

183. Dumbacher JP, Spande TF, Daly JW. Batrachotoxin alkaloids from passerine birds: a second toxic bird genus (*Ifrita kowaldi*) from New Guinea. *Proc Natl Acad Sci U S A.* 2000; 97:12970–12975.

184. Dumbacher JP, Beehler BM, Spande TF, Garraffo HM, Daly JW. Homobatrachotoxin in the genus Pitohui: chemical defense in birds? *Science*. 1992;258:799–801.

185. Meyers CW, Daly JW. A dangerously toxic new frog (*Phyllobates*) used by Embera Indians of western Colombia, with discussion of blowgun fabrication and dart poisoning. *Bull American Museum of Nat Hist*. 1977;161:309–365.

186. Cochrane CS. *Journal of a Residence and Travels in Colombia During theYears 1823 and 1824. In Two Volumes.* London, England: Henry Colbum; 1825: 406.

187. Tichy W. *Poisons: Antidotes and Anecdotes.* New York, NY: Sterling Pub; 1977: 192.

188. Catterall WA. Neurotoxins that act on voltage-sensitive sodium channels in excitable membranes. *Annu Rev Pharmacol Toxicol*. 1980;20:15–43.

189. Warnick, JE, Albuquerque EX, Onur R, et al. The pharmacology of batrachotoxin. VII. Structure-activity relationships and the effects of pH. *J Pharmacol Exp Ther*. 1975;193:232–245.

190. Catterall WA. Structure and function of voltage-sensitive ion channels. *Science*. 1988; 242:50–61.

191. Casarett LJ, Doull J, Klaassen CD. *Casarett and Doull's Toxicology: the Basic Science of Poisons*. 6th ed. New York, NY: McGraw–Hill Medical Pub Division; 2001:1236.

192. Albuquerque EX, Daly JW, Witkop B. Batrachotoxin: chemistry and pharmacology. *Science*. 1971;172:995–1002.

193. Maerki F, Witkop B. The venom of the Colombian arrow poison frog *Phyllobates bicolor*. *Experientia*. 1963;19:329–338.

194. Patockaa J, Stredab L. Brief review of natural nonprotein neurotoxins. *ASA Newsletter*. 2002;89:16.

195. Daly JW, Padgett W, Seamon KB. Activation of cyclic AMP-generating systems in brain membranes and slices by the diterpene forskolin: augmentation of receptor-mediated responses. *J Neurochem*. 1982;38:532–544.

196. US Congress, Office of Technology Assessment. *Proliferation of Weapons of Mass Destruction: Assessing the Risk.* Washington, DC: US Government Printing Office; 1993: 79–81. OTA–ISC–559.

Chapter 20

MEDICAL CHEMICAL DEFENSE ACQUISITION PROGRAMS

KEITH VESELY, DVM, PhD,* and JONATHAN NEWMARK, MD†

*Colonel, US Army; Joint Product Manager, Medical Identification and Treatment Systems, Chemical Biological Medical Systems Joint Project Management Office, 64 Thomas Johnson Drive, Frederick, Maryland 21702

†Colonel, US Army; Deputy Joint Program Executive Officer, Medical Systems, Joint Program Executive Office for Chemical/Biological Defense, Skyline #2, Suite 1609, 5203 Leesburg Pike, Falls Church, Virginia 22041; Adjunct Professor, Department of Neurology, F. Edward Hébert School of Medicine, Uniformed Services University of the Health Sciences, Bethesda, Maryland

INTRODUCTION

The Department of Defense (DoD) requires medical countermeasures to treat or mitigate illness resulting from exposure to chemical, biological, and radiological warfare agents. While medical chemical defense depends on basic and applied science to gain insight into the pathophysiology, pharmacokinetics, and pharmacodynamics of candidate countermeasures, fielding a medical countermeasure cannot occur until advanced development efforts complete full-rate production and obtain US Food and Drug Administration (FDA) approval (DoD policy stipulates that military personnel will only receive medical products approved by the FDA. Quad service doctrine, which appears in Army Regulation 40-7, states, "it is the policy of TSG [The Army Surgeon General] that drugs used will be those approved by the FDA and procured from suppliers in the United States."[1,2] This chapter will briefly describe the US military's organizations responsible for implementing advanced development and will summarize the status of current programs of record.

MEDICAL CHEMICAL ACQUISITION ORGANIZATIONS

The acquisition process may be defined as the process of developing, acquiring, fielding, maintaining, sustaining, and, when necessary, closing out any weapons or protective system in the US military. A drug, vaccine, or medical device used to protect the force against chemical or biological attack is considered a protective system, and medical countermeasures are developed and obtained using what is known as "the acquisition process." The acquisition process includes identifying requirements or capability gaps, identifying potential solutions, and developing and acquiring those solutions, whether the acquisitions are for the development of weapons systems or medical countermeasures.

Chemical and biological defense programs within the DoD are managed by a triad of equal organizations, each of which handles one aspect of the acquisition process. The Joint Requirements Office for Chemical, Biological, Radiological, and Nuclear (CBRN) defense generates and validates requirements from the field, such as the need for a skin decontaminant or for a specific chemical detector. The Defense Threat Reduction Agency, through its joint science and technology office for chemical and biological defense, conducts and supports research and development that seeks to meet these requirements and fill capability gaps. It also maintains a robust science and technology base. This chapter focuses on the third leg of the triad, the organization responsible for the acquisition of medical chemical defense items: the Joint Program Executive Office for Chemical Biological Defense (JPEO-CBD) (Figure 20-1).

In the DoD, all chemical and biological defense acquisition processes fall under the responsibility of the defense acquisition executive (the under secretary of defense for acquisition, technology, and logistics) at the DoD level. Within the DoD, the Army is the executive agent for chemical and biological defense and the assistant secretary of the Army (acquisition, logistics, and technology) is the Army acquisition executive responsible for managing these programs.

DoD chemical and biological defense acquisition programs are managed by the JPEO-CBD, which is headed by a two-star general, the joint program executive officer. The JPEO-CBD manages \$1.5 billion in acquisition programs, of which approximately 85% are nonmedical programs (boots, masks, gloves, detectors, collective protection, information systems,

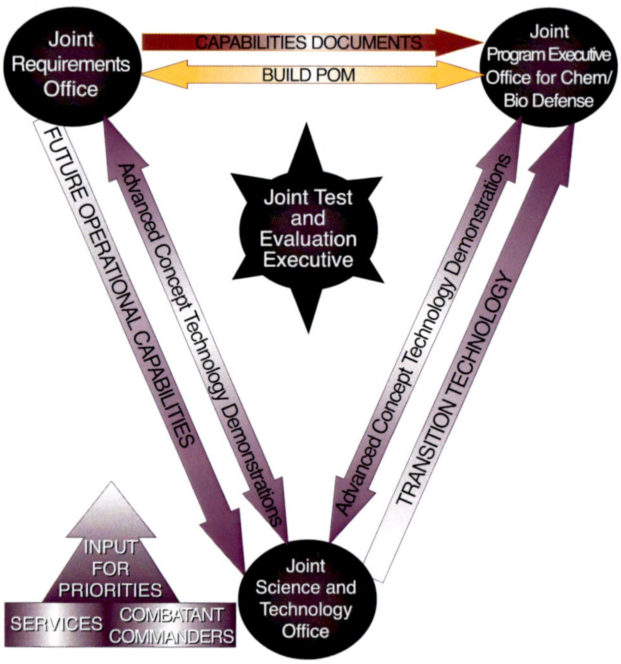

Fig. 20-1. Required capabilities, science and technology, and acquisition responsibilities and interactions.
Bio: biological
Chem: chemical
POM: program objective memorandum

equipment decontamination, etc). The JPEO-CBD is responsible for developing, acquiring, fielding, and supporting chemical and biological defense equipment and medical countermeasures that support the national military strategy.

The JPEO-CBD medical programs are managed by a subordinate organization, the chemical and biological medical systems joint project management office, headquartered at Frederick, Maryland. This office oversees three joint product management components: the joint vaccine acquisition program, the newly established transformational medical technologies initiative, and the medical identification and treatment systems joint product management office (MITS JPMO). The joint vaccine acquisition program is responsible for developing and fielding vaccines and associated products to protect military personnel against biological warfare agents. The transformational medical technologies initiative enables the DoD to protect service members from novel (and potentially genetically engineered) biological threats through the rapid development of effective therapeutic medical countermeasures, minimizing risks and saving lives. The advanced development of therapeutic and diagnostic products, which includes chemical defense programs, is managed by the MITS JPMO. The mission of the MITS program is to develop and acquire safe, effective, and FDA-approved products for the prophylaxis, treatment, and diagnosis of CBRN warfare agent exposure. The MITS JPMO is also responsible for the critical reagents program, the repository for reagents (probes and primers) and assay kits used in DoD biological detection/diagnostic systems. All MITS medical countermeasures undergoing advanced development for use against CBRN agents are fully integrated into the JPEO-CBD systems of approach to counter threat agents, thereby supporting an integrated diagnostic, prophylactic, and therapeutic capability. MITS medical countermeasures supplement and are compatible with all the equipment developed under JPEO-CBD.

MEDICAL CHEMICAL ACQUISITION PROCESSES AND CONCERNS

The major ground rules for the defense acquisition process are contained in the DoD 5000 series documents.[3,4] The federal acquisition regulations and supplements also pertain to this process.[5]

Drugs must pass through several phases of clinical trials in order to obtain FDA approval (Figure 20-2). All human research trials conducted in support of the FDA approval process must follow strict FDA regulations and guidelines ("good clinical practices"). In Phase 1 clinical trials, a new drug is first tested in a small group of healthy volunteers (usually 20–80) to evaluate its safety, determine a safe dosage range, identify side effects, and determine how the drug is absorbed, distributed in the body, metabolized, and excreted. In Phase 2 clinical trials, the study drug is given to a larger group of people (usually around several hundred subjects) to evaluate effectiveness and to further evaluate safety. In typical Phase 3 studies, the study drug is given to even larger groups of people, up to several thousand, to confirm its efficacy, monitor side effects, compare it to commonly used treatments, and collect drug safety data. However, Phase 3 studies are not used for the approval of medical chemical countermeasures because it is unethical to test the effectiveness of any drug against chemical warfare agents in people. To overcome this obstacle, the MITS JPMO plans to invoke the "animal rule" (sometimes called "the animal efficacy rule"), which allows for the testing and approval of products when human efficacy clinical trials are not feasible or are unethical,[6] as DoD accepts this means to licensure. The Phase 2 clinical trials are used as expanded safety studies for medical chemical countermeasure development and may be divided into multiple arms or studies to address all the regulatory concerns. Phase 4 (post-marketing) studies are conducted after a drug is already approved and on the market. Concurrent with the approval, the FDA may require certain post-marketing studies to delineate and document additional information about a drug's risks, benefits, and optimal use, or it may collect retrospective data on the safety and efficacy of the product if it is ever used. This is especially true for drugs approved under the animal rule. All FDA-required Phase 4 studies are the responsibility of the sponsor, whether that is the US Army Office of The Surgeon General or a system integrator.

Medical CBRN products are developed using a mix of in-house experts and commercial contractors. Within the acquisition process, drug development programs must pass through a series of gates or milestones. A milestone is a point in which a recommendation is made and approval is sought regarding starting or continuing an acquisition program.

Concept Development (Pre-Milestone A Activities)

Drug development decisions must take place earlier in the acquisition process than the typical DoD weapon system development program, requiring earlier user involvement. The DoD 5000 series does not require an analysis of alternatives for drug development efforts because they are not typically major defense

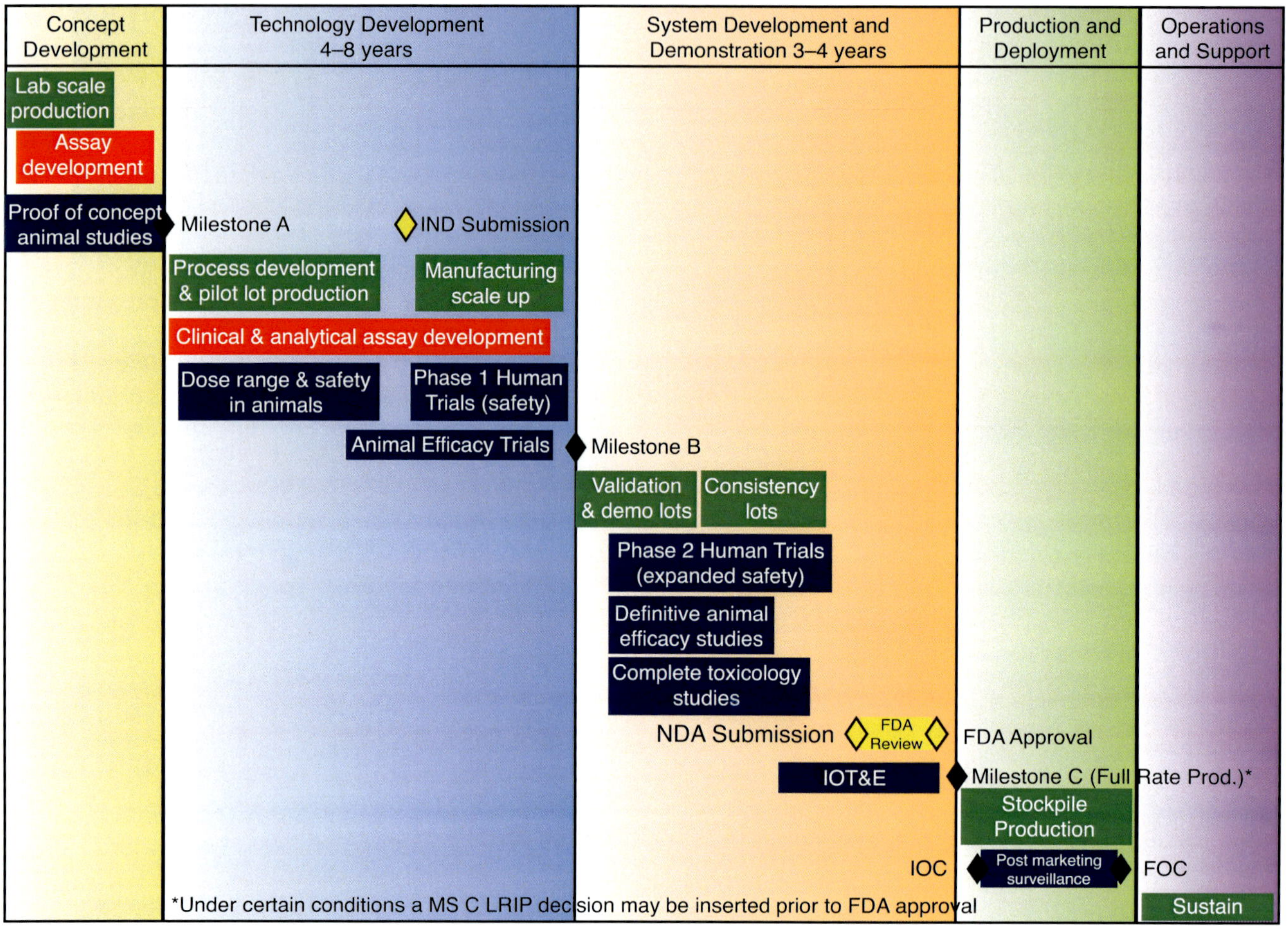

Fig. 20-2. Model for integrating pharmaceutical development, FDA regulatory, and the Department of Defense acquisition processes.
*Under certain conditions, an MS C LRIP decision may be inserted prior to FDA approval.
FDA: Food and Drug Administration
FOC: full operational capability
IND: investigational new drug
IOC: initial operational capability
IOT&E: initial operational test and evaluation
MS C LRIP: milestone C low rate initial production
NDA: new drug application
Prod: production

acquisition programs. However, an analysis addresses all alternatives (eg, prophylactics, pretreatments, therapeutics, and nonmedical countermeasures), considers risk, and performs cost and effectiveness analyses. If development of a drug product is warranted, the technology base assigns personnel, budgets, and facilities and begins basic and applied research. Activities during this phase include assay development and proof of concept animal studies.

The MITS JPMO begins coordinating early with the technology base to gain technical familiarity with potential countermeasure candidates and to ensure that advanced development funding is aligned appropriately to support a candidate at milestone A. Technology transition agreements are developed with the technology base for each product to ensure a smooth transition to advanced development.

Technology Development

Program management lead shifts from the science and technology base to the MITS JPMO at milestone A. Science and technology and advanced development funds may be used during the technology development stage, allowing MITS to engage with the science and technology base early in the process. If multiple candidates are pursued, down-selection criteria are evaluated during technology development and a down-selection recommendation is typically made at milestone B.

Between milestones A and B, the MITS JPMO pursues process development and pilots lot production of candidate drugs under current good manufacturing practices (cGMPs). Required work includes clinical and analytical assay development, dose range and safety studies in animals in accordance with good laboratory practices, investigational new drug (IND) submission to the FDA, and Phase 1 human clinical safety studies compliant with good clinical practices. Emergency use authorization may be prepared and submitted to the FDA for review with, or shortly after, IND submission.

Intellectual property rights are addressed as part of the product transition package (ie, licensure purchase, the need to trace origin to ascertain if it was government funded and, if so, claim government purpose license rights, etc). Intellectual property rights may be a concern for future products, and the MITS JPMO will examine all available options to ensure that products are developed and produced in a manner equitable to the government. Final decision on this approach will be determined by the MITS JPMO.

System Development and Demonstration

During the system development and demonstration phase, the systems integrator, in conjunction with commercial partners, develops validated processes and produces consistency lots and conducts Phase 2 (expanded safety) human studies, definitive animal efficacy studies, and complete toxicology studies. During this phase, the systems integrator files the new drug application or other necessary regulatory documentation and requests FDA submission review. Items carried by service members undergo developmental and initial operational tests and evaluations during this phase. The system development and demonstration phase concludes with FDA approval of the pharmaceutical.

Production and Deployment

As the production and deployment phase begins, products are stockpiled, and post-marketing surveillance is conducted. The MITS JPMO begins investigating post-production support plans and shelf life extension program efforts while monitoring product stability. Initial operating capability for drug development is achieved when the FDA approves the product and the contractor can ensure adequate and efficient manufacturing capability. The initial operating capability is calculated as 1/x of the troop equivalent doses required for full operating capability, with x being the threshold shelf life. Full operating capability is achieved when the required FDA-approved troop equivalent doses have been produced for the stockpile.

Operations and Support Phase

The MITS JPMO remains responsible for lifecycle management of the approved pharmaceuticals through the operations and support phase of acquisition sustainment, maintaining and safeguarding the industrial capacity to support full production, and addressing regulatory issues such as long-term human safety studies, shelf life extension, and post-marketing surveillance (ie, Phase 4 clinical trials). MITS transfers procurement and logistical management to medical logistics organizations, such as the Defense Supply Center Philadelphia or the US Army Medical Materiel Agency, once initial stockpile quantities are in place. Funding for maintaining the stockpile in the operations and support phase is the responsibility of the individual services.

Acquisition Manufacturing Strategy

The technology base develops a laboratory-scale manufacturing process that is capable of producing only small quantities of drug product. This process must be transferred to a manufacturing facility that adheres to cGMPs and development efforts initiated to ensure technology can be duplicated or new processes pursued. One or more small cGMP pilot lots are manufactured for use in the Phase 1 and 2 clinical trials and animal toxicity studies. Scaling up the manufacturing process, rather than producing additional lots at the smaller scale, can result in significant cost and schedule savings. The manufacturing process is validated and consistency lots are manufactured concurrent with Phase 2 trials. After FDA approval, replenishment lots are produced to meet requirements, depending on the shelf life approved by the FDA for each product.

Acquisition Test and Evaluation Strategy

The acquisition of medical CBRN defense products for the DoD is tailored to comply with the requirements of both the DoD and the FDA. In a memorandum dated November 21, 2003, the deputy under secretary of the Army required every chemical or biological defense program, except IND programs, to have a test and evaluation master plan. IND applications accepted by the FDA must satisfy the test and evaluation master plan requirement for drug development programs and provide authority for testing drug products in human volunteers in accordance with Army Regulation 73-1, *Test and Evaluation Policy*. For soldier-carried items, a modified test and evaluation master plan must be executed to ensure compatibility and survivability of the item and its packaging.

Acquisition Business and Contracting Strategy

The MITS JPMO is responsible for the advanced development of medical CBRN drugs. Commercial, off-the-shelf medical products are normally procured through the medical logistics system or through procurement contracts issued directly to the vendor by the servicing government contract office.

If the MITS JPMO pursues product development, it will seek a contractor to serve as the systems integrator, generally releasing a request for proposal and making it available to full and open competition. If no commercial entity is identified to serve as the systems integrator, MITS will serve as the systems integrator for products transitioning from the technology base up to milestone B, at which point a contractor will be selected.

MITS streamlines acquisition by providing a performance-based statement of objectives (in lieu of a detailed statement of work) in the request for proposal, which might impede competition because of numerous specific requirements. A performance-integrated product team, consisting of representatives from MITS, the Joint Requirements Office, and the appropriate Joint Science and Technology Office capability area program office, oversees contractor performance in accordance with best commercial and government practices. Ad-hoc members are drawn from MITS, the US Army Medical Research and Materiel Command, the test and evaluation community, JPEO-CBD, the Office of the Secretary of Defense and other DoD offices, the Department of Health Human Services and other federal agencies, the technology base, or the logistics community, as needed. Working performance-integrated product teams are formed to address issues focused on a specific requirements area pertaining to the product.

The DoD, sponsored by the US Army Office of The Surgeon General, currently holds the INDs and approvals of medical chemical defense products. The decision to allow a commercial contractor to hold the IND and drug approval for future products is made on a case-by-case basis. An approach is recommended as soon as possible, even as early as milestone A. The recommendation is based on several factors, including commercial interest, interagency discussions, and intellectual property rights.

Specific Concerns in Medical Chemical Defense

The biggest challenge in medical acquisition within the DoD is that medical development is dictated by the process of obtaining FDA approval. In this chapter, the phrase "FDA approval" broadly applies to drugs, biologics, and medical devices. In its strictest sense, the term "approval" is usually reserved for drugs, while "licensure" is used for biologics and "clearance" is used for medical devices. All drugs, vaccines, or medical devices intended for use on or in service members are regulated by the FDA. In a pharmaceutical, vaccine, or medical device company, the steps required for obtaining FDA approval drive the drug development process. Within the DoD, however, medical acquisition is embedded within the acquisition model, which was designed around planes, ships, and tanks. Thus, the challenge is to match the DoD acquisition model with the process of pharmaceutical development and FDA approval, so decisions that would be made later in the process in nonmedical military acquisition programs must be made far earlier in the medical realm, allowing INDs to be submitted to the FDA on a timely basis. The challenge, specifically for the MITS JPMO, is to integrate the FDA regulatory and DoD acquisition processes.

The need for FDA approval of any fielded product may be self-evident but deserves comment nonetheless. In civilian medicine, any licensed physician may prescribe any FDA-licensed product, whether the product is for the licensed indication or for some other symptom. Countless examples exist of "off-label" medications approved for one indication but now primarily used for others. In acute nerve agent poisoning, however, patients must be treated far forward by buddies or medics and not by licensed physicians. In that case, only an FDA-approved product used on-label can legally be given by the buddy or medic. Until full FDA approval for this indication in 2003, the use of pyridostigmine bromide as a pretreatment against soman poisoning was an off-label use, notwithstanding the over 50 years of experience using it for patients with myasthenia gravis. Until the FDA approved pyridostigmine bromide specifically for soman intoxication pretreatment, the DoD planned to institute a process of informed consent for each service member, meaning each had the right to decline to use the drug for that purpose. Once FDA approval was obtained, however, the DoD acquired the right to order its service members to take the drug.

Peculiarities of medical chemical drug development create even greater challenges. For example, unlike a naturally occurring microbial illness, the disorders caused by chemical warfare agents are not expected to occur in the general population on a regular basis. Thus, the standard model for testing drugs in clinical trials is insufficient because exposing volunteers to chemical warfare agents is unethical. Consequently, the usual route for testing and demonstrating both safety and efficacy of medical countermeasures in humans is not feasible. In 2002 the FDA recognized this problem, unique to chemical and biological warfare countermeasure development, and released the animal rule. As a result, the FDA will consider approving medical chemical, biological, and radiological countermeasures when human safety data and sufficient animal efficacy data are presented without definitive human efficacy data. This rule allows for the submission of well-controlled animal efficacy data, in multiple species, to demonstrate that the product is likely to have clinical benefits in humans, in lieu of definitive human efficacy studies. So far, only two products have been fully licensed by the FDA under this rule, pyridostigmine bromide for pretreatment against soman poisoning, approved in 2003 (see Chapter 5, Nerve Agents), and hydroxocobalamin, approved as an antidote for cyanide poisoning in 2007. So far, the animal rule has only been used for products specifically intended for medical chemical defense, but several products in advanced development include plans to use the animal rule in their regulatory development strategies as necessary.

Another challenge encountered during medical chemical drug development concerns the specific indications for which a drug is used in medical chemical defense. Although all of the classical organophosphorus nerve agents work by inhibiting the enzyme acetylcholinesterase, under a narrow reading of the statute, to obtain FDA approval for all potentially encountered battlefield nerve agents, DoD would have to obtain FDA approval against each individual nerve agent. Instead, DoD plans to seek FDA approval for a whole class of acetylcholinesterase inhibitors. As mentioned earlier, pyridostigmine bromide carries pretreatment licensed indication only against soman. This issue is a matter of present discussion with the FDA, but remains unresolved.

Specific manufacturing challenges exist and are also of concern to the FDA and the advanced developer. Stereoisomers (chiral forms of molecules) and polymorphisms (multiple crystal forms of the same molecules) must always be considered and the licensed compound's purity must be ensured. Impurities must be removed or minimized and characterized. A specific medical chemical defense challenge is that drugs must often be formulated for compatibility and bioavailability in an autoinjector delivery system, which is rarely used in other drug development programs. This challenge was met by the antidote treatment nerve agent autoinjector (ATNAA) program, in which the actual dose of atropine in the autoinjector had to be modified.

STATUS OF ACQUISITION PROGRAMS OF RECORD

The programs of record in medical chemical defense within the DoD may be divided into three categories: lifecycle management products (fielded), sustainment programs (FDA-approved products; post-marketing or Phase 4 trials required), and advanced development programs (products not yet fielded).[5]

Lifecycle Management Products

Several products have gained full FDA approval for an intended indication and are presently fielded. The Mark I (Meridian Medical Technologies Inc, Bristol, Tenn) nerve agent antidote kit descends from the AtroPen (Meridian Medical Technologies Inc), an atropine autoinjector, first developed in the 1950s for nerve agent and insecticide poisoning (see Chapter 5, Nerve Agents). The Mark I kit consists of an atropine autoinjector and a second autoinjector containing 2-pralidoxime chloride (2-PAM Cl). It achieved FDA approval in the 1980s and is the mainstay of fielded nerve agent antidotes. As such, it has a large hold on the civilian and military markets. The Mark I is being phased out and replaced with the ATNAA.

The convulsant antidote nerve agent (CANA) is an autoinjector for intramuscular administration of 10 mg of diazepam. The CANA is used as an anticonvulsant for nerve agent poisoning and was FDA approved in December 1990. It is the only approved treatment specifically for nerve-agent–induced seizures. The autoinjector has a unique shape that allows a medic or buddy to distinguish it from Mark I, ATNAA, atropine-only, and other autoinjectors in a situation of light discipline.

The medical aerosolized nerve agent antidote (MANAA) is an aerosol inhaler that contains atropine and was developed as a follow-on treatment for nerve agent casualties under medical supervision. It is intended for use after administration of either Mark I or ATNAA and after the casualty has been decontaminated and transferred to a clean environment where protective suits and masks are not required. MANAA was intended to allow a medic to supervise a group of casualties who were capable of assisting with their own care. Theoretically, MANAA could free up medical personnel to treat more severely poisoned or injured casualties in a mass casualty situation. No other aerosolized treatment for nerve agent poisoning has been licensed by the FDA. MANAA was approved by the FDA in 1990.

MANAA is approaching the end of its shelf life. The manufacturer no longer maintains the cGMP manufacturing line required to produce MANAA. Under the Montreal Protocol, an international treaty created to phase out ozone-depleting substances, aerosolized products such as MANAA must be discontinued because they contain chlorofluorocarbons. A congressionally-funded program for a dry powder inhaler atropine (DPIA) seeks to develop a product that will replace the MANAA. DPIA is being developed jointly by a team that includes MicroDose Technologies, Inc, the University of Pittsburgh, and the MITS JPMO. DPIA is anticipated to be FDA approved in 2009, with fielding anticipated the following year.

ATNAA is a product developed to replace and improve upon the Mark I. It is a dual-chambered autoinjector that delivers 2.1 mg atropine (as compared to the 2 mg atropine in the Mark I) and 600 mg 2-PAM Cl through a single needle. ATNAA was approved by the FDA in January 2002 and fielding began in 2003. ATNAA delivers antidotes faster than Mark I because it uses a single autoinjector rather than two, cutting the time needed to administer life-saving treatment to a nerve agent casualty in half. ATNAA is also smaller, easier to use, and less expensive than the Mark I.

Sustainment Programs

Other products carry FDA approval but require Phase 4 (post-marketing) studies as mandated by the FDA. For example, the Skin Exposure Reduction Paste Against Chemical Warfare Agents (SERPACWA; Fisher Bioservices, Rockville, Md) is a perfluorohydrocarbon-based barrier cream intended to pretreat vulnerable skin areas (such as the groin, neck, wrists, armpits, waistline, and boot tops) prior to donning protective overgarments. SERPACWA provides a passive barrier that protects the skin from liquid chemical agent exposure for over 8 hours. While SERPACWA is meant to be used in conjunction with mission-oriented protective posture, some Special Forces units have inquired about its use without full mission-oriented protective posture protection. The FDA approved SERPACWA in February 2000 and the US Army has purchased initial quantities. SERPACWA also protects against many natural toxins as well, including poison ivy, suggesting a possible use in civilian medicine. However, SERPACWA is currently only approved for military use.

Studies are ongoing to determine the compatibility of SERPACWA with the M291 skin decontamination kit, a pouch containing six individual decontamination packets that can provide a total of three complete skin decontaminations. SERPACWA currently has an FDA-approved, 3-year shelf life, and is included in the FDA/DoD shelf life extension program.

Another FDA-approved product awaiting Phase 4 trials is soman nerve agent pretreatment pyridostigmine, which is distributed as 30 mg pyridostigmine bromide tablets. In February 2003, this pretreatment became the first drug to be approved by the FDA via the animal rule.

The FDA has mandated the following post-marketing studies for this product:

- a human serum study to correlate dose response between pyridostigmine bromide blood levels and red cell acetylcholinesterase inhibition;
- a guinea pig study to correlate blood pyridostigmine bromide levels, red cell acetylcholinesterase inhibition, tissue acetylcholinesterase inhibition, and the direct effects upon the diaphragm;
- a nonhuman primate study to look at the same questions as in the guinea pig; and
- an in vitro human intercostal muscle study to determine if pretreatment can provide partial protection to soman exposure of the muscle.

The first two studies are complete, the remaining studies are ongoing.

Products in Advanced Development

The joint service personnel/skin decontamination system (JSPDS) program is tasked with developing an improved skin decontamination capability through open competition between commercially available products. The current skin decontamination kit, M291, which has been fielded since 1989, is based on the Ambergard resin (Rohm and Haas, LLC, Philadelphia, Pa) that adsorbs and slowly detoxifies chemical agents. The JSPDS program is under the purview of the Joint Project Management Office for Decontamination, with medical consultation from MITS JPMO. The Joint Project Management Office for Decontamination competitively chose Reactive Skin Decontamination Lotion (RSDL; E-Z-EM, Inc, Lake Success, NY), developed by the Canadian Department of National Defence under a license from the Canadian Commercial Corporation, for evaluation against the JSPDS requirements. RSDL neutralizes and removes both vesicants and nerve agents from the skin. Clinical studies completed in 2006 show that RSDL can be safely used under ambient and heat-stressed conditions. Results from limited animal studies suggest that RSDL may be safely used around wounds, which is in contrast to M291, which cannot be used around wounds.

With an anticipated shortage of Ambergard resin in 2000, the JSPDS program planned to develop RSDL as a replacement for the M291 system and compared RSDL with M291 under a DoD foreign comparative testing program, aiming to obtain FDA approval. The FDA approved RSDL in 2003. The fielding decision was expected in 2007, but as of early December, it had not been made. RSDL costs considerably more than M291. Very recently, Rohm and Haas has resumed production of Ambergard, which will require considering the pros and cons of moving to field RSDL as a substitute, continuing to field M291, or using a combination of the two.

The advanced anticonvulsant system is the acquisition program that seeks to develop midazolam in an autoinjector as a replacement for the CANA, which contains diazepam, to treat nerve-agent–induced seizures (see Chapter 5, Nerve Agents). Midazolam is presently approved for other indications and has been marketed for many years as a central nervous system depressant, but it does not carry FDA approval as an anticonvulsant, despite being used as such in many clinical contexts in an off-label fashion. Consequently, the focus of the advanced anticonvulsant system program is to obtain FDA approval for midazolam against nerve-agent–induced seizures. Midazolam's action is onset faster and lasts longer than that of diazepam. There may also be less chance of respiratory depression with midazolam. If fully developed, midazolam will be an autoinjector product like CANA.

The regulatory developmental strategy for obtaining FDA approval for midazolam as an advanced anticonvulsant system includes using the animal rule. An IND application was submitted to the FDA in April 2006. The Phase 1 clinical study is complete. Developmental concerns with midazolam include the following:

- respiratory depression (although probably less than with diazepam),
- the number of nerve agents for which on-label indication would be sought,
- Phase 2 clinical studies including drug-to-drug interactions, if any, and
- any postmarketing studies the FDA may mandate.

Approval is planned no later than 2011.

The improved nerve agent treatment system program addresses the shortcomings of 2-PAM Cl as a reactivator of acetylcholinesterase. The program has two goals. The first is to expand the on-label indications for pyridostigmine bromide against more nerve agents than it is presently approved to treat. The second aim is to develop a new oxime, MMB4 dimethanesulfonate, to replace 2-PAM Cl. MMB4 was selected because its spectrum of action is broader than that of 2-PAM Cl for reactivating nerve-agent–inhibited acetylcholinesterase.

MMB4 is not FDA approved in the United States for several reasons. For example, one reason is that many compound polymorphs are present in MMB4, causing stability and solubility concerns. Other reasons are that the number of nerve agents for which an indication for MMB4 must be determined before approval can be granted, and the design of definitive animal studies (including determining the number of agents, animals, and comparisons against 2-PAM Cl that will be needed) must be designed. The regulatory development strategy for MMB4 includes requesting the use of the animal rule. An IND application submission is anticipated in 2008, followed by approval in 2013. Postmarketing studies may also be required by the FDA.

The bioscavenger program (see Chapter 7, Nerve Agent Bioscavenger: Development of a New Approach to Protect Against Organophosphorus Exposure) consists of three separate increments. Increment I is the plasma-derived human butyrylcholinesterase, which carries few immune potential concerns because it is a human product derived from human serum. The availability of this product is limited by the supply of human serum that is suitable for manufacture of a licensed product for use in humans. In addition, manufacture of plasma-derived human butyrylcholinesterase is extremely expensive. Therefore, Increment I is considered an interim solution to the bioscavenger problem from the acquisition standpoint. The DoD will develop this product through Phase 1 clinical trials, with completion scheduled for 2007. The contractor to the DoD is Dynport Vaccine Company, with Baxter Healthcare Corporation as subcontractor; Baxter Healthcare is the sponsor of the IND application, which was submitted to the FDA in May 2006.

The Increment II program will develop a product that is more easily and economically produced than Increment I. Increment II will mitigate technical risk by transitioning two different technologies (a recombinant human butyrylcholinesterase raised in a transgenic animal and a synthetic small molecule with bioscavenging activity) through Phase 1 clinical trials. Efforts will be tailored to each technology for evaluating and maturing that technology (recombinant or small molecule) and only one technology will be selected for acquisition program initiation at milestone B. The selected product will solve the problem of short supply and consequent expense that Increment I poses, but may create challenging safety concerns. An FDA-approved product is anticipated no earlier than 2013.

Increment III is envisioned as a catalytic scavenger of nerve agent, likely to be developed with site-directed mutagenesis. No candidate is yet ready for advanced development.

SUMMARY

Good science is not enough to protect service members against the threat of chemical warfare agents. A product must be developed and approved for human use by the FDA, doctrinally on-label for the envisioned use. It must also be manufactured, stockpiled, and delivered, and the user, whether a physician or the casualty's buddy, must know how to use it, which may require extensive training. Finally, the product must be managed throughout its lifecycle and closed out if deemed necessary or if a superior product replaces it. These tasks all fall under the medical chemical acquisition mission. The average licensed product costs \$400 to \$800 million[7–9] and the vast majority, 80% to 90% by some estimates, of products in development fail to obtain full licensure. While the clinician or medical planner need not know the details of the acquisition mission or of its constituent parts, it is vital to recognize that this process is time- and resource-consuming, yet necessary if military personnel are to have proper countermeasures available should the need arise.

REFERENCES

1. US Department of Defense. *Use of Investigational New Drugs for Force Health Protection*. Washington, DC: DoD; 2000. Directive 6200.2.

2. Executive Order 13139, "Improving Health Protection of Military Personnel Participating in Particular Military Operations," *Federal Register* 64 (1999): No. 192.

3. US Department of Defense. *The Defense Acquisition System*. Washington, DC: DoD; 2003. Directive 5000.1.

4. US Department of Defense. *Operation of the Defense Acquisition System*. Washington, DC: DoD; 2003. Instruction 5000.2.

5. General Services Administration, Department of Defense, and National Aeronautics and Space Administration. *Federal Acquisition Regulation*. Washington, DC: GSA, DoD, NASA; 2005.

6. 21 CFR, Parts 314, 601, Subpart 1.

7. Hollis WW. *Test and Evaluation (T&E) Policy for Chemical and Biological Defense Program (CBDP) Systems*. US Department of the Army, Under Secretary of the Army, Operations Research; 2005. Memorandum, 29 August 2005.

8. DiMasi JA, Hansen RW, Grabowski HG. The price of innovation: new estimates of drug development costs. *J Health Eco*. 2003:22;151–185.

9. Kaitin KI, ed. Post–approval R&D raises total drug development costs to \$897 million. *Tufts Center for the Study of Drug Development Impact Report*. 2003:5:3.

10. US Government Accountability Office. *New Drug Development: Science, Business, Regulatory, and Intellectual Property Issues Cited as Hampering Drug Development Efforts*. Washington, DC: GAO; 2006. Report to Congressional Requesters. 2206.

Chapter 21

MEDICAL MANAGEMENT OF CHEMICAL TOXICITY IN PEDIATRICS

ELORA HILMAS, PharmD, BCPS*; JAMES BROSELOW, MD†; ROBERT C. LUTEN, MD‡; and COREY J. HILMAS, MD, PhD§

**Clinical Pediatric Pharmacist and Pharmacy Practice Residency Coordinator, Department of Pharmacy, Alfred I. DuPont Hospital for Children, 1600 Rockland Road, Wilmington, Delaware 19803*

†Clinical Associate Professor, Emergency Medicine, University of Florida College of Medicine, 1329 SW 16th Street, Suite 2204, Gainesville, Florida 32610

‡Professor, Emergency Medicine, University of Florida College of Medicine, 1329-SW 16th Street, Suite 2204, Gainesville, Florida 32610; Attending, Pediatric Emergency Medicine, Department of Emergency Medicine, Shands Jacksonville Medical Center, 655 West 8th Street #1, Jacksonville, Florida 32209

§Research Pharmacologist and Physician, Neurobehavioral Toxicology Branch, US Army Medical Research Institute of Chemical Defense, 3100 Ricketts Point Road, Aberdeen Proving Ground, Edgewood Arsenal, Maryland 21010-5400

INTRODUCTION

Historically, chemical attacks were limited to the battlefield, and casualties were predominantly military personnel. Thus, the majority of knowledge concerning the medical management of chemical casualties has come from treating a military population. However, the modern global political climate has increased the likelihood of a chemical attack off the battlefield.[1–29] It is therefore prudent to understand the impact of chemical agents upon the pediatric population so children can be protected and treated efficiently in the event of an attack. Although pediatric recommendations are often extrapolated from adult data, pediatric patients should not be regarded as miniature adults; they present unique vulnerabilities and special considerations should be taken to care for them.

In response to the growing possibility of a chemical agent attack affecting children, several pediatric advocacy groups and physicians have commented on the urgent need for pediatric chemical casualty research. According to some, "we must learn to manage the consequences and limit the impact on the physical and mental health of our population, particularly our children."[30(p80)] The American Academy of Pediatrics has identified five forms of terrorism that require immediate attention: thermomechanical, biological, chemical, radiological, and psychological.[31] The committees on environmental health and infectious diseases have provided the following consensus statement regarding children and chemical and biological threats:

> Because children would be disproportionately affected by a chemical or biological weapons release, pediatricians must assist in planning for a domestic chemical-biological incident. Government agencies should seek input from pediatricians and pediatric subspecialists to ensure that the situations created by multiple pediatric casualties after a chemical-biological incident are considered.[32(p662)]

Emergency planners face numerous challenges when preparing for pediatric chemical casualties. Investigating the proper treatment of children during a chemical attack can be frustrating because of the limited primary literature on the subject.[33] This chapter will guide clinicians, nurses, pharmacists, and hospital administrators in preparing for and managing pediatric chemical casualties. It will briefly review the general principles of chemical agent exposure, vulnerabilities in children exposed to chemical agents, and the unique challenges encountered while managing pediatric casualties. Specific chemical agents, their effects on children, and management of their toxicities will be discussed, along with special considerations for the decontamination of children and specific strategies that hospitals and healthcare providers can follow to prepare for pediatric chemical casualties.

HISTORY OF CHEMICAL ATTACKS INVOLVING CHILDREN

As the September 11, 2001, attacks made clear, the terrorist threat has moved away from the traditional battlefield, making civilians, including children, prime targets for terrorists attempting to destabilize governments. Although this is a relatively new concern for the US population, other countries have dealt with similar threats for decades. In World War I, German shelling of French and Belgian communities with chemicals often resulted in civilian casualties, and participants saw how ill-prepared the general population was against such weapons. School-age children in the United States were taught protective measures against chemical attacks through drills in which they donned gas masks and evacuated simulated contaminated areas.

Although cyanide was used on concentration camp inmates in World War II, chemical weapons were not used in combat on civilian populations until the Iran-Iraq War. In the spring of 1987 Saddam Hussein bombed Sardasht, a city in Northwestern Iran, with mustard munitions, resulting in thousands of civilian casualties.[12,18] Unlike nerve agents, vesicants like mustard take hours to produce visible signs of toxicity (blisters), and the number of Sardasht victims (many of whom were children) increased in local hospitals over time. Dr Syed Abbas Foroutan, an Iranian physician, provided the first descriptions of chemical agent exposure in children in his published medical notes from the Iran-Iraq War: "children of various ages with swollen eyes moaned as they clinged [*sic*] to their mothers . . . some of the children were comatose."[18(p6)] Thousands of Sardasht residents became chemical casualties and many died, including several pediatric victims who suffered chronic pulmonary sequelae or died in intensive care unit wards days later.[18]

Following the attack on Sardasht, Iraq attacked Kurd settlements in early 1988, leading to the infamous attack on Kurdish residents of Halabja in March.[3,5–8,12,18,19] Thousands of civilian ethnic Kurds perished during the attacks, 75% of whom were women and children. Mustard and nerve agents were dropped on civilians from helicopters and planes, and eyewitnesses reported that large smoke clouds caused morbidity and mortality among children.[6]

In the 1990s the Japanese Aum Shinrikyo cult manufactured and used nerve agents to target civilians of Matsumoto and Tokyo (see Chapter 4).[24,26–28,32,34] In 1995 the Aum deployed the nerve agent sarin in a Tokyo subway attack, and approximately 5,000 people, ranging from 3 to 86 years old, sought medical attention.[32] Around the same time, the Federal Bureau of Investigation uncovered a terrorist plot to release a chlorine gas bomb at Disneyland.[32] These events confirm that chemical weapons pose a threat to the US pediatric population.

GENERAL PRINCIPLES OF CHEMICAL EXPOSURE

Chemical weapons include nerve agents, vesicating or blistering agents, choking or pulmonary irritants, cyanides, vomiting agents, incapacitating agents, and riot control agents.[35] The most important agents used for terrorism are nerve agents (tabun, sarin, soman, VX), vesicants (mustards, lewisite), pulmonary agents (phosgene, chlorine), and cyanide. Injury from each agent is related to its chemical properties (eg, volatility, persistence), route of entry, and dose.[36] Volatility, or an agent's tendency to vaporize, is affected by temperature, wind, and delivery method. Persistence, or the tendency of a liquid agent to remain in the environment, is affected by temperature and surface texture. The major routes of agent entry are inhalation, cutaneous absorption, ingestion, and injection. Exposure through inhalation, which often occurs with toxic agents like sarin and chlorine, may result in asphyxia, lung damage, and upper airway obstruction. Their higher metabolic and respiratory rates put children at increased risk for toxicity after chemical agent exposure, and their diminutive stature exposes children to toxic agents that concentrate closer to the ground.

The extent of an agent's toxicity is determined by the concentration of the agent in the air and the amount of time a person is exposed. Low doses of agent can cause symptoms such as airway irritation, bronchospasm, and increased secretions, exacerbating underlying lung diseases. High doses can result in airway edema, obstruction, and copious secretions. Direct alveolar damage from pulmonary toxicants, such as chlorine or phosgene, can result in pulmonary edema. When managing affected patients, it is necessary to anticipate the need for emergency intubation; children's smaller airway calibers put them at greater risk for airway obstruction and lead to more rapid progression of narrowing and impending airway obstruction.

Cutaneous exposure affects the eyes and skin, and corrosive chemicals can cause ischemic necrosis that results in small vessel thrombosis, especially in the eyes. Acidic or alkali chemical burns can result in coagulation necrosis or liquefaction. Skin absorption can lead to systemic toxicity, and when skin is damaged, transepidermal water loss is inevitable. This is especially concerning because hypovolemic shock can occur when water loss is excessive. Extensive skin loss, prolonged exposure, and the temperature of the water used for decontamination can rapidly lead to hypothermia in children, whose surface-to-volume ratio is greater than that of adults.

Negative pressure, full-face gas mask use by untrained civilians is not a recommended method of preventing chemical toxicity.[37] Gas masks and respirators increase the work of breathing and physiologic dead space, factors that tend to reduce alveolar ventilation. Also, respirators require a proper fit and filter canister maintenance to adequately protect users, and canister integrity can be altered by handling, water damage, and excessive breathing pressure. In Israel, improper use of gas masks led to 13 suffocation deaths in adults when the filter caps were not removed, and 114 adult deaths from cardiorespiratory arrest when the masks were used in sealed rooms.[37]

In general, managing children exposed to chemical agents may be challenging. For example, it may be difficult to obtain vascular access in children because they have smaller caliber blood vessels than adults. Urinary catherization may also be challenging. Healthcare practitioners should be aware of and appropriately prepare for these issues by maintaining trained staff and a supply inventory that includes a range of equipment sizes; because there is no single pediatric size, a range of appropriate pediatric-sized equipment must be available.

CHALLENGES TO MANAGING PEDIATRIC CHEMICAL CASUALTIES

Managing pediatric victims of chemical terrorism is especially difficult. In addition to the obvious physiological and anatomical differences between children and adults (Table 21-1), there are important psychological and behavioral differences that put children at risk.[33] Anecdotal reports have claimed that children are likely to be the first to manifest symptoms, to develop more severe manifestations, and to be hospitalized for other related illnesses after chemical agent exposure. Children's smaller mass reduces the dose of toxic agent needed

TABLE 21-1

PEDIATRIC VULNERABILITIES AND IMPLICATIONS FOR CLINICAL MANAGEMENT

	Unique Vulnerability in Children	Implications and Impact From Chemical Toxicity
Body composition	• Larger BSA compared to body mass • Lower total lipid / fat content	• Greater dermal absorption • Less partitioning of lipid-soluble components
Volume status	• More prone to dehydration • Chemical agents lead to diarrhea and vomiting	• Can be more symptomatic and show signs of severe dehydration
Respiratory	• Increased basal metabolic rate compared to greater minute volume	• Enhanced toxicity via inhalational route
Blood	• Limited serum protein binding capacity • Greater cutaneous blood flow	• Potential for greater amount of free toxicant and greater distribution • Greater percutaneous absorption
Skin	• Thinner epidermis in preterm infants • Greater cutaneous blood flow	• Increased toxicity from percutaneous absorption of chemical agents
Organ size and enzymatic function	• Larger brain mass • Immature renal function • Immature hepatic enzymes	• Greater CNS exposure • Slower elimination of renally cleared toxins, chemicals, and metabolites • Decreased metabolic clearance by hepatic phase I and II reactions
Anatomical considerations	• Short stature means breathing occurs closer to ground where aerosolized chemical agents settle • Smaller airway • Greater deposition of fine particles in the upper airway • Higher proportion of rapidly growing tissues	• Exposure to chemicals can have significant impact on bone marrow and developing CNS • Increased airway narrowing from chemical-agent–induced secretions • Mustard significantly affects rapidly growing tissues
Central nervous system	• Higher BBB permeability • Rapidly growing CNS	• Increased risk of CNS damage
Miscellaneous	• Immature cognitive function • Unable to flee emergency • Immature coping mechanisms	• Inability to discern threat, follow directions, and protect self • High risk for developing PTSD

BBB: blood-brain barrier
BSA: body surface area
CNS: central nervous system
PTSD: posttraumatic stress disorder

to cause observable or lethal effects. Studies involving organophosphates (OPs), compounds related to nerve agents, have shown greater vulnerability in immature animals than in adults. Some OPs produce the same degree of lethality in juveniles at a fraction of the dose that produces lethality in adults.[33] The increased toxicity seen in children compared to adults from various routes of exposure can be attributed to a wide variety of factors:

- differences in anatomy,
- allometric scaling factors (eg, increased surface area-to-volume ratio),
- cardiovascular status,
- permeability of the pediatric blood-brain barrier,
- dermatologic factors (eg, increased cutaneous blood flow),
- increased skin pH,
- plasma protein binding,
- volume of distribution,
- organ size and maturity, and
- pharmacokinetic maturity (eg, metabolic differences).[38–42]

These unique anatomical and physiological features cause pediatric rates of absorption, distribution, metabolism, and excretion to differ from those of adults.

Respiratory Vulnerability

Children may inhale greater doses of toxic agents than adults, as seen in some studies that demonstrate a 2-fold increase in children's respiratory tract exposure (per unit of surface area) as compared to adults. Children ages 7 to 14 have also been observed to have a higher deposition of fine particles than adults when the data are normalized by lung surface area[43] (younger children show an even greater deposition[44]). Children's higher respiratory rates and minute volumes (per respiratory surface area) means that they will inhale a greater dose of a toxic chemical vapor,[33] and children can easily become intoxicated by breathing air that is closer to the ground because many toxic chemicals display a high vapor density.[45] Additionally, children's respiratory accessory muscles can endure less than adults', putting them at greater risk for respiratory failure.

Children's respiratory systems are especially susceptible to chemical intoxication when compared to adults. Their unique anatomical differences include a greater degree of subglottic narrowing, diminished airway diameter, tendency for nose-breathing, and large tongue size relative to the mouth.[33] OP nerve agents induce bronchospasm and copious glandular secretions during a cholinergic crisis, which would further restrict airflow.

Volume Status Vulnerability

Children's circulatory systems can be severely affected by chemical attacks[33] because they have lower fluid reserves than adults, and small fluid volume losses can cause significant effects. For example, a 5-kg child experiencing severe dehydration (15% body weight loss), loses 750 mL of fluid. The significant loss of fluid from the gastrointestinal tract that results from chemical-induced glandular secretions can affect intravascular volume. Also, children are more prone to vomiting and diarrhea than adults. Overall, children may dehydrate faster during a chemical event.[45]

Neurological Vulnerability

Children's immature central nervous systems (CNSs) can also make them more susceptible to chemical toxicity than adults.[33] Toxic agents can traverse children's immature blood-brain barriers. Infants and children are already at greater risk of seizures than adults, which is concerning because seizures are common in cases of moderate to severe nerve agent intoxication. Infants are at the highest risk from chemical toxicity because of their susceptibility to neurotransmitter system imbalances. Prolonged seizures, or status epilepticus, can cause neuronal injury and deficits in the normal brain development of children.

Dermatologic Vulnerabilities

Barrier thickness, cutaneous blood flow, surface-to-volume ratio, temperature, hydration, and skin pH are important factors to consider when assessing pediatric dermatologic vulnerabilities. Newborns' skin, while appearing vulnerable, has the same histologic features of adult skin, with some differences, including immaturity of collagen, hair follicles, and sebaceous glands. Although newborns and young children are often described as having thinner skin than adults, and even though the stratum corneum, the most superficial layer of the skin, is thinner in premature infants compared to full-term infants, children, or adults,[46–50] children's skin does not differ significantly compared to that of adults when measuring its physiological parameters (eg, transepidermal water loss, skin pH, and stratum corneum capacitance and conductance).[38] Three-month-old children have the same abdominal skin stratum corneum thickness as older children and adults.[42]

However, children have larger surface-area-to-volume (mass) ratios, resulting in greater potential for chemical absorption, and the skin surface area of infants and toddlers is especially large compared to their body weight. A typical infant weighs about one twentieth of a 70-kg adult male, and has a surface area about one eighth as great; therefore the total skin surface area exposed per kilogram of body weight in infants is 2.5 times that of adults.[36] Burns that result in extensive skin loss, as seen with certain chemical exposures, can cause significant water loss and toxicity in children.[36]

Plasma Protein Binding, Volume of Distribution, and Organ Maturity

Children may experience increased effects from chemical toxicity because they have lower levels of plasma proteins. Neonates have a low protein binding capacity for albumin and alpha-1-glycoprotein[51–53] and a decreased ability to conjugate and excrete bilirubin, which binds to plasma proteins. This can lead to a smaller pool of available protein binding sites in plasma.[54] A lower serum protein binding capacity equates to a greater fraction of free chemical available in the circulation and increased toxicity.

The volume of distribution (liters per kilogram of body weight) of chemicals and drugs is also an important factor to consider in pediatric patients. Water-soluble chemicals may tend to have a larger volume of distribution in newborns and infants because of their relatively large water content. On the other hand, toxic lipophilic agents, such as nerve agents, are decreased in their partitioning to fat because of the lower body lipid content in young children compared to older children and adults.[52,53,55] Lower fat stores may cause lipophilic agents to reach higher concentrations in children's plasma than they would in adults'.

Organ size relative to body weight is another factor affecting the tissue distribution of chemicals in children. Young children's brains are disproportionately large and their blood-brain barriers are relatively permeable, which leads to higher concentrations of some chemicals in the brain.[56] Liver mass relative to body weight is greatest in the early postnatal period, and other tissues (eg, liver, kidney, lung, and brain) undergo rapid growth during the first 2 years of life;[57] these organs are all at increased risk from toxicity because of children's disproportionately larger size relative to body weight.

Renal clearance is particularly diminished in children compared to adults. Glomerular filtration rate and transporter (secretory) systems in the proximal convoluted tubule are decreased at birth.[52,55] In addition, although cardiac output is higher in children than in adults, a lower percentage of the output reaches the kidneys,[54] decreasing renal clearance even further and leading to greater plasma levels of toxic agent. The parental forms of nerve agents and their metabolites undergo hydrolysis with predominantly renal elimination; however, renal clearance is faster in children compared to adults because of allometric scaling differences. According to the rules of allometric scaling, smaller organisms have greater respiratory rates, cardiac output, nutrient and oxygen demands, and basal metabolic rates compared to larger organisms. This appears to be true for children, although faster metabolic rates are not seen in neonates because of hepatic enzyme immaturity and reduced hepatic clearance (which lead to a prolonged toxic agent half-life and duration of action).

Metabolic Vulnerability

Children are unable to detoxify as efficiently as adults because they have less mature metabolic systems.[33] In particular, phase I oxidative systems, phase II conjugating systems, and other systems (eg, serum esterases, hydrolases, dehydrogenases) are all immature in children compared to adults. Neonates and children up to 1 year old are most affected in their maturing enzymatic function, with the greatest effect seen in the first 2 months of life. This leads to slower metabolic clearance of many drugs, toxic chemicals, and activated metabolites.[54] In addition, several authors have reported a reduced activity of acetylcholinesterases (AChEs), pseudocholinesterases, and arylesterases (eg, paraoxonase, the enzyme that detoxifies OP pesticides) in premature and full–term newborns.[55–61] These levels do not reach adult levels until a child is about 1 year old.[62] Newborns possess half the paraoxonase found in an average adult.[33] Other studies suggest that newborns have paraoxonase levels 4-fold lower and activities 3-fold lower than their mothers.[63]

Traumatic Injury Vulnerability

Because chemical agents are often dispersed through explosive devices, trauma and injury frequently accompany chemical attacks.[64] Traumatic injury patterns differ in children compared to adults; because of their smaller size, multiple trauma occurs more frequently in children than in adults after a chemical attack. Children often sustain more head trauma because of their relatively larger head size and weaker supportive musculature, and their more compliant skeletal systems provide less protection to internal organs, leading to greater internal injuries without overlying fractures.

Neurobehavioral Vulnerability

Immature cognitive function can also put children at risk during a chemical attack.[33] Children often lack the ability to discern threat and to protect themselves, and infants, toddlers, and young children do not have the motor skills to flee from incident sites.[32] This can adversely impact their avoidance of a contaminated area and can interrupt decontamination in the event of exposure. During decontamination, healthcare workers and emergency personnel must have a plan for dealing with children who have been separated from their caregivers. Children may need to be guided through the decontamination process.[65]

Psychological Vulnerability

Children have fewer coping skills when sustaining or witnessing injury that can produce short- or long-term psychological trauma, such as parental or sibling death.[66] Children involved in attacks often suffer from posttraumatic stress disorder (PTSD).[32] Adult reactions to a chemical event can also make managing children difficult. Children are often influenced by the emotional states of their caregivers, so providers must try to remain calm. Also, fear or discomfort may cause children to disobey or act out against care providers (Table 21-2).[31]

TABLE 21-2

MARK I* KIT DOSING FOR CHILDREN WITH SEVERE, LIFE-THREATENING NERVE AGENT TOXICITY†

Approximate Age (in years)	Approximate Weight	Number of Kits to Use	Atropine Dosage Range (mg/kg)	Pralidoxime Dosage Range (mg/kg)
3–7	13–25 kg	1	0.08–0.13	24–46
8–14	26–50 kg	2	0.08–0.13	24–46
> 14	> 51 kg	3	0.11 or less	35 or less

*Meridian Medical Technologies Inc, Bristol, Tenn.
†If an adult Mark I kit is the only available source of atropine and pralidoxime, it should not be withheld even from children under 3 years old.
Data source: Columbia University Mailman School of Public Health. Atropine use in children after nerve gas exposure. *Info Brief.* 2004;1(1):1–8.

Decontamination Equipment and Treatment Supplies

Decontamination equipment is another barrier to emergency management because it is not necessarily designed for use on children. High-pressure hoses and cold water used to decontaminate victims can expose children to significant risk,[45] resulting in hypothermia and skin damage. Also, emergency care providers often need to wear bulky, full-protective suits when treating victims, and these suits make it difficult to manage small children requiring intricate procedures, such as blood draws.

In addition to inappropriate decontamination equipment, antidotes for chemical agents are not often available in ready-to-administer pediatric dosages. In the event of a chemical attack, pediatric healthcare centers may be overwhelmed, and the ability to expand the number of pediatric hospital beds may be limited.[32] Additionally, most healthcare workers are not fully aware of the signs and symptoms of chemical agent exposure. This problem is exacerbated because children typically present differently than adults.

For certain toxic agents, such as nerve agents, children present a clinical picture that can be very different than that observed in adults. For example, children in cholinergic crisis may not necessarily manifest with miosis (constriction of pupils).[33] One case series demonstrated the absence of miosis in 43% of pediatric victims. Studies involving pediatric exposure to OPs have suggested the appearance of isolated CNS effects (such as stupor and coma) in the absence of peripheral muscarinic effects. Pediatric victims of OP intoxication display significant muscular weakness and hypotonia in the absence of glandular secretions in 70% to 100% of cases involving moderate to severe levels of exposure.[33] The presentation of central intoxication (weakness and hypotonia) from OPs without peripheral muscarinic signs and symptoms is atypical in adults.

EFFECTS OF SPECIFIC AGENTS ON A PEDIATRIC POPULATION

Nerve Agents

Nerve agent exposure can quickly incapacitate victims and can lead to mortality if not recognized and treated promptly (Exhibit 21-1). Nerve agent toxicity can be enhanced in children because of their unique pediatric vulnerabilities, and it is important to recognize the different ways children may present with toxicity compared to adults.

Nerve agents include tabun, sarin, cyclosarin, soman, and VX. These agents are clear, colorless, tasteless, and in most cases, odorless. They have been demonstrated to penetrate clothing and skin and are highly toxic (as little as 10 mg of VX on the skin is considered to be the median lethal dose in adults).[33] In addition, nerve agents produce toxicity rapidly compared to biological agents. Most G-series nerve agents (sarin, designated "GB" by the North Atlantic Treaty Organization [NATO]; cyclosarin, NATO designation "GF"; tabun, NATO designation "GA"; and soman, NATO designation "GD") are highly volatile and can be dispersed into aerosols and inhaled by victims. Nerve agents may also be disseminated in liquid form. Treatment for dermal exposure begins with rapid topical decontamination.

Although military experience managing nerve agent toxicity is limited, exposures to related chemicals, such as the OP class, occur commonly each year in the United States (in 2000 there were approximately 10,000 OP exposures across the country).[67] OPs, such as malathion, are commonly used as pesticides, and toxicity manifests similarly to nerve agent toxicity,

EXHIBIT 21-1

CASE HISTORY: NERVE AGENT EXPOSURE IN NAZHMAR, IRAN

One victim of the March 22, 1988, attack on the village of Nazhmar was a young child of unreported age and weight. He presented immediately with marked miosis and was comatose. His breathing was irregular and foamy secretions were protruding from his mouth and nose. The patient was working very hard to breathe and was noted to be using his accessory muscles of respiration. Wheezing was obvious on auscultation, and he showed obvious difficulty on exhalation. Upon suction removal of oral and nasal secretions, the patient was noted to have progressively rigid extremities; finding venous access became difficult. His secretions became bloody. Over a 15-minute period, a total of 7.5 mg atropine was administered in three treatments. The patient was noted to improve, opening his eyes, moaning, and using two-word phrases. As his muscle tone decreased, his breathing improved, but wheezing was still evident. The child was decontaminated after treatment and subsequently discharged after an hour. At the time of discharge, his secretions were not completely dried up, but his pupils were fully dilated and reactive to light.

Data source: Foroutan SA. Medical notes concerning chemical warfare, Part IX. *Kowsar Med J*. 1996;3(3):1–16.

though OPs are considerably less toxic. One case series of 16 children who experienced OP poisonings confirmed that pediatric patients present with toxicity differently than adults; they often do not manifest the classic muscarinic effects, such as salivary secretions and diarrhea, seen in adults.[68]

Mechanism of Toxicity

Nerve agents inhibit esterase enzymes, especially AChE,[33] preventing the hydrolysis of acetylcholine. When acetylcholine accumulates in the synaptic space of neurons, muscarinic and nicotinic receptors are over stimulated, resulting in cholinergic crisis. The nerve-agent–AChE bond also undergoes a reaction called "aging,"[69] irreversibly inactivating the enzyme. Prompt therapy is needed to prevent irreversible toxicity.

Clinical Presentation

The signs and symptoms of cholinergic crisis range from lacrimation and urination to seizure activity (Exhibit 21-2).[33] Cholinergic crisis manifests individually depending on the dose, route of exposure, and the duration of exposure. Death from nerve agent exposure is primarily attributed to respiratory failure; nerve agents cause central apnea, flaccid neuromuscular paralysis, bronchoconstriction, and profound glandular secretions.

Children in cholinergic crisis may not exhibit constricted pupils, salivation, diarrhea, or miosis, but may present with isolated CNS effects. Because there is no literature detailing the long-term effects of nerve agent poisoning in children, speculations must be extrapolated from what has been observed in the adult population.[33] Surveillance of victims of the sarin attacks in Japan revealed a wide range of sequelae, such as continued respiratory problems, vision disturbances, headache, and fatigue. Neuropsychiatric problems have also been reported as a delayed effect.

Laboratory Findings

Use of cholinesterase levels to confirm and treat nerve agent toxicity is limited,[33] so casualty treatment should not be delayed for the results of these studies or until cholinesterase levels return to normal. Levels should be used after exposure only to confirm diagnosis (after treatment has begun), to monitor recovery, or for forensic investigation.

EXHIBIT 21-2

MNEMONIC FOR CHOLINERGIC CRISIS

BAG the PUDDLES

- **B**: bronchoconstriction
- **A**: apnea
- **G**: graying/dimming of vision
- **P**: pupillary constriction (miosis)
- **U**: urination
- **D**: diaphoresis
- **D**: defecation
- **L**: lacrimation
- **E**: emesis
- **S**: seizures

Data source: Rotenberg JS, Newmark J. Nerve agent attacks on children: diagnosis and management. *Pediatrics*. 2003;112:648–658.

Pediatric Vulnerability

A child's smaller mass alone reduces the dose of nerve agent needed to cause symptoms or lethality. For volatile nerve agents, children are especially at risk for respiratory effects from toxicity. Their smaller airways can become compromised by copious secretions and by bronchospasm after nerve agent exposure. Also, a greater dose of nerve agent is inhaled by children than adults because of their higher respiratory rates and minute volumes.

Treatment

The overall approach to treating nerve agent exposure focuses on airway and ventilatory support, aggressive use of antidotes (atropine and pralidoxime), prompt control of seizures, and decontamination, as necessary.[70] Atropine is used for its antimuscarinic effects, and oxime is used to reactivate AChE. The combination of atropine and pralidoxime chloride (2-PAM Cl) is recommended for the prompt treatment of all serious cases, and timing atropine and 2-PAM Cl administration is critical; the faster these antidotes are given, the better the outcome. Oxime therapy is rendered ineffective if given after the enzyme aging process has been completed,[69] so autoinjectors have been developed to rapidly administer intramuscular (IM) doses of these medications. However, the US Food and Drug Administration (FDA) has yet to approve a pediatric 2-PAM Cl autoinjector. Other administration routes and methods include intravenous (IV) or intraosseous administration for atropine, and slow IV or continuous infusion for 2-PAM Cl. Data show that plasma concentrations of autoinjector medications peak in less than 5 minutes, as opposed to 25 minutes for IM administration using a needle and syringe.[33] Adult nerve intoxication therapy typically includes the use of an autoinjector set that provides both antidotes, called the Mark I kit (Meridian Medical Technologies Inc, Bristol, Tenn; see Chapter 5, Nerve Agents). The Mark I kit delivers 600 mg of 2-PAM Cl and 2 mg of atropine (via an autoinjector called the AtroPen [Meridian Medical Technologies Inc, Bristol, Tenn]) in seconds. It was originally developed for administration to soldiers. The autoinjector uses a spring-loaded needle to disperse medication in an "all-or-nothing" fashion, so it is impossible to give partial doses of an autoinjector for children, but Mark I kits can be given in their entirety to children beginning at age 3 (see Table 21-2). Drug dosing of atropine and 2-PAM Cl in pediatrics is primarily weight based, so a standard dose cannot be used. Pediatric versions of the Mark I kit are available overseas but are not currently available in the United States.[71] In June 2003 the FDA approved pediatric doses of the AtroPen to respond to the lack of pediatric-specific therapy.[72] The AtroPen is now available in four dosages, 0.25 mg, 0.5 mg, 1 mg, and 2 mg (Figure 21-1). The autoinjector needle length is 0.8 inches, with a gauge of 22. Because the AtroPen delivers only atropine and not 2-PAM Cl, the prompt treatment of pediatric nerve agent casualties remains limited. This has caused groups such as the pediatric expert advisory panel from the National Center for Disaster Preparedness to recommend the adult Mark I kit (which contains atropine and 2-PAM Cl) before use of the pediatric AtroPen alone.[71] Meridian Medical Technologies has recently received FDA approval for a dual-chambered autoinjector called the "ATNAA" (antidote treatment nerve agent autoinjector) for the military, and Duodote (Figure 21-2) for civilian emergency medical technicians and first responders. Each autoinjector contains 2 mg of atropine sulfate and 600 mg of 2-PAM Cl, which are injected sequentially.

In 1992 Amitai et al reviewed 240 instances of accidental pediatric atropine injections using adult-dose–based autoinjectors.[73] The study authors found a low incidence of toxicity and no seizures, arrhythmias,

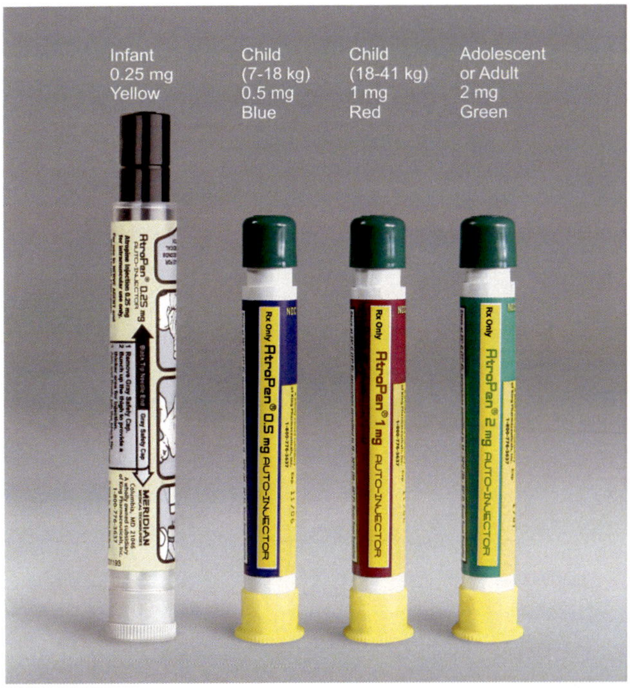

Figure 21-1. The AtroPen pediatric autoinjector, manufactured by Meridian Medical Technologies Inc, Bristol, Tenn. Dose sizes range from 0.25 mg for infants to 0.5 mg for children 7–18 kg, 1 mg for children 18–41 kg, and 2 mg for adolescents and adults.

Reproduced with permission from: Meridian Medical Technologies Inc, Bristol, Tenn.

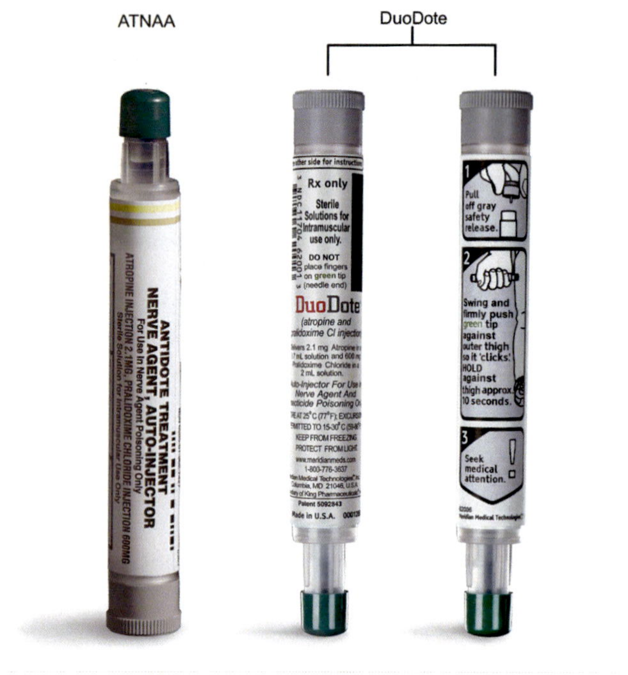

Fig. 21-2. Antidote treatment nerve agent autoinjector (ATNAA) and Duodote.
Reproduced with permission from: Meridian Medical Technologies Inc, Bristol, Tenn.

or death. Subsequently, several pediatric guidelines have suggested that adult-dose atropine and 2-PAM Cl autoinjectors can be safely used in children larger than 13 kg and inserted to 0.8 inches.

Atropine and 2-PAM Cl must be administered cautiously.[33] Atropine can cause increased heart rate and dry mouth and skin, and near vision can be affected for up to 1 day. It can also prevent sweating, so elevated temperatures and heat stress may be observed. 2-PAM Cl can cause double or blurred vision and dizziness, and doses must be reduced with renal insufficiency. Laryngospasm and rigidity can occur if the medication is given too quickly via IV. Higher doses can cause hypertension, while lower doses can cause minor electrocardiogram changes.

Benzodiazepines are not considered antidotes to nerve agent poisoning; however, because status epilepticus often occurs as nerve agent crosses the blood-brain barrier and causes irritation, they are the only agents that have been proven to treat nerve-agent–induced seizures and should be used for both prevention and treatment.[33] Benzodiazepines should be quickly administered if consciousness or more than one organ is impaired or if there is muscle twitching. The US military uses the benzodiazepine diazepam, administered via an autoinjector, to prevent and treat status epilepticus (Figure 21-3). Israel is moving toward using midazolam for its population. Some physicians recommend using lorazepam in the pediatric population. Regardless of which medication is administered, repeated dosing may be needed. Benzodiazepines should be considered for the pediatric population if seizure activity is suspected. However, nonconvulsive status epilepticus and subtle seizures are common in infants and children, making it difficult for healthcare providers to recognize these as signs of nerve agent toxicity.

Each of the medications used to treat nerve agent toxicity recommend weight-based dosing for pediatric patients (Tables 21-3 and 21-4). The exact dosing for a specific patient depends on two factors: the severity of the exposure and the weight or age of the patient.

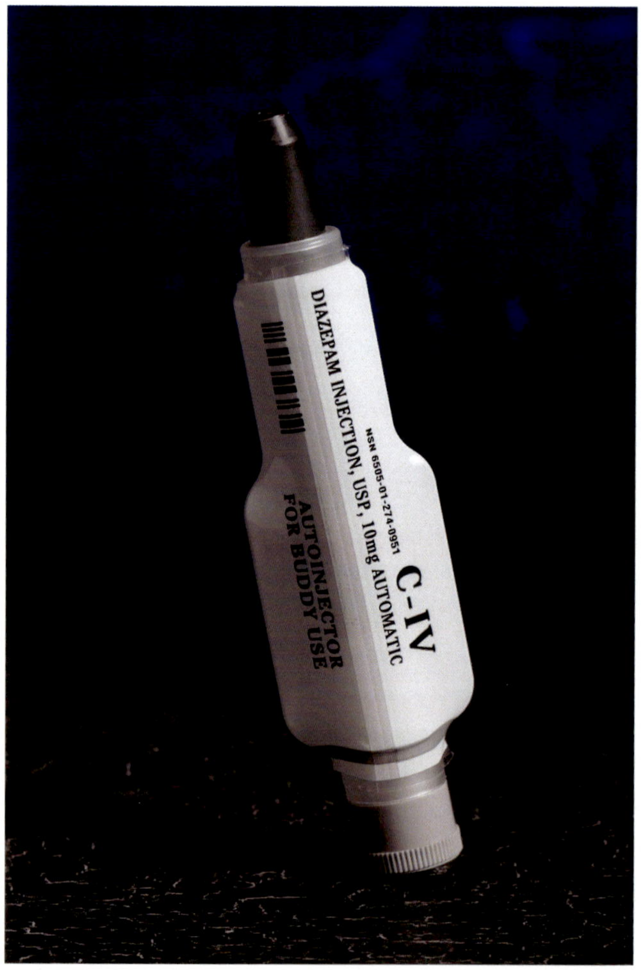

Fig. 21-3. The diazepam autoinjector.
Reproduced with permission from: Meridian Medical Technologies Inc, Bristol, Tenn.

TABLE 21-3

MANAGEMENT OF MILD TO MODERATE NERVE AGENT EXPOSURES

		Management			
		Antidotes[*]		Benzodiazepines (if neurological signs)	
Nerve Agents	Symptoms	Age	Dose	Age	Dose
• Tabun • Sarin • Cyclosarin • Soman • VX	• Localized sweating • Muscle fasciculations • Nausea • Vomiting • Weakness/floppiness • Dyspnea • Constricted pupils and blurred vision • Rhinorrhea • Excessive tears • Excessive salivation • Chest tightness • Stomach cramps • Tachycardia or bradycardia	Neonates and infants up to 6 months old	**Atropine** 0.05 mg/kg IM/IV/IO to max 4 mg or 0.25 mg AtroPen[†] and **2-PAM** 15 mg/kg IM or IV slowly to max 2 g/hr	Neonates	**Diazepam** 0.1–0.3 mg/kg/dose IV to a max dose of 2 mg, or **Lorazepam** 0.05 mg/kg slow IV
		Young children (6 months old–4 yrs old)	**Atropine** 0.05 mg/kg IM/IV/IO to max 4 mg or 0.5 mg AtroPen and **2-PAM** 25 mg/kg IM or IV slowly to max 2 g/hr	Young children (30 days old–5 yrs old)	**Diazepam** 0.05–0.3 mg/kg IV to a max of 5 mg/dose or **Lorazepam** 0.1 mg/kg slow IV not to exceed 4 mg
		Older children (4–10 yrs old)	**Atropine** 0.05 mg/kg IV/IM/IO to max 4 mg or 1 mg AtroPen and **2-PAM** 25–50 mg/kg IM or IV slowly to max 2 g/hr	Children (≥ 5 yrs old)	**Diazepam** 0.05–0.3 mg/kg IV to a max of 10 mg/dose or **Lorazepam** 0.1 mg/kg slow IV not to exceed 4 mg
		Adolescents (≥ 10 yrs old) and adults	**Atropine** 0.05 mg/kg IV/IM/IO to max 4 mg or 2 mg AtroPen and **2-PAM** 25–50 mg/kg IM or IV slowly to max 2 g/hr	Adolescents and adults	**Diazepam** 5–10 mg up to 30 mg in 8 hr period or **Lorazepam** 0.07 mg/kg slow IV not to exceed 4 mg

2-PAM: 2-pralidoxime
IM: intramuscular
IO: intraosseous
IV: intraveneous
PDH: Pediatrics Dosage Handbook
*In general, pralidoxime should be administered as soon as possible, no longer than 36 hours after the termination of exposure. Pralidoxime can be diluted to 300 mg/mL for ease of intramuscular administration. Maintenance infusion of 2-PAM at 10–20 mg/kg/hr (max 2 g/hr) has been described. Repeat atropine as needed every 5–10 minutes until pulmonary resistance improves, secretions resolve, or dyspnea decreases in a conscious patient. Hypoxia must be corrected as soon as possible.
†Meridian Medical Technologies Inc, Bristol, Tenn.
Data sources: (1) Rotenberg JS, Newmark J. Nerve agent attacks on children: diagnosis and management. *Pediatrics*. 2003;112:648–658. (2) Pralidoxime [package insert]. Bristol, Tenn: Meridian Medical Technologies, Inc; 2002. (3) AtropPen (atropine autoinjector) [package insert]. Bristol, Tenn: Meridian Medical Technologies, Inc; 2004. (4) Henretig FM, Cieslak TJ, Eitzen Jr EM. Medical progress: biological and chemical terrorism. *J Pediatr*. 2002;141(3):311–326. (5) Taketomo CK, Hodding JH, Kraus DM. *American Pharmacists Association: Pediatric Dosage Handbook*. 13th ed. Hudson, Ohio; Lexi-Comp Inc: 2006.

Perioperative Care of Children with Nerve Agent Intoxication

Chemical exposures and trauma often occur simultaneously, and surgical intervention is sometimes required. However, many drugs used for perioperative management can exacerbate the side effects of nerve agent exposure. For example, nerve agents can interact with medications typically used for resuscitative efforts.[74] Anesthetics, such as sodium pentothal and propofol, cause cardiac depression, which is intensified by the excessive muscarinic activity induced by nerve agents. Doses of these drugs may need to be reduced. Volatile anesthetics may be preferable because they

TABLE 21-4

MANAGEMENT OF SEVERE NERVE AGENT EXPOSURE

		Management			
		Antidotes*		Benzodiazepines (if neurological signs)	
Nerve Agents	Severe Symptoms	Age	Dose	Age	Dose
• Tabun • Sarin • Cyclosarin • Soman • VX	• Convulsions • Loss of consciousness • Apnea • Flaccid paralysis • Cardio-pulmonary arrest • Strange and confused behavior • Severe difficulty breathing • Involuntary urination and defecation	Neonates and infants up to 6 months old	**Atropine** 0.1 mg/kg IM/IV/IO or 3 doses of 0.25mg AtroPen[†] (administer in rapid succession) and **2-PAM** 25 mg/kg IM or IV slowly, or 1 Mark I[†] kit (atropine and 2-PAM) if no other options exist	Neonates	**Diazepam** 0.1–0.3 mg/kg/dose IV to a max dose of 2 mg, or **Lorazepam** 0.05 mg/kg slow IV
		Young children (6 months old–4 yrs old)	**Atropine** 0.1 mg/kg IV/IM/IO or 3 doses of 0.5mg AtroPen (administer in rapid succession) and **2-PAM** 25–50 mg/kg IM or IV slowly, or 1 Mark I kit (atropine and 2-PAM) if no other options exist	Young children (30 days old–5 yrs and adults	**Diazepam** 0.05–0.3 mg/kg IV to a max of 5 mg/dose, or **Lorazepam** 0.1 mg/kg slow IV not to exceed 4 mg
		Older children (4–10 yrs old)	**Atropine** 0.1 mg/kg IV/IM/IO or 3 doses of 1mg AtroPen (administer in rapid succession) and **2-PAM** 25–50 mg/kg IM or IV slowly, 1 Mark I kit (atropine and 2-PAM) up to age 7, 2 Mark I kits for ages > 7–10 yrs	Children (≥ 5 yrs old)	**Diazepam** 0.05-0.3 mg/kg IV to a max of 10 mg/dose, or **Lorazepam** 0.1 mg/kg slow IV not to exceed 4 mg
		Adolescents (≥ 10 yrs old) and adults	**Atropine** 6 mg IM or 3 doses of 2 mg AtroPen (administer in rapid succession) and **2-PAM** 1800 mg IV/IM/IO, or 2 Mark I kits (atropine and 2-PAM) up to age 14, 3 Mark I kits for ages ≥ 14 yrs	Adolescents and adults	**Diazepam** 5–10 mg up to 30 mg in 8-hr period, or **Lorazepam** 0.07 mg/kg slow IV not to exceed 4 mg

IM: intramuscular
IO: intraosseous
IV: intravenous

*In general, pralidoxime should be administered as soon as possible, no longer than 36 hours after the termination of exposure. Pralidoxime can be diluted to 300 mg/mL for ease of intramuscular administration. Maintenance infusion of 2-PAM at 10–20 mg/kg/hr (max 2 g/hr) has been described. Repeat atropine as needed every 5–10 min until pulmonary resistance improves, secretions resolve, or dyspnea decreases in a conscious patient. Hypoxia must be corrected as soon as possible. [†]Meridian Medical Technologies Inc, Bristol, Tenn.

Data sources: (1) Rotenberg JS, Newmark J. Nerve agent attacks on children: diagnosis and management. *Pediatrics*. 2003;112:648–658. (2) Pralidoxime [package insert]. Bristol, Tenn: Meridian Medical Technologies, Inc; 2002. (3) AtroPen (atropine autoinjector) [package insert]. Bristol, Tenn: Meridian Medical Technologies, Inc; 2004. (4) Henretig FM, Cieslak TJ, Eitzen Jr EM. Medical progress: biological and chemical terrorism. *J Pediatr*. 2002;141(3):311–326. (5) Taketomo CK, Hodding JH, Kraus DM. *American Pharmacists Association: Pediatric Dosage Handbook*. 13th ed. Hudson, Ohio: Lexi-Comp Inc; 2006.

bronchodilate and reduce the need for nondepolarizing drugs, which are often reversed by the use of neostigmine. Halothane should be avoided in infants because the cardiac side effects can be accentuated in the presence of nerve agents. Depression of the cardiovascular system by halothane may cause further bradycardia, hypotension, and reduction in cardiac output. In general, the use of muscle relaxants is not recommended in patients exposed to nerve agents. Nerve agents provide a depolarizing block, and in the presence of inhibited AChE activity, drugs such as succinylcholine can have longer effects than expected.[75]

Analgesia must be used carefully when caring for victims of nerve agent exposure.[74] In general, opioids are considered safe to use because they do not act on the cholinergic system directly. However, some side effects of the drugs, such as histamine release and rare muscle rigidity, can cause difficulty in patient management, making careful dose titration and side-effect monitoring critical. The potent opiod remifentanyl contains an ester linkage susceptible to hydrolysis because it is partially metabolized by plasma cholinesterase. This is the same enzyme that is inactivated by nerve agents, resulting in a prolonged duration of action for remifentanyl. Therefore, using remifentanyl in the postoperative care of nerve-agent–exposed victims is not recommended.[75]

Vesicants

Vesicants, or blister agents, are chemicals that cause blister or vesicle formation upon dermal contact (Exhibits 21-3 and 21-4). Agents such as mustards or lewisite have been used in chemical warfare in the past,[76] and although vesicants are less toxic than nerve agents, they cause prolonged morbidity. There are two types of mustard: sulfur mustard (also known as "HD") and nitrogen mustard (also known as "HN"). Sulfur mustard caused more casualties in World War I than any other chemical weapon. It also caused a significant number of casualties, both civilian and military, during the Iran-Iraq War in the 1980s. Sulfur mustard vapor is the vesicant most likely to be used by terror groups.[76] It affects multiple organ systems including skin, eyes, respiratory and gastrointestinal tracts, and bone marrow.[76] Nitrogen mustards, on the other hand, have never been used on the battlefield, probably because they are harder to make than sulfur mustards; thus, their potential use in a terrorist attack is unlikely.

Lewisite, a vesicant with sulfur-mustard–like properties, causes similar signs and symptoms involving the skin, eyes, and airways, as well as systemic effects (eg, increased capillary permeability) after absorption. However, lewisite does not suppress the immune system like mustard. Lewisite exposure can be treated with an antidote, British Anti-Lewisite. The mechanism of action, clinical effects, and treatment of lewisite injury are not discussed further in this chapter because they are reviewed elsewhere in this textbook (see Chapter 8: Vesicants).

Mechanism of Toxicity

Sulfur mustard rapidly penetrates cells and generates a highly toxic reaction that disrupts cell function and eventually causes cell death.[77] It is classified as an alkylating agent and targets poorly differentiated and rapidly reproducing cells.[76] Death results from massive pulmonary damage complicated by infection (see Chapter 8: Vesicants).

Clinical Presentation

Mustard can cause local effects on skin, airways, and eyes; however, large doses can cause fatal systemic effects.[76] In a study of clinical findings among children exposed to vesicants, the most prevalent signs of toxicity were ocular, cutaneous, and respiratory (Table 21-5).[78] Erythema occurs 4 to 8 hours after exposure, and pruritus can occur with or prior to erythema.[76,78] Over the 24 hours following exposure, large yellowish blisters form in areas of thin skin, such as the groin and underarms.[76] Eye damage can occur, ranging in spectrum from pain and irritation to blindness.[76,77] Mustard also causes clinical effects that can be delayed

EXHIBIT 21-3

CASE HISTORY: MUSTARD GAS EXPOSURE IN 14 CHILDREN AND TEENAGERS FROM HALABJA, IRAQ

Mustard gas was used on the civilian population during the Iraq-Iran War (1980–1988). A case series of 14 children and teenagers affected by mustard gas was reported by Momeni et al. They found that facial involvement was the most frequent disorder (78%), followed by genital (42%), trunkal and axillar lesions (both 14%). The most prominent laboratory abnormality was eosinophilia (12% of patients). Skin lesions appeared 4–18 hours after exposure and erythema developed within 20–30 hours. Blisters appeared after the erythema. The authors concluded that the time of toxicity onset was shorter and more severe in children and teenagers than in adults.

Data source: Momeni A, Aminjavaheri M. Skin manifestations of mustard gas in a group of 14 children and teenagers: a clinical study. *Inter J Dermatol*. 1994:33(3):184–187.

EXHIBIT 21-4

CLINICAL CASES OF MUSTARD EXPOSURE FROM MOFID MEDICAL CENTER FOLLOWING THE HALABJA, IRAQ, ATTACK ON MARCH 17, 1988

A 3-year-old male presented to Mofid Medical Center 8 days after the Halabja chemical attack with fever (39.5°C), tachycardia (HR 140 bpm), and tachypnea (RR 60). Cutaneous skin lesions were mild, but erythema and edema covered 45% of his skin surface area. Laboratory findings were unremarkable except for a mild anemia. Chest roentograms revealed hilar congestion and consolidation bilaterally. The fever continued despite antibiotic therapy. On day 10 of admission (18 days after exposure), the patient developed leukocytosis with 82% PMNs and worsening respiratory distress. The patient died 21 days after exposure.

An 8-year-old Iranian male presented at 5:30 PM with fever (40°C), severe agitation, delirium, and somnolence 24 hours after exposure to chemical agents. His blood pressure was 110/70 mmHg and the patient was notably tachycardic (HR 120 bpm) and tachypneic (RR 42). The patient was noted to have serious dermatologic, ocular, and respiratory impairment. Erythema, vesicles, erosions, bullae, ulcerations, and edema were present on 35% of his body. Ocular manifestations included conjunctivitis and palpebral edema. At that point, the patient was working hard to breathe, as evidenced from accessory muscles of respiration (sternocleidomastoid). On physical examination of the lungs, wheezing and crepitation were noted throughout all lung fields. Laboratory findings were the following:

- Na+: 139,
- K+: 4.1 mEq/l,
- BUN: 25 mg/dl,
- calcium: 7.3 mg/dl, and
- white blood cell count: 9900/mm^3 with 90% neutrophils.

Arterial blood gases were as follows:

- pH: 7.30,
- pCO_2: 31,
- pO_2: 65, and
- HCO_3: 15.1.

Chest roentograms showed bilateral infiltrates. The patient died 24 hours after admission and 48 hours after exposure, despite receiving supportive care.

A 12-year-old female presented 1 day after exposure with fever (40°C), agitation, somnolence and the following vitals:

- BP: 90/40,
- HR: 106 bpm, and
- RR: 36.

Skin erythema, edema, and lesions covered 45% of her body. Upon admission, labs revealed the following:

- Na+: 133,
- K+ 5.8: mEq/L,
- Calcium: 8.3 mg/dL,
- BUN: 51 mg/dL,
- Hematocrit: 50%, and
- white blood cell count: 20,000/mm^3 with 93% neutrophils.

(**Exhibit 21-4** *continues*)

Exhibit 21-4 *continued*

Arterial blood gases were as follows:

- pH: 7.27,
- pCO_2: 14,
- pO_2: 83, and
- HCO_3: 6.3.

Chest X-ray showed bilateral, diffuse infiltrates. Bone marrow hypoplasia developed within a few days. On day 5 of admission, hematocrit dropped to 23%, white blood cell count fell to 2100 mm^3 with 82% neutrophils and 18% lymphocytes, and blood cultures grew coagulase-positive staphylococci. The patient died 7 days after exposure despite antibiotic therapy and supportive treatment.

BP: blood pressure
bpm: beats per minute
BUN: blood urea nitrogen
HR: heart rate
K+: potassium ion
Na+: sodium ion
PMN: polymorphonucleocytes
RR: respiratory rate
Data source: Azizi MD, Amid MH. Clinical presentation of chemical warfare injuries in children and teenagers. *Med J Islamic Rep Iran*. 1990; 4(2):103–108.

for hours,[76–78] so victims may not recognize toxicity until well after exposure. During this time, sulfur works subclinically to damage the skin. Mustard exposure can affect the CNS and bone marrow, as displayed by symptoms of fatigue, headache, and depression.[77] It can also lead to pneumonia, which was the cause of death for many mustard casualties during World War I in the absence of antibiotics.[77] A leukopenic pneumonia can develop between 6 and 10 days after mustard exposure. The manifestation of leukopenia (specifically lymphopenia) results from the myelosuppressive effects of mustard agents.[77]

Laboratory Findings

Although there is no confirmatory diagnostic test for mustard exposure, some laboratory tests can prove useful. Erythrocyte sedimentation rate has been shown to be elevated in pediatric patients after mustard exposure.[79] CBCs (complete blood cell counts) may show abnormalities, depending on the severity of the vapor inhalation or exposure,[76,78] and may show low hematocrit and leukopenia if the exposure was severe. White blood cell count may show only a transient decrease and subsequent recovery.[76,78] In pediatric cases of mustard vapor exposure, decreases in hematocrit or white blood cell count were likely to occur in the first 2 weeks, with the lowest levels of hemoglobin, hematocrit, white blood cells, and neutrophils observed in the samples taken 6 to 10 days after exposure.[78] These pediatric patients also suffered from hypoxemia and renal failure,[78] but serum creatinine and renal function tests were not found in this particular study's charts. Arterial blood gases may provide useful information, but they may show a varied picture. In one pediatric study of mustard casualties, most cases (43%) showed a simple metabolic acidosis.[78] The other groups showed the following:

- mixed metabolic acidosis and respiratory alkalosis (29%),
- simple respiratory alkalosis (14%),
- mixed metabolic and respiratory acidosis (7%), and
- mixed metabolic alkalosis and respiratory acidosis (7%).[78]

Blood urea nitrogen can be elevated in pediatric casualties from severe mustard exposure cases; however, it does not predict mortality. Rather, it is a marker of mustard exposure in children. Increased blood urea nitrogen will normalize in pediatric patients that survive severe mustard exposure. In one case report, elevated blood urea nitrogen levels returned to normal in three, while the other three died.[78]

Pediatric Vulnerability

Sulfur mustard exposure affects children more severely than adults.[76] Because premature infants have thinner skin, and because their dermal-epidermal

TABLE 21-5

PEDIATRIC SIGNS OF MUSTARD EXPOSURE

Ocular	Cutaneous	Respiratory	Other
Conjunctivitis (94%)	Erythema (94%)	Dry cough (81%)	Sore throat
Eye burning	Hyperpigmentation (75%)	Dyspnea (63%)	Sneezing
Palpebral edema (81%)	Ulceration (69%)	Crepitation (50%)	Nasal secretions
Apraxia of eyelid opening (63%)	Erosion (63%)	Wheezing (25%)	Dysphonia
Keratitis (38%)	Blister (56%)	Burning sensation of the upper respiratory tract	
Blepharospasm (25%)	Edema (50%)		
Corneal ulceration (19%)	Vesicles (31%)		
Chemosis (6%)	Hypopigmentation (13%)		
Photophobia	Dermal pain and burning		
Lacrimation			
Ophthalmodynia			
Diplopia			
Itchy eyes			

Data source: Azizi MD, Amid MH. Clinical presentation of chemical warfare injuries in children and teenagers. *Med J Islamic Rep Iran*. 1990;4(2):103–108.

junctions are not fully developed,[46–50] the time between exposure and the onset of blisters is shortened in children, and the number and severity of blisters increases.[76] Ocular symptoms tend to be more pronounced in children because of their inability to protect themselves and their tendency to rub their eyes.[76,78] Children are also more susceptible to pulmonary injury for reasons previously discussed.[76,78] One case report looked at the long-term effects of mustard exposure in a child.[10] The child suffered a severe chemical pneumonia and chronic bronchiolitis. Finally, signs of gastrointestinal toxicity may be greater in children because of fluid loss and lower intravascular volume reserves.[76]

The decision to evacuate and hospitalize adult mustard casualties is based on the extent of exposure (total body surface area affected > 5% requires hospitalization), severity of the skin lesions, and the extent of multiple organ involvement,[80] but the threshold to hospitalize children with mustard injuries should be lower.

Treatment

Decontamination and supportive therapy are the mainstays of treatment for mustard exposure; antidotes do not exist.[76] Adult decontamination may include bleach solutions; however, this method can cause greater toxicity in children, so soap and water are the preferred agents to use for decontaminating children (Table 21-6).[76] Supportive care consists of managing pulmonary and skin manifestations with medications such as cough suppressants and topical silver sulfadiazine.[76–78]

There are currently no standardized guidelines of casualty management nor drugs available to prevent mustard's effects on skin and mucous membranes.[77,80] Treatment includes prompt decontamination, blister aspiration or deroofing (epidermal removal), physical debridement, irrigation, topical antibiotics, and sterile dressing for cutaneous mustard injuries.[77,80] Current treatment strategies rely on symptomatic management to relieve symptoms, prevent infections, and promote healing. The general recommendations for treating mustard casualties are described in Chapter 8 of this textbook, the *Medical Management of Chemical Casualties Handbook*,[81] the *Field Management of Chemical Casualties Handbook*,[82] the *NATO Handbook on the Medical Aspects of NBC Defensive Operations*,[83] and other references.[80] Iranian physicians treating pediatric casualties of mustard vapor during the Iran-Iraq War found that most pediatric casualties presented with multiple organ system involvement (skin, ocular, gastrointestinal, bone marrow, respiratory, etc).[78]

Dermatological Management. The goal of blister management is to keep the patient comfortable and the lesions clean and to prevent infection. Because children are especially anxious at the sight of bullae and erythema, in addition to the burning, pruritus, and allodynia associated with mustard blisters, anxiolytics may be appropriate to calm pediatric casualties and prevent them from picking at bullae.[77] Burning and itching associated with erythema can be relieved by calamine lotion or soothing creams, such as 0.25% camphor, menthol corticosteroids, antipruritics (ie, diphenhydramine), and silver sulfadiazine cream.[77,78] Pain and discomfort can be relieved with systemic analgesics, such as morphine, which should be given liberally before manipulation of the burned area.[77,78]

Vapor mustard typically causes a first- or second-degree burn, while liquid mustard produces damage similar to a third-degree burn. In any case, tense bullae are the hallmark of mustard injuries. Bullae are typically dome-shaped, thin-walled, 0.5 to 5.0 cm in diameter, superficial, translucent, yellowish, multiloculated, honeycombed,[84] and surrounded by erythema.[77] Preventing children from breaking the blisters can be challenging, especially when constant friction from clothing and blankets are irritating to the skin. Effected areas should be wrapped in protective dressings. According to Graham et al, there is a reservoir of unbound mustard in human skin following a vapor[85] or liquid exposure, leading to an off-gassing period. This period can last for 24 to 36 hours, during which application of an occlusive dressing is not beneficial due to vapor build up.[80]

It is recommended that small blisters (< 1 cm) be left alone on children, but the immediately surrounding area should be cleaned, irrigated daily, and covered with topical antibiotic.[77] Petroleum gauze bandage dressings should be wrapped around unbroken blisters and changed every few days.[77] Larger blisters (> 1 cm) should be unroofed and irrigated several times a day with saline, sterile water, clean soapy water, or Dakin's solution, and covered with topical antibiotic cream or ointment. Blister fluid does not contain mustard[86] and therefore is not hazardous to healthcare workers.[77] Options for topical antibiotic creams in children include silver sulfadiazine and triple combination antibiotic (bacitracin, neomycin sulfate, and polymyxin B sulfate).[77] Topical antibiotics should be applied to the area of bullae and surrounding areas of erythema. There is no information comparing use of triple antibiotic topical ointment in children with use in other age groups.

Mafenide acetate, a sulfonamide used to prevent bacteria and fungal infections in burn victims, is

TABLE 21-6

MANAGEMENT OF VESICANT EXPOSURES

Agent	Symptoms	Antidotes and Treatment
Mustard	• Skin erythema and pruritis • Development of large yellow blisters leading to ulcers • Eye damage • Hoarseness and cough • Mucosal necrosis • Toneless voice • Nausea • Vomiting	**Decontamination:** soap, water, no bleach; copious water irrigation for eyes **Pulmonary management:** cough suppressants, throat lozenges **Skin management:** topical agents used for burns (1% silver sulfadiazine), antibiotics for secondary infections (bacitracin, neomycin, and polymyxin B), antihistamines for itching (diphenhydramine 1 mg/kg/dose orally q6–8h, max 300 mg/day, hydroxyzine 0.5 mg/kg/dose orally q6–8h) **Immune system management**: G-CSF(filgrastim) 5–10 µg/kg/day subcutaneous for neutropenia
Lewisite	• Shock • Pulmonary injury • Blisters	**Decontamination:** soap, water, no bleach **Antidote:** BAL-dimercaprol may decrease systemic effects of lewisite **Pulmonary management:** BAL 3–5 mg/kg deep IM q4h x 4 doses (dose depends on severity of exposure and symptoms) **Skin management:** BAL ointment **Eye management:** BAL ophthalmic ointment

BAL: British Anti-Lewisite
G-CSF: granulocyte-colony stimulating factor
IM: intramuscular
Data sources: (1) Momeni A, Aminjavaheri M. Skin manifestations of mustard gas in a group of 14 children and teenagers: a clinical study. *Inter J Dermatol*. 1994:33(3):184–187. (2) Yu CE, Burklow TR, Madsen JM. Vesicant agents and children. *Pediatric Annals*. 2003;32(4):254–257. (3) Taketomo CK, Hodding JH, Kraus DM. *American Pharmacists Association: Pediatric Dosage Handbook*. 13th ed. Hudson, Ohio: Lexi-Comp Inc; 2006.

recommended for adult use as a 5% mafenide cream[77,80]; however, it is not recommended in premature or newborn infants up to 2 months old because it may lead to liver problems.[87,88] Mafenide acetate caused methemoglobinemia in two 2-year-old children treated with the cream for 50% surface area burns.[87,88] One of the patients died from the exposure to mafenide. Furthermore, a burned 12-year-old patient who was treated with 5% mafenide acetate solution to eradicate pseudomonas aeruginosa growth reportedly developed methemoglobinemia.[89] The patient's methemoglobin level was 34.5% 24 hours after application of 5% mafenide acetate cream. Mafenide may also be unsuitable in pediatrics because it can cause severe pain when applied to partial-thickness wounds and burns,[80] and it is contraindicated for patients with metabolic acidosis. If mafenide is used for pediatric burns, the healthcare provider should be aware of this rare, lethal complication in the pediatric population and should monitor methemoglobin levels concurrently.

While skin healing can take months, pigment changes (hyper- or hypopigmentation) can persist.[77,80] Not all burn injuries require treatment at a burn center, but patients will require aggressive pain management and close observation for the systemic effects of mustard exposure wherever they are treated. Skin grafting, although rare, has been successfully used for deep burns.[90]

Ophthalmology. Ophthalmologic consultation for pediatric mustard injuries will contribute to prevention of ocular scarring and infection.[77] Eyes exposed to mustard should be irrigated to remove traces of vesicant. Severe ocular involvement requires topical antibiotics (tobramycin OD) applied several times a day.[77] Topical steroids may be useful in the first 48 hours after exposure. Temporary vision loss may also occur after mustard exposure[77–79] because of palpebral edema and not corneal damage.[77]

Respiratory System. Pulmonary examination is necessary because the conducting and ventilation portions of the respiratory tract are affected by mustard vapor.[10,77,78] Bronchodilators diminish hyperreactive airways and should be used if a prior history of asthma or hyperreactive airways is documented. Further support with humidified oxygen may be required. Ventilatory support may be required for severe cases of mustard vapor exposure before laryngeal spasm makes intubation difficult. Bronchoscopy is critical for diagnosis, therapeutic dilation for mustard-induced tracheobronchial stenosis, and removal of pseudomembranes that cause airway obstruction.[77]

Antibiotic therapy should not be given during the first 3 to 4 days after mustard exposure because the toxic bronchitis produced by mustard is nonbacterial.[77] Sputum must be continually monitored with Gram's stains and culture growth to identify the specific organism responsible for any late-developing superinfection.[77] Leukopenia in children, a grave sign of mustard exposure, necessitates aggressive support with combination antibiotic treatment.[77]

Gastrointestinal Tract. Atropine or common antiemetics can be given to provide relief from nausea and vomiting, which are early signs of mustard intoxication.[76] The best choices for pediatric-specific antiemetics include medications such as promethazine, metoclopramide, and ondansetron.[77] Persistent vomiting and diarrhea are a later sign of systemic toxicity and require prompt fluid replacement.[76,77]

Bone Marrow Suppression. Mustard, a radiometric, affects rapidly dividing tissues like bone marrow, in addition to the gastrointestinal tract.[77,80] It also destroys hematopoietic precursor cells; white blood cells have the shortest lifespan and decrease in number first, followed by red blood cells and thrombocytes.[77] Resultant bone marrow suppression can be treated with filgrastim injections,[77,80] which stimulate marrow to create and release white blood cells.

Other Treatment Considerations. Fluid status, electrolytes, and urine output should be monitored in mustard-intoxicated patients. Tetanus prophylaxis should also be administered because tetanus may be fatal even after a small partial-thickness burn.[91]

Pulmonary Agents

In January 2002 a Central Intelligence Agency report stated that terrorist groups may have less interest in biological weapons compared to chemicals such as cyanide, chlorine, and phosgene, which can contaminate food and water supplies.[92] Industrial chemicals, such as chlorine and phosgene, have advantages that make them likely candidates to be used by terrorists in the future. Additionally, both are fairly easy to manufacture and handle. In the United States, millions of tons of chlorine and phosgene are produced annually to manufacture various products.[92] A detailed discussion of the general mechanisms of chlorine and phosgene toxicity can be found in Chapter 10, Toxic Inhalational Injury and Toxic Industrial Chemicals.

Clinical Presentation

Pediatric signs and symptoms of chlorine gas exposure include predominantly ocular, nasal, oropharyngeal, and pulmonary membrane irritation.[92] Respiratory complaints are the hallmark of intoxication by these choking agents.[92] Minor chlorine exposure can lead to burning of the eyes and throat, which is indicative of mucous membrane irritation. More severely exposed patients may complain of cough, choking, sore throat, shortness of breath, chest tightness, difficulty breathing, and other respiratory-related issues.[92] Clinical findings may also include lacrimation, rhinorrhea, laryngeal edema, hoarseness, aphonia, stridor, expiratory wheezing, tracheitis, and cyanosis.[93,94] Tachypnea may develop as a direct result of pulmonary irritation, and tachycardia has been demonstrated in some case reports.[93,94] Many pediatric patients with prior histories of reactive airway disease are at increased risk of chlorine-induced bronchospasm.[92]

Pulse oximetry may indicate low oxygen saturation in patients exposed to pulmonary agents.[94] While arterial blood gases usually indicate hypoxemia, carbon dioxide levels have been shown to be decreased, increased, or normal.[93,94] A hyperchloremic metabolic acidosis may be seen on blood chemistries due to systemic absorption of hydrochloric acid.[94]

Pulmonary edema, the most significant morbidity of pulmonary agents, can be seen on chest roentograms.[92] It may develop as early as 2 to 4 hours after exposure; radiographic evidence typically appears later. Pulmonary edema may produce Kerley B lines on chest X-rays.[92] These lines resemble the rungs of a ladder running perpendicular to the lateral margin of the lungs, beginning at the costophrenic angle. Chest radiographs often show opacities of acute lung injury. Pneumomediastinum has also been reported in chlorine gas exposure.[94]

Pulmonary function tests are not helpful when confirming or treating pulmonary agent exposure.[94,95] A study of school children exposed to a chlorine gas leak reported a predominantly obstructive pattern on pulmonary function tests.[95] This could be explained by the children's smaller airways or congestion and edema narrowing the central airways.

Pediatric Vulnerability

Chlorine is a pungent, green-yellow gas, twice as heavy as air, that settles near the ground.[92–94] This poses a particular problem for children, whose short stature places them closer to the ground. Children are most commonly exposed after inhaling chlorine vapors at swimming pools,[92] encountering household bleach (sodium hypochlorite) mixed with acidic cleaning agents,[94] and experiencing industrial accidents.[95] Phosgene, a dense gas that is also heavier than air, is a more lethal pulmonary agent than chlorine. While the smell of chlorine is associated with swimming pools, phosgene odor is similar to that of freshly mown hay.[92]

Initially, both chlorine and phosgene cause coughing and intense mucosal membrane irritation, typically followed by a feeling of suffocation.[92–94] Morbidity from pulmonary agents is the direct result of pulmonary edema, appearing between 2 and 4 hours after chlorine exposure. Pulmonary edema can cause rapid dehydration or even shock in children because they have a smaller fluid reserve.[92]

Treatment

The first line of treatment for children exposed to pulmonary agents is decontamination. Decontamination can be as simple as removing the victim from the source to fresh air, followed by removing contaminated clothing.[92] Supportive care includes administering humidified air and supplemental oxygen, irrigation with water, and delivering high-flow oxygen via positive pressure for pulmonary edema.[92,94] Further treatment may include surgical debridement and supportive care with medications, such as albuterol for bronchospasm, corticosteroids for inflammation, and antibiotics for secondary bacterial infections (Table 21-7).[92,94] Antidotes or specific postexposure treatments do not exist for this class of agents.

Cyanide

Cyanide is used in processing plastic, electroplating metals, tempering metals, and extracting gold and silver. It is found in fumigants, vehicle exhaust, tobacco smoke, certain fruit pits, and bitter almonds, and is used in photographic development.[96,97] Cyanide is liberated during the combustion or metabolism of natural and synthetic nitrogen-containing polymers.[98] Cyanides can be lethal through inhalation or ingestion,[99] and although cyanide exposure leads to death in minutes, it can be effectively treated with antidotes if diagnosed early.[96,97] Pediatricians, medical first responders, and firefighters need to recognize victims of cyanide poisoning in order to initiate immediate intervention.[96,97] Cyanide is one of the few chemicals for which an effective antidote exists.

Mechanism of Toxicity

The cyanide ion kills mammalian organisms by shutting down oxidative phosphorylation in the mitochondria and, therefore, the utilization of oxygen in cells.[97,98] Cyanide has a propensity to affect certain organs (eg, brain, heart, and lungs) more than others.[96,97] Significant exposure can lead to central respiratory arrest and myocardial depression.[97] Cyanide also acts as a direct neurotoxin, disrupting cell membranes and causing excitatory injury in the CNS.[96–98]

TABLE 21-7

MANAGING PULMONARY AGENT EXPOSURES

Agent	Symptoms	Treatment
Chlorine	• Lacrimation • Rhinorrhea • Conjunctival irritation • Cough • Sore throat • Hoarseness • Laryngeal edema • Dyspnea • Stridor • Acute respiratory distress syndrome • Pulmonary edema	**Decontamination**: copious water irrigation of the skin, eyes, and mucosal membranes to prevent continued irritation and injury **Symptomatic care (no antidote):** warm/moist air, supplemental oxygen, positive pressure oxygen for pulmonary edema **Bronchospasm:** beta-agonists (albuterol) **Severe bronchospasm:** corticosteroids (prednisone; also used for patients with history of asthma but use unproven) **Analgesia and cough:** nebulized lidocaine (4% topical solution) or nebulized sodium bicarbonate (use unproven)
Phosgene	• Transient irritation (eyes, nose, throat, and sinus) • Bronchospasm • Pulmonary edema • Apnea • Hypoxia	**Decontamination:** wash away all residual liquid with copious water, remove clothing **Symptomatic care:** maintain patient's airway, breathing, and circulation, hydrate, positive pressure oxygen for pulmonary edema **Bronchospasm:** beta-agonists (albuterol), corticosteroids INH/IV, Furosemide is contraindicated **Hypoxia:** oxygen

INH/IV: inhaler/intravenous solution
Data source: Burklow TR, Yu CE, Madsen JM. Industrial chemicals: terrorist weapons of opportunity. *Pediatr Ann*. 2003;32(4):230–234.

Clinical Presentation

Cyanide intoxication is an uncommon cause of childhood poisoning;[96] the pediatric population (< 19 years old) represented only 7.8% of cyanide poisonings reported in 2000.[67] Because signs of toxicity are similar to carbon monoxide poisoning (which accounts for the largest group of poisoning deaths among children), clinicians must have a high index of suspicion to make a diagnosis of cyanide poisoning.[98,99] Rotenberg describes a typical toxidrome induced by cyanide, which includes a rapid progression from hyperpnea, anxiety, restlessness, unconsciousness, seizures, apnea, and finally death.[96] Skin, blood, and fundi may be cherry red upon physical examination[96–99] because of the inability of mitochondria to extract oxygen (Exhibit 21-5).

Laboratory Findings

Arterial blood gases can provide clues to verify cyanide exposure. Classic cases present with severe metabolic acidosis, elevated anion gap, and high lactate concentrations.[96] Impaired cellular respiration leads to a high oxygen content in venous blood[96,98]; thus, a reduced arterial-venous oxygen saturation difference suggests cyanide poisoning. Blood cyanide levels are confirmatory but delay the diagnosis, which must be based on the initial clinical presentation.[96–98] An almond-like odor on the breath may indicate that a person has been exposed to cyanide, but up to 40% of the general population is unable to detect this odor.[96]

Pediatric Vulnerability

Children are especially vulnerable to cyanide attacks because of their higher respiratory rates and surface-to-volume ratios.[96] Additionally, cyanide liquid is rapidly absorbed in greater amounts when it comes in contact with children's immature skin barriers.[96] The initial symptoms described in a case report of 10 children who ingested cyanide included abdominal pain, nausea, restlessness, and giddiness.[99] Cyanosis and drowsiness were also noted, but the signature cherry-red skin color was not reported. Postmortem examination of two children that died following exposure showed bright red blood and congested tissues. These children consumed powder packets of potassium cyanide mixed in water, while the other 8 children only licked the powder. The survivors were managed with aggressive supportive care, including gastric lavage, oxygen, and IV fluids.

Treatment

In the United States, the mainstay of treatment for cyanide poisoning consists of supportive treatment and use of a multistage antidote kit that contains

EXHIBIT 21-5

MNEMONIC FOR RECOGNITION OF CYANIDE TOXICITY

FAT RED CATS

- F: flushing of skin
- A: almonds (bitter almond smell)
- T: tachycardia
- R: red (red/pink skin, bright red retinal vessels)
- E: excitation of nervous system
- D: dizziness, death, recent depression history
- C: confusion, coma, convulsions
- A: acidosis (metabolic or lactic), anion gap
- T: tachypnea
- S: soot in nose

amyl nitrite, sodium nitrite, and sodium thiosulfate (Table 21-8).[96–98] Antidotes should be provided only for significantly symptomatic patients, such as those with impaired consciousness, seizures, acidosis, hypotension, hyperkalemia, or unstable vital signs.[100] Even when patients are rendered comatose by inhaling hydrogen cyanide gas, antidotes may not be necessary if the exposure is rapidly terminated, the patient has regained consciousness on arrival at the hospital, and there is no acidosis or vital sign abnormality.[101]

Supportive Therapy. Regardless of the antidote, treatment always consists of supportive therapy,[96] which alone may reverse the effects of cyanide even in the face of apnea.[96,97,101] Supportive therapy includes decontamination, oxygen, hydration, and administration of anticonvulsants.[96–98,101] Decontamination measures should take place prior to patient transport to a medical center. First responders and healthcare professionals should take precautions not to intoxicate themselves through direct mouth-to-mouth resuscitative efforts.[98] They must also wear personal protective equipment when transporting the victims to areas with adequate ventilation.[96] Clothes are an obvious source of recontamination and must be removed from the victim. The victim's skin should be flushed with copious volumes of water,[96,97] the temperature of which becomes a consideration for children who may not tolerate extremes of cold or hot. Timely supportive care is important because antidote kits may not be available.

Antidotal Therapy. The US standard cyanide antidote kit uses a small inhaled dose of amyl nitrite followed by IV sodium nitrite and sodium thiosulfate.[96,102] This antidote converts a portion of the hemoglobin

TABLE 21-8

MULTISTAGE ANTIDOTE KIT TREATMENT FOR MANAGING UNCONSCIOUS, CYANIDE-EXPOSED PATIENTS*

Amyl Nitrite Ampules	Sodium Nitrite (for Hb = 12)	Sodium Thiosulfate (for Hb = 12)
For children ≤ 30 kg: • Crush 1 amp in gauze close to the mouth and nose of breathing victim • Inhale fore 15 secs, rest for 15 secs • Replace pearls every 30 secs until sodium nitrite can be administered	For children ≤ 30 kg: • 0.19–0.39 mL/kg not to exceed 10 mL of 3% solution to slow IV over less than 5 mins or slower if hypotension develops • For every 1 g/dL increase or decrease change in Hb, change dose by approximately 0.03 mL/kg accordingly • May repeat dose at half the original dose in 30 min if needed	For children ≤ 30 kg: • 0.95–1.95 mL/kg not to exceed 50 mL of 25% solution IV over 10–20 min • For every increase or decrease change in Hb of 1 g/dL, change sodium thiosulfate by 0.15 mL/kg accordingly • May repeat dose at half original dose in 30 min if needed
For adults: • See above	For adults: • 10 mL of 3% solution slow IV over no less than 5 min or slower if hypotension develops	For adults: • 50 mL of 25% solution IV over 10–20 min

*Other treatments include evacuation, decontamination, administration of 100% oxygen, and correction of acidosis, hypovolemia, and seizures.
Hb: hemoglobin
IV: intravenous
Data sources: (1) Cyanide antidote [package insert]. Buffalo Grove, Ill: Taylor Pharmaceuticals; 1998. (2) Berlin CM. The treatment of cyanide poisoning in children. *Pediatrics*. 1970;46:793–796. (3) Hall AH, Rumack BH. Clinical toxicology of cyanide. *Ann Emerg Med*. 1986;15:1067–1074.

TABLE 21-9

VARIATION OF SODIUM NITRITE AND SODIUM THIOSULFATE DOSE WITH HEMOGLOBIN CONCENTRATION

Hemoglobin (g/dL)	Initial Intravenous Dose of Sodium Nitrite 3% (mL/kg)*	Initial Intravenous Dose of Sodium Thiosulfate 25% (mL/kg)†
7	0.19	0.95
8	0.22	1.10
9	0.25	1.25
10	0.27	1.35
11	0.3	1.50
12	0.33	1.65
13	0.36	1.80
14	0.39	1.95

*Not to exceed 10 mL total dose
†Not to exceed 50 mL total dose
Data sources: (1) Cyanide antidote [package insert]. Buffalo Grove, Ill: Taylor Pharmaceuticals; 1998. (2) Berlin CM. The treatment of cyanide poisoning in children. *Pediatrics*. 1970;46:793–796. (3) Hall AH, Rumack BH. Clinical toxicology of cyanide. *Ann Emerg Med*. 1986;15:1067–1074.

iron from ferrous iron to ferric iron, changing the hemoglobin into methemoglobin.[96,97,102,103] Cyanide is more strongly drawn to methemoglobin than to the cytochrome oxidase of cells, effectively pulling the cyanide off the cells and onto the methemoglobin.[97,103] Once bound with the cyanide, the methemoglobin becomes cyanmethemoglobin.[102] Therapy with nitrites alone is ineffective because methemoglobin cannot transport oxygen in the blood. Adult doses can potentially cause a fatal methemoglobinemia in children[103] or may cause profound hypotension.[96] Treatment for children intoxicated by cyanide must be individualized and is based on the child's body weight and hemoglobin concentration.[96,102,104] An ampule of amyl nitrite should be broken into a handkerchief and the contents should be held in front of the patient's mouth for 15 seconds, followed by 15 seconds of rest.[102] This should be repeated only until sodium nitrite can be administered; continuous use of amyl nitrite may prevent adequate oxygenation.[102] Taylor Pharmaceuticals, the manufacturer of the kit, recommends a sodium nitrite dose of 6 to 8 mL/m^2 (approximately 0.2 mL/kg body weight) for children, not to exceed the adult dose of 10 mL of a 3% solution (approximately 300 mg).[102] While excessive sodium nitrite can cause methemoglobinemia, it should be noted that in the 70-year history of using the kit, the only reported fatality of methemoglobinemia from its use involved a child without serious cyanide poisoning who was given two adult doses of sodium nitrite.[103,104] The scientific literature recommends pediatric dosing based on monitoring hemoglobin levels.[103,104]

The next step in the cyanide antidote kit is to administer sodium thiosulfate intravenously.[96,97,102,104] The sodium thiosulfate and cyanmethemoglobin become thiocyanate and release the hemoglobin, and the thiocyanate is excreted by the kidneys. Hemoglobin levels should be continuously monitored while administering safe doses of sodium nitrite and sodium thiosulfate (Table 21-9).[102–104] If, after inquiring about a patient's medical history, a healthcare provider is concerned about anemia in a patient, doses should be decreased.[96,103,104] Methemoglobin levels must be monitored sequentially in children and should not exceed 20%.[96]

Alternative Strategies. Alternative methods of treating cyanide intoxication are used in other countries. For example, the method in France uses hydroxycobalamin (a form of vitamin B_{12}), which combines with cyanide to form the harmless vitamin B_{12a} cyanocobalamin.[96,97] On December 15, 2006, the FDA approved hydroxocobalamin for use in the United States to treat cyanide-exposed victims in a product called the "Cyanokit" (EMD Pharmaceuticals Inc, Durham, NC; see Chapter 11, Cyanide Poisoning).

DECONTAMINATING CHILDREN

Decontamination after a chemical terrorist attack needs to be well-planned, efficient, and cognizant of children's special needs. Children's unique vulnerabilities may lead to a disproportionate number of pediatric victims after a chemical attack. The potential for a high number of preventable pediatric casualties increases when a proper decontamination plan is not in place. Pediatricians must be involved in developing hospitals' plans for decontamination. Over the last several years, many advances have been made in managing critically injured children. Studies have shown that children managed in pediatric intensive care units have better outcomes than children managed in adult intensive care units.[65] Despite the lack of a pediatric intensive care unit, hospitals should be prepared to provide initial resuscitation and stabilization for pediatric victims of a terrorist attack. Community hospitals and centers that specialize in pediatric care should create written transfer agreements to allow the rapid transport of critically injured children to the sites that can ensure the best outcomes.

The first step in the decontamination process is to appropriately triage patients.[91] If this step is done quickly and accurately, patients will be appropriately managed and outcomes will improve. The key to triage is the ability to ration care when resources are limited. Victims are usually classified into tiered categories; classic battlefield categories include minimal, delayed, immediate, and expectant. Patients in the minimal category have minor injuries that may not require medical care or that can be managed with self-care; however, self-care may be difficult for children. The delayed category includes patients that have injuries requiring medical intervention, but their injuries are not immediately life threatening. The immediate category describes patients who are critically injured and need medical intervention to save life or limb, and the expectant category includes patients who are so critically injured that they are not expected to survive. The expectant category poses a special challenge to civilian healthcare workers who are used to expending vast resources to maximize survival. In a mass casualty event, this kind of effort may not be realistic. Although the classic categories of triage are fairly well known, they are not consistently used among hospitals. Some categories have been developed to specifically address chemical attacks. For example, at the University of Maryland Medical Center, the biochemical response triage categories differentiate between "exposed" and "not exposed" individuals. Furthermore, because not all exposed individuals will necessarily be symptomatic but may still need to be isolated, the categories are subdivided into those who are asymptomatic, exposed and symptomatic, exposed and asymptomatic, and those with unrelated emergent conditions. Regardless of the categories used, appropriately identifying the causative agent is critical; however, that can be challenging because full identification is often delayed.

The decontamination process should begin after triage.[65] All workers involved in decontamination must be appropriately protected with butyl rubber aprons and gloves, double layers of latex gloves, waterproof aprons, and chemical-resistant jumpsuits. Personal protective equipment should also include an appropriately selected air-purifying or atmosphere-supplying respirator, depending on how the threat environment has been categorized.

The construction and use of the decontamination area must be carefully planned. Often, the area is split into different zones.[105] At a minimum, there must be a dirty, contaminated zone and a clean, decontaminated zone, and traffic must go one way between them. This eliminates the possibility of a clean patient becoming cross-contaminated or an exposed patient entering a healthcare facility before being decontaminated. As patients enter the clean zone, a secondary triage is needed to allow them to receive antidotes or be referred for further care. For severely ill patients, antidote administration may precede decontamination.

It is also important to select the appropriate decontamination agent; plain water is usually the most effective.[105] Other agents that have been used for decontamination include carbonaceous adsorbent powder, dilute (0.5%) hypochlorite solution, water with soap, and dry decontaminants, such as flour or talcum powder. For children, water or water with soap are the preferred decontamination agents; bleach or hypochlorite solutions can irritate or damage children's skin.[105] Water should be at a comfortable temperature because children, especially newborns and infants, are prone to hypothermia and hemodynamic instability from cold water. Blankets can be used to quickly warm pediatric patients after water decontamination. In some situations, indoor sprinkler systems have been used to decontaminate patients when outdoor conditions were unsatisfactory. Patients should also change clothing and shower, and those who have encountered chemicals in the gaseous form should be exposed to fresh air.

Triage clinicians need to understand how chemical toxicities manifest in children and should understand what normal vital signs should be for a child. Pediatric-specific triage tools consider different vital signs, such as heart rate and respiratory rate parameters and the differing ability of patients to communicate. It is important for triage to include an examination of the child's mouth and eyes because of the frequent hand-to-mouth and hand-to-eye activity common in children. If antidote administration is needed, pediatric references should be readily available and medical personnel should understand pediatric dosing. When personnel lack experience with managing children, the otherwise efficient decontamination process can get bogged down. Some hospitals have set up pediatric-specific areas to address the specific needs of children.

Clinicians may also need to handle uncooperative or nonverbal children. This becomes especially challenging when an IV line needs to be started. Placing a line in a child while in full protective equipment can be difficult, and the unfamiliar presence of a clinician in full personal protective equipment can cause fear and distress in a child. Children undergoing decontamination will benefit from a guardian to guide them through the process and reassure them. For those children who present alone, a guardian should be appointed and a system for parental identification should be in place. Hospitals need to plan for this extra resource; a model may be based on the system developed by an Israeli hospital that employs social workers to manage disaster patient and family needs, including psychological distress.[106] Parents and children should not be separated during a crisis, so plans should be made for the decontamination and treatment of parent-child pairs.[105]

A variety of specially sized equipment, ranging from pediatric-sized emergency equipment to supplies for basic needs (eg, formula and diapers), is needed to appropriately manage children. Because decontamination often includes disrobing, pediatric-sized clothing is needed, and toys are useful to divert children when they need to be observed for long periods of time.

PREPARING FOR A CHEMICAL EVENT

The first step in preparing for a chemical event is understanding the chemical agents used for terrorism and knowing how to manage their toxicity. Preparedness assessments should identify deficits and be used to forge partnerships among community members.[31] For example, after its assessment exercise, the University of Maryland Medical Center decided to partner with the local fire department to coordinate water decontamination outside of the medical center entrance. Planning for an attack begins with developing local health resources because time to borrow resources from nearby communities after an attack is limited. Because most children spend the majority of the day at school, community preparation for a threat should include the local educational system and focus on developing a rapid evacuation plan and in-school shelters.

Healthcare facilities responsible for treating pediatric victims of a chemical or biological event may be easily strained and overwhelmed. Alternative areas, such as auditoriums and arenas, are often needed to triage patients after a large-scale chemical or biological incident, and these areas need to be staffed with personnel who know how to manage pediatric victims.[32] First responders must be able to recognize pediatric signs and symptoms from each chemical agent, correctly don protective gear in the face of persistent agents, handle pediatric patients, and manage field decontamination. Adequate supplies of protective gear must also be available. When planning decontamination procedures, pediatric vulnerabilities and challenges need to be considered.

Another key element to appropriate preparedness is the development of a pharmaceutical cache of antidotes, antibiotics, and vaccines. Although the Strategic National Stockpile is now in place throughout the United States, it may be several hours before supplies can reach hospitals from this cache and be divided among sites. Efforts have been made to include pediatric-ready medications, such as suspensions and solutions, in the Strategic National Stockpile. Local pharmaceutical caches should also try to address pediatric needs (Table 21-10).

Pediatricians are uniquely trained to manage pediatric casualties and to advocate for children so that their needs are addressed in emergency planning.[32,107] Pediatricians can assist in educating first responders so pediatric triage and management is appropriate. Patients and families are also critical advocates for children. Through grass-roots efforts, political interest can be generated to address deficits and encourage collaboration among groups to mobilize important resources. Parents can also prepare for an event by developing a family emergency plan (Exhibit 21-6).

In addition to developing a family emergency plan, parents must recognize that children will be deeply psychologically affected after an attack.[108,109] Terrorism causes strong emotional responses that can easily lead to panic; media coverage of an event is often real-time and frequently graphic, making fear inevitable. Because psychological and emotional impact is the predominant morbidity of an attack, some hospitals have included guidelines for managing serious psychological distress under special disaster preparation plans. Children can be expected to be among both the direct and the secondary psychological victims of a terrorist event. Somatic complaints, such as headaches and abdominal pain, may be common. Pediatric providers can help families address the underlying psychological origin of physical complaints. How children respond to a terrorist event depends on maturity, prior experience, preexisting mental health, and coping skills. Family support and community resources for stress management also play a strong role in helping pediatric victims cope. Children may demonstrate fear, manifesting as

TABLE 21-10

EXAMPLE OF A PEDIATRIC-SPECIFIC HOSPITAL EMERGENCY DRUG CACHE

Drug	Strength	Dosage Form	Pediatric Dosing	Therapy or Prophylaxis	Disease
Albuterol MDI	17gm	INH	2–4 puffs q4h	Respiratory distress from chemical agents	Chemical exposure
Amoxicillin oral suspension	400 mg/5 mL 100 mL	Oral suspension	27 mg/kg q8h–up to 40kg > 40kg 500 mg q8h	Chemoprophylaxis	Anthrax
Atropine	1 mg/mL	Injection	See dosing table	Chemotherapy	Nerve agent exposure
Ciprofloxacin oral suspension	250 mg/5 mL 100 mL	Oral suspension	20–30 mg/kg/ day divided q12h for 60 days	Chemoprophylaxis	Anthrax, plague
Clindamycin	600 mg/NS 50 mL	IV	30 mg/kg/day q8h (max 4.8 g/day)	Chemotherapy	Anthrax
Cyanide antidote package	1 kit	kit	See dosing table	Chemotherapy	Cyanide poisoning
Diazepam IV	5 mg/mL x 2 mL	Injection	See dosing table	Seizures post chemical exposure	Seizures post chemical exposure
Doxycycline oral suspension	25 mg/5 mL 60 mL	Oral suspension	2.5 mg/kg q12h– up to 40 kg, > 40 kg 100 mg q12h for 60 days	Chemoprophylaxis	Anthrax, cholera, brucellosis, plague
Oseltamivir suspension	12 mg/mL 25 mL	Suspension	For children ≥ 1–12 years old: ≤ 15 kg: 2 mg/kg/dose (max 30 mg) BID x 5 days > 15–23kg: 45 mg/dose BID x 5 days > 23–40 kg: 60 mg/dose BID x 5 days > 40 kg 75 mg/dose BID x 5 days	Chemotherapy	Avian influenza
Potassium iodide	65 mg	Tablet	For children 4–18 yrs: 65 mg; For children 1 m–3 yrs: 32.5 mg; For children < 1 mo: 16.25 mg	Chemotherapy	Radiation emergency
Pralidoxime	1 gm/20 mL vial	Powder for injection	See dosing table	Chemotherapy	Nerve agent exposure
Ribavirin solution	40 mg/mL 100 mL	Solution	LD 30 mg/kg followed by 15 mg/kg/day BID x 10 days	Chemotherapy	Viral hemorrhagic fever
Rifampin solution	20 mg/mL 100 mL	Compounded solution	10–20 mg/kg/day q12h (max daily dose 600 mg)	Chemotherapy	Anthrax, brucellosis
Triple antibiotic ointment	0.9 g	Tube	Apply as needed	Chemotherapy	Skin chemical exposure

BID: bis in di´e (twice a day)
INH: inhaler
IV: intravenous solution
LD: loading dose
NS: normal saline

EXHIBIT 21-6

DEVELOPING A FAMILY EMERGENCY PLAN

- Discuss, prepare, and practice for various types of disasters with those who share your residence.
- Formulate a plan to stay in contact if separated (eg, specify at least two meeting places as alternatives to your home and your neighborhood).
- Select an out-of-state contact that all the family members can call to provide location and personal situation information.
- Post emergency numbers at home and also have all the family members carry them when away from home.
- Practice turning off water, power, and gas at home.
- Install and check smoke detectors.
- Obtain battery-operated radios.
- Ready battery-operated flashlights to avoid using matches to see when electricity fails.
- Prepare supply kits with water, food, first aid supplies, tools, clothing, bedding, batteries for radios and flashlights, and other special items, such as medication, baby formula, or diapers. (It may be appropriate to have a kit at home and in automobiles.)

Data source: Bradley BJ, Gresham LS, Sidelinger DE, et al. Pediatric health professionals and public health response. *Pediatric Ann.* 2003;32(2):87–94.

nightmares, insomnia, fear of the dark, or separation anxiety. Under stress, they may regress developmentally and adopt the behaviors of a younger child or sibling. Parents and teachers should be taught that these behaviors may signify children are having difficulty coping. Older children may manifest with depression, pessimism, and substance abuse. Some children may be diagnosed with PTSD. PTSD is diagnosed when a patient demonstrates symptoms of increased arousal, relives the event, and avoids reminders of the event for at least 1 month. Those children directly involved in an attack are at higher risk of developing PTSD.

In responding to an event, it is important to talk to children to help them understand what has occurred and to allow them to express their feelings. Even young children should be kept informed because they can sense that a serious event has occurred and can become concerned when the issue is not explained. It may be helpful to limit children's television viewing and assure them of their safety after a disaster (Exhibit 21-7). Pediatricians and parents play a critical role in identifying coping mechanisms among children and providing the support they need to adjust to the aftermath of a terrorist attack.

EXHIBIT 21-7

STRATEGIES TO HELP CHILDREN COPE WITH TERRORIST EVENTS

- Inform children about a terrorist even as soon as possible.
- Help children understand the event by stating the basic facts in simple, direct, and clear terms.
- Limit television viewing to avoid exposing children to detailed information and graphic images.
- Reassure children they should feel safe in their schools, homes, and communities.
- Reassure children of their complete lack of responsibility.
- Watch for signs of guilt and anger.
- Act as a role model by sharing feelings of fear, sadness, and empathy.
- Offer to discuss terrorist events with older children and adolescents, but do not force conversations.
- Anticipate delayed and anniversary reactions (sadness or fear on the anniversary of a tragic event).
- Provide concrete advice on how to make participation in commemorative events meaningful.

Data source: Schonfeld DJ. Supporting children after terrorist events: potential roles for pediatricians. *Pediatr Ann.* 2003;32(3):182–187.

HELPFUL RESOURCES

Various groups have provided guidance and expertise on managing chemical threats to children. Important contributions have come from the Chemical Warfare Involving Kids (CWiK) Response Project, the Program for Pediatric Preparedness from the National Center for Disaster Preparedness, and the "Children, Terrorism, and Disasters" Web site of the American Academy of Pediatrics. The Duke University Health System has also provided pediatric mass casualty incident guidelines on the Web that include instructions for managing chemical exposures.[110]

The Chemical Warfare Involving Kids Response Project

Doctors Robert Luten and James Broselow developed a system for managing pediatric chemical exposures. The system is called "The Chemical Warfare Involving Kids (CWiK) Response Project" and its purpose is 3-fold:

1. to create resuscitation aids specifically designed to address pediatric medication dosing problems of chemical terrorism,
2. to provide a focused review of clinically significant pediatric issues in victim treatment, and
3. to disseminate these tools to help prepare to care for children.

The project aims to distribute information about pediatric vulnerabilities and antidote preparation and administration. In addition, an "antidote for chemical warfare" card was developed as a quick reference for providers managing pediatric chemical casualties. These cards are intended to be used during a chemical event and provide precalculated medication doses. Separate from this initiative, pediatric-specific dosing cards have been developed that provide medication dose ranges for each chemical agent.

Broselow-Luten System: a Systematic Approach with Color Coding

A major difficulty of managing disasters is that they may occur in areas that have limited pediatric resources. Even in areas with optimal resources for everyday practice, an acute presentation of multiple victims with a disproportionate number of affected children may be overwhelming. Healthcare providers trained to treat adults may suddenly be confronted with large numbers of acutely ill or injured children, as has been seen in areas like Afghanistan and Iraq. One solution that has been proposed is the Broselow-Luten system, which uses color-coded therapeutic pathways; children are entered into a color category according to weight (or length, measured by Broselow tape, when weight cannot be obtained). The color categories provide information on standardized therapeutic pathways and display doses of medications in milligrams and their volumetric equivalents. In addition to chemical weapons antidotes, this approach encompasses the entire spectrum of acute pediatric care (eg, fluid resuscitation, dehydration and electrolyte problems, pain management, antibiotics, equipment selection, burns), which may be a part of the care of pediatric disaster victims.

Meeting the Generic Needs of Children in a Disaster Situation

According to a recent review of the pediatric resuscitation process, an increase in logistical time is inherent in treating pediatric emergencies as opposed to adult emergencies.[111] One of the reasons for this increase is the age- and size-related variations unique to children, which introduce the need for more complex, nonautomatic or "knowledge-based" mental activities, such as calculating drug doses and selecting equipment. These detract from other important mental activities such as assessment, evaluation, prioritization, and synthesis of information, which can be referred to in the resuscitative process as "critical thinking activity." These logistical difficulties lead to inevitable time delays and a corresponding increase in the potential for decision-making errors in the pediatric resuscitative process. This is in sharp contrast to adult resuscitation. Medications used frequently in adults, such as epinephrine, atropine, glucose, bicarbonate, and lidocaine, are packaged in prefilled syringes containing the exact adult dose, making their ordering and administration automatic. The same concept is seen in equipment selection when the necessary equipment is laid out for immediate access and use. The adult provider does not need to recall formulas and calculations. The use of appropriate aids in pediatric resuscitation (those that contain precalculated doses, drug volumes, and other size-related variables) significantly reduces the cognitive load otherwise caused by obligatory calculations of dosage and equipment selection, and relegates these activities to a lower order of mental function referred to as automatic or "rule-based," increasing critical thinking time. The Broselow-Luten system has been commercially available for over 10 years and is stocked in several emergency departments across the country.[112] It has become the "standard of care" in the United States and abroad. This system is recommended in textbooks such as *Emergency Medicine* and *Pediatric Emergency Medicine* and by the American Heart Association's Pediatric Advanced Life Support Course.[113] It has been validated in several studies that have proven that the weights estimated from the measuring tape correlate with the actual weight of children up to 25 kg, and the system improves the ability to estimate a pediatric patient's weight over visual inspection or age-based equations.[114,115] Being able to obtain an accurate weight is critical to appropriately calculating medication doses. The system's color-coded chart has also been shown to improve the ability to select the right size intubation supplies and nasogastric tubes and to reduce the time to make those selections.[116] It reduces error, facilitates task completion, and saves time and resources (Figure 21-4).[111] The tools of the Broselow-Luten system, based on core concepts such as color-coding, arm bands, and chart stickers, are demonstrated visually in the chemical warfare antidote drug card for pediatric dosing of atropine (Figure 21-5). The system is being implemented in Afghanistan and Iraq to evaluate its effectiveness in a forward situation.

Meeting the Specific Needs of Children in a Chemical Disaster

Depending on the level of care, a provider may be involved in the ordering phase (physicians), the preparation and administration phase (nurses), or in both (prehospital personnel). With this in mind, tools need to be developed that are appropriate for both phases.

Drug cards and posters that contain color-coded, precalculated doses of antidotes to chemical agents and summary information on the particular needs of exposed children often give doses and drug volumes for IV, intraosseous, and IM drug administration (see Figure 21-4). Although 2-PAM Cl is recommended for both IV and IM use, the package insert only gives reconstitution directions for IV use. The insert recommends dilution of the 1 gm vial with 20 mL of sterile water to obtain a concentration of 50 mg/mL for injection.[117] No mention is made of a more concentrated dilution for IM use. However, sources have recommended 2-PAM Cl doses for both the IV and IM routes[33] because it is highly water-soluble.[118] Sidell described the preparation of a 30% solution of 2-PAM Cl for IM use,[119] implying that a dilution of 1 gm in 3 mL water (300 mg/mL) is a reasonable method of preparing 2-PAM Cl for IM delivery. This is critical information for safe administration to pediatric patients in which fluid overload could lead to toxicity.

The other route for administration is via autoinjector. Two options have recently been recommended for the use of adult autoinjectors in children. They do not address the potential morbidity from the injector needle, which is unknown, so the recommendations are based on theoretical assumptions and therefore lack supporting clinical data. Option 1 is based on the milligram-per-kilogram dose of atropine and 2-PAM Cl

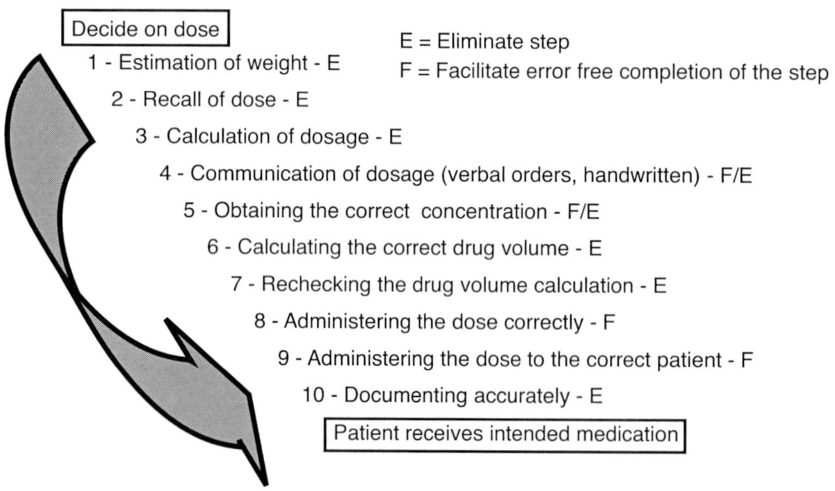

Fig. 21-4. Steps involved in administering a dose of medication. Using the Broselow-Luten color-coded standard dosing system can eliminate problematic areas such as calculations, and, if not totally eliminate, at least facilitate the error-free completion of other steps.

PEDIATRIC ANTIDOTES FOR CHEMICAL WARFARE DRUG VOLUMES (in mLs)											
DRUGS	3 kg	4 kg	5 kg	PINK	RED	PURPLE	YELLOW	WHITE	BLUE	ORANGE	GREEN
ATROPINE IV/IM	0.15 mg	0.2 mg	0.25 mg	0.3 mg	0.4 mg	0.5 mg	0.65 mg	0.8 mg	1 mg	1.3 mg	1.6 mg
0.05 mg/mL** conc	3	4	5	6	8	10	13	16	20	26	32
0.1 mg/mL** conc	1.5	2	2.5	3	4	5	6.5	8	10	13	16
0.4 mg/mL conc	0.4	0.5	0.6	0.8	1	1.3	1.6	2	2.5	3.2	4
0.5 mg/mL conc	0.3	0.4	0.5	0.6	0.8	1	1.3	1.6	2	2.6	3.2
0.8 mg/mL conc	0.2	0.25	0.3	0.4	0.5	0.6	0.8	1	1.2	1.6	2
1 mg/mL conc	0.15	0.2	0.25	0.3	0.4	0.5	0.65	0.8	1	1.3	1.6
2PAM	75 mg	100 mg	125 mg	165 mg	215 mg	265 mg	325 mg	415 mg	525 mg	665 mg	825 mg
IV 50 mg/mL	1.5	2	2.5	3.3	4.3	5.3	6.5	8.3	10.5	13.3	16.5
IM 300 mg/mL	0.25	0.33	0.42	0.55	0.7	0.9	1.1	1.4	1.8	2.2	2.8
IV DRIP 20 mg/mL	1.5-3 mL/hr	2-4 mL/hr	2.5-5 mL/hr	3.3-6.5 mL/hr	4.3-8.5 mL/hr	5.3-10.5 mL/hr	6.5-13 mL/hr	8.3-17 mL/hr	11-21 mL/hr	13-27 mL/hr	17-33 mL/hr
2PAM MEDICATION PREPARATION	IV 1 gm vial + 20 mL Sterile Water = 50 mg/mL				IM 1 gm vial + 3 mL Sterile Water = 300 mg/mL				IV DRIP Reconstitute the 1 gm vial with 20 mL NS, then dilute with 30 mL NS to a total volume of 50 mL		

**Concentrations are too dilute for IM injection in most patients. All IV medications may be given IO.

Fig. 21-5. Antidote drug card for pediatric dosing of atropine; close-up of drug chart component.

as a result of a single Mark I injection (2 mg atropine, and 600 mg 2-PAM Cl), which has been extrapolated to the weight zones of the color-coded system,[70] suggesting that children in the yellow zone (3 years old) or higher may receive one Mark I autoinjector.[70,71] Option 2 is based on the comparison of the total milligram-per-kilogram dose an adult would normally receive over 60 to 90 minutes versus the milligram-per-kilogram amount that would be received with a single Mark I injection, even in a smaller child.[71] This suggests that in the absence of another option, one Mark I may be given to any child in extremis, regardless of size. Baum, Henretig, and Wiley are developing a comprehensive color-coded toolkit for the management of both biological and chemical agents in children based on these philosophies.

Other Pediatric Resources

Another group instrumental in providing guidance on terrorism in children is the Program for Pediatric Preparedness of the National Center for Disaster Preparedness at Columbia University. This group was established to determine appropriate management and intervention for children in all types of disasters, including chemical emergencies. The program has five main goals:

1. to assess pediatric preparedness at the community, facility, local, regional, and national levels;
2. to conduct and foster research on pediatric disaster, terrorism, and public health emergency preparedness and response;
3. to provide resources to children, parents, communities, and governmental and nongovernmental agencies on pediatric preparedness;
4. to build collaboration among disciplines and occupations that must work together to care for children during an emergency; and
5. to advocate for children in all forums related to preparedness.

To achieve these goals, the group produces a quarterly newsletter on pediatric issues and preparedness, distributes informational bulletins on pediatric issues, has developed an expert advisory board to help guide development of preparedness tools, and has created a Web site to share its resources. The group also initiated a pediatric preparedness national consensus conference. The first conference was held in Washington, DC, in February 2003, and led to recommendations and treatment guidelines.[120]

The American Academy of Pediatrics also continually provides updated and valuable resources regarding children, terrorism, and disaster planning. It provides an updated bibliography of literature related to chemical casualty management in pediatrics.

The Regional Emergency Medical Advisory Committee of New York City, the City of New York Fire Department, and the City of New York Bureau of Emergency Medical Services, in collaboration with the Center for Pediatric Emergency Medicine of the New York University School of Medicine and the Bellevue Hospital Center, have developed and published a pediatric nerve agent antidote dosing schedule.[121] Dosing cards for the treatment of children exposed to weapons of mass destruction have been developed by US Public Health Service pharmacist officers.[122]

SUMMARY

Much progress has been made in understanding how to manage pediatric patients affected by chemical agents. Several pediatric organizations, such as the American Academy of Pediatrics, have offered guidance on handling these situations. Gathering information about pediatric chemical casualties is challenging because experience is limited; further research and resources are needed to fully understand all the physical and psychological impacts a terror attack has on children. In a chemical attack, prior preparation and planning will make a difference in whether lives are saved or lost. Efforts must be made to learn how to best manage chemical attacks and how to best prepare to protect the pediatric population.

Acknowledgment

The authors wish to thank Keyvan Rafei, MD (University of Maryland Medical Center, Baltimore, Maryland) and Major Scott Willens, DVM (USAMRICD) for providing insightful suggestions and comments throughout the preparation of this chapter.

REFERENCES

1. United Nations Security Council. *Report of the Specialists Appointed by the Secretary-General to Investigate Allegations by the Islamic Republic of Iran Concerning the Use of Chemical Weapons.* UN Security Council: New York, NY; 1984. Report S/16433.

2. United Nations Security Council. *Report of the Mission Dispatched by the Secretary-General to Investigate Allegations of the Use of Chemical Weapons in the Conflict Between the Islamic Republic of Iran and Iraq.* UN Security Council: New York, NY; 1986. Report S/17911.

3. Hu H, Cook-Deegan R, Shukri A. The use of chemical weapons: conducting an investigation using survey epidemiology. *JAMA.* 1989;262(5):640–643.

4. Hay A, Roberts G. The use of poison gas against the Iraqi Kurds: analysis of bomb fragments, soil, and wool samples. *JAMA.* 1990;263(8):1065–1066.

5. Kelly L, Dewar D, Curry B. Experiencing chemical warfare: two physicians tell their story of Halabja in Northern Iraq. *Can J Rural Med.* 2004;9(3):178–181.

6. Goldberg J. The great terror. *New Yorker.* March 25, 2002: 52–75.

7. O'Leary CA. The Kurds of Iraq: recent history, future prospects. *Middle East Rev Int Affairs J.* 2002;6(4):17–29.

8. Mohamed-Ali H. Late lesions due to poison gas in survivors of the Iraqi poison warfare against the Kurdish people. *Wien Med Wochenschr.* 1992;142(1):8–15.

9. Gosden C, Amitay M, Gardener D, Amin B. Examining long-term severe health consequences of CBW use against civilian populations. *Bull UN Institute Disarm Res (UNIDIR).* 1999;Disarmament Forum Three.

10. Dompeling E, Jobsis Q, Vandevijver NMA, et al. Chronic bronchiolitis in a 5-yr-old child after exposure to sulfur mustard gas. *Eur Respir J.* 2004;23:343–346.

11. Momeni A, Aminjavaheri M. Skin manifestations of mustard gas in a group of 14 children and teenagers: a clinical study. *Inter J Dermatol*. 1994:33(3):184–187.

12. Foroutan SA. Medical notes concerning chemical warfare, Part I. *Kowsar Med J*. 1996; 1(1):1–8.

13. Foroutan SA. Medical notes concerning chemical warfare, Part II. *Kowsar Med J*. 1996; (2):1–23.

14. Foroutan SA. Medical notes concerning chemical warfare, Part III. *Kowsar Med J*. 1997;2(1):1–15.

15. Foroutan SA. Medical notes concerning chemical warfare, Part IV. *Kowsar Med J*. 1997;2(2):1–15.

16. Foroutan SA. Medical notes concerning chemical warfare, Part V. *Kowsar Med J*. 1997;2(3):1–9.

17. Foroutan SA. Medical notes concerning chemical warfare, Part VI. *Kowsar Med J*. 1998;2(4):1–18.

18. Foroutan SA. Medical notes concerning chemical warfare, Part VII. *Kowsar Med J*. 1998;3(1):1–10.

19. Foroutan SA. Medical notes concerning chemical warfare, Part IX. *Kowsar Med J*. 1996;3(3):1–16.

20. Foroutan SA. Medical notes concerning chemical warfare, Part X. *Kowsar Med J*. 1999;3(4):1–12.

21. Foroutan SA. Medical notes concerning chemical warfare, Part XI. *Kowsar Med J*. 1999;4(1):1–7.

22. Vogel FJ. *The Chemical Weapons Convention: Strategic Implications for the United States*. Monograph. The Strategic Studies Institute at the US Army War College: Carlisle, Penn; 1997.

23. Sidell FR. Chemical agent terrorism. *Ann Emerg Med*. 1996;28(2):223–224.

24. Nagao M, Takatori T, Matsuda Y, Nakajima M, Iwase H, Iwadate K. Definitive evidence for the acute sarin poisoning diagnosis in the Tokyo subway. *Toxic Appl Pharm*. 1997;144:198–203.

25. Tsuchihashi H, Katagi M, Nishikawa M, Tatsuno M. Identification of metabolites of nerve agent VX in serum collected from a victim. *J Anal Toxicol*. 1998;22(5):383–388.

26. Matsuda Y, Nagao M, Takatori T, Niijima H, Nakajima M, Iwase H, et al. Detection of the sarin hydrolysis product in formalin-fixed brain tissues of victims of the Tokyo subway terrorist attack. *Toxicol Appl Pharm*. 1998;150:310–320.

27. Solberg Y, Nachtomi-Shick O, Shemer Y, Alcalay M. Terror in Japan: mass-intoxication with the nerve-agent sarin. *Harefuah*. 1998;135(7–8):268–271.

28. Okudera H. Clinical features on nerve gas terrorism in Matsumoto. *J Clin Neurosci*. 2002;9(1):17–21.

29. Yanagisawa N, Morita H, Nakajima T. Sarin experiences in Japan: acute toxicity and long-term effects. *J Neurol Sci*. 2006;249:76–85.

30. Blaschke GS, Lynch J. Terrorism: its impact on primary pediatrics, Part I. *Pediatr Ann*. 2003;32(2):80–84.

31. Blaschke GS, Palfrey JS, Lynch J. Advocating for children during uncertain times. *Pediatr Ann*. 2003;32(4):271–274.

32. Committee on Environmental Health and Committee on Infectious Diseases. Chemical-biological terrorism and its impact on children: a subject review. *Pediatrics*. 2000;105:662–670.

33. Rotenberg JS, Newmark J. Nerve agent attacks on children: diagnosis and management. *Pediatrics*. 2003;112:648–658.

34. Brackett DW. *Holy Terror Armageddon in Tokyo*. New York, NY: Weatherhill, Inc; 1996.

35. Sidell FR, Takafuji ET, Franz DR, eds. *Medical Aspects of Chemical and Biological Warfare*. In: Zajtchuk R, Bellamy RF, eds. *Textbooks of Military Medicine*. Washington, DC: Department of the Army, Office of the Surgeon General, Borden Institute; 1997.

36. Lynch EL, Thomas TL. Pediatric considerations in chemical exposures: are we prepared? *Pediatr Emerg Care*. 2004;20(3):198–205.

37. Abramowicz M, ed. Prevention and treatment of injury from chemical warfare agents. *Med Letter*. 2002;44:1–4.

38. Fluhr JW, Pfisterer S, Gloor M. Direct comparison of skin physiology in children and adults with bioengineering methods. *Pediatr Dermatol*. 2000;17(6):436–439.

39. Simonen P, O'Brien M, Hamilton C, Ashcroft J, Denham J. Normal variation in cutaneous blood content and red blood cell velocity in humans. *Physiol Meas*. 1997;18(3):155–170.

40. Fluhr JW, Behne MJ, Brown BE, Moskowitz DG, Selden C, Mao-Wiang M, et al. Stratum corneum acidification in neonatal skin: secretory phospholipase A2 and the sodium/hydrogen antiporter-1 acidify neonatal rat stratum corneum. *J Invest Dermatol*. 2004;122(2):320–329.

41. Behrendt H, Green M. Skin pH pattern in the newborn infant. *AMA J Dis Child*. 1958;95(1):35–41.

42. Fairley JA, Rasmussen JE. Comparison of stratum corneum thickness in children and adults. *J Am Acad Dermatol*. 1983;8(5):652–654.

43. Bennett WD, Zeman KL. Deposition of fine particles in children spontaneously breathing at rest. *Inhalation Toxicol*. 1998;10:831–842.

44. Martonen TB, Musante CJ, Sega RA, et al. Lung models: strengths and weaknesses. *Respir Care*. 2000;45(6):712–736.

45. Children more vulnerable than adults in the event of a chemical spill or chemical weapons attack. *Cedars-Sinai Medical Center News*. July 14, 2003.

46. Rutter N, Hull D. Water loss from the skin of term and preterm babies. *Arch Dis Child*. 1979;54:858–868.

47. Harpin VA, Rutter N. Barrier properties of the newborn infants' skin. *J Pediatr*. 1983;102:419–425.

48. Nopper AJ, Horii KA, Sookdeo-Drost S, Wang TH, Mancini AJ, Lane AT. Topical ointment therapy benefits premature infants. *J Pediatr*. 1996;128(5):660–669.

49. Seidenari S, Giusti G, Bertoni L, Magnoni C, Pellacani G. Thickness and echogenicity of the skin in children as assessed by 20-MHz ultrasound. *Dermatology*. 2000;201(3):218–222.

50. Mancini AJ. Skin. *Pediatrics*. 2004;113(4 Suppl):114–1119.

51. Besunder JB, Reed MD, Blumer JL. Principles of drug biodisposition in the neonate. A critical evaluation of the pharmacokinetic-pharmacodynamic interface. Part I. *Clin Pharmacokinet*. 1988;14(5):261–286.

52. Kearns GL, Reed MD. Clinical pharmacokinetics in infants and children. A reappraisal. *Clin Pharmacokinet*. 1989;17(Suppl 1):29–67.

53. Clewell HJ, Teeguarden J, McDonald T, et al. Review and evaluation of the potential impact of age- and gender-specific pharmacokinetic differences on tissue dosimetry. *Crit Rev Toxicol*. 2002;32(5):329–389.

54. Ginsberg G, Hattis D, Sonawane B. Incorporating pharmacokinetic differences between children and adults in assessing children's risks to environmental toxicants. *Toxicol Appl Pharmacol*. 2004;198(2):164–183.

55. Morselli PL. Clinical pharmacology of the perinatal period and early infancy. *Clin Pharmacokinet*. 1989;17(Suppl 1):13–28.

56. Saunders NR, Knott GW, Dziegielewska KM. Barriers in the immature brain. *Cell Mol Neurobiol*. 2000;20(1):29–40.

57. National Research Council Committee on Pesticides in the Diets of Infants and Children. *Pesticides in the diets of infants and children*. Washington, DC: National Academy Press; 1993.

58. Stead AL. The response of the newborn infant to muscle relaxant. *Br J Anaesth*. 1955;27(3):124–130.

59. Lehmann H, Cook J, Ryan E. Pseudocholinesterase in early infancy. *Proc R Soc Med*. 1957;50(3):147–150.

60. Augustinsson KB, Brody S. Plasma arylesterase activity in adults and newborn infants. *Clin Chim Acta*. 1962;7:560–565.

61. Ecobichon DJ, Stephens DS. Perinatal development of human blood esterases. *Clin Pharmacol Ther*. 1973;14(1):41–47.

62. Morselli PL. Clinical pharmacokinetics in neonates. *Clin Pharmacokinet*. 1976;1(2):81–98.

63. Holland N, Furlong C, Bastaki M, et al. Paraxonase polymorphisms, haplotypes, and enzyme activity in Latino mothers and newborns. *Environ Health Perspect*. 2006;114(7):985–991.

64. Abraham RB, Rudick V, Weinbroum AA. Practical guidelines for acute care of victims of bioterrorism: conventional injuries and concomitant nerve agent intoxication. *Anesthesiology*. 2002;97(4): 989–1004.

65. Wheeler DS, Poss WB. Mass casualty management in a changing world. *Pediatr Ann*. 2003;32(2):98–105.

66. Henretig FM, Cieslak TJ, Eitzen Jr EM. Medical progress: biological and chemical terrorism erratum. *J Pediatr*. 2002;141(5):743–746.

67. Litovitz TL, Klein-Schwartz W, White S, et al. 2000 annual report of the American Association of Poison Control Centers Toxic Exposure Surveillance System. *Amer J Emerg Med*. 2001;19(5):337–395.

68. Lifshitz M, Shahak E, Sofer S. Carbamate and organophosphate poisonings in young children. *Pediatr Emerg Care*. 1999;15(2):102–103.

69. Dunn MA, Sidell FR. Progress in medical defense against nerve agents. *JAMA*. 1989;262(5):649–652.

70. Henretig F, Cieslak TJ, Eitzen EM. Medical progress: biological and chemical terrorism. *J Pediatr*. 2002;141(3):311–326.

71. Columbia University Mailman School of Public Health. Atropine use in children after nerve gas exposure. *Info Brief*. 2004;1(1):1–8.

72. Meadows M. The FDA and the fight against terrorism. *FDA Consum*. 2004;38(1):20–27.

73. Amitai Y, Almog S, Singer R, Hammer R, Bentur Y, Danon YL. Atropine poisoning in children during the Persian Gulf crisis: a national survey in Israel. *JAMA*. 1992;268:630–632.

74. Abraham RB, Weinbroum AA, Rudick V, Paret G. Perioperative care of children with nerve agent intoxication. *Paediatr Anaesthesia*. 2001;11:643–649.

75. Rotenberg JS. Diagnosis and management of nerve agent exposure. *Pediatr Ann*. 2003;32(4):242–250.

76. Yu CE, Burklow TR, Madsen JM. Vesicant agents and children. *Pediatr Ann*. 2003;32(4):254–257.

77. Sidell FR, Urbanetti JS, Smith WJ, Hurst CG. Vesicants. In: Sidell FR, Takafuji ET, Franz DR, eds. *Medical Aspects of Chemical and Biological Warfare*. In: Zajtchuk R, Bellamy RF, eds. *Textbooks of Military Medicine*. Washington, DC: Department of the Army, Office of the Surgeon General, Borden Institute; 1997.

78. Azizi MD, Amid MH. Clinical presentation of chemical warfare injuries in children and teenagers. *Med J Islamic Rep Iran*. 1990;4(2):103–108.

79. Motakallem MH. Evaluation of 17 patients severely injured with sulfur mustard. *Med J Islamic Rep Iran*. 1988;2(2):99–104.

80. Graham JS, Chilcott RP, Rice P, Milner SM, Hurst CG, Maliner BI. Wound healing of cutaneous sulfur mustard injuries: strategies for the development of improved therapies. *J Burns Wounds*. 2005;4:e1.

81. US Army Medical Research Institute of Chemical Defense. *Medical Management of Chemical Casualties Handbook*. 3rd ed. Aberdeen Proving Ground, Md: USAMRICD; 2000.

82. US Army Medical Research Institute of Chemical Defense. *Field Management of Chemical Casualties Handbook*. 2nd ed. Aberdeen Proving Ground, Md: USAMRICD; 2000.

83. Department of the Army. Vesicants (blister agents). In: *NATO Handbook on the Medical Aspects of NBC Defensive Operations AMedP-6(B)*. Part III: Chemical. Washington, DC: DA; 1996.

84. Moradi A, Sodeifi M, Abdollahi B, Pakdaman A, Vessal K. Clinical presentation of chemical warfare injuries. *Iran J Med Sci*. 1986;13:1–5.

85. Logan TP, Graham JS, Martin JL, Zallnick JE, Jakubowski EM, Braue EH. Detection and measurement of sulfur mustard (HD) offgassing from the weanling pig following exposure to saturated sulfur mustard vapor. *J Appl Toxicol*. 2000;20:S199–S204.

86. Buscher H, Conway N, trans. *Green and Yellow Cross*. Cincinnati, Ohio: Kettering Laboratory of Applied Physiology, University of Cincinnati; 1944.

87. Geffner ME, Powars DR, Choctaw WT. Acquired methemoglobinemia. *West J Med*. 1981;134:7–10.

88. Ohlgisser M, Adler M, Ben-Dov D, Taitelman U, Birkhan HJ, Bursztein S. Methaemoglobinaemia induced by mafenide acetate in children. *Br J Anaesth*. 1978;50:299–301.

89. Fullerton JK, Smith CE, Neumeister MW. Methemoglobinemia induced by 5% mafenide acetate solution and topical lidocaine spray in a pediatric burn patient: a case report. *J Burns & Surg Wound Care*. 2002;1(1):14.

90. Ruhl CM, Park DJ, Danisa O, et al. A serious skin sulfur mustard burn from an artillery shell. *J Emerg Med*. 1994;12(2):159–166.

91. Marshall JH, Bromberg BE, Adrizzo JR, Heurich AE, Samet CM. Fatal tetanus complicating a small partial-thickness burn. *J Trauma*. 1972;12(1):91–93.

92. Burklow TR, Yu CE, Madsen JM. Industrial chemicals: terrorist weapons of opportunity. *Pediatr Ann*. 2003;32(4):230–234.

93. Güloğlu C, Kara IH, Erten PG. Acute accidental exposure to chlorine gas in the southeast of Turkey: a study of 106 cases. *Environ Res*. 2002;88:89–93.

94. Traub SJ, Hoffman RS, Nelson LS. Case report and literature review of chlorine gas toxicity. *Vet Human Toxicol*. 2002;44(4):235–239.

95. Pherwani AV, Khanna SA, Patel RB. Effect of chlorine gas leak on the pulmonary functions of school children. *Indian J Pediatr*. 1989;56:125–128.

96. Rotenberg JS. Cyanide as a weapon of terror. *Pediatr Ann*. 2003;32(4):236–240.

97. Baskin SI, Brewer TG. Cyanide poisoning. In: Sidell FR, Takafuji ET, Franz DR, eds. *Medical Aspects of Chemical and Biological Warfare*. In: Zajtchuk R, Bellamy RF, eds. *Textbooks of Military Medicine*. Washington, DC: Department of the Army, Office of the Surgeon General, Borden Institute; 1997.

98. Riordan M, Rylance G, Berry K. Poisoning in children: 5 rare and dangerous poisons. *Arch Dis Child*. 2002;87:407–410.

99. Prajapati NC, Puri RK, Sarangi MP, Yadav S, Khalil A. Potassium cyanide poisoning. *Indian Pediatr*. 1992;29:903–905.

100. Goldfrank LR, Flomenbaum NE, Lewin NA. Cyanide and hydrogen sulfide. In: Goldfrank LR, Flomenbaum NE, Lewin NA, Weisman RS, Howland MA, Hoffman RS, eds. *Goldfrank's Toxicologic Emergencies*. 6th ed. Stamford, Conn: Appleton & Lange; 1998.

101. Peden NR, Taha A, McSorley. Industrial exposure to hydrogen cyanide: implications for treatment. *Br Med J*. 1986;293:538.

102. Cyanide antidote [package insert]. Buffalo Grove, Ill: Taylor Pharmaceuticals; 1998.

103. Berlin CM. The treatment of cyanide poisoning in children. *Pediatrics*. 1970;46:793–796.

104. Hall AH, Rumack BH. Clinical toxicology of cyanide. *Ann Emerg Med*. 1986;15:1067–1074.

105. Rotenberg JS, Burklow TR, Selanikio JS. Weapons of mass destruction: the decontamination of children. *Pediatr Ann*. 2003;32(4):261–267.

106. Rosenbaum C. Chemical warfare: disaster preparation in an Israeli hospital. *Soc Work Health Care*. 1993;18:137–145.

107. Bradley BJ, Gresham LS, Sidelinger DE, Hartstein BH. Pediatric health professionals and public health response. *Pediatr Ann*. 2003;32:87–94.

108. Schonfeld DJ. Potential roles for pediatricians. *Pediatr Ann*. 2003;32:182–187.

109. *Effects of the World Trade Center Attack on NYC Public School Students: Initial Report to the New York City Board of Education*. New York, NY: New York City Department of Education; 2002.

110. Frush K, Hohenhaus S. Pediatric Mass Casualty Incident Guidelines. Durham, NC: Duke University Health System Emergency Medical Services for Children; 2004. Available at: http://www.wnysmart.org/References/MCI_Duke_Protocol_April04.pdf. Accessed February 29, 2008.

111. Luten R, Wears RL, Broselow J, Croskerry P, Joseph MM, Frush K. Managing the unique size-related issues of pediatric resuscitation: reducing cognitive load with resuscitation aids. *Acad Emerg Med*. 2002;9;840–847.

112. Frush K, Hohenhaus S, Luo X, Gerardi M, Wiebe RA. Evaluation of a Web-based education program on reducing medication dosing error: a multicenter, randomized controlled trial. *Ped Emerg Care*. 2006;22:62–70.

113. Luten R, Broselow J. Rainbow care: the Broselow-Luten system. Implications for pediatric patient safety. *Ambul Outreach*. 1999;fall:14–16.

114. Lubitz DS, Seidel JS, Chameides L, Luten RC, Zaritsky AL, Campbell FW. A rapid method for estimating weight and resuscitation drug dosages from length in the pediatric age group. *Ann Emerg Med*. 1988;17:576–581.

115. Vilke GM, Marino A, Fisher R, Chan TC. Estimation of pediatric patient weight by EMT-PS. *J Emerg Med*. 2001;21:125–128.

116. Agarwal S, Swanson S, Murphy A, Yaeger K, Sharek P, Halamek LP. Comparing the utility of a standard pediatric resuscitation cart with a pediatric resuscitation cart based on the Broselow tape: a randomized, controlled, crossover trial involving simulated resuscitation scenarios. *Pediatrics*. 2005;116:326–333.

117. Pralidoxime [package insert]. Bristol, Tenn: Meridian Medical Technologies, Inc; 2002.

118. Remington JP, Gennaro AR. *Remington: the Science and Practice of Pharmacy*. 19th ed. Easton, Pa: Mack Publishing Co; 1995.

119. Sidell FR. Clinical considerations in nerve agent intoxication. In: Somani SM, ed. *Chemical Warfare Agents*. San Francisco, Calif: Academic Press, Inc; 1992.

120. Markenson D, Redlener I. Pediatric terrorism preparedness national guidelines and recommendations: findings of an evidenced-based consensus process. *Biosecur Bioterror*. 2004;2:301–309.

121. Foltin G, Tunik M, Curran J, et al. Pediatric nerve agent poisoning: medical and operational considerations for emergency medical services in a large American city. *Pediatr Emerg Care*. 2006;22:239–244.

122. Montello MJ, Tarosky M, Pincock L, et al. Dosing cards for treatment of children exposed to weapons of mass destruction. *Am J Health Syst Pharm*. 2006;63:944–949.

Chapter 22

MEDICAL DIAGNOSTICS

BENEDICT R. CAPACIO, PhD*; J. RICHARD SMITH†; RICHARD K. GORDON, PhD‡; JULIAN R. HAIGH, PhD§; JOHN R. BARR, PhD¥; AND GENNADY E. PLATOFF JR, PhD¶

*Chief, Medical Diagnostic and Chemical Branch, Analytical Toxicology Division, US Army Medical Research Institute of Chemical Defense, 3100 Rickets Point Road, Aberdeen Proving Ground, Maryland 21010-5400

†Chemist, Medical Diagnostic and Chemical Branch, Analytical Toxicology Division, US Army Medical Research Institute of Chemical Defense, 3100 Rickets Point Road, Aberdeen Proving Ground, Maryland 21010-5400

‡Chief, Department of Biochemical Pharmacology, Biochemistry Division, Walter Reed Army Institute of Research, 503 Robert Grant Road, Silver Spring, Maryland 20910-7500

§Research Scientist, Department of Biochemical Pharmacology, Biochemistry Division, Walter Reed Army Institute of Research, 503 Robert Grant Road, Silver Spring, Maryland 20910-7500

¥Lead Research Chemist, Centers for Disease Control and Prevention, 4770 Buford Highway, Mailstop F47, Atlanta, Georgia 30341

¶Colonel, US Army (Retired); Scientific Advisor, Office of Biodefense Research, National Institute of Allergies and Infectious Disease, National Institutes of Health, 6610 Rockledge Drive, Room 4069, Bethesda, Maryland 20892-6612

INTRODUCTION

In the past, issues associated with chemical warfare agents, including developing and implementing medical countermeasures, field detection, verification of human exposures, triage, and treatment, have primarily been a concern of the military community because most prior experience with chemical warfare agents was limited to the battlefield. However, chemical agents have been increasingly employed against civilian populations, such as in Iraqi attacks against the Kurds and the attacks organized by the Aum Shinrikyo cult in Matsumoto City and the Tokyo subway. The attacks on the World Trade Center in New York City and the Pentagon in Washington, DC, in 2001 have increased concern about the potential large-scale use of chemical warfare agents in a civilian sector. Incidents involving large numbers of civilians have shown that to facilitate appropriate treatment, it is critical to identify not only those exposed, but those who have not been exposed, as well. In addition to health issues associated with exposure, the political and legal ramifications of a chemical warfare attack can be enormous. It is therefore essential that testing for exposure be accurate, sensitive, and rapid.

For the most part, monitoring for the presence of chemical warfare agents in humans, or "biomonitoring," involves examining specimens to determine if an exposure has occurred. Assays that provide definitive evidence of agent exposure commonly target metabolites, such as hydrolysis products and adducts formed following binding to biomolecular entities. Unlike drug efficacy studies in which blood/plasma levels usually focus on the parent compounds, assay techniques for verifying chemical agent exposure rarely target the intact agent because of its limited longevity in vivo. Following exposure, many agents are rapidly converted and appear in the blood as hydrolysis products (resulting from reactions with water) and are excreted in urine. Because of rapid formation and subsequent urinary excretion, the use of these products as markers provides a limited window of opportunity to collect a sample with measurable product. More long-lived markers tend to be those that result from agent interactions with large-molecular–weight targets, such as proteins and DNA. These result from covalent binding of the agent or agent moiety to form macromolecular adducts. As such, the protein acts as a depot for the adducted agent and the residence time is similar to the half-life of the target molecule.

Blood/blood components, urine, and, in rare instances, tissue specimens, termed "sample matrices" or "biomedical samples," can be used to verify chemical agent exposure. However, any sample obtained from an exposed individual may be considered as a potential matrix (eg, blister fluid from sulfur mustard [North Atlantic Treaty Organization (NATO) designation: HD] vesication). Regardless, analyses of these types of samples are inherently difficult because of the matrix's complex composition and the presence of analyte in trace quantities.

Noninvasive urine collection does not require highly trained medical personnel or specialized equipment. Although biomarkers present in urine are usually short-lived (hours to days) metabolites, they can be present in relatively high concentrations in samples obtained shortly after exposure. The collection of blood/plasma should be performed by trained medical personnel. Blood/plasma samples offer potential benefits because both metabolites and the more long-lived adducts of a macromolecular target can be assayed. The effectiveness of using tissue to verify chemical agent exposure is generally limited to postmortem sampling. For example, formalin-fixed brain tissues from fatalities of the Tokyo subway attack were successfully used to verify sarin (NATO designation: GB) as the agent employed in that attack.[1] Other tissue samples can be obtained from the carcasses of animals at the incident site.

Methods that do not directly analyze cholinesterase (ChE) activity typically involve detection systems like mass spectrometry (MS) combined with either gas chromatography (GC) or liquid chromatography (LC) to separate the analyte from other matrix components. MS detection methods are based upon specific and characteristic fragmentation patterns of the parent molecule, making MS detection desirable because it identifies the analyte fairly reliably. Other detection systems, such as nitrogen-phosphorus detection and flame photometric detection, have also been used. Some analytes can be directly assessed, whereas others may require chemical modification (eg, derivatization) to enhance detection or make them more volatile in GC separations. More sophisticated techniques may employ GC or LC with tandem MS (MS-MS) detection systems, allowing more sensitivity and selectivity.

Validating the performance of an analytical technique subsequent to initial in-vitro method development is usually accomplished with in-vivo animal exposure models. Additional information may be gleaned from archived human samples from past exposure incidents. Samples from humans exposed to sulfur mustard during the Iran-Iraq War and a limited number of samples from the Japanese nerve agent attacks have been used to evaluate assay techniques. In the case of some agents, background marker levels are known to exist in nonexposed individuals, making it difficult to interpret the results of potential incidents. Therefore, in addition to assessing performance in animal models and archived human samples, it is essential to determine potential background levels and incidence of markers in nonexposed human populations. It should be stressed that, for the purpose of exposure verification, results from laboratory testing must be considered along with other information, such as the presentation of symptoms consistent with the agent in question and results from environmental testing.

In the late 1980s the US Army Medical Research Institute of Chemical Defense was tasked by the Department of Defense to develop methods that could confirm potential chemical warfare agent exposure. The US Army Medical Research Institute of Chemical Defense had previously published procedures for verifying exposure to nerve agents and sulfur mustard. These methods primarily focused on GC-MS analysis of hydrolysis products excreted in the urine following exposure to chemical warfare agents. Subsequently, the methods using urine or blood samples were compiled as part of Technical Bulletin Medical 296, titled "Assay Techniques for Detection of Exposure to Sulfur Mustard, Cholinesterase Inhibitors, Sarin, Soman, GF, and Cyanide."[2] The publication was intended to provide clinicians with laboratory tests to detect exposure to chemical warfare agents.

In the mid 1990s, after the publication of Technical Bulletin Medical 296, the military adapted some of the laboratory analytical methods for field-forward use. The concept was demonstrated by the US Army 520th Theater Army Medical Laboratory, which used the Test-Mate OP Kit (EQM Research Inc, Cincinnati, OH) for acetylcholinesterase (AChE) assay and a fly-away GC-MS system. The lengthy preparation of GC and MS samples for analysis in a field environment was one of the reasons that alternative methods of analysis for chemical warfare agents were later examined.

Preexposure treatments or tests to monitor potential chemical agent exposure may be warranted for military personnel and first responders who must enter or operate in chemically contaminated environments. However, laboratory testing may not be as useful for large civilian populations unless there is a clear impending chemical threat. At the same time, determining the health effects of chemical exposure is complex because it can affect the nervous system, respiratory tract, skin, eyes, and mucous membranes, as well as the gastrointestinal, cardiovascular, endocrine, and reproductive systems. Individual susceptibility, preexisting medical conditions, and age may also contribute to the severity of a chemically related illness. Chronic exposures, even at low concentrations, are another concern. In addition to development of diagnostic technologies, strategies to detect chemical agent exposure have become a public health issue.

The transition of laboratory-based analytical techniques to a far-forward field setting can generate valuable information for military or civilian clinicians. In this transition, problems such as data analysis, interpreting complex spectra, and instrument troubleshooting and repair may need addressing. As analytical methods are developed, refined, and sent farther from the laboratory, advanced telecommunication will be needed to provide a direct link between research scientists and field operators; telecommunication will become critical to confirming patient exposure and tracking patient recovery and treatment.

This chapter provides a basic outline and references for state-of-the-art analytical methods presently described in the literature. Methods of verification for exposure to nerve agents, vesicants, pulmonary toxicants, metabolic poisons, incapacitating agents, and riot control agents will be reviewed. Biological sample collection, handling, storage, shipping, and submission will be explained.

NERVE AGENTS

Background

The first organophosphorus (OP) nerve agent, tabun (NATO designation: GA) was developed shortly before and during World War II by German chemist Gerhard Schrader at IG Farbenindustrie in an attempt to develop a commercial insecticide.[3,4,5] Shortly thereafter, sarin was synthesized. Both are extremely toxic. The German government realized the compounds had potential as chemical warfare agents and began producing them and incorporating them into munitions. Subsequently, soman (NATO designation: GD) was synthesized, but only small amounts were produced by the end of the war.[4] Five of the OP compounds are generally regarded as nerve agents: tabun, sarin, soman, cyclosarin (NATO designation: GF), and Russian VX.[4] These compounds demonstrated extreme toxicity, which was attributed to long-lasting binding and inhibition of the enzyme AChE. As a result, the compounds were referred to as "irreversible" inhibitors. Related, but less toxic compounds (ie, "reversible" inhibitors), are becoming widely used therapeutically; for example, in the treatment of Alzheimer's disease. The relative description as reversible or irreversible refers to the length of the binding to the enzyme (Figure 22-1).

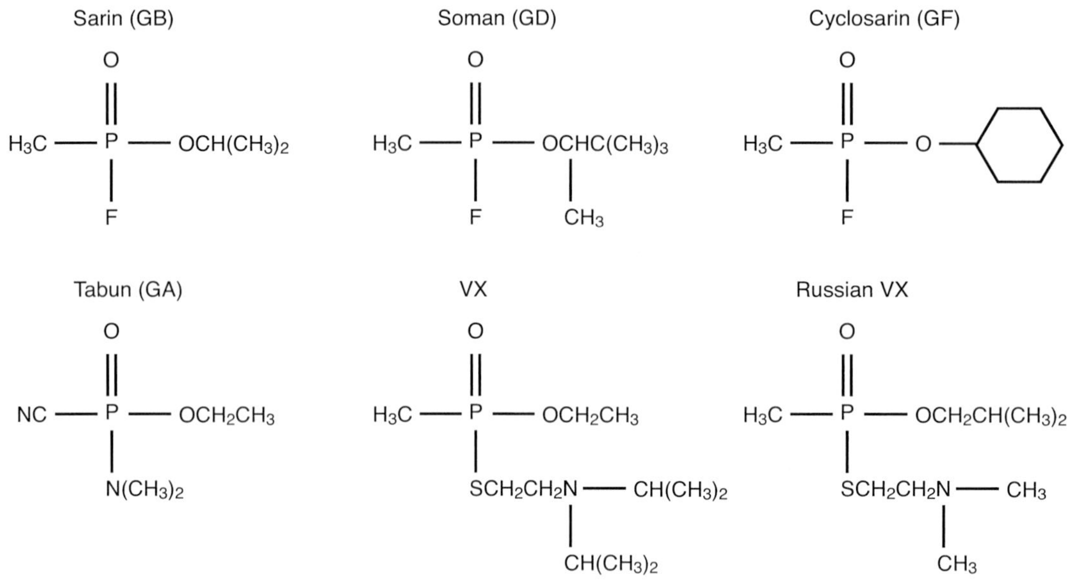

Fig. 22-1. Chemical structures of nerve agents. The nerve agents sarin (GB), soman (GD), and cyclosarin (GF) lose fluorine subsequent to binding to cholinesterase. The agents tabun (GA), VX, and Russian VX lose cyanide and the thiol groups.

Many of the assays developed for exposure verification are based on the interaction of nerve agents with ChE enzymes. Nerve agents inhibit ChE by forming a covalent bond between the phosphorus atom of the agent and the serine residue of the enzyme active site. That interaction results in the displacement or loss of fluorine from sarin, soman, and cyclosarin. The binding of tabun, VX, and Russian VX is different in that the leaving group is cyanide followed by the thiol groups (see Figure 22-1).[6] Spontaneous reactivation of the enzyme or hydrolysis reactions with water can occur to produce corresponding alkyl methylphosphonic acids (MPAs). Alternatively, the loss of the O-alkyl group while bound to the enzyme produces a highly stable organophosphoryl-ChE bond, a process referred to as "aging." Once aging has occurred, the enzyme is considered resistant to reactivation by oximes or other nucleophilic reagents.[4] The spontaneous reactivation and aging rates of the agents vary depending on the O-alkyl group. For example, VX-inhibited red blood cell (RBC) ChE reactivates at an approximate rate of 0.5% to 1% per hour for the first 48 hours, with minimal aging. On the other hand, soman-inhibited ChE does not spontaneously reactivate and has a very rapid aging rate, with a half-time of approximately 2 minutes.[4]

General Clinical Tests

With the exception of ChE analysis, there are no standard clinical assays that specifically test for nerve agent exposure. However, over the years numerous lab-based, non-ChE analytical methods have been developed, and several successfully utilized, to verify nerve agent exposure. For the most part, these employ MS with GC or LC separations. The tests are relatively labor intensive, requiring trained personnel and sophisticated instrumentation not usually available in clinical settings. Most experience using these techniques has come from animal exposure models. These assessments allow for determination of test sensitivity and biomarker longevity in experimental models. In humans, there is limited experience from accidental and terror-related exposures. This chapter will review assays for chemical warfare agent exposure that have been published in the literature and how they have been applied in potential exposure situations

Assay of Parent Compounds

Analyzing for parent nerve agents from biomedical matrices, such as blood or urine, is not a viable diagnostic technique for retrospective detection of exposure.[7] Parent agents are relatively short-lived because of rapid hydrolysis and binding to plasma and tissue proteins, imposing unrealistic time restraints on sample collection. The short residence time is especially profound with the G agents (relative to VX). Following the intravenous administration of soman at 2 times the median lethal dose (LD_{50}) results in parent agent detection at toxicologically relevant levels for 104 and 49 minutes in guinea pigs and marmosets, respectively; rapid elimination was reflected in terminal half-life rates (16.5 min for guinea pigs; 9 min for marmosets).[8] Inhalation experiments using nose-only exposure of guinea pigs to 0.8 × LCt_{50} (the vapor or aerosol exposure that is lethal to 50% of the exposed population) agent demonstrate terminal half-lives of approximately 36 and 9 minutes for sarin and soman, respectively.[9] In contrast, similar studies with VX in hairless guinea pigs and marmosets indicate VX is more persistent than the G agents.[10] These studies show that VX can be found at acutely toxic levels for 10 to 20 hours following intravenous administration at a dose one or two times the LD_{50}, with terminal elimination rates of 98 minutes (1 times the LD_{50} in hairless guinea pigs), 165 minutes (2 times the LD_{50}), and 111 minutes in marmosets (at a dose equivalent to 1 LD_{50} in hairless guinea pigs). Percutaneous administration of the LD_{50} of VX to hairless guinea pigs demonstrated relatively low blood levels (140 pg/mL), which reached a maximum after approximately 6 hours.[10] Because the route of human exposure to VX would most likely occur percutaneously, the time frame of 6 hours may be the more relevant assessment of its persistence in blood. This allows very limited time for sample collection and analysis. Others have demonstrated that VX can be assayed from spiked rat plasma.[11] These authors noted that 53% of the VX was lost in spiked plasma specimens after 2 hours. The disappearance was attributed to the enzyme action of the OP hydrolase splitting or to cleavage of the sulfur-phosphorus bond to form diisopropyl aminoethanethiol (DAET) and ethyl methylphosphonic acid (EMPA).[11]

Assay of Hydrolysis Compounds

Analytical Methods

An alternative approach to direct assay of parent nerve agents is to measure metabolic or hydrolysis products in specimens. These compounds are produced in vivo as a result of hydrolysis or detachment following spontaneous regeneration of the AChE enzyme. Studies of parent nerve agents with radioisotopically labeled phosphorus (^{32}P) or hydrogen (^{3}H) in animals suggest that agents are rapidly metabolized and hydrolyzed in the blood and appear in the urine as their respective alkyl MPAs.[12–15] This observation led to the development of assays for alkyl MPAs in biological samples,[16] the applicability of which was subsequently demonstrated in animals exposed to nerve agents.[17] The common products found are isopropyl methylphosphonic acid (IMPA), pinacolyl methylphosphonic acid, cyclohexyl methylphosphonic acid, and EMPA derived from sarin, soman, cyclosarin, and VX, respectively (Figure 22-2). Additionally for VX, hydrolysis of the sulfur-phosphorus bond occurs, yielding DAET and EMPA. The formation and assay of DAET has been reported in rat plasma spiked with VX.[11] Furthermore, the presence of diisopropyl aminoethyl methyl sulfide, presumably resulting from the in-vivo methylation of DAET, has been reported in human exposures.[18] To date, numerous variations of the alkyl MPA assay for biological fluids, such as plasma and urine, have been developed. These include GC separations with MS,[18–20] tandem MS (MS-MS),[18,19,21,22] and flame photometric detection.[23,24] Other methods involving LC with MS-MS[25] and indirect photometric detection[26] have also been reported (Table 22-1).

Application to Human Exposures

The utility of some methodologies has been demonstrated in actual human exposure incidents. Most involve assays of urine and plasma or serum. Tsuchihashi et al[18] demonstrated the presence of EMPA in the serum of an individual assassinated with VX in Osaka, Japan, in 1994. As mentioned earlier, these authors also reported the presence of diisopropyl aminoethyl methyl sulfide, which resulted from the in-vivo methylation of DAET subsequent to cleavage of the sulfur-phosphorus bond. Reported concentrations in serum collected 1 hour after exposure were 143 ng/mL diisopropyl aminoethyl methyl sulfide and 1.25 μg/mL for EMPA.

The Aum Shinrikyo cult attacked citizens twice in Japan using sarin. The first was in an apartment complex in Matsumoto City, where approximately 12 liters of sarin were released using a heater and fan. According to police reports, 600 inhabitants in the surrounding area were harmed, including 7 who were killed. In the second attack, sarin was released into the Tokyo subway, resulting in more than 5,000 casualties and 10 deaths.[27] Assay of hydrolysis products as a definitive marker were used to verify that sarin was the agent employed in these events. Minami et al[23] and Nakajima et al[24] demonstrated the presence of IMPA or MPA in victims' urine following sarin exposure in the Tokyo and Matsumoto attacks, respectively. These methods used GC separations of the prepared urine matrix coupled with flame photometric detection. In the Matsumoto incident, urinary concentrations of IMPA and MPA, as well as the total dose of the sarin exposure, were reported.[24] For one victim, MPA concentrations were 0.14 and 0.02 ug/mL on the first and third days after exposure, and 0.76, 0.08, and 0.01 ug/mL for IMPA, respectively, on the first, third, and seventh days after exposure.[24] In this case, the individual was estimated to have been exposed to 2.79 mg of sarin.

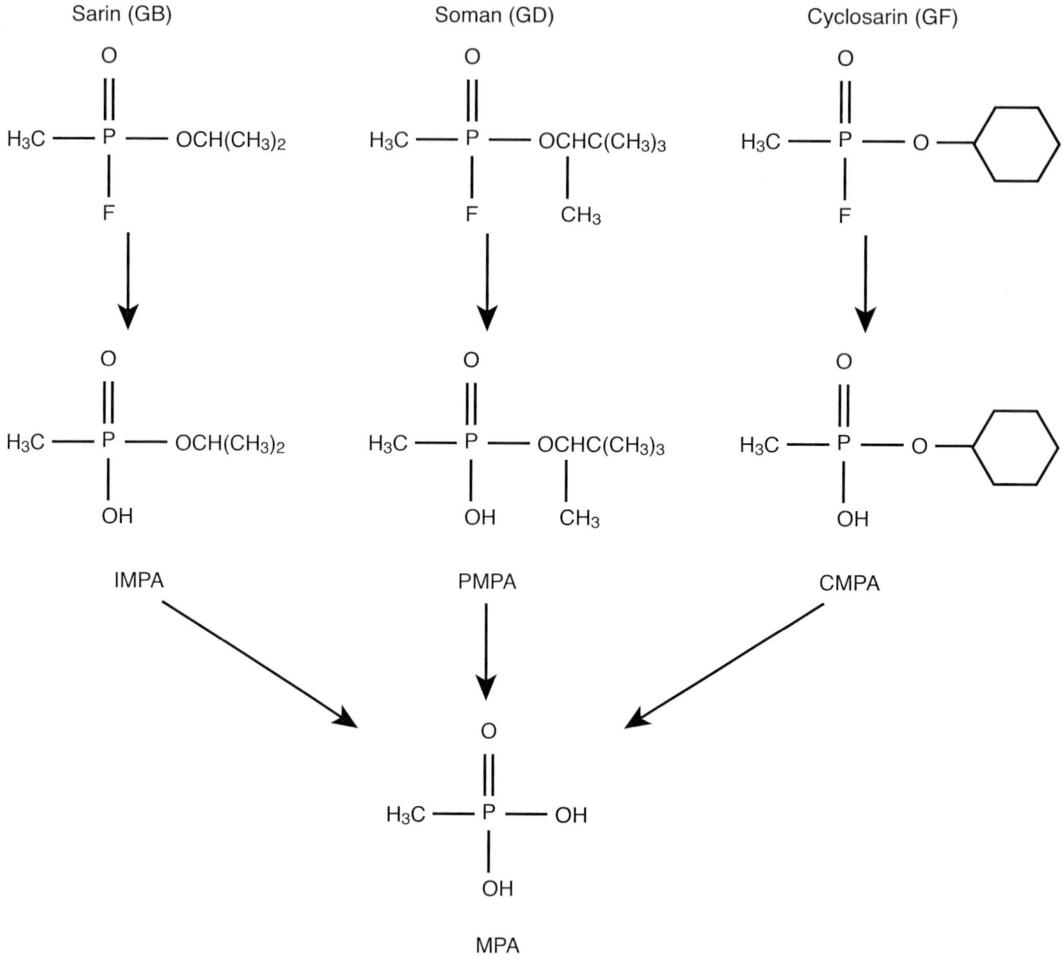

Fig. 22-2. Hydrolysis pathway of sarin (GB), soman (GD), and cyclosarin (GF). Hydrolysis pathway of nerve agents proceeds through the alkyl methylphosphonic acids IMPA, PMPA, and CMPA to MPA. Analysis of the alkyl methylphosphonic acids allows identification of the parent agent, while assay of MPA is nonspecific.
CMPA: cyclohexyl methylphosphonic acid
IMPA: isopropyl methylphosphonic acid
MPA: methylphosphonic acid
PMPA: pinacolyl methylphosphonic acid

Although the report on the Tokyo[23] incident did not directly indicate urinary concentrations, total sarin exposure was estimated. The exposure estimates in a comatose individual was 0.13 to 0.25 mg/person and 0.016 to 0.032 mg/person in a less severely exposed casualty.[23] These numbers are approximately 10-fold less than those reported by Nakajima et al[24] for a severely intoxicated patient. Consistent with rapid elimination, the maximum urinary concentration of these compounds was reported to have occurred in 12 hours of exposure. Using LC-MS-MS methods, Noort et al[25] and Polhuijs et al[28] detected IMPA in serum samples from both the Tokyo and Matsumoto incidents. This assay involves fairly sophisticated instrumentation, but allows for a simplified sample processing procedure. Reported serum concentrations ranged from 2 to 127 ng/mL and 2 to 135 ng/mL in the Tokyo and Matsumoto incidents, respectively.[25,28] Samples were obtained 1.5 hours after the incident. In some cases a second sample was obtained 2 to 2.5 hours after the incident; in those samples, the authors report significantly lower IMPA concentrations consistent with the rapid elimination of these compounds. The sarin dose in both incidences was calculated to be 0.2 to 15 mg/person.[25] These reported values for sarin exposure are in the range of those reported by Nakajima et al[24] and are approximately 10-fold greater than those reported by Minami et al.[23]

Alkyl MPAs provide a convenient marker for determining exposure to nerve agents. Numerous

TABLE 22-1

ANALYTICAL METHODS FOR ASSAY OF NERVE AGENT HYDROLYSIS PRODUCTS*

Sample Matrix	Product Identified	Analytical Method
Blood, Plasma, Urine, Lung Tissue	IMPA, CMPA, PMPA	GC-MS[1,2]
Serum, Urine	EMPA, IMPA, PMPA	GC-MS, GC-MS-MS[3]
Plasma	DAET	GC-MS[4]
Urine	EMPA, IMPA, MPA	GC-FPD[5]
Urine	IMPA, MPA	GC-FPD[6]
Serum	EMPA, DAEMS	GC-MS, GC-MS-MS[7]
Serum, Urine, Saliva	EMPA, IMPA, PMPA	GC-MS[8]
Urine	EMPA, IMPA, CMPA, PMPA, GA acid	GC-MS-MS[9]
Urine	IMPA	LC-MS-MS[10,11]
Serum	EMPA, IMPA, MPA PMPA	Indirect Photometric Detection Ion Chromatography[12]
Urine, Saliva	EMPA, IMPA, CMPA, MPA, PMPA	LC-MS-MS[13]
Urine	EMPA, RVX acid, IMPA, PMPA, CMPA, GA acid, GA diacid	GC-MS-MS[14]

* Although the sample matrices and analytical methods for some of the assays are similar, the authors specifically identified the products listed.

CMPA: cyclohexyl methylphosphonic acid
DAEMS: diisopropyl aminoethyl methyl sulfide (resulting from the metabolic methylation of DAET)
DAET: diisopropyl aminoethanethiol
EMPA: ethyl methylphosphonic acid
FPD: flame photometric detection
GA: tabun
GC: gas chromatography
IMPA: isopropyl methylphosphonic acid
LC: liquid chromatography
MPA: methylphosphonic acid
MS: mass spectrometry
PMPA: pinacolyl methylphosphonic acid
RVX: Russian VX

Data sources: (1) Shih ML, Smith JR, McMonagle JD, Dolzine TW, Gresham VC. Detection of metabolites of toxic alkylmethylphosphonates in biological samples. *Biol Mass Spectrom.* 1991;20:717–723. (2) Shih ML, McMonagle JD, Dolzine TW, Gresham VC. Metabolite pharmacokinetics of soman, sarin, and GF in rats and biological monitoring of exposure to toxic organophosphorus agents. *J Appl Toxicol.* 1994:14:195–199. (3) Fredriksson SA, Hammarström LG, Henriksson L, Lakso HA. Trace determination of alkyl methylphosphonic acids in environmental and biological samples using gas chromatography / negative-ion chemical ionization mass spectrometry and tandem mass spectrometry. *J Mass Spectrom.* 1995;30:1133–1143. (4) Bonierbale E, Debordes L, Coppet L. Application of capillary gas chromatography to the study of hydrolysis of the nerve agent VX in rat plasma. *J Chromatogr B Biomed Sci Appl.* 1997;688:255–264. (5) Minami M, Hui DM, Katsumata M, Inagaki H, Boulet CA. Method for the analysis of methylphosphonic acid metabolites of sarin and its ethanol-substituted analogue in urine as applied to the victims of the Tokyo sarin disaster. *J Chromatogr B Biomed Sci Appl.* 1997;695:237–244. (6) Nakajima T, Sasaki K, Ozawa H, Sekjima Y, Morita H, Fukushima Y, Yanagisawa N. Urinary metabolites of sarin in a patient of the Matsumoto incident. *Arch Toxicol.* 1998;72:601–603. (7) Tsuchihashi H, Katagi M, Nishikawa M, Tatsuno M. Identification of metabolites of nerve agent VX in serum collected from a victim. *J Anal Toxicol.* 1998;22:383–388. (8) Miki A, Katagi M, Tsuchihashi H, Yamashita M. Determination of alkylmethylphosphonic acids, the main metabolites of organophosphorus nerve agents, in biofluids by gas chromatography-mass spectrometry and liquid-liquid-solid-phase-transfer-catalyzed pentafluorobenzylation. *J Anal Toxicol.* 1999;23:86–93. (9) Driskell WJ, Shih M, Needham LL, Barr DB. Quantitation of organophosphorus nerve agent metabolites in human urine using isotope dilution gas chromatography-tandem mass spectrometry. *J Anal Toxicol.* 2002;26:6–10. (10) Noort D, Hulst AG, Platenburg DH, Polhuijs M, Benschop H. Quantitative analysis of O-isopropyl methylphosphonic acid in serum samples of Japanese citizens allegedly exposed to sarin: estimation of internal dosage. *Arch Toxicol.* 1998;72:671–675. (11) Polhuijs M, Langenberg JP, Noort D, Hulst AG, Benschop HP. Retrospective detection of exposure to organophosphates: analyses in blood of human beings and rhesus monkeys. In: Sohns T, Voicu VA, eds. *NBC Risks: Current Capabilities and Future Perspectives for Protection.* Dordrecht, Holland, Netherlands: Kluwer Academic Publishers; 1999:513–521. (12) Katagi M, Nishikawa M, Tatsuno M, Tsuchihashi H. Determination of the main hydrolysis products of organophosphorus nerve agents, methylphosphonic acids, in human serum by indirect photometric detection ion chromatography. *J Chromatogr B Biomed Sci Appl.* 1997;698:81–88. (13) Hayes TL, Kenny DV, Hernon-Kenny L. Feasibility of direct analysis of saliva and urine for phosphonic acids and thiodiglycol-related species associated with exposure to chemical warfare agents using LC-MS / MS. *J Med Chem Def.* 2004;2:1-23. (14) Barr JR, Driskell WJ, Aston LS, Martinez RA. Quantitation of metabolites of the nerve agents sarin, soman, cyclosarin, VX, and Russian VX in human urine using isotope-dilution gas chromatography-tandem mass spectrometry. *J Anal Toxicol.* 2004;28:371–378.

modifications of the assay for these compounds have been developed, and several have been applied to human exposure cases. Important factors to consider when anticipating using this test are the extent of exposure and time elapsed since the event. In most cases, hydrolysis products are not expected to be present for more than 24 to 48 hours following exposure; however, one of the most severely poisoned victims of the Matsumoto sarin attack had measurable IMPA in the urine on the seventh day after the incident. In this particular case, extremely depressed AChE values, in range of 5% to 8% of normal,[24] further indicated the extent of exposure (Table 22-2).

Assay of Adducts to Biomolecules

The relatively rapid excretion and short-lived presence of urinary hydrolysis products imposes time restrictions for collecting a viable sample. Efforts to increase the sampling window have taken advantage of the interactions between chemical warfare agents and biological targets with large molecular weights (adducts to biomolecules), such as proteins. The reaction of chemical agents with large molecules provides a pool of bound compound that can be tested to verify exposure. Theoretically, the longevity of the marker is consistent with the in-vivo half-life of the target molecule, provided that the binding affinity is high enough to prevent spontaneous reactivation. Binding of nerve agents to ChE targets has been one of the primary interactions leveraged in assay development. Several assays have been developed based on variations of this concept.

Analytical Methods

Polhuijs et al[29] developed an assay technique based on observations of earlier findings that sarin-inhibited ChE could be reactivated with fluoride ions.[30–32] The displacement of covalently bound sarin to butyrylcholinesterase (BChE) was accomplished by incubating inhibited plasma with fluoride to form free enzyme

TABLE 22-2

METHODS USED TO CONFIRM HUMAN EXPOSURES TO NERVE AGENTS VIA ASSAY OF HYDROLYSIS PRODUCTS

Agent/Incident	Sample Matrix	Product Identified	Concentration Reported	Analytical Method
GB, Tokyo, Japan	Urine	EMPA, IMPA, MPA	NR	GC-FPD[1]
GB, Matsumoto, Japan	Urine	IMPA MPA	0.76–0 .01 μg/mL 0.14–0.02 μg/mL	GC-FPD[2]
GB, Matsumoto and Tokyo, Japan	Serum	IMPA	Matsumoto (2–135 ng/mL) Tokyo (2–127 ng/mL)	LC-MS-MS[3,4]
VX, Osaka, Japan	Serum	EMPA, diisopropylaminoethyl methyl sulfide	1.25 μg/mL 143 ng/mL	GC-MS, GC-MS-MS[5]

EMPA: ethyl methylphosphonic acid
FPD: flame photometric detection
GB: sarin
GC: gas chromatography
IMPA: isopropyl methylphosphonic acid
LC: liquid chromatography
MPA: methylphosphonic acid
MS: mass spectrometry
NR: not reported
Data sources: (1) Minami M, Hui DM, Katsumata M, Inagaki H, Boulet CA. Method for the analysis of methylphosphonic acid metabolites of sarin and its ethanol-substituted analogue in urine as applied to the victims of the Tokyo sarin disaster. *J Chromatogr B Biomed Sci Appl.* 1997;695:237–244. (2) Nakajima T, Sasaki K, Ozawa H, Sekjima Y, Morita H, Fukushima Y, Yanagisawa N. Urinary metabolites of sarin in a patient of the Matsumoto incident. *Arch Toxicol.* 1998;72:601–603. (3) Noort D, Hulst AG, Platenburg DH, Polhuijs M, Benschop H. Quantitative analysis of O-isopropyl methylphosphonic acid in serum samples of Japanese citizens allegedly exposed to sarin: estimation of internal dosage. *Arch Toxicol.* 1998;72:671–675. (4) Polhuijs M, Langenberg JP, Noort D, Hulst AG, Benschop HP. Retrospective detection of exposure to organophosphates: analyses in blood of human beings and rhesus monkeys. In: Sohns T, Voicu VA, eds. *NBC Risks: Current Capabilities and Future Perspectives for Protection.* Dordrecht, Holland, Netherlands: Kluwer Academic Publishers; 1999:513–521. (5) Tsuchihashi H, Katagi M, Nishikawa M, Tatsuno M. Identification of metabolites of nerve agent VX in serum collected from a victim. *J Anal Toxicol.* 1998;22:383–388.

plus the parent agent (isopropyl methylphosphonofluoridate). Following isolation from the matrix with solid phase extraction techniques, the agent was then analyzed using GC with MS or other appropriate detection systems. Other research has demonstrated conceptually similar approaches for detecting tabun[28] and VX.[33] In the case of tabun, the cyanide group, which is initially lost upon binding to the enzyme, is replaced with fluorine, leading to the formation of O-ethyl N,N-dimethyl-phosphoramidofluoridate, a fluorinated analog of tabun.[28] Similarly, the thiol group in VX, which is initially lost upon binding to the enzyme, is replaced by fluorine, resulting in a fluorinated analog of VX (ethyl methyl-phosphonofluoridate; VX-G).[33] Variations and improvements of the fluoride regeneration procedure have evolved to enhance test sensitivity by optimizing agent extraction, increasing injection volumes (thermal desorption and large volume injector), and using alternate detection formats (eg, flame photometric detection, positive ion chemical ionization, and high-resolution electron impact MS).[6,33] Additionally, Jakubowski et al[34] have successfully applied the procedure to RBCs.

With regard to the ability of a fluoride ion to regenerate soman bound to BChE, it is well known that the process of aging would preclude release from the enzyme. However, studies have indicated that the fluoride ion regeneration process, as applied to soman-poisoned animals, has produced contrary results.[35] These studies suggest that soman can be displaced from sites where aging does not play a significant role. Black et al[36] have demonstrated that both sarin and soman bind to tyrosine residues of human serum albumin. The observation that the alkyl group remained intact, in particular for soman, argues that binding to this site does not result in aging as seen with ChEs.[36] Similarly, carboxylesterase, known to exist in high quantities in rats and mice, has been shown to form adducts with soman.[37–41] Moreover, soman formation has been demonstrated via fluoride-induced regeneration of soman-inhibited carboxylesterase in rat plasma[37] and purified human albumin.[35] Although the presence of carboxylesterase in significant amounts is questionable in humans, the albumin provides a potential source of the protein from which the agent can be regenerated. Currently the utility of fluoride regeneration in human exposures involving soman is unclear. More studies are needed to clarify the utility of fluoride regeneration in humans with soman exposure following confirmed events.

Nagao et al[42,43] employed a different approach, exploiting sarin bound to AChE, using blood as the matrix. This procedure detected IMPA, following its release from the sarin-AChE complex, using an alkaline phosphatase digestion process. The analytical technique used is similar to numerous other GC-MS assays for hydrolysis products.

Another approach based on OP binding to BChE has been reported by Fidder et al.[44] This method involves digesting BChE to produce nonapeptide fragments containing the serine-198 residue to which nerve agents bind. Analyzing nonapeptides employs LC-MS-MS techniques. The utility of this method was demonstrated by analyzing two archived samples from the Tokyo subway terrorist attack. The authors reported results similar to a previous analysis of those samples, in this case using the fluoride regeneration procedure.[44] A reported advantage of this technique is that aged or nonaged OPs can be successfully identified. In the case of sarin-inhibited enzyme, the serine-198 is conjugated to IMPA; for soman following loss of the pinacolyl alkyl group (ie, aging), MPA was found bound to the serine residue. In addition, the procedure was useful for detecting BChE adducted to OP pesticides as well as non-OP anti-ChEs, such as pyridostigmine.[44] A limitation of the assay is that agent identity is needed for MS analysis.[45] For this reason, an extension of this procedure was developed that uses a generic approach.[45] The method employed a chemical modification of the phosphyl group on the serine residue to a common nonapeptide, regardless of the specific agent involved.[45] Because a common nonapeptide is the outcome, a single MS method was employed in the analysis (Table 22-3).[45]

Application to Human Exposures

The fluoride ion regeneration procedure[29] was used to analyze serum from exposed individuals in the Aum Shinrikyo terrorist attacks at Matsumoto and in the Tokyo subway. As previously indicated, this procedure is based upon the use of fluoride ion to regenerate the parent agent and free BChE. The amount of regenerated sarin from serum ranged from 1.8 to 2.7 ng/mL in the Matsumoto incident and 0.2 to 4.1 ng/mL in the Tokyo attacks.[29]

Although unable to detect MPA or IMPA directly from the blood of victims of the Tokyo subway attack, Nagao et al[42,43] detected these compounds after alkaline phosphatase digestion of the sarin-AChE complex. However, the authors did not report MPA or IMPA concentrations. Although not directly relevant to diagnostic testing, a conceptually similar approach was also applied to formalin-fixed brain tissues (GB-bound AChE) from victims of the Tokyo subway attack.[1] The assays conducted on frozen cerebral cortex did not detect MPA or IMPA. Similar studies with formalin-fixed cerebellum tissue resulted in detecting only MPA. The

TABLE 22-3

ANALYTICAL METHODS USING ADDUCTS TO BIOMOLECULES

Sample Matrix	Product Identified	Analytical Method
Plasma/serum	GA, GB	GC-NPD[1,2]
Red blood cell	IMPA, MPA	GC-MS[3,4]
Brain (cerebellum)	MPA	GC-MS[5]
Plasma/serum	VX-G	GC-FPD/GC-MS[6]
Plasma/serum	Phosphylated nonapeptides from BChE	LC-MS-MS[7]
Plasma/serum	GA, GB, GF, VX-G	GC-MS/GC-MS(HR)[8]
Plasma/serum/red blood cell	GB	GC-MS[9]
Plasma/serum	Phosphylated nonapeptides from BChE- derivatized	LC-MS-MS[10]

BChE: butyrylcholinesterase
FPD: flame photometric detection
GA: tabun
GB: sarin
GC: gas chromatography
GF: cyclosarin
HR: high resolution
IMPA: isopropyl methylphosphonic acid
LC: liquid chromatography
MPA: methylphosphonic acid
MS: mass spectrometry
NPD: nitrogen-phosphorus detector
VX-G : ethyl methylphosphonofluoridate

Data sources: (1) Polhuijs M, Langenberg JP, Benschop HP. New method for retrospective detection of exposure to organophosphorus anticholinesterases: application to alleged sarin victims of Japanese terrorists. *Toxicol Appl Pharmacol.* 1997;146:156–161. (2) Polhuijs M, Langenberg JP, Noort D, Hulst AG, Benschop HP. Retrospective detection of exposure to organophosphates: analyses in blood of human beings and rhesus monkeys. In: Sohns T, Voicu VA, eds. *NBC Risks: Current Capabilities and Future Perspectives for Protection*. Dordrecht, Holland, Netherlands: Kluwer Academic Publishers; 1999:513–21. (3) Nagao M, Takatori T, Matsuda Y, et al. Detection of sarin hydrolysis products from sarin-like organophosphorus agent-exposed human erythrocytes. *J Chromatogr B Biomed Sci Appl.* 1997;701:9–17. (4) Nagao M, Takatori T, Matsuda Y, Nakajima M, Iwase H, Iwadate K. Definitive evidence for the acute sarin poisoning diagnosis in the Tokyo subway. *Toxicol Appl Pharmacol.* 1997;144:198–203. (5) Matsuda Y, Nagao M, Takatori T, et al. Detection of the sarin hydrolysis product in formalin-fixed brain tissues of victims of the Tokyo subway terrorist attack. *Toxicol Appl Pharmacol.* 1998;150:310–320. (6) Jakubowski EM, Heykamp LS, Durst HD, Thompson SA. Preliminary studies in the formation of ethyl methylphosphonofluoridate from rat and human serum exposed to VX and treated with fluoride ion. *Anal Lett.* 2001;34:727–737. (7) Fidder A, Hulst AG, Noort D, et al. Retrospective detection of exposure to organophosphorus anti-cholinesterases: mass spectrometric analysis of phosphylated human butyrylcholinesterase. *Chem Res Toxicol.* 2002;15:582–590. (8) Degenhardt CE, Pleijsier K, van der Schans MJ, et al. Improvements of the fluoride reactivation method for the verification of nerve agent exposure. *J Anal Toxicol.* 2004;28:364–371. (9) Jakubowski EM, McGuire JM, Evans RA, et al. Quantitation of fluoride ion released sarin in red blood cell samples by gas chromatography-chemical ionization mass spectrometry using isoptope dilution and large-volume injection. *J Anal Toxicol.* 2004;28:357–363. (10) Noort D, Fidder A, van der Schans MJ, Hulst AG. Verification of exposure to organophosphates: generic mass spectrometric method for detection of human butyrylcholinesterase adducts. *Anal Chem.* 2006;78:6640–6644.

inability to detect IMPA was due to hydrolysis during the 2-year storage period. The inability to detect hydrolysis products in the cerebral cortex as opposed to the cerebellum was reportedly consistent with the relative AChE activity detected in each tissue. The study authors state that this is the first verification of nerve agent exposure using formalin-fixed brains.[1]

Due to the limited number of human exposures to nerve agents, it is difficult to fully ascertain the advantages and disadvantages of various definitive testing methodologies. Numerous assays to detect hydrolysis products in blood or urine have been developed; some have been employed in exposure incidents. The disadvantage of these methods stems from the relatively rapid agent elimination and resultant limited opportunity to obtain specimens. The advantage of using adducts formed with large-molecular–weight targets (AChE or BChE) is a longer time frame (relative to that of hydrolysis products) to verify exposures. Some investigations have indicated that methods employing BChE provide benefits over those with AChE because BChE is more abundant in blood.[44] Assays involving BChE digestion with subsequent assay of nonapeptide fragments facilitate identification of aged or nonaged adduct at the phosphylated serine-198 residue; therefore they are potentially useful in detecting agents such as soman. Few methods have been published that use the assay of adducts to biomolecules to verify chemical warfare agent exposure in humans (Table 22-4).

Cholinesterase Analysis

OP chemical warfare agents are potent and irreversible inhibitors. Exposure results in excessive accumulation of acetylcholine that hyperstimulates cholinergic tissues and organs and ultimately leads to life-threatening cholinergic crises in humans.[3] The mechanism of OP toxicity is the inhibition of AChE and BChE involved in the termination of neurotransmission in cholinergic synapses and neuromuscular junctions of the central nervous system.[46] Synaptic AChE is not amenable to direct measurement, but because of functional similarities between synaptic and erythrocyte AChE, the activity of AChE in whole blood can be used as a reliable surrogate biomarker of central and peripheral nervous system activity.[47] Exposure to OP nerve agents, carbamates, pesticides, anesthetics, and drugs (such as cocaine) selectively reduces AChE and BChE activity.[3] Thus, it is crucial to diagnose OP exposure or intoxication early, and blood ChE activity (usually RBC-AChE) can be exploited as a tool for confirming exposure to these agents and commencing antidotal (oxime) therapy.[48,49] Because these ChE inhibitors comprise a group of structurally diverse compounds with a wide range of relative specificities for RBC-AChE and plasma BChE, a complete profile of inhibition is probably more accurately reflected if both ChEs are measured.

Exposure to OP nerve agents or pesticides that results in inhibition of less than about 20% AChE or BChE (especially if clinical symptoms are absent) may not easily be detected because of considerable inter- and intraindividual variations in AChE and (especially) BChE activities.[50] Moderate clinical symptoms of poisoning will be apparent at 50% to 70% AChE inhibition, with severe toxicity seen at greater than 90% inhibition.[51] While general measurement of ChE activity in blood is not specific for exposure to any OP nerve agent, carbamate, or pesticide, laboratory measurements by MS techniques can positively

TABLE 22-4

METHODS USED TO CONFIRM HUMAN EXPOSURES TO NERVE AGENT ADDUCTS TO BIOMOLECULES

Agent/Incident	Sample Matrix	Product Identified	Concentration Reported	Analytical Method
GB, Matsumoto and Tokyo, Japan	Serum	GB	Matsumoto (1.8–2.7 ng/mL) Tokyo (0.2–4.1 ng/mL)	GC-NPD[1,2]
GB, Tokyo, Japan	Red Blood Cell	IMPA, MPA	NR	GC-MS[3,4]
GB, Tokyo, Japan	Brain (cerebellum)	MPA	NR	GC-MS[5]
GB, Tokyo, Japan (selected samples)	Plasma/Serum	Phosphylated nonapeptides from BChE	10–20 pmol inhibited BChE/mL	LC-MS-MS[6]

BChE: butyrylcholinesterase
GB: sarin
GC: gas chromatography
IMPA: isopropyl methylphosphonic acid
LC: liquid chromatography
MPA: methylphosphonic acid
MS: mass spectrometric
NPD: nitrogen-phosphorus detector
NR: not reported
Data sources: (1) Polhuijs M, Langenberg JP, Benschop HP. New method for retrospective detection of exposure to organophosphorus anticholinesterases: application to alleged sarin victims of Japanese terrorists. *Toxicol Appl Pharmacol.* 1997;146:156–161. (2) Polhuijs M, Langenberg JP, Noort D, Hulst AG, Benschop HP. Retrospective detection of exposure to organophosphates: analyses in blood of human beings and rhesus monkeys. In: Sohns T, Voicu VA, eds. *NBC Risks: Current Capabilities and Future Perspectives for Protection.* Dordrecht, Holland, the Netherlands: Kluwer Academic Publishers; 1999:513–521. (3) Nagao M, Takatori T, Matsuda Y, et al. Detection of sarin hydrolysis products from sarin-like organophosphorus agent-exposed human erythrocytes. *J Chromatogr B Biomed Sci Appl.* 1997;701:9–17. (4) Nagao M, Takatori T, Matsuda Y, Nakajima M, Iwase H, Iwadate K. Definitive evidence for the acute sarin poisoning diagnosis in the Tokyo subway. *Toxicol Appl Pharmacol.* 1997;144:198–203. (5) Matsuda Y, Nagao M, Takatori T, et al. Detection of the sarin hydrolysis product in formalin-fixed brain tissues of victims of the Tokyo subway terrorist attack. *Toxicol Appl Pharmacol.* 1998;150:310–320. (6) Fidder A, Hulst AG, Noort D, et al. Retrospective detection of exposure to organophosphorus anti-cholinesterases: mass spectrometric analysis of phosphylated human butyrylcholinesterase. *Chem Res Toxicol.* 2002;15:582–590.

identify many OPs by evaluating their leaving group from fluoride-reactivated proteins.[28] Thus, the determination of an individual's ChE status can be important prior to decisions regarding oxime therapy and confirmation of OP poisoning, particularly in the case of long-lasting (eg, VX), rapidly aging (eg, soman) nerve agents and the surprising persistence of soman in blood and tissues.[52]

Although plasma BChE activity is measured in occupational and clinical toxicology laboratories, it should be noted that BChE exhibits different kinetic properties with nerve agents and pesticides than does RBC-AChE.[53] In humans, pesticide toxicity is well documented,[54] and completely different profiles of RBC-AChE and plasma BChE activities in pesticide-poisoned individuals have been reported.[55] Because decreased serum BChE often precedes a decline in RBC-AChE, an assay that measures both ChEs is more valuable for detecting initial (and smaller) changes in ChE levels that may signify exposure.

Several sensitive and specific assays for measuring AChE activity in blood have been developed for use in clinical and toxicology laboratories. For routine use, however, a number of drawbacks are apparent, including time-consuming sample preparation and long turn-around times. There is also a lack of standardization because of the difficulty comparing results between laboratories that use different ChE assays and report values in different or nonstandard units. None of the widely used methods has been approved by the US Food and Drug Administration (FDA). Clinical determination of AChE and BChE activities in blood commonly uses several techniques (colorimetric, electrometric, and radiometric) and normally measures either RBC-AChE or serum BChE concentrations, but usually not both.[56]

Colorimetric ChE Assays in the Clinical Laboratory

Several ChE assays are based on the enzyme-linked production of colored products. For these assays, monitoring color production as a function of time directly reflects enzyme activity or the ability of the enzyme to turn over substrate. Decreased enzyme turnover is reflected in less color production per unit time.

Ellman Assay. The Ellman method[57] is a popular colorimetric procedure for detecting and monitoring pesticide exposure. The breakdown of thiocholine substrates (acetylthiocholine and butyrylthiocholine) by AChE and BChE is detected kinetically using the Ellman reagent DTNB (5,5′-dithio-bis-2-nitrobenzoate). This assay is accurate, reliable, and inexpensive. However, the absorption maxima (412 nm) of the resulting yellow TNB^- (3-carboxy-4-nitrobenzenethiolate dianion) coincides with the Soret band of hemoglobin, resulting in interference and reduced assay sensitivity. By increasing the wavelength from 412 nm to 436 nm, hemoglobin interference can be reduced by 75% and assay sensitivity improved without significant sacrifice of the indicator (TNB^-) absorption.[58] Additionally, the molar extinction coefficient for TNB ($13.6 \times 10^3\ M^{-1}\ cm^{-1}$) used in the original Ellman assay[57] has been widely applied to calculate ChE activities, however, this value may vary depending on temperature, wavelength, and buffer conditions.[59] Changes in these experimental parameters can alter the extinction coefficient, resulting in different ChE activities from various laboratories. There are many published variations of the original cuvette-based Ellman assay, including the 96-well microtiter plate format.[60]

Walter Reed Army Institute of Research Whole Blood Assay. An important variation of the Ellman ChE assay is the Walter Reed Army Institute of Research Whole Blood Assay,[61] which uses 4,4′-dithiopyridine instead of DTNB as a chromogenic indicator and three thiocholine substrates (acetyl-, butyryl-, and propionyl-thiocholine). The absorption maxima in the ultraviolet range (324 nm) of the 4-thiopyridone formed yields a high signal-to-noise ratio because hemoglobin interference is minimal.[62] The use of three substrates in this assay rapidly and simultaneously provides redundancy and independent measurement of the RBC-AChE activities and plasma BChE in a small sample of unprocessed whole blood, using a 96-well microtiter plate spectrophotometer. The method is not labor intensive, and although it can be performed manually, it has been semi-automated using a Beckman-Coulter robotic platform for high sample throughput. A unique feature of the Walter Reed Army Institute of Research method is that the blood is not treated prior to assay (Figure 22-3). Thus, both AChE and BChE activities can be obtained without centrifugation or the use of inhibitors for whole, frozen, or lysed blood specimens.[62]

Test-Mate Assay. In addition to the laboratory-based methods, a field-deployable test unit is commercially available, the Test-Mate ChE system (EQM Research Inc, Cincinnati, OH). Further information (instructions, description, clinical trial date, etc) on the kit is available through the manufacturer.[63] The method is also based on the Ellman procedure and is supplied as a kit containing reagents to measure erythrocyte AChE and plasma BChE separately using a battery-operated photometric analyzer.[64] A specific serum BChE inhibitor (As1397, or 10-[α-diethylaminopropionyl]-phenothiazone) is included in the kit and is required to measure AChE (after a period of incubation). Two capillary tubes containing whole blood samples are

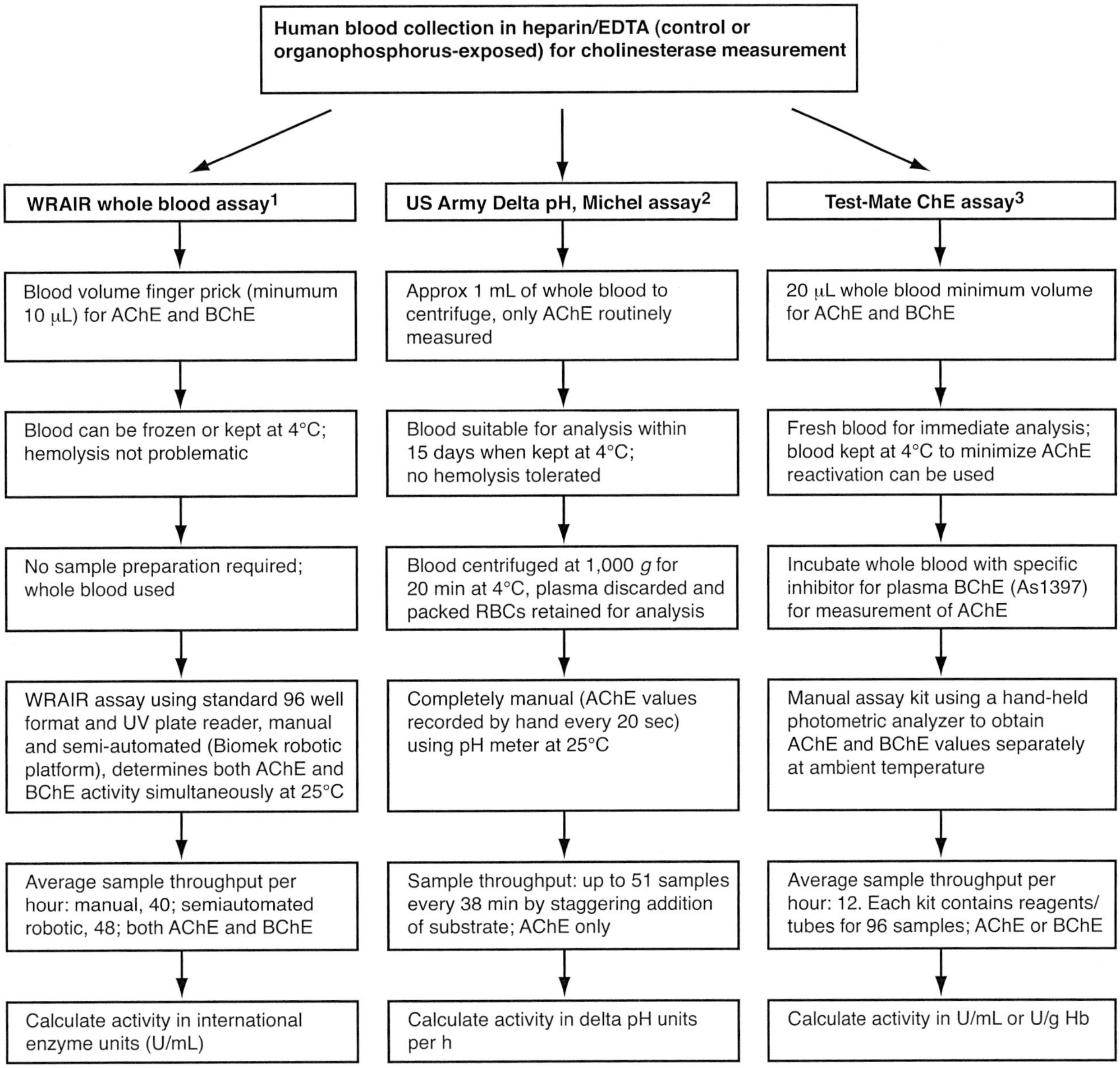

Fig. 22-3: Laboratory and field cholinesterase assays routinely used by the US Army and their required blood processing.
AChE: acetylcholinesterase
As1397: 10-(α-diethylaminopropionyl)-phenothiazone
BChE: butyrylcholinesterase
ChE: cholinesterase
EDTA: ethylenediaminetetraacetic acid
g: gravity
Hb: hemoglobin
RBCs: red blood cells
UV: ultraviolet
Data sources: (1) Gordon RK, Haigh JR, Garcia GE, et al. Oral administration of pyridostigmine bromide and huperzine A protects human whole blood cholinesterases from ex vivo exposure to soman. *Chemico Biol Interact.* 2005;157–158:239–246. (2) Ellin RI, Burkhardt BH, Hart RD. A time-modified method for measuring red blood cell cholinesterase activity. *Arch Environ Health.* 1973;27:48–49. (3) Taylor PW, Lukey BJ, Clark CR, Lee RB, Roussel RR. Field verification of Test-mate ChE. *Mil Med.* 2003;168:314–319.

necessary for AChE and BChE determination (and correction for hemoglobin content, which is also measured in each blood sample; see Figure 22-3). The kit is easy to use by a relatively untrained operator and matches the sensitivity of the laboratory-based Ellman methods, but has relatively low throughput because it is performed manually. Although the Test-Mate ChE kit is designed primarily for field use, where it is widely used for monitoring pesticide exposure in agricultural workers, longer processing times are required for complete AChE and BChE screening and hemoglobin measurement.

Electrometric ChE Assay (delta pH)

A manual method still widely used by the US Department of Defense to measure RBC-AChE is a modification[65] of the end-point delta pH method originally described by Michel.[66] This assay monitors the decrease in pH (using a simple pH electrode and pH meter) that occurs when AChE catalyzes the hydrolysis of acetylcholine to choline and acetic acid. The assay is initiated by the addition of substrate (acetylcholine) and the change in pH is monitored over 17 minutes. This method is slow and laborious, although throughput can be increased by staggering addition of substrate to each sample (see Figure 22-3). Up to 51 blood samples can be analyzed in 38 minutes, and the RBC-AChE activity is reported as a change (delta) in pH units per hour.[67] However, the delta pH method requires centrifugation of blood to pellet RBCs, followed by removal of the plasma (containing BChE) prior to analyzing AChE activity. Lysis of the blood sample is precluded, so blood must be iced (not frozen) before centrifugation and AChE analysis. Furthermore, because plasma BChE is not determined, the complete spectrum of blood inhibition is unknown. Although this technique was developed nearly 60 years ago, it is reliable, and the US Army (through the Department of Defense Cholinesterase Reference Laboratory) has a quality assurance testing program for primary RBC-AChE monitoring of more than 25,000 military personnel per year.[68]

Pretreatment Therapy for Nerve Agent Poisoning: Protection and Sequestering of Cholinesterase

Pyridostigmine Bromide. The US Army's current pretreatment against potential nerve agent poisoning is the reversible and fairly short-acting AChE inhibitor pyridostigmine bromide (PB), which was reviewed earlier.[69] PB is a quaternary ammonium compound that provides temporary protection (by carbamylation) of peripheral tissue and RBC-AChE. However, PB does not penetrate the blood-brain barrier, and thus does not afford protection against seizures and subsequent neuropathological states induced by a nerve agent such as soman.[70] During the Gulf War (1990–1991), more than 100,000 US and allied troops received PB (a single oral dose of 30 mg given every 8 h) as a pretreatment against exposure to soman. This method of pretreatment was demonstrated[62] in an FDA-supported clinical trial of human volunteers given PB as a single 30-mg dose (Table 22-5). Maximal RBC-AChE inhibition of about 27% was seen after 2.5 hours, with recovery of activity to almost 100% after 24 hours. To demonstrate protection and sequestering of AChE, the volunteers' PB-pretreated blood was exposed ex vivo to soman, followed by PB and soman removal from the blood using a small spin column, and monitoring the recovery of RBC-AChE (decarbamylation) (Figure 22-4). All of the AChE activity protected by PB pretreatment was restored to control levels within 3 hours. Plasma BChE was also inhibited in the same volunteers, albeit to a lesser extent (approximately 11%, about one third of the inhibition observed for AChE).[62] Although it was formally approved by the FDA as a specific pretreatment for soman poisoning in February 2003,[71] PB was not ordered to be taken by troops during the 2003 Iraq war.

Huperzine A: Potential Next Generation Peripherally and Centrally Acting Protection and Sequestering of Cholinesterase. Another pretreatment drug, physostigmine, can cross the blood-brain barrier and protect brain ChE in addition to RBC-AChE. However, psychological and behavioral side effects (although partially offset by a low dose of scopolamine to block muscarinic cholinergic receptors) preclude its use as an effective pretreatment against OP exposure. Furthermore, its use as an Alzheimer's drug to improve short-term memory has been discontinued because of multiple unwanted side effects, including nausea, dizziness, headaches, and sweating.

In contrast to PB, huperzine A (Hup A), an alkaloid isolated from the moss *Huperzia serrata*, is a reversible AChE inhibitor in both the peripheral and central nervous systems.[72,73] Hup A has been shown to be superior to physostigmine in its anti-ChE activity and has a longer biological half-life in humans and animals. Hup A is currently undergoing extensive clinical trials in the United States as a drug for Alzheimer's disease (it is already used for this purpose in China), though it is already sold as an over-the-counter nutraceutical supplement for memory enhancement (FDA approval is not required for this type of sale). Pretreatment with Hup A (in addition to postexposure treatment

TABLE 22-5

RED BLOOD CELL AND ACETYLCHOLINESTERASE PROTECTION STUDIES USING PYRIDOSTIGMINE BROMIDE AND HUPERZINE A AFTER EX-VIVO EXPOSURE TO SOMAN

Procedure*†	Techniques and Rationale
1) Obtain blood samples from human volunteers	Aliquot blood from subjects administered oral dose of 30 mg pyridostigmine bromide, 200 μg huperzine A, or no drug
2) Ex-vivo exposure to soman	Incubated blood with 1 μM soman for 10 min at room temperature; incubate control samples (no soman) with saline
3) Remove free drug and soman	Centrifuge samples through a C_{18} chromatography spin column to bind drug and remove from the blood
4) Allow time for AChE decarbamylation (PB) or dissociation (Hup A)	Maintain postcolumn samples at room temperature for up to 24 hours
5) Monitor time for regeneration of AChE after decarbamylation of PB or reversible inhibition by Hup A	Aliquot samples collected for AChE activity assay at indicated times postcolumn
6) Measure AChE activity	Use WRAIR whole blood ChE assay to determine recovered enzyme activity

*Acetylcholinesterase and pyridostigmine bromide or huperzine A yield an acetylcholinesterase-drug complex in procedures 1 and 2. This reaction demonstrates sequestered enzyme, which temporarily inhibits the active site.

†Over time, the acetylcholinesterase-drug complex becomes acetylcholinesterase plus pyridostigmine bromide (the decarbamylated form of acetylcholinesterase) or dissociated huperzine A in procedures 3 and 4. These reactions demonstrate the sequestered and then restored enzyme activity.

AChE: acetylcholinesterase
ChE: cholinesterase
PB: pyridostigmine bromide
Hup A: huperzine A

with atropine and an oxime) may represent a superior treatment strategy for protection against chemical warfare agent exposure and should be investigated further.

Animal studies have been used to examine the efficacy of high doses of Hup A against OP nerve agent toxicity. A dose of Hup A (500 μg/kg) significantly reduces soman lethality (protective ratios of 2–3 when used alone) and inhibits blood and brain AChE by 60% to 70%.[74] Unlike PB, Hup A can cross the blood-brain barrier and in rats protects brain AChE from inhibition by soman, thus preventing build-up of excessive acetylcholine leading to seizures and associated neuropathological damage. In guinea pig hippocampus, natural Hup A in subchronic doses (yielding 20%–30% inhibition of RBC-AChE) has little or no affinity for muscarinic, nicotinic, or *N*-methyl-D-aspartate excitatory amino acid receptors, and does not induce neuropathological damage.

Because Hup A reversibly binds to AChE, thus protecting the enzyme from reaction with OPs, the activity of the Hup-A–protected but inhibited AChE is restored once the drug-AChE complex spontaneously dissociates, which occurs after soman is cleared from the blood. To illustrate this, Hup-A– inhibited blood (drawn 1.5 h after human volunteers were given a dose of 200 μg Hup A; Figure 22-5) was exposed ex vivo to soman.[62] Blood samples were then rapidly centrifuged through a small column to remove any free soman and Hup A, the latter binding to the column matrix while allowing AChE and BChE to pass through the column. Under these circumstances, any RBC-AChE not protected by Hup A would be irreversibly inhibited by soman. In contrast, the RBC-AChE protected by Hup A would dissociate over time, and the AChE activity would eventually be restored. In one study, after soman treatment, no AChE activity was observed by the Walter Reed Army Institute of Research Whole Blood Assay in either the placebo- or drug-treated volunteers (see Figure 22-5). After the spin column removal of free Hup A and soman, and a 4-hour period to allow for complete dissociation, the Hup-A–inhibited AChE was restored to the level that was initially inhibited by the drug (about 60% inhibition by the drug before the column compared to 54% returned AChE activity after the column). AChE inhibition and sequestering

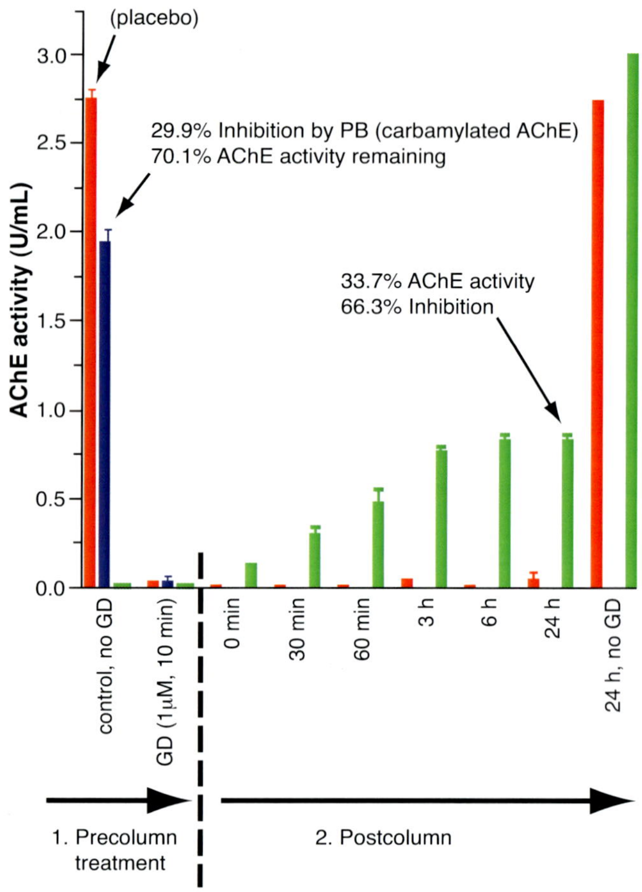

Fig. 22-4. Effects of soman (GD) on acetylcholinesterase (AChE) activity in whole blood from human volunteers who had taken pyridostigmine bromide (PB; 30 mg tablet). Blood was drawn 2.5 hours after dosing, when red blood cell (RBC) AChE is maximally inhibited by PB (blue bar, left of dashed line). After GD exposure, PB and GD were removed using a C_{18} chromatography spin column (postcolumn treatment). The PB-protected (carbamylated and sequestered) AChE activity returned by 6 hours postcolumn. Green bars show the correlation between the initial percent inhibition of RBC-AChE by PB (solid red line) and the subsequent return of AChE activity due to decarbamylation of the protected enzyme after removing PB and GD (green bars). While there was about 29.9% inhibition of RBC-AChE by PB before GD exposure (blue bar with arrow), at 24 hours (the green bar with arrow) there was about 33.7% return in activity after the column, demonstrating protection of RBC-AChE by PB pretreatment. Error bars represent the mean plus or minus the standard error of the mean.
AChE: acetylcholinesterase
GD: soman
PB: pyridostigmine bromide
RBC: red blood cell

by Hup A increased, compared to PB. Thus, Hup A is highly effective in protecting RBC-AChE from ex-vivo soman exposure.

As a pretreatment, Hup A is a specific and highly selective RBC-AChE inhibitor, with serum BChE remaining unaffected at physiological concentrations.[75] Thus, after exposure to an OP nerve agent, the effective bioscavenging capacity for serum BChE is preserved.[76] This lack of BChE inhibition represents an additional advantage of Hup A in preventing OP toxicity, and helps explain increased tolerance of Hup-A–pretreated animals to soman in comparison to animals pretreated with PB.

Studies of toxicology and treatment for nerve agent exposure have predominantly focused on lethal and supralethal doses of the agent. The acute and long-term effects of sarin in humans were well documented following the terrorist attacks in Japan in 1994 and 1995. Several severely poisoned victims (in cardiopulmonary arrest or in comas with generalized convulsions) had plasma BChE activities of 20% of normal (80% inhibited).[77] However, information regarding the delayed or long-term subclinical effects of low-level or trace amounts of sarin and other nerve agents, insecticides, and a variety of environmental chemicals (to which individuals may be asymptomatic) is relatively scarce, both in military and civilian environments. Potential scenarios can be envisioned in which low or trace exposures become significant. Given the possibility of urban terrorism involving chemical warfare OP agents, federal, state, and local authorities now have a variety of sensitive and accurate ChE and OP detection assays to initiate appropriate containment, decontamination, and treatment measures.

SULFUR MUSTARD

Background

Analysis of specimens, such as blood or urine, following a suspected chemical warfare agent exposure has been rare. Historically, biomedical samples collected after a suspected exposure were used for standard clinical assays and not preserved for later analysis. Highly sophisticated analytical methods required to verify chemical warfare agent exposure were not a part of the clinical laboratory methods inventory. More recently, a large portion of the biomedical samples obtained from casualties of suspected exposure to sulfur mustard have come from the Iran-Iraq war in the 1980s. Many victims of that conflict who exhibited clinical signs consistent with exposure to sulfur mustard were transported to hospitals in Europe for medical treatment. Prior to 1995 laboratory analysis of these specimens used methods to measure unmetabolized sulfur mustard or thiodiglycol (TDG), a hydrolysis product of sulfur mustard. Fortunately, some of the blood components and urine specimens were frozen and reanalyzed years later, after newer analytical methods were developed. Recently reported methods of analysis generally indicate greater levels of sensitivity than previous methods or target other biomarkers of sulfur mustard exposure. In addition to samples from

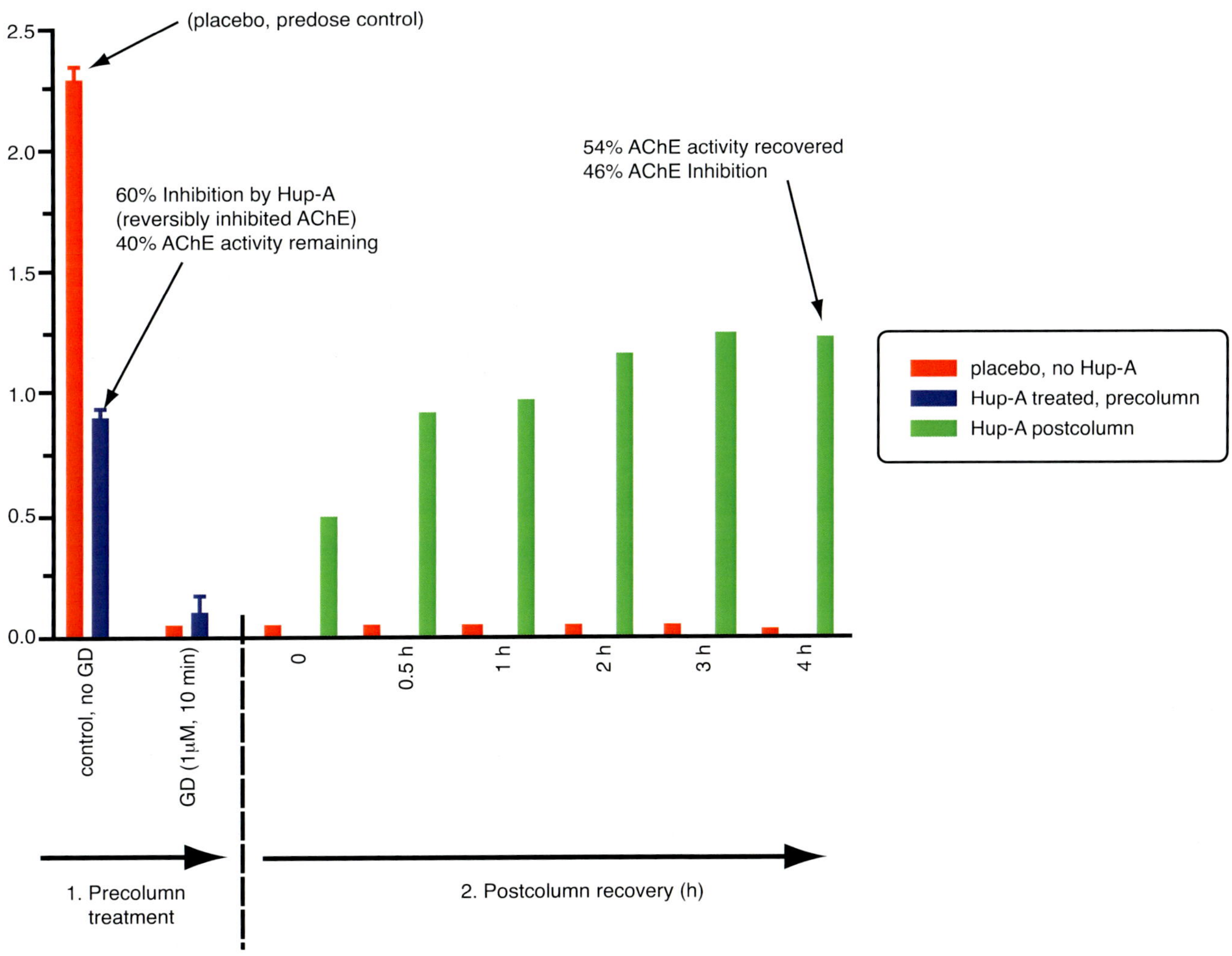

Fig. 22-5. Effects of soman (GD) on acetylcholinesterase (AChE) activity in whole blood from human volunteers who were given an increasing dose of huperzine A (Hup A). Blood was drawn 1.5 hours after the final 200-μg dose (blue bar, left of dashed line). The red bars represent red blood cell AChE from volunteers prior to receiving a placebo, while the blue bars represent AChE from an individual receiving the 200-μg Hup A dose. In the first part, after soman treatment, no AChE activity is observed by the Walter Reed Army Institute of Research assay in either the placebo- or drug-treated volunteers (red bars, close to 0 U/mL). However, after the spin column removal of free Hup A and soman, and a 4-hour period to allow for complete dissociation, the Hup-A–inhibited AChE is restored to the level that was initially inhibited by the drug (green bar with arrow, about 60% inhibition by the drug before the column versus 54% returned AChE activity after the column). Error bars represent the mean plus or minus the standard error of the mean. Note the increased inhibition and sequestering of AChE by Hup A compared to pyridostigmine bromide (see Fig. 22-4).
AChE: acetylcholinesterase
Hup A: huperzine A

the Iran-Iraq war, a small number of samples from individuals exposed to sulfur mustard in laboratory and field situations were collected, stored, and analyzed using more recently developed methods.

Some of sulfur mustard's physical properties and biochemical reactions are addressed in this volume (see Chapter 8, Vesicants) and have been reviewed extensively elsewhere.[78] Of primary importance in the development of assays for sulfur mustard is the formation of a highly reactive sulfonium ion that is produced following cyclization of an ethylene group of sulfur mustard. The sulfonium ion readily reacts with nucleophiles, such as water, or combines with a variety of nucleophilic sites in macromolecules. The resulting chemical reactions are able to produce a number of free metabolites and stable adducts that can be exploited for analysis in blood, urine, and tissue samples.[7,79,80] This section focuses primarily on metabolites that have been identified in biomedical samples from sulfur mustard casualties.

Before the early 1990s analytical methods for verifying exposure to sulfur mustard consisted of assays for the unmetabolized compound or the hydrolysis product TDG. Since 1995 a number of significant advances have occurred. Many new metabolites have been identified from specimens of sulfur-mustard–exposed individuals, and instrument advances, such as the ability to interface LC with MS and the use of tandem MS, have resulted in significant increases in test sensitivity and selectivity. Most newer methods of verifying exposure to sulfur mustard require extensive sample processing prior to introduction into the analytical system. The use of MS has enabled the incorporation of isotopically labeled forms of analytes for use as internal standards during the earliest stages of sample preparation. This has resulted in greater reproducibility of assays and made them more amenable to quantitative analysis. Although the laboratory methods presented in this section are not considered routine or standard, the efforts by a small number of laboratories worldwide that are active in this area of research have made the methods more attainable to a wider range of laboratories.

Analysis of Urine Samples

There are currently five urinary metabolites of primary interest in verifying exposure to sulfur mustard. Two of the metabolites, TDG and thiodiglycol sulfoxide (TDG-sulfoxide), are derived from chemical hydrolysis reactions (Figure 22-6). The other three products are formed following sulfur mustard's reaction with glutathione (GSH). Each of the five analytes has been identified in the urine of sulfur-mustard–exposed individuals.

Analytical Methods

Efforts to analyze specific biomarkers of sulfur mustard exposure in urine samples prior to 1995 targeted either unmetabolized sulfur mustard or TDG (Table 22-6). Vycudilik prepared urine samples by initially saturating them with sodium chloride followed by organic extraction using diethylether. The organic portion was evaporated under nitrogen and reconstituted with methylene chloride. After the addition of silica gel, the methylene chloride was evaporated under nitrogen, reconstituted with solvent, and analyzed using GC-MS.[81] Vycudilik later modified the method to isolate possible conjugates of sulfur mustard.[82] The primary difference in the latter study was the addition of strong acid to the urine samples. Urine samples were mixed with an equal amount of concentrated hydrochloric acid and saturated with sodium chloride. Using steam distillation, the distillate was collected in ether. Following sodium chloride saturation of the aqueous layer, the ether layer was dried and the residue dissolved in methylene chloride and silica gel. Samples were analyzed using GC and high-resolution MS. Vycudilik reported that the methods could not distinguish between sulfur mustard and its hydroxyethyl metabolites present in the urine samples.[82]

Wils et al treated urine with concentrated hydrochloric acid to convert TDG back to sulfur mustard.[83,84] Two methods were reported, only the later method is described here. The urine was passed through two C18 solid phase extraction cartridges. Next, a solution

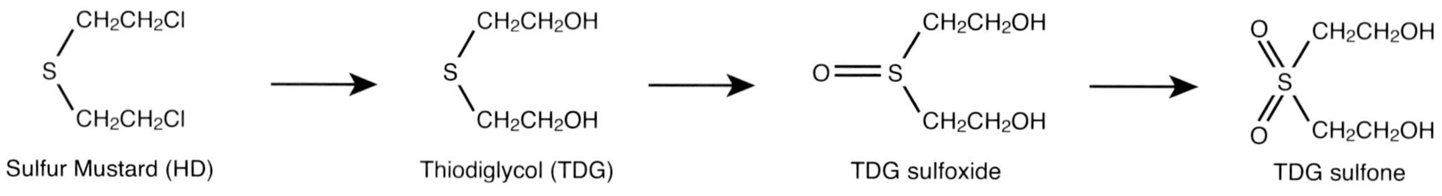

Fig. 22-6. Hydrolysis of sulfur mustard to produce thiodiglycol, followed by oxidation reactions.
HD: sulfur mustard
TDG: thiodiglycol

of deuterated TDG was passed through the same cartridges. The purified urine was mixed with concentrated hydrogen chloride (HCl) and heated. Sulfur mustard was purged from the solution and trapped onto a Tenax-TA adsorption tube. Analysis was performed using a thermodesorption cold trap injector interfaced with GC-MS. Analysis of urine samples obtained from a control group of patients found levels of TDG at low nanogram-to-milliliter concentrations. While most of the control levels were approximately 5 ng/mL, two individuals had levels that exceeded 20 ng/mL. These high background levels probably indicate that the method was also converting another analyte, in addition to TDG, into sulfur mustard (see below).

TABLE 22-6

REPORTS PUBLISHED PRIOR TO 1995 SHOWING LABORATORY ANALYSIS OF HUMAN BIOMEDICAL SAMPLES FOLLOWING SUSPECTED EXPOSURE TO SULFUR MUSTARD

Patient Sample Information*	Unmetabolized Sulfur Mustard	Hydrolysis Product†
Urine samples from 2 Iran-Iraq War casualties treated at Vienna hospital; collected 7 days after incident (no date given)[1]	Patient 1: 1.0 ng/mL Patient 2: 1.5 ng/mL	NM
Urine samples from 5 Iranian casualties treated at Ghent hospital; collected 10 days after incident (March 9, 1984)[2]	NM	Patient C1: 90 ng/mL Patient C2: 45 ng/mL Patient C3: 40 ng/mL Patient C4: 40 ng/mL Patient C5: 15 ng/mL Control samples: 3–55 ng/mL
Urine samples from 5 Iranian casualties treated at Utrecht hospital; collected 10 days after incident (March 9, 1984)[2]	NM	Patient range: 3–140 ng/mL Control samples: 3–55 ng/mL
Hair samples from 2 Iranian casualties; collected 1 day after incident (Feb 27, 1986)[3]	Patient 1: 0.5–1.0 µg/gram Patient 2: not detected	NM
Autopsy specimens (tissues and body fluids) from Iranian casualty treated at Munich hospital; collected 7 days after incident (1985)[4]	Urine: not detected; Fat, Skin, Brain, Kidney: 5–15 mg/kg; Muscle, Liver, Spleen, Lung: 1–2 mg/kg	NM
Urine samples from 12 Iran-Iraq War casualties (1986); no other details provided[5]	1–30 ng/mL for 6 individuals; not detected in 6 individuals	NM
Urine samples from 7 Iranian casualties treated at Ghent hospital; collected 5–6 and 18–19 days after incident (Feb 12–13, 1986)[6]	NM	5–6 days postexposure: range 7–336 ng/mL; 18–19 days postexposure: range 3–7 ng/mL
Urine samples from 3 Iranian casualties treated at Ghent hospital; collected 18–19 days after incident (Feb 12–13, 1986)[6]	NM	Patient range: 4–8 ng/mL Control samples: 1–21 ng/mL
Urine samples from 8 Iranian casualties treated at Utrecht hospital; collected 8–9 days after incident (Feb 12–13, 1986)[6]	NM	Patient range: 5–76 ng/mL Control samples: 1–21 ng/mL

*These are the known details of the incident and sample collection time after suspected exposure.
†The hydrolysis product was thiodiglycol.
NM: not measured
Data sources: (1) Vycudilik W. Detection of mustard gas bis(2-chloroethyl)-sulfide in urine. *Forensic Sci Int.* 1985;28:131–136. (2) Wils ERJ, Hulst AG, de Jong AL, Verweij A, Boter HL. Analysis of thiodiglycol in urine of victims of an alleged attack with mustard gas. *J Anal Toxicol.* 1985;9:254–257. (3) United Nations Security Council. *Report of the mission dispatched by the Secretary-General to investigate allegations of the use of chemical weapons in the conflict between the Islamic Republic of Iran and Iraq.* New York, NY: UN; 1986. Report S/17911. (4) Drasch G, Kretschmer E, Kauert G, von Meyer L. Concentrations of mustard gas [bis(2-chloroethyl)sulfide] in the tissues of a victim of a vesicant exposure. *J Forensic Sci.* 1987;32:1788–1793. (5) Vycudilik W. Detection of bis(2-chloroethyl)-sulfide (Yperite) in urine by high resolution gas chromatography-mass spectrometry. *Forensic Sci Int.* 1987;35:67–71. (6) Wils ERJ, Hulst AG, van Laar J. Analysis of thiodiglycol in urine of victims of an alleged attack with mustard gas, part II. *J Anal Toxicol.* 1988;12:15–19.

Drasch et al examined urine samples for unmetabolized sulfur mustard. Following organic extraction, thin-layer chromatography, and derivativation with gold, the extracts were analyzed using electrothermal atomic absorption spectroscopy.[85]

More recently, additional methods have been developed for trace level analysis of TDG and TDG-sulfoxide in urine.[86–89] There are a number of characteristics common to the methods (Table 22-7). They all use GC in association with some form of MS analysis, use a derivatizing agent to make the analyte more amenable to GC analysis and to increase sensitivity, and incorporate an isotopically labeled form of TDG as an internal standard. Most of the methods use a solid phase extraction cartridge for sample preparation. Some of the methods incubate the urine samples with glucuronidase with sulfatase activity to release any glucuronide-bound conjugates. Some of the methods use titanium trichloride in hydrochloric acid to reduce TDG-sulfoxide to TDG. The strong acid also hydrolyzes acid-labile esters of TDG and TDG-sulfoxide (Table 22-8). Ultimately, each of the methods converts all target analytes into the single analyte TDG for analysis. All of the methods have similar limits of detection, approximately 0.5 to 1 ng/mL. Although an assay has been developed to analyze TDG-sulfoxide separately without a conversion to TDG, the method is complicated by the high polarity of the analyte.[90] Consequently, the more common approach is to use the reducing agent titanium trichloride.

Unfortunately, regardless of the analytical method used, background levels have consistently been found in urine samples obtained from nonexposed individuals. In the most extensive study of background levels, urine samples from 105 individuals were examined for sulfur mustard metabolites using an assay that incorporates both a deconjugation process and a reduction step (ie, the assay measures free and bound forms of both TDG and of TDG-sulfoxide).[89] Quantifiable background levels were observed in 82% of the samples. Nearly 60% of the samples had observed levels of TDG in the 0.5- to 2.0-ng/mL range, while approximately 9% had levels in the 10- to 20-ng/mL range. When urine samples with higher background

TABLE 22-7

ANALYSIS METHODS FOR URINE SAMPLES TO MEASURE THIODIGLYCOL OR THIODIGLYCOL AND THIODIGLYCOL-SULFOXIDE

Instrumentation	Derivativizing Agent	SPE Cartridge	Glucuronidase Incubation	$TiCl_3$ Reduction	Internal Standard	Detection Limit
Negative ion chemical ionization GC-MS	Pentafluorobenzoyl chloride	Florisil	Yes	No	$^2H_4$-TDG	~ 1 ng/mL[1]
Electron impact GC-MS	Heptafluorobutyric anhydride	None	Yes	No	$^2H_8$-TDG	~ 1 ng/mL[2]
Negative ion chemical ionization GC-MS-MS	Pentafluorobenzoyl chloride	Florisil	No	Yes	$^2H_4$-TDG	< 1 ng/mL[3]
Positive chemical ionization GC-MS-MS	Heptafluorobutyric anhydride	Oasis HLB	Yes	Yes	$^{13}C_4$-TDG	0.5 ng/mL[4]

$^{13}C_4$: isotopically labeled carbon
$^2H_4$: isotopically labeled hydrogen or deuterium
$^2H_8$: isotopically labeled hydrogen or deuterium
GC: gas chromatography
HLB: hydrophilic-lipophilic-balanced
MS: mass spectrometry
SPE: solid phase extraction
TDG: thiodiglycol
$TiCl_3$: titanium trichloride

Data sources: (1) Black RM, Read RW. Detection of trace levels of thiodiglycol in blood, plasma and urine using gas chromatography-electron-capture negative-ion chemical ionisation mass spectrometry. *J Chromatogr.* 1988;449:261–270. (2) Jakubowski EM, Woodard CL, Mershon MM, Dolzine TW. Quantification of thiodiglycol in urine by electron ionization gas chromatography-mass spectrometry. *J Chromatogr.* 1990;528:184–190. (3) Black RM, Read RW. Improved methodology for the detection and quantitation of urinary metabolites of sulphur mustard using gas chromatography-tandem mass spectrometry. *J Chromatogr B Biomed Appl.* 1995;665:97–105. (4) Boyer AE, Ash D, Barr DB, et al. Quantitation of the sulfur mustard metabolites 1,1'-sulfonylbis[2-(methylthio)ethane] and thiodiglycol in urine using isotope-dilution gas chromatography-tandem mass spectrometry. *J Anal Toxicol.* 2004;28:327–332.

TABLE 22-8

TARGET ANALYTES FOR ANALYSIS METHODS OUTLINED IN TABLE 22-7

TDG			TDG-Sulfoxide		
Free	Glucuronide-bound conjugates	Acid-labile esters	Free	Glucuronide-bound conjugates	Acid-labile esters
Yes	Yes	No	No	No	No[1]
Yes	Yes	No	No	No	No[2]
Yes	No	Yes	Yes	No	Yes[3]
Yes	Yes	Yes	Yes	Yes	Yes[4]

TDG: thiodiglycol

Data sources: (1) Black RM, Read RW. Detection of trace levels of thiodiglycol in blood, plasma and urine using gas chromatography-electron-capture negative-ion chemical ionisation mass spectrometry. *J Chromatogr.* 1988;449:261–270. (2) Jakubowski EM, Woodard CL, Mershon MM, Dolzine TW. Quantification of thiodiglycol in urine by electron ionization gas chromatography-mass spectrometry. *J Chromatogr.* 1990;528:184–190. (3) Black RM, Read RW. Improved methodology for the detection and quantitation of urinary metabolites of sulphur mustard using gas chromatography-tandem mass spectrometry. *J Chromatogr B Biomed Appl.* 1995;665:97–105. (4) Boyer AE, Ash D, Barr DB, et al. Quantitation of the sulfur mustard metabolites 1,1′-sulfonylbis[2-(methylthio)ethane] and thiodiglycol in urine using isotope-dilution gas chromatography-tandem mass spectrometry. *J Anal Toxicol.* 2004;28:327–332.

levels were reanalyzed without the reduction step, the TDG level in all the samples was less than 2.5 ng/mL. This indicates that the free and bound forms of the TDG-sulfoxide, rather than the free and bound forms of TDG, are responsible for a larger portion of the observed background levels in the nonexposed human urine samples. These results are consistent with those found in other, smaller studies of background levels.[86,87,90,91] Boyer et al discovered that storage condition of urine samples must also be considered when analyzing samples for TDG and TDG-sulfoxide.[89] In a study of urine samples stored at – 20°C for an 8-month period, they found that all free and conjugated TDG in the samples had oxidized to free and conjugated TDG-sulfoxide. Consequently, the use of a reducing agent was shown to be critical for the analysis of samples that had been frozen for any length of time.

Black et al identified a series of metabolites formed from sulfur mustard's reaction with GSH, a small-molecular–weight tripeptide that acts as a free radical scavenger (Figure 22-7).[91–93] While a large number of metabolites were identified in animal experiments, there are three verified reaction products in urine samples obtained from individuals exposed to sulfur mustard. One set of reaction products is believed to result from metabolism of the sulfur-mustard–GSH conjugate by the β-lyase enzyme (see Figure 22-7d). Two β-lyase metabolites have been identified in the urine from exposed individuals:

- 1-methylsulfinyl-2-[2-(methylthio)ethylsulfonyl]ethane (MSMTESE) and
- 1,1′-sulfonylbis[2-(methylsulfinyl)ethane] (SBMSE).

MSMTESE and SBMSE can be reduced using titanium chloride and analyzed by GC-MS-MS as a single analyte: 1,1′-sulfonylbis[2-(methylthio)ethane] (SBMTE; Exhibit 22-1).[94,95] Black et al reported a limit of detection of 0.1 ng/mL,[94] while Young et al extended the lower limit of detection to 0.038 ng/mL.[95] To date, no background levels have been found in the urine of unexposed individuals, including studies where urine samples from over 100 individuals were analyzed using two different assay methods.[89,95] Alternatively, MSMTESE and SBMSE can be analyzed individually without reducing the two analytes to single analyte using electrospray LC-MS-MS.[96] Lower limits of detection were 0.1 to 0.5 ng/mL for each of the analytes.

The final urinary biomarker to be discussed is also a reaction product of sulfur mustard with GSH: 1,1′-sulfonylbis[2-S-(N-acetylcysteinyl)ethane] (see Figure 22-7e; Table 22-9). Using solid phase extraction for sample cleanup and analyte concentration, followed by analysis with negative ion electrospray LC-MS-MS, Read and Black were able to achieve detection limits of 0.5 to 1.0 ng/mL.[97]

Assays for several other potential urinary analytes have been developed, but these analytes have yet to be confirmed in human-exposed samples. N7-(2-hydroxyethylthioethyl) guanine is a breakdown product from alkylated DNA that has been observed in animal studies. Fidder et al developed both a GC-MS method that requires derivatization of the analyte and an

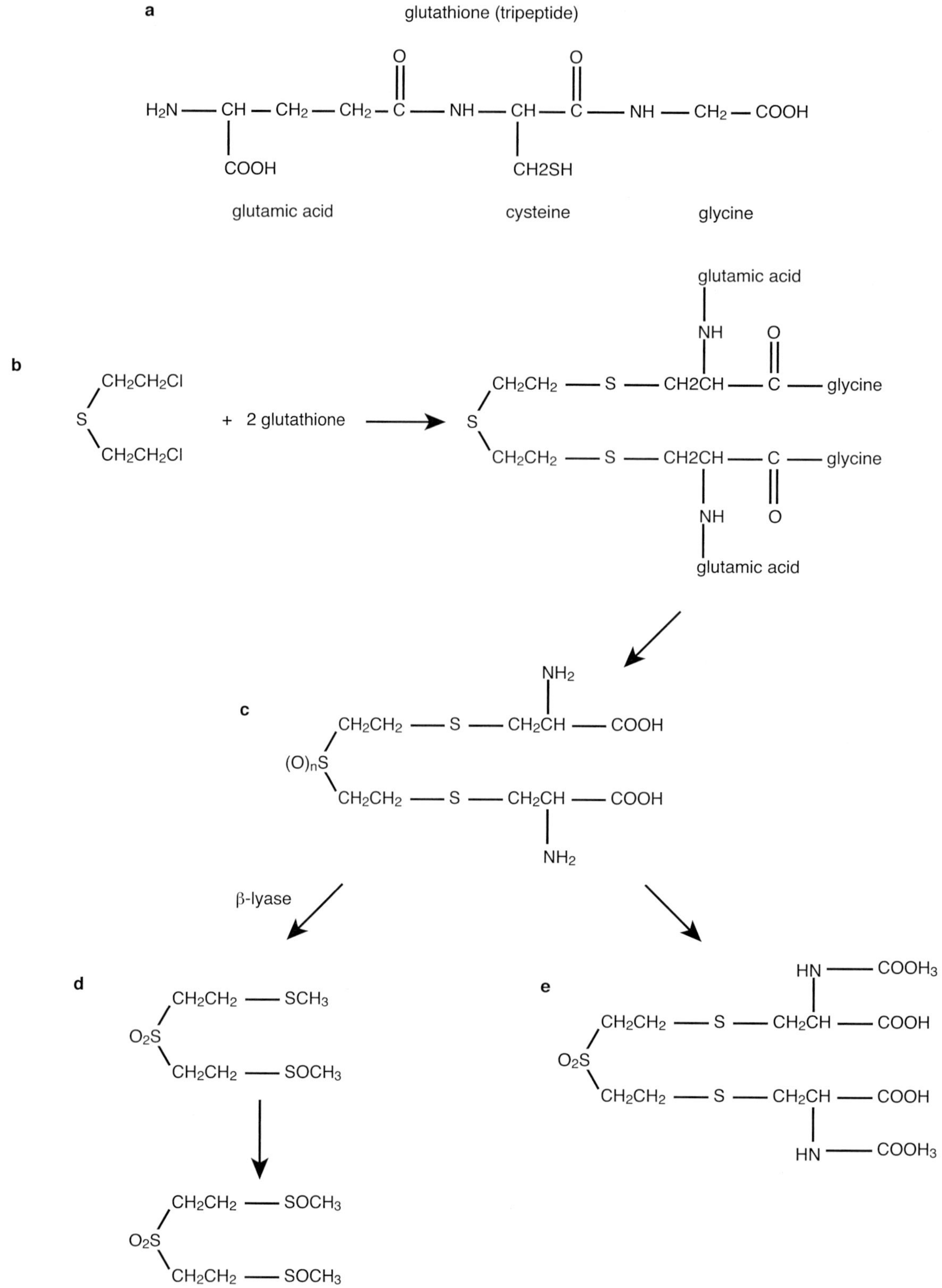

Fig. 22-7. Reaction pathway proposed by Black et al (1992). **(a)** Structure of glutathione. **(b)** Reaction of sulfur mustard and glutathione. **(c)** Intermediate product. **(d)** β-lyase metabolites 1-methylsulfinyl-2-[2-(methylthio)ethylsulfonyl]ethane (MSMTESE) and 1,1′-sulfonylbis[2-(methylsulfinyl)ethane] (SBMSE). **(e)** Bis-mercapturic acid conjugate of mustard sulfone.
Data source: Black RM, Brewster K, Clarke RJ, Hambrook JL, Harrison JM, Howells DJ. Biological fate of sulphur mustard, 1,1′-thiobis(2-chloroethane): isolation and identification of urinary metabolites following intraperitoneal administration to rat. *Xenobiotica*. 1992;22:405–418.

LC-MS-MS method that can analyze the compound directly.[98] Other possible urinary analytes are an imidazole derivative formed from sulfur mustard's reaction with protein histidine residues[99] and sulfur mustard adducts to metallothionien.[100]

Application to Human Exposure

Vycudilik analyzed urine samples from two casualties of the Iran-Iraq War who were brought to a hospital in Vienna, Austria, for treatment of suspected exposure to sulfur mustard.[81] The exposure was believed to have occurred 1 week prior to their arrival in Vienna. No clinical description of the patients' injuries was provided in the report. The concentration of sulfur mustard found in their urine samples using GC-MS was approximately 1.0 ng/mL and 1.5 ng/mL. Additional urine samples were obtained from the patients several days after admission to the hospital. Analysis using the same method produced negative results for all samples.

Vycudilik also analyzed urine samples obtained from 12 Iran-Iraq War casualties.[82] The only clinical description of the patients was the observation that they had severe skin lesions resulting from an alleged mustard gas attack. Urine samples from six of the patients produced positive results for sulfur mustard. Concentrations found ranged from 1 to 30 ng/mL. The method could not distinguish between sulfur mustard or its hydroxyethyl metabolites present in the urine samples.

Wils et al examined a large number of urine samples for TDG concentrations. The samples were obtained from Iranian casualties of the Iran-Iraq War transported to western European hospitals in Ghent and Utrecht for treatment.[83,84] The majority of the urine samples

EXHIBIT 22-1

SAMPLE PREPARATION METHODS FOR THE GAS CHROMATOGRAPHIC/MASS SPECTROMETRIC/MASS SPECTROMETRIC ANALYSIS OF THE SULFUR MUSTARD URINARY β-LYASE METABOLITES

Procedure of Black et al:

- Add the internal standard deuterated 1,1′-sulfonylbis[2-(methylsulfinyl)ethane] to 1 mL of urine.
- Add 0.4 mL of titanium trichloride.
- Incubate sample at 40°C overnight (16 hours).
- Filter solution through a preconditioned C_8 Bond Elut solid-phase extraction cartridge.
- Wash cartridge with water followed by a methanol and water mixture.
- Allow cartridge to dry.
- Elute analytes with acetone.
- Evaporate to dryness under nitrogen and dissolve in toluene.
- Analyze using GC-MS-MS with ammonia chemical ionization.[1]

Procedure of Young et al:

- Place 0.5 mL of urine into a 15 mL tube.
- Add the internal standard ^{13}C-1,1′-sulfonylbis[2-(methythio)ethane] to the urine.
- Add 1 mL of titanium trichloride.
- Incubate sample at 75°C for 1 hour.
- Add 2 mL of 6N sodium hydroxide and mix.
- Centrifuge samples for 5 minutes.
- Pour supernatant into a Chem Elut column.
- Elute analytes with 16 mL of dichloromethane and acetonitrile mixture.
- Evaporate to dryness under nitrogen and dissolve in toluene.
- Analyze using GC-MS-MS with isobutane chemical ionization.[2]

GC: gas chromatography
MS: mass spectrometry
Data sources: (1) Black RM, Clarke RJ, Read RW. Analysis of 1,1′-sulphonylbis[2-(methylsulphinyl)ethane] and 1-methylsulphinyl-2-[2-(methylthio)ethylsulphonyl]ethane, metabolites of sulphur mustard, in urine using gas chromatography-mass spectrometry. *J Chromatogr.* 1991;558:405–414. (2) Young CL, Ash D, Driskell WJ, et al. A rapid, sensitive method for the quantitation of specific metabolites of sulfur mustard in human urine using isotope-dilution gas chromatography-tandem mass spectrometry. *J Anal Toxicol.* 2004;28:339–345.

TABLE 22-9

ANALYTICAL METHODS USED TO VERIFY EXPOSURE TO SULFUR MUSTARD IN BIOMEDICAL SAMPLES

Sample Matrix	Biomarker	Sample Preparation	Analytical Method	LOD
Urine, blood, plasma	TDG	Enzyme incubation, derivatization	Negative ion chemical ionization GC-MS	~ 1 ng/mL[1]
Urine	TDG	Enzyme incubation, derivatization	Electron impact GC-MS	~ 1 ng/mL[2]
Urine	TDG, TDG-sulfoxide	$TiCl_3$ reduction, derivatization	Negative ion chemical ionization GC-MS-MS	< 1 ng/mL[3]
Urine	TDG, TDG-sulfoxide	Enzyme incubation, $TiCl_3$ reduction, derivatization	Positive ion chemical ionization GC-MS	0.5 ng/mL[4]
Urine	TDG-sulfoxide	Derivatization	Negative ion chemical ionization GC-MS	2 ng/mL[5]
Urine	SBMTE	$TiCl_3$ reduction	Positive ion chemical ionization GC-MS-MS	0.1 ng/mL[6]
Urine	SBMTE	$TiCl_3$ reduction	Positive ion chemical ionization GC-MS-MS	0.04 ng/mL[7]
Urine	MSMTESE	SPE cartridge extraction	Positive ion electrospray LC-MS-MS	0.1–0.5 ng/mL[8]
Urine	SBMSE	SPE cartridge extraction	Positive ion electrospray LC-MS-MS	0.1–0.5 ng/mL[8]
Urine	Bis-(N-acetyl cysteine) conjugate	SPE cartridge extraction	Negative ion electrospray LC-MS-MS	0.5–1 ng/mL[9]
Blood	Hemoglobin valine adduct	Globin isolation, valine cleavage by Edman degradation, derivatization	Negative ion chemical ionization GC-MS	100 nM whole blood exposure[10,11]
Blood	Hemoglobin valine adduct	Globin isolation, valine cleavage by Edman degradation	High-resolution negative ion chemical ionization GC-MS	0.5 pmol adduct/mL[12]
Blood	Hemoglobin histidine adduct	Acid hydrolysis of globin, derivatization	Positive ion electrospray LC-MS-MS	Not reported[12]
Blood	Hemoglobin histidine adduct	Acid hydrolysis of globin, derivatization	Positive ion electrospray LC-MS-MS	10 μM whole blood exposure[13]
Plasma	Albumin cysteine adduct	Albumin isolation, pronase digestion	Positive ion electrospray LC-MS-MS	10 nM whole blood exposure[14,15]
Blood, plasma	Protein adducts	Protein precipitation, alkaline hydrolysis, derivatization, SPE extraction	Negative ion chemical ionization GC-MS	25 nM plasma exposure[16]
Blood	DNA adducts	WBC isolation, lysis, extraction, treatment with RNase and proteinase K	Immunuslotblot assay	50 nM whole blood exposure[17]
Skin	DNA adducts	Epidermal layer isolation, lysis, extraction, treatment with RNase and proteinase K	Immunuslotblot assay	1 sec skin exposure to saturated vapor[17]
Skin	Keratin adducts	Alkaline hydrolysis, derivatization	LC-radiometric detector	Not reported[18]

(**Table 22-9** *continues*)

Table 22-9 *continued*

CI: chemical ionization
DNA: deoxyribonucleic acid
GC: gas chromatography
LC: liquid chromatography
LOD: limit of detection
MS: mass spectrometry
MSMTESE: 1-methylsulfinyl-2-[2-(methylthio)ethylsulfonyl]ethane
RNase: ribonuclease
SBMSE: 1,1′-sulfonylbis[2-(methylsulfinyl)ethane]
SBMTE: 1,1′-sulfonylbis[2-(methylthio)ethane]
SPE: solid phase extraction
TDG: thiodiglycol
$TiCl_3$: titanium trichloride
WBC: white blood cell
Data sources: (1) Black RM, Read RW. Detection of trace levels of thiodiglycol in blood, plasma and urine using gas chromatography-electron-capture negative-ion chemical ionisation mass spectrometry. *J Chromatogr.* 1988;449:261–270. (2) Jakubowski EM, Woodard CL, Mershon MM, Dolzine TW. Quantification of thiodiglycol in urine by electron ionization gas chromatography-mass spectrometry. *J Chromatogr.* 1990;528:184–190. (3) Black RM, Read RW. Improved methodology for the detection and quantitation of urinary metabolites of sulphur mustard using gas chromatography-tandem mass spectrometry. *J Chromatogr B Biomed Appl.* 1995;665:97–105. (4) Boyer AE, Ash D, Barr DB, et al. Quantitation of the sulfur mustard metabolites 1,1′-sulfonylbis[2-(methylthio)ethane] and thiodiglycol in urine using isotope-dilution gas chromatography-tandem mass spectrometry. *J Anal Toxicol.* 2004;28:327–332. (5) Black RM, Read RW. Methods for the analysis of thiodiglycol sulphoxide, a metabolite of sulphur mustard, in urine using gas chromatography-mass spectrometry. *J Chromatogr.* 1991;558:393–404. (6) Black RM, Clarke RJ, Read RW. Analysis of 1,1′-sulphonylbis[2-(methylsulphinyl)ethane] and 1-methylsulphinyl-2-[2-(methylthio)ethylsulphonyl]ethane, metabolites of sulphur mustard, in urine using gas chromatography-mass spectrometry. *J Chromatogr.* 1991;558:405–414. (7) Young CL, Ash D, Driskell WJ, et al. A rapid, sensitive method for the quantitation of specific metabolites of sulfur mustard in human urine using isotope-dilution gas chromatography-tandem mass spectrometry. *J Anal Toxicol.* 2004;28:339–345. (8) Read RW, Black RM. Analysis of beta-lyase metabolites of sulfur mustard in urine by electrospray liquid chromatography-tandem mass spectrometry. *J Anal Toxicol.* 2004;28:346–351. (9) Read RW, Black RM. Analysis of the sulfur mustard metabolite 1,1′-sulfonylbis[2-S-(N-acetylcysteinyl)ethane] in urine by negative ion electrospray liquid chromatography-tandem mass spectrometry. *J Anal Toxicol.* 2004;28:352–356. (10) Fidder A, Noort D, de Jong AL, Trap HC, de Jong LPA, Benschop HP. Monitoring of in vitro and in vivo exposure to sulfur mustard by GC/MS determination of the N-terminal valine adduct in hemoglobin after a modified Edman degradation. *Chem Res Toxicol.* 1996;9:788–792. (11) Noort D, Fidder A, Benschop HP, de Jong LP, Smith JR. Procedure for monitoring exposure to sulfur mustard based on modified Edman degradation of globin. *J Anal Toxicol.* 2004;28:311–315. (12) Black RM, Clarke RJ, Harrison JM, Read RW. Biological fate of sulphur mustard: identification of valine and histidine adducts in haemoglobin from casualties of sulphur mustard poisoning. *Xenobiotica.* 1997;27:499–512. (13) Noort D, Hulst AG, Trap HC, de Jong LPA, Benschop HP. Synthesis and mass spectrometric identification of the major amino acid adducts formed between sulphur mustard and haemoglobin in human blood. *Arch Toxicol.* 1997;71:171–178. (14) Noort D, Hulst AG, de Jong LP, Benschop HP. Alkylation of human serum albumin by sulfur mustard in vitro and in vivo: mass spectrometric analysis of a cysteine adduct as a sensitive biomarker of exposure. *Chem Res Toxicol.* 1999;12:715–721. (15) Noort D, Fidder A, Hulst AG, Woolfitt AR, Ash D, Barr JR. Retrospective detection of exposure to sulfur mustard: improvements on an assay for liquid chromatography-tandem mass spectrometry analysis of albumin-sulfur mustard adducts. *J Anal Toxicol.* 2004;28:333–338. (16) Capacio BR, Smith JR, DeLion MT, et al. Monitoring sulfur mustard exposure by gas chromatography-mass spectrometry analysis of thiodiglycol cleaved from blood proteins. *J Anal Toxicol.* 2004;28:306–310. (17) Van der Schans GP, Mars-Groenendijk R, de Jong LP, Benschop HP, Noort D. Standard operating procedure for immunoslotblot assay for analysis of DNA/sulfur mustard adducts in human blood and skin. *J Anal Toxicol.* 2004;28:316–319. (18) Noort D, Fidder A, Hulst AG, de Jong LP, Benschop HP. Diagnosis and dosimetry of exposure to sulfur mustard: development of a standard operating procedure for mass spectrometric analysis of haemoglobin adducts: exploratory research on albumin and keratin adducts. *J Appl Toxicol.* 2000;20(suppl 1):S187–S192.

were the first collected following hospital admission 5 to 10 days after the suspected exposure. Willems detailed the patients' medical histories.[101] Briefly, the injuries were described as moderate to severe and were consistent with sulfur mustard injury, including erythema and fluid-filled vesicles. Urine samples were initially analyzed for intact sulfur mustard, but were found to be negative. Following treatment of the urine samples with a strong acid to convert TDG to sulfur mustard, the samples were analyzed using GC-MS. The TDG concentrations found in the first set of samples collected at the hospital ranged between 5 to 100 ng/mL for the majority of the samples. The highest observed TDG concentration was 330 ng/mL from a casualty who died 1 day after admission. During the hospitalization, 18 to19 days after the exposure, a second set of urine samples was collected from one group. TDG levels in that set of samples were similar to observed background levels in control samples. TDG background levels were determined from urine samples obtained from nonexposed individuals and were generally less than 12 ng/mL, although two of the control samples had levels of 21 ng/mL and 55 ng/mL. Elevated background levels in control samples may indicate that this method also converts TDG-sulfoxide or some other analytes into sulfur mustard.

Drasch et al examined urine samples obtained during an autopsy of a sulfur mustard casualty for unmetabolized sulfur mustard.[85] The victim was an Iranian soldier, age 24, who died of complications from pneumonia 7 days after the suspected exposure. The patient had been transferred to an intensive care unit in Munich, Germany. Samples were taken during the autopsy and stored at – 20°C for 1 year prior to analysis. Despite very high concentrations of sulfur mustard found in autopsy tissue specimens, sulfur mustard was not detected in the urine samples.

In 1990 Jakubowski et al received urine samples from an accidental laboratory exposure to sulfur mustard.[102] A liquid flashpoint tester overheated, vaporized a mixture that was thought to contain only a deconned solution, and exposed a chemist who had attempted to shut down the reaction. Nine hours after the incident, the individual felt a burning sensation on his arms, hands, neck, and face. Medical care was sought the morning after blisters appeared on his hands and arms. The erythematous and vesicated areas were estimated to be less than 5% and 1% of the total body surface area, respectively. The patient collected his total urine output for a 2-week period. For the first 3 days, the patient's total urine output was only about a third to half that of the average adult daily output of 1.5 liters, but the patient had a normal output level over the next 10 days. The assay method used measured both free and conjugated TDG.[87] The maximum TDG urinary excretion rate was 20 μg/day on the third day. TDG concentrations of 10 ng/mL or greater were observed in some samples for up to 1 week after the exposure. A rate constant was calculated for TDG concentration from days 4 through 10 and the half-life was found to be 1.2 days. A great deal of intraday variability was noted for the TDG urine concentrations. Consequently, the collection of several urine samples per day is recommended. An attempt was also made to estimate the total amount of sulfur mustard on the patient's skin. The estimate was based on two assumptions: 1) the assay for the free and conjugated TDG represents approximately 5% of the total amount of sulfur-mustard–related products in the blood, and 2) the bioavailability factor from skin to blood is 10 (ie, 10% of the sulfur mustard on the skin penetrated into the blood). A total of 0.243 mg of TDG was recovered over a 2-week period. This represents 4.86 mg in the blood, or 48.6 mg on the skin.

There are currently four instances of human exposure to sulfur mustard in which urine samples were subjected to several different assays in order to target multiple urinary metabolites. The first report described a small subset of urine samples previously analyzed by Wils et al[83] and were later reanalyzed by Black and Read[88] after storage at – 20°C for a 5-year period. Willems provided clinical information on the five individuals and coded them C1 through C5.[101] This group of individuals was reportedly exposed to exploding bombs that generated black dust and rain. Decontamination efforts consisted only of clothing removal, although some victims may have also showered. Early symptomatology included eye and throat irritation along with respiration difficulties. Within 1 to 2 days, victims developed erythema and small blisters on the skin, edema of the eyelids, photophobia, coughing, dyspnea, and hemoptysis. The patients were admitted to a hospital 10 days after the suspected sulfur mustard exposure. Urine samples were obtained at that time. Four of the five patients were discharged 26 to 37 days after hospitalization. Patient C1 developed adult respiratory distress syndrome and was given ventilatory support, but died in cardiovascular shock 15 days after the original exposure event (5 days after hospital admission). Wils et al coded the urine sample set from individuals C1 to C5 as G1 to G5 in their report and, using the GC-MS assay described above, found concentrations of TDG at 90 ng/mL, 45 ng/mL, 40 ng/mL, 40 ng/mL, and 15 ng/mL for individuals 1 through 5, respectively.[83] Using a different method measuring TDG and TDG-sulfoxide as a single analyte followed by GC-MS-MS analysis, Black and Read found TDG and TDG-sulfoxide levels of 69 ng/mL, 28 ng/mL, and 33 ng/mL for individuals C1, C2, and C5, respectively. C3 and C4 were not assayed because their samples were insufficient. Control urine samples analyzed by Black and Read produced a background level of 11 ng/mL.[88] Urine samples from all five casualties were analyzed for β-lyase concentrations, with the highest concentration found in patient C1. The concentrations found in the urine from four of the casualties ranged between 0.5 to 5 ng/mL, while the individual who died had a β-lyase concentration of 220 ng/mL.[88]

Once again using the GC-MS-MS method that measures both TDG and TDG-sulfoxide as a single analyte, Black and Read analyzed urine samples from two casualties of an alleged sulfur mustard attack on the Kurdish town of Halabja in 1988.[88] The patients had been transferred to London for medical treatment and urine samples were collected 13 days after the alleged incident. Black and Read found combined TDG plus TDG-sulfoxide levels of 11 ng/mL for both patients, but also found similar concentration levels in control samples. Urine samples were also analyzed for β-lyase concentrations using GC-MS-MS. Although the concentration of the β-lyase metabolites found in both patients was near the limit of detection for the assay, the analytes were clearly detectable and ranged between 0.1 and 0.3 ng/mL.[88] The urine samples were later analyzed using the LC-MS-MS assay that can distinguish the individual β-lyase metabolites.[96] The monosulfoxide MSMTESE was only detected from one of the casualties and was near the limit of detection for the assay. The bissulfoxide SBMSE was detected in the urine from both casualties, but for each sample it was near the limit of detection of the assay (0.1–0.5 ng/mL).

Some of the most extensive testing of urine samples for sulfur-mustard–related metabolites involved two individuals who were accidentally exposed to a World War I munition containing sulfur mustard. The injuries were described as predominately cutaneous exposures, with both individuals exhibiting extensive skin blistering. Urine samples were collected 2 to 3 days after the individuals were exposed. Black and Read analyzed the urine using three different methods to detect metabolites of sulfur mustard hydrolysis.[91] In addition, the urine samples were examined for products of a reaction between sulfur mustard and GSH. The first assay measured TDG (free and conjugated together) and found concentrations of 2 ng/mL for each individual. The second assay targeted only free TDG-sulfoxide, and concentrations of 69 ng/mL and 45 ng/mL were found for the two individuals. Concentrations of 77 ng/mL and 54 ng/mL were found using a GC-MS-MS assay that measures TDG and TDG-sulfoxide as a single analyte. Control samples analyzed along with the patient samples for the second and third assays gave levels of 4 to 5 ng/mL, therefore the patient results were significantly higher than control values. The β-lyase metabolites were measured using both the GC-MS-MS method[91] and the LC-MS-MS method.[96] When the β-lyase metabolites were analyzed individually by LC-MS-MS, their concentrations ranged from 15 to 17 ng/mL and from 30 to 34 ng/mL for the monosulfoxide and bissulfoxide, respectively. When analyzed as the single, reduced form of SBMTE using GC-MS-MS, observed concentrations were 42 ng/mL and 56 ng/mL. Samples were also analyzed for a bis-(N-acetylcysteine) conjugate using LC-MS-MS.[97] This biomarker is also a reaction product of sulfur mustard and GSH. Although the biomarker is a major metabolite in rats exposed to sulfur mustard, it had not been reported in urine samples from exposed humans. The metabolite was found in urine samples from both exposed individuals, but concentrations were near the lower limit of detection (0.5–1 ng/mL).

The most recently reported exposure incident involved two explosive ordnance technicians who were part of a team tasked with destroying a suspected World War I 75-mm munition. The munition had been discovered in a clamshell driveway and was believed to have originated from material dredged from a seafloor dumping area. Following demolition procedures, two individuals came into contact with a brown oily liquid that was found leaking from the remnants of the munition. During the disposal operation, none of the ordnance team members complained of eye or throat irritation or breathing difficulties. The clinical sequence of events for one of the individuals has previously been reported,[103,104] but will be described in brief here. Within 2 hours of the munition destruction, one of the individuals (patient D1, a 35-year-old male) noticed a tingling sensation on one arm and then showered. The next morning (approximately 14 hours after the liquid contact), painful areas had developed on his hand, along with noticeable reddening and small blisters. He went to a local emergency room where the blisters were observed to grow and coalesce. He was subsequently transferred to a regional burn center. Blisters developed on the patient's arm, hand, ankle, and foot. The erythema and blistered area on the patient was estimated to be 6.5% of his body surface area (Figure 22-8). The patient never developed ocular or respiratory complications; consequently it appeared that his injuries were only the result of a cutaneous liquid exposure. The second individual (patient D2) had a small, single blister and was not hospitalized. Urine samples from patient D1 were collected on days 2 through 11 and 29, 35, and 42 days after exposure and from patient D2 on days 2, 4, and 7 after exposure. Reports containing preliminary analysis results mistakenly indicated that the first samples collected were 1 day post exposure.[104,105] Urine from both individuals was analyzed for hydrolysis metabolites and GSH reaction products.[104,105] Hydrolysis metabolites were determined using several different methods. Using a

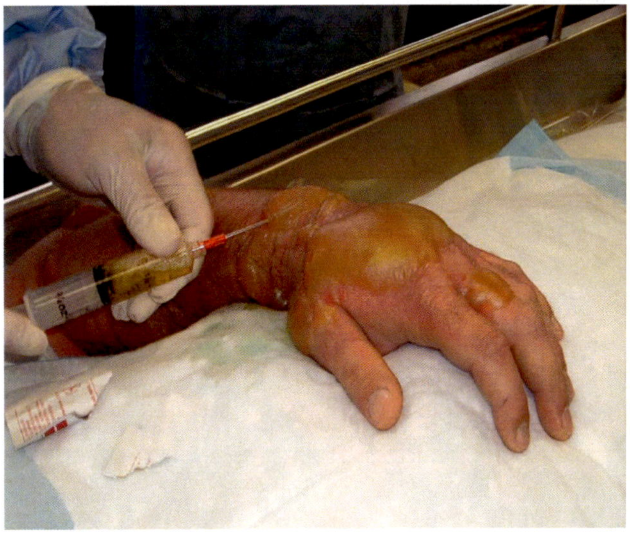

Fig. 22-8. Aspiration of blister fluid from accidental exposure to sulfur mustard.

GC-MS assay that targets free TDG and glucuronide-bound TDG,[87] detectable levels of TDG were only observed in patient D1's urine sample from day 2. Using a modified approach of the previous assay, the urine samples were incubated with concentrated HCl overnight to release acid-labile esters rather than submitted to an enzyme incubation step. TDG levels for patient D1 ranged from 40 ng/mL on day 2 to 10 ng/mL on day 6 after exposure using the modified assay.[104] TDG was not detected in urine samples beyond day 6 for patient D1 and was not detected in any of the urine samples from patient D2. Urine samples were also analyzed using a GC-MS-MS assay that measured both free and glucuronide-bound TDG.[105] There were no detectable levels in any of the urine samples from the individual with the single blister (patient D2). Patient D1 had the highest observed TDG concentration at day 2 (24 ng/mL). TDG concentrations ranged from 6 to 11 ng/mL over the next 5 days, decreased to a range of 1 to 2 ng/mL for the next 4 days, and TDG was undetected after day 11. The final method of analysis for hydrolysis metabolites was a GC-MS-MS assay that targeted free and glucuronide-bound TDG, free and glucuronide-bound TDG-sulfoxide, and acid-labile esters of TDG and TDG-sulfoxide.[105] The observed concentrations for patient D2 (2–4 ng/mL) fell within the range of concentrations previously observed in urine samples of unexposed individuals. The highest observed levels found in unexposed individuals with this assay were approximately 20 ng/mL.[89] While observed concentrations were much higher for patient D1, only days 2, 5, and 6 produced concentrations (50, 28, and 24 ng/mL, respectively) that were greater than the highest observed background control levels. β-lyase metabolites were measured as the single analyte SBMTE using GC-MS-MS.[105] Levels for both patients decreased dramatically by day 3 after exposure. Patient D2's urine SBMTE concentrations were 2.6 ng/mL, 0.8 ng/mL, and 0.08 ng/mL for samples taken 2, 4, and 7 days after exposure, respectively. Patient D1's concentrations decreased from 41 ng/mL at day 2 after exposure down to 7 ng/mL, 3.3 ng/mL, and 1.3 ng/mL over the next 3 days. For days 6 to 11, concentrations ranged between 0.07 and 0.02 ng/mL and SBMTE was not detected beyond day 11. Patient D1's urine from days 2 and 3 was also examined for the presence of the bis-(N-acetylcysteine) conjugate using LC-MS-MS. It was detected at a concentration of 3.1 ng/mL in the urine sample collected 2 days after exposure, but was not detected in the day 3 sample.

Currently the analytes of choice for assessing potential exposure to sulfur mustard in urine samples are the two β-lyase metabolites. The analytes can be measured individually using LC-MS-MS or reduced to a single analyte (SBMTE) and measured using GC-MS-MS. This has been verified in human exposure cases with sensitive and selective assays. To date, no known examples of background levels of these metabolites have been found in the urine from unexposed individuals (see Table 22-6, Table 22-10, Table 22-11).

Analysis of Blood Samples

Whereas urinary metabolites undergo relatively rapid elimination from the body, blood components offer biomarkers with potential use in verifying exposure to sulfur mustard long after the exposure incident. Three different approaches have been used for blood biomarker analysis. An intact macromolecule, such as protein or DNA, with the sulfur mustard adducts attached, can be analyzed. Currently, this approach has only been demonstrated for hemoglobin using in-vitro experiments. An alternate approach is to enzymatically digest the proteins to produce a smaller peptide with the sulfur mustard adduct still attached. Methods of this type have been developed for both hemoglobin and albumin. A third approach is to cleave the sulfur mustard adduct from the macromolecule and analyze it in a fashion similar to that used for free metabolites found in urine. The latter two approaches, described below, have both successfully verified human exposure to sulfur mustard.

Analytical Methods

Methods to measure sulfur mustard adducts to DNA in white blood cells have been developed using LC with fluorescence detection[106] and using an enzyme-linked immunosorbent assay (ELISA).[107,108] The DNA adduct that appears most abundant results from attachment of sulfur mustard to the N7 position of deoxyguaninosine (Figure 22-9a).[109] The immunochemical method used monoclonal antibodies that were raised against N7-(2-hydroxyethylthioethyl)-guanosine-5′-phosphate (Exhibit 22-2).

Hemoglobin is an abundant, long-lived protein in human blood. Alkylation reactions between sulfur mustard and hemoglobin have been shown to occur with six histidine, three glutamic acid, and two valine amino acids of hemoglobin.[110,111] Methods have been developed to analyze several of the adducts. While the histidine adducts appear to be the most abundant type, their analysis using MS techniques is problematic and the method does not appear to be as sensitive as the method for analyzing the N-terminal valine adducts.[112] Adducts to the N-terminal valine amino acids represent only a small fraction of the total alkylation of the macromolecule, but their location on the periphery of the molecule allows them to be selectively cleaved using a modified Edman degradation. Following isolation of the globin from the RBCs, the globin is reacted with pentafluorophenyl isothiocyanate to form a thiohydantoin compound, which is further derivatized before analysis (Figure 22-10). The derivatized compound can then be analyzed using negative ion chemical ionization GC-MS (Exhibit 22-3).[113,114]

Human serum albumin was found to be alkylated by sulfur mustard at the cysteine-34 position. Fol-

TABLE 22-10

PUBLISHED REPORTS (1995–2006) OF LABORATORY ANALYSIS OF HUMAN URINE SAMPLES FOR HYDROLYSIS METABOLITES FOLLOWING SUSPECTED EXPOSURE TO SULFUR MUSTARD

Patient Sample Information*	Glucuronidase Incubation†	$TiCl_3$ Reduction‡	TDG-sulfoxide	Glucuronidase Incubation & $TiCl_3$ Reduction§
Iranian casualties, 3 of 5 individuals, treated at Ghent hospital, collected 10 days after incident (March 9, 1984)[1]	NM	Patient C1: 69 ng/mL Patient C2: 28 ng/mL Patient C5: 33 ng/mL Control: 11 ng/mL	NM	NM
Kurdish casualties, 2 individuals, treated at London hospital, collected 13 days after incident (March 17, 1988)[1]	NM	Patient L1: 11 ng/mL Patient L2: 11 ng/mL Control: 11 ng/mL	NM	NM
Accidental exposure to WWI munition, 2 individuals, collected 2–3 days after incident (1992)[2]	Patient S1: 2 ng/mL Patient S2: 2 ng/mL	Patient S1: 77 ng/mL Patient S2: 54 ng/mL Control: 4.5 ng/mL	Patient S1: 69 ng/mL Patient S2: 45 ng/mL Control: 5 ng/mL	NM
Accidental laboratory exposure, 1 individual, collected 2–14 days after incident (1990)[3]	Maximum excretion rate: 20 µg/day on day 3; concentration > 10 ng/mL for 1 week postexposure	NM	NM	NM
Accidental exposure to WWI munition, 2 individuals, collected 2–42 days after incident (July 19, 2004)[4]	Patient D1: 24, 9, 5, 14, 11, 6, 2, 2, 1.5, 1.2 ng/mL for days 2 to 11 after exposure, respectively	NM	NM	Patient D1: 50, 17, 11, 28, 24, 14, 4.5, 9, 5, 6 ng/mL for days 2 to 11 after exposure, respectively
	Patient D2: not detected days 2, 4, 7	NM	NM	Patient D2: 1.8, 3, 4.4 ng/mL for days 2, 4, 7, respectively

*These are the known details of the incident and sample collection time after suspected exposure.
†Assay measures TDG (free plus glucuronide-bound).
‡Assay measures free TDG, free TDG-sulfoxide, and acid-labile esters of both.
§Assay measures TDG (free plus bound), TDG-sulfoxide (free plus bound), and acid-labile esters of both.
NM: not measured
TDG: thiodiglycol
$TiCl_3$: titanium trichloride
WWI: World War I
Data sources: (1) Black RM, Read RW. Improved methodology for the detection and quantitation of urinary metabolites of sulphur mustard using gas chromatography-tandem mass spectrometry. *J Chromatogr B Biomed Appl*. 1995;665:97–105. (2) Black RM, Read RW. Biological fate of sulphur mustard, 1,1′-thiobis(2-chloroethane): identification of beta-lyase metabolites and hydrolysis products in human urine. *Xenobiotica*. 1995;25:167–173. (3) Jakubowski EM, Sidell FR, Evans RA, et al. Quantification of thiodiglycol in human urine after an accidental sulfur mustard exposure. *Toxicol Methods*. 2000;10:143–150. (4) Barr JR, Young CL, Woolfit AR, et al. Comprehensive quantitative tandem MS analysis of urinary metabolites and albumin adducts following an accidental human exposure to sulfur mustard. In: *Proceedings of the 53rd Conference of the American Society of Mass Spectrometry*. San Antonio, Tex: June 5–9, 2005.

TABLE 22-11

PUBLISHED REPORTS (1995–2006) OF LABORATORY ANALYSIS OF HUMAN URINE SAMPLES FOR GLUTATHIONE REACTION PRODUCTS FOLLOWING A SUSPECTED EXPOSURE TO SULFUR MUSTARD

Patient Sample Information*	β-lyase Metabolites†	β-lyase Metabolites‡	Bis-(N-acetylcysteine) Conjugate§
Iranian casualties, 5 of 5 individuals. treated at Ghent hospital, collected 10 days after incident (March 9, 1984)[1]	Patient C1: 220 ng/mL Patient C2: 0.5 ng/mL Patient C3: 1 ng/mL Patient C4: 5 ng/mL Patient C5: 1 ng/mL	NM	NM
Kurdish casualties, 2 individuals, treated at London hospital, collected 13 days after incident (March 17, 1988)[1,2]	Patient L1: 0.1 ng/mL Patient L2: 0.3 ng/mL	Patient L1: MSMTESE = <0.1 ng/mL, SBMSE = ~ 0.1 ng/mL Patient L2: MSMTESE = 0.1 ng/mL, SBMSE = ~ 0.2 ng/mL	NM
Accidental exposure to WWI munition, 2 individuals, collected 2–3 days after incident (1992)[2,3,4]	Patient S1: 42 ng/mL Patient S2: 56 ng/mL	Patient S1: MSMTESE = 15 ng/mL, SBMSE = 30 ng/mL Patient S2: MSMTESE = 17 ng/mL, SBMSE = 34 ng/mL	Patient S1: 1 ng/mL Patient S2: 1 ng/mL
Accidental exposure to WWI munition, 2 individuals, collected 2–42 days after incident (July 19, 2004)[5]	Patient D1: 41, 7, 3.3, 1.3 ng/mL for days 2–5 after exposure, respectively; 0.07–0.02 ng/mL for days 6–11 after exposure Patient D2: 2.6, 0.8, 0.08 ng/mL for days 2, 4, 7, respectively	NM	Patient D1: 3.1 ng/mL

*This information includes known incident information and sample collection time after suspected exposure.
†Using GC-MS-MS analysis
‡Using LC-MS-MS analysis
§Using LC-MS-MS analysis
GC: gas chromatography
LC: liquid chromatography
MS: mass spectrometry
MSMTESE: 1-methylsulfinyl-2-[2-(methylthio)ethylsulfonyl]ethane
NM: not measured
SBMSE: 1,1′-sulfonylbis[2-(methylsulfinyl)ethane]
Data sources: (1) Black RM, Read RW. Improved methodology for the detection and quantitation of urinary metabolites of sulphur mustard using gas chromatography-tandem mass spectrometry. *J Chromatogr B Biomed Appl*. 1995;665:97–105. (2) Read RW, Black RM. Analysis of beta-lyase metabolites of sulfur mustard in urine by electrospray liquid chromatography-tandem mass spectrometry. *J Anal Toxicol.* 2004;28:346–351. (3) Black RM, Read RW. Biological fate of sulphur mustard, 1,1′-thiobis(2-chloroethane): identification of beta-lyase metabolites and hydrolysis products in human urine. *Xenobiotica*. 1995;25:167–173. (4) Read RW, Black RM. Analysis of the sulfur mustard metabolite 1,1′-sulfonylbis[2-S-(N-acetylcysteinyl)ethane] in urine by negative ion electrospray liquid chromatography-tandem mass spectrometry. *J Anal Toxicol.* 2004;28:352–356. (5) Barr JR, Young CL, Woolfit AR, et al. Comprehensive quantitative tandem MS analysis of urinary metabolites and albumin adducts following an accidental human exposure to sulfur mustard. In: *Proceedings of the 53rd Conference of the American Society of Mass Spectrometry*. San Antonio, Tex: June 5–9, 2005.

lowing isolation of the albumin from the blood, the albumin can be reacted with pronase enzyme to digest protein. One of the resulting peptide fragments is a tripeptide of the sequence cysteine-proline-phenylalanine, which contains the sulfur-mustard–alkylated cysteine-34. After solid phase extraction, the tripeptide was analyzed using LC-MS-MS.[115] The lower limit of detection for the assay (1 nM) was once again reported as an equivalent exposure level, as determined using in-vitro exposures to sulfur mustard in human whole blood. Recently, a modification to the isolation of the albumin from blood was reported using affinity chro-

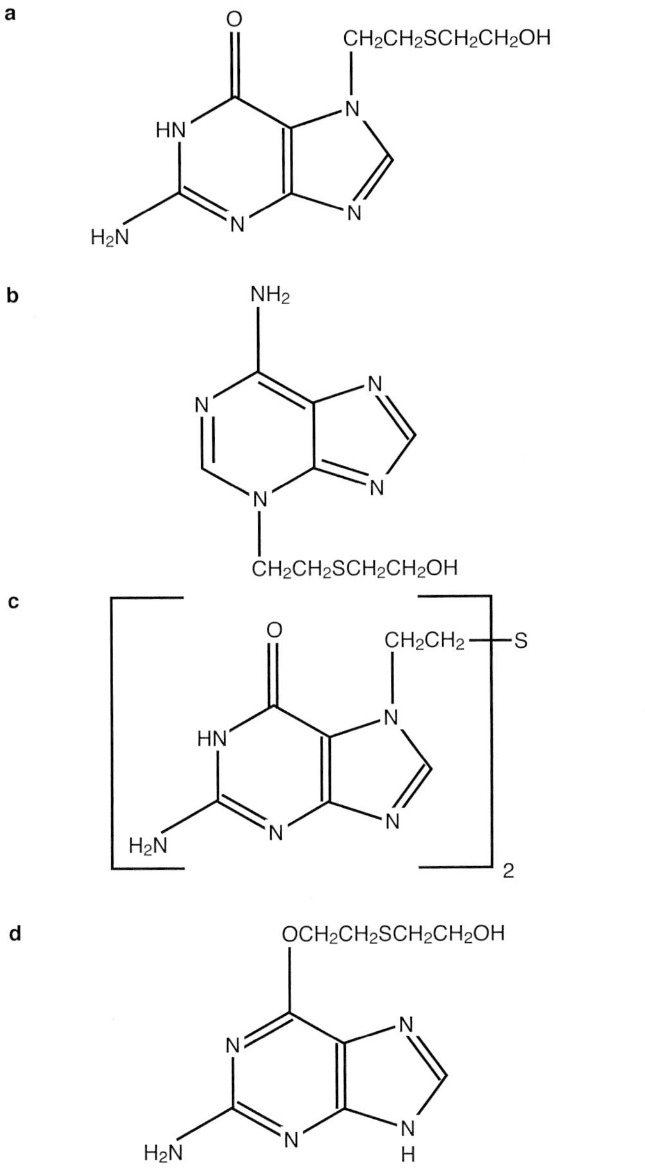

Fig. 22-9. Deoxyribonucleic acid adducts resulting from reaction with sulfur mustard. **(a)** N7-HETE-guanine. **(b)** N3-HETE-adenine. **(c)** Bis[2-(guanin-7-yl)ethyl]sulfide. **(d)** O^6-HETE-guanine.

matography rather than the precipitation procedure.[116] The modified procedure significantly reduced the sample preparation time.

The final method for analyzing blood samples to be discussed targets blood proteins in a more general approach. It was previously shown that sulfur mustard adducts of glutamic and aspartic acids to keratin could be cleaved using base.[117] Using a similar approach, precipitated proteins from plasma, whole blood, or RBCs were treated with base to liberate the sulfur mustard adduct, hydroxyethylthioethyl, from the protein. Upon release, the adduct (in the form of TDG) was derivatized and analyzed using negative-ion chemical ionization GC-MS (Figure 22-11; see Exhibit 22-3). The lower limit of detection for the assay in plasma was 25 nM, as determined using in-vitro exposures of sulfur mustard in human plasma.[118]

The limits of detection or equivalent levels of exposure to sulfur mustard reported for most of the blood assays are based on in-vitro exposures of whole blood or plasma. Quantitation of patient samples report the amount of sulfur mustard adducts that are found in the samples relative to the amount of adducts that are found from in-vitro exposures of whole blood or plasma at various known concentrations of sulfur mustard. Choosing whole blood over plasma to generate the in-vitro standard curves produces very different results because sulfur mustard readily reacts with hemoglobin. Additionally, the technique used for generating in-vitro standards can have significant effects. For example, approximately a 30% difference was observed for the generation of two in-vitro standard curves, depending on how the sulfur mustard was incubated in blood.[119] Higher adduct levels were observed when the sulfur mustard was allowed to react with the blood for 2 hours at 37°C, as opposed to 4 hours at room temperature.

Application to Human Exposure

Blood samples following a suspected human exposure to sulfur mustard rarely become available for laboratory analysis. Three of the five known reports involve the analysis of samples that were taken from casualties of the Iran-Iraq War, frozen for several years, then reanalyzed to verify exposure as new methods were developed. The other two published reports are on the analysis of blood samples obtained from three individuals who were casualties of accidental exposures to World War I munitions.

The blood from two Iranian casualties who were believed to have been exposed to sulfur mustard in 1988 was analyzed using both the ELISA method for DNA adducts and the GC-MS method for the analysis of the N-terminal valine of hemoglobin.[120] Samples were collected 22 and 26 days following the suspected exposure. One of the casualties had skin injuries that were consistent with an exposure to sulfur mustard, but the second casualty had injuries that were described as only "vaguely compatible" with sulfur mustard exposure. Both individuals had approximately the same level of hemoglobin valine adduct, equivalent to the amount observed from a 900-nM, in-vitro, sulfur mustard exposure in whole blood. ELISA DNA adduct levels observed in the granulocytes were also similar

EXHIBIT 22-2

SAMPLE PREPARATION PROCEDURE FOR SULFUR MUSTARD ADDUCTS TO DEOXYRIBONUCLEIC ACID IN BLOOD

Procedure of van der Schans et al for immunuslotblot analysis:

- Collect blood specimen in vacutube containing EDTA.
- Isolate and denature DNA using following procedure:
  - Transfer 0.3 mL of blood to Eppendorf tube.
  - Add RBC lysis solution, mix, and centrifuge.
  - Lyse pelleted WBCs with cell lysis solution containing proteinase K.
  - Shake solution for 1 hour.
  - Treat solution with RNAse.
  - Add protein precipitation solution, mix, and centrifuge.
  - Transfer supernatant to tube containing isopropanol and centrifuge.
  - Wash pellet with 70% ethanol, centrifuge, and air dry.
  - Dissolve pellet overnight in Tris buffer containing HCl and EDTA.
  - Determine DNA concentration using UV-VIS spectrometer.
  - Prepare DNA solution with formamide, formaldehyde, and Tris buffer.
  - Incubate solution at 52°C.
  - Cool rapidly on ice and store at – 20°C.
- Immunuslotblot assay procedure:
  - Dilute denatured DNA samples in PBS.
  - Spot DNA solution onto nitrocellulose filter.
  - Wash spotted sample with PBS and air-dry filter.
  - Cross-link DNA to filter using UV-gene-cross-linker.
  - Incubate filter with blocking solution.
  - Wash with PBS/Tween solution.
  - Incubate filter overnight with monoclonal antibodies that recognize N7-(2-hydroxyethylthioethyl)-2′-deoxyguanosine at 4°C with continuous shaking.
  - Wash with PBS/Tween solution.
  - Incubate filter with rabbit-anti-mouse-Ig-horseradish peroxidase antibody for 2 hours at room temperature with shaking.
  - Wash with PBS/Tween solution.
  - Blot dry filter and transfer into a luminometer cassette.
  - Measure luminescence.

DNA: deoxyribonucleic acid
EDTA: ethylenediaminetetraacetic acid
HCl: hydrochloric acid
Ig: immunoglobulin
PBS: phosphate-buffered saline
RBC: red blood cell
RNAse: ribonuclease
Tris: trishydroxymethylaminomethane
UV-VIS: ultraviolet-visible spectrophotometry
WBC: white blood cell
Data source: (1) Van der Schans GP, Mars-Groenendijk R, de Jong LP, Benschop HP, Noort D. Standard operating procedure for immunoslotblot assay for analysis of DNA/sulfur mustard adducts in human blood and skin. *J Anal Toxicol.* 2004;28:316–319.

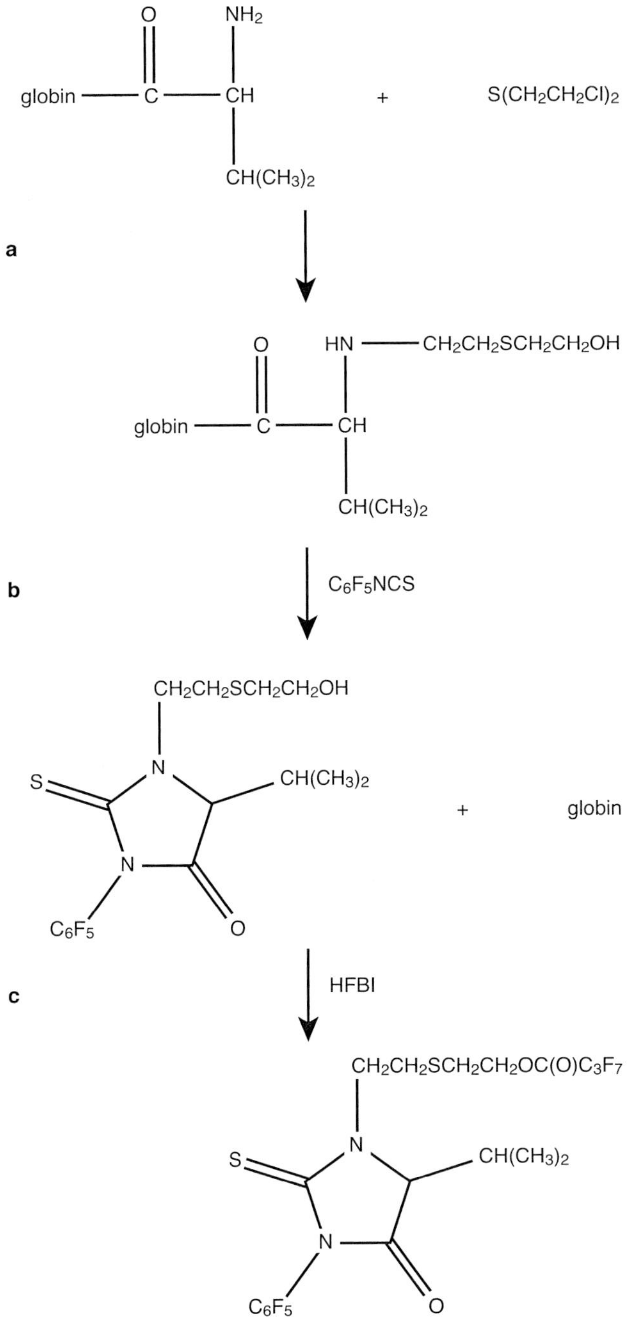

Fig. 22-10. Analytical method of Fidder et al (1996) for blood exposed to sulfur mustard. **(a)** Reaction of N-terminal valine of globin with sulfur mustard. **(b)** Modified Edman degradation of N-terminal valine-sulfur mustard adduct. **(c)** Derivatization using HFBI.
HFBI: heptafluorobutyryl imidazole
Data source: Fidder A, Noort D, de Jong AL, Trap HC, de Jong LPA, Benschop HP. Monitoring of in vitro and in vivo exposure to sulfur mustard by GC/MS determination of the N-terminal valine adduct in hemoglobin after a modified Edman degradation. *Chem Res Toxicol.* 1996;9:788–792.

for both individuals, 150 to 160 nM. The individual with the skin injuries consistent with sulfur mustard exposure had observed ELISA DNA adduct levels in the lymphocytes that were only about half that observed in the individual with injuries that were less pronounced: 220 nM and 430 nM, respectively.

Blood samples obtained in 1986 from a group of Iranian casualties that were treated at a hospital in Ghent for injuries believed to have been caused by sulfur mustard were examined years later using MS methods by Black et al for both valine and histidine adducts of hemoglobin.[114] The four individuals had blood samples collected at 5 or 10 days following the suspected exposure event. Levels of the valine adduct ranged between 0.3 and 0.8 ng/mL. Observed levels of the histidine adduct were greater than the amount of valine adduct and ranged between 0.7 and 2.5 ng/mL. Using the same methods, Black et al also examined blood from one of the two individuals who were accidentally exposed to a World War I sulfur mustard munition.[114] Several urinary metabolites were detected in specimens from this individual, indicating exposure to sulfur mustard (see above). In a blood sample obtained 2 days after the exposure, the valine and histidine hemoglobin adduct levels were 0.3 ng/mL and 2.5 ng/mL, respectively.

Blood samples obtained from nine Iranian casualties of sulfur mustard exposure were analyzed for the N-terminal valine adduct of hemoglobin using GC-MS[121] and for the albumin cysteine adduct using LC-MS-MS.[115] All nine individuals were hospitalized and had skin changes consistent with sulfur mustard exposure. Several of the casualties also had respiratory difficulties. Blood samples were collected between 8 and 9 days after the exposure incident. Exposure levels of the patient blood samples were correlated with human whole blood that was exposed to sulfur mustard in vitro. Adduct levels for both the hemoglobin valine adduct and for the albumin cysteine adduct were in very close agreement with each other. Observed exposure levels were between 0.3 and 2 μm and 0.4 and 1.8 μm for the hemoglobin and albumin adducts, respectively.

The final exposure incident to be discussed involved the two individuals who were accidentally exposed to a World War I munition in 2004. Details of the exposure were given earlier in the urine section. This particular human exposure to sulfur mustard differed from nearly all other previously reported incidents in several important aspects. The two individuals are only the second and third casualties of sulfur mustard exposure to have both urine and blood samples made available for laboratory testing. Generally, urine or

EXHIBIT 22-3

SAMPLE PREPARATION METHODS FOR THE GAS CHROMATOGRAPHIC-MASS SPECTROMETRIC ANALYSIS OF SULFUR MUSTARD ADDUCTS TO BLOOD BIOMOLECULES

Procedure of Fidder et al for sulfur mustard adduct to N-terminal valine of hemoglobin*:

- Isolate globin from blood using following procedure:
  - Centrifuge blood and remove plasma layer.
  - Wash RBCs with saline solution.
  - Lyse RBCs with water and place solution into ice water bath.
  - Centrifuge and transfer supernatant into tube containing HCl/acetone.
  - Wash the precipitate with HCl/acetone, acetone, and ether.
  - Dry precipitate.
- Mix isolated globin from blood sample with internal standard (globin isolated from blood that was previously exposed to deuterated sulfur mustard).
- Dissolve globin in formamide.
- Add pyridine and pentafluorophenyl isothiocyanate to solution.
- Incubate solution at 60°C for 2 hours.
- Add toluene, mix, centrifuge, and freeze samples in liquid nitrogen.
- Remove toluene layer and wash with water, aqueous Na_2CO_3, and water.
- Dry toluene with $MgSO_4$, evaporate to dryness, and dissolve in toluene.
- Filter solution through a preconditioned Florisil solid phase extraction cartridge.
- Wash cartridge with dichloromethane.
- Elute with methanol/dichloromethane.
- Evaporate to dryness and dissolve in toluene.
- Add heptafluorobutyryl imidazole and heat solution.
- After cooling, wash with water, aqueous Na_2CO_3, and water.
- Dry toluene with $MgSO_4$ and concentrate solution.
- Analyze using GC-MS with methane negative ion chemical ionization.[1]

Procedure of Capacio et al for sulfur mustard adducts to aspartic and glutamic acid residues of blood proteins:

- Precipitate blood proteins:
  - For plasma samples, use acetone.
  - For whole blood or RBCs, use HCl/acetone.
- Centrifuge solution and discard supernatant.
- Wash protein pellet with acetone and ether.
- Centrifuge solution and discard supernatant.
- Dry protein at room temperature.
- Add dried protein to NaOH solution.
- Heat solution at 70°C for 1.5 hours.
- Neutralize solution with HCl and dry with sodium sulfate.
- Add ethyl acetate, mix, and remove ethyl acetate layer.
- Add internal standard (deuterated thiodiglycol) to ethyl acetate and dry with sodium sulfate.
- Add pyridine and pentafluorobenzoyl chloride.
- After 10 minutes, add water and sodium bicarbonate.
- Remove ethyl acetate layer and dry with sodium sulfate.
- Pass ethyl acetate through a preconditioned silica solid-phase–extraction cartridge and collect the filtered solution.
- Pass additional ethyl acetate through cartridge, collect, and combine the two fractions.
- Analyze using GC-MS with methane negative ion chemical ionization.[2]

(Exhibit 22-3 *continues***)**

Exhibit 22-3 *continued*

*The lower limit of detection for the assay was determined using in vitro exposures of sulfur mustard in human whole blood and was determined to be equivalent to a 100 nM exposure level.[1,3] Following the administration of a single dose of sulfur mustard to a marmoset (4.1 mg/kg; intravenous), the valine adduct was still detected in blood taken 94 days later.[4] Intact hemoglobin with the sulfur mustard adducts attached have been examined using matrix-assisted laser desorption/ionization time-of-flight mass spectrometry, but to date the technique has only been utilized for in vitro experiments at relatively high concentrations of sulfur mustard.[5]

GC: gas chromatography

HCl: hydrochloric acid

MS: mass spectrometry

RBC: red blood cell

Data sources: (1) Fidder A, Noort D, de Jong AL, Trap HC, de Jong LPA, Benschop HP. Monitoring of in vitro and in vivo exposure to sulfur mustard by GC/MS determination of the N-terminal valine adduct in hemoglobin after a modified Edman degradation. *Chem Res Toxicol.* 1996;9:788–792. (2) Capacio BR, Smith JR, DeLion MT, et al. Monitoring sulfur mustard exposure by gas chromatography-mass spectrometry analysis of thiodiglycol cleaved from blood proteins. *J Anal Toxicol.* 2004;28:306–310. (3) Noort D, Fidder A, Benschop HP, de Jong LP, Smith JR. Procedure for monitoring exposure to sulfur mustard based on modified edman degradation of globin. *J Anal Toxicol.* 2004;28:311–315. (4) Noort D, Benschop HP, Black RM. Biomonitoring of exposure to chemical warfare agents: a review. *Tox Appl Pharmacol.* 2002;184:116–126. (5) Price EO, Smith JR, Clark CR, Schlager JJ, Shih ML. MALDI-ToF/MS as a diagnostic tool for the confirmation sulfur mustard exposure. *J Appl Toxicol.* 2000;20(suppl 1):S193–S197.

blood samples that are collected and made available for verifying sulfur mustard exposure are from a single time point after the exposure. In this instance, the patient with more severe injuries (patient D1, see above) had blood and urine collected almost daily for the first 10 days after exposure and then again on days 29, 35, and 42. The incident also provided an opportunity to examine blood and urine metabolite levels from individuals with very different levels of injury. Patient D1 had extensive vesication of the arm and leg, while patient D2 developed only a single small blister. (The urinary metabolite results were detailed earlier in this section.) As expected, the observed concentrations of both urine hydrolysis metabolites and GSH reaction products were much greater in patient D1. Sulfur mustard metabolite concentrations in the blood were also much greater in patient D1. Blood metabolites were assayed using two different methods. The first assay targeted the sulfur mustard adduct to cysteine-34 of albumin using pronase digestion of the protein followed by LC-MS-MS analysis.[116] Based on in-vitro exposures to sulfur mustard in human whole blood, concentrations of albumin adducts found in the plasma of patient D1 were 350 nM on day 2 after the exposure and had decreased by 74% (90 nM) on day 42.[105] The rate of decrease over that time was consistent with the reported half-life of human albumin of 21 days. Albumin adduct concentrations for patient D2 over the sample collection period of 2 to 7 days after exposure remained stable and ranged between 16 and 18 nM. The second assay targeted plasma protein adducts by cleaving the adduct with base, followed by analyzing the derivatized adduct using negative ion chemical ionization GC-MS.[118] This was the first reported use of this assay in the verification of a human exposure to sulfur mustard. Concentrations of the plasma protein adducts were 97 nM on day 2 and decreased by 76% (23 nM) by day 42, based on in-vitro exposures to sulfur mustard in human plasma instead of whole blood.[122] The assay could not detect plasma protein adducts in patient D2. The assay was modified slightly to lower the reported lower limit of detection of 25 nM, but the limited amount of plasma received did not permit

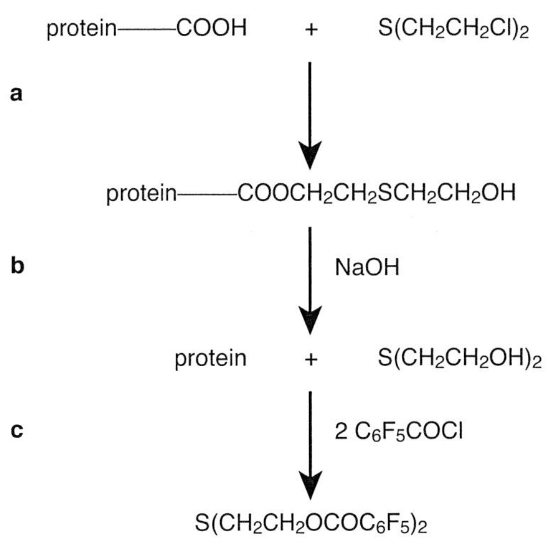

Fig. 22-11. Analytical approach of Capacio et al. **(a)** Reaction of protein carboxylic acid groups with sulfur mustard. **(b)** Hydrolysis of the ester groups to release thiodiglycol. **(c)** Derivatization of thiodiglycol using pentafluorobenzoyl chloride.

Data source: Capacio BR, Smith JR, DeLion MT, et al. Monitoring sulfur mustard exposure by gas chromatography-mass spectrometry analysis of thiodiglycol cleaved from blood proteins. *J Anal Toxicol.* 2004;28:306–310.

reanalysis for patient D2 using the modified method.

Blood provides several options for assessing potential exposure to sulfur mustard because a variety of different metabolites have been verified in human exposure cases. Most of the assays are sensitive and selective, and the majority of the methods use gas or LC combined with MS. Background levels have not been found in the blood from unexposed individuals. The time period between exposure and sample collection and the severity of the injury are probably the most important factors to consider when selecting the appropriate assay. Currently the most sensitive assay targets the alkylated cysteine of albumin, but alkylated hemoglobin should offer a biomarker of greater longevity (Table 22-12).

Analysis of Other Biomedical Sample Types (Tissue, Hair, Skin, Blister Fluid)

Urine and blood have been the traditional biomedical samples used to test for exposure to sulfur mustard; there are few reports on the analysis of other types of biomedical samples. Using the same method described in the urine methods section, Drasch et al analyzed several tissue types obtained from an autopsy for unmetabolized sulfur mustard.[85] An Iranian soldier, age 24, died of complications of pneumonia 7 days after a suspected exposure to sulfur mustard. The patient had been transferred to an intensive care unit in Munich, Germany for treatment. Tissue samples were taken during the autopsy, stored at – 20°C for 1 year, and then analyzed for unmetabolized sulfur mustard. Sulfur mustard was found in the highest concentrations in the victim's fat, skin, brain, and kidney; concentrations ranged from 5 to 15 mg/kg. Lesser amounts were found in the patient's muscle, liver, spleen, and lung and ranged from approximately 1 to 2 mg/kg.[85]

Hair specimens have been analyzed for unmetabolized sulfur mustard using a methylene chloride extraction followed by analysis with GC-MS.[123] Hair samples that were obtained from two casualties of the Iran-Iraq War in 1986 were analyzed for unmetabolized sulfur mustard.[123] The two casualties were examined by a United Nations inspection team as part of an "alleged use" investigation initiated at Iran's request. The clinical history of the patients was consistent with sulfur mustard exposure. Additionally, analysis of vapor and soil samples from the bomb site tested positive for sulfur mustard. The inspection team was presented with hair samples from two individuals that were reportedly exposed the previous day. The hair specimens were sent to the National Defence Research Institute of Sweden for analysis. One of the hair samples produced a positive response for sulfur mustard estimated to be between 0.5 and 1.0 μg/g. The second patient's hair sample tested negative for sulfur mustard.[123]

Using the urine testing method to measure TDG levels, Wils et al assayed pieces of skin that were taken from sulfur mustard casualties treated in the Ghent hospital. They found concentrations of TDG in the range of 2 to 7 μg/g in the skin samples.[84] Immunochemical detection assays for sulfur mustard adducts in human skin have been developed for keratin[124] and DNA.[108] To date, the assays have not been used on skin samples following a suspected human exposure to sulfur mustard.

Fluid removed from blisters resulting from sulfur mustard exposure has also been analyzed from two casualties. Jakubowski et al obtained a small amount of blister fluid from an accidental laboratory exposure that was detailed in the urine section above. The blister fluid was injected directly into a GC-MS for analysis. Neither unmetabolized sulfur mustard nor TDG were observed in the blister fluid, but a polymer of TDG appeared to be present.[102] The most recently reported exposure also generated blister fluid samples that were made available for analysis (see Figure 22-8). Korte et al examined blister fluid that was obtained on days 2 and 7 after exposure for both free TDG and protein-bound adducts of sulfur mustard.[122] Free TDG concentrations were 19 ng/mL and 24 ng/mL for days 2 and 7, respectively. The protein-bound adducts were measured using the same method used for plasma protein adducts.[118] The observed levels were 63 and 73 pg/mg of protein for days 2 and 7, respectively. Blister fluid from day 7 was also assayed with the albumin tripeptide LC-MS-MS method[116] previously used for plasma samples from the same individual. The concentration of the alkylated tripeptide reported using this assay was similar to the plasma concentration found for the same day.[105]

Since 1995 there has been a significant increase in the reported number of laboratory methods for verifying human exposure to sulfur mustard. Sensitivity to the analytical methods continues to improve and a number of new biomarkers have been identified and verified in biomedical samples from exposed individuals. These advances have helped verify even low doses of sulfur mustard exposure and have extended the time period from exposure event to collection. The major drawback to the current laboratory methodologies is that they require expensive instrumentation, highly trained personnel, and analytical standards that are generally not commercially available. Consequently, the time interval from sample collection, transport to an appropriate laboratory, sample preparation, instrument configuration,

TABLE 22-12

PUBLISHED REPORTS (1997–2006) OF LABORATORY ANALYSIS OF HUMAN BLOOD SAMPLES FOLLOWING SUSPECTED EXPOSURE TO SULFUR MUSTARD

Patient Sample Information*	DNA Adduct†	Hemoglobin Adduct‡	Hemoglobin Adduct§	Albumin Adduct¥	Blood Protein Adducts¶
Iranian casualties, 2 individuals, collected 22 days (Patient 1) & 26 days (Patient 2) after incident (1988)[1]	Patient 1: lymphocytes = 220 nM, granulocytes = 160 nM Patient 2: lymphocytes = 430 nM, granulocytes = 150 nM	Patient 1: 900 nM Patient 2: 900 nM	NM	NM	NM
Iranian casualties, 4 individuals, treated at Ghent hospital; collected 5 & 10 days after incident (1986)[2]	NM	Range: 0.3–0.8 ng/mL	Range: 0.7–2.5 ng/mL	NM	NM
Accidental exposure to WWI munition; 1 individual, collected 2 days after incident (1992)[2]	NM	0.3 ng/mL	2.5 ng/mL	NM	NM
Iranian casualties, 9 individuals, treated at Utrecht hospital; collected 8–9 days after incident (1986)[3,4]	NM	Range: 0.3–2 μM	NM	Range: 0.4–1.8 μM	NM
Accidental exposure to WWI munition; 2 individuals, collected 2–42 days after incident (2004)[5,6]	NM	NM	NM	Patient D1: 350 and 90 nM for days 2 & 42 after exposure respectively; Patient D2: 16–18 nM for days 2, 4, 7 after exposure	Patient D1: 97 and 23 nM for days 2 & 42 after exposure, respectively

*This information includes known incident information and sample collection time after suspected exposure.
†N7-(2-HETE)-2′-deoxyguanosine
‡(HETE)-N-terminal valine
§(HETE)-histidine
¥S-[2-(HETE)]-Cys-Pro-Phe
¶(HETE)-aspartic & glutamic acids
DNA: deoxyribonucleic acid
HETE: hydroxyethylthioethyl
NM: not measured

Data sources: (1) Benschop HP, van der Schans GP, Noort D, Fidder A, Mars-Groenendijk RH, de Jong LP. Verification of exposure to sulfur mustard in two casualties of the Iran-Iraq conflict. *J Anal Toxicol.* 1997;21:249–251. (2) Black RM, Clarke RJ, Harrison JM, Read RW. Biological fate of sulphur mustard: identification of valine and histidine adducts in haemoglobin from casualties of sulphur mustard poisoning. *Xenobiotica.* 1997;27:499–512. (3) Noort D, Hulst AG, de Jong LP, Benschop HP. Alkylation of human serum albumin by sulfur mustard in vitro and in vivo: mass spectrometric analysis of a cysteine adduct as a sensitive biomarker of exposure. *Chem Res Toxicol.* 1999;12:715–721. (4) Benschop HP, Noort D, van der Schans GP, de Jong LP. Diagnosis and dosimetry of exposure to sulfur mustard: development of standard operating procedures; further exploratory research on protein adducts. Rijswijk, The Netherlands: TNO Prins Maurits Laboratory. Final report DAMD17-97-2-7002, ADA381035, 2000. (5) Barr JR, Young CL, Woolfit AR, et al. Comprehensive quantitative tandem MS analysis of urinary metabolites and albumin adducts following an accidental human exposure to sulfur mustard. In: *Proceedings of the 53rd Conference of the American Society of Mass Spectrometry.* San Antonio, Tex: June 5–9, 2005. (6) Korte WD, Walker EM, Smith JR, et al. The determination of sulfur mustard exposure by analysis of blood protein adducts. *Wehrmed Mschr.* 2005;49:327.

and finally an analytical result is long. Because exposure to sulfur mustard can occur without overt or immediate clinical signs and the onset of symptoms can be delayed for many hours, there is interest in developing diagnostic methods for the field and patient care areas. Ongoing research in the use of immunochemical assays is one area in particular that offers hope for a field-forward assay.

LEWISITE

Background

Lewisite is an arsenical vesicant with a small molecular weight primarily found in the trans isomeric form, although it also exists in cis and geminal forms.[125] Stockpiles of lewisite or lewisite mixed with sulfur mustard reportedly exist in a number of countries and present a potential risk for accidental exposure. Most analytical methods that have been reported in the public scientific literature regarding lewisite or related compounds are for the sample preparation and analysis of environmental samples. In the past 10 years, there have only been a handful of reports regarding the analysis of biomedical samples to confirm lewisite exposure. Much like the other chemical warfare agents, lewisite is readily hydrolyzed in aqueous solutions, including biological fluids. Therefore, the likelihood of finding the parent compound in a biomedical sample, such as blood or urine, is minimal. Consequently, method development has focused on the breakdown compounds of lewisite or on products formed from its interaction with biomolecules. Until recently, most assays for lewisite have involved analyzing elemental arsenic using techniques such as atomic absorption spectroscopy. A drawback of this approach is that it lacks specificity because arsenic is ubiquitous in the environment. In addition to naturally occurring sources, arsenic is also found in some commercial products and food items (particularly marine organisms). Arsenic is also a by-product of several industrial processes.

Analysis of Urine and Blood Samples

Lewisite rapidly reacts with water to form chlorovinylarsonous acid (CVAA). CVAA slowly converts to the arsinoxide form and polymerization reactions can occur. Earlier studies indicated that animals (species not specified) exposed to lewisite either topically or via injection were found to have measurable levels of CVAA in their urine and throughout their digestive systems.[126]

Specific biomarkers of lewisite exposure are currently based on a limited number of in-vitro[127,128] and animal studies.[129,130] Wooten et al developed a solid phase microextraction headspace sampling method for urine samples, followed by GC-MS analysis.[128] It is the most sensitive method reported to date, with a lower limit of detection of 7.4 pg/mL. Animal experiments have been limited in number and scope. In one study of four animals, guinea pigs were given a subcutaneous dose of lewisite (0.5 mg/kg). Urine samples were analyzed for CVAA using both GC-MS and GC coupled with an atomic emission spectrometer set for elemental arsenic.[129] The excretion profile indicated a very rapid elimination of CVAA in the urine. The mean concentrations detected were 3.5 μg/mL, 250 ng/mL, and 50 ng/mL for the 0- to 8-hour, 8- to 16-hour, and 16- to 24-hour samples, respectively. Trace level concentrations (0–10 ng/mL) of CVAA were detected in the urine of the 24- to 32-hour and 32- to 40-hour samples. The second animal study also used a subcutaneous dose of lewisite (0.25 mg/kg) given to four guinea pigs.[130] Using GC-MS, CVAA was detected in urine samples up to 12 hours following exposure. In the same experiment, blood from the animals was also analyzed using GC-MS to detect CVAA. The amount of measured CVAA was the sum of CVAA that was displaced from hemoglobin along with free CVAA in the blood. The assay was able to detect the analyte at 10 days after the exposure, although the concentration was only 10% of that found 24 hours after exposure. Following the incubation of human blood with radiolabeled lewisite, Fidder et al found that 90% of the radioactivity was associated with the RBCs, and 25% to 50% was found with the globin.[130] Because of CVAA's reactive nature, derivatization using a thiol compound has generally been applied as part of the sample preparation process (Figure 22-12, Exhibit 22-4).

Application to Human Exposure

There are currently no reports of the collection of biomedical samples from individuals with suspected lewisite exposure. Samples from such incidents are critical to confirm the validity of assaying for the biomarkers observed in animal models. Additionally, the biomarkers that have been investigated in animal studies have indicated a rapid clearance of those biomarkers in urine and less so for blood.[130] This creates problems for the retrospective determination of lewisite exposure beyond a few days when analyzing

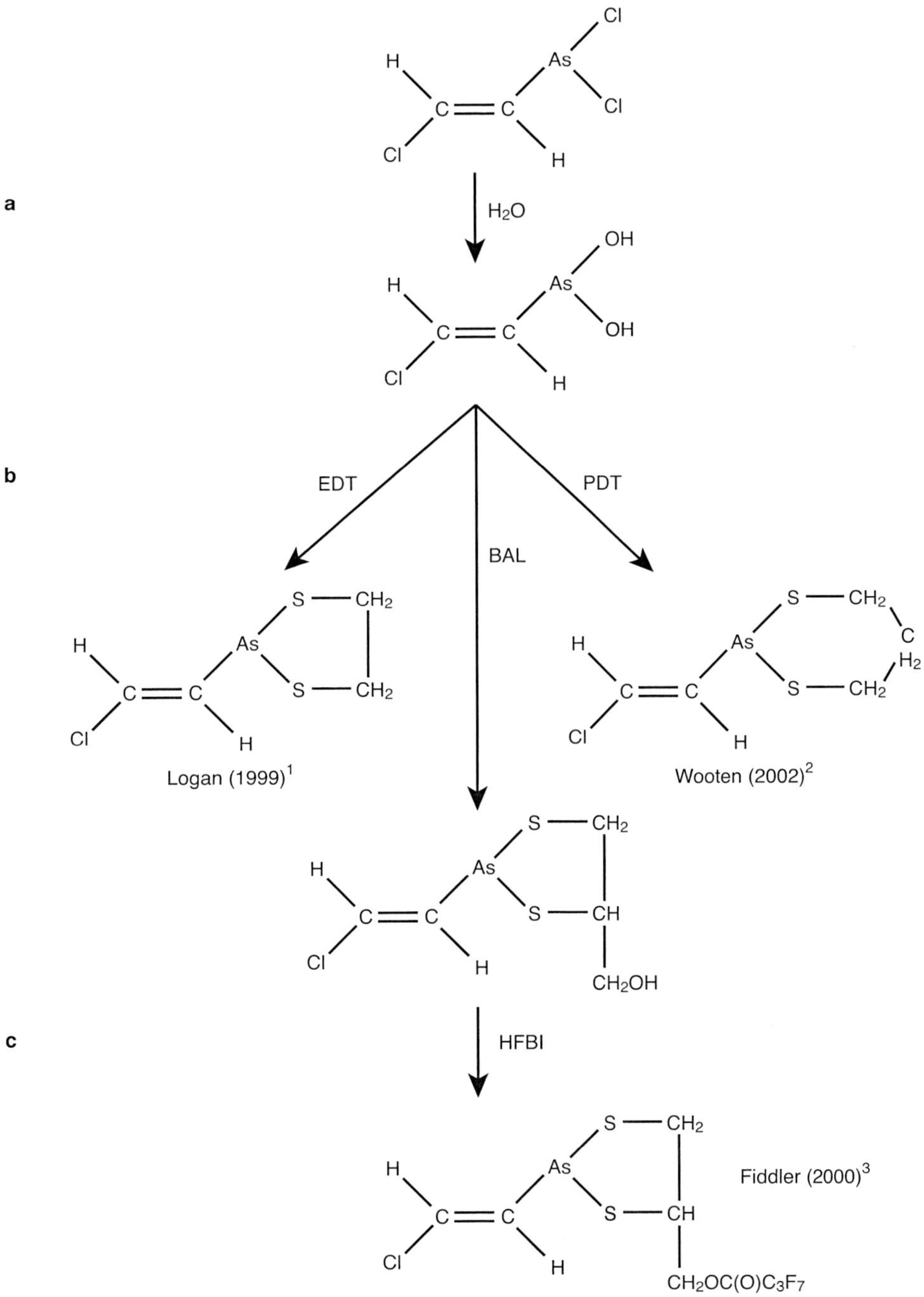

Fig. 22-12. Published analytical approaches for the analysis of chlorovinylarsonous acid in urine. **(a)** Reaction of lewisite (trans isomer shown) with water to form chlorovinylarsonous acid. **(b)** Reactions of chlorovinylarsonous acid with thiol compounds ethanedithiol, propanedithiol, and British anti-Lewisite.[1,2,3] **(c)** Derivatization using HFBI.[3]
BAL: British anti-Lewisite
EDT: ethanedithiol
H_2O: dihydrogen monoxide; water
HFBI: heptafluorobutyryl imidazole
PDT: propanedithiol
Data sources: (1) Logan TP, Smith JR, Jakubowski EM, Nielson RE. Verification of lewisite exposure by the analysis of 2-chlorovinyl arsonous acid in urine. *Toxicol Meth.* 1999;9:275–284. (2) Wooten JV, Ashley DL, Calafat AM. Quantitation of 2-chlorovinylarsonous acid in human urine by automated solid-phase microextraction-gas chromatography-mass spectrometry. *J Chromatogr B Analyt Technol Biomed Life Sci.* 2002;772:147–153. (3) Fidder A, Noort D, Hulst AG, de Jong LP, Benschop HP. Biomonitoring of exposure to lewisite based on adducts to haemoglobin. *Arch Toxicol.* 2000;74:207–214.

EXHIBIT 22-4

SAMPLE PREPARATION METHODS FOR GAS CHROMATOGRAPHIC/MASS SPECTROMETRIC ANALYSIS OF CHLOROVINYLARSONOUS ACID

SPE procedure of Logan et al for CVAA in urine:

- Precondition a C18 SPE cartridge with methanol followed by water.
- Adjust pH of 1 mL of urine to pH 6 using HCl.
- Add PAO as an internal standard.
- Transfer sample to C18 SPE cartridge for sample cleanup/extraction.
- Elute analytes using methanol.
- Evaporate to dryness under nitrogen.
- Reconstitute with ethanol containing EDT.
- Analyze using GC-MS with EI ionization.[1]

SPME headspace procedure of Wooten et al for CVAA in urine:

- Place 1 mL of urine into a 10-mL vial.
- Add ammonium acetate buffer-water solution.
- Add PAO as an internal standard.
- Add PDT in order to derivatize CVAA and PAO.
- Crimp-seal vial and heat at 70°C for 20 min.
- Insert a 100-μM poly(dimethylsiloxane) SPME fiber into the sample vial headspace for 10 min.
- Remove the SPME fiber from the vial and insert into the injection port of a GC-MS with EI ionization.[2]

SPE procedure of Fidder et al for free and bound CVAA in blood:

- Add 2,3-dimercapto-1-propanol (BAL) to a 2-mL blood sample. The BAL causes displacement of bound CVAA and derivatizes both the free and released CVAA.
- Add phenylarsine-BAL as an internal standard.
- Shake the sample at room temperature overnight.
- Dilute the sample with water.
- Transfer sample to C18 SPE cartridge for sample cleanup/extraction.
- Elute the analytes from the cartridge using dichloromethane/acetonitrile mixture.
- Concentrate the extracted sample to dryness.
- Redissolve in toluene.
- Add HFBI to derivatize the BAL hydroxyl group.
- Incubate the sample for 1 hour at 50°C and then cool to room temperature.
- Wash with water and then dry over $MgSO_4$.
- Analyze using GC-MS with EI ionization.[3]

BAL: British anti-Lewisite
CVAA: chlorovinylarsonous acid
EDT: ethanedithiol
EI: electron impact
GC: gas chromatography
HCl: hydrochloric acid
HFBI: heptafluorobutyryl imidazole
MS: mass spectrometry
PAO: phenylarsine oxide
PDT: 1,3-propanedithiol
SPE: solid phase extraction
SPME: solid phase microextraction

Data sources: (1) Logan TP, Smith JR, Jakubowski EM, Nielson RE. Verification of lewisite exposure by the analysis of 2-chlorovinyl arsonous acid in urine. *Toxicol Meth.* 1999;9:275–284. (2) Wooten JV, Ashley DL, Calafat AM. Quantitation of 2-chlorovinylarsonous acid in human urine by automated solid-phase microextraction-gas chromatography-mass spectrometry. *J Chromatogr B Analyt Technol Biomed Life Sci.* 2002;772:147–153. (3) Fidder A, Noort D, Hulst AG, de Jong LP, Benschop HP. Biomonitoring of exposure to lewisite based on adducts to haemoglobin. *Arch Toxicol.* 2000;74:207–214.

urine samples. The blood assay for both bound and free CVAA will potentially provide a longer opportunity for retrospective confirmation of exposure (based on one animal study), but also indicates a substantial decrease (90%) in concentration levels observed over a 10-day period.

CYANIDE

Background

Cyanide is an important industrial chemical that has many uses. It is produced in large quantities across the world and people are exposed to cyanide in a variety of ways. Many plants, including cassava roots, lima beans, and bamboo shoots, contain small amounts of cyanogenic glycosides.[131–133] Polymers that contain carbon and nitrogen release cyanide when burned. For example, large amounts of cyanide can be released during house and forest fires and from tobacco smoke (100–1600 parts per million [ppm]).[131] Some drugs also contain cyanide or have active ingredients that are converted to cyanide in the body, including sodium nitroprusside, which is given for the critical care of hypertension.[131] Synonyms for hydrogen cyanide (HCN) include prussic acid, formic anamminide, and fromonitrile. Deaths due to cyanide intoxication are usually due to the inhalation of HCN or the ingestion of cyanide salts. The signs of cyanide poisoning include headache, nausea, vomiting, tachypnoea, dyspnoea to convulsion, unconsciousness, and death.[131, 134–137]

Cyanide in the Human Body

Cyanide, the CN- ion, exists as HCN in the body at physiological pH. The mechanism of cyanide toxicity is believed to be the inactivation of iron III (ferric) enzymes in the body. The inhibition of cytochrome oxidase, which disrupts mitochondrial oxidative phosphorylation, is thought to be the most important mechanism for cyanide toxicity.[131, 138–141] Cyanide also binds to the hemoglobin in erythrocytes.[142] The binding of cyanide to iron III enzymes and proteins is reversible.[140,141]

At low concentrations, 93% to 99% of total cyanide is bound to methemaglobin (metHb) in the erythocytes.[131] The metHb is the deoxygenated iron III form of hemoglobin. Cyanide has a very high affinity to metHb and a low affinity to the oxygenated form of hemoglobin. Usually less than 1% of the total hemoglobin is in the metHb form, so at increased concentrations of cyanide in the blood, a larger amount is found in the serum. In tissue, cyanide binds to the heme group in mitochondrial cytochrome oxidase and inhibits electron transport.[140,141] All tissues are affected by this enzymatic inhibition, but especially those that require high amounts of oxygen and adenosine 5′-triphosphate. Other proteins and enzymes are also affected by cyanide, such as superoxide dismutase and xanthine oxidase, and may also contribute to cyanide's toxic effects.[131]

Cyanide's metabolism in the body is very rapid and can occur at 0.017 mg/min/kg.[131] The most common form of metabolism is the conversion to thiocyanate (SCN^-), which is then excreted via the kidneys.[143,144] The mitochondrial enzyme rhodanese (thiosulfate sulfur transferase) is thought to be the main catalyst for the formation of SCN^-, but β-mercaptopyruvate-cyanide transferase can transform cyanide to SCN^- through a different route.[141,145] The conversion to SCN^- is thought to be limited by the amount of thiosulfate. Cysteine, cystine, GSH, and β-mercaptopyruvic acid can also be sulfur sources.[131, 141,145] The reaction with cystine is also an important pathway leading to 15% of the total cyanide dose excreted in the urine as 2-iminothiozoline-4-carboxylic acid.[144] Other elimination pathways are the exhalation of HCN and oxidation to cyanate and reactions with vitamin B_{12} to form cyanocobalamin.[146]

Analytical Methods

Several matrices have been used to assess cyanide exposure. Whole blood is the most common, but measurements have been made in serum, plasma, saliva, tissues, gastric aspirate, and urine.

Whole Blood

Whole blood has been the matrix of choice, thus far, to determine cyanide exposure in humans. However, there are problems associated with cyanide and SCN^- measurements in blood. Sample collection, storage, and preparation are very important. Different levels of cyanide have been found in samples collected from different vessels (venous, arterial, and ventricular). Different whole blood samples can contain different amounts of metHb, which has a high affinity to cyanide. Also, free HCN may be more important because it is the form that reacts with cytochrome oxidase and causes the most significant adverse health effects.[131] Storage of the whole blood is also critical but not well understood. Some studies have shown an increase in cyanide of up to 40% upon storage of whole blood for 1 week and a 14% increase after 1 day at 4°C, while others have shown a decrease of 20% to 30% within 1

TABLE 22-13

ANALYTICAL METHODS FOR DETERMINING CYANIDE IN BIOLOGICAL SAMPLES[1]

Sample Matrix	Preparation Method	Analysis Method	LOD	Percent Recovery
Blood	Separation in MDC; derivatization	Spectrophotometry	0.1 ppm	NR[2]
Blood	Separation in MDC; derivatization	Spectrofluorometry (total CN)	0.025 ppm	NR[3]
Plasma	Deproteination with TCA; derivatization	Spectrophotometry (SCN-CN determination)	~ 0.07 ppm	96 (SCN)[4]
Erythrocyte suspension	Sample purged; absorption of HCN in NaOH; oxidation of SCN	Spectrophotometry (SCN-CN determination)	NR	93–97[5]
Blood cells	Centrifugation to separate cells; extraction; derivatization	HPLC-fluorescence detection	0.002 ppm	83[6]
Blood	Acidification	Headspace GC-NPD	~ 0.03 ppm	NR[7]
Blood	Acidification; derivatization	Headspace GC-ECD	0.1 ppm	NR[8]
Blood	Separation in MDC; color development	Spectrophotometry	~ 0.07 ppm	NR[9]
Blood	Incubation of acidified sample	GC-NPD	0.001 ppm	NR[10]
Blood	Separation in MDC; absorption in methemoglobin	Spectrophotometric (free CN)	0.4 ppm	~ 80[11]
Blood	Acidification	GC-NPD	0.014 ppm	86–99[12]
Blood	Microdiffusion, derivatization	Isotope dilution LC-MS	5 ppb	N/A[13]
Blood and liver	Sample digestion; treatment with lead acetate; absorption with NaOH	Specific ion electrode (total CN)	0.005 ppm	100–109[14]
Blood and urine	Separation in MDC; derivatization	Spectrofluorometric	0.008 ppm	66–83 (blood) 76–82 (urine)[15]
Urine	Dilution; derivatization	Spectrophotometry (SCN-CN determination)	~ 0.07 ppm	88 (SCN)[16]
Saliva	Derivatization	HPLC-UV (SCN)	2 ng (on instrument)	95–99[17]
Serum, urine, saliva	Extraction of buffered sample with isoamyl acetate	Flame AAS (SCN)	0.004 ppm	96–102[18]
Serum	Addition of acetonitrile; centrifugation; separation	Spectrophotometry (SCN)	0.3 ppm	94[19]
Urine, saliva	Basify; derivatization; extraction; back extraction	GC-ECD (SCN)	~ 0.033	83–106[20]
Urine, saliva	Dilution; filtration	Ion chromatography-UV (SCN)	0.02	95–101[21]
Urine	Ion chromatography; acidification; derivatization	Spectrophotometry (SCN)	~ 0.145 ppm (lowest reported)	NR[22]
Urine	Dilution; solid phase extraction	Suppressed ion chromatography with conductivity detection	~ 0.011 ppm	NR[23]
Urine (2-aminothiozoline-4-carboxylic acid)	Cation exchange; reduction; derivatization	Suppressed ion chromatography with fluorescence detection	~ 0.03 ppm	NR[24]
Urine (2-aminothiozoline-4-carboxylic acid)	Solid phase extraction and derivatization	Isotope dilution GC-MS	25 ppb	N/A[25]

(**Table 22-13** *continues*)

Table 22-13 *continued*

AAS: atomic absorption spectrometry
ATC: 2-amino-thiazoline-4-carboxylic acid
CN: cyanide
ECD: electron capture detection
GC: gas chromatography
GC-MSD: gas chromatography-mass selective detection
HCN: hydrogen cyanide
HPLC: high-performance liquid chromatography
LC: liquid chromatography
LOD: limit of detection
MDC: microdiffusion cell
NaOH: sodium hydroxide
NPD: nitrogen phosphorus detection
NR: not reported
ppb: parts per billion
ppm: parts per million
SCN: thiocyanate
TCA: trichloroacetic acid
UV: ultraviolet absorbance detection

Data sources: (1) US Department of Health and Human Services, Public Health Services, Agency for Toxic Substances and Disease Registry. Toxicological profile for cyanide. Atlanta, Ga: USDHHS; 1997. (2) Morgan RL, Way JL. Fluorometric determination of cyanide in biological fluids with pyrudixal. *J Anal Toxicol.* 1980;4:78–81. (3) Ganjeloo A, Isom GE, Morgan RL, Way JL. Fluorometric determination of cyanide in biological fluids with *p*-benzoquinone. 1980;55:103–107. (4) Pettigrew AR, Fell GS. Simplified colorimetric determination of thiocyanate in biological fluid, and its application to investigation of the toxic amblypias. *Clin Chem.* 1972;18:996–1000. (5) McMillan DE, Svoboda AC 4th. The role of erythrocytes in cyanide detoxification. *J Pharmacol Exp Ther.* 1982;221:37–42. (6) Sano A, Takimoto N, Takitani S. High-performance liquid chromatographic determination of cyanide in human red blood cells by pre-column fluorescence derivitization. *J Chromatogr.* 1992;582:131–135. (7) Levin BC, Rechani PR, Gruman JL, et al. Analysis of carboxyhemoglobin and cyanide in blood of victims of the DuPont Plaza Hotel fire in Puerto Rico. *J Forensic Sci.* 1990;35:151–168. (8) Odoul M, Fouillet B, Nouri B, Chambon R, Chambon P. Specific determination of cyanide in blood by headspace gas chromatography. *J Anal Toxicol.*1994;18:205–207. (9) Laforge M, Buneaux F, Houeto P, Bourgeios F, Bourdon R, Levillain P, et al. A rapid spectrophotometric blood cyanide determination applicable to emergency toxicology. *J Anal Toxicol.*1994;18:173–175. (10) Seto Y, Tsunoda N, Ohta H, et al.Determination of blood cyanide by headspace gas chromatography with nitrogen phosphorus detection and using a megabore capillary column. *Analytica Chimica Acta.*1993;276:247–259. (11) Tomoda A, Hashimoto K. The determination of cyanide in water and biological tissues by methemoglobin. *J Hazardous Materials.* 1991;28:241–249. (12) Calafat AM, Stanfill SB. Rapid quantitation of cyanide in whole blood by automated headspace gas chromatography. *J Chromatography B Analyt Technol Biomed Life Sci.* 2002;772:131–137. (13) Tracqui A, Raul JS, Geraut A, Berthelon L, Ludes B. Determination of blood cyanide by HPLC-MS. *J Anal Toxicol.* 2002;26:144–148. (14) Egekeze JO, Oehme FW. Direct potentiometric method for the determination of cyanide in biological materials. *J Anal Toxicol.* 1979;3:119–124. (15) Sano A, Takezawa M, Takitani S. Spectrofluorometric determination of cyanide in blood and urine with naphthalene-2,3-dialdehyde and taurine. *Anal Chim Acta.* 1989;225:351–358. (16) Pettigrew AR, Fell GS. Simplified colorimetric determination of thiocyanate in biological fluid, and its application to investigation of the toxic amblyopias. *Clin Chem.* 1972;18:996–1000. (17) Liu X, Yun Z. High-performance liquid chromatographic determination of thiocyanate anions by derivatization with pentafluorobenzyl bromide. *J Chromatogr A.* 1993;653:348–353. (18) Chattaraj S, Das AK. Indirect determination of thiocyanate in biological fluids using atomic absorption spectrometry. *Spectrochica.* 1992;47:675–680. (19) Li HZ, Bai G, Sun RM, Du LK. Determination of thiocyanate metabolite of sodium nitroprusside in serum by spectrophotometry. *Yao Xue Xue Bao.* 1993:28:854–858. (20) Chen SH, Wu SM, Kou HS, Wu HL. Electron-capture gas chromatographic determination of cyanide, iodide, nitrite, sulfide and thiocyanate anions by phase-transfer-catalyzed derivatization with pentafluorobenzyl bromide. *J Anal Toxicol.* 1994;18:81–85. (21) Michigami Y, Fujii K, Ueda K, Yamamoto Y. Determination of thiocyanate in human saliva and urine by ion chromatography. *Analyst.* 1992;117:1855–1858. (22) Tominaga MY, Midio AF. Modified method for the determination of thiocyanate in urine by ion-exchange chromatography and spectrophotometry. *Rev Farm Bioquim Univ Sao Paulo.* 1991;27:100–105. (23) Miura Y, Koh T. Determination of thiocyanate in human urine samples by suppressed ion chromatography. *Anal Sci 7.* 1991;(Suppl Proc Int Congr Anal Sci, 1991, Pt 1):167–170. (24) Lundquist P, Kagedal B, Nilsson L, Rosling H. Analysis of the cyanide metabolite 2-aminothiazoline-4-carboxylic acid in urine by high-performance liquid chromatography. *Anal Biochem.* 1995;228:27–34. (25) Logue BA, Kirschten NP, Petrovics I, Moser MA, Rockwood GA, Baskin SI. Determination of the cyanide metabolite 2-aminothiazole-4-carboxylic acid in urine and plasma by gas chromatography-mass spectrometry. *J Chromatogr B Analyt Technol Biomed Life Sci.* 2005;819:237–244.

day at 4°C and continued decreases over 2 weeks. A decrease in cyanide levels was seen when whole blood was stored at 2°C. Results from storage at – 20°C has been disputed, with some studies showing up to 3.5 times the original cyanide levels and others showing no change.[147] These differences appear to be independent of the original cyanide concentrations.[148]

Prior to detection, cyanide must first be separated from hemoglobin. This separation is most often done with sulfuric acid and followed by microdiffusion in a Conway cell, although there have been some problems associated with the Conway cell. Other methods use acid to release the cyanide followed by a variety of techniques. Most of these methods are colorimetric and rely on the König reaction to produce a dye that is quantified using spectrophotometry. Cyanide and SCN^- both react and must be separated using microdiffusion or distillation. Additionally, most of these methods are time consuming and lack specificity or sensitivity. Detection limits using this approach are generally in the high parts-per-billion range. There have also been assays developed that acidify the solution and then sample the head space for HCN followed by GC with a nitrogen-phosphorus detector or derivatization followed by GC with an electron capture detector. Detection limits by nitrogen-phosphorus detection and electron capture detector have been in the high parts-per-billion range. Cyanide has been measured in RBCs by high-performance LC after derivatization with fluorescence detection.

Urine, Saliva, and Serum or Plasma

Methods to detect cyanide exposure in human urine, saliva, and either serum or plasma have concentrated on SCN^-. These methods include derivatization with high-performance LC with ultraviolet detection, derivatization with spectrophotometric detection, or GC with electron capture detection. Some urine methods have measured the urinary metabolite 2-aminothiozoline-4-carboxylic acid.

Reference Range Values

Reference range values for cyanide in various matrices tend to vary greatly depending on the study and on the method of analysis. Thus, a reference range needs to be established for any method. In some of the studies, the range of blood cyanide levels in normal populations is less than 150 parts per billion and urinary SCN^- less than 1.0 mg/mL.[131] Smokers have much higher cyanide levels than nonsmokers; in some smokers blood cyanide levels as high as 500 ng/mL have been reported, which is 50 times higher than that typically reported for nonsmokers (Table 22-13).[131]

PHOSGENE

Background

Phosgene, also known as carbonyl chloride, was used extensively in World War I and caused more deaths than any other agent.[149] It is now a widely used industrial chemical. In 2002 the global production of phosgene was estimated to be over 5 million metric tons,[150] most of which is consumed at the production site.[151] The first synthesis of phosgene was performed in 1812 by exposing a mixture of chlorine and carbon monoxide (CO) to sunlight.[152] During World War I phosgene was produced in bulk by the reaction of chlorine and CO in the presence of activated carbon catalyst.[152] Phosgene is generally produced in the same way today but with higher efficiency because of newer high-surface–area catalysts.[153] Phosgene is an important intermediate in many industrial products, including insecticides, isocyanates, plastics, dyes, and resins.[150] Additionally, phosgene is formed during the combustion of chlorinated hydrocarbons during fires,[154] and by the photooxidation of chlorinated solvents in the atmosphere.[155]

At room temperature (20°C) phosgene is a fuming liquid with a vapor pressure of 1180 mm Hg and boiling point of 7.6°C. The gas is heavier than air, with a relative density ratio of 4.39 at 20°C. This density allows phosgene gas to collect in low-lying areas. Phosgene's odor is somewhat sweet and resembles that of fresh cut grass or hay. At higher concentrations the odor becomes pungent or burning and causes rapid olfactory fatigue.[156]

Exposure to phosgene gas causes irritation to the eyes, nose, throat, and respiratory tract. Higher phosgene gas exposures can lead to pulmonary edema and death. Exposure to liquid phosgene by direct skin or eye contact is rare but is thought to produce localized severe burns.[156] Inhalation is the most toxic exposure route for phosgene and the route thought to have caused most of the injuries and deaths during World War I. A patient who has inhaled phosgene requires advanced treatment techniques.

Phosgene is also a powerful acylating agent that reacts with nucleophiles such as amines, sulfides, or hydroxyls. Phosgene's toxicity was originally thought to be due to HCl generation during the reaction of phosgene with moisture in the body. Later, acylation reactions were found to be responsible for a majority of phosgene's toxic effects. Phosgene is greater than 800 times more toxic than HCl. Free amines protect against phosgene poisoning but not against the toxic effects of HCl, phosgene inhibits coenzyme I and HCl does not, and chemically similar compounds (such as ketene) that do not have chlorine to generate HCl have similar toxicity to phosgene.[157] Furthermore, phosgene's rate of reaction with free amines has been found to be much higher than its rate of reaction with water. In a solution of aniline in water, phosgene reacts almost exclusively with the aniline.[152]

Most of the data on health effects from phosgene are from inhalation exposures. The regulatory threshold limit value (8-hour, time-weighted average) for phosgene has been established by the National Institute for Occupational Safety and Health, an institute within the Centers for Disease Control and Prevention, as 0.1 ppm[158]; the 60-minute and 24-hour emergency exposure limits are 0.2 ppm and 0.02 ppm, respectively.[155]

The estimated LCt_{50} of phosgene concentration in air related to exposure time through inhalation is 500 ppm/min.[156] The aerosol exposure that is lethal to 100% of the exposed population (LCt_{100}) is estimated to range from 1,300 ppm/min to 1,600 ppm/min.[159] The nonlethal levels of phosgene are estimated to be less than 300 ppm/min, and 25 ppm/min is regarded as the threshold for lung damage.[156]

Phosgene odor can be recognized at levels greater than 1.5 ppm/min, with irritation in the mucus membranes occurring at 3 ppm/min or higher.[157] Exposure limits that cause adverse health effects can be reached either by longer exposure to lower concentration or shorter exposure to higher concentration. In one study, however, workers exposed to daily phosgene concentrations above 1 ppm but less than 50 ppm showed no difference in mortality or morbidity compared to workers in the same plant who were unexposed.[160]

The concentrations of phosgene in air that cause acute effects have been studied in many animal models. A review of previous animal studies in the literature was performed by Diller and Zante to estimate the approximate inhalation-dose–toxicity relationship for many species of animals.[161] In this report, animal LCt_{50} ranged from approximately 200 ppm/min for cats to 2000 ppm/min for goats. Guinea pigs and mice had the same approximate value as humans, 500 ppm/min. Dogs and rabbits had higher LCt_{50} values than humans (1000 ppm/min and 1500 ppm/min, respectively), while nonhuman primates and rats had estimated lower LCt_{50} values than humans (300 ppm/min and 400 ppm/min, respectively).[161]

Phosgene Metabolism and Markers for Phosgene Exposure

Phosgene is very reactive and is believed to be quickly transformed in vivo. Phosgene reacts with amino, hydroxyl, and thiol groups. In the blood, it can react with a variety of proteins, including albumin and hemoglobin. It also reacts with GSH and cysteine. Because chloroform is metabolized to phosgene in the body, it is expected that low levels of phosgene's protein adducts and metabolites can be found in the general background population because of low-level incidental exposure to chloroform. Studies are needed to accurately determine this reference range.

Glutathione and Glutathione Adducts

Because phosgene is a highly reactive acylating agent, it is expected to interact with the body's antioxidant defense system. GSH is a tripeptide thiol consisting of cysteine, glutamic acid, and glycine, which serves as both a scavenger of reactive compounds to protect cells and as a store for cysteine moieties.[162] GSH is found in general concentrations in healthy adults in the millimolar range.[162,163] GSH can be oxidized to glutathione disulfide (GSSG), a simple dimer of GSH joined by a disulfide linkage. The ratio of the GSH redox couple in vitro has been determined to be between 100:1 and 10:1 GSH to GSSG.[162,163] When depleted, GSH fails to protect cellular oxidation and leads to irreversible oxidative damage.[164]

Phosgene was found to react with GSH to form an acylated dimer, diglutathionyl dithiocarbonate (GSCOSG; Figure 22-13).[165] This marker for phosgene metabolism was first discovered by Pohl et al [165] in the metabolism of chloroform in the liver, where phosgene was believed to be generated by enzymatic action from chloroform. The bisglutathione adduct GSCOSG was detected in vivo in the bile of rats exposed to chloroform and in vitro in rat liver microsomes. Pohl et al also found a decrease in GSH levels in the rats.[165] GSCOSG was found directly by mixing phosgene with GSH in buffer solution.[166]

The in-vivo generation of GSSG and CO has also been reported in the blood of mice exposed to haloforms.[167] The observation of GSSG and CO may be linked to the further metabolism of GSCOSG after generation, but there are no studies that have identified this potential relationship.

GSH is also found in tissue, so similar reactions with GSH and phosgene are expected in the bronchoalveolar region. In the excised lung tissue from rabbits and mice inhalationally exposed to phosgene, there was

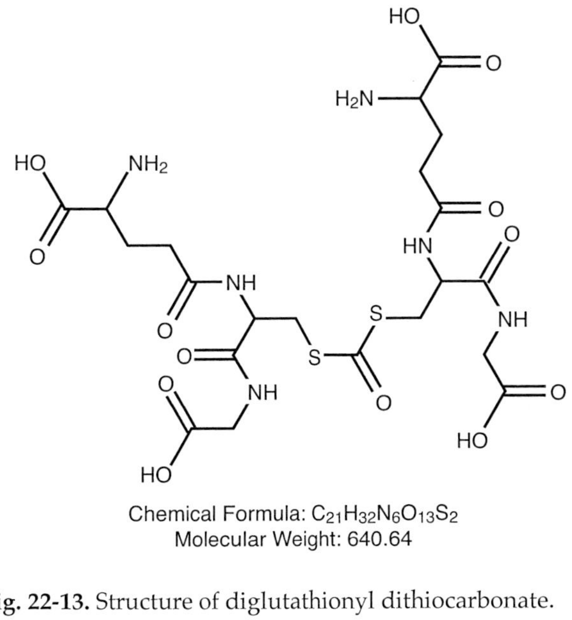

Fig. 22-13. Structure of diglutathionyl dithiocarbonate.

little change in tissue total GSH concentration, but the reduced GSH levels fell significantly and GSSG levels increased significantly.[168,169] In these studies, the reduced GSH as percent of total was 41% less than the control subject. The collection of lung tissue samples from humans that are thought to have been exposed to phosgene is impractical, but the collection of bronchoalveolar lavage fluid is possible. Sciuto has reported on the concentrations of GSSG, GSH, and total GSH in the bronchoalveolar lavage fluid of rodents with severe changes in the GSH redox state following phosgene inhalation.[170,171] Increases in total GSH levels were observed in both studies, but the redox state of the GSH was not reported. It can be anticipated that increased levels of the oxidized form of GSH would be a better indicator of phosgene exposure, but at this time only total GSH has been correlated with phosgene inhalation in lavage fluid. It should also be noted that in Sciuto's reported studies, there was no discrimination between GSSG and GSCOSG. Because these two species are similar in structure, it is unclear whether the reported detection of GSSG includes some component from GSCOSG.

The detection of GSCOSG, increased GSSG levels, and decreased GSH levels following phosgene exposure may hold promise for detecting phosgene exposure, but there are considerable obstacles to some of these approaches. The levels of total GSH and changes in GSH redox state in animal models were determined shortly after exposure to phosgene; however, the lifetime of GSCOSG is not known, and even though the levels of total GSH in mice exposed to phosgene were significantly higher than in controls up to 24 hours postexposure, the GSH levels were only marginally above controls at times up to 7 days postexposure.[171] Furthermore, there are large variations in GSH and GSSH levels in human subjects, so predetermined baseline levels should be required for each patient.[162,163] The formation of GSCOGS may be specific for phosgene (or chlorinated compounds that metabolize to phosgene). A reference range study of GSCOSG levels in people with no known exposure to phosgene is required to use this biomarker for phosgene exposure.

Cysteine Adducts

Phosgene reportedly forms an adduct with the thiol amino acid cysteine.[172] Cysteine is a building block of GSH and is the rate-limiting step in generating GSH for antioxidant tissue protection.[173] As in the case of GSH, cysteine can be reduced to the disulfide cysteine dimer cystine. Cysteine is generated in the body by the conversion of methionine through the cystathionine pathway. Average concentrations of cysteine in humans are typically lower than GSH and have been approximated at 250 μm in plasma and 400 μm in urine.[174]

The reaction of phosgene and cysteine in vitro was first reported by Kubic and Anders, and the product was identified as 2-oxothiazolidine-4-carboxylic acid (known as OTZ, OTC, or procysteine).[172] OTZ was formed by incubating hepatic microsomal fractions with chloroform, nicotinamide adenosine dinucleotide phosphate, and cysteine (Figure 22-14).[172] Isotopic studies showed that chloroform was first metabolized to phosgene by cytochrome P-450. The phosgene then reacted with cysteine to form OTZ. Synthetic routes to OTZ also have indicated the generation from cysteine and phosgene.[175]

OTZ is a prodrug of cysteine and is rapidly converted by 5-oxoprolinase to cysteine in vivo.[173] Studies have indicated that the lifetime of OTZ in the human body varies from 3 to 8 hours.[173,176] OTZ's rapid elimination limits its usefulness as a biomarker for phosgene unless samples are obtained quickly after a suspected exposure.

Other possible markers for phosgene exposure may be the reduction of cysteine to its disulfide, cystine, upon exposure to phosgene. However, this reaction is not specific to phosgene exposure. The formation of the acylated dimer cysteine-CO-cysteine has been shown in vitro when cysteine is treated with phosgene in solution, and this reaction occurs even in the presence of GSH.[166]

Small Molecule Adducts

Inhaled phosgene reportedly reacts with other components in the lungs. In 1933 treatment of lung pulp with phosgene was found to form the chlorocarbonic ester of cholesterol.[177] Kling [177] also indicated that the hydrophilic character of the fats was destroyed in the cells because of the loss of free sterols and suggested that caused acute pulmonary edema.

Phosgene forms adducts with phospholipids. In a

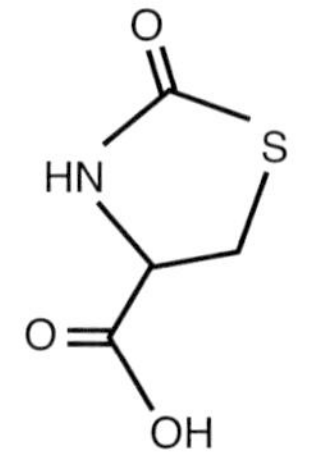

Chemical Formula: $C_4H_5NO_3S$
Molecular Weight: 147.15

Fig. 22-14. Structure of 2-oxothiazolidine-4-carboxylic acid.

study of chloroform metabolism, a single phospholipid adduct was formed and it was thought to be related to phosphatidylethanolamine (PE) because PE was the only phospholipid found to be depleted.[178] In other studies on the metabolism of chloroform, a single phosgene adduct was found and identified as an adduct of PE with the phosgene carbonyl group bound to the amine of the head group of PE.[179,180] Further work on this PE adduct characterized it as a dimer of PE, the two subsistents linked at the amine of the head group by the carbonyl from phosgene.[181] Furthermore, this adduct has been implicated as the critical alteration leading to cell death by chloroform metabolism.[182] Nonspecific increases in the phospholipid content of lavage fluid have been observed in rats 6 hours after exposure to inhalational phosgene, but specific adducts were not monitored.[183]

Macromolecule Adducts

Lung tissue damage after phosgene exposure, which leads to permeability of the blood-air barrier and pulmonary edema, is likely due, in part, to the reactions of phosgene with various macromolecules, including proteins. The permeability of the blood-air barrier also raises the possibility of phosgene entering the blood stream and forming adducts with blood proteins. Some work has been done developing methods for identifying and quantifying phosgene adducts with abundant blood proteins.

The initial evidence that phosgene reacts and forms an adduct with hemoglobin was from a study of the metabolism of chloroform. In this study, Pereira et al allowed chloroform to be metabolized with liver microsomes.[184] One of chloroform's initial metabolites is believed to be phosgene. The study authors identified N-hydroxymethyl cysteine by GC-MS, resulting from the reaction of phosgene of cysteine moiety in hemoglobin.[184] Additionally, Fabrizi et al identified phosgene adducts with petapeptides of lysozyme and the N-terminal peptide from human histone H2B, even when these peptides were treated with phosgene in solution in the presence of GSH, a known phosgene scavenger.[168] There is evidence that phosgene reacts and forms blood protein adducts in vivo. Sciuto et al reported spectrophotometric differences in plasma from mice, rats, and guinea pigs exposed to high doses of phosgene.[185] This study also suggested that phosgene could directly attack RBCs after observing the shifted fragility curve for erythrocytes.[185]

Noort et al have developed methods to detect and quantify phosgene adducts with both hemoglobin and albumin.[186] Treatment of whole blood with radioisotopically labeled phosgene showed that phosgene reacted with both albumin and hemoglobin and that there was a higher level of adduct formation with the albumin than with the hemoglobin. The analysis of the albumin-^{14}C–labeled phosgene adduct indicated that the major site of adduct formation was an intramolecular lysine-lysine adduct with a CO bridge.[186] Analysis of the hemoglobin-phosgene adduct showed the presence of a hydantoin function between the N-terminal valine and the amino portion of leucine in a fragment containing amino acids 1 to 5.[186]

Noort et al[186] were able to detect the phosgene-albumin adduct in whole blood that was treated with 1 μM phosgene and the phosgene-hemoglobin adduct in whole blood treated with 1 mM phosgene. The phosgene-albumin adduct was detectable at an order of phosgene concentration magnitude 3 times lower than the phosgene-hemoglobin adduct. The higher detection limits of the globin adduct were reportedly in part due to an interference of natural hydantoin function in the same position as the phosgene adduct.[186] Sample preparation for the more sensitive albumin-based method included isolating albumin by affinity chromatography, carboxymethylation, dialysis, and tryptic digestion. LC-MS-MS analysis was done using either a high-resolution MS instrument or by multiple reaction monitoring on a triple quadrupole mass spectrometer. The multiple reaction monitoring experiment observed the fragmentation of the doubly charged ion at 861 daltons (da) to both the 747.5 da and 773.6 da transitions. Noort et al estimate that the method in vivo should be able to detect a 320 mg/min/m^3 exposure, assuming 10% absorption of the dose by the blood, resulting in an adduct concentration of 1.3 μm, just above the detection limit for the albumin adduct.[186]

Other Indicators of Phosgene Exposure

Inhalational exposure to phosgene causes severe inflammation and tissue damage. There are many indicators for the biochemical changes caused by phosgene exposure that measure the biochemical changes in the tissues that are damaged by phosgene. These types of markers are not as specific for phosgene exposure as small molecule or protein adduct markers, but they can suggest that an individual has been exposed to phosgene and indicate the severity of the exposure.

Some of the most important nonspecific indicators for phosgene-mediated tissue damage are associated with inflammation. Sciuto et al reported that interleukin (IL)-6 levels were highly elevated in the bronchoalveolar lavage fluid from rodents exposed to phosgene compared to levels in controls.[185] Levels of IL-6 were 16-fold higher 4 hours after the phosgene exposure, peaked at 12 hours, and were still over 100-fold higher than in controls 72 hours after phosgene exposure. Macrophage inflammatory protein was also affected in the rodents exposed to phosgene, showing a 10-fold increase compared to the control rodents 8 and 10 hours after the exposure, but macrophage inflammatory protein levels returned to near-normal levels 24 hours after the phosgene exposure.[185] Sciuto et al reported that changes in IL-4, IL-10, tumor necrosis factor, and IL-1β levels were minimal after phosgene exposure as compared to changes in IL-6 levels.[185]

Sciuto et al also studied changes in fluid electrolyte levels in blood and bronchoalveolar lavage fluid from mice following exposure to phosgene.[187] Blood levels of sodium, chloride, and calcium were unchanged after exposure to phosgene compared to controls, but the levels of potassium increased drastically and approached physiologically dangerous levels. In the bronchoalveolar lavage fluid, chloride levels were unchanged, sodium dropped between 4 and 12 hours, and both potassium and calcium levels increased significantly after 4 hours and by a factor of 3 after 8 hours, compared to nonexposed controls. The simplicity of determining electrolyte levels offers promise for suggesting exposure to phosgene, but is not specific for phosgene exposure and requires supporting analyses.

Because phosgene reacts rapidly with GSH, it is expected that enzymes responsible for maintaining GSH levels may also be affected, and their levels can be monitored to suggest phosgene exposure. Sciuto et al found levels of GSH peroxidase and GSH reductase significantly increased in the bronchoalveolar lavage fluid of mice exposed to 160 to 220 ppm/min phosgene.[171] The levels of GSH peroxidase and GSH reductase were measured by ELISA and were elevated up to 72 hours after exposure.[171]

The amount of total protein in bronchoalveolar lavage fluid may also be a marker for the extent of lung damage after a phosgene exposure. Sciuto found that levels of total protein in the lavage fluid of mice was dramatically increased following phosgene exposure and remained significantly elevated up to 7 days postexposure. Other reports by Sciuto have indicated similar increases in protein levels in bronchoalveolar lavage fluid and have suggested they are due to increased permeability of the blood-air barrier.[170] In an earlier study, Currie et al found significant increases in the concentration of bronchoalveolar lavage fluid protein immediately after a relatively low exposure (60 ppm/min).[188] Total protein levels in bronchoalveolar lavage fluid are not specific for phosgene exposure, but may be helpful to determine the extent of lung damage caused by it. A simple spectrophotometric assay is suitable to determine protein levels because the amount of protein in lavage fluid is nonspecific and measures only total protein levels.

3-QUINUCLIDINYL BENZILATE

Background

Commonly termed "QNB," 3-quinuclidinyl benzilate (BZ) is an anticholinergic glycolate that has been designated "agent BZ" by the military. BZ is the only known incapacitating agent that has ever been weaponized for use by the US military. That occurred in the early 1960s when BZ was produced at the Pine Bluff Arsenal between 1962 and 1965. BZ was subsequently dropped from the chemical arsenal for several reasons, including concerns about variable and unpredictable effects.

BZ's action is very similar to other anticholinergics such as atropine and scopolamine, differing mainly in potency and duration of effect. The lethal dose of an infectious organism required to produce infection in 50% of the population (ID_{50}) for BZ is about 6.2 μg/kg (about 500 ng/person). BZ is about 25 times as potent as atropine, but only about 3-fold more active than scopolamine. However, BZ's duration of action is typically much longer, and the uptake by an oral route is about 80% that of intravenous or intramuscular routes. Under optimum conditions, BZ is also about 40% to 50% as effective by inhalation as by injection. Initial symptoms typically occur 30 minutes to 4 hours after exposure. Full recovery may require 3 to 4 days.

BZ has a molecular weight of 337 g/mol and a melting point of 168°C. It is solid at room temperature and has a negligible vapor pressure. BZ is relatively stable and moderately resistant to air oxidation and moderate temperatures, and it undergoes hydrolysis in aqueous solution to produce benzylic acid and 3-quinuclidinol.

3-Quinuclidinyl Benzilate in the Human Body

Information on BZ in the body is limited. It can take 3 to 4 days before symptoms of BZ intoxication resolve. Apparently, most BZ is excreted by the kidneys and urine is the preferred analysis matrix. Benzylic acid and 3-quinuclidinol are the probable main metabolites

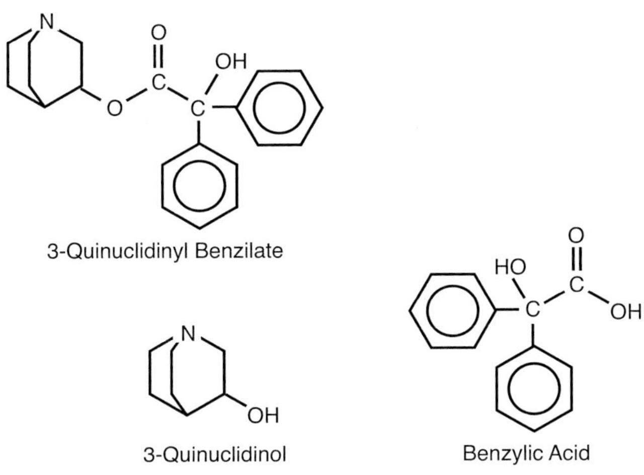

Fig. 22-15. Structure of 3-quinuclidinyl benzilate and the main metabolites 3-quinuclidinol and benzylic acid.

(Figure 22-15). It has been estimated that 3% of BZ in the body is excreted as the parent compound.

Analytical Methods

There are few references to the analysis of BZ in humans. BZ is frequently used by neuropharmacologists as a marker, but these methods are often not quantitative. In 1988 the United States began work on demilitarization of BZ stockpiles. As part of that work, the National Institute of Standards and Technology and the US Army Research and Development laboratory at Fort Detrick, Maryland, developed a method for monitoring workers. The method was based on GC-MS of the trimethylsilyl (TMS) derivatives and monitored all three analytes (BZ, benzylic acid, and 3-quinuclidinol). Detection limits were 0.5 ng/mL for BZ and 5 ng/mL for the hydrolysis products.[189]

SAMPLE CONSIDERATIONS

General

The following section describes the field collection, shipment, and storage of biomedical samples according to the guidance from the Centers for Disease Control and the United States Army Medical Research Institute of Chemical Defense. In most instances, blood (serum, plasma) and urine are the most commonly collected samples. Samples to be collected depend upon the specific method required by the assay. The information provided in this section is intended to provide general guidelines for sample collection, shipment, and storage and is not intended to be comprehensive. In all cases, questions regarding specific procedures to obtain and ship samples should be directed to the receiving laboratory by calling the laboratory or consulting its Web site before collecting the sample.

Urine

The collection of urine samples should be done under the close supervision of a healthcare provider or an unbiased observer to preclude the possibility of sample tampering. Care should be taken to ensure appropriate handling so as to minimize the chances for contamination from the environment or handling personnel. The urine should be collected immediately following the suspected exposure or at the earliest possible time. A midstream urine collection is desirable. If follow up is anticipated, additional samples should be obtained at 24 hours. Urine should be collected in clean urine cups or screw-capped plastic containers that can withstand freezing temperatures without splitting. A minimum of 25 to 30 mL should be collected. Urine samples should be frozen immediately (– 70°C or dry ice is preferred).

Whole Blood

It is recommended that samples of whole blood be handled cautiously from the start of the collection to maintain integrity and preclude the possibility of contamination, tampering, or mislabeling. All samples should be collected under the close supervision of a healthcare provider or physician and witnessed by an unbiased observer if possible. Samples should be obtained as soon as possible following the suspected exposure. Additional samples may be obtained for follow up. Blood should be collected in 5- or 7-mL blood tubes. Specific methods may require specific types of tubes, such as purple-top (ethylenediamine tetraacetic acid) tubes for plasma or the red-top, unopened, vacuum-fill tubes for serum.

For methods that analyze serum or plasma, it is useful to process whole blood samples by centrifugation followed by separation of the plasma or serum from the RBC pellet. The plasma or serum components can then be frozen (– 70°C or dry ice is preferred) and stored or shipped on dry ice. When on-site blood processing is not convenient, unprocessed whole blood samples should be stored immediately at 4°C. Packed RBCs may be stored at 4°C or frozen, depending on the properties of the analyte and the needs of the analytical method to be performed.

Preparing, Shipping, and Storing Specimens

Care must be taken not only when gathering samples for testing but when preparing them for transport. What follows are the basic guidelines for readying, transporting, and storing samples.

Labeling

Specimens should be labeled in accordance with the standing operating procedures of the receiving laboratory to ensure forensic integrity. The labels should be as comprehensive as possible and double-checked for accuracy. Label samples with the facility of origin and clear markings resistant to water and refrigeration or freezing conditions. Labels should also include patient identification information (name or other specific identifiers), date and time of collection, specimen identity, and some identification of the collector. A list of samples with the corresponding names of individuals should be maintained at the facility of origin and should also be included with the samples if they are shipped. Wrap each sample top with waterproof, tamper-evident, forensic evidence tape, being careful not to cover the sample identification labels.

Packaging

For blood, separate each tube from the others or wrap individually to prevent direct contact. Tubes should be placed in secondary packages, such as a divided box wrapped with absorbent material and sealed inside a plastic bag, other sealable containers, or individually wrapped tubes sealed inside a plastic bag. Place absorbent material between the primary receptacle and the secondary packaging. Use enough absorbent material to absorb the entire contents of primary receptacles. To facilitate processing and identification, package blood tubes so that similar tubes are packaged together (eg, all purple tops together). For urine, wrap frozen cups with absorbent material and place them into sealable secondary packaging, such as those described for blood. Do not ship frozen urine and blood in the same package.

Shipping Container

The shipping container should be a sealable, polystyrene foam or other insulated container capable of maintaining the contents at the preferred temperature for the specimens. For cushioning, place additional absorbent material in the bottom of the outer containers. For samples that require refrigeration conditions, such as whole blood, add a layer of frozen cold packs and place the secondary containers on top of the cold packs. Place additional cold packs or absorbent material between the secondary containers to reduce movement within the container. Lastly, place a layer of frozen cold packs on top of the secondary containers. When shipping frozen samples (plasma, serum, urine), add a layer of dry ice on top of the cushioning material in the bottom of the shipping container. Do not use large chunks of dry ice for shipment because they could shatter items during transport. Place additional absorbent material between wrapped urine cups to reduce their movement within the outer container. Finally, add an additional layer of dry ice.

Documentation (Shipping Manifest, Incident Report, Chain-of-Custody)

Prepare separate documentation for each container shipped. Prepare and place a shipping manifest designating sample identification numbers, quantity, and type in a zippered plastic bag on top of the specimens before closing and sealing the container. Maintain a copy of the manifest at the point of origin. Enclose an incident report form with as much information as possible describing the incident, providing the date and time of suspected exposure, detailing the onset and description of symptoms, sample collection time, and suspected agent involved. Include patient information, such as name, social security number, age, and gender, as well as a point of contact. The incident report form should be stored in a zippered plastic bag on top of the specimens before closing and sealing the container. A chain-of-custody form must also be included. Prepare a separate chain-of-custody form for samples in each container. Indicate sample identity, any pertinent descriptors, and the number of samples. Place the completed chain-of-custody forms in a plastic zippered bag on the outside of the shipping container.

Shipping

Close and secure the outer container with filamentous shipping or strapping tape. Affix labels and markings. Place a label on the outer container that indicates the proper name, "Diagnostic Specimens." For those containers with dry ice, place a Class 9 (dry ice) label on the outer container. This label must indicate the amount of dry ice in the container, the address of the shipper, and the address of the recipient. This label must be placed on the same side of the container as the "Diagnostic Specimens" label.

Storage

Upon arrival, the receiving laboratory should maintain a proper chain of custody. If the samples are not processed immediately, they should be stored as soon as possible after arriving at the receiving laboratory. Storing samples either before or after they are shipped should be in accordance with conditions dictated by the sample type. Blood should be stored refrigerated at 4°C. Plasma or serum should be stored frozen at –70°C. RBCs can be stored refrigerated at 4°C or frozen at –70°C; freezing is preferred for long-term storage. Avoid repeated cycles that move samples from frozen to thawed or refrigerated to room temperature.

SUMMARY

The general class of agents involved in severe intoxication (ie, OP nerve agents, vesicants, etc) can often be recognized by symptom presentation. However, testing is necessary to identify the specific agent involved. In cases where poisoning is suspected at low levels and symptoms do not clearly indicate intoxication with a specific chemical warfare agent, testing can provide additional information to help consider or rule out an exposure. In general, confirmatory analyses should not be initiated in the absence of other information that suggests a potential exposure has taken place; other evidence, such as patient signs or symptoms, environmental monitoring and testing, and threat intelligence information should also be considered. This information should be used to guide decisions about what agent or class of agents should be the focus of testing and it should ultimately be used in conjunction with test results to determine whether or not an exposure has occurred.

Analytical methods for verifying chemical agent exposure do not employ instrumentation that is routinely used for standard clinical testing, such as automated clinical analyzers. With the exception of cholinesterase analysis, instrumentation typically involves MS systems with either GC or LC techniques to separate the analyte from other matrix components. Although the methods are desirable because they afford a high level of confidence for identifying the analyte, they are time and labor intensive. Consequently the turnaround time for analyses is greater than that expected for standard clinical tests.

Chemical warfare agents have been used against both military and civilian populations. In many of these cases, healthcare providers have learned that it is critical to rapidly identify exposed personnel to facilitate appropriate medical treatment and support. Incidents involving large numbers of personnel have shown that is also important to determine those not exposed to avoid unnecessary psychological stress and overburdening the medical system. In addition to medical issues, the political and legal ramifications of chemical agent use by rogue nations or terrorist organizations can be devastating. Therefore, it is important that accurate and sensitive analytical techniques be employed and appropriately interpreted.

REFERENCES

1. Matsuda Y, Nagao M, Takatori T, et al. Detection of the sarin hydrolysis product in formalin-fixed brain tissues of victims of the Tokyo subway terrorist attack. *Toxicol Appl Pharmacol.* 1998;150:310–320.

2. Department of the US Army. *Assay Techniques for Detection of Exposure to Sulfur Mustard, Cholinesterase Inhibitors, Sarin, Soman, GF, and Cyanide.* Washington, DC: DA; 1996. Technical Bulletin Medical 296.

3. Taylor P. Anticholinesterase agents. In: Brunton LL, Lazo JS, Parker KL, eds. *Goodman and Gilman's the Pharmacological Basis of Therapeutics.* 11th ed. New York, NY: McGraw-Hill; 2006:201–216.

4. Sidell FR. Nerve agents. In: Sidell FR, Takafuji ET, Franz DR, eds. *Medical Aspects of Chemical and Biological Warfare.* In: Zajtchuk R, Bellamy RF, eds. *The Textbooks of Military Medicine.* Part I. Washington, DC: Borden Institute; 1997:129–179.

5. Harris R, Paxman J. *A Higher Form of Killing: the Secret Story of Chemical and Biological Warfare.* New York, NY: Hill and Wang; 1982: 53.

6. Degenhardt CE, Pleijsier K, van der Schans MJ, et al. Improvements of the fluoride reactivation method for the verification of nerve agent exposure. *J Anal Toxicol.* 2004;28:364–371.

7. Noort D, Benschop HP, Black RM. Biomonitoring of exposure to chemical warfare agents: a review. *Tox Appl Pharmacol.* 2002;184:116–126.

8. Benschop HP, De Jong LP. Toxicokinetics of soman: species variation and stereospecificity in elimination pathways. *Neurosci Biobehav Rev.* 1991;15:73–77.

9. Benschop HP, de Jong LP. Toxicokinetics of nerve agents. In: Somani SM, Romano JA, eds. *Chemical Warfare Agents: Toxicity at Low Levels.* Boca Raton, Fla: CRC Press; 2000:25–81. Chapter 2.

10. Van der Schans MJ, Lander BJ, van der Wiel, H, Langenberg JP, Benschop HP. Toxicokinetics of the nerve agent (±) -VX in anesthetized and atropinized hairless guinea pigs and marmosets after intravenous and percutaneous administration. *Tox Appl Pharmacol.* 2003;191:48–62.

11. Bonierbale E, Debordes L, Coppet L. Application of capillary gas chromatography to the study of hydrolysis of the nerve agent VX in rat plasma. *J Chromatogr B Biomed Sci Appl.* 1997;688:255–264.

12. Harris LW, Braswell LM, Fleisher JP, Cliff WJ. Metabolites of pinacolyl methylphosphonofluoridate (soman) after enzymatic hydrolysis in vitro. *Biochem Pharmacol.* 1964;13:1129–1136.

13. Polak RL, Cohen EM. The influence of oximes on the distribution of 32P in the body of the rat after injection of 32P-sarin. *Biochem Pharmacol.* 1970;19:865–876.

14. Reynolds ML, Little PJ, Thomas BF, Bagley RB, Martin BR. Relationship between the biodisposition of [3H]soman and its pharmacological effects in mice. *Toxicol Appl Pharmacol.* 1985;80:409–420.

15. Little PJ, Reynolds ML, Bowman ER, Martin BR. Tissue disposition of [3H]sarin and its metabolites in mice. *Toxicol Appl Pharmacol.* 1986;83:412–419.

16. Shih ML, Smith JR, McMonagle JD, Dolzine TW, Gresham VC. Detection of metabolites of toxic alkylmethylphosphonates in biological samples. *Biol Mass Spectrom.* 1991;20:717–723.

17. Shih ML, McMonagle JD, Dolzine TW, Gresham VC. Metabolite pharmacokinetics of soman, sarin, and GF in rats and biological monitoring of exposure to toxic organophosphorus agents. *J Appl Toxicol.* 1994:14:195–199.

18. Tsuchihashi H, Katagi M, Nishikawa M, Tatsuno M. Identification of metabolites of nerve agent VX in serum collected from a victim. *J Anal Toxicol.* 1998;22:383–388.

19. Fredriksson SA, Hammarström LG, Henriksson L, Lakso HA. Trace determination of alkyl methylphosphonic acids in environmental and biological samples using gas chromatography / negative-ion chemical ionization mass spectrometry and tandem mass spectrometry. *J Mass Spectrom.* 1995;30:1133–1143.

20. Miki A, Katagi M, Tsuchihashi H, Yamashita M. Determination of alkylmethylphosphonic acids, the main metabolites of organophosphorus nerve agents, in biofluids by gas chromatography-mass spectrometry and liquid-liquid-solid-phase-transfer-catalyzed pentafluorobenzylation. *J Anal Toxicol.* 1999;23:86–93.

21. Driskell WJ, Shih M, Needham LL, Barr DB. Quantitation of organophosphorus nerve agent metabolites in human urine using isotope dilution gas chromatography-tandem mass spectrometry. *J Anal Toxicol.* 2002;26:6–10.

22. Barr JR, Driskell WJ, Aston LS, Martinez RA. Quantitation of metabolites of the nerve agents sarin, soman, cyclosarin, VX, and Russian VX in human urine using isotope-dilution gas chromatography-tandem mass spectrometry. *J Anal Toxicol.* 2004;28:371–378.

23. Minami M, Hui DM, Katsumata M, Inagaki H, Boulet CA. Method for the analysis of methylphosphonic acid metabolites of sarin and its ethanol-substituted analogue in urine as applied to the victims of the Tokyo sarin disaster. *J Chromatogr B Biomed Sci Appl.* 1997;695:237–244.

24. Nakajima T, Sasaki K, Ozawa H, Sekjima Y, Morita H, Fukushima Y, Yanagisawa N. Urinary metabolites of sarin in a patient of the Matsumoto incident. *Arch Toxicol.* 1998;72:601–603.

25. Noort D, Hulst AG, Platenburg DH, Polhuijs M, Benschop H. Quantitative analysis of O-isopropyl methylphosphonic acid in serum samples of Japanese citizens allegedly exposed to sarin: estimation of internal dosage. *Arch Toxicol.* 1998;72:671–675.

26. Katagi M, Nishikawa M, Tatsuno M, Tsuchihashi H. Determination of the main hydrolysis products of organophosphorus nerve agents, methylphosphonic acids, in human serum by indirect photometric detection ion chromatography. *J Chromatogr B Biomed Sci Appl.* 1997;698:81–88.

27. Suzuki T, Morita H, Ono K, Maekawa K, Nagai R, Yazaki Y. Sarin poisoning in Tokyo subway. *Lancet.* 1995;345:980.

28. Polhuijs M, Langenberg JP, Noort D, Hulst AG, Benschop HP. Retrospective detection of exposure to organophosphates: analyses in blood of human beings and rhesus monkeys. In: Sohns T, Voicu VA, eds. *NBC risks: Current Capabilities and Future Perspectives for Protection.* Dordrecht, Holland, the Netherlands: Kluwer Academic Publishers; 1999:513–521.

29. Polhuijs M, Langenberg JP, Benschop HP. New method for retrospective detection of exposure to organophosphorus anticholinesterases: application to alleged sarin victims of Japanese terrorists. *Toxicol Appl Pharmacol.* 1997;146:156–161.

30. Heilbronn E. The effect of sodium fluoride on sarin inhibited blood cholinesterase. *Acta Chem Scand.* 1964;18:2410.

31. Heilbronn E. Action of fluoride on cholinesterase. II. In vitro reactivation of cholinesterases inhibited by organophosphorus compounds. *Biochem Pharmacol.* 1965;14:1363–1373.

32. Albanus L, Heilbeonn E, Sundwall A. Antidote effect of sodium fluoride in organophosphorus anticholinesterase poisoning. *Biochem Pharmacol.* 1965;14:1375–1381.

33. Jakubowski EM, Heykamp LS, Durst HD, Thompson SA. Preliminary studies in the formation of ethyl methylphosphonofluoridate from rat and human serum exposed to VX and treated with fluoride ion. *Anal Lett.* 2001;34:727–737.

34. Jakubowski EM, McGuire JM, Evans RA, et al. Quantitation of fluoride ion released sarin in red blood cell samples by gas chromatography-chemical ionization mass spectrometry using isoptope dilution and large-volume injection. *J Anal Toxicol.* 2004;28:357–363.

35. Adams TK, Capacio BR, Smith JR, Whalley CE, Korte WD. The application of the fluoride reactivation process to the detection of sarin and soman nerve agent exposures in biological samples. *Drug Chem Toxicol.* 2004;27:77–91.

36. Black RM, Harrison JM, Read RW. The interaction of sarin and soman with plasma proteins: the identification of a novel phosphonylation site. *Arch Toxicol.* 1999;73:123–126.

37. DeJong LP, van Dijk C. Formation of soman (1,2,2-trimethylpropyl-methylphosphonofluoridate) via fluoride-induced reactivation of soman-inhibited aliesterase in rat plasma. *Biochem Pharmacol.* 1984;33:663–669.

38. Clement JG. Importance of aliesterase as a detoxification mechanism for soman (pinacolyl methylphosphonofluoridate) in mice. *Biochem Pharmacol.* 1984;33:3807–3811.

39. Clement JG, Benschop HP, DeJong LP, Wolthuis OL. Stereoisomers of soman (pinacolyl methylphosphonofluoridate): inhibition of serum carboxylic ester hydrolase and potentiation of their toxicity by CBDP (2-2-methylphenoxy)-4H-1,3,2-benzodioxaphosphorin-2-oxide) in mice. *Toxicol Appl Pharmacol.* 1987;89:141–143.

40. Maxwell DM, Brecht KM, O'Neill BL. The effect of carboxylesterase inhibition on interspecies differences in soman toxicity. *Toxicol Lett.* 1987;39:35–42.

41. Maxwell DM, Brecht KM. Carboxylesterase: specificity and spontaneous reactivation of an endogenous scavenger for organophosphorus compounds. *J Appl Toxicol.* 2001;21(suppl 1):S103–S107.

42. Nagao M, Takatori T, Matsuda Y, et al. Detection of sarin hydrolysis products from sarin-like organophosphorus agent-exposed human erythrocytes. *J Chromatogr B Biomed Sci Appl.* 1997;701:9–17.

43. Nagao M, Takatori T, Matsuda Y, Nakajima M, Iwase H, Iwadate K. Definitive evidence for the acute sarin poisoning diagnosis in the Tokyo subway. *Toxicol Appl Pharmacol.* 1997;144:198–203.

44. Fidder A, Hulst AG, Noort D, et al. Retrospective detection of exposure to organophosphorus anti-cholinesterases: mass spectrometric analysis of phosphylated human butyrylcholinesterase. *Chem Res Toxicol.* 2002;15:582–590.

45. Noort D, Fidder A, van der Schans MJ, Hulst AG. Verification of exposure to organophosphates: generic mass spectrometric method for detection of human butyrylcholinesterase adducts. *Anal Chem.* 2006;78:6640–6644.

46. Silver A. *The Biology of Cholinesterases.* Amsterdam, North Holland, the Netherlands: North Holland Publishing Company; 1974:58–67.

47. Mortensen SR, Brimijoin S, Hooper MJ, Padilla S. Comparison of the in vitro sensitivity of rat acetylcholinesterase to chlorpyrifos-oxon: what do tissue IC_{50} values represent? *Toxicol Appl Pharmacol.* 1998;148:46–49.

48. Wilson BW, Sanborn JR, O'Malley MA, Henderson JD, Billitti JR. Monitoring the pesticide-exposed worker. *Occup Med.* 1997;12(2):347–363.

49. Nigg HN, Knaak JB. Blood cholinesterases as human biomarkers of organophosphorus pesticide exposure. *Rev Environ Contam Toxicol.* 2000;163:29–111.

50. Lotti M. Cholinesterase inhibition: complexities in interpretation. *Clin Chem.* 1995;41:1814–1818.

51. Sidell FR. Clinical considerations in nerve agent intoxication. In: Somani SM, ed. *Chemical Warfare Agents.* San Diego, Calif: Academic Press; 1992:163.

52. Wolthuis OL, Benschop HP, Berends F. Persistence of the anti-cholinesterase soman in rats; antagonism with a non-toxic simulator of this organophosphate. *Eur J Pharmacol.* 1981;69:379–383.

53. Worek F, Eyer P, Szinicz L. Inhibition, reactivation and aging kinetics of cyclohexylmethylphosphonofluoridate-inhibited human cholinesterases. *Arch Toxicol.* 1998;72:580–587.

54. Lockridge O, Masson P. Pesticides and susceptible populations: people with butyrylcholinesterase genetic variants may be at risk. *Neurotoxicology.* 2000;21:113–126.

55. Wilson BW, Henderson JD. Blood esterase determinations as markers of exposure. *Rev Environ Contam Toxicol.* 1992;128:55–69.

56. St Omer VEV, Rottinghaus GE. Biochemical determination of cholinesterase activity in biological fluids and tissues. In: Ballantyne B, Marrs TC, eds. *Clinical and Experimental Toxicology of Organophosphates and Carbamates.* Oxford, Oxfordshire, England: Butterworth & Heinemann; 1992: 15–27.

57. Ellman GL, Courtney KD, Anders V Jr, Feather-stone RM. A new and rapid colorimetric determination of acetylcholinesterase activity. *Biochem Pharmacol.* 1961;7:88–95.

58. Worek F, Mast U, Kiderlen D, Diepold C, Eyer P. Improved determination of acetylcholinesterase activity in human whole blood. *Clin Chem Acta.* 1999;288:73–90.

59. Eyer P, Worek F, Kiderlen D,et al. Molar absorption coefficients for the reduced Ellman reagent: reassessment. *Anal Biochem.* 2003;312:224–227.

60. Doctor BP, Toker L, Roth E, Silman I. Microtiter assay for acetylcholinesterase. *Anal Biochem.* 1987;166:399–403.

61. Walter Reed Army Institute of Research. Whole Blood Assay. US patent 6,746,850. June 8, 2004.

62. Gordon RK, Haigh JR, Garcia GE, et al. Oral administration of pyridostigmine bromide and huperzine A protects human whole blood cholinesterases from ex vivo exposure to soman. *Chemico Biol Interact.* 2005;157–158:239–246.

63. EQM Research, Inc. Test-mate ChE Cholinesterase Test System. Web site. Available at http://www.eqmresearch.com/. Accessed January 19, 2007.

64. Taylor PW, Lukey BJ, Clark CR, Lee RB, Roussel RR. Field verification of Test-mate ChE. *Mil Med.* 2003;168:314–319.

65. Ellin RI, Burkhardt BH, Hart RD. A time-modified method for measuring red blood cell cholinesterase activity. *Arch Environ Health.* 1973;27:48–49.

66. Michel HO. An electrometric method for the determination of red blood cell and plasma cholinesterase activity. *J Lab Clinical Med.* 1949;34:1564–1568.

67. US Department of Defense Cholinesterase Reference Laboratory. *Standard operating procedure for the seventeen minute red blood cell acetylcholinesterase procedure.* US Army Center for Health Promotion and Preventative Medicine: Aberdeen Proving Ground, Md; 2002. SOP CRL 40-2.7.

68. US Department of Defense Cholinesterase Monitoring Program, Cholinesterase Reference Laboratory. Web site. Available at http://chppm-www.apgea.army.mil/dls/CHOLIN.HTM. Accessed January 19, 2007.

69. Dunn MA, Hackley BE, Sidell, FR. Pretreatment for nerve agent exposure. In: Sidell FR, Takafuji ET, Franz DR, eds. *Medical Aspects of Chemical and Biological Warfare.* In: Zajtchuk R, Bellamy RF, eds. *The Textbooks of Military Medicine.* Part I. Washington, DC: Department of the Army, Office of The Surgeon General, Borden Institute; 1997: 181–196.

70. Triggle DJ, Mitchell JM, Filler R. The pharmacology of physostigmine. *CNS Drug Rev.* 1998;4:87–136.

71. US Department of Health and Human Services. US Food and Drug Administration Web site. FDA approves pyridostigmine bromide as pretreatment against nerve gas. *FDA News.* PO3-08, February 5, 2003. Available at http://www.fda.gov/bbs/topics/NEWS/2003/NEW00870.html. Accessed: January 19, 2007.

72. Grunwald J, Raveh L, Doctor BP, Ashani Y. Huperzine A as a pretreatment candidate drug against nerve agent toxicity. *Life Sci.* 1994;54:991–997.

73. Jiang H, Luo X, Bai D. Progress in clinical, pharmacological, chemical and structural biological studies of huperzine A: a drug of traditional medicine origin for the treatment of Alzheimer's disease. *Curr Med Chem.* 2003;10:2231–2252.

74. Lallement G, Baille V, Baubichon D, et al. Review of the value of huperzine as pretreatment of organophosphate poisoning. *Neurotoxicology.* 2002;23:1–5.

75. Wang R, Yan H, Tang XC. Progress in studies of huperzine A, a natural cholinesterase inhibitor from Chinese herbal medicine. *Acta Pharmacol Sin.* 2006;27:1–26.

76. Raveh L, Grunwald J, Marcus D, Papier Y, Cohen, E, Ashani Y. Human butyrylcholinesterase as a general prophylactic antidote for nerve agent toxicity. In vitro and in vivo quantitative characterization. *Biochem Pharmacol.* 1993;45:2465–2474.

77. Yanagisawa N, Morita H, Nakajima T. Sarin experiences in Japan: acute toxicity and long-term effects. *J Neurol Sci.* 2006;249:76–85.

78. Papirmeister B, Feister AJ, Robinson SI, Ford RD. *Medical Defense Against Mustard Gas: Toxic Mechanisms and Pharmacological Implications*, Boca Raton, Fla: CRC Press; 1991: 91–122.

79. Black RM, Noort D. Methods for the retrospective detection of exposure to toxic scheduled chemicals. Part A: analysis of free metabolites. In: Mesilaakso M, ed. *Chemical Weapons Convention Chemicals Analysis: Sample Collection, Preparation, and Analytical Methods.* Chichester, West Sussex, England: John Wiley & Sons; 2005: 403–431.

80. Noort D, Black RM. Methods for the retrospective detection of exposure to toxic scheduled chemicals. Part B: mass spectrometric and immunochemical analysis of covalent adducts to proteins and DNA. In: Mesilaakso M, ed. *Chemical Weapons Convention Chemicals Analysis: Sample Collection, Preparation, and Analytical Methods.* Chichester, West Sussex, England: John Wiley & Sons; 2005: 433–451.

81. Vycudilik W. Detection of mustard gas bis(2-chloroethyl)-sulfide in urine. *Forensic Sci Int.* 1985;28:131–136.

82. Vycudilik W. Detection of bis(2-chloroethyl)-sulfide (Yperite) in urine by high resolution gas chromatography-mass spectrometry. *Forensic Sci Int.* 1987;35:67–71.

83. Wils ERJ, Hulst AG, de Jong AL, Verweij A, Boter HL. Analysis of thiodiglycol in urine of victims of an alleged attack with mustard gas. *J Anal Toxicol.* 1985;9:254–257.

84. Wils ERJ, Hulst AG, van Laar J. Analysis of thiodiglycol in urine of victims of an alleged attack with mustard gas, part II. *J Anal Toxicol.* 1988;12:15–19.

85. Drasch G, Kretschmer E, Kauert G, von Meyer L. Concentrations of mustard gas [bis(2-chloroethyl)sulfide] in the tissues of a victim of a vesicant exposure. *J Forensic Sci.* 1987;32:1788–1793.

86. Black RM, Read RW. Detection of trace levels of thiodiglycol in blood, plasma and urine using gas chromatography-electron-capture negative-ion chemical ionisation mass spectrometry. *J Chromatogr.* 1988;449: 261–270.

87. Jakubowski EM, Woodard CL, Mershon MM, Dolzine TW. Quantification of thiodiglycol in urine by electron ionization gas chromatography-mass spectrometry. *J Chromatogr.* 1990;528:184–190.

88. Black RM, Read RW. Improved methodology for the detection and quantitation of urinary metabolites of sulphur mustard using gas chromatography-tandem mass spectrometry. *J Chromatogr B Biomed Appl.* 1995;665:97–105.

89. Boyer AE, Ash D, Barr DB, et al. Quantitation of the sulfur mustard metabolites 1,1′-sulfonylbis[2-(methylthio)ethane] and thiodiglycol in urine using isotope-dilution gas chromatography-tandem mass spectrometry. *J Anal Toxicol.* 2004;28:327–332.

90. Black RM, Read RW. Methods for the analysis of thiodiglycol sulphoxide, a metabolite of sulphur mustard, in urine using gas chromatography-mass spectrometry. *J Chromatogr.* 1991;558:393–404.

91. Black RM, Read RW. Biological fate of sulphur mustard, 1,1′-thiobis(2-chloroethane): identification of beta-lyase metabolites and hydrolysis products in human urine. *Xenobiotica.* 1995;25:167–173.

92. Black RM, Brewster K, Clarke RJ, Hambrook JL, Harrison JM, Howells DJ. Biological fate of sulphur mustard, 1,1′-thiobis(2-chloroethane): isolation and identification of urinary metabolites following intraperitoneal administration to rat. *Xenobiotica.* 1992;22:405–418.

93. Black RM, Hambrook JL, Howells DJ, Read RW. Biological fate of sulfur mustard, 1,1′-thiobis(2-chloroethane). Urinary excretion profiles of hydrolysis products and beta-lyase metabolites of sulfur mustard after cutaneous application in rats. *J Anal Toxicol.* 1992;16:79–84.

94. Black RM, Clarke RJ, Read RW. Analysis of 1,1′-sulphonylbis[2-(methylsulphinyl)ethane] and 1-methylsulphinyl-2-[2-(methylthio)ethylsulphonyl]ethane, metabolites of sulphur mustard, in urine using gas chromatography-mass spectrometry. *J Chromatogr.* 1991;558:405–414.

95. Young CL, Ash D, Driskell WJ, et al. A rapid, sensitive method for the quantitation of specific metabolites of sulfur mustard in human urine using isotope-dilution gas chromatography-tandem mass spectrometry. *J Anal Toxicol.* 2004;28:339–345.

96. Read RW, Black RM. Analysis of beta-lyase metabolites of sulfur mustard in urine by electrospray liquid chromatography-tandem mass spectrometry. *J Anal Toxicol.* 2004;28:346–351.

97. Read RW, Black RM. Analysis of the sulfur mustard metabolite 1,1′-sulfonylbis[2-S-(N-acetylcysteinyl)ethane] in urine by negative ion electrospray liquid chromatography-tandem mass spectrometry. *J Anal Toxicol.* 2004;28:352–356.

98. Fidder A, Noort D, de Jong LP, Benschop HP, Hulst AG. N7-(2-hydroxyethylthioethyl)-guanine: a novel urinary metabolite following exposure to sulphur mustard. *Arch Toxicol.* 1996;70:854–855.

99. Sandelowsky I, Simon GA, Bel P, Barak R, Vincze A. N1-(2-hydroxyethylthioethyl)-4-methyl imidazole (4-met-1-imid-thiodiglycol) in plasma and urine: a novel metabolite following dermal exposure to sulphur mustard. *Arch Toxicol.* 1992;66:296–297.

100. Price EO, Smith JR, Clark CR, Schlager JJ, Shih ML. MALDI-ToF/MS as a diagnostic tool for the confirmation sulfur mustard exposure. *J Appl Toxicol.* 2000;20(suppl 1):S193–S197.

101. Willems JL. Clinical management of mustard gas casualties. *Ann Med Milit (Belgium).* 1989;3(suppl):1–61.

102. Jakubowski EM, Sidell FR, Evans RA, et al. Quantification of thiodiglycol in human urine after an accidental sulfur mustard exposure. *Toxicol Methods.* 2000;10:143–150.

103. Carroll LS. Sulfur mustard: cutaneous exposure. *Clin Toxicol (Phila).* 2005;43(1):55.

104. Newmark J, Langer JM, Capacio B, Barr J, McIntosh RG. Liquid sulfur mustard exposure. *Mil Med.* 2007;172(2):196–198.

105. Barr JR, Young CL, Woolfit AR, et al. Comprehensive quantitative tandem MS analysis of urinary metabolites and albumin adducts following an accidental human exposure to sulfur mustard. In: *Proceedings of the 53rd Conference of the American Society of Mass Spectrometry.* San Antonio, Tex: June 5–9, 2005.

106. Ludlum DB, Austin-Ritchie P, Hagopian M, Niu TQ, Yu D. Detection of sulfur mustard-induced DNA modifications. *Chem Biol Interact.* 1994;91:39–49.

107. Van der Schans GP, Scheffer AG, Mars-Groenendijk RH, Fidder A, Benschop HP, Baan RA. Immunochemical detection of adducts of sulfur mustard to DNA of calf thymus and human white blood cells. *Chem Res Toxicol.* 1994;7:408–413.

108. Van der Schans GP, Mars-Groenendijk R, de Jong LP, Benschop HP, Noort D. Standard operating procedure for immunoslotblot assay for analysis of DNA/sulfur mustard adducts in human blood and skin. *J Anal Toxicol.* 2004;28:316–319.

109. Fidder A, Moes GWH, Scheffer AG, et al. Synthesis, characterization, and quantitation of the major adducts formed between sulfur mustard and DNA of calf thymus and human blood. *Chem Res Toxicol.* 1994;7:199–204.

110. Noort D, Verheij ER, Hulst AG, de Jong LP, Benschop HP. Characterization of sulfur mustard induced structural modifications in human hemoglobin by liquid chromatography-tandem mass spectrometry. *Chem Res Toxicol.* 1996;9:781–787.

111. Black RM, Harrison JM, Read RW. Biological fate of sulphur mustard: in vitro alkylation of human haemoglobin by sulphur mustard. *Xenobiotica.* 1997;27:11–32.

112. Noort D, Hulst AG, Trap HC, de Jong LPA, Benschop HP. Synthesis and mass spectrometric identification of the major amino acid adducts formed between sulphur mustard and haemoglobin in human blood. *Arch Toxicol.* 1997;71:171–178.

113. Fidder A, Noort D, de Jong AL, Trap HC, de Jong LPA, Benschop HP. Monitoring of in vitro and in vivo exposure to sulfur mustard by GC/MS determination of the N-terminal valine adduct in hemoglobin after a modified Edman degradation. *Chem Res Toxicol.* 1996;9:788–792.

114. Black RM, Clarke RJ, Harrison JM, Read RW. Biological fate of sulphur mustard: identification of valine and histidine adducts in haemoglobin from casualties of sulphur mustard poisoning. *Xenobiotica.* 1997;27:499–512.

115. Noort D, Hulst AG, de Jong LP, Benschop HP. Alkylation of human serum albumin by sulfur mustard in vitro and in vivo: mass spectrometric analysis of a cysteine adduct as a sensitive biomarker of exposure. *Chem Res Toxicol.* 1999;12:715–721.

116. Noort D, Fidder A, Hulst AG, Woolfitt AR, Ash D, Barr JR. Retrospective detection of exposure to sulfur mustard: improvements on an assay for liquid chromatography-tandem mass spectrometry analysis of albumin-sulfur mustard adducts. *J Anal Toxicol.* 2004;28:333–338.

117. Noort D, Fidder A, Hulst AG, de Jong LP, Benschop HP. Diagnosis and dosimetry of exposure to sulfur mustard: development of a standard operating procedure for mass spectrometric analysis of haemoglobin adducts: exploratory research on albumin and keratin adducts. *J Appl Toxicol.* 2000;20(suppl 1):S187–S192.

118. Capacio BR, Smith JR, DeLion MT, et al. Monitoring sulfur mustard exposure by gas chromatography-mass spectrometry analysis of thiodiglycol cleaved from blood proteins. *J Anal Toxicol.* 2004;28:306–310.

119. Noort D, Fidder A, Benschop HP, de Jong LP, Smith JR. Procedure for monitoring exposure to sulfur mustard based on modified edman degradation of globin. *J Anal Toxicol.* 2004;28:311–315.

120. Benschop HP, van der Schans GP, Noort D, Fidder A, Mars-Groenendijk RH, de Jong LP. Verification of exposure to sulfur mustard in two casualties of the Iran-Iraq conflict. *J Anal Toxicol.* 1997;21:249–251.

121. Benschop HP, Noort D, van der Schans GP, de Jong LP. Diagnosis and dosimetry of exposure to sulfur mustard: development of standard operating procedures; further exploratory research on protein adducts. Rijswijk, The Netherlands: TNO Prins Maurits Laboratory; 2000. Final report DAMD17-97-2-7002, ADA381035.

122. Korte WD, Walker EM, Smith JR, et al. The determination of sulfur mustard exposure by analysis of blood protein adducts. *Wehrmed Mschr.* 2005;49:327.

123. United Nations Security Council. *Report of the mission dispatched by the Secretary-General to investigate allegations of the use of chemical weapons in the conflict between the Islamic Republic of Iran and Iraq.* New York, NY: UN; 1986. Report S/17911.

124. Van der Schans GP, Noort D, Mars-Groenendijk RH, et al. Immunochemical detection of sulfur mustard adducts with keratins in the stratum corneum of human skin. *Chem Res Toxicol.* 2002;15:21–25.

125. Smith JR, Logan TP, Szafraniec LL, Jakubowski EM. Spectroscopic characterization of the geminal isomer of Lewisite. *Anal Lett.* 1995;28:1541–1554.

126. Waters WA, Williams JH. Hydrolyses and derivatives of some vesicant arsenicals. *J Chem Soc.* 1950; 18–22.

127. Jakubowski EM, Smith JR, Logan TP, et al. Verification of Lewisite exposure: quantification of chlorovinylarsonous acid in biological samples. In: *Proceedings of the 1993 Medical Defense Bioscience Review.* Aberdeen Proving Ground, Md: US Army Medical Research Institute of Chemical Defense; 1993. AD A275667.

128. Wooten JV, Ashley DL, Calafat AM. Quantitation of 2-chlorovinylarsonous acid in human urine by automated solid-phase microextraction-gas chromatography-mass spectrometry. *J Chromatogr B Analyt Technol Biomed Life Sci.* 2002;772:147–153.

129. Logan TP, Smith JR, Jakubowski EM, Nielson RE. Verification of lewisite exposure by the analysis of 2-chlorovinyl arsonous acid in urine. *Toxicol Meth.* 1999;9:275–284.

130. Fidder A, Noort D, Hulst AG, de Jong LP, Benschop HP. Biomonitoring of exposure to lewisite based on adducts to haemoglobin. *Arch Toxicol.* 2000;74:207–214.

131. US Department of Health and Human Services, Public Health Service, Agency for Toxic Substances and Disease Registry. Toxicological profile for cyanide. Atlanta, Ga: USDHHS; 1997.

132. Hibbs CM. Cyanide and nitrate toxicoses of cattle. *Vet Hum Toxicol.* 1979;21:401–403.

133. Conn EE. Introduction. In: Evered D, Harnett S, eds. *Cyanide Compounds in Biology.* Chichester, West Sussex, England: John Wiley & Sons; 1988: 1–2.

134. Purser DA, Grimshaw P, Berrill KR. Intoxication of cyanide in fires: a study in monkeys using polyacrylonitrile. *Arch Environ Health.* 1984:39:394–400.

135. Blanc P, Hogan M, Mallin K, Hryhorczuk D, Hessl S, Bernard B. Cyanide intoxication among silver-reclaiming workers. *JAMA.* 1985;253:367–371.

136. Izraeli S, Israeli A, Danon Y. Pharmacological treatment of cyanide poisoning. *Harefuah.* 1988;114:338–342.

137. Kirk RL, Stenhouse NS. Ability to smell solutions of potassium cyanide. *Nature.* 1953;171:698–699.

138. Warburg O. Inhibition of the action of prussic acid in living cells. *Hoppe-Seyler's Z Physiol Chem.* 1911;76:331–346.

139. Keilin D. Cytochrome and respiratory enzymes. *Proc R Soc Lond B Biol Sci.* 1929;104:206–251.

140. DiPalma JR. Noxious gases and vapers: I. Carbon monoxide, cyanide, methemoglobin, and sulfhemoglobin. In: *Drills Pharmacology in Medicine.* New York, NY: McGraw-Hill; 1971: 1189–1205.

141. Way JL. Cyanide intoxication and its mechanism of antagonism. *Annu Rev Pharmacol Toxicol.* 1984;24:451–481.

142. Farooqui MY, Ahmed AE. Molecular interaction of acrylonitrile and potassium cyanide with rat blood. *Chem Biol Interact.* 1982;38:145–159.

143. Blakley RL, Coop IE. The metabolism and toxicity of cyanides and cyanogenic blycosides in sheep. *NZ J Sci Technol.* 1949;31A(3):1–16.

144. Wood JL, Cooley SL. Detoxification of cyanide by cystine. *J Biol Chem.* 1956;218:449–457.

145. Smith RP. Toxic responses of the blood. In: Casarett LJ, Amdur MO, Doull J, Klaassen CD, eds. *Casarett & Doull's Toxicology: The Basic Science of Poisons.* 10th ed. McGraw-Hill; 1995: 335–354.

146. Ansell M, Lewis FA. A review of cyanide concentrations found in human organs. A survey of literature concerning cyanide metabolism, 'normal', non-fatal, and fatal cyanide levels. *J Forensic Med.*1970;17:148–155.

147. Seto Y. Stability and spontaneous production of blood cyanide during heating. *J Forensic Sci.* 1996;41:465–468.

148. Ballantyne C. Artifacts in the definition of toxicity by cyanides and cyanogens. *Fundam Appl Toxicol.* 1983;3:400-408.

149. Mathur BB, Krishna G. Toxicodynamics of phosgene. In: Somani S, ed. *Chemical Warfare Agents.* San Diego, Calif: Academic Press, Inc; 1992: 237–254.

150. Malveda M. CEH Product review: phosgene. In: SRI International. *Chemical Economics Handbook.* Menlo Park, Calif: SRI International; 2003: 687.

151. Focused on phosgene. *Chemistry Business.* 2002;30–31.

152. Sartori M. *The War Gases.* New York, NY: D Van Nostrand; 1939.

153. Parshall, GW. Trends in processing and manufacturing that will affect implementation of the Chemical Weapons Convention. *Pure Appl Chem.* 2002;74:2259–2263.

154. Diller WF. Medical phosgene problems and their possible solution. *J Occup Med.* 1978;20:189–193.

155. US National Research Council Committee on Toxicology. *Emergency and Continuous Exposure Limits for Selected Airborne Contaminants.* Vol 1. Washington, DC: National Academy Press; 1984.

156. Borak J, Diller WF. Phosgene exposure: mechanisms of injury and treatment strategies. *J Occup Environ Med.* 2001;43:110–119.

157. Diller WF. Pathogenesis of phosgene poisoning. *Toxicol Ind Health.* 1985;1:7–15.

158. National Institute for Occupational Health and Safety. *Pocket Guide to Chemical Hazards.* Washington, DC: NIOSH; 2004.

159. Cucinell SA. Review of the toxicity of long-term phosgene exposure. *Arch Environ Health.* 1974;28:272–275.

160. Polednak AP. Mortality among men occupationally exposed to phosgene in 1943–1945. *Environ Res.* 1980;22:357–367.

161. Diller WF, Zante R. Dose-effect relations in the effects of phosgene on man and animals. Literature review. *Zentralblatt fuer Arbeitsmedizin, Arbeitsschutz, Prophylaxe Ergonomie.* 1982;32:360–4, 366–368.

162. Pastore A, Federici G, Bertini E, Piemonte F. Analysis of glutathione: implication in redox and detoxification. *Clin Chim Acta.* 2003;333:19–39.

163. Richie JP Jr, Skowronski L, Abraham P, Leutzinger Y. Blood glutathione concentrations in a large-scale human study. *Clin Chem.* 1996;42:64–70.

164. Reed DJ, Fariss MW. Glutathione depletion and susceptibility. *Pharmacol Rev.* 1994;36(suppl 2):25–33.

165. Pohl LR., Branchflower RV, Highest RJ, et al. The formation of diglutathionyl dithiocarbonate as a metabolite of chloroform, bromotrichloromethane, and carbon tetrachloride. *Drug Metab Dispos.* 1981;9:334–339.

166. Fabrizi L, Taylor GW, Edwards RJ, Boobis AR. Adducts of the chloroform metabolite phosgene. *Adv Exp Med Biol.* 2001;500:129–132.

167. Anders MW, Stevens JL, Sprague RW, Shaath, Z, Ahmed AE. Metabolism of haloforms to carbon monoxide. II. In vivo studies. *Drug Metab Dispos.* 1978:6:556–560.

168. Sciuto AM, Strickland PT, Kennedy TP, Gurtner GH. Postexposure treatment with aminophylline protects against phosgene-induced acute lung injury. *Exp Lung Res.* 1997;23:317–332.

169. Sciuto AM, Hurt HH. Therapeutic treatments of phosgene-induced lung injury. *Inhal Toxicol.* 2004;16:565–580.

170. Sciuto AM. Assessment of early acute lung injury in rodents exposed to phosgene. *Arch Toxicol.* 1998;72:283–288.

171. Sciuto AM, Cascio MB, Moran TS, Forster JS. The fate of antioxidant enzymes in bronchoalveolar lavage fluid over 7 days in mice with acute lung injury. *Inhal Toxicol.* 2003;15:675–685.

172. Kubic VL, Anders MW. Metabolism of carbon tetrachloride to phosgene. *Life Sci.* 1980;26:2151–2155.

173. Gwilt PR, Radick LE, Li XY, Whalen JJ, Leaf CD. Pharmacokinetics of 2-oxothiazolidine-4-carboxylate, a cysteine prodrug, and cysteine. *J Clin Pharmacol.* 1998;38:945–950.

174. Pastore A, Massoud R, Motti C, et al. Fully automated assay for total homocysteine, cysteine, cysteinylglycine, glutathione, cysteamine and 2-mercaptopropionylglycine in plasma and urine. *Clin Chem.* 1998;44:825–832.

175. Boettcher B, Meister A. Synthesis of L-2-oxothiazolidine-4-carboxylic acid. *Anal Biochem.* 1984;138:449–450.

176. Porta P, Aebi S, Summer K, Lauterburg BH. L-2-oxothiazolidine-4-carboxylic acid, a cysteine prodrug: pharmacokinetics and effects on thiols in plasma and lymphocytes in human. *J Pharmacol Exp Ther.* 1991;257:331–334.

177. Kling A. Acute pulmonary edema following exposure to war gases. *Comptes Rendus De L'Academie des Sciences.* 1933;197:1782–1784.

178. Cowlen MS, Hewitt WR, Schroeder F. 2-hexanone potentiation of [14C]chloroform hepatotoxicity: covalent interaction of a reactive intermediate with rat liver phospholipid. *Toxicol Appl Pharmacol.* 1984;73:478–491.

179. De Biasi A, Sbraccia M, Keizer J, Testai E, Vittozzi L. The regioselective binding of CHCI3 reactive intermediates to microsomal phospholipids. *Chem Biol Interact.* 1992;85:229–242.

180. Guastadisegni C, Guidoni L, Balduzzi M, Viti V, Di Consiglio E, Vittozzi L. Characterization of a phospholipid adduct formed in Sprague Dawley rats by chloroform metabolism: NMR studies. *J Biochem Mol Toxicol.* 1998;12:93–102.

181. Guastadisegni C, Balduzzi M, Mancuso MT, Di Consiglio E. Liver mitochondria alterations in chloroform-treated Sprague-Dawley rats. *J Toxicol Environ Health A*. 1999;57:415–429.

182. Di Consiglio E, De Angelis G, Testai E, Vittozzi L. Correlation of a specific mitochondrial phospholipid-phosgene adduct with chloroform acute toxicity. *Toxicology*. 2001;159:43–53.

183. Jugg B, Jenner J, Rice P. The effect of perfluoroisobutene and phosgene on rat lavage fluid surfactant phospholipids. *Hum Exp Toxicol*. 1999;18:659–668.

184. Pereira MA, Chang LW, Ferguson JL, Couri D. Binding of chloroform to the cysteine of hemoglobin. *Chem Biol Interact*. 1984;51:115–124.

185. Sciuto AM, Stotts RR, Chittenden V, Choung E, Heflin MD. Changes in absorbance at 413 nm in plasma from three rodent species exposed to phosgene. *Biochem Biophys Res Commun*. 1996;226:906–911.

186. Noort D, Hulst AG, Fidder A, van Gurp RA, de Jong LP, Benschop HP. In vitro adduct formation of phosgene with albumin and hemoglobin in human blood. *Chem Res Toxicol*. 2000;13:719–726.

187. Sciuto AM, Carpin LB, Moran TS, Forster JS. Chronological changes in electrolyte levels in arterial blood and bronchoalveolar lavage fluid in mice after exposure to an edemagenic gas. *Inhal Toxicol*. 2003;15:663–674.

188. Currie WD, Hatch GE, Frosolono MF. Pulmonary alterations in rats due to acute phosgene inhalation. *Fundam Appl Toxicol*. 1987;8:107–114.

189. Byrd GD, Paule RC, Sander LC, Sniegoski LT, White E 5th, Bausum HT. Determination of 3-quinuclidinyl benzilate (QNB) and its major metabolites in urine by isotope dilution gas chromatography/mass spectrometry. *J Anal Toxicol*. 1992;16:182–187.

Chapter 23

DOMESTIC PREPAREDNESS

CAROL A. BOSSONE, DVM, PhD*; KENNETH DESPAIN, DVM†; and SHIRLEY D. TUORINSKY, MSN‡

*Lieutenant Colonel, US Army; Director of Toxicology, United States Army Center for Health Promotion and Preventive Medicine, 5158 Blackhawk Drive, Aberdeen Proving Ground, Maryland 21010

†Lieutenant Colonel, US Army; Commander, Rocky Mountain District Veterinary Command, 1661 O'Connell Boulevard, Building 1012, Fort Carson, Colorado 80913-5108

‡Lieutenant Colonel, AN, US Army; Executive Officer, Combat Casualty Care Division, United States Army Medical Research Institute of Chemical Defense, 3100 Ricketts Point Road, Aberdeen Proving Ground, Maryland 21010

INTRODUCTION

Major emergencies like the terrorist attacks of September 11, 2001, and the following anthrax mailings, as well as the devastating effects of Hurricane Katrina and the emerging threat of avian influenza are currently fresh in Americans' memories. Military healthcare providers have a role in responding to national events, whether terrorist attacks, natural disasters, or emerging diseases. This chapter outlines the organizational framework within which military healthcare providers will operate. The following pages will discuss how military healthcare providers are expected to interact with local, state, and federal agencies while remaining in a military chain of command when reacting to national emergencies. The strategy and primary goal of federal and civilian counterterrorism agencies is to deter attacks. Natural catastrophes and human-made accidents require diligence in awareness and preparedness activities to coordinate operations, prevent and safeguard lives, and protect economic interests and commodities.

This is an introduction to national measures and policies as well as to medical resources, training, and exercises available to military healthcare providers. Effective information flow is crucial to the success of a proper and well-organized emergency response for chemical, biological, radiological, nuclear, or explosive (CBRNE) incidents. Learning about the military healthcare provider's role in preparing for such an event and becoming familiar with the organizational framework and expectations of disaster preparedness results in a healthcare force that is prepared to assist in the biomedical arena of national defense.

NATIONAL CIVILIAN PREPAREDNESS (1990–2001)

The fundamental tenet of disaster response in the United States is that disasters are local. As a result, local authorities are primarily responsible for responding to incidents, whether natural or human-made. However, state and regional authorities and assets can assist upon request from the local governing body and federal assets can assist upon request of the state governor. Most states authorize either a city council, board of supervisors, or other authority sanctioned by a local ordinance to request help should a local government be unable to handle a disaster. This local governing body, or "incident command system," can request state aid. Prior to 2001 domestic preparedness efforts at local, state, and federal levels were often poorly coordinated and disruptive because of disputes over authority, particularly when legal and recovery priorities clashed. Existing federal legislation and policy was comprehensive but inconsistent and did not adequately address the full range of antiterrorism and counterterrorism actions necessary to deal with the risk of, or recovery from, a major terrorist action using chemical, biological, or nuclear weapons of mass destruction (WMDs). Disasters and terrorist attacks can take on many forms and preparedness plans require measuring risk against the potential for damage.

Incidents such as the bombings of the World Trade Center in 1993, Oklahoma City's Murrah Federal Building in 1995, and Atlanta's Olympic Centennial Park in 1996 and the Tokyo sarin attack in 1995 all highlighted inadequacies in capability and readiness to avert and manage large-scale terrorist events. Review of the events resulted in agencies understanding the importance of a coordinated response and the impact of proper communication on positive outcomes. The above experiences led to a series of policies designed to ensure interagency coordination and communication. However, these policies are complicated, which may partially explain the degraded state of coordination and communication between agencies when the September 11, 2001, attacks occurred.

After the sarin gas attacks in Tokyo and the Oklahoma City bombing, President Bill Clinton signed presidential decision directives 39 and 62.[1,2] These directives outline policy for deterring and responding to terrorism through detecting, preventing, and managing WMD incidents. *Presidential Decision Directive 39* also defines domestic and international threats and separates the nation's response to these events into what are called "crisis responses" and "consequence management responses." Crisis responses involve proactive, preventative operations intended to avert incidents and support post-event law enforcement activities for legal action against the perpetrators. Consequence management refers to operations focused on post-incident activities intended to assist in damage recovery. This phase of recovery includes tasks such as restoring public services, safeguarding public health, offering emergency relief, providing security to protect casualties, staffing response agencies, and guaranteeing information flow and infrastructure stability.

In Public Law 104-201 (the National Defense Authorization Act for Fiscal Year 1997, Title XIV, "Defense against Weapons of Mass Destruction," commonly referred to as the "Nunn-Lugar-Domenici legislation"), Congress implemented presidential decision directives 39 and 62, which directed and supported an enhanced federal effort toward preventing and responding to terrorist incidents.[3] One of these efforts led to the formation of a senior interagency group on terrorism, chaired by the Federal Emergency Management Agency (FEMA). This group coordinated federal policy issues among agencies and with state and local governments.[4] At this time the Department of Defense (DoD) outlined its responsibilities, oversight, and execution plan aimed at preparedness and response.

Section 1412 of Title XIV directed and equipped the secretary of defense to carry out a program providing civilian personnel of federal, state, and local agencies with training and expert advice regarding emergency responses to the use or threatened use of a WMD or related materials.[3] This policy became known as the "120 Cities Program" and focused on improving coordination between emergency response planners and executors at the 120 largest metropolitan centers in the United States. Section 1413 directed and equipped the secretary of defense to coordinate DoD assistance to federal, state, and local officials when responding to threats involving biological or chemical weapons (or related materials or technologies) and to coordinate with the Department of Energy for similar assistance with nuclear weapons and related materials.[3] Section 1415 directed and equipped the secretary of defense to develop and carry out a program for testing and improving federal, state, and local responses to emergencies involving biological weapons and related materials. Section 1416 directed limited DoD support to the attorney general and civilian law enforcement in emergency situations involving biological or chemical weapons.[3] The preexisting Federal Response Plan assigned specific emergency support functions (ESFs) to the DoD in the event of a local incident of sufficient magnitude to involve federal assets. Public Law 104-102 therefore expanded and clarified the DoD's responsibilities to prepare the nation's emergency response assets for a chemical, biological, or radiological incident and also clarified the nature of the DoD's cooperative relationships with other agencies. In 1999 many of those responsibilities transferred to the US Department of Justice.

DOMESTIC PREPAREDNESS AFTER SEPTEMBER 11, 2001

By September 11, 2001, many domestic preparedness initiatives and programs were already in place, but a coordinated response effort was lacking.[3,5,6] The response following September 11, 2001, demonstrated gaps in existing policy and practice as well as the need for a more expanded approach, more unified structure, and closer coordination. Creating the White House Office of Homeland Security on Oct 8, 2001, was the first step toward improving the US emergency response posture. The office published the *National Strategy for Homeland Security* in July 2002. This strategy provides guidelines and a framework by which the federal, state, and local governments, as well private companies and civilians, can organize a more cohesive response network for the nation. As part of the strategy, President George W Bush established the US Department of Homeland Security (DHS) in June 2002 to unite efforts across different agencies involved in homeland security and "clarify lines of responsibility for Homeland Security in the Executive Branch."[7]

National Strategy for Homeland Security and Homeland Security Presidential Directives

On October 29, 2001, *Homeland Security Presidential Directive 1* was issued, becoming one of the first directives to increase the security of US citizens by organizing a homeland security council.[8] The homeland security council's overarching role is to ensure there is coordination between all executive agencies (eg, secretary of defense, US Department of Health and Human Services [DHHS], US Federal Bureau of Investigation, DHS, etc) involved in activities related to homeland security. *Homeland Security Presidential Directive 3* was issued in March 2002, directing the homeland security advisory system to provide a comprehensive means to disseminate information regarding terrorist acts.[9] This system, administered by the DHS, provides current information related to threats and vulnerabilities and provides the information to the public. The DHS communicated this information by means of a color-coded threat condition chart (Figure 23-1).[9]

With more than 87,000 distinct jurisdictions, the United States faces a unique challenge when coordinating efforts across federal, state, and local governments. In February 2003 the president issued *Homeland Security Presidential Directive 5*.[10] This directive established the DHS as the lead federal agency for domestic incident management and homeland security. The secretary of homeland security coordinates the federal government's resources to prevent, prepare for, respond to, and recover from natural and human-made disasters. The *National Strategy for Homeland Security* provides the direction and framework for all government agencies to follow that have roles in homeland security.[7]

National Incident Management System and the National Response Plan

In 2003, under *Homeland Security Presidential Directive 5*, the secretary of homeland security was tasked to develop and administer the National Incident

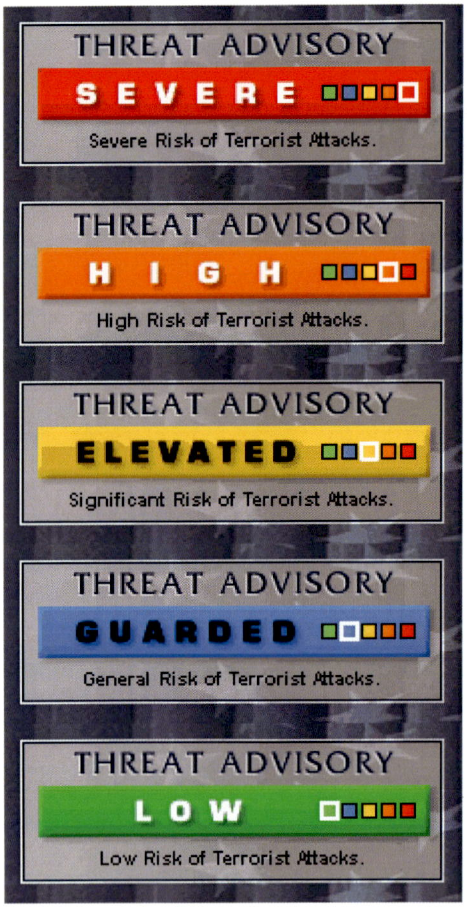
THREAT ADVISORY
SEVERE
Severe Risk of Terrorist Attacks.
THREAT ADVISORY
HIGH
High Risk of Terrorist Attacks.
THREAT ADVISORY
ELEVATED
Significant Risk of Terrorist Attacks.
THREAT ADVISORY
GUARDED
General Risk of Terrorist Attacks.
THREAT ADVISORY
LOW
Low Risk of Terrorist Attacks.

Fig. 23-1. The National Homeland Security Advisory System. The five threat conditions are outlined in Homeland Security Presidential Directive 3.
Reproduced from: US Office of Homeland Security. Homeland Security Advisory System. Washington, DC: Office of the Press Secretary; 2002. Homeland Security Presidential Directive 3.

Management System (NIMS)[10,11] and the National Response Plan (NRP).[12] The NIMS outlines how federal, state, local, and tribal communities will prevent, prepare for, respond to, and recover from domestic incidents. The NRP encompasses the NIMS and provides the structure and operational direction for the coordinated effort. All federal agencies are required to use NIMS in their domestic incident management and emergency programs. NIMS outlines a nationwide approach for federal, state, and local governments and agencies for use in command and multiagency coordination systems. It also outlines training and plans for resource management, as well as components that are used to facilitate responses to domestic incidents. These components include command and management, preparedness, resource management, and communications and information management.[11]

The command and management component of NIMS emphasizes structure (incident command systems) and organization (multiagency coordination systems) and has an additional role in informing the public of an incident. These systems involve every level of government, including DoD, with the optimum goal of facilitating management and operations. The overall structure and template for the command and management section outlines a unified command under an incident command and staff. With a unified command, no agency's legal authority is compromised and a joint effort across all agencies is achieved.

This "national domestic all-hazards preparedness goal" provides for incident-specific resources.[13] The preparedness component of NIMS is made up of activities that include planning, training, exercises, personnel qualification and certification, equipment acquisition and certification, mutual aid, and publications management. This component represents the focus of many jurisdictional levels and crosses many agencies that are responsible for incident management.[11]

NIMS unifies incident-management and resource-allocation. Under NIMS, preparedness encompasses the full range of deliberate and critical activities necessary to build, sustain, and improve the operational capability to prevent, protect against, respond to, and recover from domestic incidents. Preparedness, in the context of an actual or potential incident, involves actions to enhance readiness and minimize impacts; it includes hazard-mitigation measures to save lives and protect property from the impacts of events such as terrorism and natural disasters.[12]

Preparedness requires a well-conceived plan that encompasses emergency operations plans and procedures. NIMS outlines how personnel, equipment, and resources will be used to support incident management.[11] The plan includes all entities and functions that are critical to incident management, such as priorities and the availability of resources.[11,12] NIMS training and exercise activities outline multiagency standard courses that cross both agent-specific and discipline-specific areas. Exercises focus on all actively participating jurisdictions and agencies and on disciplines working and coordinating efforts and optimizing resources. These kinds of exercises allow for improvements built on experience.[11–13]

The NRP superseded the Federal Response Plan and several other earlier plans and provided for a more unified effort.[12] The NRP outlined and integrated the federal government's domestic prevention, preparedness, response, and recovery plans across many disciplines and hazards.

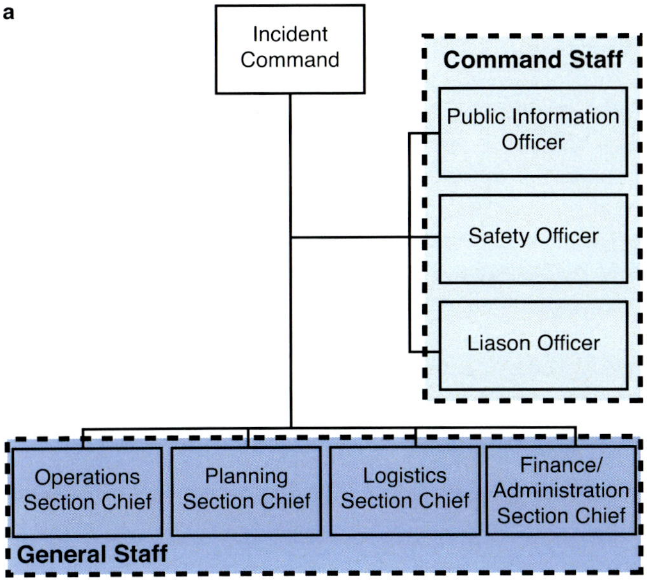

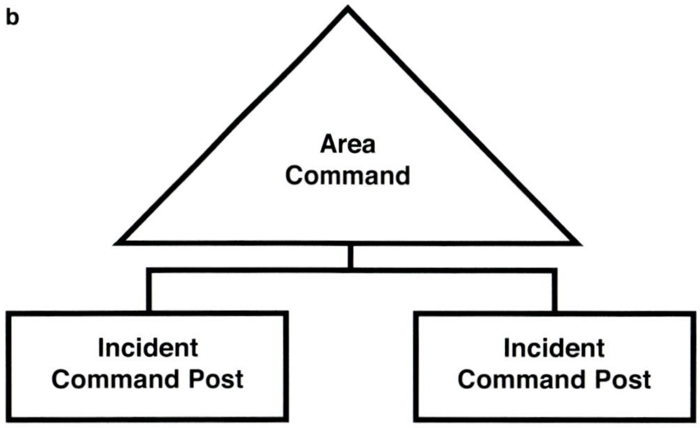

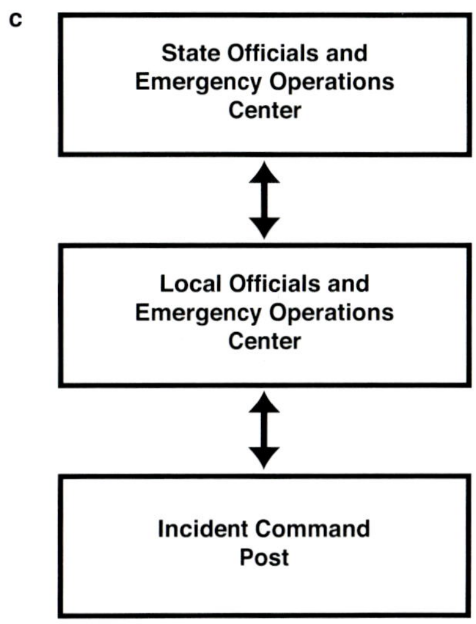

Fig. 23-2. Organizational outline for incident management command. The structures address local, field, state and joint field office national incident response organization. **(a)** Local responders use the incident command structure. **(b)** Field-level area command structure. **(c)** State and emergency operations center. **(d)** Overview of the joint field office and its key components
Reproduced from: US Department of Homeland Security. *National Response Framework*. Washington, DC: DHS; 2008.

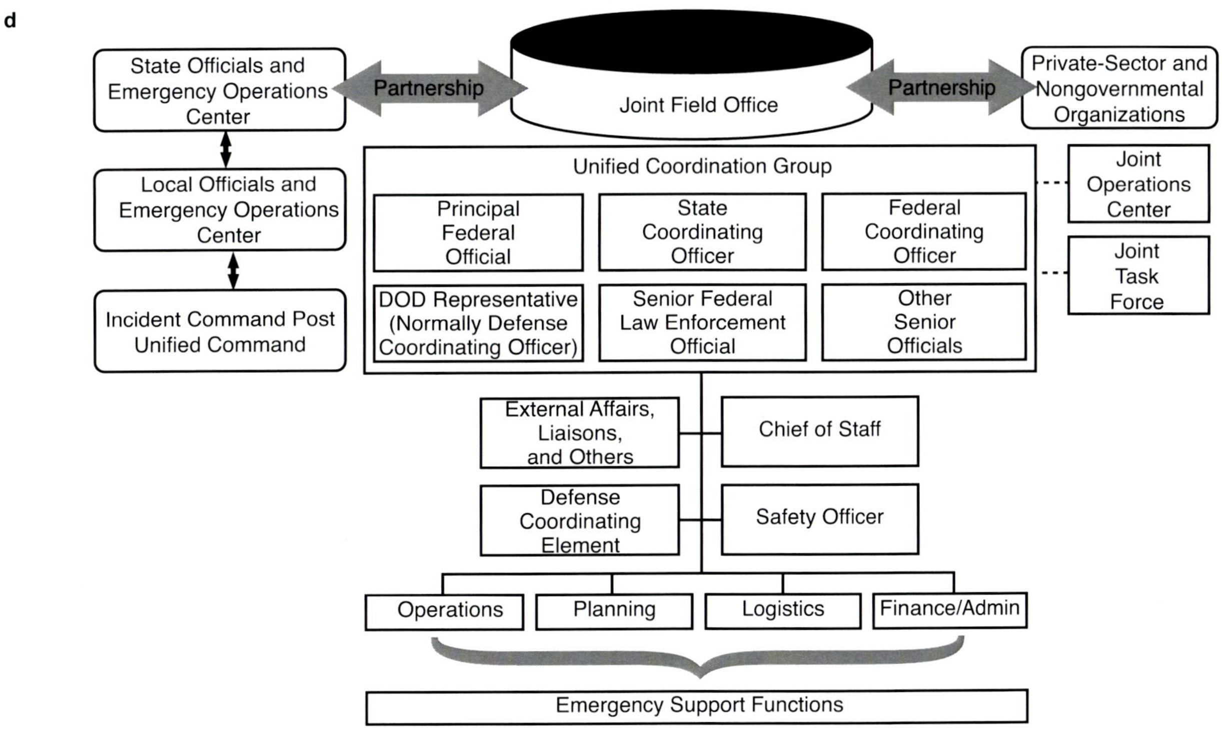

National Response Framework

In 2008 the NRP will be replaced by National Response Framework (NRF), which will guide the nation in incident response. The NRF ensures that government executives and nongovernment organizations, leaders, emergency management personnel, and the private segments across the country understand domestic incident response roles.

The NRF provides a structure for implementing national-level policy and operational coordination for domestic incident response. The NRF addresses actual or potential emergencies, hazard events (ranging from accidents to natural disasters), and actual or potential terrorist attacks. These incidents could range from modest events that are contained within a single community to ones that are catastrophic and create national consequences.

The NRF includes a wider incident audience than the NRP, including executive leadership, emergency management personnel at all government levels, and private community organizations and other nongovernmental organizations. It has expanded the focus on partnership, affirming that an effective national response requires layered and mutually supporting capabilities. Local communities, tribes, and states are primarily responsible for the safety and security of their citizens. Therefore local leaders will build the foundation for response and communities will prepare individuals and families.

The NRF has made many changes to the NRP, including updating the planning section and improving annexes and appendices. It clarifies the roles and responsibilities of the principal federal official, federal coordinating officer, senior federal law enforcement official, and the joint task force commander (Figure 23-2). The NRF describes organizational structures that have been developed, tested, and refined that are applicable to all support levels. The response structures are based on the NIMS and they promote on-the-scene initiative and resource sharing by all levels of government and private sectors. At the field level, local responders use the incident command structure to manage response operations (see Figure 23-2a). There may be a need for an area command structure at this level, which may be established to assess the agency administrator or executive in overseeing the management of multiple incidents (see Figure 23-2b). On-scene incident command and management organizations are located at an incident command post at the tactical level. State emergency operations centers are located where multiagency coordination can occur and they are configured to expand as needed to manage state-level events (see Figure 23-2c).

The joint field office is the primary federal incident management field structure and is composed of multiple agencies. It serves as a temporary facility for coordinating federal, state, local, tribal, public, and private agencies responsible for response and recovery. The joint field office is organized in a manner consistent with NIMS principles and is led by the unified coordination group (Figure 23-3). It focuses on providing support to on-the-scene efforts and supporting operations beyond the incident site.[13]

DEPARTMENT OF DEFENSE ROLES FOR DOMESTIC PREPAREDNESS AND RESPONSE

The *Quadrennial Defense Review Report* of 2006 outlines new challenges facing the DoD. This report examines four priority areas of homeland defense and protection against WMDs.[14] The DoD has unique capabilities and resources that can be used to support a federal response should an incident occur. Within the roles and responsibilities of the NRF, the secretary of defense, as directed by the president, can authorize defense support for civil authorities (in the form of an official request for assistance during a domestic incident).[13] Although the secretary of homeland security is the principal federal agent during an incident of national significance, command and control authority for military assets remains within military chains of command.

The DoD, through the secretary of defense, has two roles with respect to domestic preparedness. First, the DoD's mission is to defend US territory and its interests. Its second role is providing military support to civilian authorities when directed by the president, who can authorize the military to defend nonDoD assets that are designated as critical. The *Strategy for Homeland Defense and Civil Support* guides DoD action in each role.[15] This document builds on several others, including the *National Defense Strategy of the United States of America*,[16] the *National Strategy for Homeland Security*,[7] and the *National Security Strategy of the United States of America*.[17] The *Strategy for Homeland Defense and Civil Support* has several objectives. These include interdicting and defeating threats at a safe distance, providing mission assurance, supporting civil authorities in CBRNE attacks, and improving capabilities for homeland defense and security.[15] Overall, policy guidance and supervision to homeland defense activities are the responsibility of the assistant secretary of defense for homeland defense.

In the case of an emergency of national significance, the NRP outlines federal department or agency support to state or local governments.[12] The actions of federal agencies are dictated by the Stafford Act

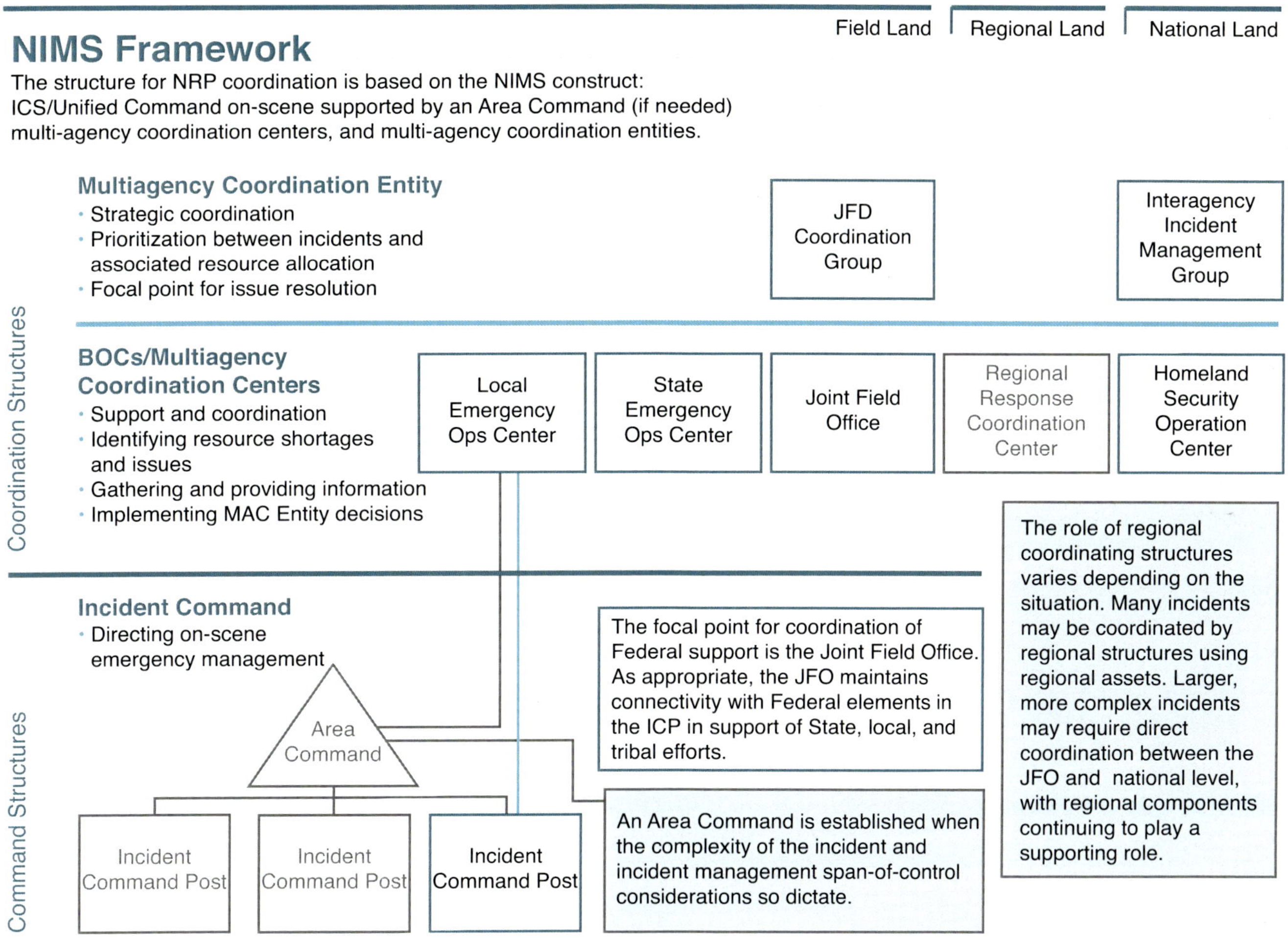

Fig. 23-3. Organizational outline for incident management command and coordinating centers. The structure addresses local (or field) to national incident management. Gray areas are established when the complexity of the incident has expanded. Blue areas indicate the national structure for managing the incident, establishing a clear progression of coordination and communication from the local level to the national headquarters level.

Reproduced from: US Department of Homeland Security. National Response Plan. Washington, DC: DHS; 2004.

EOC: emergency operations center
ICS: incident command system
JFO: joint field office
MAC: multiagency coordination
NIMS: National Incident Management System
NRP: National Response Plan
Ops: operations

(Figure 23-4).[12,18] The initial response is handled locally using available resources. After expending those resources, the local jurisdictions notify the state. State officials review the situation and respond by mobilizing state resources, keeping DHS and FEMA regional offices informed. When the situation becomes of such a magnitude that the governor requests a presidential directive for more support, regional staffing is coordinated using deployments, such as emergency response teams. A federal coordinating officer from the DHS identifies requirements and coordinates the overall federal interagency management.[12]

DoD's role in a domestic emergency depends on the scope of the incident, but it executes its responsibilities under the NRP, either as lead agency or in support of other lead agencies.[12] The DoD may first become involved in a limited role in small contingency missions, working with or under leading agencies. If the emergency is more serious (eg, a major natural disaster or a terrorist event), large-scale or specific, the DoD will

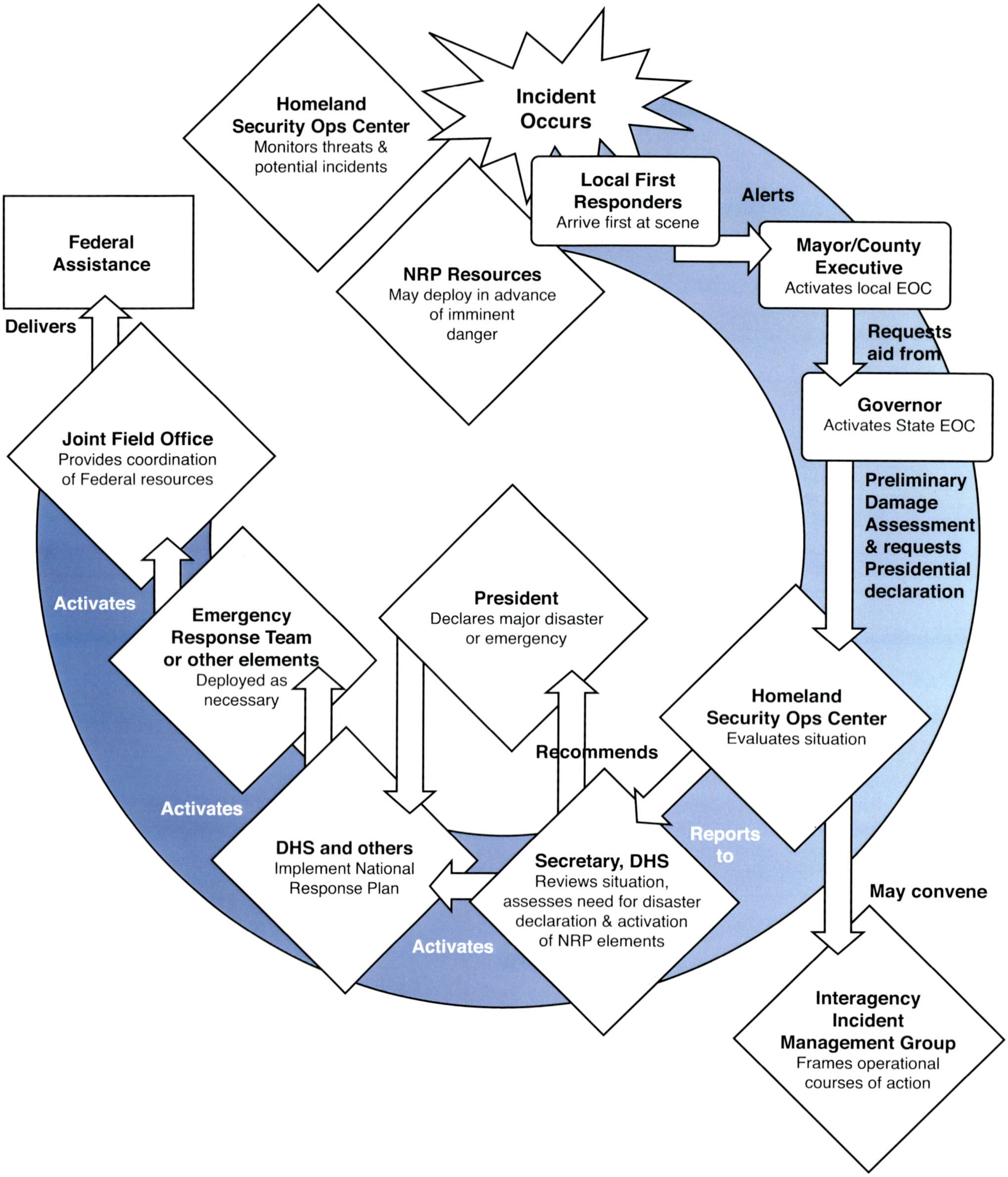

Fig. 23-4. Overview of initial federal involvement under the Stafford Act. The flowchart illustrates a course of action local and state governments may take during an emergency to request assistance from federal agencies.
Reproduced from: US Department of Homeland Security. *National Response Plan*. Washington, DC: DHS; 2004.
EOC: emergency operations center
NRP: National Response Plan
Ops: Operations

most likely be required to respond and may be asked to provide its unique capabilities to assist other agencies.

For emergencies involving chemical or biological weapons that overwhelm the capabilities of local, state, or other federal agencies, the DoD directly supports and assists in the areas of monitoring, identifying, containing, decontaminating, and disposing of the weapon. Specific NRP incidence annexes outline contingency plans for response to incidents involving biological, radiological, or chemical agents and toxic industrial chemicals and materials.[12] Although the coordinating agency may not be the DoD, the department is involved in these incidents because of its specialized training and capabilities. These unique DoD capabilities, specifically in the areas of programs and assets, are the focus of the remainder of this chapter.

THE DEPARTMENT OF DEFENSE'S SUPPORT TO CIVIL AUTHORITIES

The events of the 1995 sarin gas attack in the Tokyo subway, as well as threats against the United States and its allies, substantiated the need for planning to mitigate a chemical attack on the United States. This need became more evident with the continued threat and possible use of chemical weapons by Iraq and the former Soviet Union. The potential for exposure exists because many countries still maintain access to, or stockpiles of, chemical warfare agents. The continued threat of accidental or intentional incidents resulting from human-made disasters following the release of toxic industrial chemicals or materials has necessitated efforts to develop streamlined, rapid responses to chemical events. In an effort to provide information to the public, other agencies, and authorities, the Centers for Disease Control and Prevention (CDC) has complied a comprehensive and extensive list of toxic chemicals and chemical agents, chemical characteristics, and medical first aid and antidote treatment.[19] The anthrax attacks of 2001 and the potential use of biological weapons make emergency planning necessary. Multiagency planning is also required to prepare for potential nuclear incidents.

The DoD is uniquely capable of responding to these events because of wartime experience, continued research to counteract WMDs, and ongoing training in protective measures. Since the use of chemical weapons in World War I and the establishment of a chemical warfare service in 1918, the DoD has continued to be involved in developing countermeasures (antidotes, protective equipment, etc) through research, training, and initiating new programs, resources, and centers of authority.[20] Today challenges for the DoD include incorporating these capabilities into homeland security and coordinating these efforts with other agencies and the civilian incident commands.

The National Response Framework ESF 8 ("Health and Medical Services") outlines coordination guidelines for the DHHS, the lead agency during a domestic incident, as well as all signatory supporting agencies, including the DoD.[4,13] The NRF states that the DHHS and the US Department of Agriculture are the coordinating agencies for the food and agriculture incident annex. In this capacity, the military contributes only a supporting role to civilian authority. The DoD military operations that have priority over disaster relief[12,13,16,21] are also defined in ESF 8 (Figure 23-5).

Defense support in a domestic incident can involve federal military forces and DoD civilians and contractors, as well as other DoD components. The executive authority for military support is through the secretary of defense, who can authorize defense support of civil authorities. The secretary of defense retains the command of military forces throughout operations.[16,21] The secretary of defense also designates the secretary of the Army as the DoD executive agent for military support to civil authorities, and the point of contact for the DoD executive agent is the defense coordinating officer. This individual is the DoD's representative at the joint field office. For a domestic incident in which DoD assistance is needed, the defense coordinating officer forwards a request for assistance to the US Army Northern Command, which passes the request to the US Army Medical Command (MEDCOM) and the commander of the US Army Forces Command. If the disaster exceeds the defense coordinating officer's command and control, a supporting military commander-in-chief establishes a joint task force or response task force to control DoD assets and resources (including personnel).[21]

The DoD's role in supporting emergency response operations depends on well-trained, readily available, fully qualified personnel. These personnel are often from different commands and services within the DoD. In addition, active, reserve, and National Guard components can be made available for domestic support, depending on the extent and nature of the incident and the forces' current deployment missions throughout other regions of the world.

The capabilities of the DoD and the military to react to a CBRNE event are described in terms of "detection and response" and "reach-back response."[15] The detection and response capability provides teams trained in detection, initial response, and medical response. The initial response to a domestic incident is often the most crucial step and sets the stage for a well-executed and effective overall response. These

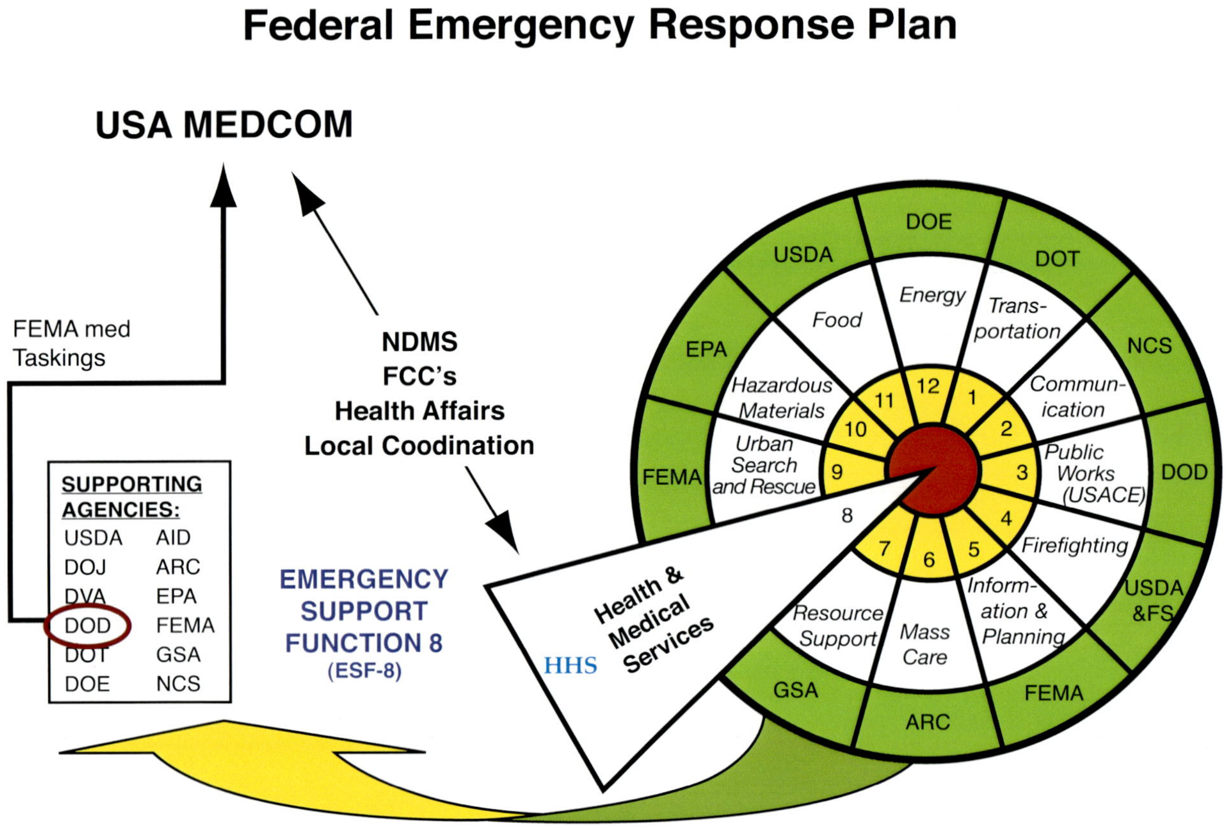

Fig. 23-5. Federal emergency response plan outlining federal government departments and their interactions with supporting agencies, such as the Department of Defense.
Reproduced from: US Department of the Army. Medical Emergency Management Planning. Washington, DC: DA; 2003. MEDCOM Pam 525-1.
AID: Agency for International Development
ARC: American Red Cross
DoD: Department of Defense
DOE: Department of Energy
DOJ: Department of Justice
DOT: Department of Transportation
DVA: Department of Veteran's Affairs
EPA: Environmental Protection Agency
FCC: federal coordinating center
FEMA: Federal Emergency Management Association
FS: Forest Service
GSA: General Services Administration
HHS: Department of Health and Human Services
NCS: National Communications System
NDMS: National Disaster Medical System
USACE: United States Army Corps of Engineers
USA MEDCOM: US Army Medical Command
USDA: US Department of Agriculture

military first responders are important assets in supporting homeland defense.

In 1996, based on *Presidential Decision Directive 39*, the Marine Corps developed a task force uniquely trained for CBRNE incidents.[1,22] This forward-support task force, called the "chemical/biological incident response force" (CBIRF), is a mobile, self-sufficient response force capable of deploying rapidly.[1] CBIRF focuses its efforts on consequence management. The team is trained to function in several roles as initial responder; for example, it is trained in decontamination, security, and medical responder assistance during specific or unique incidents, such as CBRNE events.[22–24] Currently CBIRF is located in the national capital region.

CBIRF is a consequence management force that can deploy on short notice when directed by the national command authority. The force consists of several elements, including reconnaissance (with a nuclear, biological, and chemical [NBC] element), decontamination, medical support, security, and service support. Each element includes up to 120 Marines (eg, a security element), but most elements consist of about 30 personnel. CBIRF's medical element is made up of 6 officers (3 physicians, 1 environmental health officer, 1 physician assistant, and 1 nurse) and

17 corpsmen. All elements train and certify in their respective areas. They are required to attend unique training, such as the Medical Management of Chemical and Biological Casualties Course or the Contaminated Casualty Decontamination Course given through the US Army Medical Research Institute of Chemical Defense (USAMRICD) in conjunction with US Army Medical Institute of Infectious Disease (USAMRIID). CBIRF members are also NBC-qualified by the US Marine Corps Forces, NBC School in Atlanta, Georgia. The CBIRF can provide expert advice to an incident commander by means of a reach-back capability to military and civilian scientific experts.[22–24] This means that through networking and communication, CBIRF elements "reach back" to other DoD assets or consulting experts on specific information related to chemical or biological threats. This reach-back capability results in rapid and coordinated effort.[22–24]

The National Guard's role in a domestic CBRNE event is to support state governors and fully integrate within CBRNE operations.[15] The Army National Guard is currently composed of over 360,000 individuals, while the Air National Guard has approximately 109,000. The National Guard, organized by the DoD, also coordinates its efforts across many other federal agencies.[25] When called up by the state governor, the guard provides initial security and response for up to 24 hours, after which WMD civil support teams mobilize. The National Guard has at least 55 WMD civil support teams that are equipped and trained to detect CBRNE agents. These teams are early entry forces equipped with diagnostic equipment for detecting CBRNE weapons, they are trained and equipped for decontamination, and they can provide emergency medical treatment. Depending on the mission, they can also assist other early responders and advise the incident commander.[22,25]

In March 2004 the joint chiefs of staff and the commander of the US Army Northern Command supported forming National Guard CBRNE-enhanced response force packages for CBRNE missions. The packages use existing capabilities combined with specialized training and equipment and are designed to support domestic missions for state governors, but are also able to support joint expeditionary capabilities.[23,25] The future vision for these integrated CBRNE forces is for them to work closely with other agents within the DoD, including the chemical corps, Northern Command, and other state and federal agencies. The National Guard is committed to supporting civil authorities in homeland security missions as well as serving as a first-line military capability to support homeland defense.[25]

The 20th Support Command was initiated in October 2004 and is structured out of the forces command under the US Joint Forces Command. The 20th supports a wide spectrum of CBRNE operations with fully trained forces. It is capable of exercising command and control in these operations. The 20th Support Command includes personnel from the chemical corps, technical escort unit, and the explosive ordnance disposal. Within this command structure, support continues to come from and go to MEDCOM.[26,27] There is currently an ongoing effort within the DoD to expand the 20th Support Command to serve as a joint task force capable of immediate deployment on WMD elimination and exploitation missions.[14]

The US Army's First and Ninth area medical laboratories (AMLs) also support forces' command missions. These two units, based out of Aberdeen Proving Ground, Maryland, are capable of deploying anywhere in the world on short notice to conduct health-hazard surveillance. The units draw on the scientific expertise of surrounding organizations in many areas, such as the US Army Center for Health Promotion and Preventive Medicine (USACHPPM), USAMRICD, and USAMRIID.

The AMLs conduct health-hazard surveillance for biological, chemical, nuclear, radiological, occupational and environmental health, and endemic disease threats at the theater level to protect and sustain the health of forces throughout military and domestic support operations. Using sophisticated analytical instruments combined with health risk assessment by medical and scientific professionals, the AMLs confirm environmental exposures in the field associated with the contemporary operating environment. The execution of this mission provides combat commanders with critical information that can assist in mitigating or eliminating health threats during the operational risk management process.

The AMLs are composed of personnel with military occupational specialties from the areas of occupational and environmental health, NBC exposure, and endemic disease.[27,28] The AMLs were structured from the original 520th Theater Army Medical Laboratory and maintain a chain of command through the 44th MEDCOM. This structure enables the units to provide comprehensive health hazard surveillance typically associated with MEDCOM-fixed facilities.[26,28]

The occupational and environmental health section of the AML provides comprehensive environmental health threat assessments by conducting air, water, soil, entomological, epidemiological, and radiological surveillance and laboratory analyses. In support of this mission, the occupational and environmental health section conducts analysis in four areas: environmental health, industrial hygiene, radiological assessment, and entomology.[27,28]

Some of the capabilities of the NBC section include cholinesterase activity measurement, microbial identification, and gas chromatography with mass selective detector. Other instrumentation capabilities include an electron capture and flame photometric detector, a mobile laboratory, and telechemistry. These capabilities allow the section to identify microbial organisms and monitor for chemical WMDs as well as for a wide variety of toxic industrial chemicals. The technicians of the NBC section work in an isolation facility. Soldiers set up the isolation facility using a tactical, expandable, two-sided, shelter attached to two sections of an extendable, modular, personnel tent (called a "TEMPER"), and some of the capabilities can be executed in the mobile laboratory mounted in a shelter unit on the back of a M1097 HMMWV troop carrier.[29–31]

Upon request, the endemic disease section deploys worldwide to conduct health threat surveillance for biological warfare agents and endemic disease threats at the theater level and provides and sustains force health protection. The section sets up its laboratory in an isolation facility that is nearly identical to that of the NBC section. This section is self-supporting and capable of transporting tactical and technical equipment, providing environmental control, and using power generation equipment in order to complete assigned missions. The endemic disease section relies primarily on nucleic acid and antigen-detection–based technologies, along with basic microbiological techniques, to detect, identify, and analyze naturally occurring infections and biological warfare agents that may be encountered during deployments.

The endemic disease section often includes professional officer filler information system (PROFIS) personnel, such as veterinary pathologists, veterinary microbiologists, preventative medicine physicians, and infectious disease physicians. The PROFIS system is designed to provide high-quality medical care through trained medical personnel. Medical personnel are required to provide healthcare to fixed medical treatment facilities and deploying units. PROFIS personnel within the 20th Support Command serve as subject matter experts on issues regarding infectious disease and biological warfare agents. They also provide laboratory support for infectious disease outbreak investigations and process and analyze potentially dangerous infectious specimens.[28]

MILITARY HEALTHCARE'S ROLE IN DOMESTIC PREPAREDNESS

MEDCOM also has multiple resources that can assist in responding to domestic incidents, such as those described in MEDCOM pamphlets 525-1 and 525-4.[21,32] These regulations outline potential medical support to civil authorities and provide guidance on developing plans for MEDCOM's response to emergencies related to WMDs (see Figure 22-5). In the case of a major disaster or emergency, DHHS, as the primary agency for health and medical services, would notify all supporting agencies under ESF 8. Each agency would be responsible for supplying sufficient support to any activities tasked against it and must therefore have a support individual or individuals knowledgeable in the resources and capabilities of its respective agency.[21]

The US Joint Forces Command communicates with other agencies to provide requests for assistance. In addition, MEDCOM, when directed to conduct emergency medical assistance, provides personnel through PROFIS. These individuals are deployed as directed by the Northern Command via forces command and they are recalled according to their tables of organization. Additional assistance can come from other support functions, medical treatment facilities, or other DoD medical forces, active or reserve.[21]

One support function of the Army Medical Department is special medical augmentation response teams. These teams are organized at the subordinate MEDCOMs, such as USACHPPM and the US Army Medical Research and Materiel Command. There are 38 special medical augmentation response teams, two of which are particularly important in response to a chemical incident. These are the preventive medicine and the NBC teams. Teams are made up of military personnel, civilians, and DoD contractors and can be deployed within or outside the continental United States to support local, state, or federal agencies in response to an emergency within 12 hours of notification.[21,23,32]

The chemical and biological rapid response team is another asset. The National Medical Chemical and Biological Advisory Team, which serves as the principal DoD medical advisor to the commanders or political authorities in response to a threat, directs this element. Chemical and biological rapid response teams are capable of deploying within 4 hours of notification and they provide technical support by means of an advisory team that is tasked to an incident site.[22,23] Other MEDCOM support personnel include the radiological advisory medical teams located at Walter Reed Army Medical Center in Washington, DC; the disaster assistance response team located at Madigan Army Medical Center in Tacoma, Washington; and the emergency medical response team located at Tripler Army Medical Center in Honolulu, Hawaii.[21,22]

NATIONAL PREPAREDNESS PROGRAMS AND INITIATIVES

In addition to personnel and resources, there are several programs or initiatives that coordinate domestic preparedness efforts or respond proactively to incidents. Some of these include the National Disaster Medical System (NDMS), the Strategic National Stockpile (SNS), and the Laboratory Response Network.

National Disaster Medical System

The objective of the NDMS is to coordinate a cooperative agreement between federal agencies, including the DHHS, the DoD, the DHS, and the Department of Veterans Affairs, as well as state, local, public, and private resources to ensure a coordinated medical response system. The NDMS is activated in response to emergency events and provides potential assets to meet medical health services as outlined in ESF 8 in the NRP.[11,12] FEMA coordinates necessary medical care for incidents such as natural catastrophes, military contingencies, terrorist attacks, or refugee influxes. The response is federalized, with the DHHS acting as the lead federal agency. Medical care personnel include disaster medical assistance teams, disaster mortuary teams, veterinary medical assistance teams, and WMD medical response teams.[18,21] The MEDCOM NDMS coordinates efforts with the NDMS within a geographical area.

Strategic National Stockpile

The treatment of mass casualties involved in a biological or chemical terrorist attack requires not only a coordinated effort of personnel but may also include large quantities of pharmaceuticals and medical supplies. Because an attack could occur at any time or place, life-saving resources require an equally coordinated response. In most scenarios, state and local governments do not have sufficient quantities of medical items to provide for a mass-casualty event, so effective pharmaceuticals must be rapidly deployed from a central location. This need led to the creation of a national stockpile.

In 1999 Congress directed that the DHHS and the CDC establish a national repository of antibiotics, pharmaceuticals, chemical antidotes, and other medical supplies. Identified as the "National Pharmaceutical Stockpile," the mission of this repository is to provide these items during an emergency within 12 hours of a federal decision to deploy.[33] With the approval and passage of the Homeland Security Act of 2002, the role of determining the goals and requirements of the National Pharmaceutical Stockpile shifted to the DHS. In March of 2003 the act's name was changed to the "Strategic National Stockpile Program," and oversight and guidance of the pharmaceuticals and the program transferred returned to the DHHS and the CDC to ensure that there are enough life-saving pharmaceuticals and medical supplies available in an emergency.

The SNS supplements the initial actions of first responders from state and local public health agencies. "Push packages" of pharmaceuticals and supplies are deployed within 12 hours of a request. The 12-hour push packages are composed of broad-spectrum items that can treat or provide symptomatic relief from a variety of ill-defined or yet-to-be-determined illnesses. If required, additional supplies or products specific to an incident can be obtained through a vendor-managed inventory. These items can be shipped to the community or incident site within 24 to 36 hours.

Both the DHHS and CDC determine and maintain the SNS assets. Decisions on which treatments or antidotes to maintain are based on intelligence reports, vulnerability of the population, availability of a commodity, and ease of dissemination. Inventory, continual rotation, and quarterly quality inspections guarantee quality control. A request generates shipping of a preconfigured push package via ground or air to state and local authorities. A technical advisory response unit can also be deployed with the SNS assets for advice and assistance. The SNS was used successfully in New York City following the September 11 attacks and again in response to the anthrax attacks of 2001.

The SNS program staffs, trains, and educates providers, responders, and others in disaster preparedness. In addition, the program continually works with other agencies, including regional coordinators, the Department of Veterans Affairs, the DoD, and FEMA to improve and coordinate efforts. Improvements are ongoing within the program. These developments include expanding the capability to respond to new and emerging threats, working with state and local authorities on preparedness plans, and addressing operational issues when responding to terrorist threats. The SNS is currently striving to increase city readiness; its goal is to be able to provide oral medications to 100% of the population of selected cities within 48 hours of an event.

Laboratory Response Network

Another national resource for both information and collaboration is the Laboratory Response Network. This network coordinates multiagency laboratories into an integrated communication and response plan.

The network first became operational in 1999 in accordance with *Presidential Decision Directive 39* under the DHHS and CDC.[1] The network brings together experts from various agencies to coordinate sample testing and to increase laboratory capability. Agencies participating in this program include the CDC, the DHS, the US Environmental Protection Agency, the US Department of Agriculture, the US Food and Drug Administration, the DoD, the DHHS, and other federal agencies, as well as international, state, and local public health laboratories. There are currently over 100 laboratories participating in the network.[33]

Laboratories are categorized according to their capabilities and responses into sentinel, reference, and national laboratories. Sentinel laboratories process samples for routine diagnostic purposes and determine if the samples should be shipped to reference and national laboratories. Reference laboratories (there are approximately 140) are federal, military, and international laboratories that specialize in veterinary, agricultural, food, water, or soil testing. National laboratories (eg, the CDC or military labs) perform definitive testing when required.[33] Some examples of these tests include cholinesterase testing done at USACHPPM, thiodiglycol testing at USAMRICD, and several biological tests performed at the CDC and USAMRIID.

CHEMICAL PREPAREDNESS PROGRAMS AND INITIATIVES

In 1985 Congress mandated destroying all the US chemical agent and munitions stockpiles. The original date of completion for this project was 1994; however, the date was extended to 2007 after the US Senate ratified the destruction of chemical weapons during the Chemical Weapons Convention in April 1997. Congress also directed that the well being and safety of the environment and the general public be protected in and around the areas of the eight chemical weapons storage sites. This direction led to the Chemical Stockpile Emergency Preparedness Program (CSEPP), established in 1988 and revised in 1995.[34]

A memorandum of understanding (MOU), issued in March 2004, directs the Department of the Army and DHS (through FEMA) to identify their respective roles and efforts in emergency response preparedness in the areas surrounding the remaining seven stockpile sites of chemical munitions.[35,36] The Army is the custodian for these stockpiles and FEMA provides guidance, funding, resources, and training. Other agencies lend support as needed through expert consultants. These agencies include the US Environmental Protection Agency and the DHHS. Currently the Army stockpiles sites are:

- Anniston Chemical Activity (Anniston, Alabama)
- Blue Grass Chemical Activity (Richmond, Kentucky)
- Newport Chemical Depot (Newport, Indiana)
- Pine Bluff Chemical Activity (Pine Bluff Arsenal, Arkansas)
- Pueblo Chemical Depot (Pueblo, Colorado)
- Tooele Chemical Activity (Tooele Army Depot, Utah)
- Umatilla Chemical Depot (Hermiston, Oregon)

The risk to the local communities in and around the seven chemical storage sites in the United States remains. The greatest risk is a natural or human-made event that causes the release of chemical agents from these storage facilities. There is a direct link between destroying the stockpiles under the chemical demilitarization program (see Chapter 4, History of the Chemical Threat, Chemical Terrorism, and Its Implications for Military Medicine) and the emergency preparedness plan. Officials in states and counties where these demilitarization sites are located must have emergency preparedness initiatives in place before destruction operations begin. Budgeting and funding for CSEPP are primarily approved through the Army after funding requirements are outlined by the states and counties. The Army, FEMA, and state and local communities need a constant, proactive approach to disaster preparedness. Several areas of continuous improvement are crucial to the success of the demilitarization program, such as applying lessons learned, having better relations with state and local communities, and providing assistance and guidance to states on technical assistance and leadership.[36]

These chemical depot communities exercise preparedness and assess the effectiveness and capabilities of federal, state, and local response organizations. CSEPP exercises consist of two types: federally managed exercises and alternative year exercises. Federally managed exercises, led by Army and FEMA co-directors, involve mobilization of emergency facilities, command posts, and communications centers and are federally mandated evaluations of a community's capability to respond to a chemical accident or incident. The alternative year exercise is used by the community to assess its training needs, review standard operating procedures, and evaluate resources, equipment, and personnel. Other exercises include tabletop remediation and recovery exercises and Army-mandated, quarterly chemical accident or incident response and assistance exercises.[37] All exercises are evaluated and analyzed to assess performance. The evaluations compare performance based on criteria from Army Regulation 50-6[37,38] and the applicable portions of the Code of Federal Regulations.

Emergency procedures are in place in the communities surrounding chemical stockpiles and the procedures are published. Through the CSEPP program, the communities work with FEMA and the Army to enhance their preparedness and will continue to do so until the stockpiles no longer exist. CSEPP's successes have been nationally recognized. The community risk has been significantly reduced in Aberdeen, Anniston, and Tooele, demonstrating to other communities that applying the lessons learned is beneficial.[39] Some lessons learned that have contributed to decreased risk include advances in building and improving public warning systems, increasing public awareness, and adding more trained medical personnel and responders.

Another valuable chemical countermeasure resource is the Chemical Security Analysis Center. The center provides threat awareness and assessment on a variety of chemical-related threats (eg, chemical warfare agents, toxic industrial chemicals) through a forum for subject matter experts. It supports information management, reach-back capability, and threat characterization. A similar project was developed in 2004 for the center's biological counterpart, the National Bio-Defense Analysis and Countermeasure Center. Currently the Chemical Security Analysis Center is planned for a central location and is to provide easy access to the database. These efforts aim to prevent and mitigate the consequences of chemical or biological threats by preparing ahead.

TRAINING AND EDUCATION

Training and education are an integral part of any community response to an emergency, including an act of terrorism. The ability to respond safely and effectively to incidents of chemical, biological, or radiological terrorism resulting in large numbers of casualties requires disaster education and preparedness training. This unique training, required for military response teams and healthcare providers (particularly those involved in CBRNE), has been a valuable asset in domestic preparedness. Increasing awareness and training in CBRNE will continue be important. By building on knowledge, increasing awareness, training in CBRNE, and applying lessons learned, military and civilian medical providers and first responders will become more proactive in preventing and deterring attacks and minimizing the effects of a human-made or natural disaster. In 2001 the Joint Commission on Accreditation of Healthcare Organizations challenged healthcare providers to obtain the proper training and education to decrease vulnerabilities of a catastrophic incident and improve communications between agencies for a more efficient and rapid response through emergency planning and training exercises.[40]

CBRNE training for the DoD is multiservice and single-service oriented. Although each service may have its own defense CBRNE doctrine, all US military services support the joint doctrine. The goals of these efforts are to ensure publications are up to date, coordinated across services, and relevant. For example several of the Army's field manuals[41,42] are part of multiservice doctrines. These Army manuals have Air Force, Navy, and Marine counterpart manuals that are service-specific, but that all support joint publications that are currently available or under development.[23,42,43]

Across the services, initial entry training for CBRNE events on the battlefield begins with first aid, self aid, and buddy aid. This training is augmented with rigorous instruction on employing the various mission-oriented protective posture levels and conducting personnel and equipment decontamination. Equipping service members with mission-oriented protective posture gear, pyridostigmine bromide pretreatment tablets, atropine and 2-pralidoxime chloride autoinjectors, diazepam, decontamination kits, chemical agent detection paper, and training on the use of these supplies is the foundation from which to build. Operationally, US Army Medical Department, US Army Chemical Corps, and US Army Ordinance Corps personnel with specialized training in CBRNE are a valued training resource. Effective training is essential for handling mass casualty situations, treating field casualties expediently, and managing unique aspects related to treating CBRNE casualties. The challenge of decreasing vulnerabilities and improving preparedness becomes one of improving communication between agencies for a more efficient and rapid response so that the right materials and individuals are present at the right time and place.

There have been many changes in disaster preparedness since the attacks on the World Trade Center and the Pentagon in 2001. Above all, the military healthcare system has improved medical readiness. The position of assistant secretary of defense for acquisition, technology, and logistics was established by DoD Directive 2000.12 on August 18, 2003, to direct CBRNE readiness for military medical education and training. Military education and training ensures that medical services and personnel can perform optimally in all types of disaster environments. The Office of The Surgeon General oversees and integrates the medical aspects of CBRNE programs, including materiel development, testing, evaluation, and medical oversight of nonmedical programs for all Army medical personnel. However, whoever commands and oversees these programs today could change tomorrow, so military medical personnel need to be ready for the next catastrophic event.

In their domestic preparedness roles, today's DoD healthcare providers must be capable of managing military casualties and may also be required to work with civilian healthcare agencies and providers as well as other civilian first responders and support personnel. Training for catastrophic chemical incidents has become a joint effort as well as an exchange of knowledge and emergency medical training. The US Army Medical Department has addressed the training and education of healthcare providers in the medical management of CBRNE illness or injuries in Army Regulation 40-68.[43] This regulation states that for clinical privileges or staff appointment approval, providers must be educated in the medical diagnoses and appropriate management of CBRNE casualties. In 2003 the Force Health Protection Council endorsed standards of proficiency training as a requirement for all medical personnel throughout the DoD.[44]

The Defense Medical Readiness Training Institute in San Antonio, Texas, was tasked to conduct a CBRNE training gap analysis by the assistant secretary of health affairs in 2004. In 2002 the joint staff and the deputy assistant secretary of affairs for force health protection and readiness tasked the defense medical readiness training institute to develop a tri-service CBRNE training program. This is a distance learning training program for all DoD employees. The program was developed with core competencies for clinical, medical, and specialty areas for all DoD medical employees. The program consists of a basic course, an operators' and responders' course, a clinical course, and an executive and commander course. Course levels include initial, sustainment, and advanced.[45]

Training for CBRNE and medical force health protection is conducted at the Army Medical Department Center and School, USAMRICD, USAMRIID, the Armed Forces Radiobiology Research Institute, and USACHPPM. The Web sites of the DHS, FEMA, the Navy, the Air Force, and the Army also offer training courses. The Uniformed Services University of the Health Sciences conducts a chemical warfare and consequence management course that brings together leading chemical warfare authorities from the DoD and federal, state, and local governments. The course addresses some potentially controversial topics that may be faced when making policy decisions.

In 2001 the US General Accounting Office stated in its report to the chairman of the Subcommittee on National Security, Veterans Affairs, and International Relations, Committee on Government Reform, House of Representatives, that the "gold standard" programs for medical training and education were the Medical Management of Chemical and Biological Casualties Course, the Field Management of Chemical and Biological Casualties Course,[46] and the Hospital Management of CBRNE Incidents Course developed soon after.[23]

The Medical Management of Chemical and Biological Casualties Course is conducted by USAMRICD and USAMRIID. The course is designed for US Army Medical Corps, Nurse Corps, and Medical Service Corps officers, physician assistants, and other selected medical professionals. Classroom instruction and laboratory and field exercises prepare students to effectively manage the casualties of chemical and biological agent exposure. Classroom discussion includes the history and current threat of chemical and biological agent use, the characteristics of threat agents, the pathophysiology and treatment of agent exposure, and the principles of field management of threat agent casualties. In the field, attendees practice the principles of personal protection, triage, treatment, and decontamination of chemical casualties. During this exercise, attendees learn the capabilities and limitations of mission-oriented protective posture when treating casualties in a simulated contaminated environment. Continuing medical education credits are available for this training.[23]

The Field Management of Chemical and Biological Casualties Course is conducted by USAMRICD at Aberdeen Proving Ground, Maryland. The course is designed for Medical Service Corps officers, Chemical Corps officers, and noncommissioned officers in medical or chemical specialties. Classroom instruction and laboratory and field exercises prepare students to become trainers in the first echelon management of chemical and biological agent casualties. There are small-group computer and briefing exercises that reinforce casualty management principles. During the 2 days of field training, attendees establish a casualty decontamination site and use the site during scenario-based exercises to manage litter and ambulatory casualties. Attendees practice the principles of personal protection, agent detection, triage, emergency treatment, and decontamination of chemical casualties at the site.[23]

The Hospital Management of CBRNE Incidents Course is conducted jointly by USAMRICD, USAMRIID, and the Armed Forces Radiobiology Research Institute. The course is designed for hospital-based medical professionals, including healthcare professionals, hospital administrators, medical planners, and others who plan, conduct, or are responsible for hospital management of mass-casualty incidents or terrorism preparedness. The course consists of classroom instruction, scenarios, and tabletop exercises with military and civilian hospital-based medical and management professionals with skills, knowledge, and information resources to carry out the full spectrum of healthcare facility responsibilities required by a CBRNE event.

Nonmedical NBC and CBRNE courses offered to the military include leadership courses in homeland security, antiterrorism and force protection, and consequence management, in addition to the ongoing developmental courses available to both enlisted service members and officers (eg, officer and noncommissioned officer basic and advanced courses). Opportunities also exist for certain individuals in CBRNE defense specialist training from the US Army Chemical School and the Defense Threat Reduction Agency Defense Nuclear Weapons School. Other professional military, nonmedical education includes the US Army CBRN Defense Professional Training at Fort Leonard Wood, Missouri.[23]

In addition to specialized, credentialed medical training, there are other opportunities for civilian and military individuals to obtain further education in general homeland security training. After September 11, 2001, courses on homeland security, preparedness, consequence management, and response were offered at colleges and universities across the nation. Courses range from introductory levels and information awareness to full-credit courses. These courses introduce students to topics including policy, legislation, security, management, operations, and planning.

Online distance learning and educational information are also easily accessible. The Web sites of the DHS, the CDC, and the DHHS have several valuable links that can be used to find resources for planning preparedness operations, online courses for accreditation, and reference materials for responders and medical personnel. FEMA offers an online course covering the incident command system, starting with a basic course and advancing through the NIMS and the NRP. Students are entered into a national database as trained individuals upon graduation.[47] In addition, the DHS and other federal agencies offer several assistance programs, grants and training courses to states and localities on terrorism preparedness and healthcare emergency services.[48–50]

Finally, there are several informational resources worth noting. The CDC, for example, has numerous references on topics related to chemicals and chemical emergencies. Its emergency preparedness and response Web site has a wide variety of information for both healthcare professionals and the general public.[50] Another valuable source of information from the DHHS is the Agency for Toxic Substances and Disease Registry.[19] This is a health registry of the DHHS and CDC that is available to the public and provides valuable information on toxic profiles of potentially hazardous substances and their health effects, if known. The substances are ranked according to their potential risk for exposure. The information is easy to read and understand and is updated by peer review. Currently there are 289 toxicological profiles that can be used by emergency responders.[19]

The Agency for Toxic Substances and Disease Registry is capable of assisting local, state, and federal agencies in responding to chemical terrorist acts by analyzing biological and environmental samples. The registry offers an emergency hotline service, maintains a Web site, and provides training, exercises, and qualification certification to improve laboratories.[19,50]

Exercises

Exercises are the best test of the effectiveness of preparedness plans, policies, and training. These practices measure agency and interagency abilities to respond to incidents and are critical tools that can be used to enhance coordination. Exercises also provide a way to initiate policy change, review lessons learned, and give quantifiable performance measurements that can be used for certification purposes and improvement. Exercises can be conducted at many levels, from local to national.

The first step in conducting an exercise is to train the trainers, and that process usually begins with tabletop exercises that are conducted with representatives from participating agencies. Local, state, and federal systems are tested addressing local and state response and how well that response integrates with federal support. The final step in practical exercise is usually a full-scale exercise, such as a mock event, that includes first responders, private individuals, businesses, and local, state, and federal agencies. The goal of training should be to provide immediate feedback to participants, reinforce training, and evaluate a particular method's effectiveness. An additional goal is to learn from the exercise to improve the preparedness plan for the next exercise or real event. Exercises should test the system to evaluate alternative solutions, approaches, and personnel as well as equipment needs.

The DHS Office for Domestic Preparedness has developed government-based emergency preparedness exercises involving multiple agencies. These top-official, national-level, terrorism exercises involve a specific event and are geared toward senior-level officials at all levels of government. The exercises evaluate emergency preparedness, response, and consequence management. They were congressionally mandated in May 2000 and they continue to strengthen the nation's capabilities in responding to, preparing for, and recovering from a full-scale terrorist attack. The fourth (and largest) top-official exercise took place October 15 to 19, 2007.

SUMMARY

The 2006 *Quadrennial Defense Review Report* outlines the vision for forces of the DoD to "be organized, trained, equipped, and resourced to deal with all aspects of the threat posed by weapons of mass destruction."[14] In order to accomplish this goal, military healthcare providers must be able to anticipate and respond to certain threats. Today's military healthcare providers must be capable of managing casualties within a broad, multiagency framework that adapts according to the scope and specifics of an incident. In addition to the traditional patient-provider role, military healthcare providers, logisticians, and leaders must be trained and equipped to assume a variety of other roles, from advising to involvement in specific response teams. Beyond understanding the nature of the hazards and medical management of casualties, today's military healthcare provider must understand national policies, the overall structure of a disaster response, and the DoD's role in support of civilian authorities during the consequence management phase of recovery from an incident. This can be accomplished with the knowledge acquired through research, technology development, awareness of the role of military healthcare providers within DoD and the military healthcare system, and training, including joint exercises with other agencies. Through continued learning, practice, and shared lessons learned, military healthcare providers expand their ability to respond effectively and efficiently in the event of an incident. Should one occur, a well-trained, fully prepared military medical community can alter the outcome of a major CBRNE event.

Acknowledgment

The authors wish to thank the following individuals for their assistance with this chapter: Patrick Taylor, Beverly Maliner (USACHPPM), Martha J (Max) Despain, and Joseph Perugino (Kirk US Army Health Clinic).

REFERENCES

1. US Office of the Press Secretary, White House. *US Policy on Counterterrorism*. Washington, DC: The White House; 1995. Presidential Decision Directive 39. Unclassified.

2. US Office of the Press Secretary, White House. *Combating Terrorism*. Washington, DC: The White House; 1998. Presidential Decision Directive 62. Unclassified.

3. National Defense Authorization Act for Fiscal Year 1997. Pub L 104-201. 23 September 1996.

4. US Department of Defense. *Domestic Preparedness Program in the Defense against Weapons of Mass Destruction*. Washington, DC: DoD; 1997. Report to Congress.

5. Moore DH, Alexander SM. Emergency response to a chemical warfare agent incident: domestic preparedness, first response, and public health considerations. In: Somani S, Romano J, eds. *Chemical Warfare Agents: Toxicity at Low Levels*. Boca Raton, Fla: CRC Press; 2001: 409–435.

6. Institute of Medicine and National Research Council. Introduction. In: *Chemical and Biological Terrorism, Research and Development to Improve Civilian Medical Response*. Washington, DC: National Academy Press; 1999: 15–28.

7. US Office of Homeland Security. *National Strategy for Homeland Security*. Washington, DC: OHS; 2002.

8. US Office of Homeland Security. *Organization and Operation of the Homeland Security Council*. Washington, DC: Office of the Press Secretary; 2001. Homeland Security Presidential Directive 1.

9. US Office of Homeland Security. *Homeland Security Advisory System*. Washington, DC: Office of the Press Secretary; 2002. Homeland Security Presidential Directive 3.

10. US Office of Homeland Security. *Management of Domestic Incidents*. Washington, DC: Office of the Press Secretary; 2003. Homeland Security Presidential Directive 5.

11. US Department of Homeland Security. *National Incident Management System*. Washington, DC: DHS; 2003.

12. US Department of Homeland Security. *National Response Plan*. Washington, DC: DHS; 2004.

13. US Office of Homeland Security. *National Preparedness*. Washington, DC: Office of the Press Secretary; 2003. Homeland Security Presidential Directive 8.

14. US Department of Defense. *Quadrennial Defense Review Report*. Washington, DC: DoD; 2006.

15. US Department of Defense. *Strategy for Homeland Defense and Civil Support*. Washington, DC: DoD; 2005.

16. US Department of Defense. *The National Defense Strategy of the United States of America*. Washington, DC: DoD; 2005.

17. The White House. National Security Strategy of the United States of America. Washington, DC: Office of the Press Secretary; 2002.

18. Bea K. *Federal Stafford Act Disaster Assistance: Presidential Declarations, Eligible Activities, and Funding*. Washington, DC: Congressional Research Service; 2005. CRS report for Congress, Order Code RL33053.

19. US Department of Health and Human Services. Agency for Toxic Substances and Disease Registry Web site. Available at: http://www.atsdr.cdc.gov/. Accessed 2006.

20. Smart JK. History of chemical and biological warfare: an American perspective. In: Zajtchuk R, ed. *Medical Aspects of Chemical and Biological Warfare*. Washington, DC: Department of the Army, Office of The Surgeon General, Borden Institute; 1997: 9–86.

21. US Department of the Army. *Medical Emergency Management Planning*. Washington, DC: DA; 2003. MEDCOM Pam 525-1.

22. Bea K. *Organization and Mission of the Emergency Preparedness and Response Directorate: Issues and Options for the 109th Congress*. Washington, DC: Congressional Research Service; 2005. CRS Report for Congress, Order Code RL33064.

23. US Office of the Deputy Assistant Secretary of Defense for Chemical and Biological Defense. *Department of Defense Chemical, Biological, Radiological and Nuclear Defense Program*. Washington, DC: DoD; 2005. Annual report to Congress.

24. Global Security Military Web site. Available at: www.globalsecurity.org/military/agency/usmc. Accessed November 2006.

25. Christmas W, Todd M. Chemical corps efforts to support the National Guard in its role as responders for CBRNE missions. *Army Chemical Review*. 2005:7–12.

26. US Department of the Army. *Mission Training Plan for the Area Medical Laboratory*. Washington, DC: DA; Dec 2002. ARTEP 8-668 (MRI)-30-MTP.

27. US Department of the Army. *Health Service Support in Corps and Echelon above Corps*. Washington, DC: DA; 2004. Field Manual 4.02-12.

28. Taylor PW, Gordon SW, Hall TL, Kimm GL, Tyner SP, VanHorn GT. Force health protection through laboratory analysis and health risk assessment. *US Army Medical Department Journal*. 2006:66–72.

29. Taylor P, Lukey B, Clark C, Lee R, Roussel R. Field verification of Test-Mate ChE. *Mil Med*. 2003;168:314–319.

30. Shippee RL. The TAML / AML concept: lessons / learned prescription for change. *US Army Medical Department Journal*. 2004;July–Sep:65–68.

31. Slife H, Winston J. Telechemistry, projecting laboratory expertise to a deployed area medical laboratory. *Mil Med Tech*. 2005;9.3:39–42.

32. US Department of the Army. *MEDCOM Emergency Management*. Washington, DC: DA; 2000. US Army Medical Command Regulation 525-4.

33. US Department of Health and Human Services, Centers for Disease Control and Prevention. *The Public Health Response to Biological and Chemical Terrorism: Interim Planning Guidance for State Public Health Officials*. Washington, DC: DHHS; 2001.

34. US Department of Health and Human Services, Centers for Disease Control and Prevention. CDC recommendations for civilian communities near chemical weapons depots: guidelines for medical preparedness. 60 *Federal Register* 123 (June 27, 1995): 3308–3312.

35. US Department of the Army, Office of the Assistant Secretary of the Army (Acquisition, Logistics and Technology) and Department of Homeland Security Emergency Preparedness and Response Directorate. *Exercise Policy and Guidance for the Chemical Stockpile Emergency Preparedness Program*. Washington, DC: DA; 2004.

36. US General Accounting Office. *Chemical Weapons: FEMA and Army must be Proactive in Preparing States for Emergencies*. Washington, DC: GAO; 2001. Report to Congress GAO-01-850.

37. US Department of the Army. *Chemical Accident or Incident Response and Assistance (CAIRA) Operations*. Washington, DC: DA; 2003. DA PAM 50-6.

38. US Department of the Army. *Chemical Surety*. Washington, DC: DA; 2001. Army Regulation 50-6.

39. US Department of the Army, US Department of Homeland Security, US Federal Emergency Management Agency. *CSEPP Update*. Washington, DC: DA, DHS, FEMA; 2004. Publication no. III.

40. Rubin J. Recurring pitfalls in hospital preparedness and response. *Journal of Homeland Security*. 2004.

41. US Department of the Army. *Multiservice Tactics, Techniques, and Procedures for Chemical, Biological, Radiological, and Nuclear Contamination Avoidance*. Washington, DC: DA; 2006. Army Field Manual 3-11.3.

42. US Department of the Army. *Multiservice Tactics, Techniques, and Procedures for Nuclear, Biological, and Chemical Aspects of Consequence Management*. Washington, DC: DA; 1978. Army Field Manual 3-11.21.

43. US Department of the Army. *Medical Services, Clinical Quality Management*. Washington, DC: DA; 2004. Army Regulation 40-68.

44. Winkenwerder W, Assistant Secretary of Defense for Health Affairs. *Chemical, Biological, Radiological, Nuclear, and (High Yield) Explosives Training for Military Medical Personnel*. Washington, DC: DoD; 2004.

45. Pueschel M. Core DoD response skills targeted. *US Medicine Information Central*. 2003;54:article 730.

46. US General Accounting Office. *Chemical and Biological Defense: DoD Needs to Clarify Expectations for Medical NBC Readiness*. Washington, DC: GAO; 2001. Report to the Chairman, Subcommittee on National Security, Veterans Affairs, and International Relations, Committee on Government Reform, House of Representatives GAO-02-38.

47. Federal Emergency Management Agency Independent Study Program Web site. Available at: http://training.fema.gov/IS/. Accessed November 2006.

48. US Federal Emergency Management Agency. US Fire Administration Training Courses and Schedules Web site. Available at: www.usfa.dhs.gov/applications/nfacsd. Accessed November 28, 2006.

49. US Department of Health and Human Services, Centers for Disease Control and Prevention. Emergency Preparedness and Response: Chemical Emergencies Web site. Available at: www.bt.cdc.gov/chemical. Accessed November 2006.

50. US Department of Health and Human Services, Health Resources and Services Administration. Grants: Find, Apply, Review, Manage, Report Web site. Available at: www.hrsa.gov/grants/. Accessed November 2006.

ABBREVIATIONS AND ACRONYMS

A

AA: arachidonic acid
AC: hydrogen cyanide
ACGIH: American Conference of Governmental Industrial Hygienists
Ach: acetylcholine
AChE: acetylcholinesterase
ADMS: assistant director of medical services
AEF: American Expeditionary Forces
AEGL: acute exposure guidance level
AML: area medical laboratory
AMN: atropine methylnitrate
AR: Army Regulation
ARC: American Red Cross
ARDS: acute respiratory distress syndrome
ATCA: 2-aminothiazoline-4-carboxylic acid
ATNAA: antidote treatment nerve agent autoinjector
ATP: adenosine triphosphate
aTSP: active topical skin protectant
A-V: atrial-ventricular

B

BA: bromoacetone
BAL: British anti-Lewisite (dimercaprol)
BALF: bronchoalveolar lavage fluid
BAS: battalion aid station
BBC: bromobenzyl cyanide
BChE: butyrylcholinesterase
BEF: British Expeditionary Forces
BMZ: basement membrane zone
BTX: batrachotoxin
BZ: 3-quinuclidinyl benzilate

C

CA: bromobenzyl cyanide
CaE: carboxylesterase
CAI: chemical accident or incident
CAIRA: chemical accident or incident response and assistance
cAMP: adenosine 3′,5′-cyclic monophosphate
CANA: convulsive antidote, nerve agent
CAS: Chemical Abstracts Service
CB: chemical-biological
CBIRF: Chemical/Biological Incident Response Force
CBR: chemical, biological, and radiological
CBRN: chemical, biological radiological, and nuclear
CBRNE: chemical, biological, radiological, nuclear, explosive
CBRRT: chemical biological rapid response team
CDC: Centers for Disease Control and Prevention
CEA: cultured epidermal autograft
cGMP: current Good Manufacturing Practice
CHASE (Operation): Cut Holes and Sink 'Em
ChE: cholinesterase
CK: cyanogen chloride
CN^-: cyanide anion
CN: chloroacetophenone
CNO^-: cyanate
CNS: central nervous system
COLPRO: collective protection
CP EMEDS: collectively protected expeditionary medical support
CPRP: chemical personnel reliability program
CR: dibenz(*b,f*)(1,4)oxazepine
CS: *o*-chlorobenzylidene malononitrile
CSA: The Covenant, the Sword, and the Arm of the Lord
CSEPP: Chemical Stockpile Emergency Preparedness Program
CSF: colony-stimulating factor
CSMSPD: chemical surety medical support program director
C*t*: concentration (C) of agent vapor or aerosol in air multiplied by time (*t*) of exposure
CWA: chemical warfare agent
CWC: Chemical Weapons Convention (1993)
CWS: US Army Chemical Warfare Service

D

DA PAM: Department of the Army pamphlet
DA: diphenylchloroarsine
DC: diphenylcyanoarsine
DCE: defense coordinating element
DEET: N,N-diethyl-meta-toluamide
DEPMEDS: deployable medical system
DFP: diisopropyl phosphorofluoridate
DHHS: Department of Health and Human Services
DHP: diisopropylfluorophosphate
DHS: Department of Homeland Security
DM: diphenylaminoarsine
4-DMAP: 4-dimethylaminophenol
DMS: director of medical services
DNA: deoxyribonucleic acid
DoD: Department of Defense
DOE: Department of Energy
DOJ: Department of Justice
DOT: Department of Transportation
DVA: Department of Veterans Affairs

E

ECG: electrocardiogram
EDTA: ethylenediaminetetraacetate
EEG: electroencephalogram
EKG: electrocardiogram
EMEDS: expeditionary medical support
EMS: emergency medical service
EMT: emergency medical technician
EOC: emergency operations center
EPA: Environmental Protection Agency
Eq: equine
ER: endoplasmic reticulum
Er: YAG: erbium: yttrium-aluminium-garnet
ESF: emergency support function

F

FBI: Federal Bureau of Investigation
FBS: fetal bovine serum
FCC: federal coordinating center
FDA: Food and Drug Administration
FEMA: Federal Emergency Management Agency
FHP: force health protection
FOC: full operational capability
FRC: forward resuscitation care

G

GA: tabun
GABA(A): gamma-aminobutyric A
GB: sarin
GD: soman
GF: cyclosarin
GK-11: gacyclidine
GM1: monosialotetrahexosylganglioside
GSA: General Services Administration
GSH: glutathione

H

H: mustard
H_2O_2: hydrogen peroxide
H_2S: hydrogen sulfide
HAZMAT: hazardous materials
HAZWOPER: hazardous waste operations and emergency response
HC: hexachloroethane
HCN: hydrogen cyanide
HD: mustard (distilled)
HE: high explosives
HHS: Department of Health and Human Services
HN2: nitrogen mustard
HSS: health service support
Hu PON1: human paraoxonase 1
HWA: Heereswaffenamt

I

ICAM: improved chemical agent monitor
ICG: indocyanine green
ICS: incident command system
IDLH: immediately dangerous to life or health
IgG: immunogammaglobulin
IL: interleukin
IM: intramuscular
IMA: installation medical authority
IND: investigational new drug
IOC: initial operational capability
IOT&E: initial operational test and evaluation
IP: intraperitoneal injection
IPE: individual protective ensemble/equipment
IV: intravenous

J

JFO: joint field office
JPEO: joint program executive office
JPEO-CBD: Joint Program Executive Office for Chemical Biological Defense
JPMO: joint product management office
JSGPM: joint service general purpose mask
JSLIST: joint service lightweight integrated suit technology
JSMLT: joint service mask leakage tester
JSPDS: joint service personnel skin decontamination system
JTF: joint task force

K

KCN: potassium cyanide
K_m: a measure of the strength of binding of a substrate to an enzyme

L

LCt_{50}: the vapor or aerosol exposure that is lethal to 50% of the exposed population
LD_{50}: median lethal dose
LDPI: laser Doppler perfusion imaging
LHON: Leber hereditary optic neuropathy
LPS: lipopolysaccharide
LSD: lysergic acid diethylamide

M

MAC: multiagency coordination
MANAA: medical aerosolized nerve agent antidote
MCE: maximum credible event
MDMA: 3, 4-methylene-dioxymethylamphetamine
MEDCOM: medical command
MEDEVAC: medical evacuation
MITS: medical identification and treatment systems
MO: medical officer
MOPP: mission-oriented protective posture
MPE: most probable event
MRI: magnetic resonance imaging
MRT: mean residence time
MRT: medical response team
MS C LRIP: milestone C low rate initial production
MT: metric ton
MTF: medical treatment facility
MULO: multipurpose overboot

N

N_2O: nitrogen oxide
N_2O_4: nitrogen tetroxide
NAAG: N-acetyl-aspartyl-glutamate
NaCN: sodium cyanide
NAD^+ : nicotinamide adenine dinucleotide
$NaNO_2$: sodium nitrite
NATO: North Atlantic Treaty Organization
NBC: nuclear, biological, chemical
NCO: noncommissioned officer
NCS: National Communications System
NDA: new drug application
NDMS: National Disaster Medical System
NF: number facility
NIMS: National Incident Management System
NIOSH: National Institute for Occupational Safety and Health
NMDA: *N*-methyl D-aspartate
NO: nitric oxide
NO_2: nitrogen dioxide
NORTHCOM: Northern Command
NRP: National Response Plan
NSAID: nonsteroidal antiinflammatory drug
NSP: neurotoxic shellfish poisoning

O

OC: oleoresin capsicum
OH: hydroxyl radical
OP: organophosphorus
OPCW: Organization for the Prohibition of Chemical Weapons
OPIDN: organophosphorus ester–induced delayed neurotoxicity
Ops: operations
OSHA: Occupational Safety and Health Administration

P

PADPRP: poly(adenosine diphosphate-ribose) polymerase
PAF: platelet-aggregating factor
2-PAM Cl: 2-pralidoxime chloride
2-PAM: 2-pralidoxime
PAPP: p-aminopropiophenone
PARP: poly(ADP-ribose) polymerase
PATS: protection assessment test system
PB: pyridostigmine bromide
PBN: alpha-phenyl-N-tert-butylnitrone
PBN: N-tert-butyl-alfa-phenylnitrone
PbTx: brevetoxin
PCP: phencyclidine
PFIB: perfluoroisobutylene
pHu: plasma-derived human
PKC: protein kinase C
PLA_2: phospholypase A2
pMo: plasma-derived mouse
2-PMPA: 2-pentanedioic acid
POM: program objective memorandum
PPE: personal protective equipment
PR: protective ratio
PS: chloropicrin
PTSD: posttraumatic stress disorder
PTX: palytoxin

R

RADS: reactive airways dysfunction syndrome
RBC-ChE: red blood cell cholinesterase
RCA: riot control agent
RD_{50}: dose required to cause a 50% decrease in respiration
REM: rapid eye movement
RH: relative humidity
rHu BChE: recombinant human butyrylcholinesterase
RNA: ribonucleic acid
RPM: respiratory rate, pulse, and motor function
RSDL: Reactive Skin Decontamination Lotion

S

SCN^-: thiocyanate
SE: status epilepticus
SERPACWA: skin exposure reduction paste against chemical warfare agents
SMART: special medical augmentation response team
SNS: strategic national stockpile
SRBD: seizure-related brain damage
SS: Schutzstaffel
START: simple triage and rapid treatment
STEL: short-term exposure limit
STM: Sacco triage method
STX: saxitoxin

T

TBSA: total body surface area
TEN: toxic epidermal necrosis
TIC: toxic industrial chemical
TIM: toxic industrial material
TNF: tumor necrosis factor
TRP: transient receptor potential
TTX: tetrodotoxin
TWA: time-weighted average

U

UN: United Nations
USACHPPM: US Army Center for Health Promotion and Preventive Medicine
USAMRICD: US Army Medical Research Institute of Chemical Defense
USAMRIID: US Army Medical Research Institute of Infectious Diseases
USDA: US Department of Agriculture
USJCOM: US Joint Forces Command
USMC: US Marine Corps

V

V/Q: ventilation profusion ratio
VAC: Vacuum-Assisted Closure Therapy
VR1: vallinoid receptor subtype 1

W

WBGT: wet-bulb globe temperature
WMD: weapons of mass destruction

INDEX

A

C

D

I

J

K

L

M

N

O

P

Q

R

S

U

V

W

X

Y

Z

Dedicated to the Memory of Brennie E. Hackley, Jr, and Frederick R. Sidell

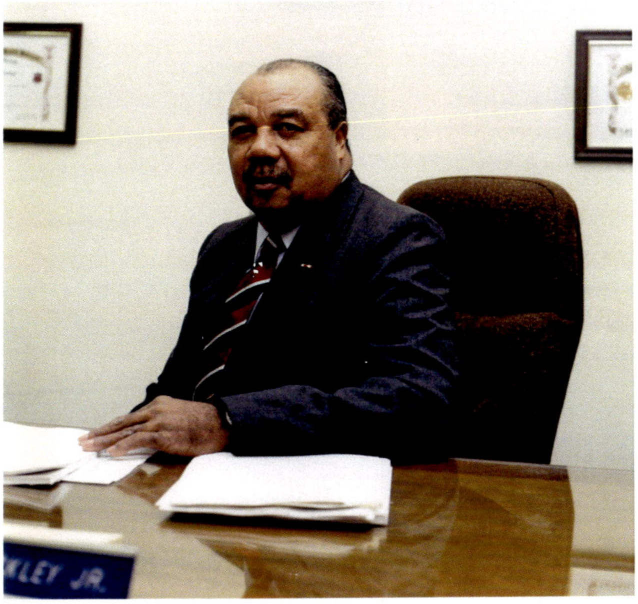

DR BRENNIE E. HACKLEY, JR

Chemist, Teacher, Scientific Advisor

July 29, 1924 – November 5, 2006

Dr Hackley received a BS in chemistry from Wilberforce University in 1946. Following graduation, he enlisted in the US Army and was later commissioned as an officer. After more than 30 years' service, he retired from the US Army Reserve Corps in 1981 at the rank of colonel. Dr Hackley began his civilian career in 1952 as an organic research chemist in the Medicinal Chemistry Branch of the Army Chemical Center and went on to earn advanced degrees in chemistry from the University of Delaware, including a PhD in 1957. During his career, Dr Hackley studied the relationship between chemical structures and chemotherapeutic activity in reference to efficacy against toxic agents. He contributed to the elucidation of mechanisms of reactions of nucleophiles with organophosphorus compounds and synthesized a number of oximes, for which he held 18 patents. One oxime synthesized by Dr Hackley, toxogonin, was adopted as an antidote against chemical nerve agents by the US Air Force.

In 1984 Dr Hackley was designated Chief Scientist and Scientific Advisor to the Commander of the US Army Medical Research Institute of Chemical Defense (USAMRICD). During Operation Desert Storm, Dr Hackley responded to emergency calls by combat divisions for predeployment briefings on medical management of chemical casualties, initiating a traveling training program that prepared deploying medical personnel to treat soldiers on the battlefield if chemical weapons were employed. As an instructor and course director for USAMRICD's Medical Management of Chemical and Biological Casualties course, Dr Hackley delivered lectures in Saudi Arabia; Johnston Island, Hawaii; Okinawa, Japan; and Germany on pulmonary agents, cyanide, vesicants, and nerve agent threats.

While serving as chairman of the Scientific Steering Committee on Nerve Agent Antidotes, he advised the Command that one of the precursors for the then current synthesis of the oxime HI-6, under consideration as a replacement for the fielded 2-PAM chloride, was carcinogenic and would not pass scrutiny by the Food and Drug Administration. Additionally, Dr Hackley convinced the Command that HI-6 wasn't cost effective, and that its effectiveness compared to 2-PAM chloride was not great enough to justify its replacement.

Dr Hackley represented the US Army Medical research program competently and effectively for almost 6 decades. His efforts significantly improved communication and relationships between the Chemical and Medical Corps and strengthened USAMRICD's image as the lead laboratory for the development of medical countermeasures for chemical threat agents.

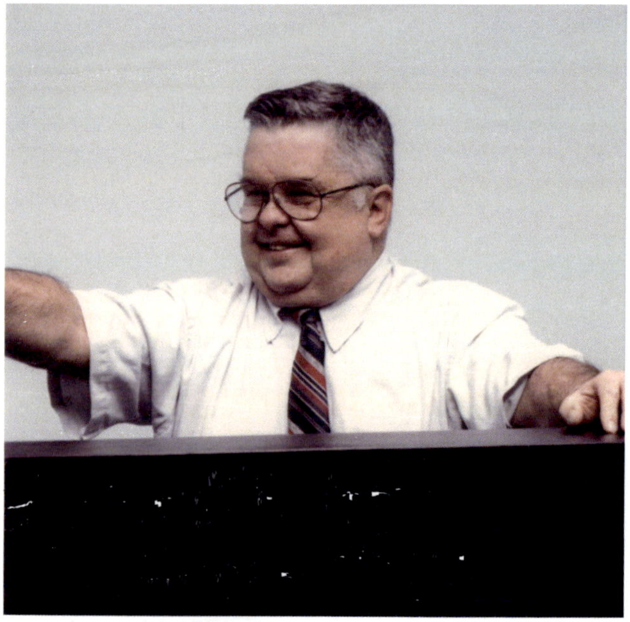

DR FREDERICK R. SIDELL

Physician, Teacher, Scientist

July 27, 1934 – February 14, 2006

No physician has contributed more to the US Army Medical Department's chemical defense training and education programs than Dr Frederick Sidell. Dr Sidell graduated from Marietta College in Marietta, Ohio, in 1956, and also later from the New York University School of Medicine. He completed his internship and residency in internal medicine at Cleveland Metropolitan General Hospital. Dr Sidell initially served 2 years on active duty with the Army Medical Corps in the rank of captain. He was stationed at Edgewood Arsenal in Maryland, an assignment that would determine his future in medicine and lead to his subsequent employment with the Department of Defense. While with the Department of Defense Dr Sidell became one of the world's leading experts and educators in the field of medical effects of chemical warfare agents. He retired in 1995 after 30 years in government service.

In the late 1960s, when training in medical chemical defense was very limited, Dr Sidell and some of his colleagues recognized the need for specialty training and developed a course for military medical personnel on the medical management of chemical agent casualties. Dr Sidell guided the development of this new training program and served as the course director for many years. Eventually, such training was expanded to additional courses for nonmedical personnel and military leaders. Dr Sidell also prepared and updated detailed educational materials addressing nerve agents, vesicants, cyanide, and pulmonary agents, and provided education and training for the Chemical Stockpile Emergency Preparedness Program and the Domestic Preparedness Program.

Dr Sidell's expertise was nationally and internationally recognized, and he was often called upon for highly sensitive assignments that required technical expertise. These included a trip to southeast Asia in 1979 to investigate the alleged use of "yellow rain" against the Hmong in Laos. In 1988, he examined Kurdish civilian casualties who were victims of chemical warfare in their homeland. He traveled to Japan in 1995 to assist and advise Japanese physicians on the care of causalities from a terrorist-led sarin nerve agent incident in the Tokyo subway system.

Dr Sidell was the lead editor of the first edition of *Medical Aspects of Chemical and Biological Warfare*, published in 1997, contributing to many of the chapters on chemical warfare agents. His research and studies have been published in over 100 reports and articles, and he also wrote several handbooks on the treatment of chemical casualties. Following his official retirement, Dr Sidell continued providing education and training in the management of chemical agents and casualty treatment to civilian first responders, including many emergency medical treatment units throughout the United States.

In addition to the many achievement awards and commander's medals received by Dr Sidell, a new building at the Edgewood area of the Aberdeen Proving Ground was named the Sidell Learning Center in 2002 in recognition of his great contribution to medical education and training. In 2003 Dr Sidell was inducted into the Marietta College Hall of Honor, becoming one of only 24 people to be so recognized at that time. Dr Sidell's knowledge, experience, and dedication contributed greatly to the development of the outstanding medical training programs throughout the Department of Defense today. His insight and pragmatic views have guided the development of medical policy against weapons of mass destruction and medical research on safe and effective medical countermeasures against current and future chemical threats facing the military.

ISBN 978-0-16-081532-4